Small Animal Veterinary Psychiatry

Small Animal Veterinary Psychiatry

Edited by

Sagi Denenberg

Langford Vets, University of Bristol, UK;

North Toronto Veterinary Behaviour Specialty Clinic, Toronto, Canada

CABI

CABI is a trading name of CAB International

CABI
Nosworthy Way
Wallingford
Oxfordshire OX10 8DE
UK

Tel: +44 (0)1491 832111
Fax: +44 (0)1491 833508
E-mail: info@cabi.org
Website: www.cabi.org

CABI
WeWork
One Lincoln St
24th Floor
Boston, MA 02111
USA

Tel: +1 (617)682-9015
E-mail: cabi-nao@cabi.org

References to internet websites (URLs) were accurate at the time of writing.

A catalogue record for this book is available from the British Library, London.

Library of Congress Control Number: 2020949979

ISBN: 978 1 78639 4552 (hardback)
978 1 78639 4569 (ePDF)
978 1 78639 4576 (ePub)

Commissioning Editor: Alexandra Lainsbury
Editorial Assistant: Ali Thompson
Production Editor: Tim Kapp

Typeset by Exeter Premedia Services Pvt Ltd, Chennai, India
Printed and bound in the UK by Severn, Gloucester

Contents

Preface

Approximately 400 years ago, the 'father of modern philosophy', René Descartes (1596–1650), declared that animals have no soul or consciousness. He reasoned that, unlike humans, animals cannot feel pain and have no emotions. As a result, animals have suffered for centuries (if not millennia). Even when their physical needs were met, their emotional needs were often completely ignored. Animals were castrated without appropriate anaesthesia and analgesia, mothers were separated from their offspring at birth, or shortly after, and experiments and testing were carried out for the benefit, and on the whim of, humans.

Things are changing, albeit slowly. Animals continue to suffer (primarily food animals), but there is now the recognition, increasingly, that they are sentient beings. I hope that this book will represent the complete opposite approach to Descartes' assertion about animals. While the book deals only with cats and dogs, the concept of thoughts and emotions is not limited to these two species.

The decision to name this text 'Veterinary Psychiatry', rather than using the older and more commonly used term 'veterinary behaviour', stems from our growing understanding of our role. If we wish to help animals that struggle, especially within human societies, we must address their emotional and cognitive needs. The behaviours we see, and of which pets' owners complain, are the result of how animals feel and think, genetics and environmental influences. Even the words psyche (breathing soul) and anima (soul) are self-explanatory. As I write the words 'veterinary psychiatry', I know that there are those who would resist the term for different reasons. Harry Harlow (1905–1981) was convinced that the infant monkey has no emotional needs. The infant rhesus proved him wrong.

In line with this approach, I have tried to steer away from description diagnoses and have focused on emotional and cognitive causes. With the help of my co-authors I feel that we have created a complete text addressing the problems owners may face with their cats and dogs. I tried approaching the book in the same way that the veterinary surgeon would approach a clinical case. We start by addressing cases in the first-opinion practice, including communication with owners and practice design (Chapter 1). Next we must rule out physical disorders, including internal medicine, neurology, dermatology and pain, which may lead to or exacerbate abnormal behaviour (Chapters 2 and 3). Once we have addressed physical health, we can approach mental and emotional health. The first step here is to know what normal behaviour is in cats (Chapter 4) and dogs (Chapter 5). We also discuss the need for an optimal start in kittens and puppies, providing them and their owners with the tools to succeed in life (Chapter 6). At this point we turn our attention to the process of diagnosis of mental and emotional disorders in cats and dogs (Chapter 7). Here we address emotions such as anxiety, phobia and the much-underestimated frustration. Once we establish a diagnosis, we can address the problem. We describe learning principles and behaviour modification, environmental management, and training (Chapter 8). As part of the management, the use of medication is often necessary (Chapter 9). The latter part of the book addresses most of the concerns that owners may have, starting with management problems (Chapter 10), aggression (Chapters 11 and 12), affective disorders (Chapter 13), elimination disorders (Chapter 14), abnormal and repetitive behaviours (Chapter 15) and ageing-related problems in cats and dogs (Chapter 16).

I have included many handouts in the appendices. These can be printed out and used within the practice or given to owners in order to help the veterinary surgeon manage cases.

I wish to thank all my co-authors for their contributions. They have given them voluntarily without any remuneration other than my thanks and appreciation. I am sure that, like me, the reader will appreciate and benefit from their contributions. Their knowledge and experience are priceless and lend this book a global view.

It has been a long road, with many twists and turns, but I am glad I took it and the opportunity to work on this book. Since graduating, and even while in veterinary school, I have learned, modified and adapted my approach to veterinary psychiatry. I could not have done it without my instructors, colleagues, owners and their pets, as well as my family. There are too many to name, but I would like to name a few:

Juraj Halagan, my physiology professor from Kosice, Slovakia, who supported me through my veterinary education. He went out of his way to help me foster my desire and learn more about veterinary psychiatry.

Gary Landsberg, who agreed to have me as an external student first, later as a resident and finally as a business partner. For nearly twenty years, Gary has been there when I needed an answer. Looking back, I would not have made it to this point without his support.

Finally, I thank my family – my wife Magdalena and my daughter Gabriela, who suffered my impatience and absences throughout the process of writing. I could not have done this without their support.

Sagi Denenberg
February 2020
Bristol, UK &
Toronto, Canada

About the Editor

Sagi Denenberg is a diplomate of the American College of Veterinary Behaviorists and the European College of Animal Welfare and Behavioural Medicine (Behaviour). He is also an RVCS Recognised Specialist in Veterinary Behaviour Medicine and has passed the membership examination of the Australia and New Zealand College of Veterinary Scientists. Dr Denenberg graduated from the veterinary school in Kosice, Slovakia. After graduation he relocated from Israel (his homeland) to Canada to pursue his specialization.

In 2015 he joined Langford Vets, University of Bristol, UK, to provide veterinary psychiatry services to owners and their pets, as well as to teach at the Bristol Veterinary School. He has a veterinary psychiatry service at the North Toronto Veterinary Behaviour Specialty Clinic, Toronto. He is also a consultant for the Veterinary Information Network, providing expert advice to veterinarians.

Dr Denenberg has written and co-authored many book chapters, including the *Merck Manual*, the *BSAVA Manual of Canine and Feline Behavioural Medicine*, *Blackwell's Five-minute Veterinary Consult: Canine and Feline Behavior*, and *Feline Behavioral Health and Welfare*. He has published many papers including 'Feline play pattern', for which he received the American Veterinary Society of Animal Behavior Award. He is a frequent lecturer around the world.

When not working, Sagi enjoys spending time with his wife and daughter (mostly building Lego with Gabi!), walking the dog, DIY projects, reading and photography.

Contributors

Alison Blaxter
BA, BVM&S, PhD, Dip CABC, MRCVS
Bristol Vet School, University of Bristol, UK
Alison.Blaxter@Bristol.ac.uk

Alex Darvill
MRICS, MCIOB, MAPM, RMaps
ACD Projects Ltd
Newmarket, UK
alex@acdprojects.com

Ed Hall
VetMB, MA, PhD, Dip ECVIM-CA, FRCVS
Emeritus Professor of Small Animal Internal Medicine, University of Bristol, UK
dred.hall@bristol.ac.uk

Tom Harcourt-Brown
VetMB, MA, CertVDI, Dip ECVN, MRCVS
Langford Vets, University of Bristol
Bristol, UK
tom.harcourt-brown@bristol.ac.uk

Lynn Hewison
BSc MSc
Joseph Banks Laboratories
University of Lincoln, UK
lhewison@lincoln.ac.uk

Angie Hibbert
BVSc, CertSAM, Dip ECVIM-CA, MRCVS
The Feline Centre, Langford Vets, University of Bristol, UK
angie.hibbert@bristol.ac.uk

Katherine Houpt
BS, VMD, PhD, Dip ACVB
Professor Emeritus, Cornell University
Ithaca, New York
kah3@cornell.edu

Jacqui Ley
BVSc (Hons), PhD, Dip ECAWBM, FANZCVS (Veterinary Behaviour)
Registered Specialist in Veterinary Behavioural Medicine
Melbourne Veterinary Specialist Centre
Glen Waverley, Australia
drjacquiley@msn.com

Samantha Lindley
BVSc, MRCVS
Associate Lecturer
Glasgow University Veterinary School
c/o Small Animal Hospital
Glasgow, UK
samanthalindley@btinternet.com

Sarah L. Liversage
MSc (Clinical Animal Behaviour), RVN
Certified Canine Rehabilitation Practitioner
Langford Vets, University of Bristol, UK
sarah.liversage@bristol.ac.uk

Daniel S. Mills
BVSc, PhD, CBiol, FRSB, FHEA, CCAB Dip, Dip ECAWBM(BM) FRCVS
European & RCVS Recognised Specialist in Veterinary Behavioural Medicine
Joseph Banks Laboratories
School of Life Sciences, University of Lincoln, UK
DMills@lincoln.ac.uk

Carlo Siracusa
DVM, MS, PhD, Dip ACVB, Dip ECAWBM(BM)
Associate Professor of Clinical Animal Behavior and Welfare
Department of Clinical Sciences and Advanced Medicine
School of Veterinary Medicine
University of Pennsylvania, USA
siracusa@vet.upenn.edu

Stephen Waisglass
BSc, DVM, MRCVS, CertSAD, Dip ACVD
Veterinary Emergency Clinic of Toronto
Toronto, Canada
dermvet@rogers.com

Helen Zulch
BVSc (Hons), Dip ECAWBM(BM), MRCVS
RCVS Recognised Specialist in Veterinary Behavioural Medicine
Head of Professional Development in Canine Behaviour, Dogs Trust UK, London
Helen.Zulch@dogstrust.org.uk

1 Addressing Mental and Emotional Health in the Veterinary Practice

Alison Blaxter[1], Alex Darvill[2] and Sagi Denenberg[3,4]*

[1]Bristol Vet School, University of Bristol, Bristol, UK; [2]ACD Projects Ltd, Newmarket, Suffolk, UK; [3]Langford Vets, University of Bristol, Langford, UK; [4]North Toronto Veterinary Behaviour Specialty Clinic, Toronto, Canada

1.1 Introduction

Behaviour problems in dogs and cats are among the leading reasons for relinquishment and euthanasia. Given that the behaviour of the dog or cat is the main reason for the human–animal bond, any behaviour changes ultimately will affect this bond.

It is critical to understand that the behaviour we see is the result of mental and emotional, and biological (physiological) drives (Panksepp, 2016). Therefore, when addressing 'behaviour problems' we must realize that there are several possibilities under this umbrella term. These include psychiatric disorder (e.g. mental and emotional), excessive presentations of normal behaviours (e.g. excessive vocalization, scratching, certain aspects of house soiling, and jumping), and physiological and physical conditions (e.g. pain, gastrointestinal and neurological conditions). The term 'behaviour problems' may not be accurate; we can change behaviours; however, if we do not change the underlying motivation, a new problem will arise later.

To address this range of possibilities, the clinician must first know what is the normal (i.e. biological) behaviour of cats (see Chapter 4) and dogs (see Chapter 5). If the behaviour of the patient is truly excessive or abnormal, the clinician should first rule out physical conditions such as dermatological, neurological or metabolic diseases (see Chapter 2) or pain (see Chapter 3).

The next step is to establish a diagnosis (see Chapter 7). Then we must manage the problem(s) using behaviour modification tools that are based on teaching the animal alternative behaviours or changing its motivation (see Chapter 8). Finally, in some cases, especially where a true pathology exists, the use of psychiatric medications is necessary (see Chapter 9).

1.1.1 Addressing owners' concerns

The process of addressing these problems can be complex. When an owner presents a dog or a cat with 'behaviour problems' the clinician must first determine if the behaviour in question is truly a problem the patient is presenting or an owner's subjective assessment. The latter, while it may not be a 'true' problem, is nevertheless an important aspect. Owners may not be aware of what is normal, and, in fact, only see what is common. For example, many dogs excessively follow their owners around the house and, as a result, do not sleep well. Owners may not be aware that this behaviour represents an abnormality, as this behaviour is common.

1.1.1.1 Subjective?

Often, owners will present a dog or a cat with an undesired behaviour that is not a true pathology (see Chapter 10). It is as important to manage these problems, and to help owners, as it is to manage true pathologies. At the end of the day, it is the owner that takes the patient home and must be happy with it. All too often, owners relinquish their pets due to conditions that other owners may see as normal, or they cope well. For example, a barking dog may not be a concern for the owner until they have a new baby at home who cannot sleep well.

*Corresponding author: s.denenberg@bristol.ac.uk

DOI: 10.1079/9781786394552.0001

1.1.1.2 Helping owners

Patients do not arrive at us on their own; owners bring them when they have concerns about them. Aside from helping patients, we must help the owners. It may be frustrating at times to address certain cases when we feel that the owner should have come earlier, or should have managed the problem differently (e.g. without punishment). However, we should not be quick to pass judgement on owners. Owners try helping their pets in most cases, even when, in hindsight, they have chosen the wrong approach.

In most cases, it suffices to review the timeline of the problem. Owners are often reactive; they only try to intervene once the problem has started. Infrequently, owners are proactive. Therefore, even when owners use punishment, they do so after the problem has started. We may criticize owners for aggravating a situation, but not always for creating it.

Also, most owners feel guilty for using these techniques or not doing something appropriately. We must avoid the tendency to blame them; giving them a 'guilt trip' is not helpful for them or any of the involved parties. Owners are not more likely to be active if they feel guilty. We must foster a partnership with owners through trust, education, encouragement and honesty (even when we disagree with their approach).

1.1.2 Whole-practice approach

Addressing behavioural problems, especially those with underlying psychiatric disorders, is time-consuming and may not always be possible during routine visits to the practice. Therefore, involving more staff members, questionnaires and follow-up appointments is necessary.

It is important to recognize that often owners will not discuss their pet's behaviours with veterinarians as they either think that veterinarians are not knowledgeable about the behaviour of animals or they are concerned about the recommendations. Therefore, veterinarians must not only ask, they must also inform owners that they can and want to help. Questionnaires and handouts are a useful method to inform owners about the service and care the veterinarian can provide.

1.1.2.1 Questionnaires

Questionnaires are good screening tools to use in the practice. While waiting at the practice, owners can fill in a questionnaire (see Handouts A1 – GP Questionnaire – Cat; and A2 – GP Questionnaire – Dog). Questionnaires should be designed to be simple to fill in and read. The veterinarian can quickly read the questionnaire as the owner enters the room and then review any concerns with the owner. These questionnaires should then be filed in the patient's file.

Questionnaires should be adjusted to the patient's age because its needs and behaviours change as it moves from one age group to the next. Time should be allotted through each routine visit to review the patient's behaviour.

1.1.2.2 Handouts

Following discussions with owners about their pet's behaviours, we must provide them with information. At times, a referral is necessary. However, even when owners decide not to pursue referral we should attempt to help them. Providing handouts helps, as we can give them concise information while maintaining a routine visits schedule. For more information on available resources see Handout A11.

1.1.2.3 Routine visits

Patients' needs should be assessed during each routine visit. Just as you would evaluate the patient's physical health, you should also evaluate its mental and emotional health.

Puppy visits should include discussions on socialization, training, identifying concerns and pathologies, and addressing emerging concerns. Starting correctly with puppies and kittens may alleviate future problems and prevent relinquishment or euthanasia (see Chapter 6).

Adult and ageing patients (see Chapter 16) should also be screened during routine visits. Their behaviour may have changed as well, especially since the juvenile state. Many, if not most, problems arise as the patient reaches social maturity and develops into an adult animal (see Chapter 6).

1.1.2.4 Veterinarians

The role of the veterinarian is to diagnose and prescribe a treatment for these problems. Aside from ruling out any physical disorder that contributes to the development and maintenance of the problem, veterinarians can offer information on its management.

Once physical disorder is ruled out (see Chapters 2 and 3), the first step is to ensure that the problem is not progressing. This can be achieved through the prevention of triggers, implementing safety, and environmental management.

Safety is not just for possible victims of aggression; it is also for the patient itself. Not only might the patient suffer injuries in a possible fight (when aggression is the presentation) but it may also self-inflict injuries in some cases of compulsive behaviours, trying to escape different situations or running after the owner. A known side-effect of psychiatric disorder is euthanasia.

When we attempt to manage psychiatric disorder in the first-opinion practice, time is a concern. We may need to schedule a follow-up appointment to address and manage the problem more thoroughly. Another option is to appoint a staff member who can address owners' concerns, offer basic training and management advice. The veterinarian can supervise the management and prescribe medications when necessary.

Veterinarians who seek more knowledge and training can pursue continuing education, seminars, online training, university degrees and clinical specialization.

1.1.2.5 Nurses

Nurses are in a unique position to help the veterinarian in the management of behavioural disorders. Nurses not only possess basic medical knowledge but they may also have more time to spend with owners, collecting information and designing a management plan. Moreover, many owners feel more comfortable talking to nurses about their pet's behaviour than they do talking to veterinarians.

Nurse clinics can be scheduled, allowing nurses to provide owners with preventative information, especially with puppies and kittens. Also, nurses can hold socialization classes in the practice for both puppies and kittens (see Chapter 6).

Today, nurses can pursue more education in animal behaviour, including online training, seminars, university degrees and specialization training.

1.1.2.6 Reception and kennel staff

To aid veterinarians and nurses, reception and kennel staff can be trained to offer basic advice. Owners often spend time in the reception area discussing their pet's behaviour. Therefore, reception staff should try to flag any concerns the owner mentions.

Reception staff can offer preventative advice, and information about products the practice carries for both prevention and management of the problem. However, staff members should be aware that 'cookbook' advice is not always helpful and might even be harmful. They should avoid offering immediate advice without allowing the veterinarian to rule out other options.

Reception staff can provide owners with questionnaires and handouts and inform owners that veterinarians and nurses are there to help with behavioural or other concerns.

1.1.2.7 Ancillary help

At times, you may want to refer patients to a trainer or an individual with a certification or accreditation in animal behaviour in your area. It is essential to recognize that not all trainers are created equally; unfortunately there are trainers who still believe in outdated learning philosophies and dominance theories. Trainers who use terms such as 'correction', 'balanced approach', 'pack leader' and 'dominance' are best avoided.

When recommending a trainer or other individual, it would be helpful to discuss the matter with this person and review their approach. Also, you should review their credentials and ask for references. If possible, attend some of their training or management sessions.

The best approach is to use humane techniques that are based on reinforcement. While it is impossible to avoid certain aspects of punishment (see Chapter 8), the emphasis should be on reinforcement.

When a problem exists, it is best to address the patient on their own at first. Therefore, classes or group sessions are best avoided until later stages. Also, sending a dog to a 'board-and-train' facility is not recommended. First, the problem may not appear in a different setting; second, the dog may not behave the same way when the owner is not present; and third, it is not always possible to know how an animal is being trained when the owner is not present. Ideal training should take place in the animal's home environment, including the surrounding area, with the owner present to handle the animal.

1.1.2.8 Veterinary specialist

When a referral is necessary, you should seek a veterinary specialist in your area. If there are no options in your area, telephone and online consultations may be available. These individuals are trained in both veterinary medicine and animal behaviour.

After completion of a veterinary degree, these individuals must take at least a one-year internship, followed by a residency programme (see dacvb.org, ecawbm.com or anzcvs.org.au for more information). This residency includes training in normal species-typical behaviour, comparative animal behaviour, the principles of learning and behaviour modification, psychology, abnormal behaviour, psychopharmacology, and the effects of disease on behaviour. The practical aspect includes at least three years seeing cases under the mentorship of a board-certified behaviourist. Publications, presentations to other veterinarians, case histories and an extensive four-part examination are all then required to achieve board certification. It takes approximately 12 years of post-secondary education to achieve the level of veterinary psychiatrist.

1.2 Communication Skills for Conversations about Behaviour

1.2.1 Role of communication in behaviour consultations or conversations

Effective communication is essential for all veterinary conversations. It could be argued that communication skills are of greater importance when dealing with problem behaviours in companion animals than in any other veterinary context. Achieving effective case outcomes is highly dependent on the vet's skills as an effective and highly attuned communicator.

Part of being an effective communicator involves self-awareness and a profound sensitivity towards others. We must ask personal questions of an owner about their family structure, daily routines and emotional life, as well as biomedical questions, to be able to, for example, investigate why a cat has started to urinate inappropriately indoors. To effectively have such conversations with owners, we need to be aware of the impact of our personal communication style and the role that specific skills can have on case outcomes.

There has been an acknowledged 'paradigm shift' in the vet–owner–patient dynamic in the last two decades, and the concept of relationship-centred care has emerged (Gray and Moffett, 2010). Expanding our enquiry beyond the biomedical, considering the consultation as a partnership and encouraging owner participation will improve health outcomes in veterinary conversations. This is nowhere more apparent than when discussing the behaviours and emotions of animals who inhabit our homes.

1.2.2 What this section is about and what it is not about

Communication in the setting of a veterinary consultation can be described as a two-way process. We, the senders, give a message that is received by owners, the receivers, and allows dialogue and discussion (Kirwan, 2010). As individuals, we develop varying styles of communication and sets of skills that serve us well, both personally and in the context of veterinary consultations and conversations. We need to be aware that the 'receiver' of our questioning or information will also have a preferred style of communication. This chapter explores the possible styles and skills we can use in our consultations, any evidence behind their use, and aims to expand the reader's skills to enable them to meet the communication preferences and needs of diverse owners.

Furthermore, communication can be divided into two distinct areas: it concerns the message or content of the enquiry, but also how this is done. For specific details of the content of history-taking and instructions for owners, you need to consider the wider content of this book. This chapter concentrates on the process of communication.

1.2.3 What are the universal components of communication?

In general, communication skills can be divided into two distinct areas: verbal and non-verbal. The components of non-verbal skills for medical communication have been described extensively elsewhere (Kurtz *et al.*, 2003). They are summarized in Box 1.1.

An overview of the skills of verbal communication when questioning and giving information in veterinary interactions is given in Box 1.2.

Box 1.1 The components of non-verbal communication skills for face-to-face interactions.

- Eye contact
- The proximity between the speaker and the listener
- The orientation between participants and the awareness of personal space
- Facial expressions
- Posture
- Movements and gesture – hand, head, body
- Physical touch
- Paralinguistic features – the 'music' of speech (i.e. tone, volume, pace, pitch, emphasis, fluency)
- Timing and the use of pause/silence

Non-verbal communication is powerful. If non-verbal and verbal communication 'messages' disagree, the listener will believe the non-verbal message (Kirwan, 2010). This means that if we say we are interested in an owner's experience with their dog but do not appear actively interested with eye contact, appropriate intonation and facial expressions, they will not believe we care.

The key differences between verbal and non-verbal communication are given in Box 1.3.

1.2.4 Can communication skills be learnt?

Evidence confirms that we can learn how to communicate more effectively in a professional context (Maguire and Pitceathly, 2002). Consequently, veterinary curricula have communication skills development as a key component of training (von Fragstein *et al.*, 2008; Mossop *et al.*, 2015). There is also evidence that the most effective way to develop face-to-face communication skills in a veterinary setting is through a process of experiential learning where feedback is provided (Latham and Morris, 2007), as in Fig. 1.1. The implication of this is that we should strive to develop our skills in communication, as with other skills required for professional life, and seek feedback from our owners and colleagues on the way we communicate.

1.2.5 When do behaviour conversations happen in practice?

Conversations can be planned as part of consultations that are booked solely to discuss mental and emotional concerns. These are often preceded by the owner completing a questionnaire and a significant amount of time being booked to deal with these cases, either in a referral setting or as part of extended services to owners in primary care clinics. However, most conversations about behaviour in general practice are components of other health consultations. Managing the time pressures and limitations associated with these is discussed in Section 1.2.12.1.

1.2.6 What are the goals of communication in consultations?

There are three primary goals:

- Fact-finding: the first set of goals relate to gathering information. In general, we will need to ask questions about the patient, their developmental and clinical histories, normal routines, activity and lifestyle. We then move on to problem behaviours: What initiated them, and how did they develop? What is the current situation? Finally, we need to determine

Box 1.2. Important aspects of the verbal component of communication in veterinary interactions.

Language choice – this includes:

- register – formal and informal
- use of technical terms or jargon
- use of pronouns, euphemisms and humour
- questioning techniques – open and closed questioning
- structures for giving information – paraphrasing, repetition and summarizing

Box 1.3. Key differences between non-verbal and verbal communication.

- Verbal communication involves the use of words, while signs and utterances which are not words constitute non-verbal communication.
- Non-verbal communication conveys emotions and feelings to a greater degree than verbal communication.
- Verbal communication may be more exact than non-verbal messaging in terms of identifying and transmitting an intended message.
- Non-verbal communication tends to override verbal messages if there is disagreement between the two.

the owner's perspective on the problem behaviours, their understanding of their animal's motivations and actions, and the strategies they have already employed to manage unwanted behaviours.

- Giving information: in this area of the consultation, we aim to provide explanations of the problem behaviours, which are often normal species-specific behaviours but unacceptable in their setting, and suggestions as to management, amelioration or resolution of the issues for the benefit of our patient and owner.
- Shared decision making: to maximize compliance and success, our goal must also be to facilitate collaborative decision making with the owner.

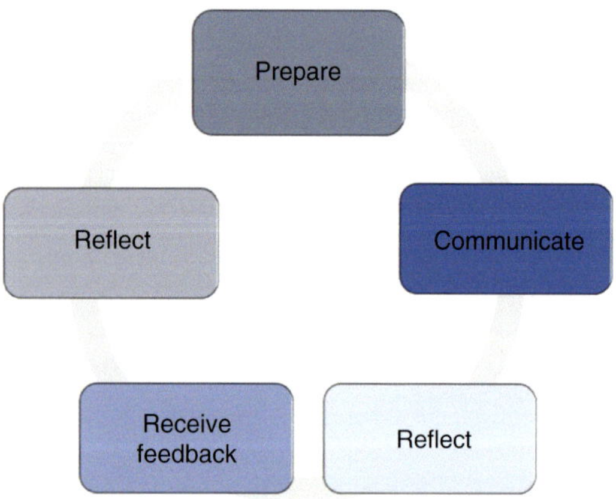

Fig. 1.1. Experiential learning in developing communication skills.

1.2.7 Models of communication/counselling valid for behaviour consults

1.2.7.1 The adapted Veterinary Calgary Cambridge Model (VCCM) (Radford et al., 2006)

This model was developed from a human medicine model and is widely used as a tool to examine the communication skills within a consultation, allowing learners access to specific skills in a tangible form. It is not intended to be linear or prescriptive but is a framework in which dialogue about skills and processes can be achieved. Readers are encouraged to view the complete form of the model, which has three specific iterations. An overview of the process is given in Fig. 1.2. the second version is a description of the goals of each phase, and the third iteration matches the phases with a specific list of over 50 skills. These provide an excellent checklist for behavioural contexts.

1.2.7.2 Motivational interviewing (MI)

This approach is an established evidence-based communication methodology used in human medicine to effect behaviour change (Miller and Rollnick, 2013). The primary principle of MI is that it is through engaging with and facilitating an individual's intrinsic motivation that behaviour change results. The concept of motivational interviewing evolved from experience in the treatment of alcoholism and addiction (Miller and Rollnick, 2013), now widely applied to a range of psychiatric disorders (Treasure, 2004), and is the National Institute for Health Care and Excellence's recommended treatment for a range of addictive disorders (NICE (National Institute for Health Care and Excellence), 2019). It is also used to improve general health by eliciting change in maladaptive features of lifestyle

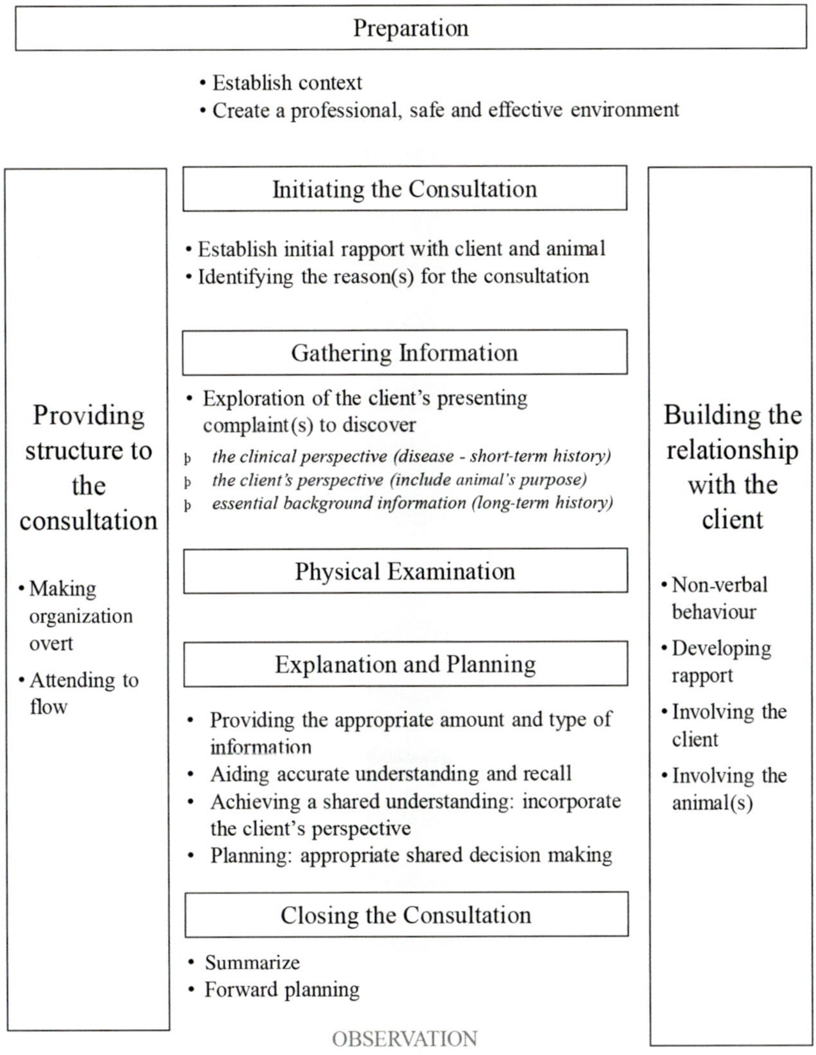

Fig. 1.2. A summary flow diagram of the guide to the veterinary consultation based on the Calgary-Cambridge model. (Adapted from Radford *et al.*, 2006)

such as smoking, excessive weight gain and inadequate exercise (Rubak *et al.*, 2005).

MI has obvious applications to veterinary behavioural medicine. Its particular use may be where we advise a change in owner behaviour that is challenging to implement. In these contexts, MI specifically focuses on exploring and resolving the psychological ambivalence that is common in complex decision making to wholly engage owners with veterinary recommendations.

1.2.7.3 The ORAS (open question, reflection, affirmation and summary) model

This is a set of interactive skills developed within MI (Miller and Rollnick, 2013). It focuses on the four basic skills of verbally displaying empathy: asking open questions, reflective listening, affirming the owner's emotions and actions, and using summary. Its value in behaviour consultations is that it provides a distinct set of skills to achieve a partnership with owners and positive outcomes for them and their animals.

1.2.8 Getting ready to discuss behaviour

1.2.8.1 Preparation

Preparation is a vital prelude to effective behavioural consultations. Attention to the physical setting, particularly considering the use of computers in consulting rooms, improves the interaction between consultants and owners (Silverman and Kinnersley, 2010). Removing the physical barrier of consulting tables and computer screens, facilitating both professionals and owners to be seated, and ensuring the conversation is private and undisturbed will all aid effective face-to-face interaction. Our physical appearance and the professionalism of the surroundings may also play a role.

In terms of non-verbal communication, a useful acronym to have in mind for body movement and posture as we prepare to communicate is SOLER (Egan, 1998) to demonstrate interest, and active listening, illustrated in Box 1.4.

1.2.8.2 Managing the patient in the room

Animals with emotional or mental disorders can be challenging to manage in a consulting room, so thought must be given to reducing their distress and the anxiety and frustration of the owner to allow effective discourse. Practically, it is difficult to conduct a conversation with an owner whose dog is continually seeking attention or vocalizing. Demonstrating to the owner appropriate human behaviour, such as responding to an attention-seeking dog with avoidance of eye contact and touch until the attention-seeking wanes, and then rewarding settled and quiet behaviour in the room, has two significant results: it will model training to the owner and allow a space in which you can interact. Having tools such as food-delivery toys and treats to reward positive behaviours are good strategies, as is the use of auditory training aids such as 'clickers' (Mills, 2002).

1.2.8.3 Initiating the conversation

This involves greeting the owner, conveying respect and warmth towards them and introducing ourselves. We may wish to overtly state the limitations of the interaction in terms of available time, our qualifications and our experience in behaviour counselling. We should indicate probable consequences of the interview in terms of requirements for the owner to modify their behaviour or the home environment, and instigating training.

1.2.9 Skills for gathering information

1.2.9.1 Questioning techniques

The way we ask questions determines the quality of information we collect. Open questions generally result in a greater and better quality of gathered information (Silverman *et al.*, 2006), particularly at the onset of a consultation (Burack and Carpenter, 1983). Open questioning must be accompanied by facilitation, with non-verbal encouragement and active listening skills. Interrupting the owner's narrative after an opening question may result in inadequate or disjointed information (Dysart *et al.*, 2011). The order in which people present issues is not always prioritized, so if we interrupt we do not get an overview of the problems, and the longer we wait before we interrupt the greater number of issues and concerns will be revealed (Beckman and

Box 1.4. Application of the SOLER model (adapted from Egan, 1998) to the veterinary consultation.

- S: Sit – ideally at a slight angle in relation to the owner.
- O: Maintain an open position with your legs and arms uncrossed.
- L: Lean slightly forward.
- E: Maintain appropriate eye contact without staring.
- R: Relax and avoid fidgeting.

Table 1.1. Types of questions for use in behaviour consultations with examples of their use.

Type of question	Examples
Open	When has Buddy been aggressive? What did you notice? Who was there when it happened? Why do you think the episodes occurred?
Probing	Could you tell me more about why the last episode was different?
Clarifying	To be clear, could you run through the order in which things happened?
Closed	Has Buddy ever bitten someone?

Frankel, 1984). Open questioning also prompts thought processes and is considered key to stimulating reflection and deeper consideration, which is an ideal outcome in a complex behavioural conundrum (Miller and Rose, 2009), in addition to engendering satisfaction and trust in the clinician (Haidet and Paterniti, 2003).

Open questioning employs words such as 'when', 'why', 'where', 'what', 'how' and 'who' and encourages the owner to identify and voice the observations and interpretations they have made without judgement. Probing and clarifying questions explore statements made, and closed questions are useful for gaining details of the specifics about situations and observations. Examples of questions are

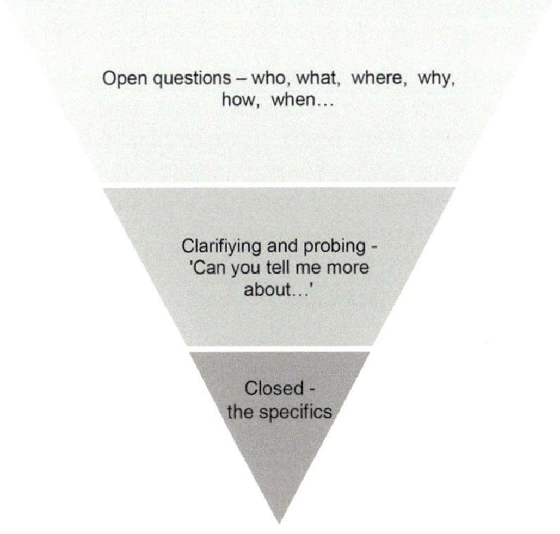

Fig. 1.3. The inverted pyramid model for effective questioning in history taking.

Table 1.2. Questions for exploring owners' ideas, concerns and expectations.

Ideas	Why do you think Tom has suddenly started to urinate inside? How would you rank the issues we have identified in terms of their importance? How would Tom rank these issues?
Concerns	How confident do you feel about keeping the cats separately in the house? What is the attitude of the rest of the family to the situation?
Expectations	What options do you think you have for Tom if treatment is not successful?

given in Table 1.1. The shape of questioning can be viewed as an inverted pyramid as in Fig. 1.3.

Care should be taken not to ask multiple questions at once as owners are not consistent in choosing which to answer. So although 'open', a question such as 'What does he eat and drink?' should be avoided and each aspect of the question explored singly.

1.2.9.2 Gaining an understanding of the owner's point of view

For behavioural contexts this is vital, as providing explanations and management plans requires an understanding of the owner's ideas, concerns and expectations (Little, 2013). Skills to use in determining these include asking the owner directly why they believe the issues have developed, inviting them to prioritize the issues identified in terms of importance to them and to their animal, asking them to rate their confidence in being able to implement any training, and asking specifically what options they feel they have if treatment is not effective. Suggestions as to how to phrase these are given in Table 1.2.

1.2.9.3 How do owners know they have been truly heard?

Being truly heard is an essential component of conversations where owners divulge personal and highly significant aspects of their lives. Being curious rather than judgemental is essential, and we need to demonstrate bravery and empathy in picking up the

Box 1.5. Skills that demonstrate active listening and facilitate the concluding of questioning.

- Non-verbal skills – head nodding, maintaining eye contact, engaged facial expression, encouraging sounds
- Curiosity – 'I'd just like to understand ...'; 'I'm interested in what you do when...'
- Verbal reflection and summary – reflecting what's been heard, summarizing for the owner and requesting they continue
- Paraphrasing and identifying key issues – reflecting on the emotions or major issues: 'It sounds like...'
- Validation – stating the justification for the lived experience of the owner and the animal: 'It is entirely reasonable to have acted/felt...'
- Identifying an agenda collaboratively to provide a springboard for the next stage of the conversation

subtle verbal and non-verbal cues of the story beneath the headlines given, as illustrated in Box 1.5.

1.2.10 Skills for giving information – providing explanations

1.2.10.1 Structure

The structure in which we give information will influence how it is received. If we explain in advance to our listeners what we are going to say, they can pace themselves, gaining something tangible to structure their memories of the process after the conversation is over. Skills to use are: 'signposting', as described in the VCC model ('I'm going to talk about the aggression first and then about the recall issues you've been having'); overt categorization, such as dividing the causes into predisposing, precipitating and perpetuating factors; and using visual aids such as diagrams and flow charts.

Overtly prioritizing what we say is important to avoid overloading our listeners. Pacing the conversation by summarizing periodically with a specific time to allow the owner to ask questions before tackling the next stage is a useful skill and often termed 'chunking and checking'. Silence and pauses are highly important when emotional or complex information is being delivered.

1.2.10.2 Terminology choice

We need to strive for clarity. Choosing terminology that does not patronize but also does not alienate can be challenging. Taking care to notice your owner's words and phrases is a good strategy to allow mirroring their language use, as is routinely defining technical phrases after you have given them. For example: 'I'm suggesting we desensitize Barney – that is, gradually expose him to the noise that causes his fear.'

1.2.10.3 How do we know they have heard?

We must gauge whether our owner has heard and understood our explanations for their animal's behaviour and the principles and options for ongoing management. We can ask them directly to tell us in their own words what they have understood from our communication but this can feel patronizing and awkward and more subtle ways of assessing owners' understanding may be appropriate. Being highly sensitive to visual and verbal cues will let us know our owner's emotional response and whether they are continuing to concentrate on the issues presented (Carson, 2007). If we notice changes, we need to stop and positively ask permission to go on, acknowledging that there has been a change in the listener's attitude. For example, 'You look confused, would you like me to repeat that description?' Putting the onus on the professional's ability to explain is a far better strategy than relying on the listener to admit that they have not understood: 'I think I said that very quickly, so I'll go through it again'. Offering summaries – 'Is it OK if I summarize what we've just talked through?' – is more likely to be acceptable to an owner.

1.2.11 Making shared decisions

1.2.11.1 Collaboration

A spectrum of communication styles in veterinary professionals has been described (Shaw *et al.*, 2006; Cornell and Kopcha, 2007). Put together, these could be viewed as a spectrum with the concept of the veterinarian as paternalistic, providing

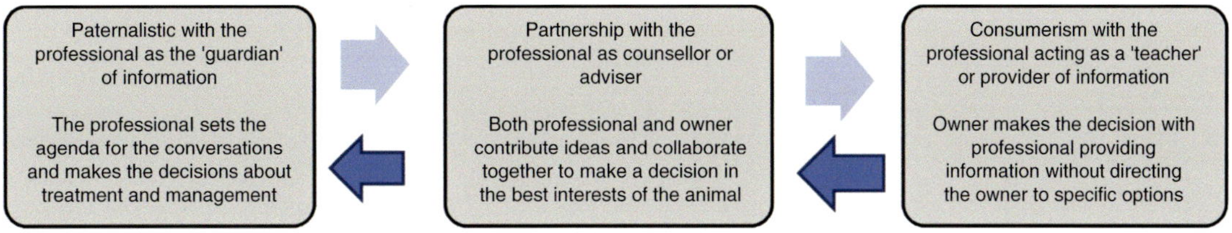

Fig. 1.4. Communication styles for professional–owner interaction in behaviour conversations. (Adapted from Shaw *et al.*, 2006 and Cornell and Kopcha, 2007.)

information and making decisions on behalf of the owner and patient at one end, and the owner being wholly responsible for the decision making at the other, the veterinarian having a passive or detached role of providing detailed and accurate information. The middle ground could be viewed as the collaborative one where both owner and veterinarian contribute ideas and together create a plan, with the role of the professional being one of advisor or counsellor as described in Fig. 1.4.

In veterinary psychiatry, although we prescribe medications to modify emotions and mental processes, these are usually in conjunction with behavioural modification programmes delivered by the owner. Without owner compliance the prognosis for cases is poor. The relationship between owner and clinician is therefore best suited to the collaborative or partnership approach.

1.2.11.2 Empathy

Empathy has been defined as 'the ability to enter into and understand the world of another person and communicate this understanding' (Egan, 1998). This is the set of skills at the very heart of our ability to truly support our owners and care for the animals under our care. It is important to note its dual dimension. It is not enough to care and feel sympathetic towards the owner and animal; we must also convey that level of care and desire to understand to the owner.

It must be truthful. At times we may be shocked or saddened by what we hear, but within this it is usually possible to find something positive to empathize with that is truthful. The non-verbal signals we give when we are telling owners untruths will always undermine the positive suggestions we voice for managing situations.

Empathy is not without risk, and although shared decision making leads to improved clinician satisfaction (Coe *et al.*, 2008), there is a significant impact on clinicians in terms of well-being (Riess, 2015).

1.2.11.3 So what are the skills required for collaborative working with owners?

These are summarized in Table 1.3.

This incorporates MI's Open Questioning (O), Affirming (A), Reflective Listening (R) and Summarizing (S).

1.2.12 The specific challenges of conversations around mental and emotional health of small animals

1.2.12.1 Time and resource limitations

We should be overt with owners and indicate at the outset the time and cost implications of consultations. This is especially true in first-opinion practices. Strategies such as using post-consultation questionnaires to gather more information, booking sequential appointments to further discuss behaviour, using phone conversations to maximize the value of face-to-face time, employing pre-prepared supporting literature, and utilizing existing services such as nurse-led clinics are positive options.

1.2.12.2 Managing owner expectations

Owners can have unrealistic expectations of us to deal with their animal's mental and emotional disorders, often reflecting how much is at stake. These disorders can be life-threatening to the patient when euthanasia is an option. Again, ensuring that we are overt and realistic about the prognosis for resolution and change is key. Prognoses differ. For example, in inter-cat aggression in a household, even with excellent owner compliance, the prognosis for the cats tolerating each other's presence to the extent owners often desire can be poor, while

Table 1.3. Communication strategies for shared or collaborative decision making.

Skill	Function	Example
Be curious	Open-questioning techniques will allow owners to feel listened to. **O**	'Are you able to tell me more about what has been most difficult for you?'
Notice and reflect what you see	Noticing and naming discomfort around specific topics will help you and owners focus on the important issues. **R**	'You looked uncomfortable when talking about your children and Tiger. Could you tell me how they get on with him?'
Reflect	Hearing you reflect, owners will feel understood and listened to. Going on to reflect the emotions behind statements is even more powerful for owners. **R**	'So last week Tiger snapped at one of the children and left a mark on her skin...and this is worrying to you.'
Legitimize	Legitimizing actions or emotions is a powerful way of expressing empathy. **A**	'It's understandable how worried you are as you don't want your daughter to be bitten, and you can see how upset Tiger is by the change in how you talk to him.'
Validate	Being praised or validated will engender a co-operative response. **A**	'You were right to come and ask for help.' 'Although Tiger is still aggressive, you were correct in noticing he was scared.'
Ask for the owner's ideas	MI has identified that people are more motivated by solutions they have found themselves than ones imposed on them.	'Have you any ideas about how you could keep Tiger away from the front door while we get the training established?'
Acknowledge the relationship between owner and their animal	This is the key to owners seeking help and reflecting this will engender trust in you from the owner. **A**	'You care about Tiger, and he hasn't left your side since you came in, so he obviously loves you.' 'I can see how much Tiger means to your family and how loyal you've been to him.'
Ask permission	Being asked if they will accept ideas validates your owners' personal sense of autonomy.	'Is it OK if I give you the perspective of why I believe Tiger has started to be aggressive towards you and the children?'
Offer choices	Suggesting flexibility and a desire to find the right solution for the owner conveys a positive, caring approach. **O**	'There are several possible ways we could manage the situation. What feels the most feasible way forward for you?'
Summarize	Summarizing demonstrates your ability to actively listen and empathize with the situation, particularly if you include the emotions in the situation. It allows a point in the conversation to take stock and redirect the discussion. **S**	'So, in summary, Tiger has now bitten you three times and recently also mouthed one of the children. You are frightened for your children's safety but also for Tiger as you can't have him in your family if he bites. You know he's scared by something and feel torn, trying to keep both Tiger and the children safe.'
Offer partnership	Using the pronoun 'we' suggests that you and the owners are working together to solve an issue and shows partnership and support.	'What I suggest is that we, together, put forward a plan for managing Tiger.'
Offer support	Offering practical support can make a task less daunting to owners.	'I'm going to make sure all the instructions are written down and that you can come and see the nurse in a week for some help with the clicker training.'

Continued

Table 1.3. Continued

Skill	Function	Example
Sensitivity	Financial or ethical dilemmas are challenging and require extreme sensitivity. Reflecting the challenging nature of these areas without necessarily offering solutions is a good starting point.	'I can see that the cost of seeing a dog trainer is going to be challenging.' 'Your family has an extremely difficult decision to make.'
'Safety netting' (giving specific suggestions as to when owners should contact you)	Making sure your owner feels 'held' by you or the practice is an empathetic response.	'Remember that someone is on the other end of the phone every day. Although I think it's unlikely that Tiger will bite again, now that we have some strategies in place, I would like you to call me immediately if he does.'

the prognosis for desensitization to a noise phobia is generally good. We need to ensure that we always talk through options associated with failure of therapy: 'What do you feel your options are if this treatment fails?' This question gives us greater insight into the owner's motivation to resolve the issues.

1.2.12.3 Dealing with self-blame

During a conversation, it may dawn on the owner that it is their behaviour that has contributed to the development or perpetuation of the difficult animal's behaviour. Examples of this would be the inadvertent reinforcement of undesired behaviours with reassurance and physical rewards, or with punishment. Similarly, a perceived lack of ability to change the environment, or lack of resources, can lead to self-blame. Being empathetic and aware of the likelihood of such emotions is the first step. Being brave enough to notice and name them is the next: 'I sense you are feeling guilty that by punishing Buddy for being aggressive to other dogs you may have made him even more fearful when he meets them.' Making an overt empathetic statement and then lightly suggesting that the important thing is now to move forward would be a worthwhile strategy: 'I can sense that you feel you have let him down, but by coming here and learning how to do things differently you can make a huge difference.'

1.2.12.4 Poor motivation for personal behaviour change in owners

Some owners constantly offer barriers to our treatment suggestions. They imply that any suggestion to change the environment or their lifestyle in order to instigate treatment is flawed or impossible. MI techniques would be highly appropriate.

The essence of MI is that arguments for change are more persuasive when the owner hears themselves making them. We all have the drive to identify an animal's and an owner's problems and then immediately offer solutions to 'fix' these by getting them to listen to the evidence behind our suggestions and the rationality of the arguments. This is sometimes termed the 'righting reflex' and is a human desire to help. However, puzzlingly, it can have the opposite effect. The explanation given for this is that when people are ambivalent about change, they often see the arguments both for and against changing. When we hear one side of what we know is a two-sided argument, we tend to defend and align with the alternative viewpoint. So by using the 'righting reflex' we inadvertently push owners into an opposing viewpoint. MI suggests we look for opportunities where the owner voices the reasons for change, and our role is to note and guide the 'change talk' to a positive conclusion (Miller and Rollnick, 2013). Readers interested in this counselling technique are encouraged to witness the process on the British Medical Association's learning section, which allows access for veterinary professionals (British Medical Association, 2019).

1.2.12.5 Differing ethical points of view

It is challenging when we discover that our owner has an ethical stance at odds with our own. Being professional initially involves listening and being curious, and remaining non-judgemental. A useful strategy is to ask permission of an owner to express and explore an alternative point of view:

'I can understand that you believe that Delilah should have a litter every year and that her behaviour makes this problematic. I differ in my viewpoint. Would it be OK for me to explain this?' If we believe the animal's welfare is compromised, we have a duty of care to also explore this with the owner in a clear and empathetic manner. One of the most powerful messages we have at this point, after developing rapport and using our ORAS skills to engage with the owner, is to state clearly the withdrawal of our support. For example, 'I can see that caging Bella solves the problem for you, but I am very concerned about her. I realize that all the suggestions I have made are not feasible for you. However, I don't feel I can support you in continuing to manage her like this.' Beyond this, asking for a second opinion from another professional and involving welfare organizations, such as the SPCA in your area, may be the appropriate, but difficult, steps to take (Mullan and Fawcett, 2017).

1.2.12.6 Quality-of-life discussions

Euthanasia is always an option in veterinary medicine. In discussing prognosis, the 'What if this can't be resolved?' question begins to open the way to discuss quality-of-life issues with, for example, owners of very fearful or anxious individuals. Keys to the discussion in assessing quality of life with companion animal owners are a holistic view of an animal's life, beyond health and physical concerns. Mullan and Main (2007) developed a screening tool asking carers to plot, on visual analogue scales, points corresponding to their dog 'at the moment' and also 'when at their best'. They also advise asking about an animal's preferences: 'What would Buster's ideal day consist of?', and then comparing this with the owner to the actuality of the animal's lived daily experience. Whether steps could be made towards the ideal can then be discussed. The responsibility we hold for our pets, and the high motivation required for owners to seek help for behavioural concerns rather than abandon animals, makes this a difficult topic.

1.2.12.7 Talking to children

Many children consider the family pet to be among the most important individuals in their lives (Melson, 2003). Contemplating issues that may result in relinquishment or euthanasia of an animal may, for a child, be intensely emotional. The death may be a child's first experience of loss, and so the child may show a profound level of grief (Sharkin and Knox, 2003).

In terms of preparation, asking the parents/carers how much they want their children to be involved and what they have already told them will promote clarity. Similarly, enquiring about the age of the child, discussion of likely cognitive developmental level, and, if appropriate, their understanding of concepts of life and death, will aid in the choice of language and approach. There are many theories associated with child development, and there are innate differences in individual ability, but Table 1.4 provides a guide.

This information aids us in formulating how to give information to children. We need to give honest, accurate and clear responses to questions. Avoid using euphemisms; for example, the phrase 'put to sleep'. Give younger children very clear and concrete details and try to incorporate the child's perspective when being empathetic.

1.2.12.8 Dealing with multiple owners

Dealing with owners who have differing views, memories and expectations of an animal's behaviour is not uncommon. Skills that are likely to be useful are: providing reflections to both sides; highlighting differences between the two views while remaining non-partisan and uncommitted to a single viewpoint. If one partner is more attached to the animal, appealing to the other to assist with help to solve the problem and validating their skills to do this may be a useful approach. Actions that may be helpful are: asking both owners, separately, to fill out questionnaires to describe the issues; asking how they can help the other in their approach; and carefully negotiating a shared decision. Offering to see absent family members or talk to them on the phone or by video call may be appropriate.

1.2.13 Conclusions

Conversations about behaviour are challenging but they allow us to use and refine our communication skills creatively to engage with owners. Skills can be learnt, and effective application of them will lead to positive outcomes for our patients, their owners and ourselves.

Table 1.4. The main ideas around understanding death. (Adapted from information provided in Piaget, 1964 and Panagiotaki *et al.*, 2018)

Approximate age	Piaget's stages of cognitive development (Piaget, 1964) Children think...	Development of understanding of death (Panagiotaki *et al.*, 2018) Children develop an understanding of:
1–2 years	Sensory motor stage ... that things continue to exist even though they cannot be seen ...they are separate beings from the people and objects around them ...their actions can cause things to happen in the world around them	
2–5 years	Pre-operational or intuitive stage	
5–7 years	...using symbols, words and pictures to represent objects ...egocentric ... struggle to see things from the perspective of others ...in concrete terms	Inevitability (living things will eventually die) Permanency (death is permanent)
Around 7 years	Concrete operations stage ...more logically and in a more organized form, although still in concrete terms ...using inductive logic, or reasoning from specific information to a general principle	Universality (all physiological and mental functions will stop with death) Cessation (all mental and physiological functions cease)
8–11 years		Causality (death is caused by the failure of normal bodily processes)
Over 11 years	Formal operations stage ...abstractly, and reasoning about hypothetical problems ...more about moral, philosophical, ethical, social and political issues that require theoretical and abstract reasoning ...using deductive logic, or reasoning from a general principle to specific information	

1.3 Building or Modifying Your Practice to Reduce Patient Stress

When designing a practice, there are numerous factors to consider and the complexity can sometimes be overwhelming. The layout must suit the workflow and the staff, and support a low-stress environment. Patients are often fearful of the practice based on past experiences, other patients' behaviour and their reaction to unfamiliar people. Also, many patients are in pain or are sick when arriving at the practice, which adds to their overall anxiety.

When considering a rebuild of an existing practice, or designing a new practice, in addition to the minimum requirements from the local regulatory body and building regulations, the design must also address options to reduce the fear of patients while in the practice. Undoubtedly there will be financial constraints and, in an existing practice, space and structural limitations.

1.3.1 Planning

When considering building a new practice, or remodelling an existing one, the first step is to outline the goals. These include, for example, the number of consulting rooms, theatres and wards, and access to them. Further, it is critical to decide which patients you are going to see (e.g. dogs and cats, or cats only) before starting the work.

It is essential to identify possible problems in the existing practice, by reviewing other practices, or areas that lead to reduced efficiency or increased anxiety for patients. Soliciting the opinions of different staff members (e.g. vets, nurses, reception or kennel assistants) may help to identify such areas.

Also, consulting with experienced architects and project managers is highly valuable. Not only can they provide ideas on workflow efficiency and what is structurally possible, but they can also provide examples of past projects.

A pivotal point to consider is that the veterinary practice is a threatening place for most patients. The practice includes many possible triggers such as smells, sounds, lights, surfaces and unfamiliar people. Planning the practice to address these factors will increase the likelihood of reducing fear during visits and stays.

The average veterinary practice has two simple workflows. The outpatient: owners and patients arrive at the reception and then move into the consulting room and back to the reception before leaving. The inpatient: owners bring their patients into the reception and then possibly into the consulting room. Then the owner leaves while the patient is left with staff members and taken to the wards. From there, the patient is taken into the treatment area for surgical preparation, theatre, recovery, and then back to the wards before being discharged at the reception. When designing the practice, these workflows must be considered for possible pitfalls such as patients passing each other in a narrow hallway, anxious and vocal patients housed near patients recovering from surgery, or dogs and cats having to wait in the same area.

1.3.2 Entrance and reception areas

The journey in the practice starts at the car park. When possible, consider having several spaces allocated not only for owners with physical disabilities but also for owners of senior dogs or dogs with difficulties in walking into the practice. A newer practice design might even divide the practice and the car park into separate areas for dogs and cats, with separate parking areas and entrances. Try to avoid stairs at the entrance to the practice or provide a ramp.

The reception area is the first bottleneck to consider. When many owners arrive at the same time, the result could be anxious patients standing next to each other, with dogs near cats or other species. Some of these patients might also be aggressive. Scheduling (known) aggressive or fearful patients appropriately or asking owners to leave the patient in the car while registering and then waiting in the car helps to reduce fear and aggression in the reception area (Fig. 1.5.).

Ideally, the reception and waiting areas would separate the different species; cats appear to be distressed when next to dogs and unable to avoid the situation (McCobb *et al.*, 2005; Volk *et al.*, 2011McCobb *et al.*, 2005). When possible, two different rooms or areas should be allotted (see Fig. 1.5C). If this is not possible, the existing area should be divided using visual barriers such as shelves with products or stands. In the cat waiting areas, stands for cat crates should be provided to keep the cats above floor level (Fig. 1.6.) and separate from each other. When stands are not available, cats should be kept on the seat next to the owner, and the crates should be covered with a blanket to minimize exposure. For more information on cats' waiting areas, see the recommended standards by the International Society of Feline Medicine (catfriendlyclinic.org).

Sliding doors at the entrance are beneficial when owners carry their patients in a carrier or when wheeling a sick patient into the practice. However, motion sensors might also react to patients and people walking by the door. The opening and closing might scare some patients, and those who are not controlled well with a lead may escape. One option is to install sliding doors that are activated using a button, or two doors with a vestibule in-between.

Having a separate entrance for anxious or aggressive patients can be very useful. Similarly, having direct access to the consulting room from the outside allows owners of fearful or aggressive patients to go into the room and then back out to the car without meeting other patients or people, apart from the veterinary surgeon and nurse.

For many dogs, walking onto and standing on the scale is threatening (Hernander, 2008). Better than a typical stand-on scale at the corner of the room is a scale in the hallway, or along a wall (but not in the corner) that the patient walks through. The scale should be buried at the floor level, creating a continuous path (see Fig. 1.7.).

Consideration should be given to a retail area in the reception. While having tasty treats and food is part of the practice, it is essential to remember that the smell of aromatic treats may be negative. Some patients that are brought to the practice are sick and nauseous. The smell may aggravate this feeling. Also, the smell of a tasty treat present while the patient is anxious may create conflict, leading to higher arousal. Therefore treats should be kept in

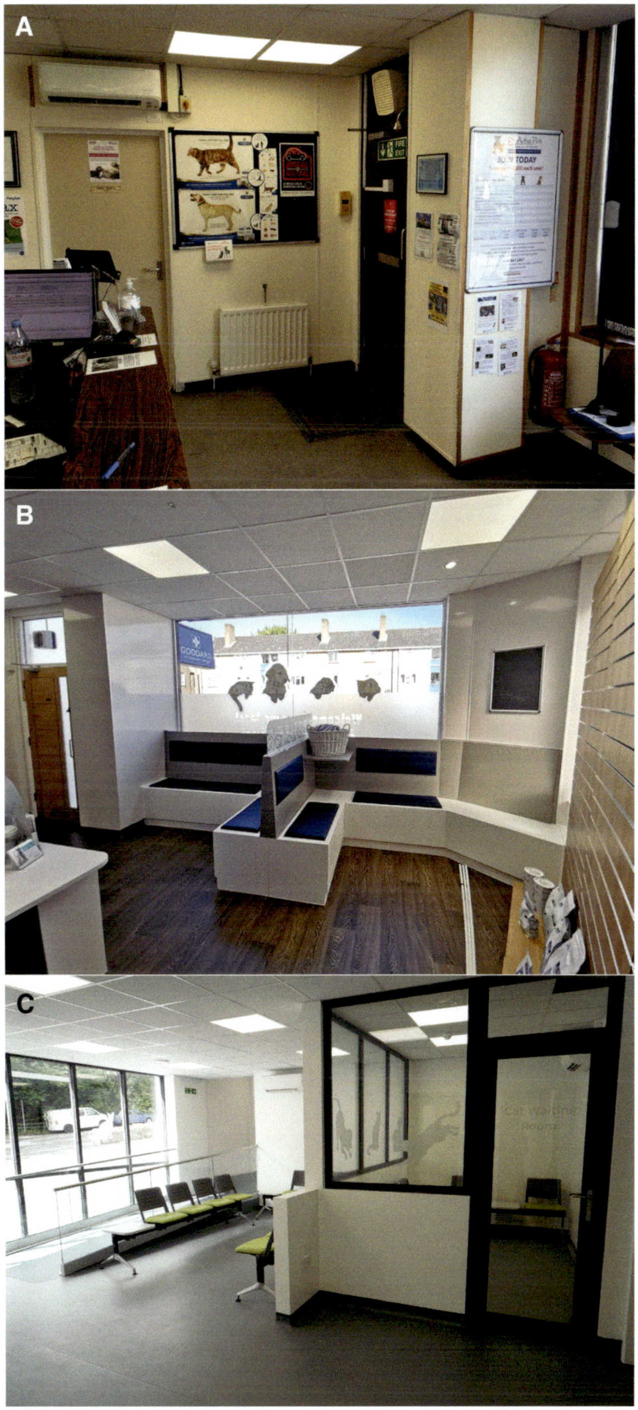

Fig. 1.5. (A) Reception area before renovation and adaptation to a more 'patient-friendly' area (photo courtesy of Mark Gill, Goddard Veterinary Group); (B) Same reception area after renovation (photo courtesy of Mark Gill); (C) When possible, try creating separated waiting areas for dogs and cats (photo courtesy of Jeremy Voakes, Archway Vets).

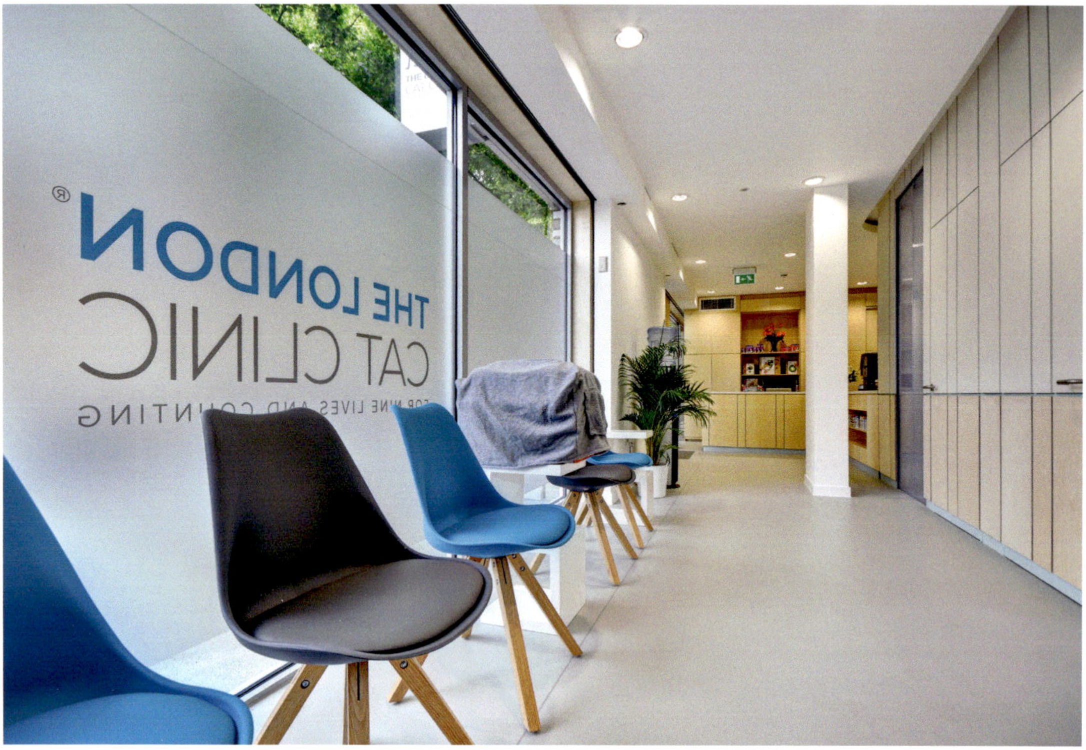

Fig. 1.6. Placing cats above floor level and covering the crate can help to minimise exposure to potentially threatening stimuli. (Photo courtesy of Dr Jeremy Campbell, The London Cat Clinic.)

a closed container and offered by owners to their patients when appropriate.

Reception areas can be designed to look like a living-room. Instead of chairs or benches, a sofa could be placed. The sofa can be made from an easy-to-clean material such as leather. The use of towels or blankets would allow dogs to settle on the floor while waiting. However, these should be replaced regularly and washed carefully to prevent the transfer of infectious diseases.

The reception desk should not be too high if using a counter; it should have space to place down carriers of small patients, especially cats. This would prevent the need to leave the carrier on the floor where cats might be exposed to other patients, in particular large dogs. The cat might feel that it cannot avoid them, thus becoming more anxious. Alternatively, a crate stand could be placed next to the reception counter.

1.3.3 Consulting rooms

This is where most patients' fear level peaks as they are being handled and manipulated by unfamiliar people. Also, some of these patients are in pain or are sick. Thus their negative bias is high. This can be exaggerated by negative memories of previous visits to the same room (or similar), causing many patients to refuse to walk into the room.

Consulting rooms should have two doors when possible; one for the owner and patient to come in, and the second for the staff. The inner door should lead to the wards and treatment areas. It also helps to have all of the necessary materials and tools for a routine examination prepared and in place in the room. This means that staff do not have to keep leaving and returning to the room.

Most dogs and cats try to avoid the examination table (Döring *et al.*, 2009). A simple metal or wood table is the most common design in practices. While it is easy to clean, it is not a comfortable surface

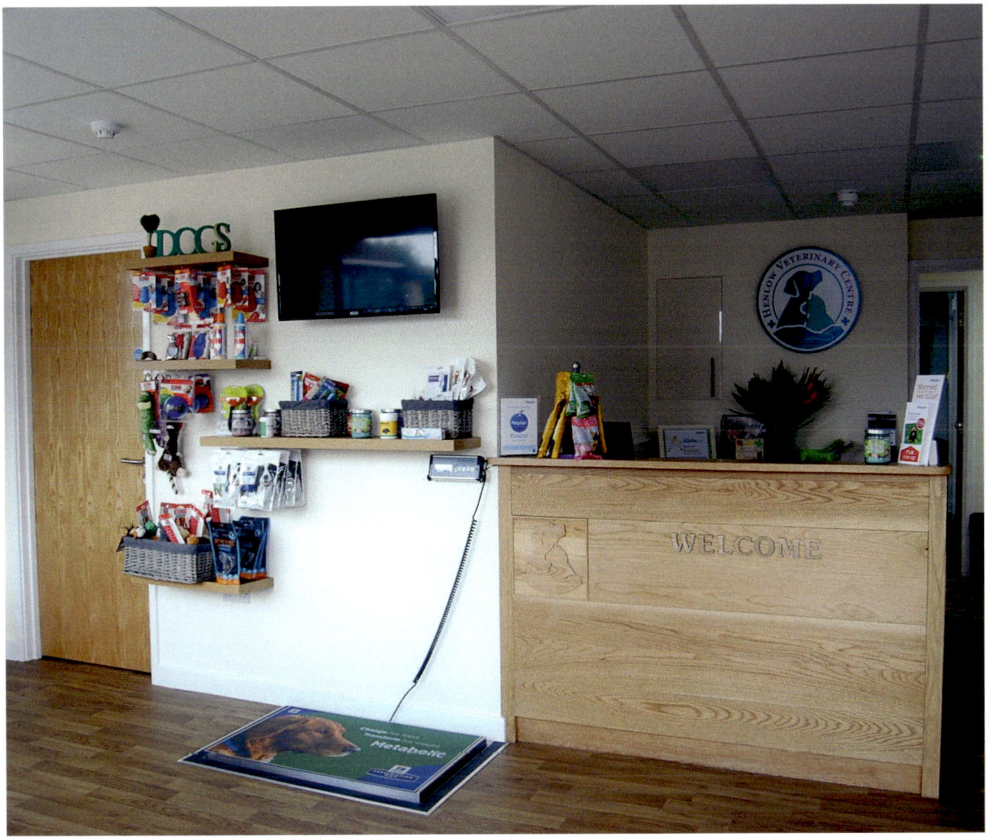

Fig. 1.7. Scales in the corner can cause more anxiety. Placing the scale along a walking path allows the dog to walk on it on its way towards the consulting room or reception. (Photo courtesy of Graeme Mason, Henlow Vets.)

for the patient to stand on and feel stable. Placing a rubber mattress or plastic mat can help the patient feel more stable and is easy to clean and disinfect. When possible, the examination, especially with large dogs or cats who refuse to come out of their crate, should be on the floor or in a crate whose top half has been removed. Therefore, installing examination tables that can be folded up to the wall or easily removed from the room gives the advantage of space and makes the room appear less like an examination room. (See Fig. 1.8.)

Providing high areas for cats to explore, perch or hide inside can be useful as well. This must be balanced with the ability to examine the cat and finish the examination on time. Thus, perching spaces should not be higher than where the staff can easily reach and have access to the cat or to clean appropriately (see Fig. 1.9).

If space allows, designating species-specific examination rooms can prevent the transfer of odours. When using the same consulting room for different species, attention must be given to appropriate cleaning and ventilation before the next patient. Alternatively, it might be possible to divide the practice schedule so that certain patients are examined at specific times. For example, cat consultations could take place in the morning, with dog consultations in the afternoon. This routine would allow for appropriate cleaning.

1.3.4 Wards

This is where patients spend most of their time in the hospital without their owners when they are sick. Also, human and patient traffic and the number of patients in the area is generally high. Kennels

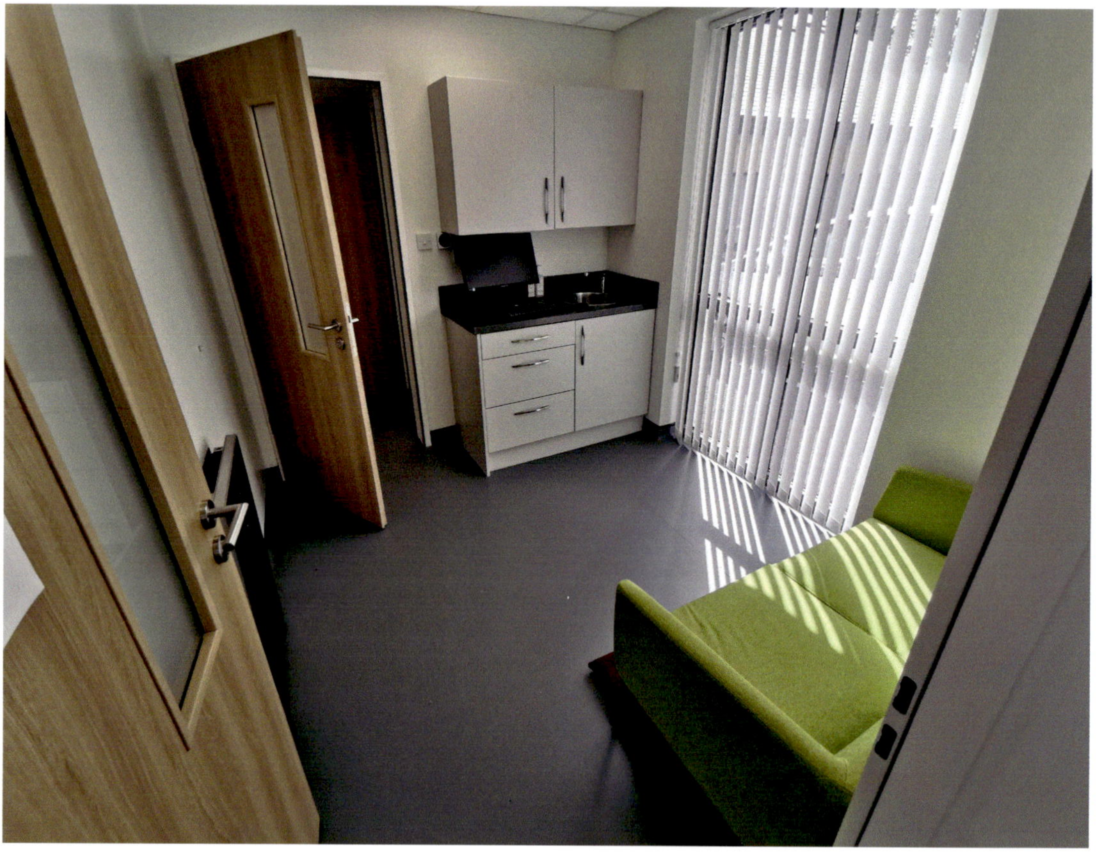

Fig. 1.8. Placing easy-to-remove examination tables helps increase space in the consultation room. Some pets respond better to a physical examination on the chair, the floor or in their owner's arms or crate. (Photo courtesy of Jeremy Voakes, Archway Vets.)

should, therefore, be designed in such a way as to reduce the anxiety of the patient.

Dog kennels should vary in size based on the size of the dog. Cats' kennels should have sufficient space for a litter tray and a hiding box. Ideally, a cat kennel should be high enough internally to allow for a perch to be mounted within it. The patient should have sufficient space to stand up, circle, lie down comfortably, and fully stretch. The floor of the kennel should have a comfortable surface for the patient to lie down on and walk (Fig. 1.10A and B).

An ideal design is to stagger kennels at a 45-degree angle to the entrance to the room. This design allows staff in the ward to observe multiple patients at once and, at the same time, reduces the ability of the patients to see each other, which can lead to increased fear (Kry and Casey, 2007) (Fig. 1.11).

Another option is to place barriers in front of the kennel or on the kennel door, to block the view of anxious patients. This is also important at night when patients need to sleep, yet the staff need light.

Some patients, especially geriatric, orthopaedic or neurological large and giant breed dogs may have mobility problems or find the floors slippery. Installing an overhead crane and support system can assist the staff and patient to move into and outside the kennels and the wards (see Fig. 1.12).

1.3.5 Treatment area and surgical preparation

These are busy areas of the practice, and often only minimal consideration is given to the patient's

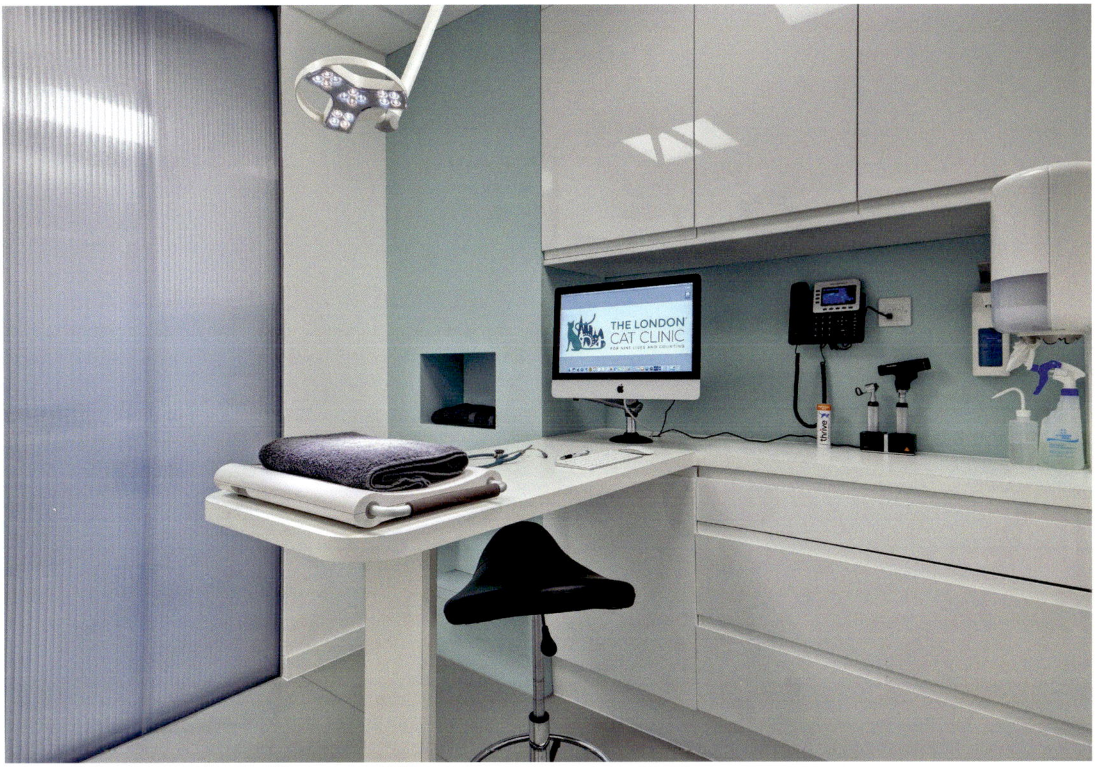

Fig. 1.9. Cats may want to hide or perch while you talk to the owners. Providing an appropriate option helps reduce anxiety and facilitates easier examination. (Photo courtesy of Dr Jeremy Campbell, The London Cat Clinic.)

emotional needs in these areas. As much thought and consideration should be taken when designing treatment rooms and preparation areas as it is for the consulting rooms. When possible, handling patients in the treatment area should be done when no other patients are present. If more than one patient is treated at the same time, the area should be divided into isolated pods (see Fig. 1.13A and B).

The surface of the treatment table should be covered with a rubber mat to allow the patient to stand comfortably on a non-slippery surface. If different species are handled in the same area, ideally, this should be done at different times to allow appropriate cleaning and ventilation.

1.3.6 Other species

When working with patients other than dogs and cats, similar considerations of species-specific adjustments are necessary. Cats are the natural predators of many other patient species such as rats, guinea pigs and birds. Thus, when examining or hospitalizing any of these patients, all cat odours and sight of cats should be avoided. When space and finance allow, a separate waiting area, consulting room, ward and treatment area should be available. The kennels in wards should allow for the patient carrier to be placed inside without taking the patient out of its carrier.

1.3.7 Practice-wide approach

The following sections detail different factors that apply to all areas within the practice. These factors are meant to reduce the anxiety and fear of patients while ensuring that the workflow and hygiene are maximized.

1.3.7.1 Vision

The practice should appear pleasant not only to owners but also their patients. The colour scheme,

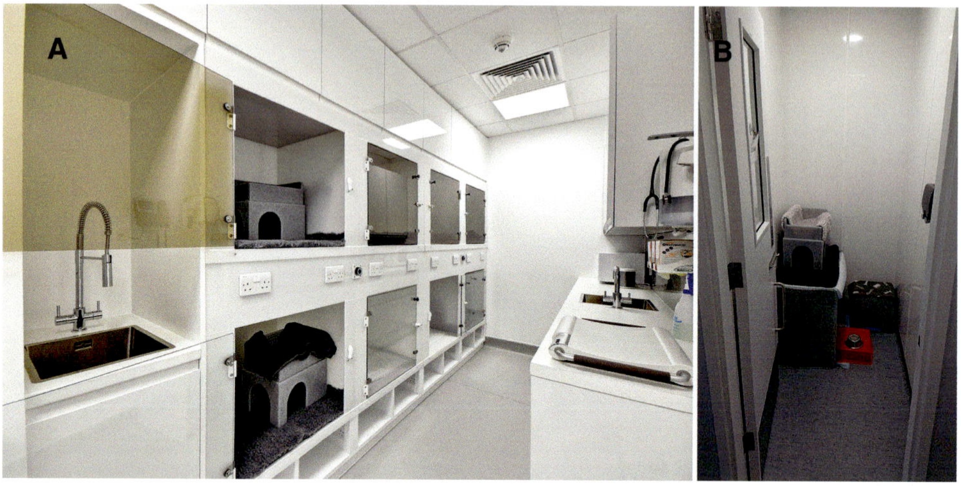

Fig. 1.10. (A) Cat kennels for hospitalized patients. The kennel is sufficiently large to allow the cat to walk inside, lie comfortably, and eat. Also, a litter tray can be placed inside while allowing the cat to rest high on a perch or hide. Note the tinted doors of the upper kennels – it helps cats to rest better while allowing staff members to observe the patient; (B) Larger units allow placement of more hiding boxes and vertical stimulation. These are useful for longer-stay patients. (Photos courtesy of Sagi Denenberg, Langford Vets.)

lighting and scent all have an impact on the patient. Dogs have a dichromatic vision, and while they can see most of the range of colours that humans can, they cannot easily distinguish wavelengths between green and orange (Neitz *et al.*, 1989). Cats' vision is trichromatic, although with less colour precision than humans, and they also discern the blue and violet end of the spectrum better than the red end. Both species can see into the ultraviolet spectrum and many surfaces and materials can appear fluorescent to them. Both dogs and cats see better in low light compared to a human. Therefore

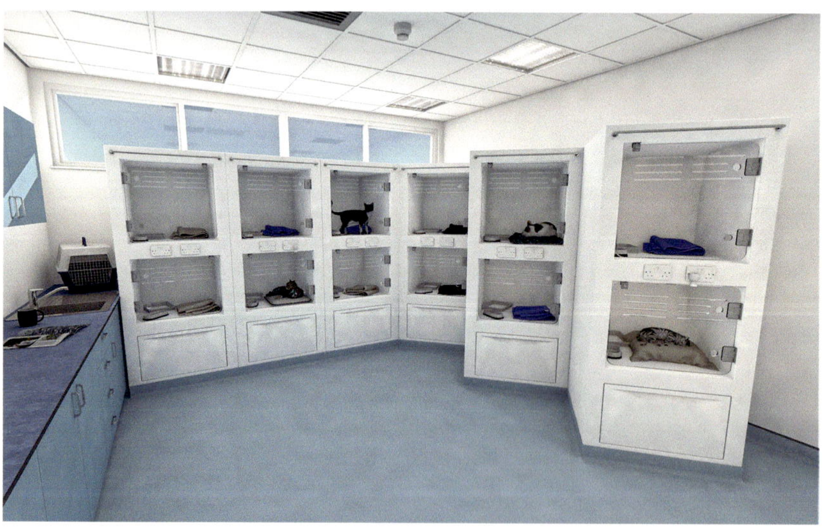

Fig. 1.11. Staggering kennels at a 45-degree angle allows staff members to see all hospitalized patients while preventing the patients from seeing each other. Also, airflow is likely to be more optimal for ventilation. (Photo courtesy of Alex Darvill, ACD Projects.)

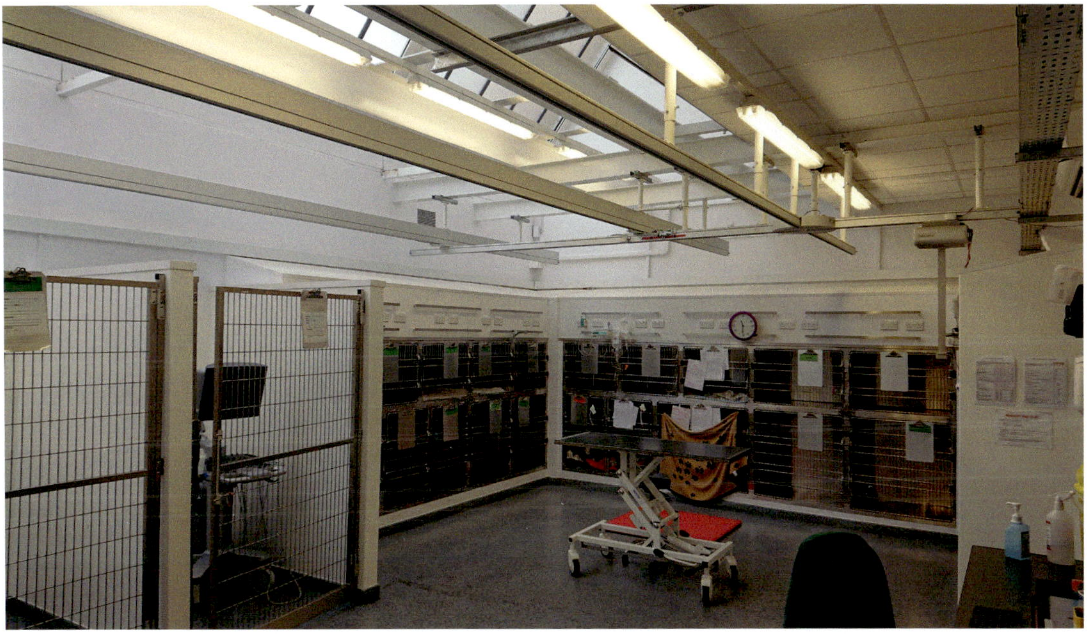

Fig. 1.12. Having kennels in different sizes allows the management of different-sized patients efficiently. Placing rubber mats on the floor allows patients to stand on a slippery surface. Note the overhead crane system to harness large dogs who cannot move well. (Photo courtesy of Sagi Denenberg, Langford Vets.)

it is preferable to avoid bright colours like whites, reds and oranges, and darker colours are generally better. Making more use of pastel shades of blue can create a calmer environment (Lewis, 2015). Unfortunately, white plastic is often used for frequently cleaned areas as the dirt is easier to see, and the white material is usually cheaper than coloured versions.

1.3.7.2 Sound

Our patients hear exceptionally well, so reducing noise throughout the practice should be a key focus in your design and material specification. The wards are where the highest concentration of dogs will be at any one time and the most likely place for any excess noise to be generated. As dogs are most likely to bark when they are disturbed, attention must be paid to reducing disturbance as much as possible.

The use of music in veterinary hospitals has been investigated; however, no conclusive data exist. It might be that classical music is more soothing for the dog, especially with slower rhythm (McConnell, 1990; Wells *et al.*, 2002; Kogan *et al.*, 2012; McConnell, 2013). It is also possible that playing audiobooks is even more helpful (Brayley and Montrose, 2016). Cats appear to respond better to music of a higher tempo and pitch than dogs (Snowdon *et al.*, 2015). Therefore, during the planning of the practice, consideration should be given to installing speakers and having the connecting cables buried in the walls to prevent patients from chewing them, and also to reduce surface area for cleaning. Alternatively, the use of wireless speakers is recommended.

In addition to playing music and trying to maintain a quiet environment, considering suppression and retention of sound is essential. For example, sound-absorbing ceiling tiles, insulation and double-glazed windows can dramatically reduce noise reverberation (Moser, 2004).

1.3.7.3 Odours

Dogs and cats rely on olfaction as one of their primary senses. When designing and, later, maintaining a practice, care must be given not to overlook olfaction. Much thought also needs to be given to the ventilation, cooling, heating and reclaimed air

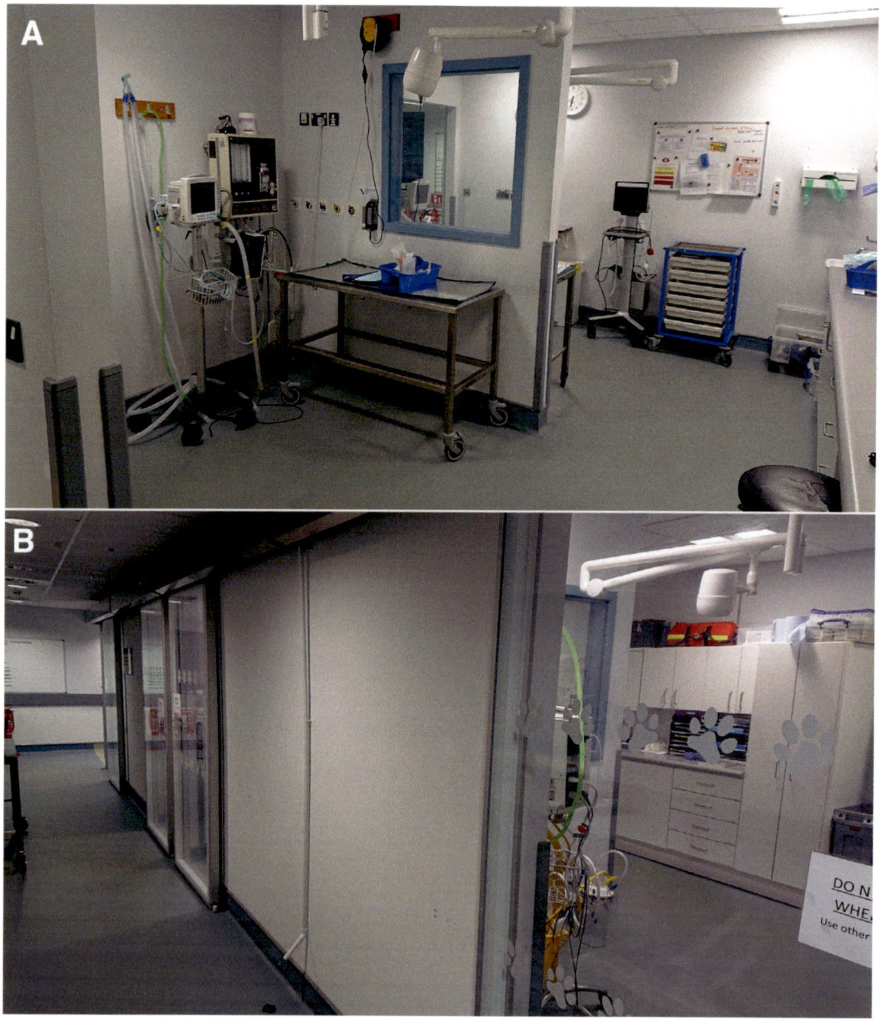

Fig. 1.13. (A) Treatment and anaesthetic induction areas divided into individual units. This design allows the staff to work efficiently while separating patients who might be distressed or agitated. (B) Showing separate entrances to each unit. Patients do not have to be in contact or close to other patients. (Photos courtesy of Sagi Denenberg, Langford Vets.)

throughout the practice. Investing in the right air filtration and handling equipment can make it more comfortable for the staff and patients, ensuring it's not too hot in the summer or too cold in the winter. It is also more economical in the long term for the business, and it will mean cleaner air, if the transfer of disease and spread of odours is prevented. Furthermore, a good filtration system will eliminate vapours of caustic materials. For example, it is common practice to clean and disinfect kennels and treatment areas using solutions containing sodium hypochlorite, sodium perborate or hydrogen peroxide. These solutions are strong oxidizing liquids that adhere to surfaces and leave vapours. Sudden exposure of a dog or a cat to these vapours, for example when immediately placing a patient inside a recently cleaned kennel, can result in damage to the nasal mucosa (olfactory neurons), reducing the patient's olfactory abilities. This has the effect of disabling the patient's ability to perceive information accurately, which can also lead to the patient becoming more anxious.

1.3.7.4 Surfaces

Surface materials in veterinary practices should always be easy to clean and disinfect. The most commonly used surface is a simple and standard vinyl, which is a ruberoid or plastic material. Rubber surfaces can be used, as well as polyurethanes and epoxy resin floorings. These all come in an abundance of different slip resistances, and they should, therefore, be considered during your build. Ceramic tiles are another alternative. However, if choosing ceramics, you must consider the durability of the grout and adhesive used. As with epoxy resins and polyurethanes, you have to go into great detail with application and type of broadcasting required to achieve a slip resistance. You must also be aware of the substrate underneath the flooring as this often has detrimental effects by cracking these sprayed-on surfaces. Linoleum should be avoided as it is not necessarily a waterproof product and cannot handle the amount of washing required, especially those with hessian backing.

There is a balance to be found in terms of slip resistance and cleanliness. Those surfaces which are most easy to maintain can also be slippery and may increase the anxiety of patients, especially those who are sick or have mobility issues. A simple solution could, of course, be to provide slip-resistant shoes for staff and washable mats for patients to walk on, instead of changing the flooring to a non-slip material that is harder to clean.

1.3.8 Exercise area

Where possible, you should always provide an external exercise area for you to take the dogs for short breaks outside the veterinary practice. This could be for walks, exercise, rehabilitation or just for them to relieve themselves.

Grassed areas are not always possible and, of course, if they are used a lot in wet weather they will deteriorate fast and turn into mud baths. Many vets prefer concrete or even tarmac, laid with a slight fall to a channel drain, which is always useful as this will then facilitate hosing down.

Concrete and tarmac are fine finishes for dogs, though not particularly stimulating for them. Tarmac would last longer, especially if washed down frequently, but both of these surfaces have small pitted areas which could harbour disease unless cleaned down thoroughly.

Astroturf is also very common, although when deciding to use this material you should avoid the high-pile version as there are many short finishes on the market, which are easier to clean and can also be washed down. This material can, therefore, be cleaned and will not deteriorate like natural grass.

The fencing that surrounds these areas can be as simple as timber fencing, although try to avoid this as much as possible as timber on its own could easily rot, break or harbour pathogens such as fungi (e.g. ringworm).

Another option would be to cover timber fencing with white plastic sheeting to give an aseptic and easy-clean finish. This only needs to be to approximately 1400 mm from the ground, and if the Astroturf comes up the wall by 100 mm, you can overlap the Astroturf, thus providing a good finish. Alternatively, a brick finish with smooth joints, or even rendered, would suffice.

References

Beckman, H.B. and Frankel, R.M. (1984) The effect of physician behavior on the collection of data. *Annals of Internal Medicine* 101(5), 692–696. DOI: 10.7326/0003-4819-101-5-692.

Brayley, C. and Montrose, V.T. (2016) The effects of audiobooks on the behaviour of dogs at a rehoming kennels. *Applied Animal Behaviour Science* 174, 111–115. DOI: 10.1016/j.applanim.2015.11.008.

British Medical Association (2019) Motivational interviewing in brief consultations. Available at: https://learning.bmj.com/learning/module-intro/.html?moduleId=10051582 (accessed 2 September 2019).

Burack, R.C. and Carpenter, R.R. (1983) The predictive value of the presenting complaint. *The Journal of Family Practice* 16(4), 749–754.

Carson, C.A. (2007) Nonverbal communication in veterinary practice. *Veterinary Clinics of North America: Small Animal Practice* 37(1), 49–63. DOI: 10.1016/j.cvsm.2006.10.001.

Coe, J.B., Adams, C.L. and Bonnett, B.N. (2008) A focus group study of veterinarians' and PET owners' perceptions of veterinarian-client communication in companion animal practice. *Journal of the American Veterinary Medical Association* 233(7), 1072–1080. DOI: 10.2460/javma.233.7.1072.

Cornell, K.K. and Kopcha, M. (2007) Client-veterinarian communication: skills for client centered dialogue and shared decision making. *Veterinary Clinics of North America: Small Animal Practice* 37(1), 37–47. DOI: 10.1016/j.cvsm.2006.10.005.

Döring, D., Roscher, A., Scheipl, F., Küchenhoff, H. and Erhard, M.H. (2009) Fear-related behaviour of dogs in veterinary practice. *The Veterinary Journal* 182(1), 38–43. DOI: 10.1016/j.tvjl.2008.05.006.

Dysart, L.M.A., Coe, J.B. and Adams, C.L. (2011) Analysis of solicitation of client concerns in companion animal practice. *Journal of the American Veterinary Medical Association* 238(12), 1609–1615. DOI: 10.2460/javma.238.12.1609.

Egan, G. (1998) Attending, listening and understanding. In: Egan, G. (ed.) *The Skilled Helper: A Problem Management Approach to Helping*, 6th edn. Brooks/Cole Publishing Company, California, pp. 61–78.

Gray, G. and Moffett, J. (2010) Introduction: the veterinarian-owner-patient relationship. In: Gray, G. and Moffett, J. (eds) *Handbook of Veterinary Communication Skills*. Wiley-Blackwell, Chichester, UK.

Haidet, P. and Paterniti, D.A. (2003) "Building" a history rather than "taking" one: a perspective on information sharing during the medical interview. *Archives of Internal Medicine* 163(10), 1134–1140. DOI: 10.1001/archinte.163.10.1134.

Hernander, L. (2008) *Factors Influencing Dogs' Stress Level in the Waiting Room at a Veterinary Clinic*. Student Report. Swedish University of Agricultural Sciences, Department of Animal Environment and Health, Ethology and Animal Welfare Programme. Available at: http://ex-epsilon.slu.se/3006/1/huvudversion_klar_lollo.pdf

Kirwan, M. (2010) Basic communication skills. In: Gray, G. and Moffett, J. (eds) *Handbook of Veterinary Communication Skills*. Wiley-Blackwell, Chichester, UK, pp. 1–22.

Kogan, L.R., Schoenfeld-Tacher, R. and Simon, A.A. (2012) Behavioral effects of auditory stimulation on kenneled dogs. *Journal of Veterinary Behavior* 7(5), 268–275. DOI: 10.1016/j.jveb.2011.11.002.

Kry, K. and Casey, R. (2007) The effect of hiding enrichment on stress levels and behaviour of domestic cats (*Felis sylvestris catus*) in a shelter setting and the implications for adoption potential. *Animal Welfare* 16, 375–383.

Kurtz, S.M., Silverman, J.D. and Draper, J. (2003) *Teaching and Learning Communication Skills in Medicine*, 2nd edn. Radcliffe Medical Press, Oxford, UK.

Latham, C.E. and Morris, A. (2007) Effects of formal training in communication skills on the ability of veterinary students to communicate with clients. *Veterinary Record* 160(6), 181–186. DOI: 10.1136/vr.160.6.181.

Lewis, H. (2015) Fear-free: what you see is not what the cat or dog gets. Available at: http://veterinaryhospitaldesign.dvm360.com/fear-free-what-you-see-not-what-cat-or-dog-gets (accessed August 2019).

Little, G. (2013) How to talk so that clients will listen. *Veterinary Record* 173(17), i. DOI: 10.1136/vr.f6588.

Maguire, P. and Pitceathly, C. (2002) Key communication skills and how to acquire them. *BMJ* 325(7366), 697–700. DOI: 10.1136/bmj.325.7366.697.

McCobb, E.C., Patronek, G.J., Marder, A., Dinnage, J.D. and Stone, M.S. (2005) Assessment of stress levels among cats in four animal shelters. *Journal of the American Veterinary Medical Association* 226(4), 548–555. DOI: 10.2460/javma.2005.226.548.

McConnell, P.B. (1990) Acoustic structure and receiver response in domestic dogs, *Canis familiaris*. *Animal Behaviour* 39(5), 897–904. DOI: 10.1016/S0003-3472(05)80954-6.

McConnell, P. (2013) New research on dogs and music. Available at: https://www.patriciamcconnell.com/theotherendoftheleash/new-research-on-dogs-and-music (accessed August 2019).

Melson, G.F. (2003) Child development and the human-companion animal bond. *American Behavioral Scientist* 47(1), 31–39. DOI: 10.1177/0002764203255210.

Miller, B. and Rollnick, S. (2013) (eds) Motivational interviewing. In: *Helping People Change*, 3rd edn. The Guilford Press, New York.

Miller, W.R. and Rose, G.S. (2009) Toward a theory of motivational interviewing. *American Psychologist* 64(6), 527–537. DOI: 10.1037/a0016830.

Mills, D.S. (2002) Learning, training and behaviour modification techniques. In: Horwitz, D.F. and Mills, D.S. (eds) *BSAVA Manual of Canine and Feline Behavioural Medicine*. BSAVA publications, UK.

Moser, S.A. (2004) Combatting noise and odor. Available at: http://veterinaryhospitaldesign.dvm360. com/combatting-noise-and-odor (accessed August 2019).

Mossop, L., Gray, C., Blaxter, A., Gardiner, A., MacEachern, K. *et al.* (2015) Communication skills training: what the vet schools are doing. *Veterinary Record* 176(5), 114–117. DOI: 10.1136/vr.h425.

Mullan, S. and Fawcett, A. (2017) *Veterinary Ethics: Navigating Tough Cases*, 1st edn. 5m Publishing, Sheffield, UK.

Mullan, S. and Main, D. (2007) Preliminary evaluation of a quality-of-life screening programme for pet dogs. *Journal of Small Animal Practice* 48(6), 314–322. DOI: 10.1111/j.1748-5827.2007.00322.x.

Neitz, J., Geist, T. and Jacobs, G.H. (1989) Color vision in the dog. *Visual Neuroscience* 3(2), 119–125. DOI: 10.1017/S0952523800004430.

NICE (National Institute for Health Care and Excellence) (2019) Guidance for mental health and behavioural conditions. Available at: https://www.nice.org.uk/search?q=motivational+interviewing (accessed 2 September 2019).

Panagiotaki, G., Hopkins, M., Nobes, G., Ward, E. and Griffiths, D. (2018) Children's and adults' understanding of death: cognitive, parental, and experiential influences. *Journal of Experimental Child Psychology* 166, 96–115. DOI: 10.1016/j.jecp.2017.07.014.

Panksepp, J. (2016) The Psycho-neurology of cross-species affective/social neuroscience: understanding animal affective states as a guide to development of novel psychiatric treatments. In: Wöhr, M. and Krach, S. (eds) *Social Behavior from Rodents to Humans. Current Topics in Behavioral Neurosciences*. Springer International Publishing, pp. 109–125.

Piaget, J. (1964) Cognitive development in children. *Journal of Research in Science Teaching* 2, 176–186.

Radford, A., Stockley, P., Silverman, J., Taylor, I., Turner, R. *et al*. (2006) Development, teaching, and evaluation of a consultation structure model for use in veterinary education. *Journal of Veterinary Medical Education* 33(1), 38–44. DOI: 10.3138/jvme.33.1.38.

Riess, H. (2015) The impact of clinical empathy on patients and clinicians: understanding empathy's side effects. *AJOB Neuroscience* 6(3), 51–53. DOI: 10.1080/21507740.2015.1052591.

Rubak, S., Sandbaek, A., Lauritzen, T. and Christensen, B. (2005) Motivational interviewing: a systematic review and meta-analysis. *The British Journal of General Practitioners* 55(513), 305–312.

Sharkin, B.S. and Knox, D. (2003) Pet loss: issues and implications for the psychologist. *Professional Psychology: Research and Practice* 34(4), 414–421. DOI: 10.1037/0735-7028.34.4.414.

Shaw, J.R., Bonnett, B.N., Adams, C.L. and Roter, D.L. (2006) Veterinarian-client-patient communication patterns used during clinical appointments in companion animal practice. *Journal of the American Veterinary Medical Association* 228(5), 714–721. DOI: 10.2460/javma.228.5.714.

Silverman, J. and Kinnersley, P. (2010) Doctors' non-verbal behaviour in consultations: look at the patient before you look at the computer. *British Journal of General Practice* 60(571), 76–78. DOI: 10.3399/bjgp10X482293.

Silverman, J., Kurtz, S. and Draper, J. (2006) *Skills for Communicating with Patients*, 2nd edn. Radcliffe Medical, Abingdon, UK.

Snowdon, C.T., Teie, D. and Savage, M. (2015) Cats prefer species-appropriate music. *Applied Animal Behaviour Science* 166, 106–111. DOI: 10.1016/j.applanim.2015.02.012.

Treasure, J. (2004) Motivational interviewing. *Advances in Psychiatric Treatment* 10(5), 331–337. DOI: 10.1192/apt.10.5.331.

Volk, J.O., Felsted, K.E., Thomas, J.G. and Siren, C.W. (2011) Executive summary of the Bayer veterinary care usage study. *Journal of the American Veterinary Medical Association* 238(10), 1275–1282. DOI: 10.2460/javma.238.10.1275.

von Fragstein, M., Silverman, J., Cushing, A., Quilligan, S., Salisbury, H. *et al*. (2008) UK consensus statement on the content of communication curricula in undergraduate medical education. *Medical Education* 42(11), 1100–1107. DOI: 10.1111/j.1365-2923.2008.03137.x.

Wells, D.L., Graham, L. and Hepper, P.G. (2002) The influence of auditory stimulation on the behaviour of dogs housed in a rescue shelter. *Animal Welfare* 11, 385–393.

2 Ruling Out Physical Disorders Leading to Behavioural Changes

Ed Hall[1], Tom Harcourt-Brown[1], Angie Hibbert[2], Stephen Waisglass[3] and Sagi Denenberg[1,3*]

[1]Langford Vets, University of Bristol, Langford, Bristol, UK; [2]The Feline Centre, Langford Vets, University of Bristol, Bristol, UK; [3]Veterinary Emergency Clinic of Toronto, Toronto, Ontario, Canada

2.1 Introduction

When presented with a pet with suspected psychiatric disease, the first step is to rule out or confirm and treat physical diseases. Changes in a pet's behaviour are often the first, if not the only, sign of physical abnormalities. At times, a misdiagnosis of a physical disease leads to the assumption that the underlying problem is a mental health problem. This assumption may lead to reduced welfare of the pet and, possibly, aggravation of the existing physical disease.

Further, there are cases where the pet is presented with both physical and mental abnormalities. In this case, whether the physical disease led to mental disease (e.g. cystitis leading to house soiling) or psychiatric disease led to physical disease (e.g. compulsive licking leading to acral lick dermatitis), both conditions must be addressed concurrently. Of course, in some pets, the presence of a concurrent physical disease might be unrelated to the reported changes in behaviours. Therefore, the response to treatment might help identify the involvement of the physical disease (whether treatment normalizes the behaviour).

This chapter reviews some of the most common presentations of psychiatric diseases that result from a physical disease. In addition, approaches to different patients and suggested diagnostic tests are discussed. Chapter 3 will address more specifically the interaction between painful conditions and psychiatric disorders.

2.1.1 Approach to the patient

A 'problem-solving' approach is commonly used in medicine (vs pattern recognition) and is particularly helpful in working through cases where there could be multiple potential causes of a single presenting issue. Acquiring a complete history and performing a thorough physical examination are required to be able to identify relevant problems. The history should, ideally, briefly cover access to core resources and social background at the outset, to help identify factors that could impact behaviour (see below). Providing the owner with a questionnaire to complete in the waiting room or online before the consult can be helpful. A logical approach is to ask a number of clinical questions that can be answered through a physical examination and relevant laboratory tests. These questions are part of an algorithm that you should follow when presented with a patient.

A problem list should be constructed with the information gained from the history and physical examination, and problems prioritized, with non-specific signs such as lethargy often listed lower. From this list, differential diagnoses can be considered, and a plan for investigations or treatment trials can be formulated.

2.1.2 Signalment

Breed predispositions are recognized for many medical conditions. Common cat examples include: hyperthyroidism, which is less common in pedigree cats; Siamese cats are over-represented in cases of

*Corresponding author: s.denenberg@bristol.ac.uk

DOI: 10.1079/9781786394552.0002

feline asthma; and Burmese cats are predisposed to diabetes mellitus. In dogs, common examples include portosystemic shunts in miniature schnauzers and chiari-like malformation in Cavalier King Charles spaniels.

Age may be of relevance, too; cats reaching the age of social maturity (12–24 months) and dogs (12–36 months) are more likely to be affected by social conflict, potentially leading to the development of behavioural concerns around this time point (e.g. urine marking, aggression and idiopathic cystitis). Conversely, behavioural changes in senior and geriatric pets warrant investigation of age-related diseases (e.g. hyperthyroidism, IBD, neoplasia, renal disease and hypertension).

2.1.3 History tips

- Establish a timeline of the presenting problem(s) considering the speed of onset (acute vs chronic), duration of the problem and progression (e.g. non-progressive, progressive, improving).
- Include a systems checklist after discussion of the owner's presenting complaints; for example, any vomiting or diarrhoea, any change in thirst or appetite, coughing, sneezing, nasal or ocular discharge, and any change in mobility or activity. Any neurological signs such as circling, head pressing, ataxia or loss of balance. This checklist often picks up aspects of the animal's condition that the owner may not have thought relevant to the discussion.
- Consider pre-existing surgical or medical issues.
- Determine whether the animal is receiving any current medications or supplements.
- Establish current diet.
- Consider the response to any prior prescribed treatments for the presenting problem.

2.1.4 Physical examination considerations

- Some animals may not tolerate a nose-to-tail approach. We must be flexible to be able to complete a thorough examination; for example, the oral examination is often accepted better at the end.
- Work quietly and slowly. Avoid fast hand movements, approaching the animal face-to-face and using loud voices.
- Use a cats' and dogs' pheromones-sprayed towel on the examination table; alternatively, examine the animal in the location where it is most comfortable, such as the bottom half of the carrier, on the floor or on your lap, or on the window sill. If the animal is anxious, allow time to acclimate (if possible) and provide something for the animal to hide under (e.g. partially cover with a towel), or allow it to tuck behind its owner.
- Palpate carefully for a thyroid goitre in all cats of more than five years of age; hyperthyroidism is not a disease of only senior and geriatric cats.
- Assessing gait and mobility can be challenging in the consultation room setting when many pets freeze. Use treats, toys and play-wands to encourage movement. Placing a cat on a chair gives it an opportunity to jump down and may allow observation of its mobility. Assess muscle mass carefully (see Chapter 3 for more information on gait and pain assessment).
- Retinal examination using indirect ophthalmoscopy is under-utilized but is a useful and quick way to look for evidence of hypertensive retinopathy or other retinal pathologies.
- A basic neurological examination can be carried out in less than five minutes at the end of a routine examination.

2.1.5 Basic behaviour questions to ask

- Household background – multi-pet versus single pet, any other pets, any recent changes to the household structure (pets and humans).
- The nature of interactions with other animals outside the house.
- Past and current stressors (e.g. cattery or kennel stays, visitors, attendance at a show, travel).
- Access to core resources:
  - food stations – number, separation from water bowls and access;
  - water bowls – number, location and access;
  - latrine – toileting outdoors or inside; if inside, number and type of litter boxes, and access;
  - resting places – Where does the animal choose to rest? Is a raised hiding space available/used for cats?
  - any access to play activities;
  - information about access to, and interaction with, household humans.

2.1.6 Baseline tests

For many of the problems, the following baseline tests will include:

- haematology – complete blood count and blood smear assessment;
- serum biochemistry including electrolytes;
- thyroxine level;
- urinalysis (dipstick, urine protein: creatinine ratio; culture, if signs of cystitis only); and
- systolic blood pressure measurement.

These baseline tests enable quick exclusion of common conditions, including chronic kidney disease (CKD), hyper- or hypothyroidism, anaemia, diabetes mellitus, liver disease, hypokalaemia, hypercalcaemia and hypertension.

Second-level testing commonly includes measurement of feline or canine pancreatic lipase immunoreactivity, cobalamin, folate, dynamic bile acids, faecal analysis, hormonal assays, orthopaedic and neurological examination, and imaging.

2.2 Neurological Diseases

Behaviour change is a frequent presenting complaint when a dog or a cat suffers from neurological disease. This is particularly difficult to investigate when the behaviour change is episodic and the dog or cat appears to be normal during the consultation. Using videos captured at home, history, physical examination and advanced imaging has greatly improved the clinician's ability to differentiate the various causes.

2.2.1 Animals with persistent behaviour change

One simplistic view of behaviour is that it is regulated by two areas of the brain: the forebrain (cerebral cortex) receives inputs from the body and the environment, integrates them and generates an output, while the brainstem (in particular the reticular activating system) selects which information to send up to the forebrain for processing.

Dysfunction in the forebrain or the brainstem can, therefore, cause typical and predictable behaviour changes – abnormal processing with forebrain disease and lack of information transfer to the forebrain with brainstem disease.

A neurological examination allows us to test the function of both the forebrain and the brainstem. Table 2.1 summarizes the typical behaviour changes that can be seen with persistent (i.e. non-episodic) forebrain and brainstem diseases as well as the neurological examination techniques that can be used to raise suspicion of an intracranial cause. These individual tests are described elsewhere.

Obtundation is defined as a reduced response to external stimuli; stupor is a response only to noxious stimuli and coma is no response to any stimulation. Hemineglect refers to the phenomenon where only half the world is perceived and manifests with such things as only eating food from half a bowl. The lists of differential diagnoses given are not exhaustive and only represent the more common conditions.

The menace response and the proprioceptive responses (hopping and paw placement in particular) are important screening tests for forebrain dysfunction and should be performed in every animal with behaviour change, so it is essential to be competent in these tests.

2.2.2 Episodic behaviour changes

A logical approach to these cases is critical as there may not be any inter-ictal neurological deficits to help differentiate neurological disease, so the history and examination of any videos become the only tools available. A clear process of clinical reasoning is vital to extract the important features of the events to determine the most likely underlying cause.

The most important features to extract from the history are:

1. Is there a consistent preceding event to the seizures (e.g. exercise or excitement)?
2. How long are the episodes?
3. How similar are the episodes to one another?
4. Is the animal responsive during them?
5. What are the typical features of the episodes?
6. Do they return to normal afterwards, or is there a period of altered behaviour?
7. How many can they have at a time?

It is very useful to be able to summarize these findings for the owners to ensure that they agree with the clinical picture. Often owners do not see the full clinical picture as they focus on the episodes themselves. Reviewing the information together with the owners helps them see the clinical picture and remember further details that help to obtain most of the information. Once all the information is available we can apply a clinical reasoning framework to it. The process we use is

Table 2.1. Typical findings with diseases affecting different neurolocalizations.

Neuro-anatomical location	Typical behaviour changes	Other tests that may be affected	Possible differential diagnoses
Focal forebrain	Obtundation Compulsive walking or circling Hemineglect Seizures	Contralateral menace response Contralateral proprioceptive responses (e.g. paw placement) Contralateral nasal mucosal sensation	Neoplasia Infectious or autoimmune encephalitis Haemorrhagic or ischaemic infarction
Diffuse forebrain	Oscillating mania/ hyperactivity with obtundation Compulsive walking or circling Seizures	Bilateral menace responses Bilateral proprioceptive responses Bilateral nasal mucosal sensation	Metabolic or toxic encephalopathies (e.g. hepatic encephalopathy) Hydrocephalus Neurodegenerative disease (Neoplasia) (Encephalitis)
Rostral brainstem (thalamus)	Obtundation	May be no other neurological abnormalities except profound obtundation Usually bradycardia and hypothermia Blindness with loss of pupillary light reflex (PLR) Abnormal palpebral reflex/ facial movement	Pituitary tumours Other neoplasia Infectious or immune-mediated encephalitis
Mid to caudal brainstem	Obtundation	Anisocoria Head tilt Nystagmus (may only be evident in dorsal recumbency) Facial paralysis Masticatory atrophy Dysphagia/Dysphonia	Neoplasia Infectious or immune-mediated encephalitis Haemorrhagic or ischaemic infarction

summarized in Fig. 2.1 and described below in more detail.

2.2.3 Physiological conditions

We define these conditions as those where the behavioural response is appropriate for the inciting cause. These tend to be associated with intermittent or waxing and waning acute pain or discomfort; for example, disc disease, abdominal pain or severe dermatitis.

Acute pain episodes can last minutes to hours and happen several times a day. The behaviour adopted is similar, but not identical, each time, and as a general rule animals with episodic pain move less, not more, during the episode and adopt a posture change to protect the painful area (e.g. kyphosis or lifting a limb). Animals that show increased activity during an abnormal episode are unlikely to be painful.

It is very unusual for an animal to be in pain enough to cause severe episodic behaviour change, but not then have some evidence of pain on physical examination, in its history or on video. We cannot definitively rule out that an animal is in pain, and this can be an emotive point for owners. However, if there is no response to manipulation during the examination and the animal can perform a full range of activities (e.g. jumping, running and climbing stairs) without a problem in-between the episodes, we would consider an acute pain condition unlikely.

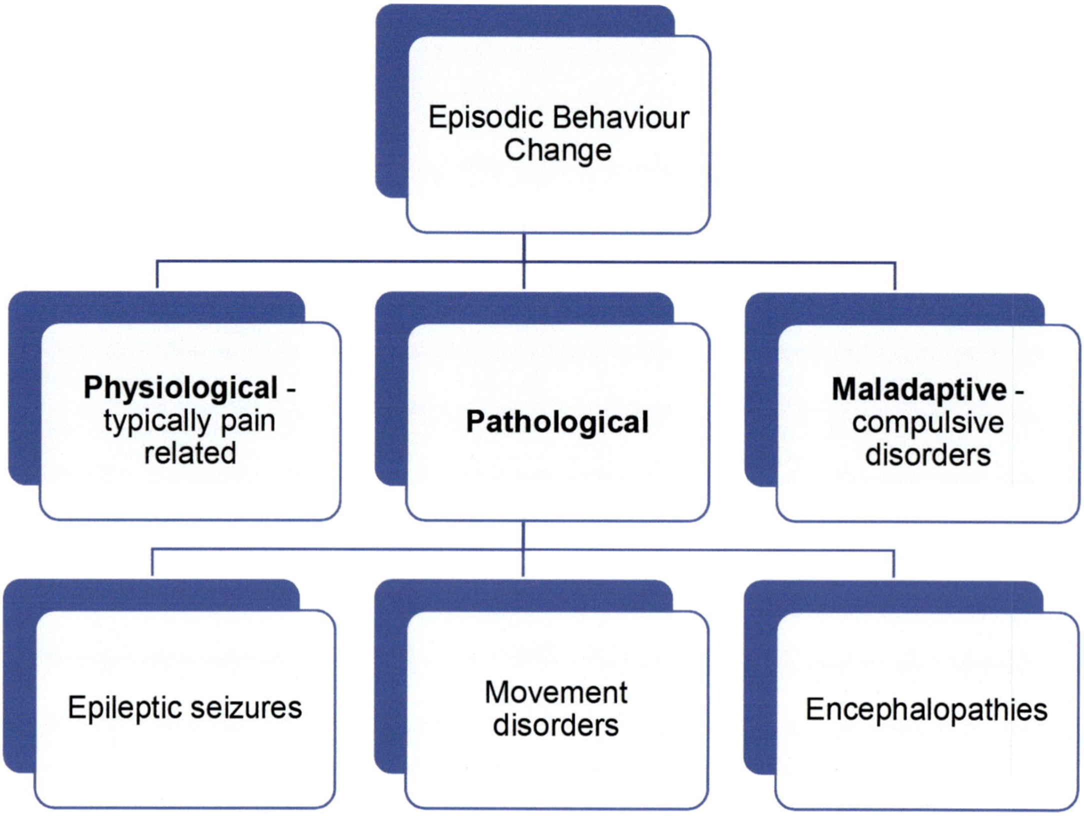

Fig. 2.1. Clinical reasoning framework to episodic behaviour changes.

2.2.4 Pathological conditions

Pathological conditions encompass diseases where the brain is malfunctioning to cause abnormal behaviour. The three most common categories are epileptic seizures, movement diseases (also called paroxysmal dyskinesia) and encephalopathies. Cataplexy, narcolepsy and paroxysmal vestibular episodes are much less common episodic diseases.

Epileptic seizures and movement diseases commonly have no identifiable underlying cause, and all diagnostic tests appear normal. This makes the description of the events (their semiology) crucial as it may be the only factor with which a diagnosis can be made.

2.2.4.1 Epileptic seizures

These are the result of excessive synchronous activity of neurons in the cerebral cortex. They can manifest in almost any form, but we would consider them to have three key defining features:

- They should be stereotypical so that the ictal phase follows an almost identical pattern each time.
- The ictal phase should last less than 5 minutes.
- There is a post-ictal phase of behaviour change that gradually resolves and can last minutes to hours (or even days).

Supportive, but not essential, features that exist in most epileptic seizures are:

- increased muscle tone or rhythmic movement of at least one body area;
- a mixture of autonomic signs (e.g. salivation, urination, pupil dilation) with skeletal motor signs (e.g. movement and tone); and
- altered or no response to external stimuli suggesting alteration or loss of consciousness.

2.2.4.2 Movement diseases

These have several names; the most common is paroxysmal dyskinesia, but also hyperkinesis, cramping or episodic falling are used. Their cause is unknown in most cases, but they are thought to arise when the areas of the brain responsible for planning and regulating movement temporarily malfunction, possibly due to a very localized seizure activity. Movement diseases, typically, do not affect the cerebral cortex or the autonomic areas, so the response to the environment and autonomic function should be unaffected.

These used to be considered rare diseases but now appear to be reasonably frequent and were probably previously misdiagnosed as focal epileptic seizures, prior to using videos provided by owners.

Their key features are:

- sustained abnormal movement with increased tone and over-flexion of joints in the affected limbs; this manifests as a very abnormal gait and posture, frequently causing the affected animals to be unable to walk;
- episodes can last minutes to hours with multiple episodes in a day;
- episodes are similar but not identical each time with some variation around a central theme;
- immediate return to normal after an episode with no post-ictal phase; and
- episodes are not terminated by interaction with affected animals, but an appropriate response to the external environment is preserved. For example, the animal will try eating food that we offer despite having very abnormal movement.

2.2.4.3 Encephalopathies

Encephalopathies characteristically cause persistent behaviour change, as outlined above. However, some encephalopathies (particularly hepatic encephalopathy) can cause seizures alone or have subtle behaviour changes that are not apparent to the owners in-between much more dramatic behaviour changes, so they appear episodic.

Most structural, intracranial encephalopathies can be excluded by looking for the neurological abnormalities outlined in Table 2.1. The most common causes of episodic encephalopathy that may not have clinical signs in-between are:

- hepatic encephalopathy (dogs or cats at any age but, commonly, younger animals);
- hypoglycaemic encephalopathy (primarily in older dogs, very young dogs or toy breeds); exercise or fasting is the most common cause of these encephalopathies; and
- cardiac syncope (usually associated with exercise intolerance in dogs, but may have no other signs in cats).

Because of this, all animals with episodic behaviour change and no other identified cause should have their post-prandial bile acids and fasting glucose measured, as well as prolonged auscultation for rhythm abnormalities.

2.2.5 Maladaptive conditions

We define these as conditions where there is a trigger for the behaviour (as in physiological conditions) but the response is inappropriate. This category generally includes compulsive disorders. The key features that differentiate this category are:

- episodes are similar, but not stereotypical behaviour changes that have core similarities (e.g. fly biting) but which vary over time in their duration and severity;
- episodes can last minutes to hours;
- there is no post-ictal phase;
- animals may be distracted from the events when the disease starts (although this may change with time); and
- there may be an inciting factor.

2.3 Internal Medicine of Cats

Cats are often presented to the veterinarian with vague clinical signs. These signs may be non-specific, such as lethargy or inappetence; however, they are usually recognized by owners because they represent a change from the cat's normal behaviour. Determining quickly whether the origin of the problem is medical or behavioural can be challenging in some scenarios for several reasons: commonly, there is overlap in physical and psychiatric diseases presenting with systemic signs, for example periuria (toileting outside of the litter box), which could be caused by a urinary tract infection, cystoliths, neoplasia, idiopathic cystitis or marking (see Table 2.2). Further, it is not unusual for feline patients to present acutely ill, with earlier signs of illness or stress potentially missed by the owner, due to the cat's inherent nature of hiding illness or

Table 2.2. Presenting signs with behavioural and medical disease overlap in cats. The lists of differential diagnoses given are not exhaustive and only represent the more common conditions. (Adapted from Horwitz and Rodan, 2018)

Behaviour change	Presenting sign	Examples of common physical pathologies	Behavioural, mental and environmental considerations
Appetite	Inappetence	Pain, nausea, pyrexia, primary gastrointestinal disease (e.g. food or steroid-responsive enteropathy, lymphoma), pancreatitis, oesophageal disease, hepatopathy, oral disease, periodontal disease, neoplasia, kidney disease, neurological disease, cardiac disease	Access to food bowls (e.g. location and cat's ability to reach the bowl, effects of social conflict on access), recent changes in diet, stress or anxiety associated with hospitalization or home environment
	Polyphagia	Hyperthyroidism, malabsorption, maldigestion (e.g. EPI – exocrine pancreatic insufficiency), diabetes mellitus, acromegaly, adrenal neoplasia	Diet quality and form, competition between household cats for food
	Pica	Anaemia, malabsorption, maldigestion, iron deficiency	Substrate preference, any prior history of pica
Drinking	Polydipsia	Diabetes mellitus, CKD	Compulsive disorder
Activity	Inactivity	As for inappetence plus musculoskeletal disease (e.g. DJD – degenerative joint disease), anaemia, cardiorespiratory disease, hypertension	Social relationships at home (inter-cat and human–cat) as potential stressor or cause of anxiety; access to toys, play activities, food presentation (bowls vs puzzle feeder), recent changes to the household structure (e.g. environment, pets and humans)
	Hyperactivity	Hyperthyroidism, pruritus, partial seizures	
	Pacing	Hyperthyroidism, hypertension, brain disease (e.g. cognitive dysfunction, neoplasia), abdominal pain, toxin ingestion	
Vocalization	Increased vocalization	Hyperthyroidism, pain, hypertension, cognitive dysfunction, deafness	Context of vocalization; any conflict in social relationships, resource availability
Elimination	Undesirable toileting– periuria	Feline idiopathic cystitis, lower urinary tract infection, urolithiasis, bladder neoplasia, pyelonephritis, incontinence, causes of polydipsia/ polyuria including CKD – chronic kidney disease, and diabetes mellitus	Distinguish urine marking (spraying) from undesirable toileting. Ability to access litter box or outside the area to toilet (consider location, cat's mobility, social conflict in the household), litter substrate, any change to litter substrate, litter box hygiene
	Undesirable toileting – defecation	Constipation, enteropathy (e.g. colitis- associated with urgency and tenesmus), musculoskeletal disease, cognitive dysfunction	As above

Continued

Table 2.2. Continued

Behaviour change	Presenting sign	Examples of common physical pathologies	Behavioural, mental and environmental considerations
Social interactions	Aggression towards the owner, other pets	Pain, nausea, fear, acute stress response, hepatic encephalopathy, hyperthyroidism, hypertension, musculoskeletal disease, brain disease (e.g. neoplasia and cognitive dysfunction)	Social relationship structure between household pets, neighbouring cats and cat–human (any changes in structure, any known conflict), resource access
Grooming	Increased grooming	Ectoparasites, food responsive dermatopathy, atopy	Compulsive, anxiety
	Decreased grooming	Pain, degenerative joint disease, hyperthyroidism, obesity	Anxiety, depression
Miscellaneous	Lip licking	Nausea, acute stress response, oral pathology	Anxiety, pain, fear
	Panting	Acute stress response, pain, cardiomyopathy, feline asthma, hyperthyroidism, pyrexia	Fear, phobia
	Ptyalism	Hepatic encephalopathy, nausea, pain, fear, oral pathology (e.g. periodontal disease, gingivostomatitis, and feline calici virus-associated ulceration)	Anxiety

distress, an evolutionary survival tactic (Bradshaw, 2016). Finally, the impact of stress of the clinic visit may hamper patient assessment in the consultation. A logical approach is required to expedite reaching a diagnosis.

In many cases, psychiatric diseases are diagnosed following the exclusion of medical causes. However, it is crucial to consider that some patients have coexisting psychiatric and physical diseases. Psychiatric diseases also have the potential to exacerbate concurrent physical diseases, for example feline herpes infection, feline oral pain syndrome or a geriatric cat with osteoarthritis that begins to struggle to use a high-sided litter tray due to orthopaedic pain; reluctance to enter the litter box could consequently lead to constipation. When considering the interplay between physical and mental health, it is necessary to include a basic behavioural assessment when approaching any feline patient.

2.3.1 Night vocalization

Night vocalization is often described by owners of senior and geriatric cats. Possible physical causes include pain, hyperthyroidism, hypertension, CKD, cognitive dysfunction, visual and hearing defects and brain neoplasia.

Historical features may help to narrow the list down, for example by identification of polyuria/polydipsia in CKD or polyphagia in hyperthyroidism. Physical examination may identify potential sources of pain; assess for orthopaedic disease by checking muscle mass, joint range of movement and mobility in the consulting room. However, a normal examination does not fully exclude pain (orthopaedic and other; see Chapter 3) in feline patients, and a therapeutic analgesic trial may be required, e.g. using transmucosal buprenorphine or NSAID (if no contra-indications).

Clues towards hyperthyroidism include the presence of thyroid goitre, unkempt coat, tachycardia, arrhythmias or heart murmur, along with reduced body condition and muscle mass (review for changes in the cat's weight, muscle and body condition score).

Palpation of the kidneys may reveal contour irregularity and reduction in size in chronic kidney disease; asymmetric kidneys could indicate ureteral disease. Hyperthyroidism and CKD can usually be quickly diagnosed with measurement of urea, creatinine +/- SDMA, thyroxine measurement and urinalysis.

Measurement of systolic blood pressure and examination of the retinas can establish whether hypertension is present. Retinal blood vessel tortuosity, haemorrhage and retinal detachment may be present in hypertensive cats. Overcoming situational hypertension (previously known as the 'white coat' effect) to obtain a realistic reading may require allowing more time for the cat to acclimate in the room, using Feliway™ pheromone-sprayed towels, or remeasuring following dosing with gabapentin, to alleviate hospital-induced anxiety; persistent readings >160 mmHg are considered significantly elevated and warrant treatment (Acierno *et al.*, 2018).

The next step is to exclude visual, hearing and neurological deficits by performing a neurological and ophthalmic examination. If these are normal, the differential diagnoses can be narrowed to cognitive dysfunction and psychiatric disease, leading to more in-depth evaluation of the patient's behaviour and environment.

2.3.2 Periuria

Differential diagnoses for periuria include feline lower urinary tract disease (FLUTD), manifesting as cystitis, incontinence and emotional causes such as anxiety leading to marking, and undesirable toileting habits due to developed aversions or preferences. FLUTD comprises several conditions including urinary tract infection (UTI), urolithiasis, neoplasia and feline idiopathic cystitis (FIC). In conjunction with the routine history, establishing details regarding the voiding behaviour can help narrow the list of differentials. As a first step, you should determine the size of void, posture, location and the cat's behaviour during micturition.

Cystitis is typically associated with passing small frequent voids of urine (pollakiuria), pain and difficulty in voiding (e.g. stranguria or dysuria) and haematuria. The cat may frequently groom the perineum and vocalize during voiding. Periuria may be associated with cystitis due to the cat associating the pain of voiding with the litter box. The cat usually adopts a typical squatting posture and voids urine on horizontal surfaces (unlike urine marking where the cat often, but not always, holds the tail erect and sprays onto a vertical surface (Heath, 2019)).

An examination may reveal either a large turgid bladder if the cat is experiencing concurrent urethral obstruction or a small uncomfortable bladder. Serum biochemistry, haematology, complete urinalysis (e.g. dipstick, specific gravity, urine protein: creatinine ratio, sediment examination and culture) and abdominal imaging can be used to assess the urinary tract for uroliths, UTI, renal pathology and bladder neoplasia. Abdominal lateral and ventrodorsal radiographs may identify upper and lower mineralized uroliths (e.g. struvite and calcium oxalate). Abdominal ultrasound is complementary and provides information regarding the renal parenchyma, any ureteral dilation, bladder wall thickening and luminal material. Retrograde urethrography is indicated in male cats with recurrent cystitis, to search for urethral strictures, stones or urethritis.

The most common cause of cystitis in cats under the age of 6 years is FIC (Sparkes, 2018). However, this remains a diagnosis of exclusion. Once we diagnose FIC, we should evaluate for possible emotional triggers due to the understanding of the role of stressors in triggering and exacerbating the condition. Often we can identify a trigger (e.g. inter-cat conflict, and recent change in household structure) through a review of the cat's history and environment. Cystitis in older cats is more frequently secondary to other comorbidities including hyperthyroidism, CKD and diabetes mellitus. Historical and physical examination findings and baseline laboratory testing should enable a diagnosis to be reached. Finally, ureteric disease may also be associated with cystitis and is becoming increasingly recognized. Asymmetric kidneys on abdominal palpation may be a clue.

Incontinence, a further cause of periuria, may manifest as voiding medium-to-large volumes when the cat is at rest or the cat may dribble urine unconsciously. We can exclude the causes of polyuria and polydipsia using serum biochemistry and urinalysis. Along with an assessment of bladder tone and residual volumes after voiding, a neurological and gait examination can help to establish whether a lower or upper motor neuron defect exists. Exclusion of cystitis and incontinence in presentations of periuria narrow the differentials to psychiatric diseases.

2.4 Internal Medicine of Dogs

All physical and behavioural investigations begin with the history and thorough physical examination. In the history, reporting of physical manifestations in association with behavioural changes are much more likely to be physical in origin. For example, a history of intermittent seizures and altered behaviour would immediately raise concerns about a structural brain or metabolic disease; vomiting and diarrhoea with altered behaviour might suggest abdominal pain altering behaviour; reluctance to jump up or climb stairs may reflect orthopaedic or joint pain (see Chapter 3). However, some signs, such as polydipsia, can be due to physical disease or psychiatric disease (see Table 2.3). Any abnormal findings and clinical signs of pain on physical examination should be investigated; they may be the cause of the altered behaviour, although they may be coincidental.

The next step in physical investigations would be a laboratory minimum database of haematology, serum biochemistry and urinalysis. Anaemia may be the primary cause of altered behaviour or merely a marker of an underlying physical condition (i.e. anaemia of chronic disease). Any significantly abnormal white blood cells (WBC) pattern, except a stress leukogram (mature neutrophilia, usually with a mild monocytosis, lymphopenia and eosinopenia), is indicative of an underlying inflammatory condition. Serum biochemistry may indicate a metabolic disease is causing changes in behaviour (e.g. polydipsia in diabetes mellitus, renal and hepatic diseases or hypercalcaemia). Urinalysis is essential in animals with either polyuria or inappropriate urination; the urine specific gravity (SG) will confirm polyuria if the urine is hyposthenuric, and sediment analysis may identify urinary tract infection.

2.4.1 Lethargy or apathy

In young dogs a major differential diagnosis would be hepatoencephalopathy related to a portosystemic shunt when there are also often changes in behaviour (e.g. lethargy, aimless wandering, resistance to physical restraint). Dynamic bile acid testing is likely to confirm hepatic insufficiency, and a definitive diagnosis is made by an abdominal ultrasound examination or CT-angiography. Lethargy and apathy are often a manifestation of pain or metabolic disease.

2.4.2 Anorexia or adipsia

Anorexia, the refusal to eat when physically capable of doing so, is most often the result of an underlying physical problem. Other clinical signs, the physical exam findings, the laboratory minimum database, and imaging findings will help diagnose the cause. Anorexia as a psychiatric disease is anecdotally reported in dogs that are supposedly grieving, in most cases where there are no localizing clues, the problem is usually neurological or gastrointestinal.

Adipsia is a very rare condition and ultimately can cause abnormal mentation and behaviour due to consequent hypernatraemia. Although thought to relate to an abnormality in the hypothalamic thirst centre, it is not a true primary psychiatric disease.

2.4.3 Pica

Pica (a depraved appetite) is sometimes seen in dogs, and the most common presentation is coprophagia. There are several hypotheses as to why dogs may be coprophagic: it may be a learned behaviour that elicits attention from the owner, whereas a nutritional deficiency is not likely. Pica can be seen in dogs with pancreatic insufficiency, or intestinal dysbiosis, although they typically have diarrhoea and lose weight. Measurement of serum TLI may confirm pancreatic insufficiency, and serum folate and cobalamin deficiencies can be markers of intestinal disease. Oral, abdominal or gastrointestinal pain might also lead to pica in dogs.

2.4.4 Polydipsia and polyuria

This presenting complaint first needs to be documented by measuring the water intake and then confirmed by finding an inappropriately low urine specific gravity (SG) by refractometry (NB dipsticks for measuring SG are unreliable). Polydipsia is defined as drinking >100 ml/kg/day although most healthy animals drink ~20–30 ml/kg/day (depending on food type, exercise, and environmental temperature) and any increase may be significant. Urine SG is normally >1.030 in dogs. Young dogs are less able to concentrate their urine, but if there is true polydipsia, a major differential diagnosis would be hepatoencephalopathy related to a portosystemic shunt (see above).

Persistent isosthenuria (SG 1.008–1.014) is most often not normal and is most likely related to chronic kidney disease, although other metabolic diseases such as diabetes mellitus, hypercalcaemia, hepatoencephalopathy and pyometra in nulliparous bitches, are quite common. The presence of glycosuria can help to screen for diabetes mellitus. Other metabolic causes are likely to be identified by the serum biochemical testing, and imaging.

Table 2.3. Presenting signs with behavioural and medical disease overlap in dogs. The lists of differential diagnoses given are not exhaustive and only represent the more common conditions.

Behaviour change	Presenting sign	Examples of common physical pathologies	Behavioural, mental and environmental considerations
Appetite	Inappetence	Pain, nausea, pyrexia, primary gastrointestinal disease (e.g. food or steroid-responsive enteropathy, lymphoma), pancreatitis, oesophageal disease, hepatopathy, oral disease, periodontal disease, neoplasia, kidney disease, neurological disease, cardiac disease	Access to food bowls, effects of social conflict on access, recent changes in diet, stress or anxiety associated with separation or home environment
	Polyphagia	Malabsorption, maldigestion (e.g. EPI – exocrine pancreatic insufficiency), diabetes mellitus, acromegaly, adrenal neoplasia	Diet quality and form, competition between household dogs for food
	Pica	Anaemia, malabsorption, maldigestion, iron deficiency	Compulsive disorder, anxiety, any prior history of pica
Drinking	Polydipsia	Diabetes mellitus, diabetes insipidus, Hyperadrenocorticism, CKD	Compulsive disorder
Activity	Inactivity	As for inappetence plus musculoskeletal disease (e.g. DJD – degenerative joint disease), anaemia, cardiorespiratory disease	Social relationships at home (inter-dog and human–dog) as potential stressor or cause of anxiety; access to toys, play activities, food presentation (bowls vs puzzle feeder), recent changes to the household structure (e.g. environment, pets and humans)
	Hyperactivity	Pruritus, partial seizures	
	Pacing	Hypertension, brain disease (e.g. cognitive dysfunction, neoplasia), abdominal pain, toxin ingestion	
Vocalization	Increased vocalization	Pain, cognitive dysfunction, deafness	Context of vocalization; any conflict in social relationships, resource availability, separation
Elimination	Undesirable toileting – urination	Infections, urolithiasis, bladder neoplasia, pyelonephritis, incontinence, causes of polydipsia/polyuria including CKD – chronic kidney disease, and diabetes mellitus	Distinguish urine marking or lack of training from undesirable toileting No access to outdoor soiling area, separation
	Undesirable toileting – defecation	Constipation, enteropathy (e.g. colitis-associated with urgency and tenesmus), musculoskeletal disease, cognitive dysfunction	As above
Social interactions	Aggression towards the owner, other pets	Pain, nausea, fear, acute stress response, hepatic encephalopathy, musculoskeletal disease, brain disease (e.g. neoplasia, adrenal neoplasia and cognitive dysfunction)	Social relationship structure between household pets, and dog–human (any changes in structure, any known conflict), resource access
Grooming	Increased grooming	Ectoparasites, food responsive dermatopathy, atopy	Compulsive
	Decreased grooming	Pain, DJD, obesity	Anxiety

Continued

Table 2.3. Continued

Behaviour change	Presenting sign	Examples of common physical pathologies	Behavioural, mental and environmental considerations
Miscellaneous	Lip licking	Nausea, pain, response, oral pathology	Fear, acute stress
	Panting	Pain, cardiomyopathy, pyrexia, nausea	Fear, phobia
	Ptyalism	Hepatic encephalopathy, nausea, pain, fear, oral pathology (e.g. periodontal disease)	Fear, phobia, panic

Hyposthenuria (SG 1.001–1.008) indicates primary polydipsia and active urine dilution, or diabetes insipidus (DI). Psychogenic polydipsia (PP) can cause this dilution; however, the diagnosis is made by exclusion of all physical disease. Hypercalcaemia is ruled out by the serum biochemistry, and diabetes mellitus by urinalysis and serum biochemistry. Suspected hepatoencephalopathy should be investigated by dynamic bile acid and plasma ammonia concentration measurements. In older dogs, hyperadrenocorticism is more likely, and is often suspected from the history (e.g. polyphagia, panting and exercise intolerance), the physical examination findings (e.g. pot belly, alopecia and comedones) and serum biochemistry (i.e. increased ALP), and can be confirmed by dynamic cortisol testing (ACTH stimulation, low-dose dexamethasone suppression) and imaging of the adrenals (and pituitary).

Only once metabolic diseases (and pyometra in intact bitches) have been ruled out, can we safely perform a water deprivation test. This test is dangerous in patients with metabolic diseases, and the results may be confusing as dogs with hypercalcaemia and hyperadrenocorticism are unable to concentrate their urine fully. A water deprivation test is used to differentiate DI from PP after ruling out other causes of polydipsia. If the modified test, with gradual reduction in water access over several days' hospitalization, is used, it often identifies PP quite quickly as the patient in a new environment often starts to concentrate their urine (>1.030) before complete water deprivation is scheduled. The patient alters their behaviour when hospitalized and voluntarily reduces its water intake. If after complete water deprivation and loss of 5% body weight the urine is still hyposthenuric, administration of DDAVP will help differentiate central from nephrogenic DI. Trial DDAVP treatment as a substitute for a water deprivation test is not reliable as it cannot always differentiate DI from PP or hyperadrenocorticism.

2.4.5 House soiling – urine

The history is critical in distinguishing between inappropriate urination in the house environment, where the patient is deliberately urinating, pollakiuria (frequent small voids of urine) and urinary incontinence. Urinalysis and urine culture are then essential to determine if a urinary tract infection is causing pollakiuria, and the possibility of polydipsia and polyuria should be considered in a previously continent animal.

2.4.6 House soiling – defecation

Defecation in the home environment in a previously house-trained animal may indicate an emotional cause, but if there are any other behaviour changes, a primary CNS disease (e.g. brain tumour) must be considered, and a neurological examination is required. During this exam, the anal tone should be checked as inadvertent soiling will occur if there is faecal incontinence. Of course, if the pet has diarrhoea, potential causes of primary gastrointestinal disease should be investigated. When the dog passes normal stools in regular frequency and pattern, we should investigate the possibility of pain as a cause.

2.4.7 Night-time waking or restlessness

While this may be a sign of cognitive dysfunction in older dogs, we must rule out painful conditions. Osteoarthritis is common, and historical clues about lethargy, stiffness or unwillingness to exercise, jump or climb stairs raise suspicions. Physical examination and relevant imaging may provide a definitive diagnosis, but an analgesic trial is often attempted first in practice.

Gastrointestinal pain may be more noticeable at night as the animal cannot settle, but does not always manifest as vomiting and diarrhoea. Reflux oesophagitis is also more common at night when the animal is lying down, and the stomach is empty. However, careful history taking may elicit information of repeated spontaneous gulping or swallowing motions and occasional regurgitation indicative of active reflux, although owners of brachycephalic breeds often believe this is normal behaviour.

2.5 Dermatological Diseases

Some of the most commonly encountered presentations are dermatological diseases labelled as psychiatric disease. Often owners and clinicians assume that a dog biting its nails or paws is bored or anxious, and a cat who over-grooms its ventral abdomen presents a compulsive disorder. A successful differentiation and therapy are dependent on a thorough dermatological diagnosis.

2.5.1 Alopecia in the absence of self-trauma

Dermatological diseases as a result of a psychiatric disease would almost invariably involve self-trauma. Therefore, in the absence of self-trauma, the likelihood of an underlying psychiatric disease is unlikely. Several questions to ask include:

- Does the hair regrow if the patient wears an Elizabethan collar? In such cases, we need to evaluate the hair follicle for structural or functional defects.
- Is the hair fractured, miniaturized or absent, or does it epilate easily?
- Are the guard hairs lost with retention of the puppy coat?
- Is the skin normal, thickened or thin? A good place to look for the presence of thin skin is on the ventral abdomen near the umbilicus; the skin may have a 'chicken skin' appearance, and blood vessels may be more visible.
- Is there any evidence of scaling or follicular casts (where scales travel up the hair shafts) that could indicate a disease of cornification?
- Is there any evidence of inflammation?
- Are there any clinical signs of disease that might suggest an endocrinopathy such as polyuria and polydipsia (hyperadrenocorticism), or lethargy, weight gain or heat-seeking behaviour (hypothyroidism)?

Skin scrapings (for Demodex) and fungal culture (dermatophytosis) are the initial tests of choice. If these tests are negative, a haematological and biochemical profile, urinalysis, endocrine test panels and a skin biopsy may be warranted.

The chronological order to consider when performing these tests is case-by-case dependent. If there are clinical signs or behaviours that are consistent with systemic disease, we should first perform blood profiles and urine evaluation. If not, we should proceed with a skin biopsy. Use a biopsy punch to collect multiple samples from the most alopecic areas and at least one sample from a normal skin as a control. These samples should be submitted to a veterinary dermatohistopathologist (preferably). If there are indications of endocrine or other systemic diseases on biopsy, appropriate blood tests are warranted.

2.5.2 Alopecia due to self-trauma

A systematic approach is needed to separate the numerous etiologies that can present as self-induced alopecia. Several questions may help to narrow the list:

- How old was the pet when the hair loss began?
- Has the pet lived in the same geographical region all its life? Most pets with environmental allergies start to traumatize their skin between six months and three years of age (Willemse, 1986; Prelaud *et al.*, 1998; Favrot *et al.*, 2010) unless they have moved from a different region later in life.
- Are any other members of the household or pets in contact affected (contagion)?
- What areas of the body are affected? Diagrams are available that show predilection sites for the various causes of pruritus (Hensel *et al.*, 2015).

2.5.2.1 *Self-trauma in cats*

Self-trauma in cats, leading to thin coat, alopecia and skin lesions, is likely to be multifactorial (Waisglass *et al.*, 2006). Common causes include atopy, adverse food reactions, parasitic hypersensitivity and environmental allergy. These disorders account for nearly 75% of self-trauma cases. A small percentage of cats (less than 15%) may have a combination of both physical and psychiatric disease (Waisglass *et al.*, 2006). Therefore, when presented with a cat who shows signs of self-trauma leading to dermatological disease, we must take a careful approach to rule out physical disease.

Flea combing is helpful to look for the presence of flea and other external parasites. We should look all over the body with emphasis on the back, from the thoracolumbar junction to the top of the tail and behind the ears. We should perform deep skin scrapings at lesional sites. However, superficial scraping at the base of the neck should also be included to rule out Demodex gatoi. This mite is found in the more superficial layers of the skin and can be contagious to other cats. Stool examination may yield information about external parasites the cat has swallowed.

Whether we find parasites or not, we should still treat the cat. The best choice is a broad-spectrum parasiticide with activity against Demodex gatoi as well as fleas, Cheyletiella and others. Even indoor cats, who never set foot outside of the house or building may have parasites.

Skin cytology will help to identify any secondary infections that need to be managed, such as a yeast or bacterial dermatitis. Samples for fungal culture should be collected using the toothbrush technique (using a sterile toothbrush to comb all areas, ending in the most affected, and pressing the bristles onto the medium). If the index of suspicion is high (e.g. owners have lesions as well), we should add a fungal PCR. Results are faster than the three weeks it could take for a culture to be positive. However, PCR results might yield a false negative result. Therefore, we should submit a sample for culture as well.

Food trials should also be part of the diagnosis. There are three steps in performing a food trial. In a study of cats presented for psychogenic alopecia, 57% of the cats in the study were diagnosed with food hypersensitivity (Waisglass *et al.*, 2006). Blood tests and saliva testing for food are not reliable; an appropriate food trial should be done.

Food trials should be performed strictly and for a period of up to eight weeks. We should obtain a good dietary history so that we can avoid items that could cross-react. Veterinary diets intended for diagnosis of food allergies are recommended; studies have shown cross-contamination with unlabelled ingredients in many commercially available pet foods (Horvath-Ungerboeck *et al.*, 2017). Re-check the animal once the diet has been fed exclusively for eight weeks and appropriate measures have been taken for external parasites (and microbial dermatitis, if indicated).

If there is a good response to the food trial, the animal is then 'challenged'. A dietary challenge involves giving the animal all of the previous foods and treats. Most animals will relapse within three to five days of chronic exposure to all the previously fed foods; some react in hours, and all food-allergic patients typically react by two to three weeks. In the event of a reaction, the diet reverts to the test hypoallergenic one until the animal is no longer pruritic.

The final stage of the food trial is re-challenge. At this stage, individual ingredients are added to the base hypoallergenic diets for up to two weeks (if no reaction) or until there is a reaction (if less than two weeks). The purpose of this provocation trial is to isolate individual ingredient(s) that should be avoided.

In cases where the response to the diet trial is incomplete, we can add steroids to the diet. By adding steroids to the treatment regime, we can assess for the possibility of both a food allergy and some other cause of pruritus (likely environmental allergies as long as parasites and microbes have been controlled).

Another test to consider is environmental allergy testing. The purpose of an allergy test is to determine the best allergens to place in the immunotherapy vaccine. A positive allergy test only confirms the presence of a reaction to the allergen, but not necessarily the cause of pruritus. If a test was positive for house dust mites, and the animal is no longer pruritic following flea treatment, immunotherapy for house dust mites is not indicated. Furthermore, some allergic patients have negative allergy tests, regardless of methodology; this is called 'atopic-like dermatitis'.

2.5.2.2 Self-trauma in dogs

In many cases, generalized pruritus in the dog is readily identified as a physical condition. However, localized self-trauma (e.g. acral lick dermatitis, nail-biting, or flank-sucking) tends to be labelled as psychogenic. In many respects, the work-up of cases of localized self-trauma in dogs follows the same diagnostic protocol as self-trauma in cats. However, dogs are more prone to long-lasting microbial dermatitis when compared to cats; deep infections in the dog may require months of antimicrobial medications.

When presented with a dog that is chewing its claws, we should collect a sample for cytology from the claws and below the claw fold. Many of these cases have an undiagnosed microbial dermatitis, especially a Malassezia paronychia. Many dogs will stop chewing when they are treated for their yeast dermatitis. If the claws are abnormal (dystrophic) and multiple claws on multiple paws are affected, consider Symmetric Lupoid Onychodystrophy. When the interdigital space is also affected, other aetiologies need to be considered including environmental and food-induced allergic dermatitis, possibly complicated by microbial dermatitis.

Acral lick dermatitis (ALD) occurs when a dog licks and bites an area on its body, leading to self-inflicted injuries (see Chapter 15). While there may be an emotional component to this condition, it is important to assess the role that physical causes play. Several conditions that can mimic ALD include lymphoblastic lymphoma, irritation secondary to an intramedullary pin, mast cell tumour, leishmaniasis and fungal disease (Denerolle *et al.*, 2007). Radiographs may help identify underlying orthopaedic pathology. Insertion of an indwelling catheter could also be a trigger.

Moreover, skin tests routinely performed in cases of ALD should include skin scraping to rule out demodicosis, cytology to assess for a surface yeast and bacterial dermatitis, culture and a food trial.

Deep infections presenting as furunculosis must be aggressively treated. Antimicrobial medications are commonly dispensed for a long course; they should be administered for one to two weeks past resolution of the lesions or when the lesion has reached a plateau and is no longer changing. Choosing the correct medications might be challenging; deep cultures match superficial cultures in only 36% of cases (Shumaker *et al.*, 2008). Two methods can help improve sample collection and, therefore, the accuracy of the culture result. In both cases, the dog should be sedated as these techniques are likely to cause pain. First, the area should be aseptically prepared. Then the lesion is squeezed until deep tissue liquid appears on the surface and is collected for culture. Another option is to collect punch biopsy tissue samples which are then submitted for culture.

2.5.3 Final note: brain–skin connection

There is an increase in disease severity in human patients with atopic dermatitis and an increase in Psoriasis Area and Severity Index and itch in stressed patients who have psoriasis (Arndt *et al.*, 2008; Verhoeven *et al.*, 2009). The increase in glucocorticoids in humans seen in stressful situations results in an inhibition of lipid synthesis. This inhibition leads to a decreased production and secretion from lamellar bodies of the keratinocytes with a resultant defective lipid barrier (Choi *et al.*, 2006). Given that atopic dermatitis in dogs is associated with an epidermal barrier defect (Marsella and Samuelson, 2009), how does stress affect our veterinary patients?

References

Acierno, M.J., Brown, S., Coleman, A.E., Jepson, R.E., Papich, M. *et al.* (2018) ACVIM consensus statement: guidelines for the identification, evaluation, and management of systemic hypertension in dogs and cats. *Journal of Veterinary Internal Medicine* 32(6), 1803–1822. DOI: 10.1111/jvim.15331.

Arndt, J., Smith, N. and Tausk, F. (2008) Stress and atopic dermatitis. *Current Allergy and Asthma Reports* 8(4), 312–317. DOI: 10.1007/s11882-008-0050-6.

Bradshaw, J. (2016) What is a cat, and why can cats become distressed? In: Sparkes, A. and Ellis, S. (eds) *ISFM Guide to Feline Stress and Health: Managing Negative Emotions to Improve Health and Wellbeing*. Tisbury, UK, pp. 16–30.

Choi, E.-H., Demerjian, M., Crumrine, D., Brown, B.E., Mauro, T. *et al.* (2006) Glucocorticoid blockade reverses psychological stress-induced abnormalities in epidermal structure and function. *American Journal of Physiology-Regulatory, Integrative and Comparative Physiology* 291(6), R1657–R1662. DOI: 10.1152/ajpregu.00010.2006.

Denerolle, P., White, S.D., Taylor, T.S. and Vandenabeele, S.I.J. (2007) Organic diseases mimicking acral lick dermatitis in six dogs. *Journal of the American Animal Hospital Association* 43(4), 215–220. DOI: 10.5326/0430215.

Favrot, C., Steffan, J., Seewald, W. and Picco, F. (2010) A prospective study on the clinical features of chronic canine atopic dermatitis and its diagnosis. *Veterinary Dermatology* 21(1), 23–31. DOI: 10.1111/j.1365-3164.2009.00758.x.

Heath, S. (2019) Unacceptable indoor elimination. *Journal of Feline Medicine and Surgery* 21(3), 199–208.

Hensel, P., Santoro, D., Favrot, C., Hill, P. and Griffin, C. (2015) Canine atopic dermatitis: detailed guidelines for diagnosis and allergen identification. *BMC Veterinary Research* 11, 196. DOI: 10.1186/s12917-015-0515-5.

Horvath-Ungerboeck, C., Widmann, K. and Handl, S. (2017) Detection of DNA from undeclared animal species in commercial elimination diets for dogs using PCR. *Veterinary Dermatology* 28(4), 373–e86. DOI: 10.1111/vde.12431.

Horwitz, D.F. and Rodan, I. (2018) Behavioral awareness in the feline consultation: understanding physical and emotional health. *Journal of Feline Medicine and Surgery* 20(5), 423–436. DOI: 10.1177/1098612X18771204.

Marsella, R. and Samuelson, D. (2009) Unravelling the skin barrier: a new paradigm for atopic dermatitis and house dust mites. *Veterinary Dermatology* 20(5-6), 533–540. DOI: 10.1111/j.1365-3164.2009.00809.x.

Prelaud, P., Guaguere, E., Alhaidari, Z., Heripret, D., Faivre, N. *et al.* (1998) Réévaluation des critères diagnostiques de la dermite topiqueé. *Revue de médecine vétérinaire* 149, 1057–1064.

Shumaker, A.K., Angus, J.C., Coyner, K.S., Loeffler, D.G., Rankin, S.C. *et al.* (2008) Microbiological and histopathological features of canine acral lick dermatitis. *Veterinary Dermatology* 19(5), 288–298. DOI: 10.1111/j.1365-3164.2008.00693.x.

Sparkes, A. (2018) Understanding feline idiopathic cystitis. *Veterinary Record* 182(17), 486. DOI: 10.1136/vr.k1848.

Verhoeven, E.W.M., Kraaimaat, F.W., de Jong, E.M.G.J., Schalkwijk, J., van de Kerkhof, P.C.M. *et al.* (2009) Individual differences in the effect of daily stressors on psoriasis: a prospective study. *British Journal of Dermatology* 161(2), 295–299. DOI: 10.1111/j.1365-2133.2009.09194.x.

Waisglass, S.E., Landsberg, G.M., Yager, J.A. and Hall, J.A. (2006) Underlying medical conditions in cats with presumptive psychogenic alopecia. *Journal of the American Veterinary Medical Association* 228(11), 1705–1709. DOI: 10.2460/javma.228.11.1705.

Willemse, T. (1986) Atopic skin disease: a review and a reconsideration of diagnostic criteria. *Journal of Small Animal Practice* 27, 771–778.

3 Addressing Pain in Veterinary Psychiatry

Samantha Lindley*

Glasgow University Veterinary School, Glasgow, UK

3.1 Introduction

Pain is an arresting sensation. It is arresting because it is frightening, and it is frightening because, in the acute phase, it signals existing or potential tissue damage. The message to the animal is to stop or avoid a specific behaviour in order to avoid further damage and threaten its survival. Pain is a common cause of behaviour changes in the veterinary species because it sends a frightening message to which the animal is compelled to pay attention.

3.2 Acute and Chronic Pain

Acute pain is adaptive, i.e. biologically useful, and it causes behaviour changes. These changes are more likely to be presented to the veterinary surgeon than are those associated with chronic pain because they are linked with sudden onset disability, lameness, injury, visceral dysfunction, and vocalization. In other words, the owner can see that their pet is unwell or in pain and will associate any behavioural change with the illness.

Acute pain may be the cause of acute onset behavioural changes when spinal pain occurs without obvious neurological signs. Sudden onset of, often, bizarre, fearful and sometimes aggressive behaviours may prompt investigation for possible brain disorders, including cognitive dysfunction in the older animal. Failure to find any specific neurological cause of these behavioural changes would indicate a strong possibility of pain as the eliciting factor.

Chronic pain is maladaptive and offers no long-term benefit to the animal. Why, then, do animals experience it? To answer this, it may be helpful to compare acute and chronic pain with fear and anxiety, respectively. The ability to experience fear and to respond to it keeps the animal alive. Anxiety (defined as chronic anticipation of threatening or negative stimulus) is of no biological use and is, in its chronic or severe form, detrimental to the organism, but the factors that lead to its development are integral to the usefulness of fear. In other words, anxiety can be seen as a 'side effect' of the life-saving emotion of fear, and chronic pain is the side effect of the life-saving sensation (and, some would argue, emotion) of acute pain. Pets do not die of chronic anxiety or chronic pain, and reproduction and nurturing of the young, although potentially impaired, can continue in the face of chronic pain and anxiety.

3.3 Pain, Fear and Stress

Animals, human and non-human, are adapted to experience fear, stress and acute pain, but these experiences must be limited so that the body and brain can return to a state of homeostasis. When such experiences are prolonged, as they are in chronic pain, anxiety and stress, fundamental changes may occur in the body and brain.

The pain–emotion connection is highly complex, and a complete review is outwith the scope of this chapter, but an excellent review of the current science (still not fully elucidated) can be found in al'Absi and Flaten (2016).

The following summary focuses particularly on the features of pain that are relevant to changes in behaviour and their impact on the emotional state of the animal.

3.3.1 Perception of pain and relevance to behaviour

All pain is perceived in the brain (see Fig. 3.1). The initial (fast pain) stimulus rapidly reaches the

*samanthalindley@btinternet.com

  Small Animal Veterinary Psychiatry (ed. S. Denenberg)
DOI: 10.1079/9781786394552.0003

Nociception ↓	Peripheral nociceptors activated by tissue damage Release of inflammatory mediators
Transduction ↓	Peripheral nociceptors convert noxious stimuli to electrical signals
Transmission ↓	Signals conducted along small myelinated and unmyelinated fibres and synapse with second order neurons in the dorsal horn of the spinal cord. These include nociceptive specific and wide dynamic range neurons
Modulation ↓	Other sensory inputs (touch and temperature) from the periphery and the influence of descending inhibitory pain pathways from the brain can inhibit or facilitate the transmission of noxious stimuli at the dorsal horn of the spinal cord
Projection ↓	Second order neurons project to third order neurons in the brain
Perception	Third order neurons project to cortical areas resulting in conscious perception of pain

Fig. 3.1. The most basic representation of pain perception.

somatosensory cortex so that the animal perceives that there is a threat (the result of which causes the animal to stop, withdraw and react), and the slow pain stimulus activates the limbic system so that the animal suffers (thereby protecting the area and learning to avoid the stimulus in future).

The painful stimulus activates multiple connections in the brain and spinal cord. The animal must pay the right amount of attention to the pain: too much, and there is over-reaction with the resulting danger of missing other important stimuli; too little, and the damage may continue, thereby threatening survival. The brain and spinal cord work together to achieve this balance and, in most normal individuals, work well to react, respond and then return the organism to normal functioning.

Problems occur, and subtle shifts in behaviour begin, when the pain stimulus continues. In simple terms, this stimulus signals to the animal:

- that it is continually under threat;
- that it must pay attention to the pain;
- that it is vulnerable and so should be hypervigilant and more defensive; and
- that it should avoid anything that makes the pain worse or appears to trigger it.

From a behavioural standpoint, when the pain stimulus continues, it could result in any or all of the behavioural problems seen in practice.

3.3.2 The components of pain

There are four main components of pain:

- Sensory (discriminative) – perceiving a pain stimulus and knowing where it originates;
- Affective (emotional) – suffering, i.e. how the pain makes one feel;
- Cognitive – how the patient thinks about their pain, including introspection and projection in humans or association and conditioning in non-human animals; and
- Motor – the postural and movement responses associated with the pain.

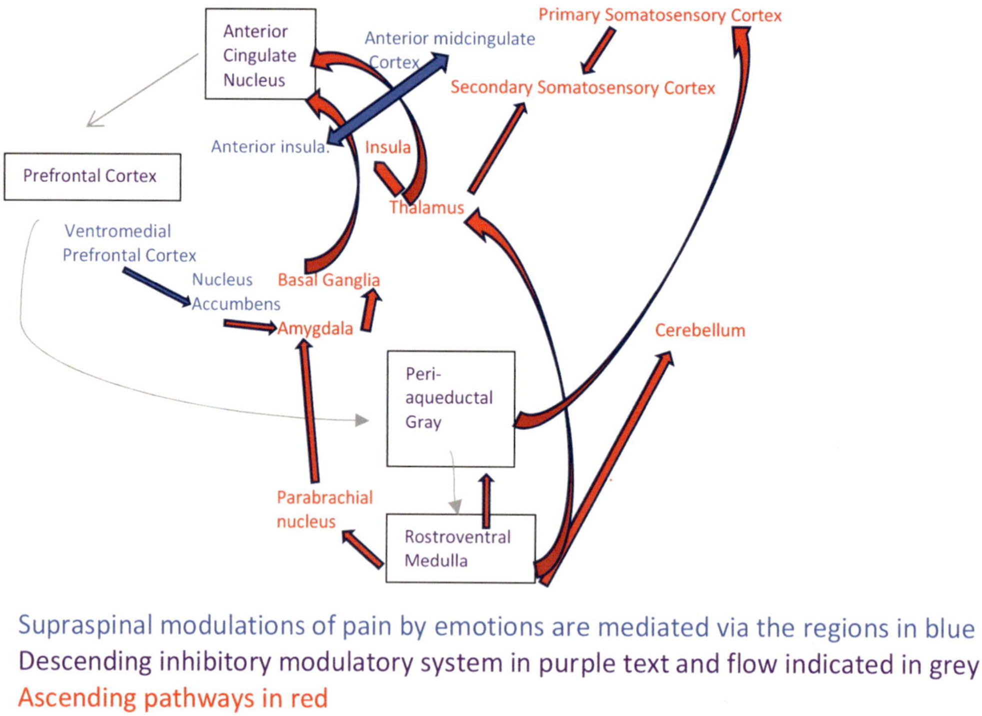

Fig. 3.2. Modulation that occurs from the ventromedial prefrontal cortex and the nucleus accumbens and between the anterior insula and the anterior midcingulate cortex. (From Wieser and Pauli, 2016.)

These components arise from the way that pain is processed, perceived and modulated in the brain and spinal cord (see Fig. 3.2).

Figure 3.2 shows the ascending pain pathways (although the term 'pathways' is a simplistic one) and the modulation of pain superimposed upon them.

3.3.3 The relevance of the pre-frontal cortex in animals and the treatment of chronic pain

Pain is modulated mainly through the descending pathways, but also supraspinal pathways, influenced in part by the prefrontal cortex. Non-human animals are less influenced by the pre-frontal cortex than are humans, and this is important to appreciate because while our patients will worry less about what pain means and, presumably, not at all about its influence on their future, it is not possible to teach them to be unafraid of their pain. Modern chronic pain medicine for humans focuses, in part, on techniques of cognitive behaviour therapy (CBT), where, essentially, patients learn not to be frightened of their pain. We cannot teach animals this, and therefore they often require more analgesic input to limit their sensation of, and suffering from, pain.

3.3.4 Central processing of pain and its influence on behaviour

Pain and emotion are inextricably linked through the structural organization of the brain.

3.3.4.1 The 'pain matrix'

The pain matrix is formed by the anterior cingulate nucleus gyrus, insula, frontal cortices, primary and secondary somatosensory cortex and amygdala.

The lateral region of the matrix gives the location and intensity of the painful stimulus. The medial region comprises the anterior cingulate cortex (ACC), which is involved in the affective component of pain (especially pain associated with fear, anxiety and depression); and the insula, which is involved with localization, affective-motivational and cognitive components of pain.

The hippocampus, in the medial temporal lobe, has an important role in pain processing and learning-related behaviours and plays an important part in chronic pain and the behaviours associated with avoidance of chronic pain.

3.3.4.2 Default mode network of the brain

The pain matrix overlaps with the concept of a default mode network (DMN) of the brain. Defined as the 'spatial coherence of resting brain activities', involved in introspection and vigilance, the DMN includes the ventral medial prefrontal cortex, posterior cingulate, precuneus, dorsal medial prefrontal cortex, inferior parietal lobe, lateral temporal cortex and hippocampus. It is related to the central modulation of chronic pain and individual responses to pain and appears to be altered in chronic pain and depressive states (Baliki *et al.*, 2008; Broyd *et al.*, 2009).

3.3.4.3 Limbic system

The pain matrix is also closely associated with the limbic system; functional MRI studies show similar overactivity in the limbic system in chronic stress and chronic pain (Fomberstein *et al.*, 2013).

The limbic system is the border between the cerebral hemispheres and the brain stem and includes the hippocampus, amygdala and nucleus accumbens. This system integrates information associated with fear, anxiety, arousal, vigilance and sympathetic autonomic activity, memory, learning, olfaction, pleasure, reward and addiction.

3.3.5 The neurotransmitters

Neurotransmitters are endogenous chemicals that transmit signals across a synapse. They are released into the synaptic cleft and bind to receptors on the post-synaptic side of the cleft (except for the endocannabinoids, which are formed in the post-synaptic cell and undergo retrograde transmission to the receptor on the pre-synaptic cell).

Neurotransmitter release is usually triggered by an incoming action potential, but may also be triggered by graded potentials, or even spontaneously. Most neurotransmitters that are associated with the modulation of pain sensation are also associated with the modulation of different behaviours.

3.3.5.1 Actions of common neurotransmitters

- Glutamate tends to be associated with fast excitatory synapses.
- Gamma-aminobutyric acid (GABA) tends to be associated with fast inhibitory synapses (and is the target for many sedative/tranquilizers).
- Acetylcholine (Ach) is the transmitter at neuromuscular junctions.
- Dopamine (DA) is associated with reward but is also implicated in motor function.
- Serotonin (SE) regulates appetite, sleep, memory, mood, temperature and learning. It may be involved in the emotional modulation of pain.
- Substance P (SP) enhances the transmission of pain.

3.3.5.2 From acute pain to sensitization

Alpha-amino-3-hydroxy-5-methyl-4-isoxazole propionic acid (AMPA) is the main receptor involved in acute pain, but when sufficient signals have unblocked the magnesium ions from the N-methyl-D-aspartate (NMDA) receptors, then these become involved in the amplification of pain that occurs during sensitization (and may result in an exaggerated and expanded pain field). Kainite (KA) channels modulate the release of GABA (reducing inhibition).

Substance P acts on neurokinin 1 (NK1) receptors and modifies the gain of pain transmission and, in persistent inflammatory states, NMDA channels are upregulated, further potentiating glutamate transmission and leading to central sensitization (also known as secondary sensitization).

Calcitonin gene-related peptide (CGRP) promotes the release of substance P and glutamate, promoting further activation of NK1 and glutamate and further sensitization.

The local release of serotonin caused by tissue damage acts on 5HT2 and 5HT3 receptors triggering thermal hyperalgesia and increased sensitization. (Bushnell *et al.*, 2013).

A small but persistent pain signal can become magnified to result in an expanded and exaggerated pain field, the impact of which bears no correlation to the severity of the original inciting stimulus. If this process continues, the result is a painful, frightened animal, but few or no definitive findings from imaging.

3.3.5.3 Endocannabinoid system

The endocannabinoid system is made up of five endocannabinoids (there may be more), two known cannabinoid (CB) receptors and enzymes involved in production and breakdown. Endocannabinoids are involved in every process in the body and maintain homeostasis. In chronic disease, this system may become depleted or it may be dysfunctional in certain individuals predisposing to chronic and persistent disease states.

CB1 receptors are in the central nervous system, primarily the amygdala, thalamus, periaqueductal gray (PAG), hippocampus and spinal cord. CB2 receptors are in the peripheral nervous system, immune system and bone. Both types are found in the liver, heart, gastrointestinal and reproductive systems and skin.

From the perspective of this chapter, they are part of the regulation of pain perception and emotional modulation (Grotenhermen, 2003).

3.4 The Stress Response

Many patients we see suffer from stress. This stress may be caused by pain or exacerbated by pain, and subjecting patients that are in pain to increased stress is likely to increase their pain.

The effects of stress on the body are mediated by the hypothalamic-pituitary-adrenal axis (HPA), the sympathetic nervous system (SNS) and the

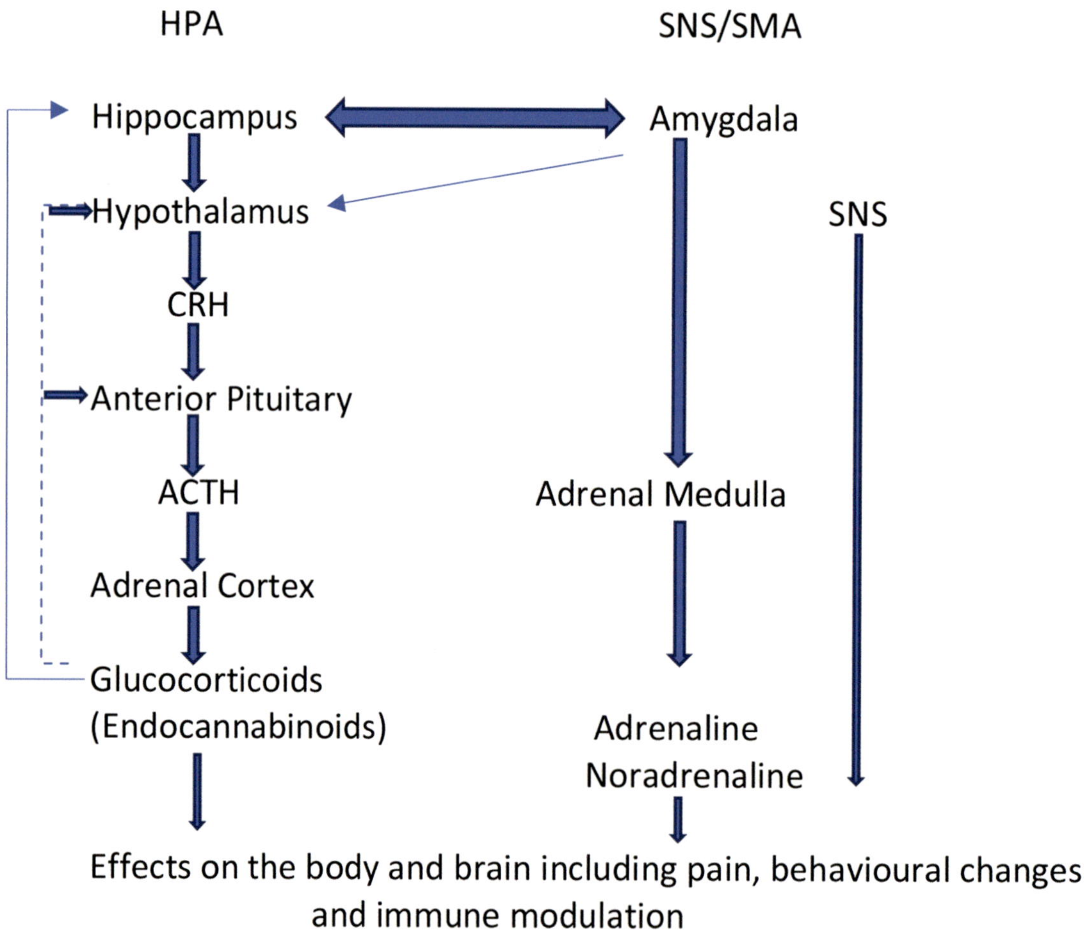

Fig. 3.3. Hypothalamic-pituitary-adrenal axis, sympathetic nervous system, and sympathomedullary-adrenal system pathways.

sympathomedullary adrenal axis (SMA) as shown in Fig. 3.3 (Murison, 2016).

Stress may produce analgesia, hypoalgesia or hyperalgesia. Stress analgesia appears to be associated with a severe threat, and this makes adaptive sense (fight or run away; do not stop to worry about injury). Hyperalgesia is associated with a moderate or low threat, where it makes sense to be hypervigilant.

Many of our patients are subject to continuous or intermittent, low or moderate threat so that hyperalgesia will be the more likely outcome; for example, cats with poor core territory or undersocialized dogs and cats having to deal daily with stimuli and social situations for which they are unprepared.

Stress-induced analgesia is mediated by cortical mechanisms including the amygdala, hypothalamus, PAG, the rostroventral medulla via so-called ‘off cells’, and the spinal cord via noradrenaline (NA), serotonin or opioids. Analgesia mediated by opioids is associated with short-term stressors and is activated by the hypothalamic-pituitary-adrenal axis.

Stress-induced hyperalgesia is associated with repeated or chronic stressors, which may be physical or psychogenic.

In human studies, it has been shown that stress exacerbates pain in chronic disorders of the bowel and fibromyalgia and that there is a high comorbidity between affective disorders and pain.

In summary, chronic pain triggers the stress response and alters the function of the brain, especially those areas associated with mood, emotion, fear, learning and sleep. Chronic stress has the same effect and will exacerbate chronic pain. Both chronic pain and chronic stress may lead to similar changes in the body and brain (Murison, 2016), including:

- hypertension;
- inhibition of gastrointestinal functions;
- immunosuppression;
- down-regulation of glucocorticoid receptors in the hippocampus and prefrontal cortex;
- corticotrophic releasing hormone (CRH) hyperdrive;
- hyperplasia and hypertrophy in the adrenals; and
- neuronal dysfunction, reduction of cognitive performance, and reduction in hippocampal volume.

3.5 Modulation of Pain

3.5.1 Descending pathways

Descending pathways are facilitatory or inhibitory, depending on the neurotransmitter involved. These are considered to be the most important in non-human animals.

The PAG has inputs from the thalamus, hypothalamus and brain stem, and projections to the locus coeruleus, rostroventromedial pathway (RVM), cell groups of the lateral reticular nucleus and nucleus tractus solitarius.

Stimulation of the PAG in the mid-brain inhibits the nociceptive dorsal horn neurons via the RVM and produces analgesia via spinal 5-hydroxytryptamine (5-HT) and alpha 2 adrenoreceptors. It also activates enkephalinergic releasing neurones that project to the raphe nucleus and release serotonin. Serotonin inhibits onward transmission.

The locus coeruleus connects directly with the spinal cord and, when stimulated, inhibits responses to noxious stimuli via the alpha 2 adrenoreceptors.

3.5.2 Supraspinal modulation

Fig. 3.2 shows modulation that occurs from the ventromedial prefrontal cortex and the nucleus accumbens and between the anterior insula and the anterior midcingulate cortex (Wieser and Pauli, 2016).

3.6 Summary of the Neurobiology of Pain and Emotion with Relevance to Behaviour

- Chronic pain is a chronic stressor and has widespread and deleterious effects on the brain and body.
- These changes will take time to reverse.
- Chronic stress and anxiety are likely to increase pain and vice versa.
- Reduction of cognitive function and hippocampal volume mean that trying to teach animals positive lessons while painful and stressed is not helpful.
- The development of chronic pain states, affective disorders and stress responses are interlinked and influenced by prenatal, neonatal and

early learning experiences as well as by genetic influences (Murison, 2016).

- The ability to control situations and develop coping mechanisms can influence the effects of stress and pain.
- Although animals have a cognitive component of pain, they do not have the introspection and projection aspects. This is both an advantage (worrying makes the pain worse) and disadvantage – we cannot teach animals not to be frightened of their pain.

3.7 The Influence of Pain on Psychiatric Diseases

3.7.1 Aggression

Pain causes a feeling of vulnerability and hypervigilance. Individuals may become aggressive in different situations depending on their genetics, experience, degree of socialization, and ability to cope with stressful situations.

Pain can also cause reactive aggression: normal greeting may change rapidly to a display of aggression because the patient associates the person or dog with the pain they have just experienced. Vulnerability might also result in resource-guarding behaviours in some dogs.

3.7.2 Anxiety

Given the links between pain and emotion in the brain discussed above, it should be a simple matter to understand how animals in pain are in a state of anxiety and feel vulnerable. Whatever the gaps are in their life experience (e.g. socialization, or, for cats, poor core territory) or whatever previous traumas they have undergone (e.g. frightened by loud noises, intolerant of another cat in their core territory), the effects of these are likely to be exacerbated by their pain.

NB Although difficult to prove, there is every reason to assume that an animal may become sensitized to the pain stimulus in the same way they become sensitized to any external stimulus. This assumption is based on cases where the palpable pain appears resolved, but the animal still reacts as strongly to the same stimuli. There would be suspicion, but not proof, since 'neuralgic' pain (pain arising from nervous tissue) cannot be palpated and is, arguably, the most frightening of all pains because it is unpredictable, sudden, sharp and lancinating.

3.7.3 Compulsive disorders

When pain cannot be attenuated by any of the animal's usual coping strategies (some dogs will want to exercise more rather than less; cats will usually withdraw or may overgroom), then the patient is conflicted. One result of a conflict that cannot be resolved is the development of compulsive disorders.

NB Pain can sometimes cause a genuine compulsive disorder or give rise to behaviours that look like compulsive disorders.

3.7.4 Attention-seeking behaviours

Many animals in pain will attempt to get comfort from their owners, and this can appear to be attention-seeking for the sake of the reward (like begging for food) rather than an emotional need for reassurance. Ignoring or punishing this behaviour is not appropriate.

3.8 Recognizing Pain as a Cause of Behaviour Changes

Although pain has been recognized as a major contributor to psychiatric diseases for some years, it is only recently that interesting figures have emerged. In this author's practice, the percentage of pain-related changes in pets has been close to 70 for the last five years; prior to that it was around the 50% mark. (Whether this difference is due to lower incidence or recognition is a moot point.)

The behaviour clinics at the University of Lincoln and the University of Bristol (D.S. Mills and S. Denenberg, respectively, 2019, personal communication) and others involved in referral behaviour consultations concur with this figure.

This is not to say, of course, that 70% of all behavioural disturbances are caused by pain. The referral population will often (but not always) have undergone numerous other interventions by the time they reach the referral clinic. Even so, it is an arresting statistic and a worrying one.

It is possible that the number of pain-related psychiatric diseases has genuinely increased. More than ever, owners involve dogs in activities whereby they cannot regulate their exercise (e.g. running, cycling, agility, toys that encourage jumping, twisting,

Table 3.1. Behavioural changes that give the suspicion of high pain index in cats.

Behaviour changes	Elements of presentations that give a high index of suspicion of pain
Aggression	Sudden onset in the absence of suboptimal core territory or environmental change or trauma or series of low-grade traumas Changes in utilization of core territory resources Changes in social relationship, grooming or activity with no environmental explanation
House soiling (urine and faeces)	Unpredictable Near the litter tray Other locations if access to tray or outside is difficult Change in posture Vocalization while eliminating Small amounts
Compulsive disorders	Excessive grooming Evidence of skin rolling or twitching with no external stimuli No identifiable cause (e.g. lesion or parasites) Vocalization
Night-time	Vocalization Pacing Lack of sleep, difficulties in lying down

and landing heavily), but dogs and cats are also living longer than they used to and are therefore more subject to the wear and tear of increasing age. Also, the function of descending modulation may decrease with age (Iwata *et al.*, 2002).

Animals adapt to chronic pain in subtle ways. This is not to say that they stop suffering from the pain, because they do not, but they do alter their behaviour in order to deal with the pain. It is when those attempts to cope break down (or the owners stop tolerating the attempts) that we see the behavioural change emerge.

3.8.1 Diagnosis of pain as a component or cause of a psychiatric disease

The diagnosis of pain as a component or the cause of a psychiatric disease is not always straightforward. Often it requires identifying isolated signs through the daily behaviours of the animal and during the consultation and combining them to a larger clinical picture. The signs must be consistent with pain, be repetitious and relevant to the presenting complaints.

Tables 3.1 and 3.2 give the common and less common behavioural changes caused by pain. However, any behavioural change, except predatory behaviour, could be caused by pain.

The first step is to determine whether the cause of the problem is physical, environmental or emotional. It could be a combination of these. (For more information, see Chapter 2.)

From the history and presentation, a physical cause for a behaviour change is likely when the behaviour:

- is of sudden onset with no environmental or emotional changes, or trauma;
- is genuinely unpredictable;
- is extreme for the animal's temperament or breed;
- is disproportionate to the eliciting stimuli;
- represents changes in multiple areas of the animal's life; and
- does not make sense from the history (no necessary and probable conditions).

Owners (and sometimes veterinary surgeons) desperately try to construct patterns of behaviour and signs that will make sense to them, but it is just as important to recognize when no pattern is present because where there is no logical pattern, a physical cause is likely.

It is, of course, possible that there may be a mixture of reasons for the behaviour and, in these cases, some behaviours will emerge as predictable and explicable, and others not.

The example of sound sensitivity exacerbated by pain falls into this category: the animal may react predictably to noises like fireworks, thunder and gunshots, but erratically to other noises or even as

Table 3.2. Behavioural changes that give the suspicion of high pain index in dogs.

Behaviour changes	Elements of presentations that give a high index of suspicion of pain
Aggression towards unfamiliar dogs	The patient is well socialized No trauma from other dogs Worse with high-energy dogs Unpredictable Aggression occurs during play Aggression occurs after a friendly greeting Aggressive to dogs that were previously greeted normally Aggression to all dogs, high-energy dogs or unfamiliar dogs suggests that pain is causing vulnerability Unpredictable aggression suggests a reaction to immediate pain, associating it with the other dog)
Aggression towards other dogs in the same household	The age, sex or breed distribution is not suggestive of conflict The dogs have lived together in genuine harmony for years No changes in the household/relationships with humans The 'antagonist' is smaller, weaker or is at a disadvantage during fights The dog being attacked repeatedly displays appropriate appeasement behaviours and does not challenge the antagonist Fights occur unpredictably but often in small/narrow spaces Fights may occur during normal play
Aggression towards the owners	The dog does not resource-guard and is generally obedient The dog usually shows appeasing behaviours The dog looks frightened, worried or appeasing after aggression The aggression may be linked to resources but is not consistent (NB The resource-guarding dog may not look appeasing after an attack and resource-guarding will often need to be addressed before it becomes clear that pain is a trigger for the behaviour)
Aggression towards unfamiliar people	The dog has been well socialized and is socially competent There have been no traumas associated with people The behaviour is worse with loud/rapidly moving people/children The behaviour is displayed towards unfamiliar people only The behaviour occurs unpredictably towards people the dog knows well and has previously been friendly with A friendly greeting turns into an attack with no warning
Noise aversion	There is no history of sound sensitivity The dog shows no problem with thunder, fireworks and other sounds The dog does not always react in the same way to the same noises Fearful behaviour occurs in the absence of noises
Separation distress	The problem is a sudden onset There is evidence that the dog can be relaxed when alone The problem is unpredictable The dog shows no signs of anxiety when the owner is present (i.e. does not follow the owner around or look anxious when the owner prepares to leave) There is no over-attachment or hyper-attachment (NB Pain can cause genuine separation distress because the dog becomes afraid of being on its own. In other situations, the anxiety occurs only when the pain is experienced and, in these cases, needs to be distinguished from external causes of alarm when the owner is not present)

Continued

Table 3.2. Continued

Behaviour changes	Elements of presentations that give a high index of suspicion of pain
Night-time behaviour	Sudden onset Dog not comforted by the presence of owners Cognitive behaviour is still normal (N.B. Many cases of 'cognitive dysfunction' are caused by or exacerbated by pain. Every one of the DISHA criteria can be caused by pain. Similarly, diagnoses of 'night terrors' or PTSD should be viewed with caution and an assumption of pain made before medication is started)
Compulsive disorders	Sudden onset No external evidence of social conflict The behaviour occurs irregularly and can sometimes be interrupted (NB Pain may appear to cause a compulsive disorder or even a complex partial seizure such as absences, fly-snapping or tail-chasing or may become a compulsive behaviour if the pain triggering the original behaviour is not resolved)

though they have heard a noise when no noise has occurred.

As well as helping to establish the cause of the problem, the history will indicate the importance of different resources to the animal and therefore the cost of removing those during treatment for pain (e.g. restriction of exercise and play).

The second stage is to rule out (as much as possible) any physical cause that might elicit or contribute to the pain (see Chapter 2). The third step is to piece together all the information to complete a clinical picture. Tables 3.1 and 3.2 give the common changes that may be expected when animals are in pain.

The fourth step is to assess the patient's gait. Videos of the animal's gait in different situations are invaluable. It is often not easy to ascertain gait abnormalities in the clinical setting or even in the house, as cats may not move around much in the presence of strangers and there may not be space to see a dog in action in a tiny garden.

Tell the owner what is needed: videos of normal movement on a flat surface, going up and down stairs, and attempts to jump (cat and dog). For the dog: movements such as running, trotting, walking, on and off the lead, are required (see Handout A8 – Pain Assessment).

Gait abnormalities might include:

- 'pacing', where the dog's or cat's ipsilateral limbs move together instead of the contralateral limbs, gives a high index of suspicion of back pain;
- 'crabbing', where the animal tends to move at a diagonal to the straight line of forwards progression, is indicative of back pain;
- 'bunny-hopping', which is where the back legs move together when the front limbs move separately, is indicative of hindquarter dysfunction;
- walking on the front legs only (not common) is a sign of back pain;
- obvious lameness is helpful, but by no mean necessarily apparent; and
- low head carriage indicates neck pain.

Evaluation of gait is not helpful if the pain is suspected to be unconnected with the locomotory system.

The fifth stage is to evaluate any physical signs and difficulties:

- moving up and down stairs: note that going at speed does not rule out pain – sometimes this reflects a loss of control and sometimes an attempt to get past the painful process;
- getting up: a normal dog will rise on all four legs together while painful animals often haul themselves up with their forelimbs or push their hindquarters up first;
- lying down, gingerly in slow sequence or crashing down;
- toileting: reduction or total failure to lift the leg in males, change in defecating pattern, wandering about, or inability to hold a squatting position;
- inability to scratch with the hindlimbs;

- reduced, or absence of, full-body shaking;
- lying or sitting down to eat;
- sudden jumping, starting and looking around at the body or attacking the body;
- chewing or licking excessively (usually at the body but sometimes excessive licking of people, floors, or soft furnishings);
- for cats especially: changes in jumping, and increased or decreased grooming;
- post-prandial behaviour changes may be associated with gastrointestinal pain as well as hepatic dysfunction.

The final step is an examination for pain:

Veterinary surgeons should train themselves, or be trained, in examination techniques beyond routine clinical skills. By the time many patients present, they will have adapted their gait and posture such that they have extensive muscular back, and sometimes spinal, pain. The development of such pain is often the point at which they fail to cope with their suffering and the behaviour problem becomes significant. It does not mean that the primary problem is back or spinal pain.

When assessing patients for psychiatric diseases, the initial goal is not to diagnose the cause of the pain but to identify that pain is present and that the history supports a probable influence of that pain. In due course a diagnosis, if possible, is desirable, but, initially, the aim is to reduce the pain and note a reduction or resolution of some or all the behaviours.

In some cases, because the animal is too aggressive or fearful, they cannot be examined, so the diagnosis is based only on the preceding stages. It is a disadvantage to work with one less clue and one less outcome measure to treatment, but it does not make progress impossible. Ideally, during the physical examination, the animal should be as relaxed as possible.

When the patient stands squarely, we can examine its weight distribution. Weight-shifting may indicate pain in one or more limbs when it is not apparent by stance or gait.

Abnormal or uneven muscle mass may indicate dysfunction of an affected limb. Hypertrophy of the shoulder girdle muscles is suggestive of chronic weight shift from the pelvic limbs.

If central sensitization is not apparent or not widespread, the most useful physical clues from palpation are myofascial trigger points (MFTrPs). These 'knots' in the muscle are located at the site of the damaged endplate (neuromuscular junctions). A leakage of Ach causes muscle fibre contraction, compromise of local blood flow, a build-up of the waste products of muscle metabolism, and consequent sensitization of the local sensory nerve, resulting in a tender band within a muscle that may be spontaneously painful and refer the pain some distance from the site. These MFTrPs arise from muscle strain and other painful somatic and visceral sources and are therefore a valuable clue to the presence of pain. However stoical the animal is, it is almost impossible to fail to elicit a response under the fingers from correct palpation of these structures (Cummings, 2016).

Additional examination techniques such as ROM of joints, depression of bony spine and neck flexion and extension should be performed, if possible, without causing distress.

3.8.2 Identifying allodynia and hyperalgesia

Allodynia is defined as a pain response to a previously non-noxious stimulus, such as touch. Recognition of allodynia would, technically, require delivery of a known and consistent pressure at one site compared with the same pressure at another site. In practice, use the flat of the hand/fingers all over the patient's body, noting subtle signs of a pain response, such as tremors or fasciculations, transient tension and moving away. Facial expression changes and turning towards the area, with or without a low, rapid appeasing tail wag might indicate allodynia or the anticipation of pain, especially when the site has been repeatedly and painfully examined.

Hyperalgesia is defined as an exaggerated pain response. It can be difficult to identify and will overlap with allodynia. Relatively light palpation of muscle, joint or bone can give rise to a painful response and is suggestive of hyperalgesia.

The presence of hyperalgesia or allodynia represents an exaggerated and expanded pain field (secondary or central sensitization) and may cover most of the animal's body or be regional.

When identifying allodynia or hyperalgesia, there is little point in going further with the examination because any structure involved in this field will appear painful, whether or not any pathological changes are involved, and all further palpation will do is hurt the patient and make subsequent examinations more difficult.

3.9 Treatment of the Painful Causes of Behavioural Changes

Treatment will usually be medical analgesia in the first instance. This is more likely to achieve a rapid response, and it is important to convince the owner of the accuracy of the diagnosis. We need to urge the owner to have patience as the initial conviction is rapidly overtaken by scepticism when there is no immediate change in behaviour. It is important to note that it can take six weeks to wind down pain. It will often take longer for changes in the brain to occur if the problem has been present for months or years.

It is as well to warn the owners that we may need to use multimodal analgesia (ideally a combination of therapies to target different elements of pain processing while keeping the dosages to a minimum) because they may perceive the addition of further medications to be a failure of treatment rather than a normal therapeutic progression.

Owners' initial responses to being told that their animal is in pain are various and may include denial, anger, shock, sadness and concern. Also, owners may have questions such as:

- Can it be fixed? As often as not, the problem will be managed.
- Should there be imaging studies (e.g. radiographs or MRI)? Sometimes, depending on the severity, breed and age of the patient; more commonly, the aim is to first establish the link between relief of pain and change of behaviour. Very often, investigations will yield nothing or at least nothing conclusive. Reasons to investigate further include failure to resolve the pain or improve beyond a certain point despite several different medications or approaches, worsening in pain or signs of pain despite medications, the breakthrough of pain despite treatment, and return of signs of pain as the medication is reduced.
- How long will my pet need medication? First, we must see whether it helps the pain, but if it does, we can later explore whether physical therapies can replace or reduce the need for medicine.
- Will my pet live a shorter life because of the medication? Not necessarily, but it is important to remember that being in chronic pain is the same as being subject to chronic stress, and that it is potentially life-shortening and certainly damaging to health.

At some point, the animal may need anxiolytics and other behaviour-modifying medications. However, this is not common when pain is the primary cause of change in the animal's behaviour. If the pain is dealt with adequately, the anxiety usually subsides and the behaviour improves. If behavioural signs continue, it is better to err on the side of assuming that the pain continues, not that the animal has learned anxiety, although, of course, this does happen, and anxiolytic trial therapy may be necessary. See Fig. 3.4 for an algorithm of the approach.

3.9.1 Approach to the treatment of pain

The following is a general guideline to addressing the selection of treatment options for chronic pain:

3.9.1.1 Classify the pain

The first step is to know the type of pain we are treating. The type of pain will indicate the treatment required:

- nociceptive or nociceptive-inflammatory;
- neuropathic pain (neuralgia);
- visceral; or
- central sensitization.

3.9.1.2 Source of pain

Next we need to identify the sources of pain, if possible, and then the classification of pain for each source:

- dermatological;
- mucosal (anal sacs, gingiva, aural or oral);
- muscle (usually myofascial in chronic pain, and less commonly muscle spasm. Myositis is usually acute progressing to chronic);
- joints and the skeletal system (synovial capsule, bone on bone impingement, fragments, microfractures or joint instability) and associated soft tissue;
- visceral;
- spinal (disc-related: inflammation or impingement; meninges; syrinx and oedema (Chiari malformation/Syringomyelia), facet joint, nerve root, or entrapment and inflammation); and

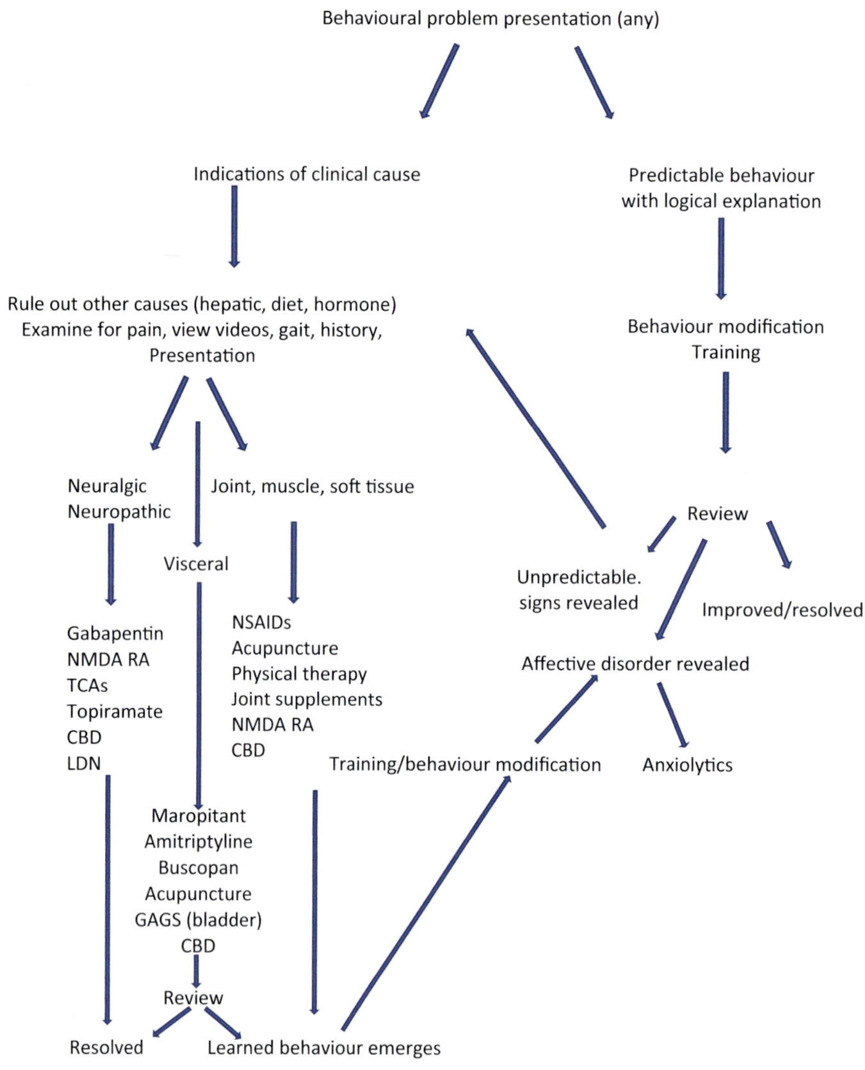

Fig. 3.4. Algorithm for the diagnosis and management of pain and emotional disorders (a simplistic view).

- no remaining pathological lesion: the pain has become the disease.

3.9.1.3 Choice of analgesia

Select the analgesia based on the likely classification of pain, the relevance of the side-effect profile and the ease of dosing for each individual (see Table 3.3).

For nociceptive or nociceptive-inflammatory disease:

- non-steroidal anti-inflammatory drugs;
- EP4 receptor antagonist (piperants);
- paracetamol (gastrointestinal and kidney-sparing NSAID) with or without codeine;
- corticosteroids;
- joint supplements;
- pentosan polysulphate (joints, bladder);
- palmitoylethanolamide (PEA) an endocannabinoid; and
- tramadol.

Table 3.3. Analgesia selection, indications and potential side effects.

Analgesic	Mechanism of action and dosage	Possible common side effects (see data sheets for full information)	Indication/comments
NSAIDs (numerous licensed)	Inhibit the cyclo-oxygenase pathway of the production of prostaglandins or the lipoxygenase pathway to leukotrienes, thereby limiting pain and inflammation Dose: as per data sheet	Vomiting, nausea, inappetence diarrhoea, haematemesis, melaena	Nociceptive/inflammatory pain Six-week trial Swapping NSAID type with an appropriate washout period may be helpful Meloxicam and robenacoxib licensed for cats
Grapiprant	EP4 receptor antagonist 2 mg/kg on an empty stomach	Vomiting, diarrhoea	Nociceptive, inflammatory pain, especially mild to moderate arthritis Dogs only
Pentosan polysulphate	Chondroprotectant Potent activator of the fibrinolytic system 3 mg/kg s/c Once weekly for 4 weeks to gauge the effect	Vomiting, dullness	Nociceptive, inflammatory pain, specifically, osteoarthritis May be useful in feline idiopathic cystitis
Paracetamol (acetaminophen) Paracetamol with codeine	NSAID but acts via peri-oxidase enzyme component of prostaglandin H2, therefore spares GI and renal mucosa Known safe dosage is 10–15 mg/kg bid Antipyretic and analgesic at this dose Some evidence to suggest anti-inflammatory effects at higher doses (20–25 mg/kg) (Single toxic dose 100 mg/kg) Data sheet 1 tablet per 12 kg (33 mg/kg) bid/tid	Vomiting, diarrhoea Toxic in cats Nausea, inappetance, constipation	A useful addition in acute flare-ups when changing from one NSAID to another during washout In some cases, appears to be as effective for pain as the other NSAIDs depending on the dose NOT IN CATS Useful for additional pain relief, especially in OA and when other NSAIDs are contraindicated Licensed for 5 days only NOT IN CATS
Tramadol	Weak mu agonist, Increases SE and inhibits the reuptake of NA 2–6 mg/kg bid to quid Primary action probably through descending inhibitory control	Dysphoria, sedation, vomiting, diarrhoea Care with primary serotonergic drugs May lower seizure threshold	Reduction of suffering Care in behavioural cases: may increase or change the context of aggression, and delayed anxiety and agitation probably due to dysphoria Use lower dose and frequency in cats: 1–4 mg/kg bid

Continued

Table 3.3. Continued

Analgesic	Mechanism of action and dosage	Possible common side effects (see data sheets for full information)	Indication/comments
Gabapentin Pregabalin	Structural analogue of GABA but does not work at GABA receptors Calcium channel stabilizer Pregabalin is gabapentin and an inactive sidearm, differences in bioavailability and therefore tolerance by the patient The initial dose for gabapentin is 5–10 mg/kg bid/tid Tolerance is common, and doses may increase to 60 mg/kg tid The initial dose for pregabalin is 2.5–5 mg/kg bid	Sedation, ataxia, vomiting, diarrhoea, polyphagia, weight gain, Less common: hair loss, dyskinesia	Acts as an antihyperalgesic Use in central (secondary sensitization) or suspected neuralgic pain (jumping/starting/hyperaesthesia) Some evidence that there may be effects on anxiety
Topiramate	Anti-convulsive, antinociceptive, neuroprotective 5–10 mg/kg bid/tid	Anorexia, ataxia, sedation, diarrhoea	Appears to be useful in neuralgic pain, including syringomyelia
Amantadine	NMDA receptor antagonists 2–6 mg/kg sid or divided dose bid	Vomiting, diarrhoea Dissociative in sensitive patients (dullness or agitation) Sedation	Useful in hyperalgesia and allodynia Suspected neuralgic pain Can take 2 weeks to work
Memantine	0.3–0.8 mg/kg sid or divided dose bid	Dissociative in sensitive patients Sedation	Hyperalgesia, allodynia, suspected neuralgic pain Can take 2 weeks to work
Ketamine	0.5 mg/kg s/c 5 days or CRI	Sedation and dissociative effects, depending on the dose	Very painful patients, pain breakthrough, acute flare-ups
Tricyclic anti-depressants: Amitriptyline Imipramine	Inhibit re-uptake of NA and SE Block cholinergic, adrenergic and histaminergic receptors More noradrenergic than serotonergic in their action For pain: 0.5–1 mg/kg bid	Contra-indicated in cardiac arrhythmia Constipation, dry eye, vomiting, diarrhoea, sedation, anxiety and agitation No concurrent use with MAOI, other TCAs, SSRIs or SNRIs Care with other drugs that increase serotonin, like tramadol because of possible serotonin syndrome	Visceral pain, neuropathic and nociceptive pain The possible negative effects on behaviour must be considered Despite the role of SE in the pain- modulation system, serotonergic drugs (including Fluoxetine) appear less useful in controlling pain, unless the emotional component has become the predominant factor

Continued

Table 3.3. Continued

Analgesic	Mechanism of action and dosage	Possible common side effects (see data sheets for full information)	Indication/comments
Duloxetine	Serotonin – noradrenaline reuptake inhibitor 1–2 mg/kg sid	Sedation, diarrhoea, vomiting, Behavioural changes No concomitant use with TCAs, SSRIs, MAOIs	Currently, use restricted to where anticonvulsants, TCAs and NMDA receptor antagonists not working or not tolerated Widespread pain, secondary sensitization, neuralgic pain NO INFORMATION RE CATS
Herbal medicines	The theory that the whole plant has beneficial actions over and above the active ingredient, including mitigating against side effects. Should be prescribed by trained veterinary surgeons	Dependent on the herb It is important to know whether the patient is taking any herbal medicine that may interact with concurrent medications, especially those with gastro-irritant or a potentially serotonergic effect	Wide variety of signs depending on the herb employed. Note that many owners confuse herbal with homoeopathic and assume that herbal medicine is completely safe. Owners may be using herbal tranquilizers/anxiolytics, which may interact with pain medication
Endocannabinoids: Cannabidiol (CBD) Palmitoylethanolamide (PEA) (THC where legal)	CBD modulates effects of other neuromodulators on CB2 receptors (allosteric modulator) Dogs 0.25–1 mg.kg bid Cats 0.1–0.5 mg/kg sid or EOD PEA acts on CB2 receptors among other actions 10–20 mg/kg si/bid THC acts on CB1 receptors should be given with CBD to counter psychoactive effects)	Sedation Some interaction with other CNS agents, antibiotics and anti-cancer treatments	CBD Refractory pain including neuropathic, visceral, cancer, inflammatory, because of the expression of CB receptors through most body systems and effects on non-cannabinoid receptors. It takes 3–4 weeks to reach a steady-state, then the dose can be decreased PEA experimental evidence looks promising (Re *et al.*, 2007) but might be better introduced earlier in the disease process. (Della Rocca, Cremona, 2018, personal communication)
Low-dose naltrexone	Transient blockade opiate receptors, release of endorphins antagonism of toll-like receptors (TLR) 0.5–4.5 mg/dog sid. No information for cats	Transient diarrhoea, night disturbances, mild agitation	Refractory pain, especially with indications of an inflammatory component

For neuropathic pain including central sensitization (secondary sensitization – an exaggerated and expanded pain field):

- anticonvulsants (Gabapentin, pregabalin, topiramate);
- NMDA receptor antagonists (memantine, amantadine, ketamine);
- tricyclic antidepressants (amitriptyline, imipramine);
- endocannabinoids (cannabidiol, palmitoylethanolamide); and
- opiate receptor antagonist (low-dose naltrexone).

Specifically, to reduce suffering and in acute flare-ups:

- opiates (methadone, tramadol and buprenorphine OTM);
- ketamine;
- maropitant (gastrointestinal pain);
- hyoscine butylbromide (gastrointestinal pain);
- amitriptyline (bladder and gastrointestinal pain); and
- glycosaminoglycans (bladder pain).

Serotonin syndrome may result from combining serotonergic drugs, especially MAOIs, SNRIs, SSRIs, some TCAs and other analgesics. This syndrome may be fatal and requires intensive care.

3.9.2 Physical therapies

There is a wide range of physical therapies available for pets (see Table 3.4). Choosing the appropriate one for a patient can be challenging. Selection can be based on suitability of the therapy to the patient's needs, the patient's 'willingness' to accept the technique, local availability and bias towards and prejudice against therapies based on personal experience, clinical outcomes, the individual's understanding, or otherwise, of the mechanism of the therapy.

When treating a patient with pain leading to behavioural changes, we should consider physical therapies when:

- pharmaceuticals have not had a sufficiently potent effect;
- pharmaceuticals have significant and unpleasant side effects for the patient;
- Pharmaceuticals have helped the pain and the problem, but the long-term view must now be to help the animal to rehabilitate, reduce the likelihood of recurrence and the need for additional medication; and
- the owner requests further input either to try to reduce or to stop the medication or because they feel that further help is required.

3.9.2.1 Is it safe?

For many physical therapies, evidence of specific effects is limited, and so the considerations for the clinician should be the safety and welfare of the patient. Safety includes:

- the inherent safety of the technique;
- additional stress to the patient in terms of travel, exposure to novel and stressful situations, discomfort, and proximity of who or what the pet might see as a threat;
- possible delay in specific diagnosis; and
- inappropriate removal or reduction of medication under the advice of the therapist.

NB It should not be assumed that these therapies are all harmless, but owners are less inclined to recognize or believe this of such treatments than they are of medication.

3.9.2.2 Are there any mechanisms by which it might work positively?

Any physical therapy should be gentle, non-aversive and preferably result in the animal becoming relaxed. Positive physical interaction with an animal is likely to reduce blood pressure and increase positive mood neurotransmitters (Odendaal, 2000).

3.9.3 Provision and the emotional cost of restriction of resources

While collecting behavioural history, we should investigate which resources are most important to the patient. These resources may be restricted by the pain and disease (cats unable to jump; dogs unable to walk far enough to socialize with other dogs) or have been restricted by the treatment of the pain (reduction of food; stopping of certain kinds of play).

Loss of these resources will have an emotional impact on the patient (see Table 3.5). Owners are often acutely aware of this and may comply less

Table 3.4. Common physical therapies, their mechanisms of action and additional comments.

Physical therapy	Mechanism of action	Frequency of treatment	Side effects and influence on behaviour
Acupuncture	Stimulates afferent nerves and modulates pain locally and at the dorsal horn of the segment stimulated Deactivates the limbic system Modulates DMN and the descending inhibitory pain pathways (Lundeberg and Lund, 2016)	Once to twice weekly for 4–6 weeks and then to effect	Temporary worsening Sedation (positive) Cautions depending on concurrent disease and needle placement Transient anxiolysis, but numerous studies on human psychiatric disease fail to show a long-term specific effect on depression
Physiotherapy	Wide range of therapies depending on the training of physiotherapists The aim is to restore an animal to optimum achievable function following disease, injury or surgery	Once weekly for 4–6 weeks and then to effect, with exercises for the owner to apply at home	Temporary worsening depending on condition and techniques used Mental stimulation and social activity may have transient beneficial effects Increased owner interaction and co-operation at home may improve bonding
Hydrotherapy	The use of the inherent qualities of water to restore or improve function and reduce pain	Once to twice a week for 4–6 weeks and then to effect	Worsening of certain conditions possible: avoid swimming with cervical pain and extended stride length in lumbosacral disease Care with atopy and IBD Elderly and frail animals should use a treadmill only Mental stimulation, endorphin release and social activity may have transient beneficial effects
Laser	Mechanisms are still controversial There are antinociceptive effects and some central effects (Baxter and McDonough, 2016)	Once or twice a week and then to effect	Class IV lasers carry a risk of burns, and anxious animals may not like the heat sensation Some evidence of central effects on depression
Chiropractic	Manual realignment of the spine and associated soft-tissue structures	Depends on the therapist – some will perform very small adjustments regularly, while others perform larger adjustments with several weeks in-between	Temporary worsening of pain Some patients actively enjoy the interaction Effects on behaviour are likely to be secondary

Continued

Table 3.4. Continued

Physical therapy	Mechanism of action	Frequency of treatment	Side effects and influence on behaviour
Osteopathy	Use of a variety of manual therapies to relieve trigger points, mobilize joints, stretch muscles	Depends on the therapist – some will perform very small adjustments regularly, while others perform larger adjustments with several weeks in-between	Temporary worsening of pain Some patients actively enjoy the interaction Effects on behaviour are likely to be secondary
Bowen therapy	The mechanism is controversial. The original intention appears to have been to provide an unusual stimulus to the body and brain in the form of gentle soft-tissue movements to trigger healing/analgesic responses	Depends on the therapist, often weekly and then to effect	Unlikely to be a worsening unless the patient is very sensitive Secondary effects on behaviour
Massage, Emmet, Galen myotherapy	The use of touch, myofascial release, stretch and gentle manipulation of soft tissues	Depends on the therapist; weekly and to effect	Any positive physical interaction is likely to have short-term anxiolytic effects

with the overall programme when they recognize the effect that this loss has on their pet.

3.10 Reducing Pain Relief – Consequences

Once the pain appears to be under control, and the behaviour returns to normal or improves, the owners will be keen to reduce or stop any medication. While this might be desirable, it is not always achievable. The weaning process should be done slowly, and we should be aware of the following:

- Pain may take 6 weeks to wind back up.
- Breakthrough pain is not always resolved by a return to previous doses of analgesics.
- The phenomenon of emotional rebound may make the behavioural change appear worse than ever. This phenomenon is where the pain, having been reduced, returns to a lesser degree, but the animal feels worse about it than they did when it was at its most severe. Our investigation may yield less pain than before; however, the patient is suffering more, probably in part due to a loss of previous coping mechanisms.

3.11 Pain and Anxiety – Where in the Vicious Cycle Is the Patient?

This is the most vexing of questions. It appears that, in many cases (where the pain is the primary component), if we can resolve the pain, then the behaviour returns to normal.

However, in some cases, especially where there are clear behavioural components (e.g. sound sensitivity) and pain that exacerbates them, then pain reduction is only part of the management, and behavioural modification with or without behaviour-modifying drugs may be necessary.

In a few cases, the palpable pain is resolved (i.e. there is no longer any pain felt on examination) and the behaviour is improved, but it remains erratic. The question here is whether this is remaining, probably neuropathic, and significant pain, or whether the patient is now sensitized to a pain stimulus that would previously have received little attention?

Table 3.5. Important resources in cats and dogs and suggestions as to how these can be modified and improved.

Resources: Cats	Effects of treatment intervention/condition	Suggestions of how to replace the resource/deal with the deficiency
Height and hiding	Cannot access high areas or hideouts – increase in stress	Use steps, ramps or strategic use of furniture to allow access to preferred areas Provide low-level hides in the form of boxes and covered tables as an alternative
Food	Restriction because of weight gain Reduction in appetite because of pain	Food toys, scatter feed, increase enrichments Increase food palatability; ensure access is easy and close enough to sleeping and hiding areas
Water	Reduction in access because of pain and debility	Increase the number of water stations and ensure they are close to the cat's preferred areas Ensure these are separate from food; use a wide and shallow dish
Scratching posts	Reduction in access because of debility Change of preference to horizontal	Change position Provide horizontal scratch pads Stop punishment of scratching
Grooming	Reduced grooming because of pain and physical ability to reach Over-grooming because of the stress response	Use gentle groomers to help improve coat quality and comfort Reduce pain and anxiety to reduce over-grooming
Social interactions	Reduced because cats withdraw when painful Change in relationships with other cats	Ensure plenty of hiding areas with accessible height in family areas Use gentle affection (if previously desired), such as stroking Increase the quality of core territory and ensure sufficient resources for all
Play	Reduced or stopped	Change the style of play so that the cat can play without having to run or jump
Toileting	Toileting outside the box because the box is too far away or too high or too awkward Toileting outside the box because squatting or covering hurts (usually indicated by toileting in multiple random areas on different substrates)	Provide a box closer to the new preferred area Use a seed tray, or cut out the side of the box, or provide a step or ramp to the box Further analgesic measures to reduce pain
Access outside	Reduced if the cat feels vulnerable Reduced if cat flap too high, heavy, awkward	Increase analgesia Look at the area immediately outside access points and improve security and ability to gain a vantage point despite the pain Change flap type, introduce a step, improve easy access

Resources: Dogs	Effects of treatment intervention or condition	Suggestions of how to replace the resource/deal with the deficiency
Food	Restriction (fat contributes directly to pain and inflammation) but stress increases the desire to eat	Food games, slow feeders, and random delivery (if not stressful for the individual) Low-calorie treats such as carrots, and satiety and metabolic diets

Continued

Table 3.5. Continued

Resources: Dogs	Effects of treatment intervention or condition	Suggestions of how to replace the resource/deal with the deficiency
Play	Reduce play and removal of a favourite type of play in order to: limit unsupported spinal flexion and extension (e.g. running, jumping, twisting in suspected spinal disease) Limit repeated concussion of joints in joint disease	Change the type of play; roll instead of throwing the ball Have the dog carry the ball Hide-and-seek with food and favourite toy Increase interactions with other dogs if appropriate Increase interest by changing routes and walking areas
Travel in car	Restriction because the dog should not be jumping in and out Anxiety because of movement of car associated with pain	Support climbing in and out of the car (e.g. ramps, boxes, steps or pillows) Use of hammocks or harnesses for support Confine in smaller spaces or deep, supportive beds
Sleep	Unable to sleep because of pain or heat (stress)	Look for qualities in a bed that match what the dog has demonstrated it needs (e.g. support, warmth, coolness) — use of cool pads or heat-reflecting beds, and support beds/bolsters and pillows
Exercise	Restriction of exercise Change of substrate to reduce concussion on joints	Vary the walks to avoid repetition Drive the dog to the park to interact with other dogs where appropriate or use a buggy Support climbing in and out of the car (e.g. ramps, boxes, steps or pillows)
Social interactions	May be reduced if the dog is not allowed on the furniture or upstairs May be reduced because of the restriction of play with other dogs May have trouble coping with floors in the house and spend more time away from the owner or seek cool areas	Support dog going up- and downstairs where necessary Use of box or ramps to access furniture Increase grooming if enjoyed Increase mentally stimulating games with the owner Visit friends, other dogs or places where the dog will receive attention Use of boots, plastic paw covers or strategic use on non-slip rugs Cool pads, heat-reflecting beds and cooling fans
Grooming	Reduced because of pain	Change the grooming device Change associations with grooming Improve analgesia

It is impossible to tell, therefore, if two or three different treatments for neuropathic pain have been tried and made no difference, whether a trial of psychiatric medications may be helpful, if rarely definitive.

In the world of pain, anxiety and stress, the veterinary surgeon must learn to embrace a certain amount of mystery even while endeavouring to take a systematic and scientific approach to each patient's care.

References

al'Absi, M. and Flaten, M.A. (2016) *The Neuroscience of Pain, Stress and Emotion: Psychological and Clinical Implications*. Elsevier, UK.

Baliki, M.N., Geha, P.Y., Apkarian, A.V. and Chialvo, D.R. (2008) Beyond feeling: chronic pain hurts the brain, disrupting the default-mode network dynamics. *Journal of Neuroscience* 28(6), 1398–1403. DOI: 10.1523/JNEUROSCI.4123-07.2008.

Baxter, G.D. and McDonough, S.M. (2016) Laser acupuncture. In: Filshie, J., White, A. and Cummings, M. (eds) *Medical Acupuncture: A Western, Scientific Approach*. Elsevier, UK, pp. 269–277.

Broyd, S.J., Demanuele, C., Debener, S., Helps, S.K., James, C.J. *et al.* (2009) Default-mode brain dysfunction in mental disorders: a systematic review. *Neuroscience & Biobehavioral Reviews* 33(3), 279–296. DOI: 10.1016/j.neubiorev.2008.09.002.

Bushnell, M.C., Čeko, M. and Low, L.A. (2013) Cognitive and emotional control of pain and its disruption in chronic pain. *Nature Reviews Neuroscience* 14(7), 502–511. DOI: 10.1038/nrn3516.

Cummings, M. (2016) Western medical acupuncture – the approach to treatment. In: Filshie, J., White, A. and Cummings, M. (eds) *Medical Acupuncture: A Western, Scientific Approach*. Elsevier, UK, pp. 102–107.

Fomberstein, K., Qadri, S. and Ramani, R. (2013) Functional MRI and pain. *Current Opinion in Anaesthesiology* 26(5), 588–593. DOI: 10.1097/01.aco.0000433060.59939.fe.

Grotenhermen, F. (2003) Pharmacokinetics and pharmacodynamics of cannabinoids. *Clinical Pharmacokinetics* 42(4), 327–360. DOI: 10.2165/00003088-200342040-00003.

Iwata, K., Fukuoka, T., Kondo, E., Tsuboi, Y., Tashiro, A. *et al.* (2002) Plastic changes in nociceptive transmission of the rat spinal cord with advancing age. *Journal of Neurophysiology* 87(2), 1086–1093. DOI: 10.1152/jn.00243.2001.

Lundeberg, T. and Lund, I. (2016) Peripheral components of acupuncture stimulation – their contribution to the specific clinical effects of acupuncture. In: Filshie, J., White, A. and Cummings, M. (eds) *Medical Acupuncture: A Western, Scientific Approach*. Elsevier, UK, pp. 22–58.

Murison, R. (2016) The neurobiology of stress. In: al'Absi, M. and Flaten, M.A. (eds) *The Neuroscience of Pain, Stress and Emotion: Psychological and Clinical Implications*, Kindle Edition. Elsevier, UK, pp. 33–44.

Odendaal, J.S. (2000) Animal-assisted therapy – magic or medicine? *Journal of Psychosomatic Research* 49(4), 275–280. DOI: 10.1016/S0022-3999(00)00183-5.

Re, G., Barbero, R., Miolo, A. and Di Marzo, V. (2007) Palmitoylethanolamide, endocannabinoids and related cannabimimetic compounds in protection against tissue inflammation and pain: potential use in companion animals. *The Veterinary Journal* 173(1), 21–30. DOI: 10.1016/j.tvjl.2005.10.003.

Wieser, M.J. and Pauli, P. (2016) The neuroscience of pain and emotion. In: al'Absi, M. and Flaten, M.A. (eds) *The Neuroscience of Pain, Stress and Emotion: Psychological and Clinical Implications,* Kindle Edition. Elsevier, UK, pp. 3–27.

4 Normal Behaviour – Cats

Katherine Houpt*

Cornell University, Ithaca, New York, USA

4.1 The Social Life of Cats

Cats are a solitary species that can adapt socially to live in large groups in places where there is a large, reliable food source. Examples are cats in fishing ports or, on a smaller scale, on farms where abundant rodents are supplemented with milk provided by the farmer. Most of the cats in these groups are related and will reject a newcomer. Females remain near their mothers, but males disperse. Tomcats have an extensive home range, which may encompass the home ranges of several females. Tomcats will mate with those females and attempt to drive away any other males. Cats within a group show affiliative behaviour especially rubbing against one another or entwining tails (Bradshaw, 1992).

When two cats approach each other aggressively, they walk on tiptoe, slowly lashing their tails about the hocks and turning their heads from side to side while making direct eye contact. This threat may intimidate a subordinate cat who will retreat. Evenly matched rivals will continue to approach one another. They will walk slightly past one another before one cat will spring, trying for a grip on the nape of the opponent's neck. The attacked cat throws itself on its back, thus protecting the nape. The two adversaries will both lie on the ground, abdomen to abdomen, while they claw, vocalize and bite at each other. After a few moments, one cat, usually the original attacker, will jump free. The other cat may adopt a defensive posture, attack or run away. The victor usually pursues the vanquished. Cats that are aggressive towards other cats are not necessarily aggressive towards people, and vice versa (Houpt, 2018).

In a home or on a farm, cats will form dominance hierarchies, but marked aggression may persist in this solitary species. Ten per cent of the cats are still aggressive a year after introduction. When feral cats, which voluntarily determine the group composition, are studied, a hierarchy emerges that varies with body size in females and age in males. Larger, older cats and male cats tend to be dominant over smaller younger female cats. Cats may divide up a house to coexist with minimal interactions. Room-mates may find that the two cats belonging to one person will group against the single cat belonging to the other.

Cats roll on their backs, but sex differences appear in this behaviour. Most female rolling occurs during oestrus and is directed toward males, whereas most rolling exhibited by young males is towards adult males and is, presumably, a sign of submission.

4.2 Territorial Behaviour

Males maintain non-overlapping territories in the non-breeding season but overlap considerably in the breeding season. Therefore, in both free-ranging and pet cats, intra-species aggression among intact male cats is a prevalent problem. Many tomcats are presented repeatedly for treatment of bite wounds and abscesses resulting from fighting behaviour. Castration is approximately 90% effective in eliminating roaming and fighting in adult male cats.

In highly concentrated populations in which cats compete for food, males are dominant over females. Cats can form harmonious social groups, but adding a new cat leads to fighting in 50% of households, and there is a higher risk of fighting if the cats are allowed access to the outdoors.

4.3 Predatory Behaviour

When hunting, the cat carries its body as close as possible to the ground (see Fig. 4.1). It moves toward its prey slowly, taking advantage of any

*kah3@cornell.edu

DOI: 10.1079/9781786394552.0004

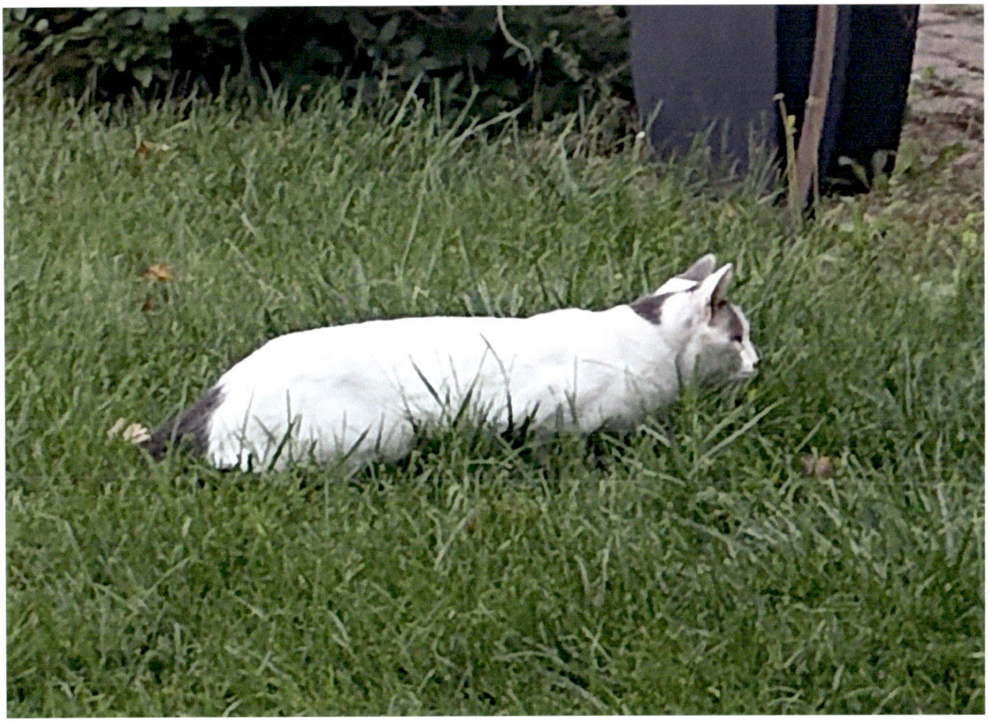

Fig. 4.1. Hunting cat. Note the ears held upwards and forward, and low body posture. (Photo courtesy of Dr Sagi Denenberg.)

natural cover. The closer the cat gets to its prey, the more slowly it advances. Almost inevitably, the cat will pause before leaping to attack; this results in many birds flying away and accounts for why cats are more successful at capturing mammals than birds. When attacking a large animal, cats try to make a nape bite to sever the spinal cord.

Predatory aggression is innate but has some learned characteristics. Kittens learn to direct various innate predatory motor patterns to the prey. One behaviour that owners abhor is playing with the dying prey they have caught. If the cat is not hungry and the prey is easily caught, they do play with it a lot, but if the prey is large and difficult to hunt, the hungry cat is more likely to eat it than to play with it.

The number of prey taken by owned cats is controversial because they are a threat to birds and endangered species. Only 20% bring prey back to their homes; they either consume or abandon it — the use of video cameras worn by the cat made possible accurate estimates of the rate of predation. House cats catch prey every other day. The species of prey will vary with the environment from amphibians in the south-eastern USA to rodents in rural England and ground-foraging birds in many areas. Feral cats kill three times more than owned cats resulting in the death of over a billion birds and seven billion mammals in the USA alone each year (Loss *et al.*, 2013). The best solution to feline predation is an outdoor containment system for cats that allows the cat to run, climb, eat grass, eliminate where it wishes, but protects the cat from dogs and cars and protects the local fauna from the cat.

4.4 Activity Patterns

4.4.1 General activity

Cats vary individually in the amount of time they spend active from 2% to 20% of 24 hours (Andrews *et al.*, 2015). Most cats show short bursts of activity (one to two hours of activity distributed throughout the day) and are more active during the day than at night. Disruption of schedule can result

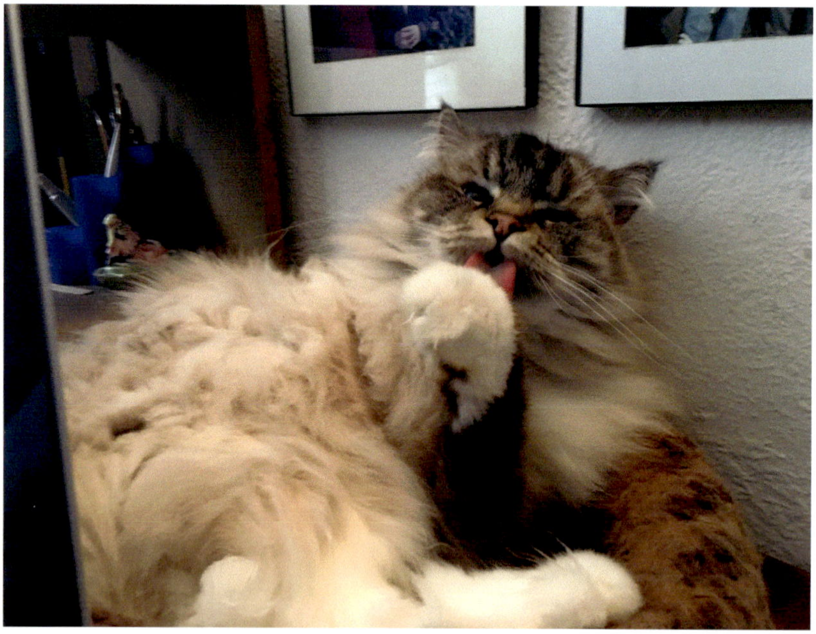

Fig. 4.2. Cat grooming. Cats must use saliva spread on a paw to reach places they cannot lick directly. (Photo courtesy of Charles Houpt.)

in sickness behaviour in cats, so consistency in the environment of cats is essential.

Grooming accounted for 4% of the overall time budget or 8% of the non-sleeping time. Cats are most apt to groom after they rest. Most grooming is with the tongue, but they also scratch with their hind limbs. Cats groom from head to tail, not in the opposite direction. Areas that they cannot reach directly with their tongues are groomed with a paw that has been coated with saliva (see Fig. 4.2). Cats cool themselves by licking their sides, but rather than lick up the saliva as they do in grooming they leave the saliva to evaporate from their coat, thus cooling them.

4.4.2 Sleep

Caged laboratory cats spend ten hours daily sleeping. Free-ranging cats may spend similar time sleeping but have not been systemically observed. Slow-wave sleep occupies 39% of the day, and REM sleep 8%. During REM sleep, the nictitating membrane covers the eye. There are two major sleep epochs at night. Drowsiness varies with the feeding schedule. Cats fed three times a day drowse more than those fed once daily, and fasted cats drowse even less. Older cats (>10 years of age) sleep more but dream less.

4.4.3 Elimination

Cats eliminate three to five times a day. They spend 12 seconds digging before elimination, sniff the litter for 18 seconds and cover for 12 seconds (Sung and Crowell-Davis, 2006). All that time spent sniffing is another indication of how important olfaction is to cats and why litter hygiene is important.

4.5 Communication and Sensory Abilities

4.5.1 Vocal

Feline domestication has resulted in more vocal cats in comparison to the wild ancestor of cats, the Libyan desert cat (*Felis sylvestris lybica*). We have selected cats to communicate with us in 'pleasant' voices in contrast to that of the desert cat. Many feline vocalizations exist; the most common are the meow, oestrous cry, caterwaul, growl, hiss, shriek and purr.

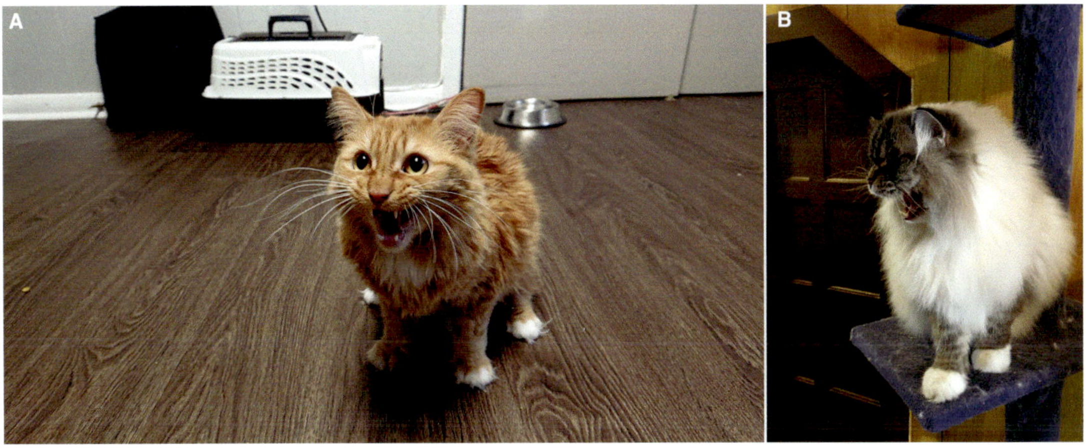

Fig. 4.3. Hissing. Note the ears to the side and large pupils. (Photos courtesy of Dr Sagi Denenberg (A) and Charles Houpt (B).)

We can encourage meowing on the part of a cat by answering it. Cats are the only domestic species to purr. Purring is produced by a rapid contraction of the muscles of the larynx. It is produced during both inspiration and expiration. Purring occurs when the cat appears to be happy, but also occurs in the dying cat, perhaps as a response to endogenous or therapeutic opiates.

Agonistic calls are longer in duration and lower in frequency than affiliative calls. People, even non-cat owners, can distinguish positive and negative affect in feline vocalizations. The caterwaul is given by cats in conflict. Cat hiss when they are frightened, and this can escalate to spitting in the highly aroused cat (see Fig. 4.3A and B). Cats sometimes chatter when they see prey out of a window. It must be a response to frustration because if a cat chattered before it pounced it would not be very successful.

4.5.2 Hearing

The absolute upper limit of hearing in cats is 60–65 kHz. This means that cats can hear high-frequency sounds that humans cannot. Presumably, this ability evolved so that cats can hear the high-frequency sounds made by rodents, their primary prey. Humans can hear 8.5 octaves; cats can hear 10 octaves. The sound is perceived within the ear, but the outside of the ear is also important. Without the external ear (the pinnae), a sound must be louder for the cat to perceive it.

Cats are not as good as humans at localizing sound. They can discriminate between sounds 5° apart, whereas humans can discriminate sounds 0.5° apart. Cats recognize their owners' voices in that they discriminate between strangers' voices and their owners.

4.5.3 Olfaction

The nose of the cat contains twice as many olfactory receptors as the human nose despite the size difference between an adult human and a cat. It is not surprising that olfaction seems to play an essential part in feline communication. Kittens use the sense of smell to find the nipple or the nest.

Cats spend a significant amount of time sniffing and will sniff another cat or dog or human as if identifying the individual by smell rather than by sight (See Fig. 4.4). Cats have many glands that could impart scents. Sebaceous glands are located on the head, between the digits, and in the perianal area. Temporal glands are located on each side of the forehead. The submental gland exists under the chin. The circumoral glands exist at the corners of a cat's lips. Some or all these glands may secrete odours deposited when the cat rubs an object, another cat or a person. Most important may be the anal glands, which contain short-chain fatty acids, because cats can distinguish anal sac secretion of one cat from another (Miyazaki *et al.*, 2018). When cats sniff one another, they often sniff the perianal area.

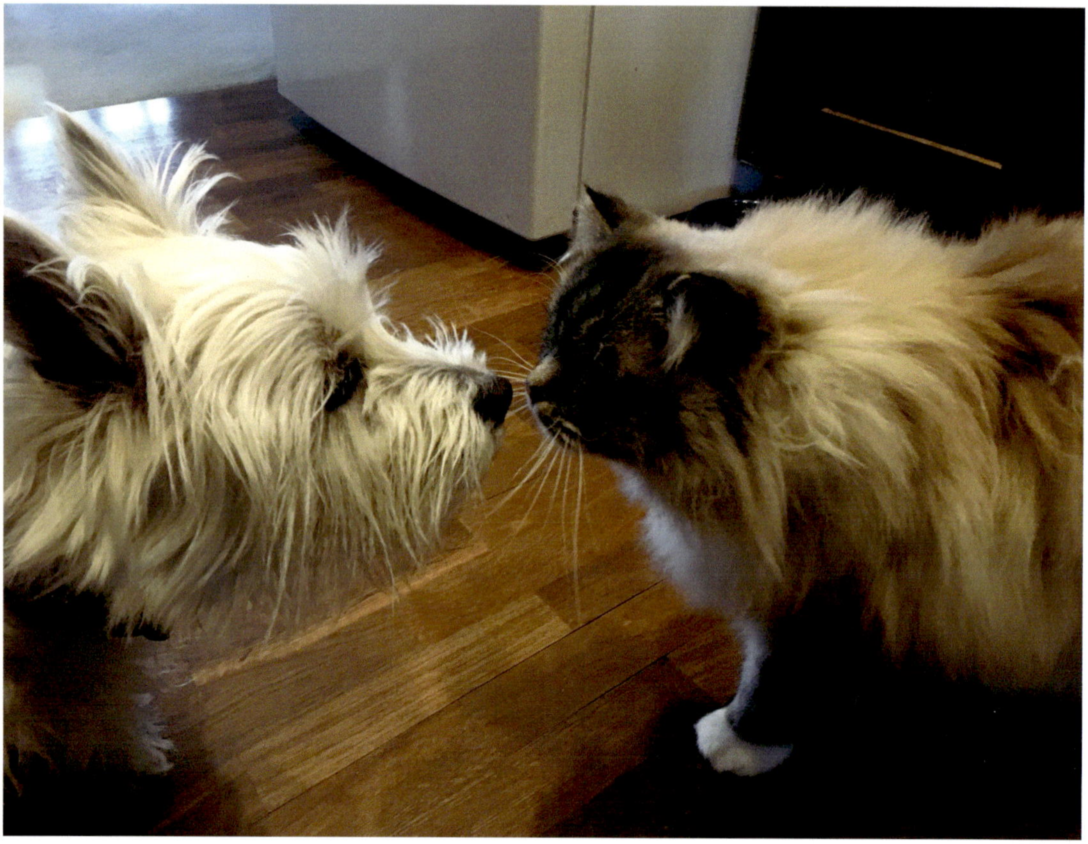

Fig. 4.4. Olfactory investigation. Note that the ears of the cat are forward. (Photo courtesy of Charles Houpt.)

If the cat smells something interesting with its nose, where the main olfactory receptors are, it may investigate more closely by touching the smelly substance with the tip of its tongue. Doing so, the cat transfers the substance to the opening of the vomeronasal organ in the roof of its mouth, just behind the upper incisors. This process allows the cat to perceive something that is non-volatile, which would not be recognized by the main olfactory system. The cat usually remains very still for a few seconds with a fixed expression during this process. This unique expression is called gape. In the vomeronasal organ are nerve endings that connect directly to the parts of the brain involved in sexual or social behaviours.

4.5.3.1 Catnip

Nepetalactone, a volatile terpenoid found in the Nepeta cataria (catnip), attracts cats and elicits behaviour similar to oestrus. Cats roll in catnip and rub. The response to catnip depends on the main olfactory system, not on the vomeronasal organ. Catnip can be used to attract cats to a scratching post, for instance, and is added to many cat toys.

4.5.4 Vision

Cats have remarkable, vertical pupils, which can increase to three times the size of human pupils in low light. They also have more rods, which are more sensitive to light, than cones, which are sensitive to colour. Cats also have a light-reflecting tapetum. These physical differences enable the cats to see up to five times better in low-light conditions than humans. However, their resolution is one tenth that of humans.

Cats have colour vision, but it is limited because they have only two visual pigments, in contrast to the human's three. They are better at the violet and blue end of the spectrum, which may explain why the orange cat sleeps on the pink blanket; it is not a clash of colour, but rather two shades of yellow (Ringo *et al.*, 1977).

Cats can see images on television and prefer to watch prey animals such as birds and mice moving or even moving balls on the screen. Although TV can be used to amuse or enrich a cat, cats in a shelter look at the screen only 6% of the time (Ellis and Wells, 2008). Free-ranging cats were proved far-sighted, whereas caged cats are near-sighted.

As a consequence of the genes for coat colour, Siamese cats have an abnormality in which some of the fibres from the retina pass to the contralateral rather than the ipsilateral side of the lateral geniculate. The strabismus of Siamese cats develops a few weeks after the eyes open and may be an adaptation to compensate for the abnormal vision.

4.5.5 Posture

The ears are probably the best indication of a cat's emotions. The ears are held upwards with the opening pointing forward when the cat is interested (Fig. 4.5) and are pressed more and more tightly to the head as the cat becomes more frightened (Fig. 4.6). In contrast, the aggressive, but not frightened, cat turns its ears backwards so the opening points back.

The next best indication is the tail. If the tail is held straight up, the cat is interested. If it is held up and piloerected, the cat is frightened but aggressive. The piloerection is caused by adrenaline release. The pupils might dilate, also due to adrenaline, at the same time. When hunting, the tail is held low and the tip twitches. The faster the cat moves, the lower the general posture, including the tail.

A cat carries its tail high when greeting, investigating or when frustrated. When walking or trotting, the tail is held out at a 40° angle to the back, but as the cat's pace increases, the tail is held lower. A relaxed cat usually stands with tail hanging, but the cat's ears are generally forward. When the cat's attention is attracted, the tail is raised, and both ears are pointed forward and held erect. When the tail is held upright and the entire tail 'vibrates' from the base to the tip, this is the posture of a cat marking vertical surfaces with urine (see Section 14.2.2 – Marking behaviour).

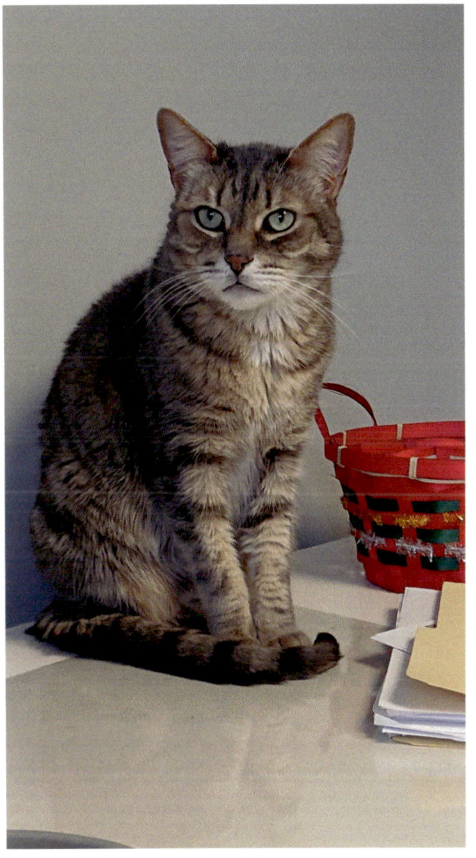

Fig. 4.5. Calm and curious. Note the ears directed forwards and narrow pupils, but the tail is curled tightly around the body, indicating some anxiety. (Photo courtesy of Dr Sagi Denenberg.)

4.5.5.1 Inter-species communication

Cats can respond to their owner's facial expression. The cats move their ears forward and relax when they see the owner smile, but they don't respond to verbal expression of emotion (Galvan and Vonk, 2016).

4.5.6 Tactile

Cats use their sense of touch when they rub on their associates, their owners or objects in their environment. They use their vibrissae (whiskers) not only to judge the width of openings but also to orientate their killing bite when hunting.

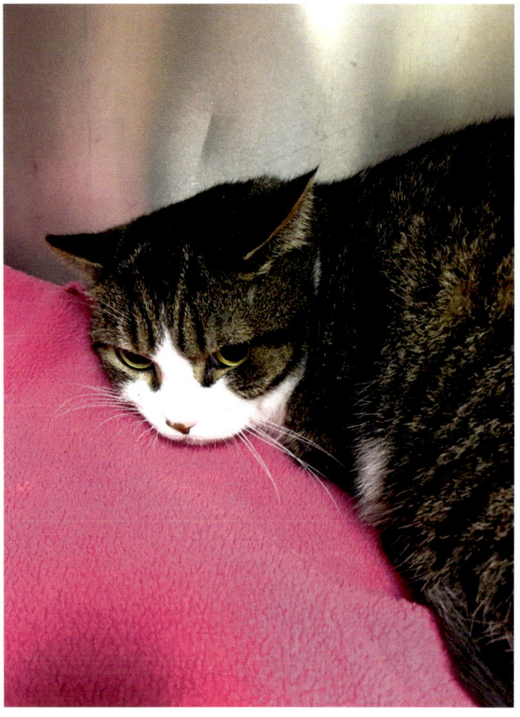

Fig. 4.6. A very frightened cat. Note the ears held down and to the side and the very large pupils. (Photo courtesy of Dr Katherine Anderson.)

Owners stimulate their cats by petting them, but not all petting is the same. Cats prefer to be petted by familiar rather than non-familiar people, and they much prefer to be patted on the head and neck rather than the back and the base of the tail (Ellis *et al.*, 2015). One can tell which areas of the cat are most sensitive by observing the representation of the cat's body in the brain. The head, especially the nose and mouth, and the paws are very well represented whereas the back and hind limbs are not.

4.6 Sexual and Maternal Behaviour

4.6.1 Free-ranging cats

In a feral situation, one oestrous female will be surrounded by a group of males. An oestrous female may show a darting behaviour in the presence of several tomcats. It will repeatedly run a short distance from the toms, and this may be the means of assessing the relative strength of the males as they chase the queen and try to displace one another.

Tomcats will knock one another off an oestrous queen or mount the tom that is mounting the female, but little overt aggression takes place during courting. A male dominance hierarchy, based on size and age, gives the dominant tom priority of access to females. Dominant males tend to be closer to oestrous females than are subordinate males, but they do not mount more frequently. Approximately 15 copulations will occur in 24 hours. Groups of cats living on farms seem to have only one sexually active tom. Although pair-bonding does not happen in the domestic cat, short-term consort behaviour usually occurs. A male and female may remain together for several hours or days, mating many times. Juvenile males tend to move away from their birth area before their third year.

4.6.2 Oestrous cycle

The queen is seasonally polyoestrous. If not bred, the cat will cycle every three weeks for several months. Actual oestrus lasts four days if the cat is bred, but nine to ten days without copulation.

The queen is an induced ovulator. Thus, conception may be accomplished whenever the female shows receptivity. This is one reason for the plethora of kittens. Females will usually reach puberty at six to ten months

There appears to be avoidance of incestuous mating in that oestrous females will travel farther from home if the closest male is related.

4.6.3 Courtship behaviour

An oestrous female will call and purr. It will be restless and show increased general motor activity. If the queen is an indoor cat, she may run from one room to the next, stopping to call at each door or window. It may be very affectionate towards the owners. Urination occurs frequently, and the queen may spray. It rubs its head and flanks on furniture; glands in these areas may produce pheromones that contain information announcing the presence of an oestrous female. The queen will crouch, and elevate the hindquarters region, thus arching her back, and treads with the rear paws. It will also tread with the forepaws, extending and retracting the claws. The queen rolls, squirms and stretches, whether or not a tomcat is present. Owners should be aware of the stages of oestrus because, although a queen in proestrus will roll and solicit the tom's attention, it will act aggressively if the male mounts. When in oestrus, queens are fully receptive, crouching in lumbar lordosis with the head held on the ground between the forelegs, tail deviated to one side, and will allow the male to mount.

4.7 Maternal Behaviour

4.7.1 Parturition

Gestation is 63–66 days in cats. Births have a seasonal distribution, with the highest number of litters being born in the summer and the least in autumn and early winter. Most cats will choose a cave-like place, such as a closet or a linen cabinet. The queen is attracted to the smell of the amniotic fluid at the birth site, so moving the kittens to a more suitable location will not entice it from a chosen spot. Extensive licking characterizes parturition in cats. The queen licks its abdomen and genital areas, the foetal fluids from itself and the area, and the kittens. The queen is responding to the fluids, rather than to the kittens, at this time. The queen seems unaware of the kittens despite bouts of licking them; it might step on them when pacing and ignores their cries.

The queen is very restless and will lie down, sit up, lick the vulva, squat, exhibit lordosis, circle, walk, roll and lie down. No consistent pattern emerges, and the behaviour of the queen varies with the endogenous stimuli (from the uterus) and exogenous stimuli (from the birth fluids and kittens). The bursts of activity are interspersed with periods of rest. The uterine contractions of labour can be distinguished from foetal movements because the raised rear legs of the queen usually flex when she is in labour.

Most cats prefer solitude, although some highly socialized ones seem to be content only when the owner is present. Cats, with the exception of Siamese, are usually quiet during parturition. The queen will eat the placenta and part of the cord with the same tilt of the head and pronounced chewing motions shown when consuming prey. In the process of eating the placenta, the queen stretches the umbilical cord, so that little bleeding occurs when the cord is severed. Eating the placenta rarely extends to cannibalism.

The interval between kitten births can range from minutes to an hour, even in normal births. Following the birth of the last kitten, the queen directs its attention to the kittens. The queen lies down with an encircling motion, positioning the legs in such a way as to form a U around the kittens. For the next 12–24 hours, the queen rarely leaves the kittens and then only for brief intervals to eat, drink and eliminate. Each time it returns, the queen arouses the kittens by licking them and then encircling and nursing them. Queens emit a specific call (chirp) when they are approaching the nest. The kittens will respond more to the queen's chirps than to those of another cat.

4.7.2 Acceptance of kittens

Cats will accept alien kittens that are not much older than their own at the time of parturition. Maternal behaviour persists much longer in cats than in ungulates, so a queen whose kittens were removed at birth will accept one kitten weeks later and encircle it. Three kittens will be avoided or attacked under the same circumstances. In general, species that produce litters are more willing to accept foster young than are those that produce a singleton or twins, probably because the mothers of litters do not discriminate between individual offspring.

4.7.3 Weaning-nutritional independence

The queen discourages kittens' attempts to suckle from the third week onwards by moving away or by licking the kittens so vigorously that they cannot attach to the nipples. A singleton will be allowed to nurse long after a larger litter would have been weaned

4.8 Development

4.8.1 Neurological development

Kittens show a dominance of flexor tone for the first two weeks of life and then a dominance of extensor tone for the second two weeks. That means that if you pick a kitten up by the scruff of the neck, it will pull its limbs in for the first two weeks and after that push its legs out when picked up. The motor cortex involved in forelimb movement develops during those first two weeks and cortical control of the rear limbs in the second two weeks. This is reflected in the locomotion of kittens. Kittens drag themselves by their forelimbs at first, but later the pushing movement of the rear limbs grows stronger. The eyes open at seven days (range 6–10 days), and visual acuity improves 16-fold between two and ten weeks of age. An orienting response to sounds appears in the first week. The ear canals are fully open by four weeks. Between the third and sixth week, cats develop the ability to land on their feet (righting reflex).

The gape response is seen in kittens older than five weeks and is similar in frequency and performance to adult gaping at seven weeks. Kittens can make ultrasonic vocalizations.

After the eyes have opened, the kittens use visual cues to find their nest; before that, they use olfaction. Very young kittens will become less active and less vocal when placed on a warm rather than cool surface, but the calming effect of thermal stimuli is lost after the first week. Isolation produces most vocalizations (four cries per minute) at three weeks of age; younger and older kittens vocalize less.

4.8.2 Sleep

Sleep in kittens also shows a developmental pattern. Although the percentage of time that kittens are awake remains constant, the percentage of active REM sleep decreases and that of quiet sleep increases. Muscle twitching, which is characteristic of REM sleep, also decreases with age. The sleep cycles are also much shorter than those of the adult cat. Kittens also pass directly from the awake state to REM sleep; adult cats almost always pass through SWS sleep before entering REM sleep. A mature sleep-wake cycle does not appear until three months of age.

4.8.3 Finding the teat

Most kittens are suckling within an hour or two of birth (Hudson *et al.*, 2009). Kittens with anaesthetized tongues can find the nipple but cannot suckle; kittens with anaesthetized lips cannot locate the nipple but can suckle. Kittens who cannot smell cannot find the teat. Newborn kittens with no suckling experience respond to the udder of lactating, but not to the udder of non-lactating, females with search behaviour and attach to nipples within minutes. Even in older kittens, nipple attachment depends on females' reproductive state. The highest attachment is to early-lactating females, followed by pregnant females, and the lowest attachment is to late-lactating females. Kittens can locate their particular, most used, nipple on their mother but not on a female of similar lactational state, even after opening their eyes. Kittens respond from birth with efficient nipple-search behaviour to olfactory cues on the mother's udder. These may be pheromones. Kittens also quickly learn olfactory cues specific to their particular nipples.

Kittens locomote by pulling themselves along with their front limbs while paddling with the weaker rear limbs. As they crawl forward, they turn their heads from side to side. When they encounter the nipple, they pull their heads back and lunge forward with open mouths. Eventually, the nipple is secured in the mouth. The position of the mother facilitates locating the mammary region. The responses of the kittens to the areola and nipple appear to be innate, almost reflex.

Prolonged experience with suckling from an artificial teat (one to three weeks) delays, but does not abolish, the kitten's ability to initiate natural suckling. Milk reinforcement is not necessary for suckling, because intra-gastric fed kittens will initiate suckling on the teats of a non-lactating cat.

4.8.4 Teat order

Within 12 hours of birth, kittens have a teat order determined, which is usually, but not always, followed. There is no relation between kittens' use of particular nipples and their weight gain, milk intake or involvement in contests during suckling, but the kittens do push one another off nipples at least once a day. The kittens ingest 1.4 grams/nursing for the first week and four grams/nursing by four weeks.

Some litters do not form a teat order. After establishing the teat order, a kitten can use the presence of its sibling on either side to help guide it to the proper nipple, though sometimes the kittens obstruct more than facilitate one another's progress. Kittens massage the udder with treading motions of the paws. Treading on soft surfaces persists in the adult cat, presumably as a pleasurable activity or in pleasurable social situations. Solitary cats do not tread.

4.8.5 Homing and retrieval

Even before the opening of their eyes, kittens can return to their nest from several feet away. They use olfactory cues; a washed floor between the kittens and the nest prevents them from finding their way back.

Feline retrieval behaviour is different from the canine form. Queens retrieve their kittens in response to auditory, not visual, signals. The more the kitten vocalizes, the more likely the queen is to retrieve it. When kittens are left alone in the nest, they will call, and the mother responds to the call by returning. Their mother responds to the calls of younger kittens more often; apparently their voices change with age.

The queen usually picks the kitten up by the scruff of the neck, though occasionally it grasps the skin of the back of the head or even the kitten's whole head. Queens can lift and jump several feet carrying large kittens. The peak of kitten carrying occurs when they are three weeks old.

Grooming plays as important a part in feline maternal behaviour. Queens lick their kittens frequently and lick the perineum to stimulate urination and defecation for the first two to three weeks of life. Anyone raising an orphan kitten must do the same using a cotton swab. The queen ingests the kittens' urine and faeces for several weeks post-partum, thereby keeping the nest clean.

4.8.6 Socialization

The sensitive period for socialization begins at two weeks and ends at seven weeks before many kittens have gone to their new homes. A litter of kittens isolated for the first month will be reluctant to approach people even if they are genetically friendly. Handling for 15 minutes per day from two to six weeks will result in friendly kittens.

Handling of kittens during their sensitive period is important. Handling kittens for less than 30 minutes twice a week, from the time the kittens are five weeks until they are eight weeks, does not increase their friendliness. More handling beginning at an earlier age does, especially if the kittens are genetically inclined to be friendly.

4.8.7 Play

Play in kittens is first seen at the beginning of the third week while the queen begins the process of weaning by repulsing the kittens' attempts to nurse. Malnourished kittens play more, especially contact play. Perhaps some of the kittens whose play is too exuberant for their new owners were deprived while suckling. Certainly, this appears to be true of hand-reared kittens.

Play in kittens begins with gentle pawing at one another. As kittens improve in co-ordination, biting, chasing and rolling replace simple pawing. One kitten is usually in the belly-up position (kitten lies on its back with all four limbs held in a semi-vertical position). Social play increases from four to 11 weeks and then declines relatively rapidly). At first, three or more kittens may play together, but by eight weeks, almost all play is between pairs of kittens. A reliable sign of play is the arched back and tail, but a definite play signal has not been defined in cats.

Usually, four play periods occur per day. Almost an hour a day is spent in play at nine weeks of age. Most kitten play bouts begin with a pounce and end with a chase. In between, the kittens frequently face-off, hunching forward with tails arched out and down. They may bat at one another. Kittens also assume a vertical stance in play, rearing back on their rear limbs, sometimes standing up by extending the limbs. Various leaps are also seen. Play bouts may have one chase per minute. Play may occupy 9% of the kitten's total time and 4–9% of its energy expenditure, indicating that play may be important, but it is not calorically costly. Play can be encouraged in adult cats by a pause of five minutes after a two-minute play bout and by changing toys.

Mothers play an active role in the development of the kittens' predatory behaviour. Mothers not only attack and eat prey in front of their kittens but also vocalize to attract the kittens' attention to these activities. These behaviours occur when the kittens are four to eight weeks old. After that, the mother defers to the kittens; it rarely kills and seldom eats the prey. The kittens are more apt to interact with the prey if the mother has been interacting with it than if a littermate has, indicating that the mother has a greater influence. Kittens also learn other tasks better from watching their mother than from watching another cat.

By two months of age, those kittens that will be frightened rather than aggressive towards prey and other cats can be identified; these same kittens are reluctant to explore and to relax with people in a new environment. Some people prefer that their cat does not hunt, and many wish their cats to be less aggressive towards other cats; but almost all owners want their cat to be friendly, even in a novel environment.

Kittens' play does not contain elements of sexual behaviour. However, sex difference appears in play behaviour. Males show more object contact than females; females with male littermates play with objects more than do females with no male littermates. Play may be more important for intra-species socialization in cats than it is in other species because

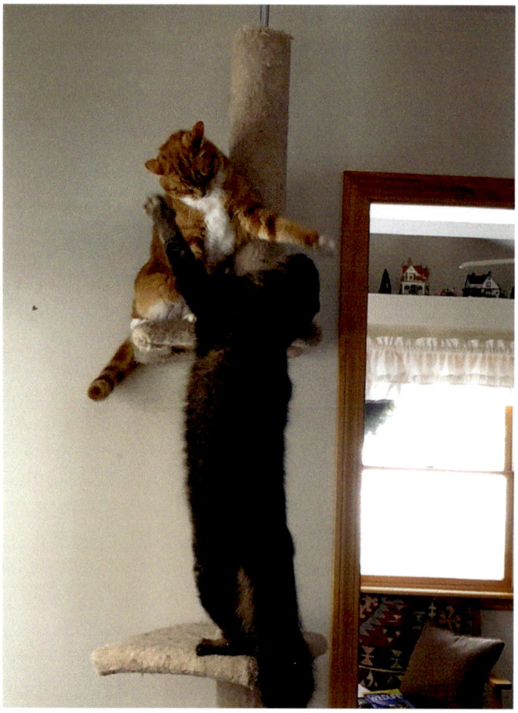

Fig. 4.7. Two young adult cats play-fighting. (Photo courtesy of Dr Pamela Perry.)

the ancestral species are solitary for much of their adult lives.

Solitary play in kittens begins to decline at four months, gradually. Kittens will chase small rolling objects or even a moving string. They particularly like to bat at suspended objects, such as window shade pulls or tassels. Solitary kittens may perform many of the pounces and face-offs of social play with 'imaginary' playmates, a mirror or their own shadow. Solitary play persists in many adult cats. Playfulness is a factor for which breeders should select because it enhances the pleasure a cat gives to its owner as well as to itself (Fig. 4.7). Social play may also occur between species. Cats will often play with familiar dogs. Inter-species play consists mostly of chases by the dog and pounces by the cat.

Several factors may contribute to the decline of play in kittens. Adolescent cats begin to sleep more during the day. Older cats tend to spend more time sitting quietly but alertly. Male kittens show non-play sexual activity by four-and-a-half months and attempt to mount and bite the scruff of females, who will reject these attempts until they reach sexual maturity a few months later.

4.8.8 Feeding

Cats eat many small meals (12) per day when given free access to food. They eat both in the light and in the dark. The caloric intake per meal is approximately equal to that contained in one mouse. A feral cat with excellent hunting skills might easily catch 12 mice (or three rats) per day.

4.8.9 Palatability

Cats are notoriously finicky. This reflects the strong influence of palatability on food intake in cats. Because of the sweet receptor gene deletion, cats do not prefer sucrose as most animals do. Cats do not show a sucrose preference for aqueous solutions of sugar, but they do prefer sucrose in salt solutions or fat. Cats will not eat foods containing medium-chain triglycerides or hydrogenated coconut oil. Cats possess lingual lipase and may break triglycerides down to fatty acids in their mouth and are markedly sensitive to bitter tastes.

Cats prefer fish to meat and novel foods to familiar ones. Maximum intake is achieved when a variety of foods are fed to the cat. If the new food is not more palatable than the familiar one, the cat will, after a few days, begin to choose the familiar food. Observation of cats' behaviour can be an indication of palatability. Cats lick their noses after encountering unpalatable food but groom their face (licked paw over the ear) after eating palatable food.

When presented with a choice between a food frequently made available to them and one that is infrequently offered, cats will choose the latter, even if both foods are dry commercial cat food. Experience may modify the choice of novel food. Farm cats avoid dry food, which is difficult to ingest, whereas pet cats avoid raw beef.

Cats may alter their food choice if preferred meat is present but unavailable (tuna inside a sealed bowl); they will choose the food closest to the sealed bowl. The presence of the 'phantom' food influences their choice (Scarpi, 2011).

Some of the risk factors for obesity in cats are neutering, confinement in an apartment and free-choice feeding of a prescription diet. Neutered males and females have a lower metabolic rate, and if the cat is fed *ad libitum* very palatable food and is not very active, obesity can result. Feeding a limited amount of a high-fibre diet results in a more significant weight loss than an equal-calorie-content low-fibre diet. Owners reported that the cats were more affectionate while their intake was limited (Levine *et al.*, 2016).

4.9 Animality

Seventeen studies of feline temperament revealed that the factors sociable, dominant and curious were most valid. A good pet cat would be sociable and curious, not fearful, and probably not dominant. Neutered female cats with the A form of the oxytocin receptor allele in the single nucleotide polymorphism G738A were more likely to be aggressive (Arahori *et al.*, 2016).

A laboratory test of sociability showed that as early as ten weeks cats differed among themselves in their reactions to unfamiliar people, rats and the aggressive vocalization of adult cats. The cats that demonstrated fearful behaviour in those three situations were classified as defensive and represented 25% of the population. These differences in animality appear to be inherited because a paternal effect has been noted. Of course, both sire and dam contribute genetically to any behaviour, and the sire does not have to nurture influence on the kittens. However, the paternal effect can be found when the kittens of a few sires and many mothers can be differentiated.

Cats that are vocal as kittens are vocal as adults. Very active kittens were less likely to spend time with people when adults.

References

Andrews, C.J., Potter, M.A. and Thomas, D.G. (2015) Quantification of activity in domestic cats (*Felis catus*) by accelerometry. *Applied Animal Behaviour Science* 173, 17–21. DOI: 10.1016/j.applanim.2015.05.006.

Arahori, M., Hori, Y., Saito, A., Chijiiwa, H., Takagi, S. *et al.* (2016) The oxytocin receptor gene (OXTR) polymorphism in cats (*Felis catus*) is associated with “Roughness” assessed by owners. *Journal of Veterinary Behavior* 11, 109–112. DOI: 10.1016/j.jveb.2015.07.039.

Bradshaw, J.W.S. (1992) *The Behaviour of the Domestic Cat*. CAB International, Wallingford, UK.

Ellis, S.L.H. and Wells, D.L. (2008) The influence of visual stimulation on the behaviour of cats housed in a rescue shelter. *Applied Animal Behaviour Science* 113(1-3), 166–174. DOI: 10.1016/j.applanim.2007.11.002.

Ellis, S.L.H., Thompson, H., Guijarro, C. and Zulch, H.E. (2015) The influence of body region, handler familiarity and order of region handled on the domestic cat's response to being stroked. *Applied Animal Behaviour Science* 173, 60–67. DOI: 10.1016/j.applanim.2014.11.002.

Galvan, M. and Vonk, J. (2016) Man's other best friend: domestic cats (*F. silvestris catus*) and their discrimination of human emotion cues. *Animal Cognition* 19(1), 193–205. DOI: 10.1007/s10071-015-0927-4.

Houpt, K.A. (2018) *Domestic Animal Behavior*, 6th ed. Wiley Blackwell, Hoboken, New Jersey.

Hudson, R., Raihani, G., González, D., Bautista, A. and Distel, H. (2009) Nipple preference and contests in suckling kittens of the domestic cat are unrelated to presumed nipple quality. *Developmental Psychobiology* 51(4), 322–332. DOI: 10.1002/dev.20371.

Levine, E.D., Erb, H.N., Schoenherr, B. and Houpt, K.A. (2016) Owner's perception of changes in behaviors associated with dieting in fat cats. *Journal of Veterinary Behavior* 11, 37–41. DOI: 10.1016/j.jveb.2015.11.004.

Loss, S.R., Will, T. and Marra, P.P. (2013) The impact of free-ranging domestic cats on wildlife of the United States. *Nature Communications* 4, 1396.

Miyazaki, T., Nishimura, T., Yamashita, T. and Miyazaki, M. (2018) Olfactory discrimination of anal sac secretions in the domestic cat and the chemical profiles of the volatile compounds. *Journal of Ethology* 36(1), 99–105. DOI: 10.1007/s10164-017-0532-x.

Ringo, J., Wolbarsht, M.L., Wagner, H.G., Crocker, R. and Amthor, F. (1977) Trichromatic vision in the cat. *Science* 198(4318), 753–755. DOI: 10.1126/science.910161.

Scarpi, D. (2011) The impact of phantom decoys on choices in cats. *Animal Cognition* 14(1), 127–136. DOI: 10.1007/s10071-010-0350-9.

Sung, W. and Crowell-Davis, S.L. (2006) Elimination behavior patterns of domestic cats (*Felis catus*) with and without elimination behavior problems. *American Journal of Veterinary Research* 67(9), 1500–1504. DOI: 10.2460/ajvr.67.9.1500.

5 Normal Behaviour – Dogs

KATHERINE HOUPT*

Cornell University, Ithaca, New York, USA

5.1 The Social Life of Dogs

Dogs form groups, but the size of the groups vary considerably. This may be a function of climate, resource availability and acceptance of free-ranging dogs. In the 1980s, people were less likely to restrain their dogs so that even owned dogs formed packs of two to five during the day and then went home to their owners in the evening. Dogs in day care may also form subgroups. A study of suburban dogs showed a core home range of about 1.7 hectares (0.0174 km^2), and the dogs usually ventured only a short distance from their home.

Behavioural thermoregulation occurs so that the dogs were most active early in the morning, avoiding the midday heat. In Baltimore, Maryland, stray dogs were more likely to be alone or in small groups, and the groups were not stable, whereas those in Rome were larger (4–12 dogs per pack) and were stable. They used wooded areas to find resting sites, refuges and dens for puppies but travelled to an open area to eat the meat provided. In the Apennine region of Italy, feral dogs lived in packs of three to fifteen. Their core home range was 12 km^2; their food source was a dump, but they spent the day sleeping elsewhere, presumably to avoid people. They were most active at dawn and dusk. One important characteristic was that new females would be allowed to join a pack, but not new males.

These dogs exhibited affiliative behaviours towards their pack mates such as tail wagging, playing, play invitation, allogrooming and resting in physical contact. The dominant dog had first access to food and an oestrous bitch (Cafazzo *et al.*, 2010). When approaching a dominant dog, the subordinate dog's posture is slightly crouched, the ears are flattened and the tail is down and wagging. Behaviours towards dominant dogs included both submission elicited by aggression and dominance behaviour (avoiding eye contact, lowering the head, lowering the tail between the rear legs, lying down on the back, yelping, fleeing, withdrawing, and interruption of feeding) and deference display during greeting (licking the muzzle of another dog or pushing the muzzle of the other dog with the nose). As noted above, subordinate dogs lick the muzzles of dominant dogs. This behaviour is probably retained from puppyhood when the pups lick their mother's muzzle, and the mother responds by regurgitating food for them.

There are two types of aggression observed in feral dogs – within the pack and between packs. Within the pack, the aggression is usually about access to food or a resting place and is relatively mild. Not everything is agonistic within a pack. They play, wag their tails and lie down together. The aggression between groups is usually at territorial boundaries and probably about access to resources. The most interesting aspect of aggression between packs is that they seem to consider the likelihood of success in a conflict. Smaller packs rarely threaten larger packs and, instead, leave the area (Bonanni *et al.*, 2010). Feral dogs in an Indian city are aggressive eight or nine times daily, usually over food, which they must steal. Both males and females are aggressive, and females are more aggressive, especially when they are raising pups (Pal, 2005).

5.2 Dog–human Interaction

Canine domestication took place tens of thousands of years ago, and over those centuries the two species have evolved a close relationship. Areas of the canine brain, in particular the temporal cortex, have been located that respond to human or dog faces (Cuaya *et al.*, 2016). Dogs associate their owner's voice with their face. When a stranger's

*kah3@cornell.edu

DOI: 10.1079/9781786394552.0005

voice is played while the owner's picture is displayed, the dogs gaze longer, indicating that there is a mismatch. A dog can match a female voice by looking at a woman, but only if the dog lives with more than one person of each sex. Dogs may or may not be able to gauge our moods, but they can be taught to distinguish smiling from blank faces. They must live with owners of both sexes to be able to distinguish expression based on photographs. This indicates that the dogs must learn about humans rather than innately being able to distinguish expressions (Nagasawa *et al.*, 2011).

Dogs will stare at photographs of humans and dogs interacting. They stare longer at humans than at dogs, whereas people stare more at dogs than at people. Both species stare more at images in which the two subjects (human and dog) interact. Dogs will whine or whimper more often if their owners stare at them but are no more likely to approach or paw at them. They will approach their owner or even strangers when they cry. When threateningly approached by a stranger, dogs will avoid or threaten, but not if the stranger approaches playfully. The owner is approached playfully even when threatening.

Oxytocin is a neurohormone involved in mother and offspring bonding as well as the physiological effects of milk letdown and uterine contraction. When a dog gazes into the eyes of its owner, the human releases oxytocin and is more affiliative to the dog, which in turn releases oxytocin. Both dog and owner release oxytocin in a positive feedback loop (Nagasawa *et al.*, 2015). Oxytocin does not always increase affiliative behaviour. When owners threateningly approached their dogs, the dogs reacted more aggressively after oxytocin treatment (Hernádi *et al.*, 2015).

When faced with a stranger, most dogs will look at the stranger and then at their owners; females do this sooner than males. Molossoid breed dogs (e.g. mastiffs, great dane, and dogue de Bordeaux) look at the stranger longer than shepherds. If the owner moves away from the stranger the dog will take longer to contact the stranger and will spend less time near the stranger; this indicates that the dog is responding to the owner's reaction (Duranton *et al.*, 2016).

Dogs have been trained in the laboratory to bark 33 times for each small food reward. Dogs learn faster when the reward is a simple contact with a passive person than when the reward is stroking or picking up (Feuerbacher and Wynne, 2015). Dogs learn more quickly for food than for petting or praise and prefer petting to verbal praise, but this applies only to the initial sit-stay training.

Anxious dogs solve a simple problem more slowly than normal dogs, indicating the influence of emotion on ability. Learning itself can result in cortisol release; shelter dogs that were clicker-trained to touch a bucket had higher cortisol than those who could not learn the task and who were depressed.

Dogs decide which person will give them food by observing that person's behaviour toward another person. This phenomenon is called 'social eavesdropping'. A dog observed two people, each with a bowl. A third person begged for food from each. One person would say, 'Take it' and share the food, and the other would say 'No' and gesture the person to retreat. The dog would approach first and spend more time with the generous person. Vocal cues were more important than visual ones. Critics have said that the dogs may have been choosing the side on which the people sat rather than their relative generosity. Another example of social eavesdropping occurs when dogs observe a person turning away from their owner rather than assisting when the owner has asked for help in opening a jar; they will not take food from that non-helpful person. The dog will take food from a person who opened the jar or from a neutral person who sat beside the owner but was not asked for help. This indicates that dogs are sensitive to human interactions and, apparently, make judgements as to whether a person can be trusted.

When faced with an insoluable task, agility-trained dogs are most likely to look at their owners and search and rescue dogs the least. Pet dogs were intermediate. Dogs respond to their owners' emotions and respond appropriately to an object the owner appears to like rather than one the owner finds disgusting.

5.3 Activity Patterns

Like most carnivores, dogs rest most of the day. Stray dogs who must forage for food in dustbins must move from one site to another but will rest several times a day. Pet dogs kept indoors show a different pattern. While their owners are gone, they usually rest. The exception is those dogs with anxiety (see Chapter 13) who may be frantically active, pacing and scratching, but even those dogs will usually stop and rest every 20 minutes or so. The pet dog who has been minimally active all day becomes animated as soon as the owner returns and will remain active until the owner goes to bed (Hansen *et al.*, 2007). In other words, the dog has entrained to the owner's schedule. Aggression is more likely to occur in the evening. This may be a result of a change in neurochemical release at night when serotonin declines and melatonin increases, or fatigue-induced irritability because the owner is stimulating the dog to be active longer and later in the day than it would normally be. Changes in sleep patterns are a hallmark of canine cognitive dysfunction (see Chapter 16).

Dogs can sleep flat on their sides or even on their backs, but most dogs eventually curl up, clockwise or counter-clockwise, but they do not remain immobile. They arise every 30 minutes or so, stand up and lie back down, sometimes changing the direction in which they curl. Undisturbed, they will sleep for ten hours.

Dogs probably dream. Their brain waves, while asleep, can be the same pattern as ours when we dream. Some dogs will run or vocalize in their sleep. We can only speculate about their dreams, but some are obviously hunting and others fighting. There is an adage 'Let sleeping dogs lie', and that is good advice because a dog disturbed while resting may bite. We do know that dogs fall asleep more quickly and have more REM sleep if they have had negative experiences, such as being threatened or being left alone, just before they were allowed to sleep (Kis *et al.*, 2017).

5.4 Movements

Dogs can move at three speeds: walk, trot and gallop or run. The trot is a two-beat gait in which the feet at the diagonally opposite ends of the body strike the ground together. Dogs can run or gallop, and in racing greyhounds this is intensified so that the front legs are in full extension forward while the rear legs are in full extension rearward. Additionally, the dog's back is folded and attains maximum overreach, or where the rear feet extend in front of the front feet, and the front feet extend behind the rear feet. When the feet pass each other, the front feet are inside of the rear feet. Greyhounds can attain speeds of 70 km/hr.

Dogs apparently align themselves on a north–south axis when eliminating, especially when defecating. The significance of that is unknown.

5.5 Communication and Sensory Abilities

5.5.1 Vocal

Some dogs are more vocal than others. Northern breed dogs – huskies and malamutes – have a large vocabulary of grunts, moans and yowls as well as howls. Hunting dogs are bred to communicate with the human hunter by howling or barking. Terriers and shelties bark a lot. Most owners can interpret their dog's barks (Pongrácz *et al.*, 2005). There is the territorial invasion bark, which is noisier, meaning it has more frequencies than the demand bark, which means, 'Give me dinner' or 'Let me out'. Howling is a vocalization selected for in some breeds. A bloodhound or a beagle is likely to howl; a poodle is not.

Growling is aggressive and seems to mean 'Stop what you are doing, or more aggression will commence'. Dogs may growl in play with one another or with people, but a growl may indicate that the play is too exciting. Adult people seem to recognize the meaning of different growls (Faragó *et al.*, 2010).

Whining or whimpering is a sound the dog makes when it wants something, usually something social such as the owner's attention.

5.5.2 Hearing

Dogs cannot localize sound as well as a human can, but they can hear higher frequencies, which is the reason that ultrasonic whistles are effective. The absolute upper limit of hearing in dogs is 45 kHz. Dogs are quieter when classical music is played but more reactive when heavy metal is played (Wells *et al.*, 2002). Dogs usually hear our commands but may choose not to obey. They may not understand commands if the pronunciation is too different from the one they originally learned. Dogs are more likely to obey a command if their name is not used.

5.5.3 Olfaction

Dogs are notorious for their excellent sense of smell, which has been estimated to be thousands of times more acute than ours. They can find people buried by an avalanche and distinguish the fingerprints of identical twins. Their acuity is matched by, and is a result of, the large number of olfactory receptors in their noses as well as their unique nasal airflow pattern. Airflow from each nostril is separated so that the dog should be able to locate the source of the odour. In addition, when the dog sniffs, rather than breathing, the airflow is directed to the receptor-rich portion of the nose (Craven *et al.*, 2009). Not all dogs have the same number of receptors and, not surprisingly, brachycephalic dogs, like the pug, have fewer receptors than dolichocephalic dogs such as the hound. When you take a dog for a walk, allow it to sniff the ground and vertical objects, which will be of much more interest than the view.

Although dogs do not appear to recognize themselves in a mirror, they recognize their odour. This was tested by presenting dogs with canisters containing their urine or that of another dog. They spent more time sniffing the other dog's urine (Horowitz, 2017).

When investigating something interesting, such as oestrous urine, a dog thrusts its tongue repeatedly just behind its incisor teeth while holding the mouth slightly open. This behaviour is called tonguing. The dog is using the tongue to move non-volatile material, urine for example, into the opening of the incisive ducts that open into the vomeronasal organ. The vomeronasal organ consists of paired tubes lying between the oral cavity and the nasal cavity. It is lined with neurons that synapse more directly with the parts of the brain involved in sexual and social behaviour than does the main olfactory system (Houpt, 2018).

Scent marking

Scent marking (lifting the leg on a vertical object) can be a clinical problem (see Section 14.2.2 – Marking behaviour) but is a part of normal canine behaviour. Mostly males mark, and it almost always is in an upright posture with the flexed rear leg lifted. Bitches also urine mark, usually while squatting, but still lift their rear leg, but do so for only about half their urinations. Feral males tend to mark during group feeding. Dogs in a shelter mark more the longer they have been there, presumably because the shelter becomes their territory. Small dogs mark more than large dogs and older dogs mark more than younger ones (McGuire, 2016).

Dogs countermark, urinating on top of (overmarking) or urinating at about 60 cm distance from another dog's urine mark (adjacent marking). Dogs that carry their tails high, who presumably are less fearful, are more likely to overmark than dogs with lowered tails (Lisberg and Snowdon, 2009). Dogs may adjacent mark, in response to unfamiliar urine. The location of the marks is important. Adjacent marking is done equally by males and females; overmarking is done exclusively by males.

5.5.4 Vision

In the Snellen system, humans have 20/20 acuity, whereas dogs have 20/85. This means that what a person could see from 85 feet a dog would have to be within 20 feet to see. Brachycephalic dogs have better vision, especially binocular vision, than the dolichocephalic breeds (McGreevy *et al.*, 2004). Dogs have a higher critical flicker fusion (the point at which a flickering light appears to be fused, or a steady light) than humans, which means that dogs can see modern, high-definition television, but in some cases, older images may appear jerky to them.

Dogs can see the view, of course, but their visual acuity and depth perception are worse than ours. They are myopic – nearsighted – but they detect movement well, and they can see better than humans in near darkness because of their tapetum lucidum. In the most carefully conducted studies, dogs appear to see the world not in shades of grey but, rather, in shades of violet, blue and yellow.

Much is made of the olfactory ability of dogs, but that functions only at short range and is dependent on airflow, so dogs, like us, must rely on visual signals to determine the mood of another dog. The best indicators are the ears, tail and general body position. Ears up indicates interest (Fig. 5.1), whereas ears down indicates fear (Fig. 5.2). Tail up is arousal, and the lower the tail the more frightened the dog is (Figs 5.2 and 5.3). In intense fear, the dog will tuck its tail between its legs. A wagging tail is not necessarily a friendly greeting; it indicates that the dog is willing to interact, but the outcome of the interaction may be aggression.

Body tension increases as the dog becomes more fearful or aggressive. On closer examination, its pupils may be dilated and the hair on the back (hackles) may stand up. The latter two changes indicate increased activation of the sympathetic nervous system (noradrenergic activation).

If the dog shows its teeth it is more aggressive. If its mouth is pulled back, exposing the back teeth, the dog is probably afraid. Dogs will lean forward when aggressive and back when frightened. A relaxed dog will have a lolling tongue; a tense dog will have its mouth closed until it is fearful enough or aggressive enough to show its teeth. Anxious dogs lick their lips and yawn. The whites of their

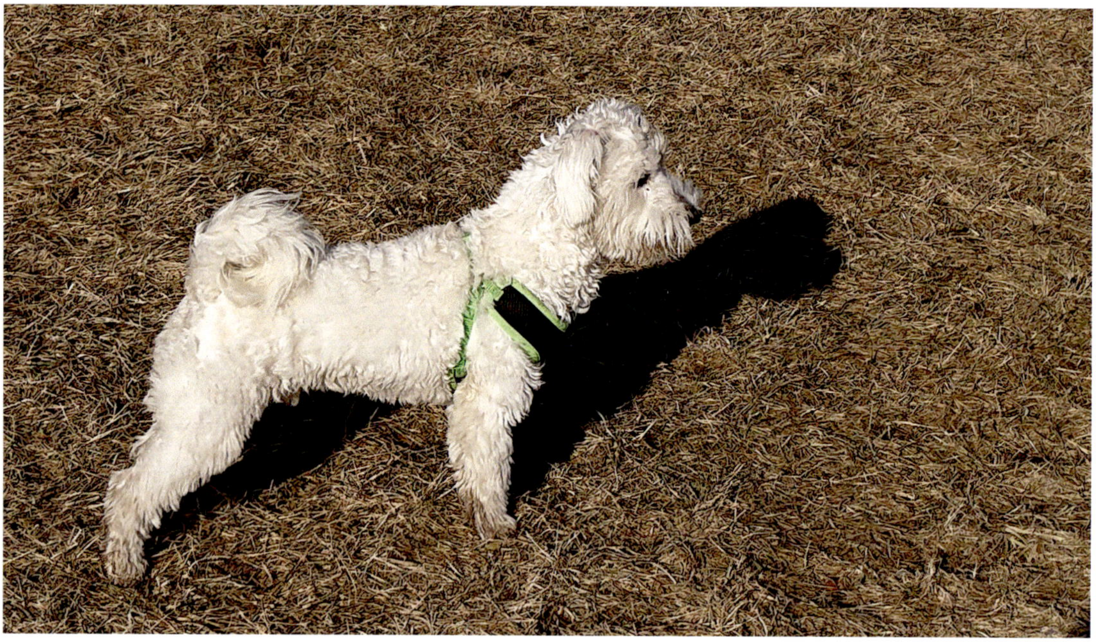

Fig. 5.1. The alert dog. Note that the ears and tail are up. (Photo courtesy of Dr Sagi Denenberg.)

eyes will show because their eyes are open wider due to adrenaline release. Instead of staring straight at another dog (or person), as an aggressive dog would, they gaze out of the corners of their eyes. When very fearful, the dog will crouch down and even lie on its side and raise its rear leg, sometimes urinating. This is termed submissive urination.

Dogs have a signal, the play bow, which indicates an intention to play, in which the rump is in the air and the forelegs on the ground. The dog will give that signal to dogs and people when it wants to play (Fig. 5.4). The most successful method of inducing a dog to play is to lunge or bow toward the dog while whispering or speaking in a high-pitched voice.

We do not think of dogs as having much facial expression. Dogs raise their eyebrows and their lower lip. They can pull the corner of their lips, stretch

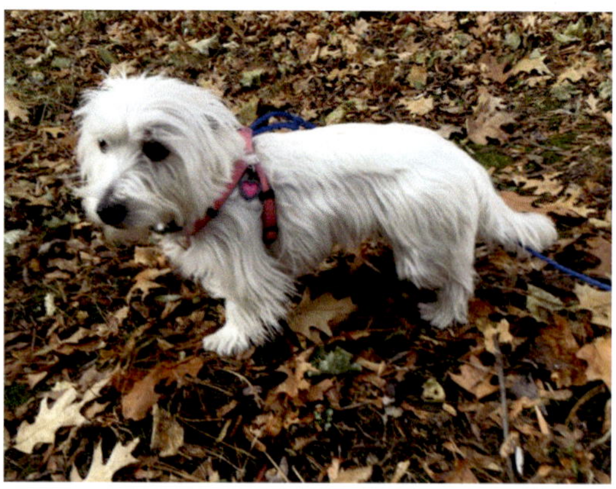

Fig. 5.2. The fearful dog. The ears and tail are down. (Photo courtesy of Charles Houpt.)

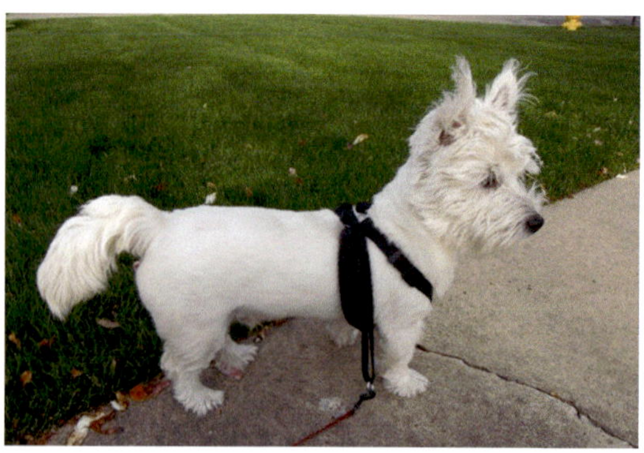

Fig. 5.3. The ambivalent dog. The tail is curved down while the ears are up. (Photo courtesy of Doris Young Saygan.)

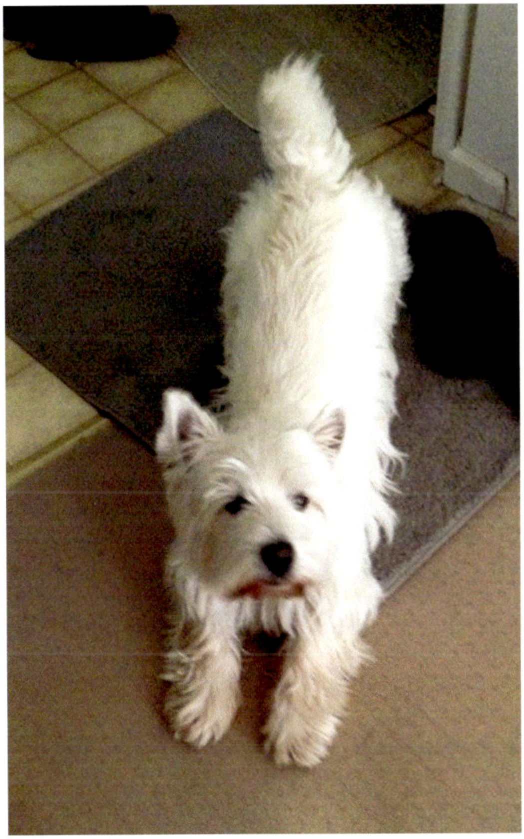

Fig. 5.4. The play bow. The rump is higher than the shoulders. (Photo courtesy of Doris Young Saygan.)

their mouth and wrinkle their noses. Some breeds of dog seem to frown, and all dogs clench their jaws when tense. They can pucker their lips. The most intriguing expression is the raised eyebrow. When only one eyebrow is raised, the dog has a quizzical expression that leads to faster adoption from a shelter (Waller *et al.*, 2013). Observation of both the change in facial expression and the vocalizations gives one a better understanding of the dog's motivation. Horizontal contraction of the lips is associated with a low level of growling and snarling. The vertical contraction of the lip is associated with the baring of teeth, especially in the case of loud growling. Because of the changes in the dog's anatomy brought about by selective breeding (or surgery), some breeds of dog are limited in their signalling ability. Dogs with no tails or very short tails cannot signal fear or aggression as easily. Dependent, floppy ears hardly move, except at the skull, so interest and fear are hard to differentiate. The more fur on the face, the more difficult it is to interpret the dog's facial expressions and hence its emotions.

5.5.5 Scratching

So far, no one has found the significance of scratching after elimination, although it is such an overt behaviour it probably has a function, particularly because it occurs in areas where other dogs have been.

5.6 Sexual and Maternal Behaviours

5.6.1 Sex differences

There are sex differences in many behaviours in addition to sexual behaviour itself. Males are more reactive, more confident and more aggressive. Females are more social than males. Females are easier to house-train, more obedient and affectionate, but less active, as indicated in surveys from several countries, whereas males are more aggressive, more active, more playful and more likely to bark and be destructive.

5.6.2 Mating

Most bitches come into oestrous twice a year. They will go through a proestrus period during which they will bleed from the vulva for a week. During the proestrus period, they are attracted to male dogs but will not allow the male to mount. When they are in oestrus (approximately a week) they will allow the male to mount and, if he is not immediately interested, they will prance in front of him, play bow and even mount him. Male dogs are attracted to oestrous females and can detect them over long distances. The odour, a pheromone or chemical produced by one animal that affects the behaviour of another one, has not been identified. In a stray or feral dog situation, several males will surround the female and vie for her. The male dog mounts the female, inserts the penis while clasping her sides with his forelegs. Dogs have a unique copulatory mechanism called the lock, in which the glans penis swells and the vagina of the bitch constricts so that the male cannot withdraw. The animals are attached for some time, usually about 20 minutes. The dog often steps over the bitch so that the two are facing in opposite directions. The pair is particularly vulnerable at that time.

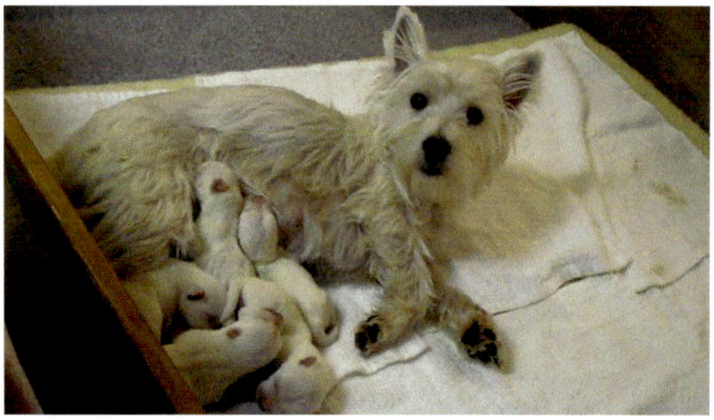

Fig. 5.5. Neonatal puppies. These three-day-old puppies cannot see or hear. They move by pulling with their forelimbs. They spend most of their time sleeping and suckling. They cannot eliminate spontaneously. The dam initiates nursing. (Photo courtesy of Doris Young Saygan.)

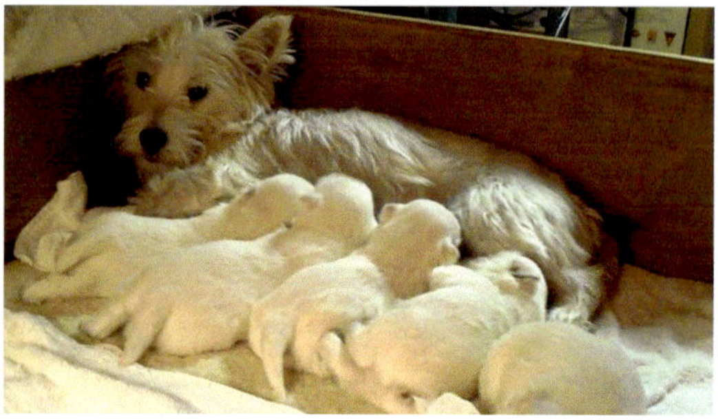

Fig. 5.6. Thirteen-day-old puppies. The puppies have doubled in size and are beginning to see and hear and use both fore and hind limbs to move. They start to initiate nursing. (Photo courtesy of Doris Young Saygan.)

The bitch can be bred several times, and one litter of puppies can contain the offspring of several sires. Bitches have individual preferences for mates. What is most interesting is that the dog a bitch chooses to mate with is not necessarily the one she chooses to spend the most time with when she is not in oestrus (Beach and LeBoeuf, 1967).

5.6.3 Maternal behaviour

After a gestation period of 63 days, a bitch will find a secluded place and deliver the puppies. She spends most of the time between births licking the fluids she has expelled, licking the fetal membranes and licking the puppy. Because dogs usually have more than one puppy, the bitch will ignore a puppy after the initial licking while it is in labour with the next, even walking over it. Once the litter is complete, the bitch will lie on its side so the puppies can suckle (Fig. 5.5). The puppies are attracted to warm hairless places. The bitch may excrete an odour from the skin surrounding the nipples that attracts them. The bitch stays with the puppies almost continuously for the first day and, only later, leaves to eat, drink and eliminate.

After the puppies are born, the dam will continue to lick the puppies and will now concentrate on the anogenital region. Puppies cannot spontaneously urinate and defecate for the first two weeks of life; anorectal licking stimulates these functions. If the puppies wander away from the nest, the bitch will retrieve them, sometimes by carrying them.

Over the next few weeks, the dam's maternal behaviour will weaken. She will nurse the pups less frequently, lick them less and direct more aggression to them if they play too violently with her, or if they persist too long in attempts to suckle. The bitch will leave them for longer and longer periods. The smaller the litter, the longer the maternal care.

Male feral dogs of India do exhibit paternal behaviour in that they will stay near their puppies and protect them from predation (Pal, 2005).

5.7 Development

The puppies' ears open at five days and their eyes open around ten days (Fig. 5.6). They can move about, pulling themselves by the forelegs, but not stand and walk until they are a month old. They spend most of the first few weeks sleeping and eating. The newborn puppy spends 96% of its time sleeping, and this drops to 30% by one month. Most of the sleep is rapid eye movement sleep, the state associated with dreaming in humans.

Social play commences at three weeks of age in feral dogs; at five weeks agonistic play appears, and at six weeks sexual play appears. Males play more than females and initiate play fighting (stalking, chasing and attacking) more often with male littermates. They initiate sexual play (mounting, clasping and pelvic thrusting) with female littermates. Social play diminishes by nine weeks but exploratory behaviour increases (Pal, 2008).

5.7.1 Socialization

There is a sensitive period between seven and 14 weeks when exposure to new sights, sounds, animals or people will have a lasting effect on the

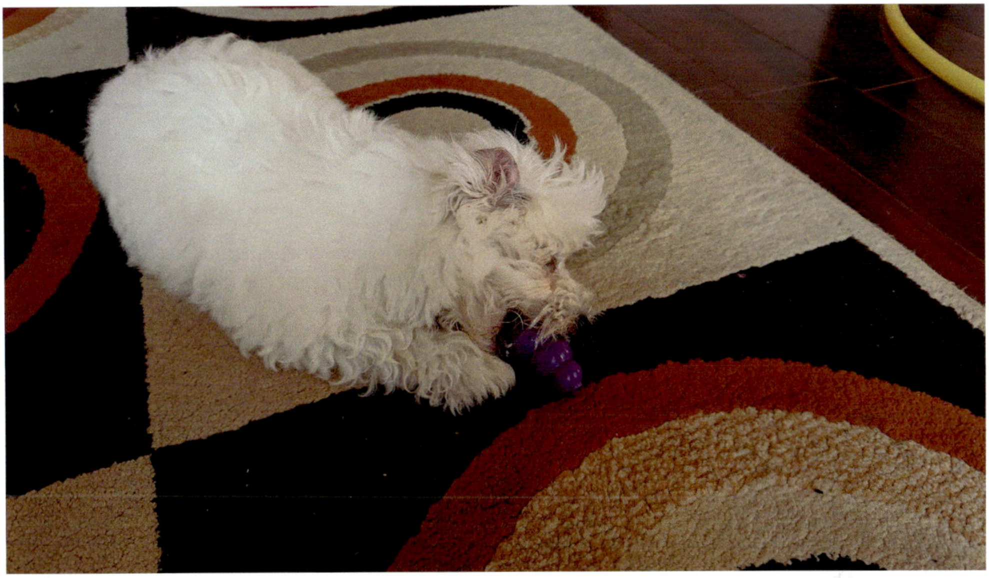

Fig. 5.7. Puppy at nine weeks. Learning to stay alone and become independent is an important skill that most dogs must learn. Using feeding toys and short periods alone helps puppies learn this. (Photo courtesy of Dr Sagi Denenberg.)

puppy's behaviour even when he reaches adulthood (see Figs 5.7 and 5.8). Exposure to people of all races, to friendly dogs, to bicycles and skateboards during this time, when most puppies are happy to see anyone or anything, will minimize the risk of developing problems in the future. Some puppies exhibit aggression towards other dogs even at a few months of age. Whether these puppies grow up to be aggressive is not known. Lack of exposure during the sensitive period probably accounts for the

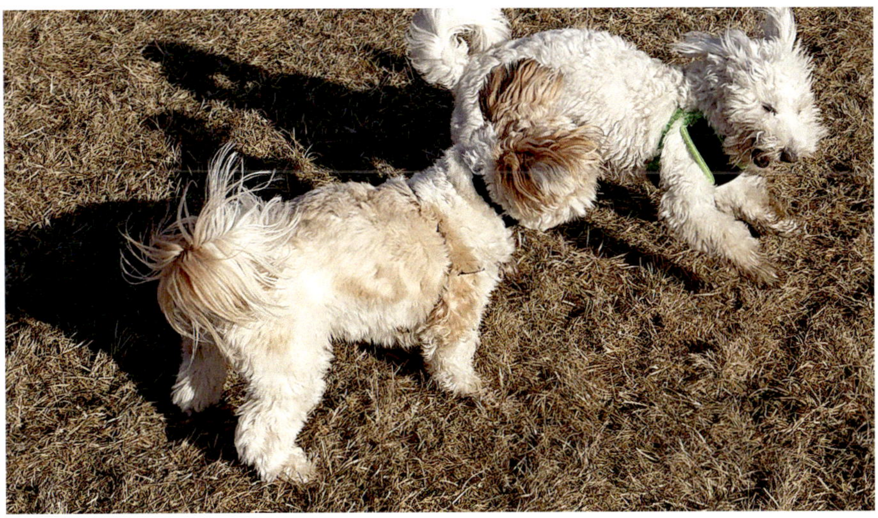

Fig. 5.8. The socialization period. Playing with other dogs helps puppies to learn about the world around them. Owners should allow puppies to interact as soon as possible. This interaction should take place under supervision and with a suitable partner. (Photo courtesy of Dr Sagi Denenberg.)

increased incidence of behaviour problems in dogs obtained as adults. One can socialize adult dogs but it takes much more time and effort. Introducing a vacuum cleaner to a puppy can prevent hours of terror (or attacks on the machine) for the dog as an adult (see Chapter 6).

Feral dogs in India disperse from their natal pack; that is, they do not remain with their mother and littermates. Young male dogs are most likely to leave the area in which they were born but they move only a kilometre or two (Pal, 2008).

5.7.2 Feeding

Pet owners feed their dogs once or more times a day with most owners feeding twice a day. A few owners leave kibble out for their dog all the time so the dog can 'graze'. When given free choice of food, beagles will eat every two hours. Free-ranging dogs may show as many variations in feeding patterns as pet dogs. Feral dogs in Italy visit a rubbish tip every night and will spend hours there, both finding food among the inedible trash and eating. They leave the dump at dawn and hide from people. Dogs that support themselves by hunting could eat 12 mice or one rabbit a day. Free-ranging urban feral dogs depend on garbage for their sustenance. Male dogs use gap widening to reach the food inside a packet, whereas females rip the packet open unless they are pregnant or lactating, in which case they use the more efficient gap widening, presumably to meet their greater caloric demands (Mangalam and Singh, 2013).

In the presence of free-choice palatable food, some dogs become obese and others do not. Obesity is a frequent problem in dogs. The reasons are the provision of very palatable and calorically dense food, lack of exercise and the dog's ability to beg.

There are signals from the body to the brain, indicating when the gastrointestinal tract contains the nutrients and when the body reserves are filled. Ghrelin is released when the stomach is empty. When the intestine contains fat or protein, hormones such as cholecystokinin, glucagon-like peptide and peptide YY are released. The latter was the basis of a drug to inhibit canine food intake. It worked well as an appetite suppressant, but the side effect of steatorrhea was unacceptable to owners.

Most of this hormonal information, along with neural information on gastrointestinal fill, is carried to the brain on the vagus nerve. These signals stimulate neuropeptide Y (NPY) and agouti-related protein (AGRP) to stimulate feeding, or cocaine and amphetamine-related transcript (CART) and melanocyte stimulating hormone (MSH) to suppress feeding by their actions in the hypothalamus. The neuropeptide orexin-A (OX-A) promotes wakefulness, and the endocannabinoid 2-arachidonoylglycerol (2-AG) promotes appetite.

Of course, the owner should regulate the caloric intake of the dog, but the pet can be persuasive in its demands for meals and snacks. High-fibre diets are somewhat effective in promoting weight loss in dogs because gastric fill can signal satiety.

Dogs have definite preferences. They prefer canned food over dry food. They prefer meat but would rather have cooked than raw meat. They like sweets. They also prefer variety and will eagerly eat a new flavour, but may tire of it after a few days if it is not innately palatable. Beef and chicken are preferred to horsemeat and pork.

Dogs drink when the osmotic pressure of their blood increases or if the volume of their blood decreases. The former is directly detected in the brain, but the latter is mediated by the release of the hormone angiotensin. In the home, dogs are most likely to drink after a meal or after a bout of panting. They may also drink if their mouth is dry, which would be after eating dry food.

5.8 Animality

5.8.1 Temperament

There have been many publications on the evaluation of canine temperament using a variety of methods from a battery of tests, experts' opinions and ratings of individual dogs by their owners. Recently, a review of previous publications concluded that temperament testing of dogs yields mediocre results at best and should not be used for any practical reasons (Patronek and Bradley, 2016). A review of over 50 studies of canine temperament revealed seven traits: reactivity, fearfulness, sociability, activity, responsiveness to training, submissiveness and aggression.

5.8.2 Animality

There are many tests of canine animality. Some studies are based on owners' descriptions, others on the opinions of experts, such as veterinarians and obedience judges, and still others on temperament tests. One extensive survey of veterinarians and obedience judges rated breeds on such traits as barking at strangers, attention-seeking, ease of house training, and aggression to strangers, owners and children. One interesting result was that, when analysed statistically, aggression to strangers and owners did not fall into the same category as snapping at children, which means that some breeds are more likely to bite children, whereas others are more likely to bite adults.

One popular temperament test involves six situations: (i) a stranger approaches the dog; (ii) the stranger approaches and tries to pet the dog; (iii) marbles are shaken in a metal bucket behind a barrier; (iv) a gun is fired; (v) the dog must walk over a grate; and (vi) the dog is threatened by a strangely dressed person. The animality description terms that occur most are: reactivity, fearfulness, sociability, activity, responsiveness to training, submissiveness and aggression. There is little evidence that the tests have validity. There is evidence for convergent validity (a measure correlates with other measures to which it should be related), but not for discriminative validity (a measure does not correlate with measures to which it is theoretically unrelated) (Jones and Gosling, 2005). Trainability, boldness, calmness and dog sociability are desirable attributes. Owners reported more positive attitudes toward their pets when the behavioural styles of their pets complemented their inter-personal styles (Zeigler-Hill and Highfill, 2010).

There have been several approaches to defining canine animality. The traits of fearfulness, activity, sociability, responsiveness to training, submissiveness and aggression resulted from a meta-analysis of 31 studies (Rayment *et al.*, 2015). The dog's personality does not seem to impact the dog–owner relationship. Only fearfulness is correlated with the relationship (Meyer and Forkman, 2014). Fear responses to less salient noises such as television or traffic may, therefore, reflect fearful animality characteristics, while those to very salient noises, such as gunshots and fireworks, may be learned. Early experience with thunder or gunshots increased the likelihood of fear of either of these noises as adults (Blackwell *et al.*, 2013). When a large number of owners were surveyed as to the trainability and boldness of their dogs, herding dogs were more trainable than hounds, working dogs, toy dogs and non-sporting dogs; sporting dogs were also more trainable than non-sporting dogs. In parallel, terriers were bolder than hounds and herding dogs. Regarding genetic relatedness, breeds with ancient breeds (Asian or African origin) were less trainable than breeds in the herding/sighthound cluster and the hunting breeds. Breeds in the mastiff/terrier cluster were bolder than the ancient breeds.

Dog breeds are typically divided according to historical usage into working, hunting, herding, hound, and terrier groups plus the toy group and, in some countries, a separate gun-dog group. When the results of a temperament test involving reactions to strangers who attempt to play tug-of-war with the dog are compared to the historical use of the dog, there is little correlation, but there is a similarity in response within a breed. Most interesting is that, considering the two most popular breeds, the golden retriever is fearful and the labrador is bold. These results suggest that the present use of a dog differs from historical use (Svartberg, 2006).

Recently, considerable interest has arisen in the temperament attribute of impulsivity. On a delayed reward choice task (press one bar and immediately get a small reward; press another bar and a more substantial reward will appear after a delay of up to 27 seconds), the dogs' performance – their ability to delay gratification – was related to their owners' subjective rating of impulsivity. In addition, the impulsivity score was correlated with serotonin and dopamine metabolites in the urine (Wright *et al.*, 2012). Impulsivity may be a component of aggression in dogs (see Chapter 12).

5.8.2.1 Optimism

Some dogs are more optimistic than others. For example, dogs with separation anxiety may not believe their owners will ever return. There is a test for optimism which consists of training the dog that of two dishes, for example, the one on the right will always contain food and the one on the left, will not. Once the dog learns that, it will go straight to the bowl on the right. The test is how fast will it approach a bowl in the centre, halfway between the one it learned would have food and the one it learned would not have food. The more optimistic it is, the faster it will approach the bowl in the centre. The drawback of this test is that you must have an optimistic group of dogs to act as a control for speed of approaching the centre bowl.

5.8.2.2 Yawning

There are three reasons why a dog may yawn: it is tired, nervous or someone else is yawning. Whether dogs yawn empathetically when a human yawns is controversial. If a person yawns for five minutes with auditory as well as visual stimuli, the dog will yawn, but if a person yawns without sound for three minutes, the dog will not yawn. Because dogs do not often yawn in response to another dog or a human yawning, anxiety is probably the main reason for canine yawning in the rested dog

5.8.2.3 Can dogs be jealous?

Almost every dog owner would answer yes, but that is hard to prove. A study showed that dogs reacted behaviourally when their owners paid attention to another dog. They got between the dog and the owner or snapped at the other dog. The other dog in this case was a stuffed one, but it was still able to elicit what appears to be jealousy from the dog (Harris and Prouvost, 2014).

5.8.2.4 Do dogs feel guilty?

Many owners claim that their dog knew it had done wrong because it acted guilty in different situations. In one study, owners brought their dog into a room where pieces of meat were presented to it. The owner told the dog not to eat the food and left the room. The experimenters picked up the food, so no dog ate it, and after a few minutes called the owners back. Half the owners were told that their dog ate the food; the other half were told that their dog did not steal the food, whereas, actually, no dog had eaten the food. The owners of dogs who had been told that their dog had taken the food said that their dog looked guilty. The owners who had been told that their dog did not steal the treat saw no signs of guilt. Either the tone of voice or general posture of the owner was a cue for the dog to act submissively with his head and tail down. That was a frightened, not a guilty, look (Ostojić *et al.*, 2015).

5.8.3 Laterality or pawedness

There are several ways to test for laterality: the paw used to remove tape from the nose, to overturn a can under which a treat had been hidden, to remove a blanket placed over the dog's head, hold a Kong toy, the first step taken downstairs, or the paw raised when the dog is told 'Give paw'. Dogs display right- and left-paw preferences. Female dogs have a higher preference for using their right paws on all tasks, but males are more inclined to use their left paw, although this is not seen in all studies. Dogs with stronger laterality are more relaxed and confident. Ambidextrous dogs are more likely to suffer from noise phobias such as a storm phobia and fear of fireworks. Ambidextrous dogs were faster at solving a manipulative task (opening a container by pushing a treadle). Because specialization of each side of the brain is part of normal development, dogs that do not show laterality may be somewhat developmentally disadvantaged (Marshall-Pescini *et al.*, 2013). Negative emotions are associated with the right hemisphere, and positive emotions are associated with the left hemisphere. Dogs wag their tails to the left when looking at a large, aggressive dog but to the right when looking at their owner (Quaranta *et al.*, 2007).

Dogs inspect the left side of photographs of human faces, whether the photographs are right side up or upside down (Guo *et al.*, 2009). They do not display similar laterality to dog faces unless the dog face displays aggression, in which case they show a left bias (Racca *et al.*, 2010). Dogs process meaningful sounds in their left brain, which they indicate by turning their head to the right; they turn toward the left when meaningless sounds are heard (Ratcliffe *et al.*, 2014). When a dog sniffs something, the information is initially transmitted to the same side of the brain, in contrast to vision, which is sent to the opposite side of the brain. Therefore, a dog may sniff at something with its left nostril and process that information in the left side of the brain. Dogs initially show a consistent right nostril bias when sniffing a veterinarian's sweat (presumably a frightening odour) and a left nostril bias when sniffing food or canine vaginal secretion, presumably pleasant stimuli (Siniscalchi *et al.*, 2011). Dogs were given cotton swabs of sweat from humans who had just seen a 15-minute horror movie or, as a control, just after a shower. The dogs sniffed the swabs from frightened people with their left nostril. This might mean that they can perceive fear in a human or at least a different smell when the human is frightened (Siniscalchi *et al.*, 2016).

There is also a side bias in tail wagging. Dogs wag their tails to the right when facing the owner or an unfamiliar person, although the amplitude of the wag is smaller to an unfamiliar person. Heart rates are lower when the dog wags to the right, indicating a positive emotional state. Dogs looking at moving video images of conspecifics showed higher cardiac activity and higher scores of anxious behaviours when observing left- rather than right-biased tail wagging. A cat also elicits a right-sided bias, but a strange dominant dog elicits a left-sided bias (Quaranta *et al.*, 2007).

References

Beach, F.A. and LeBoeuf, B.J. (1967) Coital behaviour in dogs. I. Preferential mating in the bitch. *Animal Behaviour* 15(4), 546–558. DOI: 10.1016/0003-3472(67)90057-7.

Blackwell, E.J., Bradshaw, J.W.S. and Casey, R.A. (2013) Fear responses to noises in domestic dogs: prevalence, risk factors and co-occurrence with other fear related behaviour. *Applied Animal Behaviour Science* 145(1-2), 15–25. DOI: 10.1016/j.applanim.2012.12.004.

Bonanni, R., Valsecchi, P. and Natoli, E. (2010) Pattern of individual participation and cheating in conflicts between groups of free-ranging dogs. *Animal Behaviour* 79(4), 957–968. DOI: 10.1016/j.anbehav.2010.01.016.

Cafazzo, S., Valsecchi, P., Bonanni, R. and Natoli, E. (2010) Dominance in relation to age, sex, and competitive contexts in a group of free-ranging domestic dogs. *Behavioral Ecology* 21(3), 443–455. DOI: 10.1093/beheco/arq001.

Craven, B.A., Paterson, E.G. and Settles, G.S. (2009) The fluid dynamics of canine olfaction: unique nasal airflow patterns as an explanation of macrosomia. *Journal of the Royal Society Interface* 7(47), 933–943. DOI: 10.1098/rsif.2009.0490.

Cuaya, L.V., Hernández-Pérez, R. and Concha, L. (2016) Our faces in the dog's brain: functional imaging reveals temporal cortex activation during perception of human faces. *PLOS ONE* 11(3), e0149431. DOI: 10.1371/journal.pone.0149431.

Duranton, C., Bedossa, T. and Gaunet, F. (2016) When facing an unfamiliar person, PET dogs present social referencing based on their owners' direction of movement alone. *Animal Behaviour* 113, 147–156. DOI: 10.1016/j.anbehav.2016.01.004.

Faragó, T., Pongrácz, P., Range, F., Virányi, Z. and Miklósi, Ádám. (2010) 'The bone is mine': affective and referential aspects of dog growls. *Animal Behaviour* 79(4), 917–925. DOI: 10.1016/j.anbehav.2010.01.005.

Feuerbacher, E.N. and Wynne, C.D.L. (2015) Shut up and pet me! Domestic dogs (Canis lupus familiaris) prefer petting to vocal praise in concurrent and single-alternative choice procedures. *Behavioural Processes* 110, 47–59. DOI: 10.1016/j.beproc.2014.08.019.

Guo, K., Meints, K., Hall, C., Hall, S. and Mills, D. (2009) Left gaze bias in humans, rhesus monkeys and domestic dogs. *Animal Cognition* 12(3), 409–418. DOI: 10.1007/s10071-008-0199-3.

Hansen, B.D., Lascelles, B.D.X., Keene, B.W., Adams, A.K., Thomson, A.E. *et al.* (2007) Evaluation of an accelerometer for at-home monitoring of spontaneous activity in dogs. *American Journal of Veterinary Research* 68(5), 468–475. DOI: 10.2460/ajvr.68.5.468.

Harris, C.R. and Prouvost, C. (2014) Jealousy in dogs. *PLOS ONE* 9(7), e94597. DOI: 10.1371/journal.pone.0094597.

Hernádi, A., Kis, A., Kanizsár, O., Tóth, K., Miklósi, B. *et al.* (2015) Intranasally administered oxytocin affects how dogs (*Canis familiaris*) react to the threatening approach of their owner and an unfamiliar experimenter. *Behavioural Processes* 119, 1–5. DOI: 10.1016/j.beproc.2015.07.001.

Horowitz, A. (2017) Smelling themselves: Dogs investigate their own odours longer when modified in an "olfactory mirror" test. *Behavioural Processes* 143, 17–24. DOI: 10.1016/j.beproc.2017.08.001.

Houpt, K.A. (2018) *Domestic Animal Behavior*, 6th edn. Wiley, Hoboken, New Jersey.

Jones, A.C. and Gosling, S.D. (2005) Temperament and personality in dogs (*Canis familiaris*): a review and evaluation of past research. *Applied Animal Behaviour Science* 95(1-2), 1–53. DOI: 10.1016/j.applanim.2005.04.008.

Kis, A., Gergely, A., Galambos, Ágoston., Abdai, J., Gombos, F. *et al.* (2017) Sleep macrostructure is modulated by positive and negative social experience in adult PET dogs. *Proceedings of the Royal Society B: Biological Sciences* 284(1865), 20171883. DOI: 10.1098/rspb.2017.1883.

Lisberg, A.E. and Snowdon, C.T. (2009) The effects of sex, gonadectomy and status on investigation patterns of unfamiliar conspecific urine in domestic dogs, *Canis familiaris*. *Animal Behaviour* 77(5), 1147–1154. DOI: 10.1016/j.anbehav.2008.12.033.

Mangalam, M. and Singh, M. (2013) Differential foraging strategies: motivation, perception and implementation in urban free-ranging dogs, *Canis familiaris*. *Animal Behaviour* 85(4), 763–770. DOI: 10.1016/j.anbehav.2013.01.019.

Marshall-Pescini, S., Barnard, S., Branson, N.J. and Valsecchi, P. (2013) The effect of preferential paw usage on dogs' (*Canis familiaris*) performance in a manipulative problem-solving task. *Behavioural Processes* 100, 40–43. DOI: 10.1016/j.beproc.2013.07.017.

McGreevy, P., Grassi, T.D. and Harman, A.M. (2004) A strong correlation exists between the distribution of retinal ganglion cells and nose length in the dog. *Brain, Behavior and Evolution* 63(1), 13–22. DOI: 10.1159/000073756.

McGuire, B. (2016) Scent marking in shelter dogs: effects of sex and age. *Applied Animal Behaviour Science* 182, 15–22. DOI: 10.1016/j.applanim.2016.06.001.

Meyer, I. and Forkman, B. (2014) Dog and owner characteristics affecting the dog–owner relationship. *Journal of Veterinary Behavior* 9(4), 143–150. DOI: 10.1016/j.jveb.2014.03.002.

Nagasawa, M., Murai, K., Mogi, K. and Kikusui, T. (2011) Dogs can discriminate human smiling faces from blank expressions. *Animal Cognition* 14(4), 525–533. DOI: 10.1007/s10071-011-0386-5.

Nagasawa, M., Mitsui, S., En, S., Ohtani, N., Ohta, M. *et al.* (2015) Social evolution. Oxytocin-gaze positive loop and the coevolution of human–dog bonds. *Science* 348(6232), 333–336. DOI: 10.1126/science.1261022.

Ostojić, L., Tkalčić, M. and Clayton, N.S. (2015) Are owners' reports of their dogs' 'guilty look' influenced by the dogs' action and evidence of the misdeed? *Behavioural Processes* 111, 97–100. DOI: 10.1016/j.beproc.2014.12.010.

Pal, S.K. (2005) Parental care in free-ranging dogs, *Canis familiaris*. *Applied Animal Behaviour Science* 90(1), 31–47. DOI: 10.1016/j.applanim.2004.08.002.

Pal, S.K. (2008) Maturation and development of social behaviour during early ontogeny in free-ranging dog puppies in West Bengal, India. *Applied Animal Behaviour Science* 111(1-2), 95–107. DOI: 10.1016/j.applanim.2007.05.016.

Patronek, G.J. and Bradley, J. (2016) No better than flipping a coin: reconsidering canine behavior evaluations in animal shelters. *Journal of Veterinary Behavior* 15, 66–77. DOI: 10.1016/j.jveb.2016.08.001.

Pongrácz, P., Molnár, C., Miklósi, A. and Csányi, V. (2005) Human listeners are able to classify dog (Canis familiaris) barks recorded in different situations. *Journal of Comparative Psychology* 119(2), 136–144. DOI: 10.1037/0735-7036.119.2.136.

Quaranta, A., Siniscalchi, M. and Vallortigara, G. (2007) Asymmetric tail-wagging responses by dogs to different emotive stimuli. *Current Biology* 17(6), R199–R201. DOI: 10.1016/j.cub.2007.02.008.

Racca, A., Amadei, E., Ligout, S., Guo, K., Meints, K. *et al.* (2010) Discrimination of human and dog faces and inversion responses in domestic dogs (Canis familiaris). *Animal Cognition* 13(3), 525–533. DOI: 10.1007/s10071-009-0303-3.

Ratcliffe, V.F., McComb, K. and Reby, D. (2014) Cross-modal discrimination of human gender by domestic dogs. *Animal Behaviour* 91, 127–135. DOI: 10.1016/j.anbehav.2014.03.009.

Rayment, D.J., De Groef, B., Peters, R.A. and Marston, L.C. (2015) Applied personality assessment in domestic dogs: limitations and caveats. *Applied Animal Behaviour Science* 163, 1–18. DOI: 10.1016/j.applanim.2014.11.020.

Siniscalchi, M., Sasso, R., Pepe, A.M., Dimatteo, S., Vallortigara, G. *et al.* (2011) Sniffing with the right nostril: lateralization of response to odour stimuli by dogs. *Animal Behaviour* 82(2), 399–404. DOI: 10.1016/j.anbehav.2011.05.020.

Siniscalchi, M., d'Ingeo, S. and Quaranta, A. (2016) The dog nose "KNOWS" fear: Asymmetric nostril use during sniffing at canine and human emotional stimuli. *Behavioural Brain Research* 304, 34–41. DOI: 10.1016/j.bbr.2016.02.011.

Svartberg, K. (2006) Breed-typical behaviour in dogs—Historical remnants or recent constructs? *Applied Animal Behaviour Science* 96(3-4), 293–313. DOI: 10.1016/j.applanim.2005.06.014.

Waller, B.M., Peirce, K., Caeiro, C.C., Scheider, L., Burrows, A.M. *et al.* (2013) Paedomorphic facial expressions give dogs a selective advantage. *PLOS ONE* 8(12), e82686. DOI: 10.1371/journal.pone.0082686.

Wells, D.L., Graham, L. and Hepper, P.G. (2002) The influence of auditory stimulation on the behaviour of dogs housed in a rescue shelter. *Animal Welfare* 11, 385–393.

Wright, H.F., Mills, D.S. and Pollux, P.M.J. (2012) Development and validation of a psychometric tool for assessing impulsivity in the domestic dog (Canis familiaris). *International Journal of Comparative Psychology* 24, 210–225.

Zeigler-Hill, V. and Highfill, L. (2010) Applying the interpersonal circumplex to the behavioral styles of dogs and cats. *Applied Animal Behaviour Science* 124(3-4), 104–112. DOI: 10.1016/j.applanim.2010.02.012.

6 Raising Mentally and Emotionally Healthy Pets

Helen Zulch*

Dogs Trust UK, London, UK

6.1 Introduction

The behaviour of any individual is underpinned by a combination of its genetic potential and the experiences it has through life (Wilsson, 2016). Although all experiences are likely to influence later behaviour, it is recognized that there is a sensitive period early in an animal's life where experience has the most influence. In dogs, this early sensitive period is generally believed to occur between 3 and 12 weeks of age (Horwitz *et al.*, 2009) and in cats between two and seven weeks (Bradshaw *et al.*, 2012), although literature in both species can cite some level of variation. During this time, both experiences within the litter as well as from stimuli external to the litter and maternal environment (both pre- and post-weaning) are likely to have long-term consequences for behaviour and thus should be optimized.

In addition, it is particularly important to recognize that merely signing a new puppy owner up to a puppy training course, or a kitten owner up to a kitten education course, is inadequate to maximize the chances of life-long appropriate behaviour. Owners need to understand the importance of every daily interaction that their puppy or kitten experiences for later behaviour. Veterinary practices can assist in young pet education by stressing the importance of embedding correct learning into everyday life.

However, it is also important to realize that learning does not stop at the end of the sensitive period and therefore it is recommended that behaviour and learning are carefully managed at least until social maturity has been reached (postulated to be 12–36 months of age in dogs, not known to be reported in cats) (Serpell and Duffy, 2016). A supportive veterinary practice should stress the importance of cementing appropriate learning through puberty, a time which can be particularly challenging for owners, and into social maturity.

This chapter will consider pre-weaning influences on puppies and kittens and what this means for a new pet owner selecting a dog or cat, before discussing in more detail the advice which the veterinary profession can give to minimize the risk of problem development in dogs and cats through appropriate early life experiences. Finally, the chapter will cover some critical aspects of 'behavioural first aid'; how we can intervene early when an owner reports problematic behaviour. Practices can foster owner understanding, minimize the risk of behaviours deteriorating, and maximize the opportunity for the dog or cat to develop behaviour that enables it to fit seamlessly into the owner's lifestyle and society's expectations while also experiencing appropriate welfare.

6.2 Selection of a Kitten or Puppy

Deciding to add a kitten or puppy to the family is a significant and exciting decision and usually not one which involves input from the veterinary practice. However, given the importance of this decision for setting owners up for the best possible life-long experience with a pet and the implications this has for the pet's well-being, encouraging owners to make the best decisions regarding this is something practices should endeavour to do. Simply raising awareness of practice staff's availability to discuss the decision may be enough to encourage an existing client to broach the subject of a new addition to the family.

*Helen.Zulch@dogstrust.org.uk

DOI: 10.1079/9781786394552.0006

When you are given the opportunity to offer advice, there are three areas where suggestions regarding decision making are essential:

1. the genetic background of the dog/cat concerning health parameters;
2. the genetic background of the pet relating to behaviour; and
3. the maternal environment in which the individual is raised.

Once a person has decided to acquire a puppy or kitten, generally, the next key consideration will be the breed. If we are offering advice on this topic, we need to be very careful of falling into the trap of stereotyping breeds for characteristics which are not part of the specific breed's genetic heritage or where learning and life experience is more likely to play the more significant role. This is not to say that there are no differences between breeds – of course, it will be easier to herd sheep with a Border collie than with an English pointer – but most characteristics which are shown in a pet home (e.g. aggression, trainability and playfulness) are likely to vary more within a breed than between breeds. It has also been demonstrated that, to an extent, the breed can become a self-fulfilling prophecy (Clarke *et al.*, 2013) with owners not attempting to manage a given behaviour because it is perceived as 'That's what X breed does'. Breed stereotyping is dangerous on two fronts: it can prevent owners from seeking help when it is needed from the perspective of the dog's welfare (e.g. treating a noise fear in a herding dog or tail-chasing in a bull terrier); and it can also lull people into a false sense of security (e.g. 'Labradors are friendly and therefore won't bite', and 'All ragdolls are cuddly').

The best advice we can give our clients when it comes to pet selection is, rather than to become distracted by the merits of one breed versus another, to undertake due diligence to ensure, to the best of anyone's ability, the behavioural stability of the individual chosen. This involves meeting the mother of the litter, *in situ*, with the puppies or kittens as well as, ideally, the father (Westgarth *et al.*, 2012) and, where at all possible, adult siblings from previous litters. In this way, a fuller picture of this individual's behavioural genetic potential will be obtained.

Ideally, if this step is carefully undertaken, prospective owners will not face a litter of very nervous puppies or kittens when they visit. However, should this happen, they should be armed with enough knowledge to either walk away, if they feel unable to cope with what this might mean for future behaviour, or understand the potential for remedial confidence building that may be needed. When selecting within a litter, should a novice pet owner be faced with a litter where temperament variability is seen, it is usually advised that a 'middle of the road' puppy or kitten is selected. Novice owners should stay away from puppies or kittens that appear to be extremely fearful as it is possible that these individuals will be more demanding of a new owner in order to build confidence over time.

Potential owners should be encouraged to ask questions relating to health screening for a litter when purchasing from a breeder. Anyone breeding a specific breed or cross should be undertaking the advised breed-specific screening for diseases known to have a hereditary component.

6.2.1 The importance of the maternal environment

As discussed above, puppies and kittens are born with a genetic blueprint which is then shaped or changed by their experiences throughout their lives. As altricial animals, just as age matures their physical capacities, their sensory and neurological capabilities change, too, as sense organs mature and neurological pathways develop. The critical aspect of this development in the very young neonate is the interaction which occurs between the environment and the genetically driven intrinsic maturation process. It is important to remember that there is flexibility in the genetic blueprint to enable the neonate to take advantage of environmental factors in their behavioural development. This flexibility allows us to shape development to the individual pet's advantage.

Although the importance of maternal behaviour and environment has been well recognized in other species such as rodents, we are only now beginning to understand the details of how pre-weaning experiences impact on the adult behaviour of our companion animal species (Foyer *et al.*, 2013; Guardini *et al.*, 2016). For example, studies in the pre-weaned puppy have shown that maternal environment can influence isolation behaviour in very young animals (Gazzano *et al.*, 2008a) and correlates with differences in avoidance behaviour and the likelihood of aggressive behaviour in adult dogs (Appleby *et al.*, 2002). Studies in kittens show that the number of people that a kitten interacts with pre-weaning can influence both interaction and play behaviours in adults (Bradshaw *et al.*, 2012). Further, the experiences which a kitten has with prey species while still in the nest influences future predatory behaviour (Caro, 1979, 1980). However, literature in this area, as it pertains to puppies and kittens, is still scarce.

Because we know we can shape behaviour pre-weaning, it would be best if we have contact with breeders of dogs and cats, and are available to offer sound advice regarding the rearing environment they provide. Furthermore, advising potential new owners on what to consider when looking at the rearing environment of a puppy or kitten can help them to select a pet that has had the best possible start in life.

Research has shown that puppies born and raised in the home, as opposed to in a kennel or outbuilding, are at an advantage (Appleby *et al.*, 2002). It is also generally advised that the environment provided for the young animals is enriched both concerning contact with people and the presence of inanimate objects. Ensuring that puppies and kittens are handled carefully and appropriately by a range of people (in the presence of their litter and not removed from the litter for prolonged periods when they are very young, but picked up nonetheless) is considered positive (Battaglia, 2009; Schoon and Berntsen, 2011). Specific research in kittens has demonstrated that within the first seven weeks of life, human contact of between 15 minutes and one hour per day, regularly, is recommended (Bradshaw *et al.*, 2012). Being handled by a few people rather than one person will assist cats to be more comfortable and accepting of handling by multiple people later in life (Collard, 1967).

Ensuring exposure to a range of sounds, particularly household sounds, but also vehicle noises and similar, is also positive. Presenting very young individuals with a variety of items in their whelping/kittening box is positive (different textures, shapes and odours, all safe for investigation by small mouths) and once they are mobile and leaving the safety of the nest, providing these new experiences in different areas around the home and garden is advised. All exposures need to be positive, so set up novel objects, sounds and scents in a manner that the puppy or kitten can choose to approach or not, and in a manner that ensures that they always retain a sense of safety. Do not overwhelm individuals by adding too much to the environment at once.

Once the puppies and kittens are more mobile, taking them into new environments and for short car trips as a litter, setting up obstacle courses in the wider environment (including safe climbing frames for kittens) and using equipment such as vacuum cleaners in their vicinity (but far enough away so as not to scare them) are all advised. As long as their mother is comfortable around these items, she should be with them, as a point of safety, when the novelty is introduced. Otherwise, puppies and kittens should be exposed to items using food, confident littermates and people they trust, without an anxious dam. The aim is to provide young individuals with a sense that new and different things in the environment are positive and not frightening.

6.2.2 What about kittens and puppies from other sources?

Kittens and puppies can be acquired from many sources. When an individual is sought from a breeder, we should be advising (as above) how to select a reputable breeder and dissuading purchase via the internet. Those sourcing puppies and kittens from friends and family can be given the same advice as above. However, what about the sourcing of puppies and kittens from rehoming charities?

In these cases, there is usually little information regarding the parents, unless the mother has been relinquished along with its litter, in which case some assessment of the behavioural genetic potential of the litter can be made. However, it must always be borne in mind that the behaviour exhibited by the mother in the kennel or cattery environment may be very different from that which might be displayed in a home. Probably the most crucial point to investigate when adoption from a shelter or rehoming organization is considered is the investment made into the development of the puppies and kittens while in the care of the charity. Ideally, only adopting from a charity that is offering a suitable maternal environment and pre-weaning experiences for the puppies and kittens should be considered. Practices that have relationships with such charities can assist in ensuring that the most up-to-date information is given on this front and that behavioural as well as physical health is addressed where the raising of neonates is concerned.

6.3 Homing Age and Process

There is still no undisputed evidence regarding the best age to take puppies and kittens into their new homes. Kittens are generally advised to be weaned at around seven weeks of age. Remember that at this age, exposure to people needs to have been accomplished before homing. As many breeders keep their kittens well beyond this age, the importance of appropriate interaction with people within the maternal environment cannot be overstated.

In general, the advice given regarding puppies is to home them at seven to eight weeks (Jokinen *et al.*, 2017). However, if the neonatal environment is impoverished and the new owner is skilled and can offer a better socialization experience, it may be advised to take the puppy into the new home at six to seven weeks.

6.3.1 Providing kittens and puppies with an appropriate environment

There are many books which describe preparing the home for the arrival of a new kitten or puppy, but we can help to ensure that owners have thought through meeting their new pet's psychological as well as physical needs. This includes: introducing their puppy or kitten appropriately to all family members (two- and four-legged), investigating training classes, and thinking through preparing their pet for fitting into their lives in the longer term. For example, getting their puppy used to being left alone while they are at work, or getting their kitten acclimatized to the outdoor environment.

Ensuring that every individual is provided with a safe haven where they will not be disturbed by anyone, including children or visitors, is something that needs to be considered, and in the case of a new kitten owner, it is essential to remind them that cats utilize three-dimensional space and most cats choose to rest at a height. Providing cats with high places to rest and avoid others (e.g. pets or visitors) will help reduce stress. Ensuring that some of these are semi-enclosed to provide hiding places will benefit the kitten even more. Remember in multi-cat households where not all cats have close relationships, hiding places and high resting platforms need to have at least two access points so that a cat can move away from another cat coming up to it, should it so wish.

6.4 Raising a Kitten or Puppy

The term most commonly associated with puppy raising is 'socialization'. While this is a critical component of helping puppies and kittens to develop appropriate behaviours in a human-centred world, it is not the only consideration in raising behaviourally healthy individuals. This section will, as well as discussing proper socialization and habituation of puppies and kittens, touch on a few other key areas where owners often need advice and support.

6.4.1 What is socialization/habituation?

In recent years, the term 'puppy socialization' has become ubiquitous, and most dog owners, as well as many cat owners, will be aware of the need to have an adequately socialized puppy or kitten. However, not all owners or trainers know what this means and how to undertake the process to ensure benefit to the puppy or kitten without increasing the risk of problem behaviour through inappropriate interventions.

Socialization is defined as 'the process by which animals adapt their behaviour patterns appropriate to the social environment in which they live, allowing them to coexist/interact with other individuals' (Mills *et al.*, 2010). Habituation is defined as 'learning not to respond to a stimulus' (Mills *et al.*, 2010), or in practical terms for puppies and kittens, learning to accept as a normal part of their environment all the day-to-day objects, sounds and other items that they may encounter.

Socialization and habituation are best started during the sensitive period for inter-specific socialization learning; this is generally considered to be between 3 and 12 weeks in puppies (possibly up to 16 weeks) and 2–7 weeks (possibly up to 9 weeks) in kittens.

Ideally, all young animals should be socialized/habituated to all the stimuli, animate and inanimate, that they are likely to come across later in life. This must be done in a manner that elicits a positive and appropriate emotional and behavioural response towards these stimuli. In reality, no individual is going to, during its sensitive period, meet everything that it is likely to encounter in later life, but there is a theory that introduction to sufficient variety (in the correct manner) can help to buffer the individual against a negative response to novelty in later life. Therefore, the recommendation is usually to ensure appropriate experiences early in life, with a range of stimuli, to develop in the individual an ability to cope with new stimuli added to the set later. These new items are then classified by the dog or cat as 'safe stimuli'.

Note that, although this section will repeatedly refer to experiences which are appropriate to the individual's lifestyle, care must be taken to ensure that socialization and habituation experiences are sufficiently broad. The lifestyle predicted for the puppy or kitten may be that of living with a single adult in a quiet rural environment. However, this does not mitigate against the need for the pet to be able to cope with visitors and trips to the vet, at the very least, let alone insure against the possibility, however remote, that it might need to live in a very different environment one day. As stated above, it would appear that a sufficiently wide range of experiences when young promotes the ability to deal better with novelty later in life.

Generally, the advice to new owners would be to introduce the puppy, within the first 12 weeks of life, and the kitten within the first seven weeks of life, to a range of people, other animals, objects, sounds, substrates and environments (as appropriate to the species and the individual's predicted lifestyle). However, the key is *how* these introductions are made. As far as possible, introductions should be structured to ensure that they are a positive experience and that the pet is not overwhelmed by too many exposures in quick succession. Unfortunately, no literature exists that can guide us as to how much exposure and over what period is the most appropriate, and this will likely be determined mainly by the personality of the individual. However, advising owners to take puppies out for brief periods daily, or exposing them in the home to something novel daily, should be sufficient, without overwhelming.

When puppies and kittens are introduced to novelty, try to ensure that they are given control of their proximity to the item/individual. Allow the pet to explore in its own time and observe it, ensuring that it is coping with the experience. Owners can reward appropriate interactions with treats, but do not encourage a puppy or kitten up to a novel object/person using a food lure. The risk in such a situation is that the youngster is put into a situation of motivational conflict – it wants the treat but doesn't want to approach novelty – as this can be detrimental to the learning we want (see Section 7.3.2 – Conflict) Alternatively, the pet can be so focused on the food that it is unaware of the proximity of something which, by the time it notices the object/person, is so close to it that he is worried by it. In the author's experience, most young animals find interacting with something novel and interesting sufficiently reinforcing and do not need the addition of food rewards.

It is important to encourage owners to see all interactions from the young animal's perspective as sometimes an interaction considered by an owner to be appropriate is not seen as positive by a puppy or kitten. For example, an unknown dog bouncing over to play can scare a puppy as much as an unknown dog lunging and snapping. Care must be taken to read the puppy's or kitten's body language at all times to try to gauge how it perceives the encounter. Should the puppy or kitten show concern about the novel object/person, do not force it into closer proximity. If it is happy to stay at a distance, or even move closer in its own time, allow that. However, if it is becoming more concerned, the longer it remains near the item/individual, gently remove it from the situation to minimize the risk of it having a negative experience and possibly becoming sensitized.

Although there is no good evidence for or against the benefit of taking a puppy out in the owner's arms, for example before it has had its primary vaccinations, if this is to be done it needs to be carefully considered. A puppy in an owner's arms has no control over its proximity to items or individuals, especially people who may approach to greet it. For a puppy who is worried about the approach of strangers, this inability to create distance appropriately could lead to an adverse reaction to strangers later in life. Therefore, it is best to advise that puppies in owners' arms are allowed to be viewed but not be approached. Probably a lesser risk, but a risk nonetheless, is that a puppy may become increasingly frustrated by being restrained in arms when it wants to get down to interact. In this case, again a negative emotional state can be fostered in the presence of novelty, or the puppy may even learn that frustrated behaviour pays off, i.e. if an owner decided to 'give in' and let it down at this point.

Another consideration which generally pertains more to puppies than to kittens is teaching puppies the right way to approach a new individual as well as the fact that greetings will not always be possible. Several problems with interactions in later life can be traced back to inappropriate learning early in life. A puppy being scared by someone, another dog or another animal, early in life is easy to understand as the initiating cause for a later problem; the practising of inappropriate greetings when growing up is less recognized, but just as important.

If a puppy is allowed to run up to and interact with all people or dogs when it is very young, this can set the scene for problems later. An outgoing puppy can find this an extremely reinforcing experience and can very soon develop the expectation that it can enjoy interactions with all those it sees. The first time a problem may be noted as a result of this behaviour is when, as an adolescent, it runs up to a strange dog and elicits a less than friendly reaction, but, additionally, when later an owner wants to curtail the behaviour for any reason, these puppies can become extremely frustrated at not being allowed to interact. This can manifest as inappropriate behaviour (such as lunging and barking on the lead) which is challenging in itself, but when in some situations this then leads to punitive reactions from the owner, over time a gregarious puppy can become motivationally conflicted about meeting other dogs or people, which can result in serious problems. It is thus a good idea to recommend to new owners that they manage their puppy's behaviour and expectations from young. On some occasions, encourage their puppy to walk past or away from an individual that they wish to greet using a food lure or toy distraction if needed, and reward them for moving away. Additionally, when puppies are to be allowed to greet, encourage them to remain calm as they approach, through the use of food rewards for keeping close to the owner, until they are close enough to be allowed to greet and they are likely to do so in a manner that is more controlled and appropriate.

Finally, note that research has correlated early life severe illness and hospitalization with the risk of increased fear and aggressive behaviour later in life (Jagoe, 1994). It is hypothesized that this may relate to the curtailing of appropriate socialization experiences or learning negative associations during this crucial period. For this reason, when puppies or kittens are seriously ill, or ill for a prolonged period during their early life, it is worth spending time advising their owners on appropriate remedial socialization and training experiences that may benefit them.

6.5 What Else Does a Kitten Owner Need to Know?

Raising kittens is not only to do with socialization and habituation; there are many other skills that we need to teach them to enable them to live comfortably in our modern environments, to fit into our lifestyle and to minimize the risk of problem behaviour development. The next sections will give some brief advice regarding subjects on which owners most commonly seek advice. Please note that detailed explanations are beyond the scope of this book; some additional resources for further information is included in the reading list. It is often wrongly assumed that kittens come with a full set of skills, and no training, socialization and habituation are necessary. People often believe that cats cannot be trained, but the same principles that apply to training dogs through positive reinforcement apply to cats. New owners should train the kitten to enjoy aspects of life, such as grooming and travel, and will benefit from putting in the time to teach kittens additional responses such as coming when called and waiting in particular places while food is prepared.

6.5.1 Litter trays

Most kittens will have learnt to use a litter tray before leaving their mother. To try to ensure that there is no setback in toilet training, ensure that a litter tray of adequate size (large enough for the kitten to comfortably stand and turn around in) with a sufficiently low rim and containing (at least to begin with) the same litter as they were used to, is placed in an area they can easily access (see Handout C8 – Litter Tray Training). Ensure that the litter is of adequate depth. Placing the kitten in the litter tray once or twice, or calling it over to it so that it can investigate it and quickly knows where to find it is usually sufficient for most kittens to start to use the tray immediately. Even if owners wish the kitten to use the garden as a toilet in the long term, in the early stages, providing access to a litter tray might prevent accidents and the wrong habits from developing. For kittens that are to use the outdoors from young, ensure that they have easy access to a place where they can comfortably dig (soft soil in a sheltered spot), and, again, consider taking them there a few times to investigate. If there are pot plants or areas where you do not wish the kitten to go to the toilet, in the short term you can make these less attractive by placing gravel or similar substrate in the area.

6.5.2 Destructive behaviour

Scratching is a normal cat behaviour but scratching furniture is generally unacceptable to owners.

Providing kittens with appropriate scratch posts in easy-to-access areas can help reduce scratching other objects and assist in developing the correct habits right from the beginning. Owners should provide a variety of scratchable objects which might include commercial posts, homemade posts (e.g. pieces of carpet stapled to a board), or even natural wood.

Kittens can also cause damage to the home by playing, for example, should they climb up curtains. Providing appropriate outlets for play can help to prevent this (see Section 6.5.4) and, in addition, not making the activity of climbing inappropriate objects into a fun activity (by excited human reactions) should avoid these behavioural experiments from becoming problematic behaviours.

6.5.3 Handling

All cats will need to be handled all over at some point in their life – whether it is to groom them (especially important in long-haired individuals), to medicate them or for a physical examination. Getting kittens used to gentle handling is therefore essential. When an owner starts to accustom their kitten to handling, it's best to choose a time of the day when the kitten is most likely to be calm (after a meal and a while after any games which may have excited them) and gently stroke them. Starting in areas that most cats like the most (such as around the head) (Ellis *et al.*, 2015) and gradually moving all over the body in short bouts and small increments usually works best. It can sometimes help to pair the kitten being calm and accepting of the handling with food treats, but this may make some kittens more excited. Over time, all areas of the body should be able to be handled, including the toes, the tail, the ears and mouth. If a kitten objects to handling of any areas, the owner must not get angry and tell them off, simply back off and move more slowly towards handling that area at a later stage. If some areas are very challenging to manage, advice should be sought sooner rather than later as this is not a problem that is likely to resolve on its own.

6.5.4 Play

As much fun as it is to engage in games where kittens chase and pounce on people's fingers and toes, this type of activity should be discouraged. Encouraging games with human body parts can lead to unwanted and potentially dangerous scratches and bites as the kitten gets older. All games with a human should be with toys, not rough-and-tumble play.

It is essential for owners to provide a range of toys for kittens, including toys where the owner plays with the kitten and toys for the kitten to play with alone. Anecdotally, cats tend to enjoy short bouts of play, but switching between toys can keep their interest for longer and thus extend a game. Homemade toys (e.g. toilet roll inners with treats in or crumpled up sheets of paper to chase) can be an inexpensive means of entertaining a kitten. Kitten owners should be encouraged to dedicate time every day to fostering appropriate play.

Toys which encourage chasing and catching, such as fishing rod toys and similar, are enjoyed by most cats, but it is important that the cat is allowed to 'catch' the toy sufficiently frequently to keep up its interest in the game. Catnip-filled toys are attractive to some cats but can also lead to over-excitement, which can spill over into unwanted behaviours. Should this happen, access to such toys may need to be restricted or stopped.

Toys which dispense food when manipulated are available for cats, and as long as they are of an appropriate size and difficulty level, kittens can be encouraged to use them. Particularly if kittens are to be restricted to the indoors, creating additional feeding interest and activity through the use of these feeders can be very beneficial.

6.5.5 Travel

All cats will, at some point in their lives, need to travel to the vet, a cattery or a new home. For this reason, it is important to teach kittens from young that their cat carrier, and travel itself, is not scary. This will make later travel with the cat less stressful for all. Investing in an adult-sized cat carrier that is sturdy and has a top which lifts off completely is advised. As a first step, owners should leave the carrier, with a bed in the bottom, around the house permanently. They can consider using a feline pheromone in the basket and periodically hiding treats in it so that the kitten views it as a good place to be.

After this, the door can gradually be closed for short but extending periods, and then the carrier moved short distances from place to place with the kitten inside. The kitten can be trained to enter the carrier on cue or enticed in with a treat (assuming it views the carrier as positive, or this won't work more than once or twice).

Over time, the carrier can be carried to the car, and the kitten taken for short, and then longer, drives. Always keep the experience positive by providing treats and a good experience at the end.

If this approach is not working to transport the kitten calmly, then specialist advice should be sought.

6.5.6 Multi-cat households

When introducing a new kitten into a home with other cats, owners should first ensure that the resident cat or cats have no history of animosity towards other cats, and there is a likelihood of accepting the new kitten. Further, owners should provide sufficient resources (e.g. food, water, perches, litter trays and affection) for all cats to reduce any conflicts and competition. The introduction should be gradual and controlled. Owners should first allow the cats to smell the other cat's toys, beds, litter and brushes. Then, allowing the cats to see each other through a barrier (e.g. a screen door) while taking treats helps to foster positive association. Finally, owners can allow the cats to be in close contact. However, they must be supervised, and the interactions should be short at the beginning.

Since kittens do not have a full social understanding, owners should limit the kitten more than the older resident cat. Doing so will allow the resident cat to rest and maintain its routine and environment, leading to a lower risk of conflict. Also, the older cat may not be as playful and interactive as the new kitten, while kittens might play and disturb the resident cat. For more information on social framework and interactions between cats, see Chapter 4.

6.6 What Else Do Puppies Need to Know?

As with kittens, there are many skills we need to teach puppies that will help them to live harmoniously withinthe human-centred world. Once again, the next sections will give some brief advice regarding subjects on which owners most commonly seek advice. However, please note that detailed explanations are beyond the scope of this book; some additional resources for further information are included in the reading list.

6.6.1 House training

Most puppies, at the time of adoption, will need to learn where the owner wants them to eliminate. Therefore, training new puppies is an essential part of adapting to the new home (see Handout C9 – House Training Your Puppy). Owners need to anticipate the times that their puppy may want to go to the toilet and preemptively take them out to their chosen toilet spot at these times. Key times include: immediately on waking, after eating, after playing, and every few hours in-between these events. At these times, or if the owner sees their puppy sniffing the ground or circling (signs usually preceding urination or defecation), they should gently call the puppy or lift it and carry it to the spot where they would like it to go to the toilet. After it has been to the toilet, owners should praise it and consider giving it a treat or game.

Owners should avoid punishing, verbally or physically, their puppy for soiling in the house. Instead, they should clean the area appropriately and take note of why it may have happened. Leaving the puppy outdoors unsupervised is not recommended – the puppy is likely to wait by the door to be let inside and then urinate. Moreover, the puppy may be distracted by another dog or toys and will then eliminate when back indoors. Owners should not take their puppy back indoors immediately after it has eliminated outside; prolonging the time outdoors may teach the puppy to hold on.

6.6.2 Sleeping arrangements

Owners usually have very clear ideas of where they would like their dog to sleep, and, with a few exceptions, there is no good evidence to suggest supporting one choice over another. However, it is advisable for a new owner to have a long-term plan regarding these sleeping arrangements so that they can work towards this. In general, the first couple of nights in a new home are stressful for a puppy. There is some evidence that this may be mitigated through the use of dog-appeasing pheromone (Taylor and Mills, 2007; Gaultier *et al.*, 2008) and new owners can consider the use of a diffuser or collar. Another means of helping the distress is to have the puppy sleep in a crate next to the owner's bed for the few nights where they can comfort the puppy. If the crate is just large enough for the pup to stand, lie or turn around in, and is filled with comfortable bedding, it is also less likely that it will eliminate in the crate, and when it is restless in the night it can be taken out immediately, thus helping with toilet training.

Over time, the crate can be moved out of the bedroom and into the space that the owner would like to be the pup's long-term bed area, and eventually the crate can be faded out, too, if that is the owner's desire. If the puppy is showing distress at the idea of being shut in a crate, a puppy pen can be substituted.

If the owner does not want the puppy in the bedroom at all to start with, then a plan needs to be made to settle the pup in a different room and decisions made regarding when the owner will return to the pup during the night should it become distressed. This needs to be carefully thought out as, if the puppy learns that the moment it whines it will have company, training to cope with being left to sleep alone will be undermined; but by the same token, if it is left to become distressed, this could give rise to later problems with separation-related behaviour.

If owners are struggling after the first week or so to settle their puppy into a good bedtime routine, help should be sought from a skilled trainer or behaviourist to ensure that this can be overcome as soon as possible.

6.6.3 Being left alone

Every puppy should be taught to cope with being alone as at some point in its life it is likely to need to be separated from its owners. It is also essential that it learns to be left alone as there is no guarantee that it will always be left in the presence of another dog. Ideally, from a week or so after the puppy has been brought into the new home, it needs to be introduced to the fact that being alone is a good thing. For most puppies a simple staged plan will work, for those who don't cope with this, additional help should be sought from a qualified practitioner.

The first few times a puppy is to be left, ensure that it has had an opportunity to go to the toilet, has had some exercise (but is not in an excited state immediately prior to being left), and is not hungry. Leave the puppy in a safe, enclosed space, whether this is a room, pen or crate, depending on the owner's long-term plans. However, if a crate is to be used, then before the door is closed on the puppy, correct crate training procedures need to be undertaken, so early leaving rituals should not incorporate being closed into the crate.

The puppy should be calmly taken to the space where it is to be left and provided with water, a bed, some toys that are safe, or a stuffed food toy (assuming it knows how to empty it) and some treats scattered over the area. Owners should calmly leave the puppy, close the door or gate and walk away. A critical factor in this early stage is to return within only a few minutes, ideally before or just after the pup has finished the food item or chew. We want it to have noticed the absence of people, but not become concerned about it. This leaving alone should be done daily for gradually longer periods and at different times so that, ideally, leaving becomes something the pup looks forward to as it predicts 'getting good stuff'. Upon returning, owners should calmly open the door or gate and allow the puppy to make contact again in their own time, avoiding excited greetings or excessive attention.

If the pup whines a little when left the first couple of times, ideally don't return to the puppy as it is whining. However, a judgement call needs to be made as it is counterproductive to allow the puppy to become severely distressed, and if this appears to be happening, the leaving-alone training needs to be stopped and advice sought.

6.6.4 Travel

Every dog is likely, at some stage, to need to travel, and therefore getting puppies used to travelling appropriately in a vehicle is important. In most countries, there is a requirement that dogs in cars are appropriately restrained, which may mean that they go behind a guard, in a crate or secured on the back seat via a car harness. Whichever of these is likely to be the long-term mode of travel for the dog should be established right from the start. The exception may be very small puppies who may most safely travel in a crate, and only later be introduced to a harness.

Most puppies, if the first few trips in a vehicle are kept positive – a short excursion to somewhere they like, with owners who help them stay calm and relaxed, sitting close maybe feeding them treats or providing a chew toy –will grow up finding car travel positive. For puppies who become car sick on a few trips in a row, even when they have not had a large meal prior to travel, seeking help from their vet as soon as possible is advisable as it is very easy for these puppies to grow up with an aversion to car travel.

If a puppy struggles to settle in the car and becomes highly excited by stimuli – for example people passing outside the window – using a covered crate and working on rewarding calm, relaxed behaviour is advised. For any puppy who is struggling to settle calmly in a vehicle within the first few months of life, help should be sought as this is the sort of problem that is likely to get worse with time.

6.6.5 Toys, games and training exercises

All puppies should have access to activities that give them mental stimulation and enjoyment. This includes access to appropriate toys and games, training activities (which are fun as well as teach useful skills) and, as soon as vaccination protocols allow, walks in a range of areas that allow for environmental investigation.

It is difficult to predict what type of toy a puppy will like, and trying a range of different ones is best. This also includes inexpensive homemade toys such as cardboard boxes (all staples and tape removed) into which treats or chews can be placed, with or without crumpled up paper to enable the puppy to have fun tearing this apart to access the food. It is essential that owners realize that no toy can be guaranteed to be indestructible and all new toys should be given to a puppy under supervision, initially, to determine their safety as well as how much interest a puppy shows in them.

To maintain a puppy's interest in toys, owners should not give them all to the puppy at once. They should provide a few toys and then, every day or two, rotate one or two with others they have packed away. This way, the toys retain their novelty and are fun for longer. Some toys can be held back for special games with the owner, and it may be safer only to allow unsupervised access to a subset that the puppy is unlikely to chew up and ingest when it is left alone.

When walking, ensure that the environment and length of the walk are appropriate to the age as well as the psychological and physical development of the puppy – that is how well is it likely to cope in the environment as well as how much stress is being put on developing musculoskeletal systems. The critical point of the walk is to give the puppy time to learn new things and meet its need for an investigation. Therefore, a shorter walk, where a puppy is allowed to investigate at its leisure (assuming it's safe and appropriate), is better than a longer route march where it cannot do this.

For puppies who are less inclined to spend time investigating, or those who are prone to focus on and potentially react to specific environmental stimuli, appropriate exploration can be encouraged by hiding treats in areas where you plan to take it to explore, which will encourage it to sniff. However, in general, rewarding a puppy for exploring is not necessary. Rewarding appropriate behaviour in the presence of stimuli such as people, other dogs and traffic is advisable as this sets a foundation for encouraging appropriate responses in the future.

When training basic behaviours, owners should focus on rewarding the behaviours they want and distract the puppy from, or ignore, undesired behaviour. Consistency through training allows the puppy to learn the pattern and progress faster. Owners should ensure that, between training sessions, they meet the puppy's needs and encourage calm behaviours.

Owners can refer to books and websites on trick training for suggestions of fun activities to teach as these not only can build an owner's relationship with their puppy but can also help the puppy to become more owner-focused and more likely to take an owner's directions in the future. If owners feel frustrated through training, they should stop and try engaging with play. If lack of success through training persists, the advice of a professional trainer can help.

6.6.6 Play biting

Puppies naturally explore the environment with their teeth, a fact that can give rise to both unwanted mouthing of people as well as destructive behaviours. Further, most puppy play includes biting, and people find this painful, so many puppies get into trouble for biting their family members. The key to appropriately stopping biting behaviour (assuming that it is playing- or exploration-related and not a distance-increasing behaviour) is to provide the pup with appropriate items to bite on and chew, and have these handy so that as soon as there is any indication that it is likely to bite, they can be substituted. Engaging in a game utilizing toys it can mouth at times when it wants to engage in this behaviour can very quickly teach it that the appropriate game is a fun activity. If, at the same time, all feedback for biting people is removed – people don't squeal, wave their limbs around, smack it or run away – then grabbing a person becomes devoid of fun for the pup, while grabbing a toy is greatly rewarding.

This behaviour may be more challenging in a household with children who may not be able to avoid reacting to a puppy bite. Owners should not allow puppies to interact with children unsupervised, and when a child interacts with the puppy, toys should be used to redirect biting behaviour from the child to the toy.

Teaching calm acceptance of handling will also assist in managing mouthing behaviour (see Section 6.5.3 on kitten handling for more advice).

Mouthing and biting behaviour can quickly escalate to problematic levels if it is not appropriately addressed. Therefore, specialist advice should be sought sooner rather than later if an owner is struggling.

6.6.7 Destructive behaviour

As mentioned above, puppies naturally explore the environment with their mouths. Additionally, as they teeth (from deciduous to permanent teeth), they may be more inclined to want to chew on things. It is essential that owners understand that chewing of prized possessions is not a malicious act but simply the puppy not knowing what it may and may not chew.

Owners should ensure that the puppy has appropriate chew toys; firm rubber food toys or chews are beneficial. Puppies vary in what they find attractive to chew, and therefore it is important to provide variety. Also, ensuring that these toys and chews are always available, and rewarding the puppy when it plays with them, helps to curb destructive chewing. Removing access to all items (e.g. shoes, children's toys, remote control devices) or preventing the puppy from accessing certain areas by using stairgates or doors will minimize the problem. When owners cannot control the environment, they should supervise the puppy.

If the puppy is chewing on an object that it is not supposed to, owners should not punish it. Instead, if possible (if the item is not immediately dangerous or valuable), they should try ignoring the puppy and creating a distraction which encourages it to leave the object to see what is happening elsewhere. Then the owner can remove the object and redirect the puppy to chew on a suitable item.

Chasing a puppy who has stolen a valuable or dangerous item and cornering it to remove it might turn this behaviour into a game or a sense of it needing to defend itself, both of which can lead to severe consequences later in life. Therefore, the distract-and-substitute route is usually best. In an emergency, a food lure or prized toy can be used to swap for the item it has, but this can create risks. However, it is still better than forcibly removing an item.

Over time, 'drop' and 'leave' cues can be taught, and in difficult situations specialist advice should be sought, but for most puppies the above advice works well.

6.6.8 Encouraging good behaviour

A new owner can help shape the behaviour they want by applying a few simple principles. Ensure that the puppy gets positive feedback in a way that it likes for all behaviour the owner desires. Manage situations to prevent the possibility that it can practise unwanted activities and behaviours and, where possible, should it manage to circumvent management and do something undesirable, the owner should think about whether this can be safely ignored (without leading to escalation or risk) or if they can use a distraction technique to break the behaviour. For example, leave the room and make interesting sounds out of the puppy's sight. Everyone in the family should always adhere to the same rules for the puppy as a consistent rule application means that it will find it easier to learn. Finally, ensure that, as well as having enough to do to burn physical energy and meet its needs for investigation and mental activity, it also has quiet times in its day where it is encouraged to calmly interact with its toys, chews and the environment.

6.7 What Do Owners Need to Know?

Many problems can be prevented by educating owners in what constitutes normal dog and cat behaviour, understanding how to read body language and how learning occurs (Gazzano *et al.*, 2008b).

Although teaching owners about reading dogs' and cats' communicative signals is beyond the remit of this chapter (see Section 7.3 – Body Language), research has shown that, even for owners who have had multiple dogs in the past, without good information they are not always able to correctly interpret their dog's communicative signals (Tami and Gallagher, 2009). The same is also likely for cats. Educating owners to understand signs of increasing arousal, signs of true play and affiliation, as well as distance-increasing signals, can help owners avoid putting their puppies and kittens in situations where they can't cope. It is better to take the pet away from a situation where they are demonstrating subtle distance-increasing signals or where arousal continues to rise so that unwanted behaviours are not practised. If we do not do this, we risk the pet learning that the only way out of a situation they do not like is through the use of extreme distance-increasing signals such as snapping, biting or scratching. Focus can then be put on appropriately teaching the pet to accept these situations in the future. It is critical to help owners understand that respecting their pet's feelings and calmly removing them from a situation where they are not coping, rather than 'making them do it' or 'not letting them get away with it', will, in the long term, avoid more severe problems.

Veterinary practices investing in means of educating dog and cat owners in these three areas are likely to reduce the incidence of problem behaviour development, increase pet welfare and increase owner satisfaction with their relationship with their pet (Seksel *et al.*, 1999; Duxbury *et al.*, 2003).

6.8 When Things Go Wrong

With the best intentions in the world, owners may still experience training or behaviour challenges with their puppy or kitten. Creating a practice atmosphere where owners can raise concerns regarding behaviour and where the practice actively solicits information about behaviour from owners can help ensure that behavioural concerns regarding young animals are addressed in a timely manner. We cannot overstate just how important it is that owners' concerns are addressed appropriately as soon as possible, as the alternative – an owner seeking potentially inappropriate advice from family and friends or the internet – can lead to problems worsening, becoming more resistant to modification in the long term and, potentially, leading to compromised safety and welfare of the pet and the family. The practice intervening to give good behavioural first aid advice early can sometimes be the difference between life and death for a pet.

6.8.1 Giving advice

As a first step, it is essential to educate owners that, for the most part, young animals do not 'grow out of' behaviours which owners are finding problematic or which may pose a risk or welfare concerns. The more behaviours are practised, the more difficult they will be to change in the long term. Behaviours are usually maintained because something is reinforcing them – either extrinsically or intrinsically – and thus they become learnt and more difficult to modify.

It is also important to be able to educate owners regarding normal species behaviour as some owners may not be aware of what behaviours lie within the normal range. Helping owners to be understanding can in some cases negate the need for intervention, or at least help them to be more sympathetic while they direct behaviours in a way that is more acceptable to them – for example, a kitten that is starting to scratch or bite during play or an adolescent male dog that is beginning to urine mark. However, sometimes it may be the onset of a behaviour that, if left, may develop into a true problem – for example, a puppy that is engaging in overly boisterous interactions with unfamiliar dogs or a kitten that is hiding when friends visit. This is the time to address the fact that behaviours like these won't be 'grown out of' and are likely to become more problematic.

For any behaviour which practice staff feel may lie outside of the normal range, it is important, even in a young animal, to undertake a full physical examination and rule out any possible underlying or contributory physical problems. From there on, the advice that needs to be given immediately is first aid advice; procedures to manage risk, prevent the problem from worsening and begin to improve the problem behaviour. Remember, although much of the advice given may seem to be commonsense, some owners will not have considered even basic interventions. And for owners who have, it is still essential to ensure that procedures are being implemented appropriately.

When managing risk, remember to consider the potential risk to the pet, people (owners as well as members of the public), other animals and property. When considering risk mitigation, it is important to discuss with the owner means of avoiding the situations eliciting the behaviour (in the immediate term) as well as avoiding opportunities for confrontation as these situations are likely to make the problem worse. The use of food to lure the pet away or the use of distraction techniques are all fine as short-term measures.

Preventing the problem from worsening is the crucial next approach. The following aspects should be addressed as first aid advice:

- Avoid triggers for the behaviour. If you only give one piece of behavioural advice, this should be it. Any behaviour which is practised over time will become stronger and may begin to generalize to other contexts, so preventing practice is essential. This may take some creativity, but it is worth taking time to explore with the owner options to achieve this. For example, if a dog isn't coping being left alone, can they leave it with a friend in the short term? If a dog is reacting to every person it sees on the street, consider not walking it until additional help can be sought. The latter means ensuring that the dog's needs are met in another way but giving the owner permission not to walk their dog can reduce stress in both dog and owner in the short term, mitigate risk and prevent the unwanted behaviour from being practised.
- Stop all punishment – even with the best plans to avoid the behavioural triggers, the behaviour may still occur, so explain to the owner the detrimental effects of reprimanding or otherwise punishing a dog or cat to try to suppress an unwanted behaviour should it occur. This does not mean a pet cannot be removed from a situation where a behaviour poses a risk. However, understanding that this may be perceived as punishment by the pet (with its associated fallout of increased frustration, for example) again helps owners to understand the better approach of avoiding the opportunity for the situation to arise in the first place.
- Ensure that the behaviour, if it does occur, is not reinforced. Just as punishment can give rise to numerous short- and long-term adverse consequences, inadvertently reinforcing an unwanted behaviour will strengthen it. Ensure that owners are not giving much attention when the behaviour occurs, for example. If food is being used to distract a pet from performing an unwanted behaviour, make it clear to an owner that unless it is an emergency and the pet needs to be distracted immediately, the food should be used to distract the pet to prevent the unwanted reaction, not delivered after the reaction is occurring.
- Manage incidents/behaviour appropriately. Both of the above can be summarized in this – give owners some tips on how to appropriately manage unwanted reactions – usually removing the pet as calmly and neutrally as possible from the situation is critical. Also, once the pet is out of the situation, where possible, if the pet is emotionally aroused by the incident, allowing it to calm down before expecting it to cope with anything else is essential.
- Implement the obvious. As mentioned before, sometimes people struggle to see an easy solution – for example, if a cat that has always used the outdoors as a toilet is house soiling, provide a litter tray.
- Try to ensure owners behave consistently – speak to the family about the importance of adhering to a single set of rules in all situations. If the same action from the pet will predictably elicit the same reaction from people every time, it removes from the pet a level of anxiety about interactions. This, in turn, can help the pet to feel less anxious, which can quickly improve some behaviours.

Finally, it is essential to begin to lay the foundation to start the process of behaviour change:

- Reinforce wanted behaviours – owners should start offering rewards when the pet shows desirable behaviours. For example, every time the pet is playing with its toys or otherwise appropriately amusing itself (resting quietly), offer praise or even – if it will not undermine the independent behaviour – engage with it in the activity. On a walk, if a dog that usually reacts to other dogs in a manner the owner finds inappropriate sees a dog and remains calm, praise and reward this with a food treat.
- If safe and appropriate to do so, start teaching some basic behaviours. For example, if the dog has not learnt any obedience cues, working on teaching it (using appropriate positive reinforcement techniques) to sit when asked and walk nicely on a lead can create foundations for later behaviour modification and will begin building the dog–owner relationship and training skills.
- Ensure the pet's daily needs are met – for example, if a cat doesn't have appropriate toilet facilities, sleeping places and enrichment opportunities, be sure to implement these. This starts to build a positive emotional state in the pet, which may later help with a behaviour modification plan.
- Meal feeding – this will, of course, be species- and individual-dependent, but for dogs, as food treats are commonly used to help modify behaviour, moving a dog that is fed *ad lib* to a meal schedule can help with later training.

6.8.2 Referring on and additional support

Although, for some pets, giving appropriate first aid advice that owners can and do implement may resolve the problem, or negate the need for further specialist support, there will be a number of patients for whom additional advice or a full behavioural and emotional assessment is advisable. If the practice cannot offer this service, this will necessitate a referral to a veterinary psychiatrist.

6.9 Conclusion

The veterinary practice can and should be the source of sound, appropriate and welfare-friendly advice on the acquisition and raising of puppies and kittens. If the team is aware of the range of influences which are likely to affect the adult behaviour of puppies and kittens, even before birth, they can appropriately advise both breeders and new owners on the best approach to take to shape these new young lives. This way we can maximize the chances of them settling into human society, experiencing good quality of life and contributing to human well-being.

6.10 Suggested Reading

- Bradshaw, J. and Ellis, S. (2016) *The Trainable Cat: A Practical Guide to Making Life Happier for You and Your Cat*. Basic Books, New York.
- Horwitz, D. and Mills, D. (2009) *BSAVA Manual of Canine and Feline Behavioural Medicine*. 2nd edition, Britsh Small Animal Veterinary Association.
- Mattinson, P. (2014) *The Happy Puppy Handbook: Your Definitive Guide to Puppy Care and Early Training*. Ebury Press.
- Pluijmakers, J., Appleby, J.P.D. and Bradshaw, J.W.S. (2003) Sensitive periods in the development of behavioural organization in the dog and the role of emotional homeostasis. Available at: https://www.semanticscholar.org/paper/1-SENSITIVE-PERIODS-IN-THE-DEVELOPMENT-OF-IN-THE-OF-Pluijmakers-Appleby/28c1add6b8c0eba2bcb8084f631f401ac46da5e7 (accessed 17 May 2020).
- Ryan, S. and Zulch, H. (2014) *No Walks? No Worries! Maintaining Wellbeing in Dogs on Restricted Exercise*. Hubble & Hattie, Dorchester, UK.
- Webster, S.D. (1997) Being sensitive to the sensitive period. In: Mills, D.S., Heath, S.E. and Harrington, L.J. (eds) *Proceedings of the First International Conference on Veterinary Behavioural Medicine*. Birmingham, UK, pp. 20–27.
- Zulch, H. and Mills, D. (2012) *Life Skills for Puppies: Building a Loving, Lasting Relationship*. Hubble and Hattie, Dorchester, UK.
- Zulch, H. and Mills, D. (2015) *Helping Minds Meet: Skills for a Better Life with Your Dog*. Hubble and Hattie, Dorchester, UK.

References

Appleby, D.L., Bradshaw, J.W.S. and Casey, R.A. (2002) Relationship between aggressive and avoidance behaviour by dogs and their experience in the first six months of life. *Veterinary Record* 150(14), 434–438. DOI: 10.1136/vr.150.14.434.

Battaglia, C.L. (2009) Periods of early development and the effects of stimulation and social experiences in the canine. *Journal of Veterinary Behavior* 4(5), 203–210. DOI: 10.1016/j.jveb.2009.03.003.

Bradshaw, J.W., Casey, R. and Brown, S. (2012) *The Behaviour of the Domestic Cat*, 2nd edn. CAB International, Wallingford, UK.

Caro, T.M. (1979) Relations between kitten behaviour and adult predation. *Ethology* 51(2), 158–168.

Caro, T.M. (1980) The effects of experience on the predatory patterns of cats. *Behavioral and Neural Biology* 29(1), 1–28. DOI: 10.1016/S0163-1047(80)92442-5.

Clarke, T., Cooper, J. and Mills, D. (2013) Acculturation: perceptions of breed differences in behavior of the dog (Canis familiaris). *Human-Animal Interaction Bulletin* 1(2), 16–33.

Collard, R.R. (1967) Fear of strangers and play behavior in kittens with varied social experience. *Child Development* 38(3), 877–891. DOI: 10.2307/1127265.

Duxbury, M.M., Jackson, J.A., Line, S.W. and Anderson, R.K. (2003) Evaluation of association between retention in the home and attendance at puppy socialization classes. *Journal of the American Veterinary Medical Association* 223(1), 61–66. DOI: 10.2460/javma.2003.223.61.

Ellis, S.L.H., Thompson, H., Guijarro, C. and Zulch, H.E. (2015) The influence of body region, handler familiarity and order of region handled on the domestic cat's response to being stroked. *Applied Animal Behaviour Science* 173, 60–67. DOI: 10.1016/j.applanim.2014.11.002.

Foyer, P., Wilsson, E., Wright, D. and Jensen, P. (2013) Early experiences modulate stress coping in a population of German shepherd dogs. *Applied Animal*

Behaviour Science 146(1-4), 79–87. DOI: 10.1016/j.applanim.2013.03.013.

Gaultier, E., Bonnafous, L., Vienet-Legué, D., Falewee, C., Bougrat, L. *et al.* (2008) Efficacy of dog-appeasing pheromone in reducing stress associated with social isolation in newly adopted puppies. *Veterinary Record* 163(3), 73–80. DOI: 10.1136/vr.163.3.73.

Gazzano, A., Mariti, C., Notari, L., Sighieri, C. and McBride, E.A. (2008a) Effects of early gentling and early environment on emotional development of puppies. *Applied Animal Behaviour Science* 110(3-4), 294–304. DOI: 10.1016/j.applanim.2007.05.007.

Gazzano, A., Mariti, C., Alvares, S., Cozzi, A., Tognetti, R. *et al.* (2008b) The prevention of undesirable behaviors in dogs: effectiveness of veterinary behaviorists' advice given to puppy owners. *Journal of Veterinary Behavior* 3(3), 125–133. DOI: 10.1016/j.jveb.2008.04.004.

Guardini, G., Mariti, C., Bowen, J., Fatjó, J., Ruzzante, S. *et al.* (2016) Influence of morning maternal care on the behavioural responses of 8-week-old beagle puppies to new environmental and social stimuli. *Applied Animal Behaviour Science* 181, 137–144. DOI: 10.1016/j.applanim.2016.05.006.

Jagoo, J.A. (1994) Behaviour problems in the dog: a retrospective and prospective study to identify factors influencing their development. Unpublished PhD Thesis. University of Cambridge. Reported in Jagoe, J.A. and Serpell, J. (1996) Owner characteristics and interactions and the prevalence of canine behaviour problems. *Applied Animal Behaviour Science* 47, 31–42.

Jokinen, O., Appleby, D., Sandbacka-Saxén, S., Appleby, T. and Valros, A. (2017) Homing age influences the prevalence of aggressive and avoidance-related behaviour in adult dogs. *Applied Animal Behaviour Science* 195, 87–92. DOI: 10.1016/j.applanim.2017.06.003.

Mills, D.S., Marchant-Forde, J.N., McGreevy, P.D., Morton, D.B., Nicol, C.J. *et al.* (2010) *The Encyclopedia of Applied Animal Behaviour and Welfare*. CAB International, Wallingford, UK.

Schoon, A. and Berntsen, T.G. (2011) Evaluating the effect of early neurological stimulation on the development and training of mine detection dogs. *Journal of Veterinary Behavior* 6(2), 150–157. DOI: 10.1016/j.jveb.2010.09.017.

Seksel, K., Mazurski, E.J. and Taylor, A. (1999) Puppy socialisation programs: short and long term behavioural effects. *Applied Animal Behaviour Science* 62(4), 335–349. DOI: 10.1016/S0168-1591(98)00232-9.

Serpell, J.A. and Duffy, D.L. (2016) Aspects of Juvenile and adolescent environment predict aggression and fear in 12-month-old guide dogs. *Frontiers in Veterinary Science* 3, 49. DOI: 10.3389/fvets.2016.00049.

Tami, G. and Gallagher, A. (2009) Description of the behaviour of domestic dog (*Canis familiaris*) by experienced and inexperienced people. *Applied Animal Behaviour Science* 120(3-4), 159–169. DOI: 10.1016/j.applanim.2009.06.009.

Taylor, K. and Mills, D.S. (2007) A placebo-controlled study to investigate the effect of Dog Appeasing Pheromone and other environmental and management factors on the reports of disturbance and house soiling during the night in recently adopted puppies (*Canis familiaris*). *Applied Animal Behaviour Science* 105(4), 358–368. DOI: 10.1016/j.applanim.2006.11.003.

Westgarth, C., Reevell, K. and Barclay, R. (2012) Association between prospective owner viewing of the parents of a puppy and later referral for behavioural problems. *Veterinary Record* 170(20), 517. DOI: 10.1136/vr.100138.

Wilsson, E. (2016) Nature and nurture – How different conditions affect the behavior of dogs. *Journal of Veterinary Behavior* 16, 45–52. DOI: 10.1016/j.jveb.2016.10.002.

7 Diagnosis

Daniel S. Mills[1]*, Lynn Hewison[1] and Sagi Denenberg[2,3]

[1]Joseph Banks Laboratories, School of Life Sciences, University of Lincoln, Lincoln, UK; [2]Langford Vets, University of Bristol, Langford, UK; [3]North Toronto Veterinary Behaviour Specialty Clinic, Toronto, Canada

7.1 Introduction

Reaching the correct diagnosis is, arguably, the most important aspect of veterinary psychiatry. While management is important, effective application relies on the appropriate diagnosis. Similarly, the choice of medications (when necessary) depends on knowing the underlying neurochemistry (see Chapter 9).

The terminology used for diagnosis varies and is confusing at times. It is essential to remember that if we are to provide optimal care with a good outcome, we should focus on the mechanism of the problem, not its name. A tendency exists to use descriptions of behaviours and contexts as diagnosis (e.g. aggression towards people, separation anxiety, or petting-induced aggression). A description tells us very little about the underlying mechanisms such as neurophysiological and neurochemical components, and emotions. We also need to consider other factors such as ontogeny and phylogeny, or the adaptive value of the behaviour. Diagnosing a dog with aggression towards other dogs, or a cat with redirected aggression is not a diagnosis; it is a description of a situation and is similar to diagnosing a patient as limping. The patient may show similar behaviours due to different underlying causes (e.g. damage property due to frustration, lack of stimulation, anxiety or panic).

We must follow medical diagnostic processes: collecting history and clinical signs, and examination of the patient (including observation of body language), before deciding on the likely underlying cause. As an example, limping is a clinical sign derived from pain following a rupture of the cruciate ligament amongst other lesions. To effectively treat the dog, we must know why it is limping and address the cause. Thus, if we want to practise medicine, we should reach a medical diagnosis. Changing behaviours without addressing the underlying cause is like giving pain control without investigating the cause of pain; it is not a good practice. It is worth noting that when we are unable to reach a diagnosis, we can still manage the syndrome (a group of clinical signs that commonly appear together). In these cases, we need to control the risks, attempt symptomatic care and possibly consider trial medication.

For the sake of simplicity, when communicating with owners, we can describe the context and behaviour; however, the diagnosis must be clearly communicated to the owner. For example, a dog may show separation distress due to anxiety, panic or frustration (or all of these). Using this example, we can then design a management plan that owners can implement.

To reach an accurate diagnosis, we must follow a process of collecting information (context and body language), discern between the different emotions and cognitive process, and evaluate the patient's ability to control its behaviours and emotions in the given situation. We must also rule out physical disorders eliciting or contributing to the presentation (see Chapters 2 and 3).

7.2 Context

Psychiatric disorders occur within a certain framework. This framework consists of elements such as genetics and epigenetics, triggers, environments, situations and patterns. When presented with a patient, we must first assess the context in which the problem occurs. It is essential to remember that more than one condition may exist within a patient

*Corresponding author: dmills@lincoln.ac.uk

DOI: 10.1079/9781786394552.0007

at the same time. It is usually the more salient presentation that the owner is focusing on. For example, owners often focus on a dog with an aggression problem and may overlook a separation-related problem. Other than looking at the immediate presentation, we must review the patient's environment, normal behaviours, routines, social interactions with the owner (and family), other animals, physical health, training, past attempts to manage the problem at hand, and the owners' goals.

Other than signalment, we should review the patient's past and current behaviours. Not always can owners provide all the necessary information, as in the case of adoption from shelters later in life. Unless reliable information was given to the owners at the time of adoption, we should not speculate about unknown information or reasons for relinquishment; we cannot change it at present and we might be biased in speculating. A typical example is owners believing that their dog was abused before adoption, and therefore it is fearful.

To help with gathering information, the use of questionnaires is helpful (see Handouts A3 – Behavioural Questionnaire – Cats; and A4 – Behavioural Questionnaire – Dogs). We should ask owners to fill these in and give them back before the consultation. Reviewing the questionnaires ahead of the consultation saves time and allows us to prepare. However, it is crucial to remember that questionnaires are not to be used instead of a discussion with the owners and observing the patient. Owners may not report all the necessary information for a variety of reasons, including embarrassment, not knowing what is important, or simply forgetting details. During a discussion about the patient and the problem, especially with a non-judgemental consultant, owners are likely to feel more comfortable and share more information.

Similarly, owners may interpret the situation differently and report their thoughts, not the actual presentation (see also Section 7.3.1). For example, owners may not describe aggression, believing that aggression is synonymous with a bite, or avoid the word aggression, thinking that it means the dog is 'bad' or 'vicious'.

During the consultation we should review the questionnaires with the owners and ask them to clarify and elaborate certain areas. Also, we can ask owners to describe how they feel (and observe their body language) about the problem and the patient (see also Section 1.2 – Communication Skills for Conversations about Behaviour).

7.2.1 Evaluation of what is normal

Often, but not always, the patient is presented with a suspected problem due to unmet needs. Cats (especially indoor-only cats) and dogs are captive animals; they depend on the owners for all their needs (e.g. exercise, social interactions, food, water and sleep). When their needs are not, or only partly met, the patient may become frustrated, anxious or even fearful.

All too often, owners rely on what is common rather than what is typical for animals in similar situations. This is partly the result of the plethora of information on the internet, talking to friends and neighbours, relying on experience with previous pets and soliciting the wrong advice. Examples include owners who feel that their dog sleeps adequately when it only sleeps seven to eight hours daily, or that cats do not require social interaction with their owners. For more information on normal behaviours and needs, see Chapters 4, 5 and 6.

When we review the situation, we must ensure that owners provide an optimal environment and routines. While most dog breeds (and, to a lesser extent, cats) were 'created' for a reason, it is also important to remember that some behaviours are universal (i.e. they apply to the domestic dog or domestic cat) and some are individual. Therefore, when assessing normal, we should know what is normal for dogs, for a particular breed, and for the individual. The latter is difficult. Many patients presented were never 'normal'; that is, they always displayed dysfunctional behaviours. Also, it is critical to remember that the variability within the breed is often higher than the variability between breeds.

7.2.2 Home environment

As part of each case evaluation, we should review the environment in which the patient lives. Not only the physical environment should be evaluated, but also the social environment must be assessed. Reviewing the environment may shed light on possible reasons and triggers for the problem.

When a house call is not available, owners should describe the home (videos, photos and schematics may help), including areas for feeding, sleeping and resting, play and elimination. As part of the physical environment, we should review areas where owners walk their dogs, and the presence of other animals in those areas (e.g. other cats coming into the garden).

The social environment includes the family, other pets at home and any social interactions the patient has with other animals outside the home. Questions should include the level of interaction and approach each family member has with the patient, the presence of young children and any other caretakers (e.g. dog walker, sitter or trainers).

7.2.3 Normal (daily) behaviours

It is easy to focus on the presentation (i.e. the problem) and overlook other aspects of the patient's life. This is a mistake. As part of our evaluation, we should review the patient's entire life. Reviewing the patient's feeding routine (e.g. frequency, diets, treats and chews), pattern (e.g. grazing vs 'inhaling'), sleep and rest, play, exercise and elimination, helps us ensure that the patient's needs are met and to identify any problems or triggers.

For example, many anxious animals tend to eat either too fast or show signs of anorexia. Similarly, when a patient eats well and takes treats readily, but refuses the same treat at other times, we should examine those times it refuses the treat. Similarly, the patient may stop eating as the owner approaches it. The patient may not show aggression; it may even not raise its head from the bowl. However, a closer look at the patient may indicate a tense body and the patient might be looking at the owner from the corner of its eye. This conveys information about the patient; it may be anxious or frustrated (see Fig. 7.1).

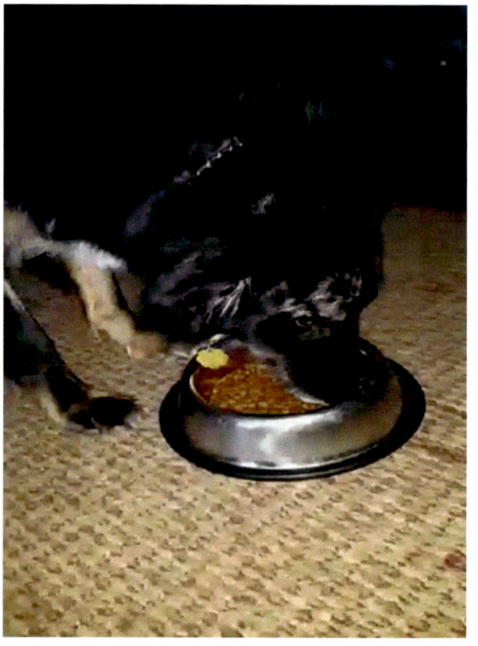

Fig. 7.1. Dogs who are anxious or frustrated when their owners (or someone else, including another animal) approaches may change their behaviour. The change may not be noticeable (e.g. aggression) but may be subtle such as staring towards the owner from the corner of its eyes without moving. (Photo courtesy of Sagi Denenberg.)

Some patients may appear to be sleeping (lying down, eyes closed and breathing calmly), but as soon as the owner exits the room, the patient immediately follows. This pattern indicates hypervigilance, mostly as a result of anxiety. When mentally healthy animals sleep, they do not wake up in response to minimal sounds and are not following the owners all over the home. Owners may describe their pet as their shadow, feeling that it is normal and even desirable. However, such behaviours often indicate an unhealthy bond between the two.

Dogs on walks use their senses, especially vision, olfaction and hearing, to acquire information from the environment. When letting dogs off the lead, the confident dog ventures away from the owner, engaging in exploration. Some owners may describe their dog as checking on them or staying by their side all the time. While these behaviours might be desired by the owners, they may also indicate anxiety, especially the dog staying close to the owner to feel more comfortable. Similarly, dogs who are not engaged with the environment but are constantly looking around (owners may describe them as 'having their head on a swivel') may be showing signs of hypervigilance.

Cats may also show over-dependency on their owners, including following them around the home and waiting for them at the door when they arrive. These behaviours, too, may indicate anxiety and the patient's need for reassurance.

7.2.4 Routine

Reviewing the daily routine allows us to evaluate if the patient's needs are met regularly. Also, we can evaluate any necessary adjustment. Each day, owners should provide the patient not only with food, water and opportunities to eliminate, but also with social interactions (e.g. affection, play and training), exercise, and sufficient time to sleep and rest.

Routine means more than a daily schedule, it also means that owners are consistent in how they interact with the patient. The schedule may vary depending on different factors such as the owner's work schedule and the day of the week. However, the routine should remain similar. That is, if the owner provides a morning walk, then it should be given daily, even if some days it is at seven in the morning and other days it is at eight. Cats and dogs are creatures of routine and have their biological rhythms adjusted after some time. Changes in routine may affect them negatively.

7.2.5 Reactivity

The next step is to review how the patient reacts in different situations or to different triggers. This is not a temperament test; many temperament tests done in an artificial environment or setting are no more than an indication of how the patient performed during the test (Patronek and Bradley, 2016). In other words, a patient that passed 'with flying colours' may still fail in real life.

We can examine the patient's typical reactivity by direct observation (or videos), when possible, or a series of questions about different situations, asking owners to describe not only the behaviour but also the patient's body language (see Section 7.3). It is important to stress to owners not to capture videos if the process places someone, including the patient, in danger when doing so.

Questions should be grouped based on the interaction. First, we should ask about the patient's interactions with the owners and the immediate family. It is important to note that people the patient meets frequently may be considered family even when there are no 'family ties' to the owners. In other words, a close friend who visits regularly is more of a family member to the patient than an owner's relative who visits once a year. Questions should include details about play behaviours, exercise, giving affection, handling (e.g. bathing, administering medications, or brushing), and greeting and departure.

The next groups of interactions to inquire about are interactions with other family pets, other people and animals, situations and environment. For example, questions should include details about the patient's behaviour during loud noises, when left alone at home, at the veterinary practice, during travel and in new environments.

Each scenario should follow a similar line of questioning. We should inquire about the patient's behaviour, body language, intensity, recovery (the time it takes the patient to return to its previous behaviour once the interaction ended) and frequency of reactivity.

7.2.6 Presentation

Once we have reviewed the patient's environment, routines, reactivity and normal behaviours, we can start focusing on the presenting complaints. It is important to let the owners describe the situation in as much detail as possible. However, we should ensure that the conversation stays on track and provides us with the necessary details. This can be achieved by asking a series of questions that help direct the discussion (see also Section 1.2). If owners have videos or photos of the patient when it presents the behaviour, we should review those at this time.

The description of the problem should follow a chronological order. The owners should describe the problem as it first started, how it evolved, and the current situation. Also, when possible, owners should attempt to describe what happens before the patient starts showing the problem, the problem itself, and the consequences.

Owners should describe the behaviour but should try staying descriptive rather than analytical. It is vital to review the patient's behaviour and body language (see Section 7.3), not the owner's interpretation. Focus on details such as body parts (e.g. eyes, ears, tail, fur), vocalization and posture. Moreover, the entire behaviour of the patient is important. We should note details such as conflict, displacement behaviours or fidgeting (see Section 7.3). Finally, we should verify if the owner can predict, based on body language, the emanating change (and therefore might be able to implement prevention).

The next group of questions should focus on possible triggers. Questions should include details about the environment, who is present (people and other animals) and frequency. When possible, owners should provide details about the intensity of the trigger. These details may include the distance from the trigger when the problem starts, the loudness of the noise, or duration of being alone before showing any changes in behaviour. These numbers can help in designing the management programme later.

7.2.7 Previous attempts

Often when patients are presented to veterinarians, particularly in referral practices, the owners have tried managing the problems already. Therefore, we should question the owners about these past attempts and why they failed (they would not come to us if they had succeeded). These attempts may, in fact, have worsened the problem.

Possibly some of these attempts would have succeeded if the owners were consistent, persistent or had more patience. Often the right approach is taken but the timing is inappropriate. Many trainers, for example, and owners tend to rush and start implementing behaviour modification techniques as soon as possible. We must remember that many of our patients are not ready, mentally and emotionally, to absorb new information and learn how to react (see Section 7.4). However, we must also appreciate that owners are doing their best, and in many cases the failure of a treatment plan can be very informative in terms of ruling out competing explanations for the behaviour; for example if the animal was anxious, this should have worked, and failure may indicate the animal is frustrated instead.

7.3 Body Language

Our patients communicate with their social environment, including their owners, us and other animals, using body postures, facial features and vocalization. Intimate knowledge of the cat's and dog's body language is imperative for an accurate diagnosis (see Handouts B1- Body Language – Cat; and, B2 – Body Language – Dog). A detailed description or observation of the patient's body language, vocalization and context is necessary to decipher the information. Furthermore, observing physiological changes is helpful. Only then can we make an inference of the underlying emotional, mental and, therefore, neurophysiological and neurochemical states, and reach the diagnosis.

Like verbal language, body language changes over time. Adults not only learn how to interact and present the appropriate signs compared to the kitten or puppy, but they also change and adapt. The patient may learn which aspects of communication help and which do not. As a result, the language the patient may presently show may differ from that in the past. For example, a dog may have given signs such as a stare and growl in the past when approached by a threatening person. With time, if the problem persists (that is, people continue to approach), the patient may stop staring and growling, realizing these signs are ineffective. Instead, the patient may lunge and bite immediately, without warning. Therefore, when reviewing body language we should also attempt to find out any past signals. Expecting the patient to follow a typical pattern of escalation might be dangerous at times.

When discussing body language with owners, we must remember two important aspects. First, it is important to avoid fallacies such as wagging tail means happiness or excitement, purring is pleasure and contentment, or growling is viciousness. Second, primarily in dogs, human-made interventions may alter the patient's ability to communicate appropriately. It is 'nice' to describe the tail, ears, mouth and body positions, or the eyes and hackles, to describe the body language, but, in reality, it might be far more complicated. Unfortunately, some dogs have docked tails, cropped ears, or they have been devocalized. Also, different breeds may have facial and body features that prevent them from communicating appropriately (see Fig. 7.2).

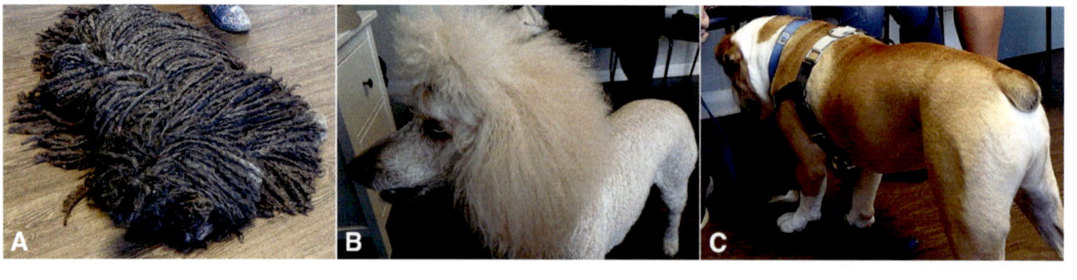

Fig. 7.2. Through many years of selective breeding, we have created breeds of dogs that significantly differ from the ancestor dog in appearance. As a result, their ability to communicate effectively might be reduced as effective communication requires certain body postures, facial features and vocalization. In some cases, we cannot see the ears, eyes or hackles of the dog. The ears (A) tail (B) or position (C) of some dogs are difficult to assess. (Photos courtesy of Sagi Denenberg.)

Finally, different grooming may alter the dog's ability to communicate (e.g. fur covering the face, or shaving that prevents us seeing hackles).

7.3.1 Anthropomorphism

As humans, we naturally tend to interpret situations and behaviours from our point of view. When we do so with animals, we engage in anthropomorphism or the attribution of human characteristics to an animal which may be invalid as we have evolved to adapt to very different environments and have very different levels of cognitive development. Examples include owners who describe their animal as 'known to have done something wrong', 'remorseful', 'guilty' or 'did it for spite'.

We must ask owners to describe the body language they see, rather than interpreting it. There is something in the body language of the patient that has led the owners to interpret it the way they did. For example, when owners return home and find that the dog caused damage, and, when they walked through the door, the dog ran to them and showed signs of 'guilt'. In many cases, the owners may describe a dog that cowers near them, ears backwards, low tail and eyes wide open.

Not only is anthropomorphism not helpful, it may lead to a negative or aversive approach during management. If owners believe their animal did something 'wrong', although it 'should have known better' or that it did it 'out of spite', the owners may elect to punish their animals. It may also lead to owner frustration at not being successful in teaching their animal to behave appropriately.

7.3.2 Conflict

When the patient is caught between *approach* and *avoidance*, it may show a *conflict-related behaviour*. The patient is expressing behaviours that are related to two (or more) incompatible motivations. For example, a stranger may offer a fearful dog a treat. The dog may want the treat; however, it also wants to stay away from the stranger (see Fig. 7.3A and B). The patient may approach a few steps and then back away, stretch towards the person but not walk to the person, or it may take the treat and run away. Other examples include growling and tail wagging, taking a treat and dropping it, circling, or sniffing a second cat but avoiding direct contact. In intense conflicts, aggression may result. During conflict situations, the patient may show vacuum activities, displacement behaviours or redirected behaviours (see below).

Conflict raises the patient's arousal level and reduces our ability to interact with the patient (see Section 7.4.3). Conflict-related behaviours also tend to confuse owners. They see their animal showing signs of willingness to interact and then may bite. It is worth noting that conflict may stretch along a temporal line. This is most likely to occur with owners. For example, owners may feed their animal, play with it, give affection and treats, and take it for walks. These are all interactions and resources

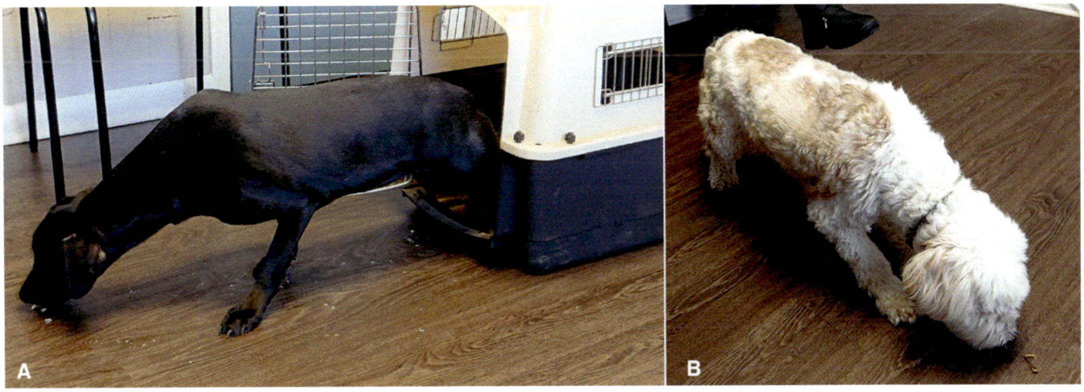

Fig. 7.3. These dogs show conflict; they want the treat in front of them, but do not want to leave the safety of the crate (A), or approach the person who offered the treat (B). Note how they stretch instead of approach. (Photos courtesy of Sagi Denenberg.)

the animal wants and, as a result, it shows positive interactions with the owner. However, owners may also do things their animal dislikes such as nail trims, brushing or punishing. These different interactions may lead the patient to show conflict when the owner approaches it.

Often, conflict depends on the patient's ability to exercise executive control of its emotions. Negative emotions, such as fear, anxiety or frustration, may lead to a negative bias (Harding *et al.*, 2004). Therefore, patients with negative emotions will show a higher degree of conflict, given that their ability to perceive information is negatively skewed.

One of the management goals is to avoid conflict whenever possible. It is difficult in many cases and nearly impossible to eliminate all conflicts. However, the approach is one of progress, not perfection. For example, owners of a patient that is fearful of unfamiliar people should not attempt to 'socialize' the patient at the early stages of the management. Similarly, veterinarians should not offer a treat to a fearful patient and a minute later 'manhandle' it and stab it with a sharp object. Owners should also attempt to minimize conflict involving them – for example, punishing and offering treats later.

7.3.3 Fixed-action pattern

Animals, like people, show different behaviours that are relatively rigid in their pattern, speed and expression. These behaviours may be a specific stimulus (or social releaser) and called a *fixed-action pattern* (Lorenz and Tinbergen, 1970). Some reflexes can be considered a fixed-action pattern. Other examples of fixed-action patterns include a dog that is lifting its leg to countermark, even though its bladder is empty, or a cat that is hunting when it sees a mouse, even though it is not hungry. When fixed-action patterns occur out of context or disconnected from their releasing signs, they indicate a high arousal level (see Fig 7.4 for some example behaviours).

7.3.3.1 Vacuum activities

When patients have a high arousal level, they may show a fixed-action pattern; however, the releasing signal is missing. The patient is then said to be showing *vacuum activity*. Examples include mounting behaviours, fly-snapping, frantic and random sprinting in the garden or at home, or scratching the floor before lying down.

7.3.3.2 Displacement behaviours

As a result of high arousal, the patient may show normal behaviours that appear out of context, also known as *displacement behaviours* (behaviours displaced from one context to another). For example, yawning when not tired, or lip-licking when no food or water are present on its lips. Four observations can help to identify whether what the owner describes is normal or displacement:

- the behaviour is out of context;
- the behaviour is repetitive;
- the behaviour occurs with other displacement behaviours (e.g. yawning and lip-licking); and
- we can reproduce the behaviour by placing the patient in a similar situation in the future.

Common displacement behaviours include yawning, lip-licking, full-body and head shaking, stretching, squinting, sneezing, 'huffing' and whole body (wet dog) shakes, and possibly flashing alterations of gaze (see Fig. 7.4).

7.3.3.3 Redirected behaviour

Inaccessible triggers may still elicit fixed-action patterns in patients. *Redirected behaviours* occur when the patient shows a fixed-action pattern towards a trigger which is not the original releasing signal. For example, a cat who cannot go outside to hunt a bird may redirect its behaviour towards another animal or person at home. Similarly, a cat that is 'bullied' by a stronger cat in the home may redirect its behaviour towards a third cat, or a dog who is herding family members, or young children when it cannot herd sheep. In this case the apparent 'aggression' may be a single swat, which then escalates.

7.4 Executive Control of Behaviour and Emotion

The brain is an active organ and so cannot be switched off as such. However, it does engage in a lot of suppression to prevent chaos. At any given time, various actions are competing for expression, and while the traditional view focuses on how certain behaviours (responses) are encouraged or triggered or stimulated by environmental events

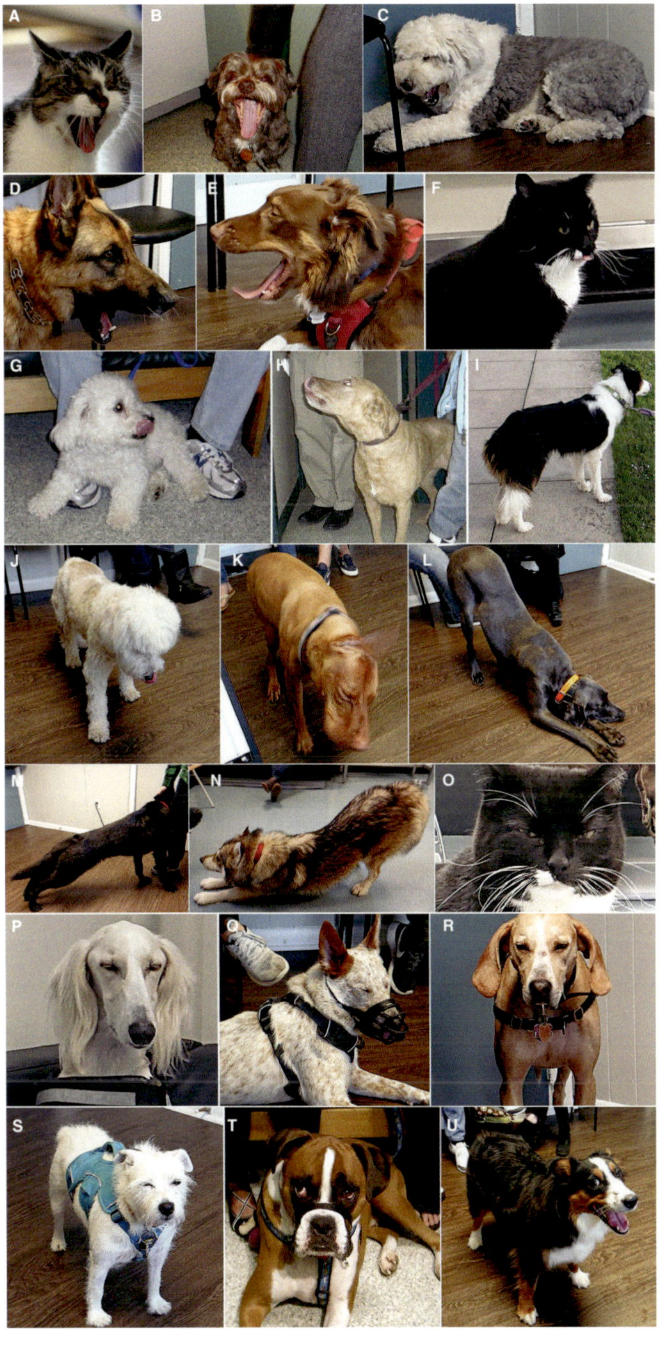

Fig. 7.4. Displacement behaviours are normal behaviour shown out of context. The patient is likely to show several of those behaviours when they are highly aroused (see Section 7.4.3). These behaviours are subconscious; the patient is not electing to show them. These behaviours are all normal; however, the appropriate releasing signal is missing Common displacement behaviours include yawning (A–E), lip licking (F–J), full body and head shake (K), stretching (L-N), squinting (O-S), and averted gaze or looking from the corner of the eyes (T and U). Presence of these behaviours should alert the owner that the patient arousal level is increasing. (Photos courtesy of Sagi Denenberg.)

(stimuli), a neurobiological perspective focuses more on understanding how these factors release inhibitions. Some behaviours have very simple associations with events, and these might be termed reflexes. However, most behaviours have a wide variety of factors affecting them, and so are subject to control by a variety of influences from both the internal and external environment, which are integrated to produce a decision. These processes of integration and behavioural control through the release of inhibition are referred to as the executive control processes governing the expression of behaviour. For example, although many animals may appear to become very aggressive at the slightest provocation, threat displays are potentially risky since they could provoke an aggressive response in return, and even if the patient wins a fight it could still be injured. It is not surprising that evolution has favoured individuals who assess many factors before making this decision (even if it is made very rapidly). Many behaviours have diverse consequences depending on the circumstances, and the subjective evaluation of these is one of the functions of emotion.

7.4.1 Impulsivity

The speed with which decisions are made about whether to respond is reflected in the animal's level of impulsivity. Thus, in general, we might say that cats are perhaps more impulsive than dogs, but certain dogs may be more impulsive than others. Impulsivity is a trait, not a condition, and refers to the tendency towards rapid, unplanned reactions to internal or external stimuli, potentially without a fully functional evaluation of the consequences of this action to the individual or others. A key feature of impulsivity is the extent to which a fully functional evaluation of the consequences of an action is often made. Thus, more impulsive individuals are, potentially, more likely to make bad decisions when there are potentially aversive consequences that are not overt. Often more impulsive individuals overestimate rewards and underestimate costs compared to less impulsive individuals. This is not a problem when the environment is safe (and there are few costs). However, when there are greater risks, such as the risk of coming into conflict with others, this can be problematic. A consequence of poor decision making is that the individual might find itself in a more tricky situation or find it is frustrated, so more impulsive individuals are often more emotionally reactive and are at greater risk of encountering situations that will lead to frustration. Unless the individual has developed appropriate skills to cope with such frustration, this can lead to a wide range of problems, such as intensive vocalization (meowing in cats and whining, barking or howling in dogs, depending on the circumstance) or aggressive displays as the animal seeks to escape from the situation. The solution to these problems lies in either teaching the individual to be less impulsive or teaching it to cope with the emotional arousal in a more acceptable way (see Chapter 8). It would be wrong to assume that impulsivity was the root of all problems relating to emotional arousal. Therefore, we will consider emotional responses in more detail first.

7.4.2 Emotions and emotional processing

The brain is presented with a mass of information every second; it must decide which information needs greater attention and processing than others. It is natural and highly adaptive to give extra weight to stimuli associated with harm, i.e. harmful stimuli (punishers) or stimuli that signal harm (conditioned punishers). However, harm is not the only important factor an animal needs to attend to; many other important qualities need to be evaluated.

In a given environment, animals will, potentially, process all this information relating to relevant stimuli and then decide on the appropriate action based on their perceptions and priorities. Emotional processes serve to allow this, and different emotions may be associated with different stimuli.

It would be a mistake to think that animals do not possess similar emotions to humans simply because we cannot ask our patients. Even in humans, it is estimated that 93% of all communication is non-verbal (Yaffe, 2011). We can see a different individual in a particular situation, and based on their body language, behaviour and tone of voice, understand how they feel. Similarly, many owners can see their animal and recognize their emotional state. This, however, may reflect a degree of anthropomorphism and we should be cautious about such claims. With the advances of science and imaging techniques such as functional magnetic resonance imaging and positron emission tomography, more and more data allow us to see that animals possess similar circuits to humans, and hence are likely to experience similar basic emotions (Berns *et al.*, 2012). Moreover, recent studies were able to differentiate facial features related to different emotional circuits, and future studies are likely to reveal more (Finka *et al.*, 2014; see also www.animalfacs.com).

To avoid anthropomorphism and to clarify the diagnosis, we regard emotions as diffuse neural networks, building on the work of the late Panksepp (1998). There are eight well-established networks, and each provides the animal with a strategy to manage through different situations it encounters. When each network is activated (aroused), the animal will respond accordingly. We should keep in mind that while these systems are relatively discrete, they are not mutually exclusive; more than one system may be activated at one time. These networks are divided into two groups: networks related to the individual (e.g. fear, frustration, pain and desire) and social networks (attachment figures, dependants, affiliates and sexual partners). There is ongoing debate about the distinctiveness of a ninth circuit associated with social exclusion.

7.4.2.1 Fear and anxiety

This network is probably the one we will encounter the most in our caseload (see Chapter 13). The main function of this system is survival. As long as the environment and routine are predictable and safe, the system will not be activated. However, once it is activated by a threatening trigger (fear) or the anticipation of such a situation (anxiety), the patient will react. This network will initiate a strategy to avoid or repulse the trigger. The exact behaviour depends on the quality and intensity of the trigger, past experiences and the environment. Whenever possible, the goal is to avoid the trigger, not to fight it. Fighting also means taking a chance of getting hurt or dying. Hence, from an evolutionary point of view, it is better to avoid it. Therefore, the patient may show an elaborate sequence of behaviours, postures and vocalization in an attempt to repulse the trigger when it cannot avoid it. For example, cats may arch their backs, hiss and growl, and show piloerections, ears pinned back and dilated pupils. Dogs may growl, snarl, bark and stare, and show raised hackles, ears backwards and low tail. It is prudent to warn owners that there are cases where there are no signs; it depends on the intensity of the trigger, the time the patient has to react and the proximity.

7.4.2.2 Frustration

Animals need different resources to maintain an optimal functional level. These resources may include food, water, toys, proximity and contact with the owner, sleeping areas and litter trays. When the animal cannot control these resources or protect them, or its access to the resource is denied, the frustration network will be activated. The result may be irritability and aggression (the rage component of the network). However, unlike aggression in the case of fear and anxiety, in the case of frustration, the body language suggests that the patient is not willing to back down. For example, cats may show straight, not arched, back, their tail will be rigid and bent downwards, ears forward or rotated to the side, and vocalize with a lower pitch. Dogs may stare directly towards the trigger, not from the corner of their eyes, snarl with partly, not fully, open mouth, their ears pointing forward. Overall, the patient appears as trying to go forward, not avoiding. When the patient cannot reach its trigger, it may redirect its behaviour towards another animal or person nearby. For more details see Chapter 13.

7.4.2.3 Pain

When a body system is damaged or becomes dysfunctional, the pain network is activated (see Chapter 3). The purpose of this system is to protect the body from further damage. The trigger may be actual damage (injury or disease) or anticipated damage. It is worth noticing that activation of this system may lead, in similar situations in the future, to activation of the fear-anxiety network.

7.4.2.4 Desire

Animals need resources such as shelter, food and water for survival. This network triggers seeking and exploration behaviours for resources the animal desires. This is not the same as desiring a mate (see Section 7.4.2.8). When this system is activated, we may see behaviours such as attention-seeking behaviours, counter-surfing (see Chapter 10) and predatory aggression. Predation is the consequence of the desire to acquire resources. Solitary play is also activated by this network, possibly as a learning experience for predation skills. Inactivity of this network may cause apathy and withdrawal from any activity to seek resources (e.g. anorexia).

7.4.2.5 Grief

This network is part of the social emotions network and concerns attachment figures and other social contacts. Even in species that are traditionally considered solitary such as the domestic cat, social interactions, especially with attachment figures (people or other animals) are important for survival. Loss of social contact leads to activation of this system. The loss could be permanent (e.g. death of a family member or pet) or temporary (e.g. owners leaving for work or vacation). Activation of this network leads the patient to show behaviours that are meant to regain social contact. These behaviours may include vocalization, trying to follow the attachment figure and restlessness. In more severe cases, a full panic may develop leading to more intense reactions such as separation distress (see Chapter 13).

7.4.2.6 Care

The purpose of this network is protecting dependants. Both females and males can display behaviours related to care. The activation of this network is mostly in the presence of dependent offspring or equivalents; however, it can be seen in other cases when the patient feels the need to protect another animal or person or in relation to inanimate objects, for example toys gathered to the nest in a case of false pregnancy. The patient may show aggression to protect the dependant, nesting, or if the system is disrupted, rejection of dependants and infanticide.

7.4.2.7 Social play

This network is responsible for social interactions such as mutual play and developing social ties with other animals. Play can be considered, especially in young animals, as learning experience directed towards adulthood. The young animal learns about its abilities to interact with other animals and people, hunt, and even mate, through social play. When this network is inhibited, the patient may show dysfunctional play patterns (e.g. too aggressive, avoiding or without appropriate signals).

7.4.2.8 Lust

The lust network organizes behaviour related to finding a mate and copulation. As a result of hormonal activation, this system is sexually dimorphic, and activation depends on the reproductive status of the patient. Those that were neutered early, before the system became active, are less likely to show behaviour related to this network. Activation of this network may lead to behaviours such as marking, aggression towards rivals, and attempts to mate.

7.4.3 Arousal

We have mentioned the word arousal many times throughout this chapter, and others. What is arousal? Arousal is a general physiological response to an emotional or physical trigger. The purpose of arousal is to prepare the individual for action. Arousal is not an emotion or thought, and does not have a positive or negative quality built in to it. Positive emotions such as joy and happiness as well as negative emotions such as fear and frustration can trigger increased arousal. The result of either can lead (if the level is too high) to problematic behaviours. The relationship between arousal and performance was first described by Yerkes and Dodson (1908) over a century ago and was further explained by (Easterbrook, 1959). The Yerkes-Dodson Law (YDL) describes two relationships between arousal level and performance. In a simple task, as the arousal level increases, the performance increases almost in a linear fashion, finally levelling. However, when the task is complicated, the trend is different. At first, the level of performance increases as arousal level increases; however, at some point, the level of arousal continues to increase, while performance decreases (creating a bell curve – see Fig. 7.5).

The basic principle of the YDL is that once arousal crosses the optimal level, the performance of the animal, or its ability to absorb information and interact with its environment decreases. This is believed to be at the core of many of the problems we see in our patients.

It is worth noting that the YDL is a simplification, considering the complex relationship between cognitive processes and emotional arousal. The assumption that the animal's ability to process information and execute cognitive functions is low when highly aroused might be incorrect (Storbeck and Clore, 2008). From an adaptive (evolutionary) point of view, it is possible that when the arousal level exceeds a certain threshold, the brain purposely blocks signals that are not relevant for survival, rather than is unable to process the information.

From the moment the animal perceives the information until the brain networks are fully activated

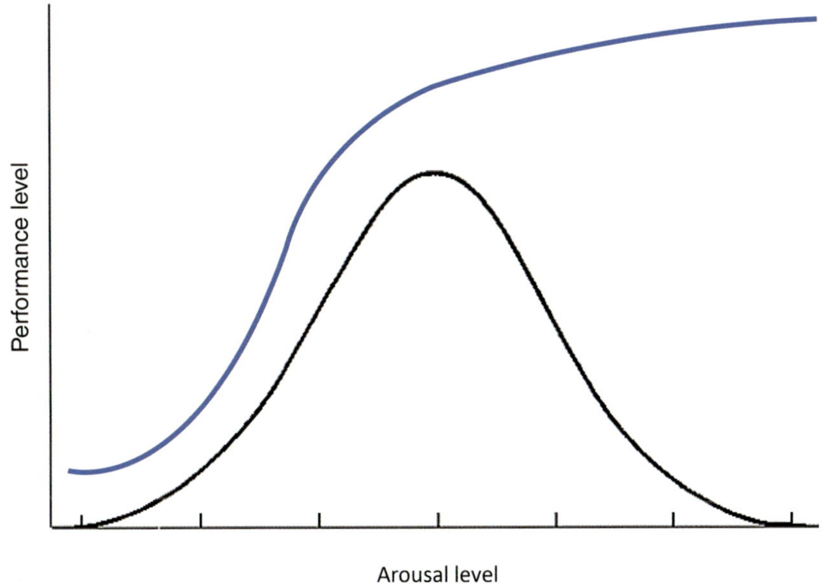

Fig. 7.5. When the task is simple, the level of performance increases with the level of arousal, until it reaches a plateau (blue line). When the task is more complicated, the level of performance initially increases as arousal increases; however, if the level of arousal continues to increase, the level of performance drops (black line). (Adapted from Yerkes and Dodson, 1908.)

(aroused), approximately three quarters of a second have passed. In contrast, it can take minutes, hours, and sometimes even longer, before the physiological and emotional levels return to preactivation level (see Fig. 7.6). The rate of reduction depends on factors such as personality, environment, the intensity of the trigger and cognitive biases.

When owners are first introduced to the concept of arousal, they may find it confusing, especially how arousal is affecting their animal. Maintaining a diary is helpful both to identify signs of increasing arousal (when and where) and to monitor future progress. A diary is also a tool to train owners to identify conflict-related behaviours, displacement

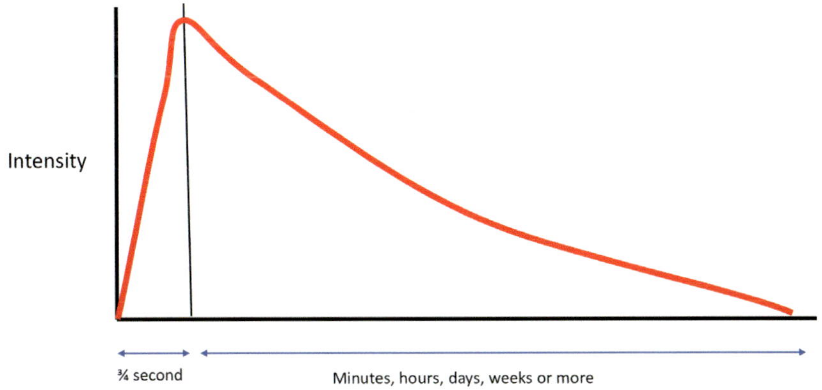

Fig. 7.6. The level of arousal increases rapidly, while the recovery period (the time it takes the animal to return to the preactivation level) may be much longer. As a result, the animal may stay alert for long periods and can be triggered faster and higher while still recovering from the previous activation. This underpins the phenomenon commonly referred to as "trigger stacking" over an extended time.

behaviours and triggers (see Handout A7 – Behaviour Diary Template).

7.4.3.1 Emotional arousal

Once one of the emotional networks (see Section 7.4.2) is activated, we consider the animal to be emotionally aroused. The activation is a result of an emotional or cognitive trigger (e.g. threat, sexual partner or food). Activation of any of those networks activates an instinctual strategy that helps the animal to choose the correct behaviour. For example, when a cat sees a threat, the fear–anxiety network is activated. Then, based on the distance, intensity of the trigger and the cat's ability to execute a behaviour (e.g. pain, disease and environmental options), a behaviour is chosen. If, say, the threat is a far-away dog, the cat is physically healthy and the environment has no limitations (e.g. closed space), the cat will choose to run away. However, if the environment limits the cat from running away, or the cat has a musculoskeletal disease that prevents it from running, it may attack instead. Similarly, a dog on-lead knows it is unable to avoid an approaching person and may elect to repulse or become inhibited, if it is afraid of the person, whereas a dog off-lead can choose to avoid, if it is afraid of the person.

7.4.3.2 Physiological arousal

When an emotional network is activated, the body must be ready to react. Therefore, the brain will initiate a physiological reaction that prepares the body for activity. Physiological arousal involves the activation of the sympathetic nervous system (SNS) and the hypothalamic-pituitary axis (HPA). The result of this activation is an alert mode of the brain and body. This reaction is mediated primarily by the locus coeruleus (LC), the main alertness-inducing nucleus (Carlson and Birkett, 2017). The LC has rich and widespread excitatory projections throughout the cerebral cortex. These include serotoninergic neurones of the dorsal raphe, cortically projecting neurones of the thalamus, and considerable inhibitory effect on the sleep-promoting GABAergic neurones in the basal forebrain and ventrolateral preoptic area. In addition, the LC has direct projections to the spinal cord, and different nuclei (e.g. vagus, ambiguus, caudal raphe and the amygdala). As a result, LC activation leads to increased activity of the SNS (see Fig. 7.7) and reduced activity of the parasympathetic system (Samuels and Szabadi, 2008).

Chronic or intense activation of physiological arousal can lead to behaviour changes such as hyposomnia or insomnia, restlessness and pacing (fidgeting), anorexia or hyperphagia, disconnecting from the owners when faced with a trigger, and conflict-related behaviours.

7.4.3.3 Thresholds

Not all triggers are equal, nor do all lead to undesired behaviours. The intensity of the trigger, the patient's emotional state and biases, and the environment join in to modulate the intensity of the arousal. It is important to remember that the patient's genetic component is critical; different individuals will respond differently in the same situation (Scott and Fuller, 1965; Reese, 1978). Epigenetic factors such as maternal care, prenatal maternal factors (e.g. malnourishment, anxiety or hyperadrenocorticism), and early separation from

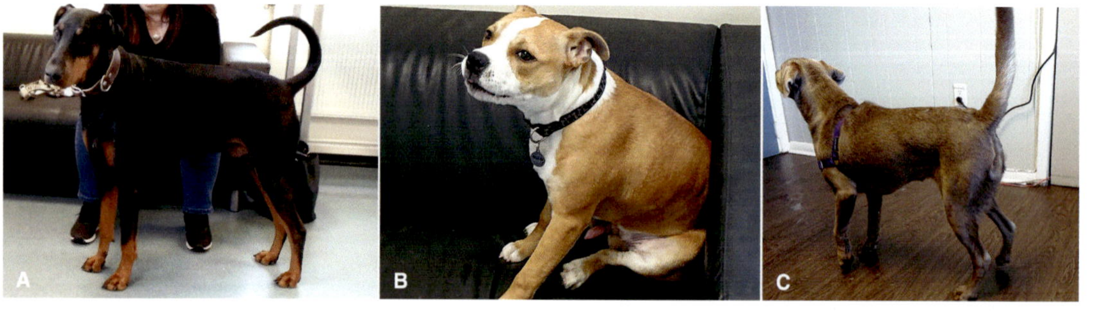

Fig. 7.7. High physiological arousal leads to changes in body language and postures such as tense muscles (A), erection (B) and piloerection (C). (Photos courtesy of Sagi Denenberg.)

the mother can also contribute to the development of future arousal responses (Pierantoni *et al.*, 2011).

Arousal is a normal response; it is meant to help the individual survive. However, when it is too high, it may lead to worsening of existing pathologies and the development of a new one.

It can be easier to understand and explain to owners by dividing the reaction into three stages: normal, high, and very high or pathological. The behaviours seen in each stage are different, and our ability to interact with the patient differs.

Figure 7.8A and B illustrate the different levels using a traffic-light analogy. There are two thresholds to note (Fig. 7.8). The lower threshold (yellow line) is the emotional and the higher threshold (red line) is the behavioural threshold. Where these thresholds are above the baseline, the gap between them varies from one situation to the other. It depends on genetics, epigenetics, learning from past situations, the environment, and the intensity of the trigger. Figure 7.8 illustrates the level of arousal animals reach. Animals in the green zone show normal behaviours as their arousal level is adaptive (normal). Their arousal will increase and decrease but will stay under the significant emotional threshold; the animal can control its emotions, and the reaction to the trigger is appropriate. Animals in the yellow zone show high arousal but are still in control of their cognitive behaviours. The animal is no longer able to control its emotions effectively. Careful observation allows us to see signs such as conflict-related behaviours, displacement behaviours, and mild signs of SNS and HPA activation (see Section 7.3). Once the patient has crossed the behavioural threshold, that is, it cannot contain its behaviours, it has entered the red zone. This is a very high arousal level. Patients in this level show what some may call 'pathological behaviours' such as affective aggression (see Chapters 11 and 12), abnormal repetitive behaviours (see Chapter 15), and may lose control over their bladder and colon (see Chapter 14).

7.4.3.4 Summation of effects

As noted earlier, the arousal response develops rapidly but takes much longer to return to baseline. One trigger may be very intense, or the patient is very sensitive to different triggers, and as a result, the arousal response will be very rapid and intense.

However, it is more likely that several triggers combine to elicit a full reaction. Figure 7.9A and B illustrate how several triggers can interplay and lead to the development of so-called pathological behaviours. If the patient has time to recover between different triggers (assuming the intensity of the trigger is the same), it is not likely to escalate (Fig. 7.9). However, if the patient does not have time to recover from one trigger before the next one is presented, it will escalate (Fig. 7.9). The next trigger will not start at the baseline (as the patient did not recover), leading to a higher level of arousal and will take longer to decrease. Each added trigger causes further escalation. The last trigger is the one to cross the behavioural threshold and elicit the pathological behaviour (e.g. aggressive response), although it may not be the most significant trigger. This is one of the reasons that owners are sometimes surprised about the patient's behaviour. They might have missed all the triggers that added to the build-up of arousal, and when they wanted to pat or brush the patient, it was the 'last straw', and the patient bites.

It is essential to note that whether it is through genetic regulation or long-term activation of the arousal systems, some patients do not return to a normal baseline. As a result, they are more reactive both in speed and intensity of the reaction. These patients are more difficult to handle and require a more intensive management programme and medications. Baselines may also be raised as a result of things like mood effects, such as occurs with chronic pain.

When reviewing Fig. 7.9, it is easier to understand the principle of the initial management of psychiatric disorders. The first step is prevention; trying to reduce the number of triggers presented to the patient. Prevention is achieved through environmental management and routine changes. However, it is not always simple to avoid triggers (e.g. not leaving the house in the case of separation distress or avoiding thunderstorms in noise-phobic patients). Therefore, the next step is to reduce the intensity of the trigger by teaching the animal how to react appropriately and using medications (especially in cases where the patient is in the red zone).

7.5 Summary

Reaching an accurate diagnosis is an essential aspect of veterinary psychiatry. Once we have a diagnosis, we can design an appropriate management programme and select medications accordingly.

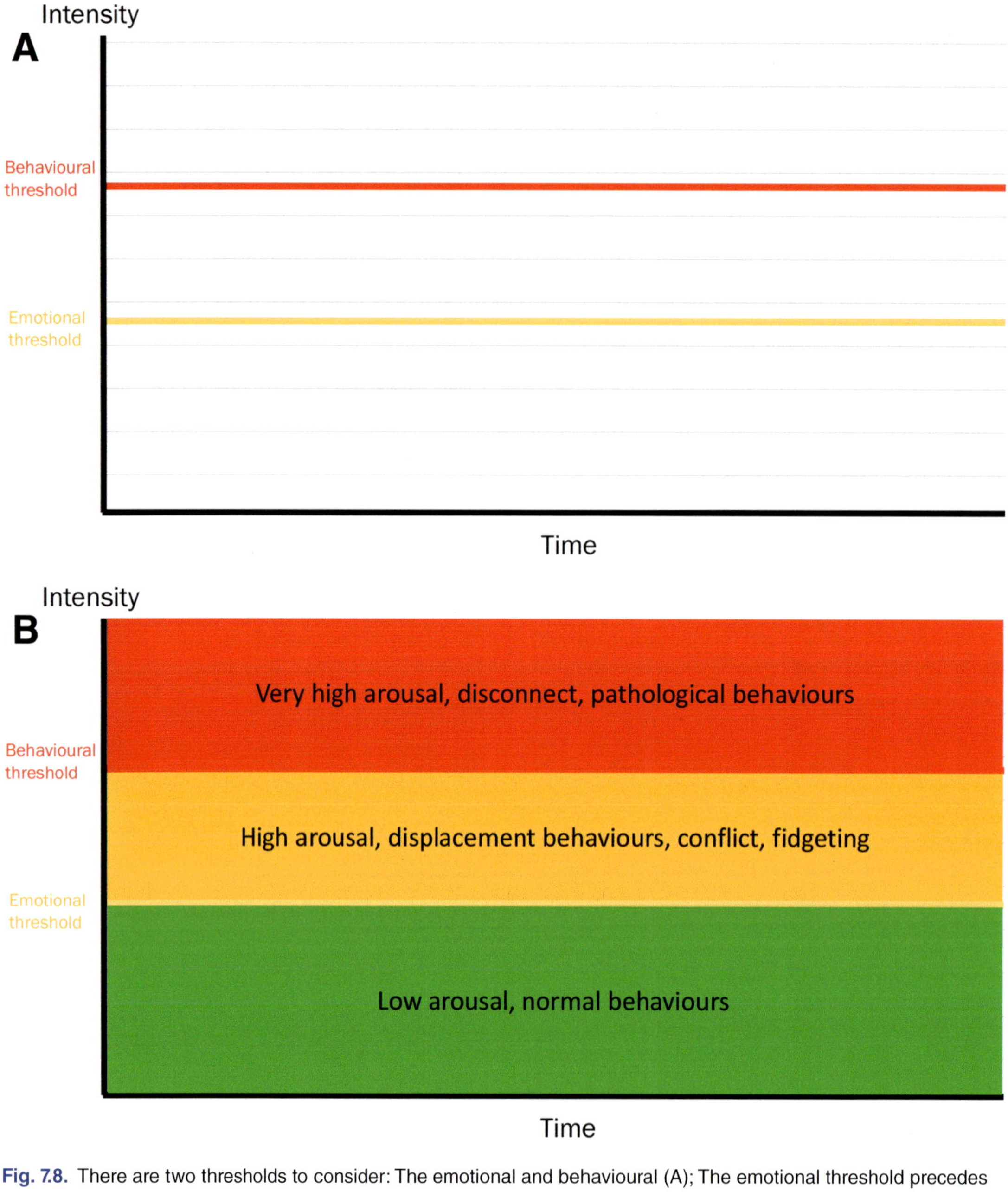

Fig. 7.8. There are two thresholds to consider: The emotional and behavioural (A); The emotional threshold precedes the behavioural one. First, the patient loses its ability to control its emotions. If the patient's arousal level continues to escalate, the patient will lose its ability to control its behaviour. The level at which each threshold is, and the gap between both thresholds, varies based on many internal (e.g. genetics) and external (e.g. environment, the trigger and distance) factors. The behaviour of the patient changes depending on the intensity of the arousal. Using a traffic-light analogy simplifies the explanation for owners (B). The goal of management is to maintain patients in the green zone with minimal crossing to the yellow zone while avoiding the red zone.

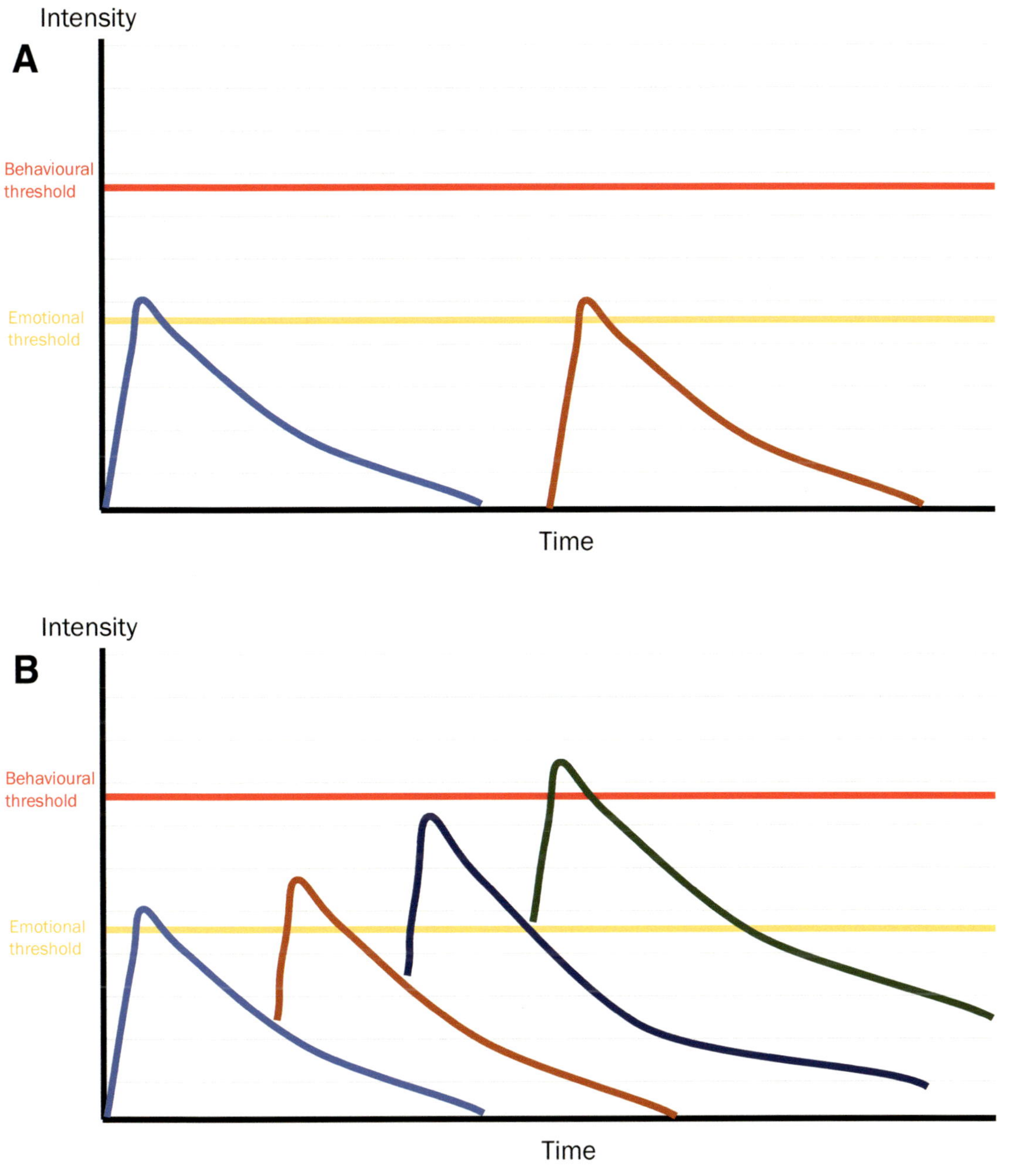

Fig. 7.9. When the patient has sufficient time to settle down following a trigger, before facing the next trigger, the reaction is likely to be more appropriate (A). However, when the patient is presented with successive triggers without sufficient time to recover, the patient's arousal level will increase and finally cross both thresholds leading to pathological behaviours (B).

Reaching a diagnosis is part of the art of medicine. First, we need to gather all the information about the patient, its environment, interactions, reactions and the problem itself. Next, we need to review the patient's behaviour and body language both during the problem situations and through normal situations. Once we know the context and the body language, we can decide what the underlying mental and emotional pathology is. Finally, we must review the level of executive control the patient has during the problem situation. Then we can decide about the management, starting from prevention, environmental and routine changes, through behaviour modification techniques and medications.

References

Berns, G.S., Brooks, A.M. and Spivak, M. (2012) Functional MRI in awake unrestrained dogs. *PLOS ONE* 7(5), e38027. DOI: 10.1371/journal.pone.0038027.

Carlson, N.R. and Birkett, M.A. (2017) *Physiology of Behavior*, 12th edn. Pearson, Harlow, UK.

Easterbrook, J.A. (1959) The effect of emotion on cue utilization and the organization of behavior. *Psychological Review* 66(3), 183–201. DOI: 10.1037/h0047707.

Finka, L., Ellis, S.L.H., Wilkinson, A. and Mills, D. (2014) The development of an emotional ethogram for *Felis silvestris* focused on FEAR and RAGE. *Journal of Veterinary Behavior* 9(6), e5. DOI: 10.1016/j.jveb.2014.09.018.

Harding, E.J., Paul, E.S. and Mendl, M. (2004) Animal behaviour: cognitive bias and affective state. *Nature* 427(6972), 312. DOI: 10.1038/427312a.

Lorenz, K. and Tinbergen, N. (1970) Taxis and instinct in egg-rolling response of the greylag goose. *Studies in Animal and Human Behavior* 1, 328–342.

Panksepp, J. (1998) *Affective Neuroscience: the Foundations of Human and Animal Emotions*. Oxford University Press, Oxford, UK.

Patronek, G.J. and Bradley, J. (2016) No better than flipping a coin: reconsidering canine behavior evaluations in animal shelters. *Journal of Veterinary Behavior* 15, 66–77. DOI: 10.1016/j.jveb.2016.08.001.

Pierantoni, L., Albertini, M. and Pirrone, F. (2011) Prevalence of owner-reported behaviours in dogs separated from the litter at two different ages. *Veterinary Record* 169(18), 468. DOI: 10.1136/vr.d4967.

Reese, W.G. (1978) Familial vulnerability for experimental neurosis. *The Pavlovian Journal of Biological Science* 13(3), 169–173. DOI: 10.1007/BF03001390.

Samuels, E.R. and Szabadi, E. (2008) Functional neuroanatomy of the noradrenergic locus coeruleus: its roles in the regulation of arousal and autonomic function. Part I: Principles of functional organisation. *Current Neuropharmacology* 6(3), 235–253. DOI: 10.2174/157015908785777229.

Scott, J.P. and Fuller, J.L. (1965) *Genetics and the Social Behaviour of the Dog*. The University of Chicago Press, Chicago, Illinois, pp. 134–136.

Storbeck, J. and Clore, G.L. (2008) Affective arousal as information: how affective arousal influences judgments, learning, and memory. *Social and Personality Psychology Compass* 2(5), 1824–1843. DOI: 10.1111/j.1751-9004.2008.00138.x.

Yaffe, P. (2011) The 7% rule: fact, fiction, or misunderstanding. *Ubiquity* October, 2011. DOI: 10.1145/2043155.2043156.

Yerkes, R.M. and Dodson, J.D. (1908) The relation of strength of stimulus to rapidity of habit-formation. *Journal of Comparative Neurology and Psychology* 18(5), 459–482. DOI: 10.1002/cne.920180503.

8 Learning Principles and Behaviour Modification

LYNN HEWISON* AND DANIEL S. MILLS

Joseph Banks Laboratories, School of Life Sciences, University of Lincoln, Lincoln, UK

8.1 Introduction

Problem behaviour often relates to clusters or degrees of behaviours, emotional states and cognitions, which the owner finds problematic (see Chapter 7). Training and behaviour therapy involve using controlled interactions and structuring of the environment to bring about change in either the motivational (specific goal) or emotional (appraisal and subsequent strategic focus) basis to the problem behaviour. Depending on the nature of the problem, it may be more efficient to focus on either the motivational or emotional element. For example, if a dog presents with food guarding and it can be established that the behaviour is limited to this particular context, then it might be hypothesized that the dog is specifically motivated to protect food for some reason (there are both potential diseases and learned reasons why this might be the case). However, if it is established that the dog is more generally protective of resources, and possibly also has broader issues associated with intrusion into its personal space (including territory), it might be indicative of a more general problem with frustration. In the former case, managing the specific factors leading to a motivation to protect food may be more efficient; however, in the latter case, rather than seeking to address each context as a separate problem, focusing on treatment to reduce the tendency for frustration might be more efficient.

This chapter considers how managing contingencies within the social and physical environment can be used to bring about predictable changes in behaviour to support the management of a range of problems. Rather than approach this issue from a 'theory first, application second' perspective, which is commonly used in many other texts (e.g. Ramirez, 1999; McGreevy and Boakes, 2007; Horwitz and Mills, 2009), the chapter is structured along the lines of considering first those practices and practical outcomes that alter the specific motivation for a behaviour (which underpins traditional training practice), and then considering how more general changes in behaviour can be brought about through the control of emotional arousal and executive function (see Section 7.4 – Executive Control of Behaviour and Emotion). We introduce technical terminology and theoretical concepts on an as-needed basis to make the chapter more accessible to those without a learning theory background. For those seeking more information on theory, we suggest the texts cited above.

8.2 Changing the Consequences of an Animal's Behaviour

Behaviour is always followed by a consequence, with the latter typically having the effect of either strengthening or weakening the behaviour it follows. Events that strengthen behaviour, thus making the behaviour more likely to occur again in the future, are termed *reinforcers*. Events that weaken behaviour, or stop it from occurring again in the future, are termed *punishers*. Thus, these two terms are defined by their consequence and not the intention of anyone contributing to the consequences of an animal's behaviour.

There are two forms of reinforcers (positive and negative) and two forms of punishers (positive and negative), which can typically occur as

*Corresponding author: lhewison@lincoln.ac.uk

DOI: 10.1079/9781786394552.0008

consequences to behaviour. The terms positive and negative refer to whether something is being added (positive) or removed (negative) to bring about the change. These are discussed further below, along with some of the important welfare and emotional considerations required before deciding what type of consequence and method of training to use. First, we must consider some ethical guidelines that should inform all management decisions.

8.2.1 Four ethical principles of behaviour modification practice

In general, those working with animals should follow the four cardinal principles guiding ethical practice:

8.2.1.1 Respect for autonomy

We should respect the decisions made by other people concerning their own lives; owners may have certain preferences for how they manage their animals, which need to be respected even if not entirely agreed with. If we feel that our standards clash with those of owners, based on trying to comply with the other's ethical principles, then we should try to counsel the owners to see the ethical argument, so they can proceed in what they consider to be the most ethical way. However, ultimately, owners have the right to insist on doing things their way so long as it is legal, and we would argue that it is unethical for consultants to walk away from owners and their animals when they are seeking professional help. To resolve this dilemma, we suggest that the consultant should make it clear in writing that while they do not agree with the proposed limits imposed by the owners, they will do their best to help them within limits applied by them. In addition, the owners should be fully briefed about additional risks, the consequences of harm arising from these risks, for both them and their animal, as well as the potential impact of their choice on the prognosis for the case. These should be included in writing with the treatment recommendations.

8.2.1.2 Beneficence

We try to bring about good in all our actions. In other words, we must always act with good intent for all. This also means that where there is good evidence for the efficacy of a particular intervention, we should favour that over one with less evidence in support of it, where both have similar welfare implications, simply because we can be more confident in the one with good evidence and so reduce the risk of delaying effective treatment.

8.2.1.3 Non-maleficence

'First, do no harm.' This means we should make a full assessment of all reasonable options for the circumstance and decide which poses the least risk *overall*. A particular treatment regime may stand the highest chance of being successful, but if there is a risk that it could cause significant harm, then it may not be the preferred course of action.

8.2.1.4 Justice

We must treat all people equally, fairly and impartially. This means we should identify everyone's needs and give equal consideration (but not necessarily weight) in our final decision. Likewise, we should not be tempted to use additional products, simply because they have just been launched and we want to see if they are any good, when there is a viable alternative.

8.2.2 Reinforcement

Reinforcement is used to strengthen behaviour and make that behaviour more likely to occur in similar situations in the future. As mentioned above, there are two forms of reinforcement:

8.2.2.1 Positive reinforcement

The provision of something of value, or something which is desired by an individual, in order to strengthen behaviour. Examples of common positive reinforcers include food, toys, games and access to interaction or attention. The value of reinforcers may vary with context and with different individuals. For example, although food is often a good initial choice, it needs to be considered that the timing of when reinforcers are given may influence their value. If the animal has just been fed, then kibble may be less valuable than it was before the meal. Thus, it is not the 'food' *per se* that is the reinforcer but the perception of it as a 'desirable thing to eat now' that is important among its reinforcing properties. This means that different reinforcers may be required at different times to achieve the same level of engagement with, or response in, each situation.

8.2.2.2 Negative reinforcement

Negative reinforcement is also a means for strengthening behaviour. This is where something the animal does not like or wishes to avoid at the time (an aversive) is removed when the desired behaviour is achieved. The removal or escape from the aversive helps to strengthen the immediately preceding behaviour in the future. An example of this may be getting a dog to sit through pushing down on the rump. When the dog sits, the pressure is taken off the body, so the dog learns to sit to avoid the pressure. From an ethical perspective even though training may lead to the generation of cues that negate the need to apply an aversive (because they reliably predict it in the case of non-compliance), negative reinforcement will require some aversion, even if mild, as in the current example, and so is less preferable than the use of positive reinforcement in terms of seeking to operate with non-maleficence. The same is true for training and behaviour modification, which is primarily focused on the use of punishment.

8.2.2.3 Schedule of reinforcement

The schedule of providing the reinforcement can affect the acquisition of a new task and maintenance of existing tasks. Reinforcing each successful task is known as a *continuous schedule of reinforcement*; for example, providing a treat after each time the owner gives the signal to sit and the dog sits. To teach an animal a new task, a continuous schedule works the best. An *intermittent schedule of reinforcement* is the best for maintaining the animal's performance of tasks it already knows; the reinforcement is given after a varying number of successful tasks. The intermittent schedule is further divided into *ratio* and *interval schedules*. In a ratio schedule, the reinforcement is given after either a fixed or variable number of repetitions of the task. In other words, the animal will receive the reward after each fourth repetition (fixed ratio of four) or once after three repetitions, and the next time after five (variable ratio of four). In an interval schedule, the reinforcement is given a fixed time after the animal performed the task (i.e. two seconds after the animal performed the task), or variable time (e.g. once after two seconds, and the next time after five seconds).

Owners mostly use continuous or variable (ratio or time) schedules, depending on their consistency and timing. Behaviours that receive reinforcement on an intermittent schedule are likely to be more difficult to extinguish. It is essential to note that many undesired behaviours are inadvertently rewarded intermittently by the owners (see Chapter 10).

8.2.3 Punishment

Punishment is used to suppress a behaviour and make that behaviour less likely to occur again in the future. As with reinforcement, there are two forms of punishment defined by whether something is being added or taken away from the situation.

8.2.3.1 Negative punishment

Negative punishment involves the withholding of something that is wanted from an individual in order to suppress the ongoing behaviour. Even if successful, this will typically result in frustration, and the associated risks need to be considered. Another important thing to appreciate is that if a trainer uses treats, then they also use negative punishment, since every time they do not give a reward that is anticipated by the animal, they are applying negative punishment. For example, if a dog is asked to sit, but the sit is either delayed or 'sloppy', the handler may not deliver the food as they wish to avoid reinforcing the poor-quality sit, even though the dog did sit. This would be an example of a negative punisher being used to reduce poor-quality responding in future. This may be both necessary and desirable to shape a desired level of response, in combination with positive reinforcement. This paradigm means that there is no such thing as 'training without punishment', or 'reinforcement-only' training, despite other claims. From a practical perspective, soon after the negatively punished response, a skilled trainer who is focused on positive reinforcement will encourage the dog to sit again, and if the dog does a better sit, he will give a positive reinforcer to the dog. In this way, the desired behaviour is identifiable with positive reinforcement. When considering the withholding of food in this context, it is important to be sensitive to how well-established the behaviour is. If this particular dog had had a lot of experience of sitting when asked, then missing one or two reinforcers periodically is unlikely to reduce the fluency or frequency of the sitting behaviour. However, if the dog is new to doing the sitting behaviour, then withholding reinforcement may not reduce the poor performance, but it may also reduce the tendency for the dog to try to sit at this time. An important point to appreciate is that punishment, unlike reinforcement, does not direct the animal towards a specific behavioural goal; it simply indicates that the current action is not beneficial. It is therefore a potentially inefficient method of training as we depend on the animal's ability to work out from all the available options what might be preferable. Therefore, in training, we should always aim to set the animal up to succeed in gaining positive reinforcement, by considering changing the environment as and when needed to enable the best course of action to be easily identifiable. This may be a particularly important consideration in the early stages of training when working with a less-experienced learner.

8.2.3.2 Positive punishment

This is the application of something the animal does not like or wishes to avoid (an aversive) to suppress the ongoing behaviour in future. An example of this may be shouting at the animal to get it to stop doing a particular behaviour. However, it is important to appreciate that punishment, like reinforcement, is defined by its long-term impact and not its immediate effect on behaviour. An animal may stop doing something immediately after a certain outcome, either because it has achieved the goal it was seeking or because the behaviour was punished. In the latter example, shouting at a dog that is 'playing up' for attention may actually make the behaviour worse in the long run as the dog has been reinforced through the provision of attention. Alternatively, the behaviour might be interrupted by the shouting if it is not perceived as being related to the behaviour but rather is seen as a distraction. Unfortunately, many owners fail to appreciate these two points as they are focused on the immediate consequences. By enquiring how effective this strategy has been for them (i.e. has it reduced the behaviour in the long term?) it may be possible to get the owner to reappraise the value of this type of response by explaining the simple principles of reinforcement and punishment in relation to their longer-term effects.

8.2.4 Perceived consequences and future behaviour: practical considerations

Behaviours are often learned in association with the consequences which follow them. When pairing a consequence with a behaviour for learning of the association to occur, the consequence should be contingent upon the behaviour it follows. For example, if a dog sits when it sees its owner holding its food bowl, then it will be more likely to receive food. The dog receiving food is contingent upon sitting. Likewise, if the owner does not wait till the dog is seated, then other behaviours, including barking, may be reinforced by delivery of the meal. Animals can quickly learn associations by pairing a behaviour with a particular consequence. When this behaviour and consequence consistently occur together through repeated exposure of the context, the animal starts to predict the behaviour that will lead to a particular consequence. This is what is meant by the term *associative learning*, and it can be manipulated by us to help modify behaviour.

8.2.4.1 Use of aversives and problem behaviour

It has been reported that owners who use positive reinforcement (focused on teaching what behaviour is wanted) are also less likely to report behaviour problems in their dogs (Blackwell *et al.*, 2008). Although we might suppose that owners who have dogs without problem behaviour may not need to use punishment, we must recognize that using positive punishment has the additional risk of damaging the relationship between the animal and the owner, with the animal becoming anxious about, or around, the owners. In this situation, owners will struggle to provide the social support that characterises a healthy dog–owner relationship (Rehn and Keeling, 2016). There is also some evidence to support the suggestion that positive punishment may increase the risk of problem behaviour, since where aversives have been applied to achieve behaviour change (positive punishment or negative reinforcement), then more aggressive behaviours towards handlers have been reported compared to when these methods were not used in training (Herron *et al.*, 2009; Arhant *et al.*, 2010). The prevalence of problem behaviours is also positively associated with owners who give rewards alongside physical punishment (Hiby *et al.*, 2004). While this might reflect the perceived need to 'correct' the animal's behaviour, it might also indicate a link to the frustration that will often develop when owners are inconsistent in the support they provide.

8.2.4.2 Obedience versus well-behavedness

Animals do not need any specific direction/manipulation from us to learn associations. When we deliberately create a particular response to a cue in a given context, we often consider this *obedience training*. However, when we create the circumstances for a dog to choose appropriate behaviour without an overt cue, we consider this *well-behavedness*. It still arises from training in that we have deliberately set up the environment to encourage the response we want, but in this circumstance the dog is using more general environmental cues rather than instructions from a human to determine its behaviour. In this way, dogs can learn to do what we want without being instructed continuously. If the owner asks the dog to sit for its meal, and it does so, then the dog is obedient, but if it sits in anticipation of the meal without being asked, the dog is well-behaved. Controlling the animal becomes less demanding for the owner. When it comes to managing problem behaviour, the skill is often to create well-behaved animals rather than obedient ones.

If an owner remarks that their dog starts to get excited and jump around because it knows when it is time for a walk, due to the shoes the owner has just put on, then the shoes become a cue for the jumping-up behaviour, which is then reinforced by the walk (a positive reinforcer). Although the dog may have associated the shoes with the walk through associative learning, the jumping-up behaviour is maintained by the association with the positive reinforcement of the walk.

8.2.5 Impact of different types of consequence

8.2.5.1 Mistaking the complaint as the problem

It should now be evident how this process of learning through association can lead to the development or exacerbation of a wide range of problem behaviours. For example, if a young dog who was already scared of fireworks (perhaps because of previous negative associations) walked into a garden at night and heard a firework, the behaviour of walking into the garden may be associated with the loud noise of the firework. The scariness of the firework is aversive, and its association with the dog walking into the garden may be sufficient positive punishment to stop the dog from using that exit from the house. What starts off as a fear of noises then develops into a dog refusing to go outside/into the garden and may actually present as a problem concerning fear of the dark or garden, because the owner fails to recognize how the problem has developed through learning and perhaps considers the fear of noises as natural, and therefore not a problem to worry about.

8.2.5.2 The power of punishment

At this point it is worth noting that when it comes to aversives, a single bad experience may be all that is required, because from an evolutionary perspective, it pays not to take a risk in future. This is why so many animals develop problems associated with negative emotions like fear. From a biological perspective, it is better to run away unnecessarily many times than fail to run away when you should have done so, as the costs of being wrong are so great, compared to the cost of running away unnecessarily. Developing this sort of association with an aversive is sometimes referred to as 'one-shot' learning and is a reason why some trainers believe using aversives are efficient and justifiable, but there are two important arguments against this:

- Although an association with punishment may be learned quickly, it simply stops the animal from doing something and does not predictably encourage desirable behaviour, and so may not be efficient if the animal chooses another problem behaviour.
- It is unethical when there are usually plenty of alternatives that do not require the use of aversives. Animals trained with a focus on punishment, as opposed to positive reinforcement, have been found to show more stress-related behaviours (Cooper *et al.*, 2014; Deldalle and Gaunet, 2014), and even if not directly associated with problem behaviour, they may predispose the individual to a range of emotional concerns.

8.2.5.3 Pros and cons of positive reinforcement

Despite the previous example, we should note that, as a general rule, the consistency of the association between a behaviour and a given consequence is often important for robust and efficient learning to occur. It is especially true when considering the use of positive reinforcement. Again, an evolutionary perspective on the behavioural tendencies created by positive reinforcers can be valuable. Once an animal has learned that a certain response reliably results in a certain reward, it is natural for the brain to test these boundaries in order to try to establish the minimum effort required to achieve the goal (this helps the animal to be efficient in the natural setting and not waste energy unnecessarily in future). It is important for those trying to train an animal to be aware of this phase of learning with reinforcers, as it will often present as the animal appearing to either forget (e.g. perhaps doing a half-sit on the sit command) or seem to play up (e.g. not coming back fully on command), just as the owner thinks they have successfully trained it. The important point is for the owner to be consistent at this time with the quality of the response they want, and then the animal will soon learn that a poorer response gets no reward. Indeed, the variability in response is an opportunity to improve the quality of response in a way that cannot be done when training with a focus on aversives. If owners only reward the best responses, the quality of the animal's responses will keep drifting upwards. This *shaping* of the response is one of the ways to achieve high performance efficiently and humanely.

8.2.5.4 Poor predictability and variety of experience

We must consider what happens when the consequences are less predictable. Suppose a behaviour occurs many times with a good consequence for the animal but only once with a relatively mild unwanted/bad consequence; then there is little consistency between the behaviour and the unwanted/bad consequence, so little chance they will be associated together. However, this will depend on both how severe the bad consequence is (this can be greatly reduced by having a supportive owner present who provides the dog with confidence in the form of social support at times of need) and not only how good the previous experience has been, but also how extensive this experience has been. If the dog has had experience in diverse settings, there will be little, if anything, to predict the bad consequence, and so the impact is likely to be minimal. An important point to note here, from a training perspective, is that it is not the number of repetitions but the variety of contexts which largely provides protection. So, when training, it is not a case that more is better, but variation of context and consistency of outcome. To return to an example of a dog who fears fireworks, suppose the dog is not predisposed to fear (i.e. does not have a fearful temperament) and it has walked into the garden many times at night before the night when a single firework bang occurs. If over the following few nights no further bangs occur when the dog is in the garden, then the dog is unlikely to generalize the learning in the same way as the fearful dog. An exception to this might be if the dog has some underlying musculoskeletal problem (possibly undiagnosed), as chronic pain related to this sort of problem may sensitize the dog or result in one-shot learning associated with pain as the dog tenses in response to the noise (Lopes Fagundes *et al.*, 2018).

Exceptions to the general protective rule of variety are often associated with particularly salient consequences (good or bad) to the individual concerned (regardless of how important an owner thinks it might be. This is why checking out things like chronic pain is essential – see Chapter 3). It is worth emphasizing again that negative consequences often carry a disproportionate weight in generating avoidance responses for the reasons discussed, and this is why so many problem behaviours occur that are associated with fear and chronic pain.

8.2.5.5 The timing of consequences

The impact of reinforcement and punishment on behaviour also relies on its timing in relation to the behaviour that occurred. Associations are more readily made with events that occur closely together in time. This applies to both punishment and reinforcement. Although a person delivering the consequence to the animal may believe they know which behaviour is associated with the consequence they think they are delivering, the animal may have a different perspective and not make the same association. For example, consider a dog who has toileted in the house while the owner was in another room or out of the house. The toileting occurred because the animal needed to empty its bladder or bowels (there could be many reasons for this, including that it has yet to learn to ask to go outside). Regardless of the reason, if the owner comes into the room later, notices the mess and physically reprimands the dog (positive punishment), they may believe they are punishing the dog because of the toileting. However, from the dog's perspective, the reprimand, especially if physical, may be associated with the owner coming into the room (a more closely related event in time), the room itself or possibly the presence of the mess (but not necessarily to the making of the mess – i.e. a spatial association rather than temporal one), or perhaps some other environmental feature such as someone else coincidently walking in at the same time (another strong temporal association). There is then the potential that the dog avoids these environments or interaction with associated individuals, but it does not learn anything useful about toileting indoors. Avoidance of interaction with someone due to an association with punishment can also encourage 'cringing'-type responses towards the individual in similar circumstances. Owners may then misinterpret 'cringing' as guilt, thus justifying the belief in the need for further punishment (Horowitz, 2009). A vicious cycle of avoidance and problem behaviour can then develop as a result of the actual timing of previous attempts to control the animal.

8.3 Motivation and Goal-directed Behaviour

While it could be justifiably argued that all training is associated with a change in motivation, we suggest that from a behaviour management perspective it is useful to distinguish between training that is focused on altering a specific behavioural motivation and training that is aimed at bringing about a more general change in behavioural predisposition (skill development and the control of emotion). The latter is the focus of a later section; here we focus on specific behaviour associations involved in training and behaviour modification.

8.3.1 The type of motivational state associated with reinforcement and punishment

The motivation for a particular behaviour depends on the trade-off of the perceived rewards and punishments for the options available at any given time. This will be affected by internal factors such as the genetic predisposition of the animal (which is reflected in aspects of its temperament and personality) and current underlying motivational state (e.g. how hungry the animal is). However, here we will focus more on the importance of the immediate factors controlling behaviour. We start by considering the relationship between motivation in a broad sense and reinforcement versus punishment.

Reinforcement serves to motivate and thus encourage a specific response directed towards a specific goal; by contrast, punishment serves to reduce the motivation for a behaviour in a given context. If a specific response does happen to develop in association with the use of punishment, it is because there has been some form of reinforcement for the particular behaviour that is now being expressed. This might arise through positive reinforcement, i.e. the animal happens to engage in a behaviour that achieves a desirable goal. However, perhaps more often, the behaviour arises as a result of negative reinforcement; an association being made between the termination of the punisher and whatever behaviour was occurring at that time.

Negative reinforcement of an escape response is a common outcome of behavioural motivation when ineffective punishments are used in training, but also when animals experience a range of other naturally occurring aversives and can give rise to a range of problem behaviours – for example, the animal who tries to run away or escape from a sudden noise. Behaviours learned through negative reinforcement are much more fixed in their form, and so, potentially, harder to alter than behaviours learned through positive reinforcement. The reason for this is again about the judgement brains make concerning the risks of being wrong. Having found a response that works with regard to escape, it is too risky to see if a lesser response is still successful as the potential cost could be enormous. With regard to the development of problem behaviour, this means that if an animal makes a massive effort to escape, perhaps from a house during a thunderstorm, when the storm naturally subsides the individual may have learnt that this level of response is associated with escape from the scary noises. So next time it is in a similar situation, it mounts another extreme response. This may be termed a phobia, but it is still a functional (albeit maladaptive) response, which has arisen from conditioning. Thunderstorms and fireworks are particularly powerful conditioners of escape responses as they often move around, and while we know it is safer to be inside than out, our pets may not be capable of such reasoning as they do not necessarily understand the nature of the cause of these moving sounds; so from their perspective, the next crash could be on top of them.

8.3.2 Training and behaviour modification focused on managing specific behavioural motivations

As already mentioned, in some circumstances, we may be presented with a problem associated with a specific motivation, in which case the associated training might need to adopt an approach focused on doing something about this. There are two common strategies used in these situations: motivate the animal to do something else in this circumstance (operant counter-conditioning) or redirect the motivation towards another substrate. These are each discussed in more detail below.

8.3.2.1 Altering the motivation in the circumstances

The best way to teach an animal to perform a specific behaviour is to motivate it to show the desired behaviour and then strengthen the tendency to perform using rewards in a variety of settings. Teaching a behaviour is often achieved effectively in practice by structuring training into incremental steps. This often involves teaching the animal the desired behaviour in a context different from the one in which it may ultimately be used. For example, consider a dog who is new to the family but who jumps up at visitors. The owners would like the dog to sit when greeting visitors arriving at the door; however, the dog has not been effectively taught a reliable sit behaviour on cue. In this situation, the dog may be excited when visitors arrive, and there are likely to be many distractions which make it challenging for the dog to concentrate and learn new behaviours successfully without a high rate of failure; trying to train the sit response at this time is likely to be frustrating for the owner. However, if the sit is first introduced at a quiet time with minimal distractions, then learning success will likely be high, and the dog will quickly learn what is required in order to get the reward. Once the behaviour is reliably performed to the desired cue, the cue-response tendency can be strengthened and a structured approach taken to introducing the use of the sit when visitors are arriving. Owners need to be aware that as the difficulty of the situation for the dog increases (e.g. more distractions or competing interests), they will probably need to support their dog and perhaps repeat a step here or there to support their animal in making the desired choice. Thus, it is important to consider not only the behaviour being taught and how this will be done, but also the environment in which the learning is occurring as adaptations to both will likely be required for efficient learning by the individual. The individual characteristics of an animal are often overlooked when designing a training plan but are important to consider as they can play a key role and may influence the approach to training or the speed taken at different steps. Therefore, the needs and character of the individual should always form an integral part of any training plan.

When teaching an animal any behaviour, we need to consider the environment and set this up so as to encourage opportunities for positive reinforcement and successful learning towards our goal. If a new behaviour is to be taught then it is best introduced incrementally at a pace suitable for the learner, not just the trainer. It is also best to choose a quiet location, low in distractions for initial teaching. Once the desired behaviour has a good reinforcement history and is performed with fluidity, then moving into more distracting environments can be considered. You should expect less reliability not only when you increase the difficulty of the situation in which you are asking for it, but also if you change quite innocuous aspects of the training context, such as changing the room of training (Braem and Mills, 2010). For example, if the dog can run to you quickly and without hesitation across 50 m between the house and garden, when out in a field away from the house you may need to be 5 m away to get the same response. It takes time to generalize a response, especially to a command word (see Mills, 2005, for a review of some of the factors affecting response to a command word). If a structured approach has been taken, the animal should be able to rapidly perform the desired behaviour, albeit with some additional support from the owner after the first few repetitions. If the animal's performance remains lower following some form of environmental difficulty, then this could be interpreted as the animal finding the situation too difficult, and, as such, they are struggling to make the desired choice. If this occurs, it is often useful to reassess the environment and associations to reduce the chances of the animal making an error. Examples of this can include moving the animal further away from a situation or having fewer distractions present. If the performance of the behaviour then improves, reevaluation for progressing training should include ways to increase difficulty in smaller increments.

To expand on the example above, if an owner wishes to teach a dog to sit before meeting visitors, the first stage may be the teaching of the sit itself. To help the animal learn, this initial stage can often be achieved quite quickly through the use of a food lure (a piece of food held close to the nose and moved so the animal follows). In following the food, the animal is also following the hand and the movement of the hand. This allows the opportunity to see if the animal can perform the behaviour to be taught. If after a few repetitions of the food being in the hand the food is left out and the hand moves as it was previously, most animals will continue to follow the hand. The food, in this case, is the reinforcer for the behaviour and can be delivered from a source close by or given from the other hand. At this stage, the behaviour will largely be under the control of the hand or some other visual cue. There needs to be fluidity and reliability in the behaviour before progressing from a hand cue to a verbal signal. If we add a verbal signal, we should introduce it just before the hand cue. The dog would then learn the new signal (verbal sit) is followed by the old cue (hand lure to sit), which elicits the behaviour which is reinforced. After more repetitions of this, the dog should start to sit on the verbal signal and the hand cue is no longer needed.

So long as the sit continues to be reinforced, it will continue to occur in the circumstances. If at any time the dog does not sit, the reinforcer (food) is withheld; and with time, particularly quick sits (or some other desirable characteristic of the behaviour) may be reinforced in preference to less desirable ones, in order to incrementally improve performance. However, if there are multiple 'failures' of the dog to perform the desired behaviour when asked, then it is worth looking at the environment in which the dog is being asked to do the behaviour. This is of particular importance if the behaviour is reliable in other, perhaps less distracting, environments. When it comes to environmental set-up, managing the immediate surroundings and choosing suitable locations to train can help to improve training efficiency. As training progresses, we can manipulate the environment to increase the difficulty gradually. As an example, with a dog learning to sit for visitors arriving, it may be beneficial to practise with a familiar person at an open door the first few times it is used with a visitor, as this will be less exciting than an unfamiliar person who cannot be seen. If the greeting of people is enjoyable for the dog, through the provision of calm praise and gentle contact, then over time the greeting itself may become the reinforcer for the sit. As the dog continues to learn to predict reinforcement from sitting when people arrive, the verbal signal may be faded out as well.

Maintaining reinforcement for desired behaviours helps to maintain the behaviour, but this must not become monotonous. Once a behaviour has a strong reinforcement history, there are, potentially, a variety of reinforcers that can be used to maintain it in a given context, and if they are delivered in association with reliable environmental cues, we may go from an obedient dog (who responds reliably to a verbal signal) to a well-behaved one (i.e. one who adopts certain desirable behaviours in the presence of certain environmental contingencies). For example, a behaviour like a sit could be requested at a kerbside, and then reinforced by the continuation of the walk, movement forwards and sniffing. A sit for mealtime could be reinforced by the delivery of a bowl with food. The throwing of a toy may reinforce a sit in the garden. If the sit is asked for, performed and then rewarded in a range of situations, such as those described above, then, over time and with repetition of these situations, the animal will learn to predict that under these conditions a sit gains reinforcement and the verbal cues are no longer required. This sort of consistency is what makes a well-behaved dog. With an established behaviour, so long as more often than not some form of reinforcement occurs in association with it (which may be simply some form of pleasurable activity and does not need to be food), the behaviour should continue to occur under those conditions.

Consistency in reinforcement and punishment is key to helping the animal understand how its behaviour is instrumental to the outcome. Suppose a dog is waiting for the food bowl to be put on the floor. If the animal has learned and has previous experience that sitting results in the bowl arriving on the floor, then the sitting should continue to occur. However, if the animal is excited due to the anticipation of the food arriving, it may jump up towards the owner. The owner could then move the food bowl further away, thus negatively punishing the jumping-up behaviour. When the dog sits again, the food bowl moves closer to the ground. The owner may be working on the contingency that the dog's bottom being on the floor is what predicts the lowering of the food bowl to the ground. The dog learns the behaviour of sitting in this situation gets reinforced by the delivery of food. Thus the behaviour is driven and shaped by the consequences immediately following it (reinforcement or punishment). Learning to change behaviour as a result of its consequences is referred to as *operant conditioning* or *instrumental learning*. When this form of learning is used to establish a behaviour that is incompatible or counter to another behaviour, the behaviour modification technique is referred to as *operant counter-conditioning*.

8.3.2.2 Altering the specific target of the motivation in the circumstances

In some situations, we may not want to create a new behaviour, but we may wish to redirect it towards a more appropriate target. For example, if a dog enjoys running and chasing, then it is important to allow these behaviours but in a controlled way, so the dog does not cause a problem. A toy or game which facilitates running and chasing is likely to be a stronger reinforcer than food in this situation. If the motivation to chase something is high for an individual and they learn they can do this in an uncontrolled way when out on a walk, although they may be rewarded by food on the return to the owner, the chase is often more reinforcing than the food and so it is likely the animal will continue to chase whatever it wants when given the opportunity. This may present as a problem in itself but also as a poor response to recall cue. In this situation, strict management is needed to ensure that the animal cannot continue to practise the undesired chasing behaviour and the pleasure of running is redirected into a recall-related activity and controlled chase. In this situation a reinforcer, which provides the opportunity to chase, such as a 'whip-it' style toy (Fig. 8.1A and B) may be necessary.

If the dog has a lot of practice of ignoring the old recall cue, it may be easier and quicker to start training to a new cue given the poor contingency between the old command and an appropriate response that can be reinforced. A new cue brings the potential to build new associations, without the difficulty of changing old associations or the lack of them! During the training of the new cue, the owner should reinforce the dog's return each time as described previously. This is so the dog learns to associate the cue with the reinforcer on offer. Training should be structured to set both the dog and owner

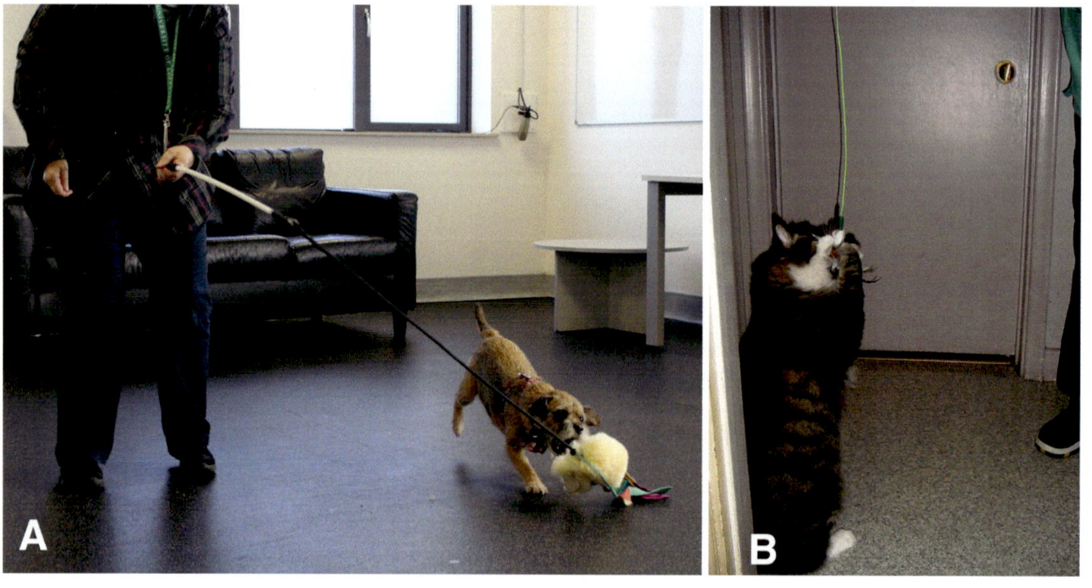

Fig. 8.1. A dog (A) and cat (B) playing by chasing a toy. Rather than try to encourage an alternative motivation for chasing, it may be easier to teach the owner to redirect the behaviour in a safe and acceptable way as illustrated here. (Fig. 8.1A courtesy of Daniel Mills, University of Lincoln. Fig. 8.1B courtesy of Sagi Denenberg.)

up for success. Considerations should include the distance the dog is being asked to recall and also the level of difficulty associated with the environment. Where the environment is more challenging, it is best to ask for a response over a decreased distance initially, only increasing the distance once reliable responses have been established. A simultaneous increase in distance and difficulty is more likely to result in poor responding. It is therefore advised to start training in low-distraction environments and gradually increase the level in which the dog is being asked to respond while managing the risk of errors. Management may include utilizing physical tools to shape the environment in favour of a positive response, such as working in fenced paddocks or using long lines on the dog.

This behaviour modification technique is often referred to as *behavioural redirection* because the behaviour that was giving rise to the problem is still allowed, but it is being increasingly reinforced when displayed towards more selected targets in order to motivate the animal to engage in this form of the behaviour rather than the problematic form. Thus the behaviour is redirected away from the problem context. A common example in cats involves training them to use a scratch post rather than the furniture for scratching.

8.4 Teaching Skills Relating to Emotional Control

For many problem behaviours, it is often the emotional element that is at the heart of the problem (see Chapter 7). For example, the cat that hisses and bites when the owner goes to pet it might be responding out of pain (in which case the response is focused on protection), or a fear of pain if petting previously was associated with pain – the cat may then have learned the response as an avoidance response, and although the pain may no longer be present, the animal is not aware of this and so continues with the relatively rigid avoidance response (as a 'safe bet'). Perhaps being petted is associated with being held on the owner's lap, and the cat wants to avoid that restriction to its autonomy (in which case the underlying emotion is associated with frustration). In this sort of scenario, it is often more efficient to aim treatment on focusing on and managing the respective emotion rather than simply focusing on changing the behaviour.

By way of further illustration of the value of focusing on emotion rather than behaviour, it is worth remembering that a scared animal will be focused on escape, while if it is frustrated, the focus will be on the resource, and these emotions may be the source of the behaviours which owners find problematic. If we want to encourage more acceptable behaviours, we need to put the animal in a more emotionally receptive state (less emotionally aroused or in a different emotional state), so we can train what the owner wants more efficiently.

Several techniques used in behaviour modification have this type of focus (even if it is not clearly acknowledged in other texts), and there are two main approaches used in this regard: changing the intensity of the emotion or changing the actual emotion associated with the context.

A critical thing to appreciate when trying to change an aspect of the emotional response is that it is not so much what the animal does, but how it feels that we are looking to change. So trying to manage the problem of a dog jumping up when meeting someone might involve deciding to train the dog to sit as described above, since if we are interested in controlling motivation, we need to specify the behaviour to be reinforced. In this case, training will involve reinforcement of sitting. However, this might result in a dog that is still very excited and liable to show some other problematic behaviour when released from this. By contrast, if we believe it is important to control the emotion, we would not simply reward 'sitting' because if the dog is in the same emotional state, it has not shown the change we desire. In this case, it is the inferred internal state which we are looking to change. Indeed, the dog may not even need to sit to be reinforced; it can simply show any relaxed behaviour to be reinforced in an appropriate way (in this case gentle contact with the owner, rather than food may be preferable).

Another outcome from this perspective is the ability to teach an animal certain skills or predispositions, which generalize not only across contexts but also to novel situations. Two common exercises taught in this way are impulse control and frustration tolerance, which we describe below, before considering the more general principles associated with emotion-control exercises. Key elements to skill development exercises compared to the specific behavioural development exercises discussed in relation to motivation are that the animal learns without a specific cue to change its behaviour and that exercises are given across a variety of contexts. If the contexts are limited, then the behaviour change is also limited, and the more general skill is not established.

8.4.1 Impulse control

We use this technique when we believe the animal may make better decisions if it was to act less impulsively. Impulsivity can be assessed and monitored in dogs using the widely validated instrument the Dog Impulsivity Assessment Scale (DIAS – Wright *et al.*, 2011; http://lincolnabc.co.uk/resources/). Our work indicates that by teaching animals to self-settle (i.e. calm down and defer to the owner without specific cues being given by the handler, but rather these coming from the environmental context as discussed above) when it wants something, then they may become less impulsive overall (for example, a self-settle before going through a door or before being fed). The key to this process is to identify a range of contexts that are commonly encountered every day where the animal can practise this sort of restraint (delayed reward gratification). With a suitable breadth of circumstances, this appears to bring about a more global change in impulsivity, rather than context-specific learning and generalization.

8.4.2 Frustration tolerance

While the exercises above also involve teaching a degree of frustration tolerance, there are situations where the focus is as much, or more, on the tendency to not act quickly, but the consequences of this can be increased frustration. In other words, the problem lies in the type of response that the animal shows when it is frustrated, and it is this which is the focus of change. In this case, we can adapt and extend the exercises described in the previous paragraph to focus specifically on coping with frustration response; however, care is necessary not to exacerbate the problem seriously. It is essential that animals are exposed to situations with which they can cope, and that tolerance is built up incrementally. It is *not* a case of exposing the animal to the stimulus until it settles down (a process known as *flooding*), which not only has its own ethical and welfare concerns but also can be dangerous, as an animal in such a state may become quite aggressive and redirect this to anyone or anything nearby. The specific exercises selected in a given case have to be chosen with care with a thorough assessment of the risks. Example contexts that might be considered to help teach frustration tolerance include self-control in relation to delayed rewards (as per the impulse-control exercises above, but also the use of certain self-control food-delivery toys like the Tug-A-Jug; Fig. 8.2A and B). Note, in this case, it is not about the toy simply providing a delayed reward, but more controlled behaviour resulting in greater reward (this makes it different to the commonly used stuffed-Kong-type activities). Other frustration tolerance exercises can be built around coping with unmet expectations such as the provision of a lower value food than expected for a given task on an intermittent basis or a smaller meal. Others might involve coping with various forms of barrier frustration and restraint such as waiting for the dog to check in with the handler when on a lead when it sees something of interest ahead (again getting the right gradient of stimuli so as not to over-arouse the dog) or coping with varying degrees of confinement. Reducing behavioural perseverance when mildly frustrated can also be helpful in some circumstances, depending on the problem. This can be achieved by using mild distractions (the key here is for the handler to show interest in something else of interest and not to offer this distraction to the dog, as it could end up reinforcing the frustration response). Other exercises related to frustration tolerance involve learning to cope with intrusions into personal space. This can vary from the animal's territory, personal space or touch, all of which are triggers of a frustration response, a simple example of one of the contexts involved in this might be teaching the animal to enjoy grooming. When undertaking this sort of training, it is particularly important to pay attention to how aroused the animal becomes and also how it copes with the arousal. Relatively high levels of arousal associated with interest are acceptable; however, the animal must learn self-restraint if it is to truly learn frustration tolerance rather than simply be desensitized to the various stimuli used in training. Exactly which exercises are chosen will vary with the focus of the frustration, but insight can be gained by profiling the dog using the canine frustration questionnaire (McPeake *et al.*, 2019; http://lincolnabc.co.uk/resources/) and this instrument can also be used to monitor progress, beyond the specific contexts selected as appropriate for training.

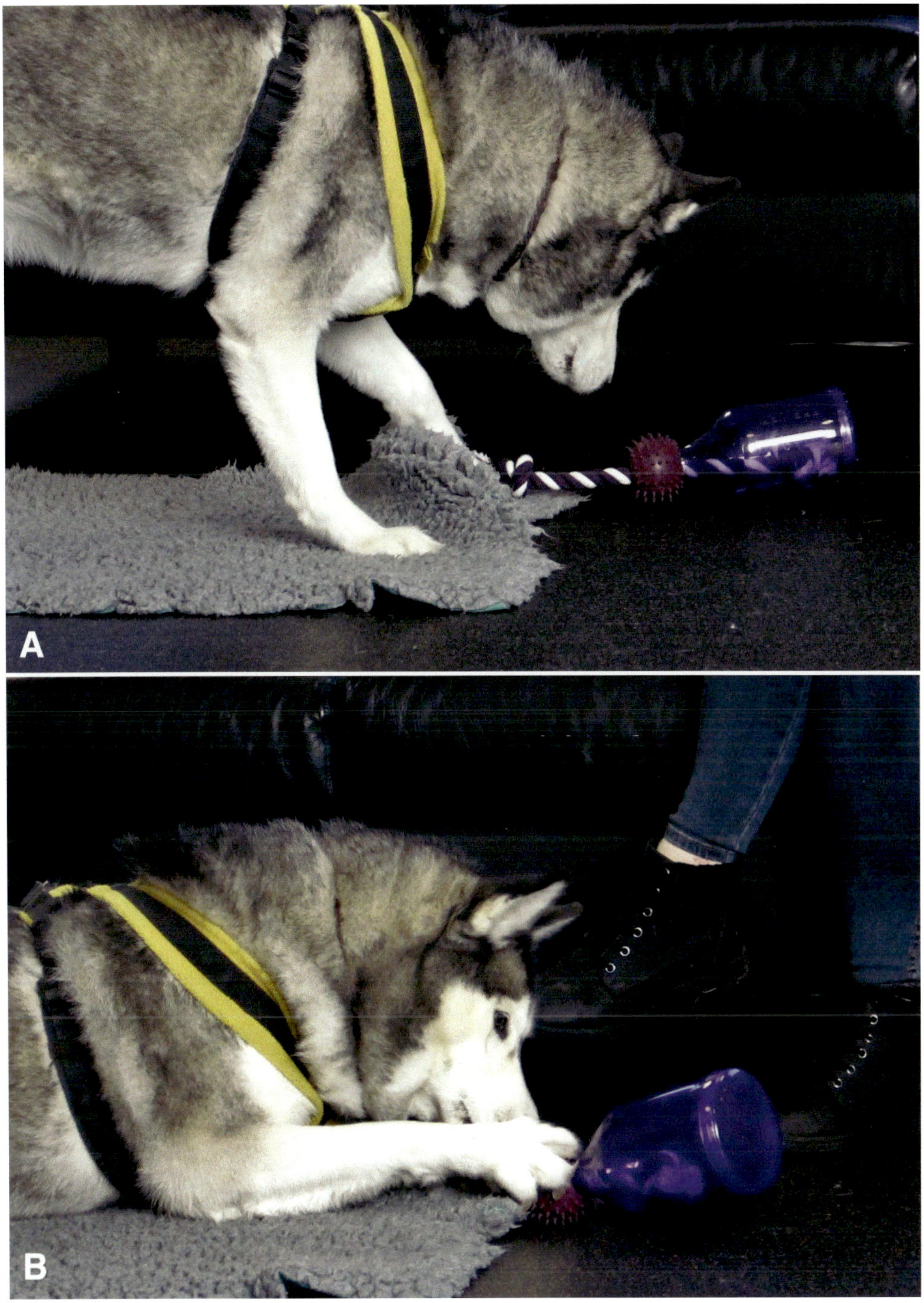

Fig. 8.2. Some toys can encourage impulse control, e.g., the Tug-A-Jug illustrated here (Fig. 8.2A) has a knotted string, which, if pulled fully, will block the release of treats contained within. The dog therefore has to learn to tip the toy in a controlled way and ensure the rope does not block the neck of the bottle in order to obtain the treats contained within (Fig. 8.2B). (Photos courtesy of Daniel Mills, University of Lincoln.)

8.5 Training and Behaviour Modification Focused on Managing Emotion

In this section we consider two general strategies used within problem behaviour management when the focus is on the emotional response of the animal. These principles are general and are adapted for the specific emotion associated with the problem and the emotional response desired as a solution.

8.5.1 Controlling the intensity of arousal if emotion-appropriate

In some situations, the animal's emotional response may be appropriate but too intense. This might be either a positive emotion (e.g. excitement at seeing someone) or negative emotion (e.g. fear concerning a sudden noise). In this instance, the goal of behaviour modification will be to reduce the intensity of the emotion rather than replace it. *Systematic desensitization* is the most widely used procedure in this context. The idea here is to expose the animal at a low enough threshold to arouse interest, but not a problematic behaviour. Through repeat exposure the animal learns (through a process commonly referred to as *habituation*) that this level of the stimulus is of no significance, and so the intensity of exposure can be increased to a slightly higher level, which now has the same original effect (i.e. creates interest but not the problem behaviour). In effect, the animal is learning to cope with the trigger of the emotion at increasingly higher intensities of exposure (this is referred to as an *exposure gradient*). This process is often combined with operant counter-conditioning (see Section 8.3.2.1). However, if we focus on the intensity of the animal's emotional response rather than precise behaviour, then we are using it to control emotion rather than motivation.

An example of this is the dog that sits or shows deference to the owner rather than jumping up when it sees a visitor. In a combined desensitization and counter-conditioning programme, we reinforce the calmer response (operant counter-conditioning) and expose the dog to the visitor stimulus at a distance with which the dog can cope (desensitization). In this situation, it is best if we teach the response and level of arousal that we want in advance and try to maintain this state during exposure, rather than wait for the animal to offer the behaviour after exposure. This means our pre-training to create the alternative desired response has to focus not only on making the response reliable to the cue but also on ensuring it can be maintained for a prolonged period (i.e. we have to create an expectation that the behaviour has to continue for a certain duration before it is reinforced). If exposure has been too intense during behaviour modification, the animal may 'break out' from the conditioned response. In this case we should reduce the intensity of the stimulus and wait for the desired behaviour to be shown (ideally without being cued, since we want the animal to learn to be well behaved rather than obedient) before reinforcing it. It is then essential to recognize that the level of exposure offered previously was too great for the dog and to go back a few stages in our gradient

8.5.2 Controlling the quality of the emotion if the emotional state associated with the problem behaviour is problematic

In the previous section, the focus was on reducing the intensity of emotion, but many behaviour problems may require changing the emotion associated with the context. There are several ways to do this. If the behaviour is being well rewarded (even if unintentionally), then it may be appropriate to use an extinction schedule before training a more appropriate response (focusing on either the emotion or behaviour). However, in other situations, we will want to replace the emotion.

8.5.2.1 Extinction

If a behaviour has been recurring over some time in a given context, then the behaviour must have some form of reinforcement, and an association will have become established between the behaviour and the reinforcer. External reinforcement is often desired in some of these circumstances and it is this desire for reinforcement which may be at the heart of the problem, in which case we may seek to remove this expectation through extinction. If the consequence is changed, the previous learning is still present, and the animal will continue to perform the behaviour in the expectation of the previous reinforcement. Over time, as the expectation is not met, there will be more variation in the behaviour and probably an increase in its intensity as the animal becomes frustrated by the lack of expected reward. The intensification can be seen as an attempt to 'try harder' to get the expected consequence. The frustration may also make the individual more predisposed to become aggressive if interfered with at this time. This persistence and increase in the intensity of the original behaviour is called an *extinction burst*. During an extinction protocol, so long as reinforcement continues to be withheld (and this must be done beyond any initial increase in behaviour), then a decrease should occur as the animal learns the behaviour will no longer be reinforced and so the desire to perform it wanes. The time taken to get to this point varies and cannot be reliably predicted. Once this desire has subsided, a new behaviour or emotional response may be developed as an alternative in ways described earlier. Needless to say, it is not appropriate to use an extinction protocol for some behaviours as the intensification may be problematic and the risk of increased aggression unacceptable. The other important risk to appreciate is that if reinforcement is obtained when the behaviour is intensified (e.g. in the case of barking for attention, perhaps because the owner cannot cope any more, and so they shout at the dog and thus give it attention), then they will have successfully trained the animal to be even more intense and persistent in its behaviour. Indeed, this is how many severe attention-seeking behaviours are built up in the first place. There are therefore many concerns with the use of simple extinction schedules, and while theoretically reasonable, they are often not very useful in practice. If an extinction protocol is to be used as part of a behaviour modification programme, it is essential to ensure that relevant individuals are counselled on the behaviours to expect when implementing this and carefully assess the risk of the individual going through the protocol, particularly concerning their expression of frustration. If there is any history of the use of aggressive behaviours in situations when the individual has become frustrated in the past, then using extinction protocols would be best avoided due to the potential risks of injury involved.

Withdrawing sources of reinforcement is often the advice given to stop issues like jumping-up behaviour. In this situation, the jumping up has often received positive reinforcement in the form of attention (verbal and physical contact) from someone. The advice is to ignore the jumping-up behaviour. However, by trying to ignore the jumping-up behaviour, it will often increase in intensity and be more varied. Over time, if all individuals are consistent in continuing to ignore the dog at this time (which might include the dog barking and potentially clawing or mouthing at the owner at the same time), the behaviour will decrease, but this sort of consistency is infrequent, and it is natural for someone to respond to a surprising event by instinctively reacting to it in some way. Consequently, this advice is not very practical and a process of operant counter-conditioning of a less intense emotional response (along the lines described in the earlier section), with the dog trained to be calmer and remaining with all four feet on the floor, is preferable. It may also be necessary to combine the training with management to prevent continued practice of the excited jumping up and make it easier to create new options.

8.5.2.2 Emotional substitution

Emotional substitution is often used when it would be preferable if there were different emotions triggered in relation to a stimulus that currently leads to the problem. In effect, what we are seeking to do is to change the animal's perception of this stimulus. This is done through a behaviour modification processes known as *respondent counter-conditioning* or a form of operant counter-conditioning. Respondent counter-conditioning is similar to operant counter-conditioning (see Section 8.3.2.1) but rather than using a learned response, we expose the animal to stimuli which elicit an unconditional emotional response. In the operant version of emotional substitution, we use a learned response with a strong positive association to replace the previous emotional response (usually a negative one). It is critical to ensure that the animal's new emotional response (whether it be respondent or operant in nature) is given more weight by the patient than the previously problematic response in the training circumstances. A common emotional response used in the context of respondent counter-conditioning is the pleasure associated with eating some tasty special treats. Likewise, treats may be associated with an operant response, such as a signalled sit. Used in this context, engaging in such an activity is incompatible with being scared, but given what we have previously said about the weight given by the brain to rewards versus aversives, it is important to appreciate that this is only likely to work when the negative state is mild. This does not mean that the problem has to be mild, as, once again, we can (and usually do) combine this sort of training with desensitization. Factors used to reduce the intensity of the problem context include increased distance, less of the stimuli or just a component of the stimuli that normally come together in the problem scenario. In essence, what we do is teach the animal that when stimuli which might have previously led to an undesired response are present, something the animal likes is now present. To build a strong contingency between the problem context and the new response, it is helpful to ensure that when the problem stimulus goes away, so should the pleasant outcome shortly afterwards. It is also best if the reinforcer (i.e. treat) is reserved for this context and not used at other times. The pleasant outcome is then consistently paired with, and contingent upon, the presence of the stimulus. Over time and with repeated exposures (at a rate the individual can cope with), the previously problematic context comes to have a different emotional meaning and the problem behaviour no longer appears, even without the reward.

Consider a dog who has been barking and lunging at other dogs. The owner reports the dog looks, then stiffens, then pulls forwards before barking, lunging and snapping. The escalation often occurs as distance reduces. It is not unusual for food or any other reinforcement to be ignored by the dog at the stage where it is barking or lunging forwards as the arousal levels are too high. In this particular case, the owner would be advised to maintain distance from other dogs. Reinforcers in the form of food may be given when the dog is stiff in the body language. Any behavioural escalation above this (lunging, barking or snapping, for example) would not want to be reinforced and *could not be reinforced as the dog would not take food anyway*. Initially, the owner may be asked to observe the body language and feed the dog as soon as it has seen other dogs. While feeding, the owner is encouraged to feed the dog slightly to the side or drop food on the floor to encourage the dog to look away from the other dog (respondent counter-conditioning). With a consistent approach from the owner, the dog should turn to the owner when it sees a dog in the distance, albeit it briefly. This change in behaviour (brief period of looking at the owner) is facilitated by the earlier intervention of feeding and enables the opportunity to ask the dog for an alternative more appropriate behaviour when seeing another dog. It might be that training the dog to give the owner eye contact on the cue 'watch me' may be helpful (operant counter-conditioning). The 'watch me' signal needs to be taught over time and strengthened in a range of situations before being used in the situation with other dogs.

8.5.3 Specific considerations concerning the use of desensitization and counter-conditioning

From the previous sections, it will be apparent that desensitization and counter-conditioning often play an important role in the management of many cases. However, depending on how it is used, it may influence behaviour either directly through a specific effect on behavioural motivation or indirectly through an effect on emotion. A typical systematic desensitization and counter-conditioning protocol needs to acknowledge the following elements:

- The alternative and more desired response needs to be elicited or taught by respondent or operant counter-conditioning, respectively, away from the stimulus which elicits the undesired behaviour.
- Only once the response is reliable for a predefined period should the animal be introduced to the problem-eliciting stimulus, and this should be done slowly and at an intensity with which the animal can cope. This may involve breaking down the eliciting stimulus into different elements. For example, a dog may react to other dogs but be worse with male dogs, or dogs of a particular size, in which case the less arousing form of dogs should be used first. Distance is often an important influence on the probability of the problematic reaction and also a way of controlling stimulus intensity during management. It is worth writing down all of the identifiable factors which affect the intensity of the response and scoring them to create a scale. The scale can be used to create a stimulus gradient with which the owner can work. Another useful point to note in this regard is that when the problematic response has become associated with a wide range of stimuli, it is generally easier to work on the learned aspects first. Although different elements of the stimulus may have been identified, it is not always possible to present each type independently of others. This needs to be borne in mind as the presentation of multiple elements may be more challenging for the individual to cope with.

- Where possible, owners should be advised to avoid any exposure to the problematic eliciting stimulus during the implementation phase of the behaviour management protocol. If exposure is inevitable, then it should be managed as far as possible so that it can be at an intensity where no significant reaction would occur. This can be difficult in practice, and unexpected exposures may occur. In these circumstances, owners should be encouraged to reinforce any response which differs positively to the undesired one, to approximate towards the desired goal over time.
- When implementing these protocols, it is important to observe the animal's body language and work at the speed of the individual, modifying the plan and approach as and when needed. The aim is to expose the animal to a level which causes interest but with which it can cope and thus respond appropriately. Setting up situations in which owners can practise may be beneficial initially to help them develop their training and observational skills. If this can be done in a safe environment where access to stimuli is more controlled, the owner is more likely to succeed later on when they are by themselves as they have developed a history of what they need to do and what they are looking for from their animal. There can sometimes be a fine line between coping and not, and it is not always possible to predict what will happen in the real world, so safety needs to be considered throughout. As such, risk-management interventions need to be considered and implemented as needed in each case. In some cases, interventions such as muzzle training may be required before starting a desensitization and counter-conditioning protocol. The impact of increased arousal also needs to be considered as although the animal may appear calm from a behavioural point of view, physiologically it may still be highly aroused. This can present as the animal being able to cope with several exposures but then reacting to another relatively mild event. It is important not to try to do too much too soon, and it is best to stop the formal exercise until the next time while things are going well.

Consider a dog who shows undesired behaviour towards people; people are considered the triggering stimulus. However, there are different elements to this stimulus which may include the noises they make, different smells, the people's interactions with the dog, types of clothing they may wear (e.g. hats, dangling jewellery, or high-visibility vests), the number of people, the ages (e.g. children, adults or elderly), and the movement (e.g. walking, running

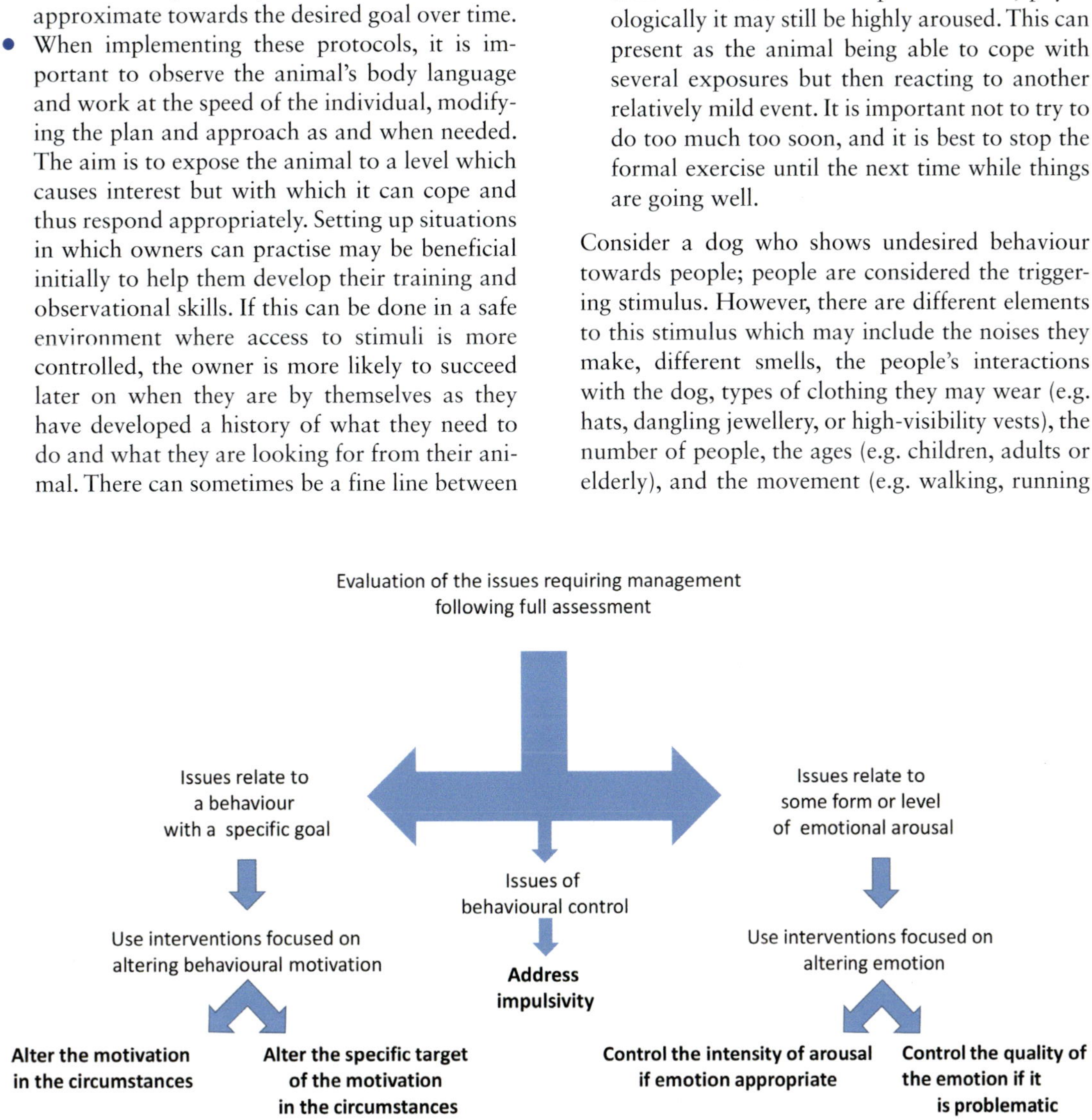

Fig. 8.3. An algorithm explaining the approach to choosing between altering the motivation or managing emotions leading to problem behaviours.

or walking-sticks). Once each of the significant elements affecting the response has been identified, these can be scored and presented gradually according to a gradient. This might involve switching exposure from one element to another, which has a similar intensity, rather than gradually working up the gradient of a given element. For example, managing certain people at a given distance may be followed by exposing the dog to noisy people at a greater distance, rather than moving to a reduced distance with quiet people.

If a dog is concerned about the presence of people in proximity at home, then working outside and away from the home initially provides more distance between the dog and the stimuli which may be more likely to facilitate desired behavioural responses from the dog. Going somewhere quiet where there may be a few people in the distance may also give the owner more time to watch the dog's body language and reward desired responses (e.g. engaging with the owner and environment, or looking away from the person in the distance). If the dog can interact with the environment (i.e. sniff and wander around) and not focus solely on the person in the distance, this would suggest the dog can cope, although there is, of course, a lot of individual variation with the response. The impact of increased arousal caused by training could be evident from the dog having seen two people pass in close proximity and appeared to have coped well, but a few minutes later another person passing by, even at a greater distance than the others, results in an undesirable response.

See Appendix C for basic training protocols and using tools such as a muzzle, head halter, and body harness. See Appendix D for a list of desensitization and counter-conditioning protocols. These handouts provide a guideline to follow when managing dogs and cats with emotional problems.

8.6 Conclusion

Animals learn through association, and this depends on the predictability and regularity of events. This requires owner consistency in the use of reinforcement, whether or not the behaviour is put on an overt cue to create obedience or associated with more general environmental events to create well-behavedness. Animals will not learn when random behaviour is just as effective as purposeful behaviour (e.g. if an owner delivers potential reinforcers freely at times outside the training or behaviour modification context). Animals will also struggle to learn when events to be associated are motivationally or emotionally irrelevant, and so attention needs to be given to the impact of a potential reinforcer, given the circumstance in which it is being used, rather than thinking that food is always best. For a social behaviour, social reinforcers like play may be best. Likewise, it should be appreciated that certain procedures, such as systematic desensitization and counter-conditioning, embrace a wide range of mechanisms to bring about a change in problem behaviour, and not all methods should be considered equivalent. By clearly distinguishing between whether it is the specific behaviour motivation that needs to be altered or the underlying emotional state, it is possible to build more effective behaviour modification programmes that also fit with an owner's goals and abilities (see Fig. 8.3).

References

Arhant, C., Bubna-Littitz, H., Bartels, A., Futschik, A. and Troxler, J. (2010) Behaviour of smaller and larger dogs: effects of training methods, inconsistency of owner behaviour and level of engagement in activities with the dog. *Applied Animal Behaviour Science* 123(3-4), 131–142. DOI: 10.1016/j.applanim.2010.01.003.

Blackwell, E.J., Twells, C., Seawright, A. and Casey, R.A. (2008) The relationship between training methods and the occurrence of behavior problems, as reported by owners, in a population of domestic dogs. *Journal of Veterinary Behavior* 3(5), 207–217. DOI: 10.1016/j.jveb.2007.10.008.

Braem, M.D. and Mills, D.S. (2010) Factors affecting response of dogs to obedience instruction: a field and experimental study. *Applied Animal Behaviour Science* 125(1-2), 47–55. DOI: 10.1016/j.applanim.2010.03.004.

Cooper, J.J., Cracknell, N., Hardiman, J., Wright, H. and Mills, D. (2014) The welfare consequences and efficacy of training pet dogs with remote electronic training collars in comparison to reward based training. *PLOS ONE* 9(9), e102722 DOI: 10.1371/journal.pone.0102722.

Deldalle, S. and Gaunet, F. (2014) Effects of 2 training methods on stress-related behaviors of the dog (*Canis familiaris*) and on the dog–owner relationship. *Journal of Veterinary Behavior* 9(2), 58–65. DOI: 10.1016/j.jveb.2013.11.004.

Herron, M.E., Shofer, F.S. and Reisner, I.R. (2009) Survey of the use and outcome of confrontational and non-confrontational training methods in client-owned dogs showing undesired behaviors. *Applied Animal*

Behaviour Science 117(1-2), 47–54. DOI: 10.1016/j.applanim.2008.12.011.

Hiby, E.F., Rooney, N.J. and Bradshaw, J.W.S. (2004) Dog training methods: their use, effectiveness and interaction with behaviour and welfare. *Animal Welfare* 13(1), 63–70.

Horowitz, A. (2009) Disambiguating the "guilty look": salient prompts to a familiar dog behaviour. *Behavioural Processes* 81(3), 447–452. DOI: 10.1016/j.beproc.2009.03.014.

Horwitz, D. and Mills, D. (2009) *BSAVA Manual of Canine and Feline Behavioural Medicine*. British Small Animal Veterinary Association, Gloucester, UK.

Lopes Fagundes, A.L., Hewison, L., McPeake, K.J., Zulch, H. and Mills, D.S. (2018) Noise sensitivities in dogs: an exploration of signs in dogs with and without musculoskeletal pain using qualitative content analysis. *Frontiers in Veterinary Science* 5, 18. DOI: 10.3389/fvets.2018.00017.

McGreevy, P.D. and Boakes, R.A. (2007) *Carrots and Sticks: Principles of Animal Training*. Cambridge University Press, Cambridge, UK.

McPeake, K.J., Collins, L.M., Zulch, H. and Mills, D.S. (2019) The Canine Frustration Questionnaire – Development of a new psychometric tool for measuring frustration in domestic dogs (*Canis familiaris*). *Frontiers in Veterinary Science* 6, 152. DOI: 10.3389/fvets.2019.00152.

Mills, D.S. (2005) What's in a word? A review of the attributes of a command affecting the performance of pet dogs. *Anthrozoös* 18(3), 208–221. DOI: 10.2752/089279305785594108.

Ramirez, K. (1999) *Animal Training: Successful Animal Management through Positive Reinforcement*. Shedd Aquarium, Chicago, Illinois.

Rehn, T. and Keeling, L.J. (2016) Measuring dog-owner relationships: crossing boundaries between animal behaviour and human psychology. *Applied Animal Behaviour Science* 183, 1–9. DOI: 10.1016/j.applanim.2016.07.003.

Wright, H.F., Mills, D.S. and Pollux, P.M. (2011) Development and validation of a psychometric tool for assessing impulsivity in the domestic dog (Canis familiaris). *International Journal of Comparative Psychology* 24(2).

9 Psychopharmacology

Sagi Denenberg*

Langford Vets, University of Bristol, Langford, UK; North Toronto Veterinary Behaviour Specialty Clinic, Toronto, Canada

9.1 Introduction

Alongside behaviour modification (see Chapter 8), psychopharmacology is an important aspect of veterinary psychiatry. When we face a patient with problem behaviours, first we must determine whether the problem is a normal behaviour that is excessive or does not meet the owner's expectation, or a result of a true pathological condition. Environmental management, routine and behaviour management, and setting realistic expectations can help manage the former. The addition of medications to the above tools can help manage the latter.

Some owners and clinicians consider the use of medication controversial. This is mostly the result of misconception about the purpose and expectation of using medications and relying on medications without behavioural therapy. It is important to remember that medications will not alter the relationship between the patient and the trigger. In other words, if a dog does not like to be around other dogs, no medications will make the dog like the situation. However, the medication can help the dog to calm down and be less intense near other dogs.

In this chapter, we review some of the most commonly used medications and several less commonly used medications (see specific sections below). For a more in-depth discussion of individual medications and their metabolism, see Crowell-Davis *et al.*, 2019.

9.2 Making a Diagnosis

The first step is to reach a diagnosis (see Chapter 7). A description of the behaviour is not a diagnosis. This is an unfortunate and commonly occurring situation that must be changed. When describing the behaviour (e.g. inter-cat aggression, aggression towards people, or house soiling), we are naming clinical signs rather than the underlying cause. Using a descriptive terminology might be helpful for owners. However, it does not help us in choosing the appropriate medication. Behaviour is the consequence of an underlying emotion, similar to limping (behaviour) as the result of pain (emotion) due to torn cruciate ligament (morphological/functional failure).

Patients' behaviour is modulated by physiological needs (e.g. thirst, hunger, procreation and thermoregulation) and emotions (e.g. fear, anxiety, frustration and caring) (Panksepp, 2016). The exact expression of the behaviour also depends on genetic and epigenetic factors, learning and the external factors including owners, other animals and the environment (Robinson *et al.*, 2008; Amat *et al.*, 2016).

The modulation of behaviour is facilitated by different neurotransmitters and electrical processes in the brain. Psychiatric medications affect one or more neurotransmitters and receptors in the brain. Therefore, establishing the diagnosis allows us to choose a medication that will affect the desired neurotransmitters and receptors (Stahl, 2013).

Furthermore, physical pathology (e.g. degenerative joint disease, hyperthyroidism in cats, pain, and otitis externa) (see Chapters 2 and 3) can alter the behaviour and must be ruled out or treated before making a psychiatric diagnosis. Finally, many physical pathologies might limit or contradict the use of psychiatric medications.

9.3 The Goals of Using Medications

Once a diagnosis and the decision to use medications are reached, the next question is 'What are the aims?'

There are several goals. First, we want to improve the well-being of the patient, to reduce its suffering.

*s.denenberg@bristol.ac.uk

DOI: 10.1079/9781786394552.0009

Medications can attenuate fears, anxieties, frustration and intensities. High levels of arousal can be detrimental to the patient and its ability to learn (see Chapter 7). The use of medications can facilitate better and faster learning by reducing arousal (Crowell-Davis *et al.*, 2019). Once we increase the patient's threshold to the trigger by using medications, the patient is less reactive and the owner can implement the necessary behavioural therapy more effectively.

Most pets with psychiatric disorders have altered biological rhythms and patterns of behaviour. For example, they might not sleep adequately (in both quantity and quality), have an abnormal appetite (anorexia or excessive) and show abnormal reactions. Also, these patients cannot habituate or learn in these situations. The use of medications can help to restore normal biological patterns. In other words, medications can help restore normal patterns by balancing levels of neurotransmitters, enhancing neuronal signals and promoting gene translation in the brain leading to improved learning, sleep–wake cycle, appetite and reduced arousal.

In some cases, the situation is very complex, and several pathologies exist, and the owner's ability to control, manage or avoid the situation is limited. For example, a dog with separation distress might show anxiety around the owner, panic when left alone at home, frustration that it cannot follow the owner and grief due to loss of social interaction. At the same time, the owner's ability to avoid these emotions is limited as the owner must leave the dog alone, at least part of the time, and cannot be there when the dog suffers the most. In these situations, the use of psychiatric medication is essential.

9.4 Choosing the Medication

Once we decide to use a medication or medications, the next challenge is the choice of medications. Reaching a diagnosis helps as it narrows down the selection based on the neurotransmitter(s) and receptors that you are attempting to manage. We first must consider several guidelines that help us choose the correct medication.

Most medications modulate the pre- and postsynaptic receptors, inhibit or enhance enzymes that either produce or degrade neurotransmitters or block re-uptake processes (see below for detailed modes of action of different medications). The monoamine (dopamine, noradrenaline and serotonin) and gamma-aminobutyric acid (GABA) are the most commonly targeted neurotransmitters in the management of behaviour problems. Other neurotransmitters such as glutamate, acetylcholine, substance P and opioids are targeted less frequently. It is essential to know the function of these neurotransmitters and their pathways in order to choose the appropriate medication and to know what to expect. Most medications will affect more than one target neurotransmitter, especially in higher doses, leading to the appearance of side effects (Ferguson, 2001).

Depending on the neurotransmitters, receptors or pathways, psychoactive medications have a broad range of effects. For example, serotonergic medications improve learning and perception, while reducing arousal, intensity and motivation to perform undesired behaviours. Dopaminergic medications can improve learning and memory and reduce depression and inactivity. GABAergic medications provide a calming effect by reducing fear and anxiety.

9.4.1 Availability

Not many medications are licensed for use in animals. Also, not all countries have the same selection. Currently, only clomipramine, fluoxetine, selegiline, imepitoin, dexmedetomidine oromucosal gel, and propentofylline are licensed and commercially available (not in all countries) for the use in dogs or cats. However, many other medications are available and can be used for patients.

In some cases, the medication might be available; however, the strength or size might be a problem. For example, in many countries, fluoxetine is available as 10 mg and 20 mg capsules. However, the average dose for a cat is approximately 5 mg. Therefore, the use of liquid or compounded form might be required. When choosing medications that are not licensed, off-label or compounded, owners must be advised and sign a consent form.

9.4.2 Frequency

An important factor in selecting the medication to use is the frequency of administration. Using once-daily dosing is likely to be easier for owners than three times daily medication. Owners' compliance is an important factor in the success of managing patients. Helping owners by minimizing their workload helps improve compliance.

Another aspect of the frequency of dosing is daily use or 'as needed' use. The decision depends primarily on the nature of the problem. When a patient presents the problem on an isolated schedule (e.g. noise phobia only through fireworks or thunder), we can choose a medication that is active within a short period and can be used only during the time needed. Conversely, when the pet is suffering from an ongoing or daily problem (e.g. separation distress each time the owner leaves, or fear of people and other dogs on daily walks), we must choose a medication that is active throughout the day, each day.

Similarly, when the patient suffers from a situational problem, but the owners cannot predict when the situation is likely to occur, and the problem is presented frequently (e.g. storm phobia during storm season), a long-term daily medication should be used.

Most medications that are used for situational problems (i.e. as needed) can also be used daily (e.g. gabapentin, trazodone or benzodiazepines). For specific indications, the frequency of administration and potential benefits, refer to the discussion on individual medications below. When prescribing medications for situational use, the author always recommends testing the medication in the owner's presence before the actual intended use. For example, the owners should give a dose a few days before an actual visit to the vet and observe the effects the medication has on the patient. Some medications may have a side effect, not be effective in the recommended dose or have a paradoxical effect (e.g. stimulating rather than calming).

9.4.3 Administration

When deciding which medication to use, other than availability and frequency, the process of administering the medication should be considered as well. If owners cannot successfully administer the medication, not only due to schedule conflict but also difficulties with the patient taking the medication, then the treatment will fail.

Most medications that are not licensed for patients are bitter. For example, most serotonergic medications (e.g. fluoxetine HCL, sertraline HCL or paroxetine HCL) are hydrochloric acid based. Most patients, especially cats, tend to avoid bitter tastes. Some owners might struggle to administer medications due to their abilities, or the pet might show aggression towards the owners (accidentally at times) who administer the medications. Therefore, using a single medication might be preferable to the use of several medications.

In some cases, owners might report side effects such as increased aggression, hiding or reduced appetite. It is essential to investigate whether these are truly side effects of the medication or related to the administration process. The patient might show aggression towards the person who administers the medication or avoids the owner or food (if the medication is hidden inside it).

The use of liquid medications might appeal to some owners as an easier route of administration. Also, it is easier to titre the desired dose using liquid preparation. However, should the patient spit out part of the liquid, the dilemma is how much to supplement. Similar to generic forms, liquid might be bitter, and the patient might refuse taking it. Finally, some liquid medications (for humans) might contain artificial sweeteners such as xylitol. Care is necessary to avoid accidental intoxication of patients.

Clinicians and owners might find transdermal preparations appealing. However, absorption and bioavailability are poor and inconsistent (Ciribassi *et al.*, 2003; Mealey *et al.*, 2004) and increasing the concentration of the preparation is not a reliable method to increase bioavailability and might lead to toxicity. Transdermal preparation may cause local irritation and lead to dermatitis (Mealey *et al.*, 2004). These preparations also depend on skin temperature for their absorption rate. In warmer environments the absorption rate might be higher, leading to an accidental overdose. Lastly, other animals may accidentally ingest transdermal preparations while grooming the patient.

9.4.4 Dosing

The next step after deciding which medication to use is the dose. We should start using the medication on a low dose. A low dose is defined as the lowest dose within the therapeutic range. In specific cases, such as geriatric patients, sick patients or patients on other medications, a lower dose can be used as a starting point. The rationale behind starting the medication on a low dose is an attempt to avoid potential side effects.

Side effects may appear within minutes to days of administration, while beneficial effects may take up to several weeks to be seen. The timing depends on the choice of medication. While in most cases side effects are mild and transient (i.e. disappear after some time), they might be distressing to the patient and the owners. Also, avoiding side effects can help to maintain owners' compliance and improve the outcome. Owners should be advised to seek help if they notice side effects. For specific information about the doses, time of onset and duration, and potential side effects, see the sections about the specific medications.

Once we choose the medication and the starting dose, we must allow sufficient time before evaluating the effect of the medication. If the dose is too low, the medication is unlikely to be effective regardless of time. For example, using clomipramine at 0.5 mg/kg twice daily is unlikely to have the desired effect on a dog even after two months. Correspondingly, using clomipramine at 2 mg/kg for one week is unlikely to have the desired effect in this time.

After selecting the medication and the dose, we should advise the owners what to expect (both beneficial and potential side effects) and the timeframes. If no beneficial effects are seen within the required timeframe (e.g. 4 weeks for fluoxetine), we should increase the dose and allow more time before re-evaluating. As long as no side effects are seen, we can increase the dose (within the reference range or slightly higher), trying to achieve beneficial effects. However, the higher the dose, the more likely it is that we see side effects (Ferguson, 2001).

If, after increasing the dose several times and reaching the maximal dose, no beneficial effects are seen, it is prudent to review the diagnosis. It is also essential to evaluate the owner's involvement: Were they able to administer the medication successfully, implement behavioural and environmental modification, and prevent when necessary?

If there are no to minimal desired effects at the highest dose, we must consider changing the medication. It cannot be assumed that when one medication is not effective the same would be true for another, even from the same class (i.e. sertraline may be useful where fluoxetine failed) (Stahl, 2013).

The author adjusts the dose based on the patient's body weight and the presentation of the medication. For example, a small cat will receive 2.5 mg of clomipramine, a middle-sized cat 5 mg, and large cats will receive 7.5 mg of clomipramine once daily as the tablet size is 5 mg. When using a liquid or compounded medication, it is easier to tailor the dose to the patient's weight.

9.5 Length of Treatment

9.5.1 Duration

The purposes of using medication as part of the management are to improve the mental and emotional well-being of the patient, reduce arousal and intensities, restore normal biological patterns and, if possible, solve the problem. In other words, if the medication helps to achieve these goals, then the patient should receive the medication for as long as necessary.

In many cases, this may mean a life-long treatment with medications. The length of treatment also depends on the ability of the owners to manage the problem, the environment and exposure to triggers. Once the owners report that the patient is feeling and behaving well over several months, and the owners feel that the problem is under control within a manageable level, it is reasonable to attempt to withdraw the medication.

9.5.2 Termination

We should follow a gradual and controlled process to wean the patient off the medication once the decision is made. The length of the process depends mainly on the type of medication and its half-life. Also, a slow process would allow owners to watch for any signs of regression. In other words, the problem might return as we wean the patient off its medication. A good rule of thumb is to reduce the dose by 25% every month for daily-used medications that were used for more than several months. Gradual withdrawal also allows for the brain chemistry and plasticity (type and number of receptors) to adjust, thus reducing the likelihood of withdrawal side effects.

In the author's experience, if the patient starts showing regression while tapering the medication, the dose should revert back to the last effective dose and remain at that level for several months. If the patient regresses during the next attempt to wean the medication, despite adequate environmental management and behaviour modification, the author will recommend leaving the patient on medication for life.

9.6 Monitoring the Effects of Medications

Following initiation of treatment using medications, we must monitor the patient and evaluate the effect of the medication(s). The first step is informing the owners what to expect. Owners may have unrealistic expectations of the medication or are worried about side effects.

Depending on the medication we choose, beneficial effects may take minutes to weeks (see below for specific medications and their pharmacokinetics). Side effects tend to appear faster than beneficial effects. In some cases, owners may interpret side effects as beneficial. For example, some medications may cause lethargy that owners might interpret as calmness. Other medications might reduce urination due to urethral muscle spasms or inhibition of the central micturition centre in the brain, rather than reducing anxiety. Therefore, the disappearance of undesired behaviours within the initial phase of the treatment should not be the sole indicator of improvement or usefulness of the medication.

Owners should be given reliable measures that they can use to evaluate the true effect of the medication. There are several parameters that owners can follow and rate to help to determine the usefulness of the medication.

9.6.1 Intensity of the behaviour

Often, the undesired behaviour will not completely disappear when using medications. This is more true when owners rely solely on the medication, or in the early stages. However, owners can be instructed to develop an 'intensity scale' that is limited to their pet for a specific problem.

For example, a dog that shows aggression near other dogs can be rated on a zero to ten scale. Zero denotes no reaction at all (including the absence of displacement behaviour, conflict or other covert signs of aggression or high arousal (see Chapter 7)). Ten denotes the most intense behaviour this particular dog has demonstrated before coming for a consultation. The owner is then instructed to rate the dog on this subjective scale, so the dog serves as its own comparison. At the beginning of the treatment, the dog is rated at ten, part or most of the time. The owner should use ongoing encounters (which ideally are avoided (see Chapter 12)) and compare them to the previous encounters. Even if this scale is not scientifically accurate, it serves the purpose; owners will be able to see the trend. Of course, some of the changes, ideally improvement, would be due to the behavioural and environmental management.

9.6.2 Recovery period

At the beginning of an incident, the patient arousal level is increasing. Once the situation has finished, the patient arousal level starts to decrease (see Chapter 7). The time it takes the patient to return to its previous state (before the incident) is termed the recovery period. Owners should be instructed to measure this time.

For example, a cat might be resting on a windowsill and then starts to show aggression when it sees the second cat outside. Once the owner removes the cat from the area, or the second cat disappears, the aggressive cat will start calming down. This is the starting point of the recovery period (T0). The owner then should start to measure how long it takes the cat to settle down until it rests again as it did before. Owners often feel that their pet calms down fast, even within several minutes. However, it is important to stress to owners that, most likely, their pet is still aroused as they cannot measure its pulse, blood pressure or cortisol level. Therefore, owners should be given information about calm body language and observe visible physiological markers such as slow breathing, loose facial and body muscles, calm body posture and calm responses to the owners. Once the cat reached this level, the owner can stop measuring the recovery period (T1). This period (T0–T1) should decrease in duration if the medication is effective.

9.6.3 Frequency of the behaviour

The last parameter to improve is the occurrence of the behaviour. Its intensity, duration and recovery period would improve faster. The question is qualitative: Does the patient show the behaviour or not? This parameter depends primarily on learning. Medications can help improve learning (also by reducing arousal) but not teach the patient how to behave. It is likely that once the medication attenuates the intensity of the situation (by reducing motivations and negative emotions), the patient would be less inclined to show the behaviour. However, owners still must teach the dog how to respond appropriately or change the behaviour completely.

For example, a dog who shows aggression as a result of anxiety might start showing less aggression or no aggression at all if it is less anxious in the presence of the trigger. However, the dog may still dislike the trigger and will continue showing a degree of undesired behaviour when faced with the trigger. It is then up to the owner to use behaviour modification to modify the dog's motivation or alter its behaviour (see Chapter 8).

9.7 Altering the Protocol

When the desired effects are not seen (at all or in full), changing the medication protocol might be necessary. Before considering a change, we must ensure that:

- we used the appropriate dose or increased when necessary;
- we have allowed sufficient time to pass (depending on the choice of medication);
- the owner was able to administer the medication as directed; and
- the owner implemented behavioural and environmental management appropriately.

If all of the above conditions are met, then we can consider changing the medication. There are two decisions to be made: changing the medication for a different one, or adding another medication (see Fig. 9.1).

9.7.1 Changing medications

Before changing from one medication to a different one, we must wean the patient off the current medication. This is especially important when changing to a different medication from the same class (neurotransmitter), for example fluoxetine to sertraline. The weaning process and length of wash-out depends on the medication we currently use.

For example, fluoxetine has an extended half-life (owing to its active metabolite norfluoxetine). When changing from fluoxetine to selegiline, a minimum of five weeks' wash-out period is recommended. However, when changing from selegiline to fluoxetine, only two weeks wash-out period is necessary.

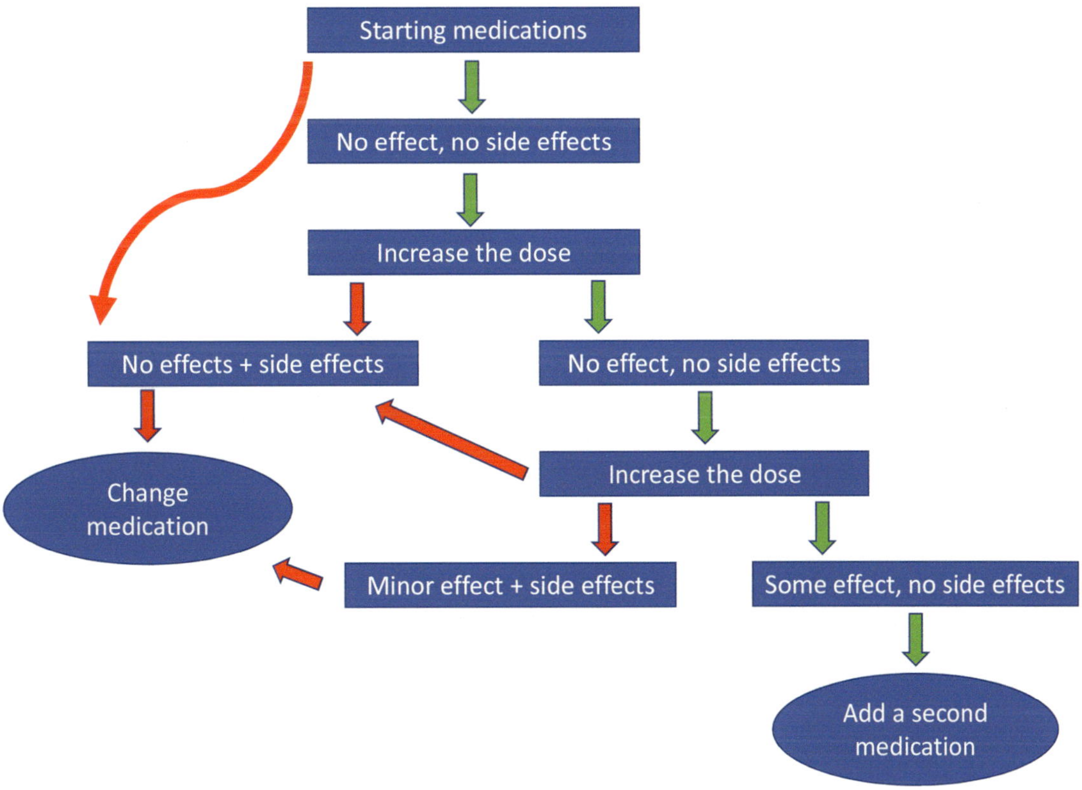

Fig. 9.1. A simple algorithm guiding the decision making in changing medication protocol.

When changing a medication from one class to a different one, no wash-out is necessary. For example, discontinuing lorazepam (GABA) and starting trazodone (serotonin) can be done immediately.

9.7.2 Augmenting medications

When we feel that we have exhausted the dose of medication but the result is not sufficient, we have the option of adding a second (and sometimes third and fourth) medication. Adding more medications might pose a difficulty to owners in both frequency of administration (e.g. once daily to three times daily), or with medicating the patient.

The purpose of adding a second medication is enhancing the overall beneficial effect without increasing side effects. There are two main advantages to adding a second medication rather than increasing the dose of the first medication even further. First, it is preferred to give several medications on a lower dose (not lower than the low reference range) than to give one medication on a very high dose. Increasing the dose of any medication may not yield beneficial effects and can lead to the emergence of side effects. Second, when adding medications, we can affect more target pathways and neurotransmitters (e.g. serotonin and adrenaline, or serotonin and GABA). Doing so helps to complement the first medication and obtain a broader effect.

When adding a second medication we should consider several guidelines:

- We should start introducing the second medication at a dose close to the lower end of the therapeutic range.
- Serotonin syndrome (see Section 9.8.1) can result from combining different serotonergic medications. Primarily, MAOI should not be used with other serotonergic medications.
- Combining medications from different classes (neurotransmitters or mode of action) is generally safe and practical.
- Synergistic and additive effects should be reviewed before starting the second medications.
- Considering the cytochrome P450 system helps in deciding which medication to choose (see below).

9.7.3 Interactions

Our patients mostly tolerate psychoactive medications well. While most medications can be used throughout the patient's life, a logical and careful approach is necessary. Current or future medications that the patient might require (e.g. analgesia, antibiotics, gastric motility modulators, or antipruritic) might interact or contradict the use of psychoactive medications. For example, tramadol, metronidazole or metoclopramide have a minor effect on serotonin. In combination with fluoxetine, the level of serotonin might increase. Similarly, clomipramine reduces the uptake of clonidine by noradrenergic receptors leading to potential hypertension.

Aside from the effect these medications have on blocking receptors or on neurotransmitters, they also interact with other medications through the cytochrome P450 (CYP) liver enzyme system. Concurrent intake of inhibitors or inducers of the CYP isozymes involved in the biotransformation of specific psychoactive medications may alter plasma concentrations of these agents. It is important to note that inducing the CYP means enhancing its effects or, in other words, decreasing the amount of the substrate. Inhibiting the CYP increases the amount of substrate. For example, fluoxetine inhibits CYPD26, and, as a result, the level of most other serotonergic medications might increase, potentially leading to serotonin syndrome (see Section 9.8.1).

Fluoxetine, paroxetine and sertraline (only in high doses) are potent inhibitors of the CYP2D6 and fluvoxamine is a potent inhibitor of CYP1A2 and CYP2C19. Citalopram, escitalopram, venlafaxine and mirtazapine are weak inhibitors of the CYP system and presumably are safer to combine with other medications (Spina *et al.*, 2008). It is important to note that most data stem from human medicine and, to a lesser degree, from animals. While we cannot assess the interaction accurately in our patients, it is prudent to take the same precautions used in human medicine. Table 9.1 illustrates some of the commonly used medications and their effect on the CYP system and substrates.

9.8 Serotonergic Medications

The most commonly used medications in veterinary psychiatry affect the serotonergic pathways (see Table 9.2). There are several different modes of action, including enhancing the release of serotonin into the synaptic cleft, blocking the re-uptake of serotonin from the synaptic cleft, or inhibiting the

Table 9.1. Cytochrome P450 enzymes, their inducers, inhibitors and substrates. These data are adopted from human medicine. While some changes are likely with our patient, it is prudent to take the information from human medicine into account.

Enzyme	Inducer	Inhibitor	Substrate
1A2	Carbamazepine Phenobarbital	Fluoroquinolones Fluoxetine Fluvoxamine Paroxetine Sertraline TCAs (most)	Duloxetine Fluvoxamine Mirtazapine Omeprazole TCAs
2C9	Carbamazepine	Fluoxetine Fluvoxamine Sertraline	Amitriptyline Fluoxetine Sertraline
2C19	Carbamazepine	Fluoxetine Fluvoxamine Sertraline	Citalopram Clomipramine Sertraline
2D6		Citalopram Duloxetine Fluoxetine Paroxetine Sertraline TCAs (most)	Citalopram Duloxetine Fluoxetine Paroxetine TCAs Trazodone Venlafaxine
3A4	Carbamazepine	Fluvoxamine TCAs	Sertraline Trazodone TCAs Venlafaxine

degradation of serotonin. Due to their effect on various serotonin receptors (e.g. pre-synaptic 5HT1A and post-synaptic 5HT2A, 5HT2C and 5HT3) and other neurotransmitters (e.g. noradrenaline, dopamine, histamine and acetylcholine), serotonergic medications have a varied range of indications in animals. Also, this broad effect explains their potential side effects.

9.8.1 Serotonin syndrome

All serotonergic medications have a potentially serious, and even fatal, side effect. This condition is the result of an excessive amount of serotonin in the brain, and mostly attributed to severe overdose. Combining several serotonergic medications or using potent inhibitors of the CYP enzymes that metabolize serotonergic medications can lead to excess serotonin in the synaptic cleft.

In the beginning, signs include agitation, restlessness and irritability (mostly seen as aggression). As the condition develops, gastrointestinal signs such as vomiting and diarrhoea might appear. At later stages, sympathetic activation (e.g. dilated pupils, hypertension, tachycardia and tachypnea) might appear, finally leading to neurological signs such as ataxia, muscles fasciculation, coma and death (Haberzettl *et al.*, 2013).

Intravenous fluids and supportive care (e.g. anticonvulsants, antiemetics and gastroprotectants) follow gastric decontamination. If treated early and aggressively, most animals survive.

9.8.2 Selective serotonin re-uptake inhibitors (SSRIs)

9.8.2.1 Mode of action and metabolism

By inhibiting the serotonin transporter (SERT, re-uptake pump) at the pre-synaptic neuron, these medications increase the level of free serotonin in the synapse (Stahl, 2013). These medications may also affect, to a lesser extent than serotonin, other neurotransmitters including dopamine, noradrenaline, histamine and acetylcholine, which can explain some of their potential side effects (Crowell-Davis

Table 9.2. Serotonergic medications doses and indications.

Medication	Class	Indications	Dose	Comments
Citalopram	SSRIs	Fear and anxiety with or without aggression, phobia, depression, apathy, compulsive behaviours, high arousal and impulsivity	Dog: 1–2 mg/kg q24 h Cat: 2.5–5 mg/cat q24 h	All SSRIs need at least 4 weeks to affect
Escitalopram	SSRIs	Same as above	Dog: 0.5–1 mg/kg q8-12 h	
Fluoxetine	SSRIs	Same as above	Dog: 1–2 mg/kg q24 h Cat: 2.5–5 mg/cat q24 h	Infrequent urethral spams; caution in cats
Fluvoxamine	SSRIs	Same as above	Dog: 1–2 mg/kg q12-24 h Cat: 2.5–5 mg/cat q24 h	
Paroxetine	SSRIs	Same as above	Dog: 1–2 mg/kg q24 h Cat: 2.5–7.5 mg/cat q24 h	Strong antihistaminic effect No active intermediate metabolite
Sertraline	SSRIs	Same as above	Dog: 1–2 mg/kg q12 h Cat: 2.5–7.5 mg/cat q24 h	Considered well-tolerated SSRI in both dogs and cats
Amitriptyline	TCAs	Compulsive behaviours involving skin disorders (e.g. acral lick dermatitis), anxiety, pain	Dog: 1–2 mg/kg q12 h Cat: 2.5–5 mg/cat q24 h	Strong antihistaminic effect: can cause drowsiness and urethral spasms
Clomipramine	TCAs	Fear and anxiety with or without aggression, phobia, depression, apathy, compulsive behaviours, high arousal and impulsivity	Dog: 1–2 mg/kg q12 h Cat: 2.5–5 mg/kg q24 h	Most potent TCA Well-tolerated by most patients Mild anticholinergic effect – may slow bladder and bowel output At least 4 weeks to affect
Doxepin	TCAs	Compulsive behaviours involving skin disorders (e.g. acral lick dermatitis), anxiety	Dog: 2–5 mg/kg q8-12 h Cat: 2.5–5 mg/cat q12-24 h	Mild sedative due to strong antihistaminic effect
Imipramine	TCAs	Same as above Also cataplexy and narcolepsy	Dog: 2–5 mg/kg q12-24 h Cat: 2.5–5 mg/cat q12-24 h	
Duloxetine	SNRIs	Anxiety, fear, phobia, pain, depression, post-traumatic stress disorder, impulsivity	Dog: 1–2 mg/kg q12-24 h	Poor bioavailability, not likely to be effective

Continued

Table 9.2. Continued

Medication	Class	Indications	Dose	Comments
Venlafaxine	SNRIs	Same as above	Dog: 1–2 mg/kg q8-12 h Cat: 2.5–5 mg/cat q12-24 h	Very short half-life, may need q8 h dosing
Buspirone	Azapirone	Mild anxiety and fear in dogs and cats. Can be combined with SSRIs and TCAs (lower dose)	Dog: 0.5–1 mg/kg q8-12 h Cat: 2.5 mg-7.5mg/cat q12-24 h	Caution when combining with SSRIs and TCAs 10–14 days to affect
Trazodone	SARI	Situational or ongoing fears and anxieties	Dog: 5–10 mg/kg q12-24 h Cat: 15–25 mg/cat q12-24 h Up to 50 mg/cat for 'as needed' use	Hypnotic at high doses May not be anxiolytic when using 'as needed'
Mirtazapine	Alpha-2 antagonist	Appetite stimulant, anxiety, depression	Dog: 0.2–0.5 mg/kg q24 h Cat: 1.25 mg-2.5mg/cat q24–48 h	Can be combined with SSRIs and TCAs, caution advised

et al., 2019). As a result of treatment using these medications, the number of both pre- and post-synaptic serotonin receptors (depending on the specific medication) can decrease. SSRIs are metabolized by the liver and will affect the CYP450 system (see Section 9.7.3), and are later excreted by the kidneys. Therefore, caution is required in patients with hepatic or renal impairment.

The level of serotonin at the somatodendritic synapses (primarily at the median raphe) increases within hours of using SSRIs and peaks within several days. This pharmacokinetic sequence explains why patients may experience side effects within the initial timeframe. As the somatodendritic synapses become saturated with serotonin (as a result of a reduced re-uptake process), the number of 5HT1A receptors decreases (also known as downregulation). The process of receptors reduction depends on genomic translation, and thus takes two to four weeks to complete. This is the timeframe when the patient starts recovering from side effects, and the medication becomes effective. Further, as the number of somatodendritic 5HT1A receptors decreases, the neuron becomes disinhibited (the main effect of serotonin is inhibitory) and starts releasing more serotonin at the axonal synapse. The increased axonal release of serotonin will lead, in turn, to downregulation of the post-synaptic receptors at the axonal synapse (Stahl, 2013).

In many chronic affective disorders such as anxiety, depression and phobia, the level of brain-derived neurotrophic factor (BDNF) decreases and may affect learning and memory (Björkholm and Monteggia, 2016). SSRIs promote gene translation, which leads to an increase in the synthesis of BDNF.

9.8.2.2 Indications

Given the role serotonin plays and its effect on the brain, SSRIs have a broad range of effects and are useful for many conditions such as anxiety disorders, fears, compulsive disorders, high arousal and depression.

Fluoxetine is the most widely used SSRI in veterinary medicine. It is licensed for use in dogs who show separation-related anxiety (Landsberg *et al.*, 2008). Other presentations include generalized anxiety (Reisner, 2003), aggression (Dodman *et al.*, 1996; Dodman, 1998) and compulsive disorders (Wynchank and Berk, 1998; Irimajiri *et al.*, 2009; Yalcin, 2010).

In cats, fluoxetine is also frequently used for urine marking (Pryor *et al.*, 2001; Hart *et al.*,

2005), aggression (Denenberg, 2015) and compulsive disorders.

Other SSRIs can be used in veterinary psychiatry as well. Citalopram (Stein *et al.*, 1998); Escitalopram, fluvoxamine, paroxetine and sertraline (Dehasse, 2001) are all available options.

9.8.2.3 Side effects and contraindications

The most common side effects are appetite reduction and gastrointestinal signs, such as nausea and diarrhoea (Sherman, 2017). An important side effect to consider, and caution the owner about, although infrequent, is urinary retention. Serotonin plays a role in regulating the central micturition nucleus, and increased serotonin levels over the first few days until a full downregulation (see Section 9.8.2.1) can inhibit the nucleus leading to urethral spasms (Thor, 2003; Ouslander, 2004; Padala *et al.*, 2006). Starting SSRIs on a low dose and increasing when necessary may help to avoid side effects.

SSRIs should be used cautiously in senior or debilitated patients, and those with renal or haptic impairment. Other contraindications include diabetes and bleeding disorders. An older contraindication is the use of SSRIs in patients with seizures. However, more recent information indicates that some SSRIs might be beneficial in patients with seizures (Robinson *et al.*, 2003; Specchio *et al.*, 2004).

9.8.2.4 Interactions with other medications

SSRIs can be combined with other medications, both psychiatric and others. However, care is required as SSRI are potent inhibitors of many CYP450 enzymes (see Section 9.7.3). Combinations with other serotonergic medications might lead to serotonin syndrome (see Section 9.8.1). Combination with medications that affect other neurotransmitters or pathways (e.g. gabapentin, benzodiazepines and clonidine) are considered safe and effective (Ibáñez and Anzola, 2009; Pineda *et al.*, 2014; Sherman, 2017).

When considering a change from one SSRIs to another, or other serotonergic medication, we should exercise caution and allow sufficient withdrawal time to avoid side effects or serotonin syndrome (Black *et al.*, 2000; Renoir, 2013).

9.8.3 Tricyclic antidepressants (TCAs)

9.8.3.1 Mode of action and metabolism

Tricyclic antidepressants, similar to SSRIs, block the SERT pump, thereby elevating the level of serotonin in the synaptic cleft. These medications are less selective to serotonin and have a stronger effect on other neurotransmitters compared with SSRIs. As a result, TCAs are likely to be less potent and have more side effects than SSRIs.

TCAs are absorbed and metabolized in the liver and excreted by the kidneys. Therefore, TCAs should be used carefully in senior patients or those with hepatic or renal diseases.

9.8.3.2 Indications

Of all TCAs, clomipramine is the most serotonin-selective. Its active metabolite (desmethylclomipramine) is mostly noradrenergic. Common indications of clomipramine in dogs include separation-related anxiety (King *et al.*, 2000, 2004), compulsive disorders (Rapoport *et al.*, 1992; Hewson *et al.*, 1998; Moon-Fanelli and Dodman, 1998) and noise aversion (Crowell-Davis *et al.*, 2003). In cats, clomipramine appears useful for anxiety and urine marking (Seksel and Lindeman, 1998; Hart *et al.*, 2005; Landsberg and Wilson, 2005).

Amitriptyline and doxepin are minor to moderate SERT inhibitors but are potently antihistaminic. Both might be beneficial for compulsive behaviour where pruritus might be present (e.g. acral lick dermatitis, psychogenic alopecia and flank sucking. Due to their antihistaminic effect, the patient might be drowsy, which the owner may interpret as calm. Clomipramine was found to be significantly more effective than amitriptyline (Overall and Dunham, 2002).

9.8.3.3 Side effects and contraindications

Owing to their effect on acetylcholine, noradrenaline or histamine, common side effects might include urine retention, slower intestinal motility, reduced appetite, keratoconjunctivitis sicca, mydriasis, hypotension and dry mouth. Side effects can be categorized based on which neurotransmitter is affected. TCAs with a strong antihistaminic effect (H1 and H2 receptors), such as amitriptyline and doxepin, can cause sedation. Equally, doxepin and amitriptyline are strong anticholinergic medications that can cause urinary retention and reduced gastrointestinal motility. TCAs, like SSRIs, are contraindicated in patients with cardiac disease, glaucoma and hyperthyroidism and should be used cautiously in patients with seizures.

As a result of an extensive side effect profile and low potency compared to SSRIs, apart from clomipramine, TCAs should not be considered as first-choice medication.

9.8.3.4 Interactions with other medications

TCAs should not be combined with SSRIs and MAOI due to the risk of serotonin syndrome. When combining TCAs with other antihistaminic or anticholinergic medications caution should be taken. TCAs such as amitriptyline are also used as analgesia and can be combined with most analgesic medications.

9.8.4 Serotonin-noradrenaline re-uptake inhibitors (SNRIs)

9.8.4.1 Mode of action and metabolism

These medications block, at the pre-synaptic cell, the re-uptake of serotonin and noradrenaline, and to a lesser extent, dopamine. To date, there are little data on the use of these medications in dogs and cats. In dogs, duloxetine appears to have poor absorption of only 5% of the administered dose (KuKanich, 2013), while the half-life of venlafaxine is only two to four hours (Howell *et al.*, 1994). The latter indicates the need for twice-, or even three-times, daily dosing of venlafaxine.

9.8.4.2 Indications

In human medicine, SNRIs are used for mood disorders such as depression and anxiety, and chronic pain. Venlafaxine and duloxetine may have similar indications in dogs and cats. Venlafaxine may also have a beneficial effect when treating narcolepsy or cataplexy (Delucchi *et al.*, 2010). In cats, venlafaxine might be useful for the treatment of urine marking when anxiety and idiopathic cystitis are present (Hopfensperger, 2016).

9.8.4.3 Side effects

Side effects of SNRIs are similar to those seen with SSRIs and TCAs. Venlafaxine seems to be tolerated well in cats, even following accidental ingestion of high doses (Pugh *et al.*, 2013).

9.8.5 Azapirones

9.8.5.1 Mode of action and metabolism

Azapirones are serotonergic (5HT1A partial agonist) and dopaminergic (minor effect as a D2 receptor agonist) medications (Peroutka, 1985; Cole and Yonkers, 2004).

Following oral administration, the bioavailability of buspirone in cats is high, while it is low following transdermal absorption (Mealey *et al.*, 2004; Chávez *et al.*, 2016). Buspirone is well tolerated in cats and dogs with minimal side effects.

9.8.5.2 Indications

Buspirone is indicated to reduce anxiety and fear and improve dullness. A fearful cat (e.g. the victim in a case of two cats fighting at home) may benefit from buspirone. While the latter is anecdotal, an increasing number of case reports and personal communication support the notion that buspirone increases confidence. Another possible indication for the use of buspirone is urine marking (anxiety-related behaviour) in cats (Hart *et al.*, 1993). It can be administered as a first-option medication although it is not as potent as some of the other serotonergic medications.

9.8.5.3 Side effects and contraindications

Lethargy or sedation was reported in some cats (Hart *et al.*, 1993). Caution is advised in patients with chronic renal or hepatic disease (Crowell-Davis *et al.*, 2019). Other side effects may include nausea, vomiting and restlessness.

9.8.5.4 Interactions with other medications

Buspirone should not be combined with monoamine oxidase inhibitors, such as selegiline (Crowell-Davis *et al.*, 2019). While combining buspirone with SSRIs or TCAs may help to enhance serotonergic pathways, the combination carries the risk of serotonin syndrome.

Combinations of buspirone with clonidine, benzodiazepines or gabapentin appear to be beneficial and safe in both dogs and cats (S. Denenberg, personal communication).

9.8.6 Serotonin antagonist re-uptake inhibitors (SARIs)

9.8.6.1 *Mode of action and metabolism*

Trazodone is the most commonly used SARI in veterinary psychiatry. SARIs block the 5HT2A and 5HT2C receptors when used at a low dose. In higher doses, these medications also block serotonin reuptake (SERT) at the pre-synaptic cell (Stahl, 2013).

9.8.6.2 *Indications*

In dogs, trazodone may be useful in the management of different anxiety disorders (Gruen and Sherman, 2008). It may also be used for travel-related anxiety, veterinary visits and noise aversion. In cats, in high doses, trazodone is also helpful in treating anxiety, fear and impulsivity, but can lead to sedation (Stevens *et al.*, 2016).

Given its sedative effect in high doses and a relatively short half-life, trazodone is a second- or third-option medication. Also, it is likely that the beneficial effects of trazodone, like other serotonergic medications, are based on genomic translation and molecular changes that require several weeks (Duman, 1998). Therefore, it is likely that the 'as needed' effect is based on mild sedation rather than calmness.

9.8.6.3 *Side effects and contraindications*

Trazodone should be used cautiously in patients with cardiac disease and may lead to hypotension (Murphy *et al.*, 2017; Fries *et al.*, 2018). Side effects may include lethargy, sedation, vomiting, increased vocalization, restlessness and agitation.

9.8.6.4 *Interactions with other medications*

Trazodone can be combined with SSRIs or TCAs, but caution should be exercised to avoid serotonin syndrome. Further, trazodone can be combined with benzodiazepines (increased sedative effect), gabapentin and clonidine.

9.8.7 Alpha-2 antagonist

9.8.7.1 *Mode of action and metabolism*

Serotonergic neurons also have pre-synaptic alpha-2 heteroreceptors. When noradrenaline binds to these receptors, the net effect is the inhibition of serotonin release (Stahl, 2013). Alpha-2 antagonists such as mirtazapine bind and block these receptors, thus increasing the release of serotonin. When binding to alpha-1 post-synaptic receptors on serotonergic neurons in the locus coeruleus, these medications block noradrenaline and increase the level of serotonin release from these neurons downstream in the cortex.

As a potent 5HT2A, 5HT2C and 5HT3 antagonist, with mild antihistamine activity, mirtazapine is a useful alpha-2 antagonist (Stahl, 2013; Ferguson *et al.*, 2016). As such, mirtazpaine may provide anxiolytic and antiemetic effects and appetite stimulation (Quimby and Lunn, 2013; Agnew and Korman, 2014).

9.8.7.2 *Indications*

Common indications include appetite stimulation, antiemetic and anxiolytic (Nobukazu *et al.*, 2009; Argüelles *et al.*, 2017).

9.8.7.3 *Side effects and contraindications*

Mirtazapine should be used cautiously in animals with suspected or confirmed cognitive impairment. Side effects may include muscle tremors, increased vocalization and hyperactivity (Agnew and Korman, 2014).

9.8.7.4 *Interactions with other medications*

Mirtazapine can be used alone or as an adjunct to SSRI or TCA in the management of anxiety, fear and high arousal in cats and dogs. Care should be taken when combining mirtazapine with other serotonergic medications. Additional combinations include benzodiazepines, gabapentin, clonidine and trazodone (with caution).

9.9 Dopaminergic Medications

These medications alter the level of dopamine, through various pathways, and, to a lesser extent, other monoamine neurotransmitters (see Table 9.3)

9.9.1 Monoamine oxidase inhibitors (MAOIs)

9.9.1.1 *Mode of action and metabolism*

The enzymes monoamine oxidase A and B deaminate (degrade) the monoamine neurotransmitters dopamine, noradrenaline and serotonin. MAOIs class-inhibit these enzymes and reduce

Table 9.3. Dopaminergic medication doses and indications.

Medication	Class	Indications	Dose	Comments
Selegiline	MOAI	Cognitive decline, anxiety, depression, apathy	Dog: 0.5–1 mg/kg q24 h Cat: 2.5–5 mg/cat q2 h	Should be given in the morning Should not be combined with serotonergic medications Four to six weeks to affect
Bupropion	DRI	Anxiety, depression, apathy	Dog: 0.5–1.5 mg/kg q24 h Cat: 2.5–5 mg/cat q24 h	Anecdotal use in dogs and cats
Bromocriptine	Ergot alkaloid derivative	Depression, apathy, cognitive decline, pseudopregnancy	Dog: 5–10 ug/kg q24 h Cat: 100–150 ug/cat q24 h	At least 4 weeks to affect
Cabergoline	Ergot alkaloid derivative	Same as above	Dog: 2–4 ug/kg q24 h Cat: 2.5–5 ug/cat q24 h	

or terminate the catabolism of the monoamine neurotransmitters. Further, MAOIs also enhance the activity of the enzymes superoxide dismutase and catalase, which decrease toxic oxygen-free radical species in the brain, thus reducing oxidative damage to the brain tissue (Knoll *et al.*, 1996). In addition, MAOIs can inhibit the re-uptake of catecholamines, stimulate the release of catecholamines and stimulate action potential-transmitter release coupling. Monoamine oxidase A is primarily active in the intestine, and catabolizes exogenous amines such as tyramine (which is found in some foods such as cheese and cured meats), whereas monoamine oxidase B is mostly active in the CNS and catabolizes catecholamines (dopamine, noradrenaline, serotonin and beta-phenylethylamine).

Selegiline is the most commonly used MAOI in dogs and cats. Selegiline is a preferential, irreversible MAOI-B with minor MAOI-A effect in high doses (Landsberg *et al.*, 2010). It is a two-step inhibition sequence. First, the inhibition is reversible, and then it becomes irreversible (Heinonen *et al.*, 1994). Its effect varies between species: it increases dopamine levels in dogs, humans and possibly cats, but not in rats (Crowell-Davis *et al.*, 2019). It also blocks the re-uptake of serotonin and noradrenaline. Selegiline should be given in the morning due to its stimulant effect.

9.9.1.2 Indications

In cats, the main indications for the use of selegiline are cognitive decline and chronic emotional disorders, although not approved for either indication in cats (Dehasse, 1999; Landsberg *et al.*, 2010).

In dogs, selegiline is licensed for chronic emotional disorders in Europe (Pobel *et al.*, 1997). In North America, selegiline is licensed for cognitive decline (Milgram *et al.*, 1993) and pituitary-dependent hyperadrenocorticism (Bruyette *et al.*, 1995). Prolactinaemia worsens chronic emotional disorder. As a dopaminergic medication, selegiline might counteract this effect, improving the well-being of the patients (Mengoli *et al.*, 2017). Selegiline may also improve learning and training in dogs (Mills and Ledger, 2001).

9.9.1.3 Side effects and contraindications

Gastrointestinal upset or restlessness and agitation are seen infrequently (Denenberg and Landsberg, 2017). Selegiline has proved safe in cats with doses up to ten times the recommended dose (Ruhel *et al.*, 1996). Side effects may include gastrointestinal upset, restlessness, agitation, lethargy and reduced hearing (Landsberg *et al.*, 2010).

Given the effects of MAOI-A in the intestine, in human medicine people are instructed to avoid eating tyramine-containing foods (e.g. hard cheese and cured meat). While selegiline is a weak MAOI-A, especially at the dose range recommended in veterinary medicine, it may be sensible to reduce or avoid treats and foods containing tyramine (Crowell-Davis *et al.*, 2019).

9.9.1.4 *Interactions with other medications*

Although a poor serotonergic, selegiline should not be used concurrently with other serotonergic medications, such as SSRIs or TCAs, due to a high risk of serotonin syndrome. An ideal wash-out period of four weeks following SSRIs, or two weeks following TCAs should take place before starting selegiline (Crowell-Davis *et al.*, 2019). Selegiline may interact with metronidazole, prednisone and trimethoprim-sulfa; therefore caution is advised

9.9.2 Dopamine re-uptake inhibitors (DRIs)

9.9.2.1 *Mode of action and metabolism*

This class of medications acts similarly to SSRIs. They block the dopamine transporter (DAT) pump of the pre-synaptic neuron, preventing absorption of dopamine with a net result of increasing the level of dopamine in the synaptic cleft (Stahl, 2013). These medications are not commonly used in veterinary psychiatry. Following absorption, bupropion reaches peak plasma levels in just under two hours (Butz *et al.*, 1981). Bupropion undergoes extensive metabolism, which reduces its bioavailability, and is excreted by the kidneys (Butz *et al.*, 1981; Welch *et al.*, 1987).

9.9.2.2 *Indications*

Bupropion may have similar indications to selegiline (e.g. chronic emotional disorder and prolactinaemia). The author has used it anecdotally in both dogs and cats. Common presentations included depression, inactivity and apathy, emotional feeding (binging), and when SSRIs, TCAs or MAOIs appeared to fail.

9.9.2.3 *Side effects and contraindications*

Side effects might include restlessness and insomnia, gastrointestinal signs and hypertension. It is recommended to measure the patient's blood pressure before starting the medication and then every two weeks while adjusting the dose. DRIs should not be used concurrently with MAOIs or other dopaminergic medications. DRIs and trazodone should not be used together to avoid increasing the toxicity of bupropion.

9.9.2.4 *Interactions with other medications*

While DRIs can be combined with SSRIs, caution should be exercised – elevated toxicity might occur. DRIs can be combined rather safely with medications such as benzodiazepines, gabapentin and imepitoin.

9.9.3 Ergot alkaloid derivatives

9.9.3.1 *Mode of action and metabolism*

These medications are dopamine receptor agonists at the post-synaptic neuron. They also inhibit prolactin release from the anterior pituitary gland (Seksel, 2008). Bromocriptine and cabergoline are used in veterinary medicine to suppress signs of pseudopregnancy (Okkens and Kooistra, 1997). Following absorption, bromocriptine, a potent D2 receptor antagonist acts on dopamine receptors both in the gut and brain (Bueno *et al.*, 1984; de Leeuw van Weenen *et al.*, 2010). It may also suppress glutamate release (Shirasaki *et al.*, 2010). Following subcutaneous injection, bromocriptine reaches plasma levels in three to five hours in dogs. In humans, it reaches peak plasma levels in one to two hours following oral administration. Steady-state plasma levels may need 10–14 days. Cabergoline is also a D2 receptor agonist with similar activity to bromocriptine.

9.9.3.2 *Indications*

Ergot alkaloid derivatives are indicated for the treatment of pseudopregnancy in dogs and cats. Other possible indications include depression, apathy and cognitive decline.

9.9.3.3 *Side effects and contraindications*

The most common side effect reported is vomiting. Other side effects may include hypotension, diarrhoea, ataxia and lethargy. Most side effects are seen following the first dose and can be overcome by administering a lower first dose.

Table 9.4. Noradrenergic medications doses and indications.

Medication	Class	Indications	Dose	Comments
Clonidine	Alpha-2 receptor agonist	Anxiety, panic, phobia	Dog: 0.01–0.05 mg/kg q8-12 h Cat: No established dose Anecdotal dose: 0.025–0.1 mg/cat q12 h	'As needed' or ongoing with TCAs and SSRIs
Dexmedetomidine	Alpha-2 receptor agonist	Anxiety, panic, phobia	Dog: 0.125–0.250 mg/m^2 prn or q12 h Cat: No established dose in cats. May be difficult to administer	Oromucosal gel Can repeat every 2 hours up to five doses May be cost-prohibitive in some countries for ongoing use
Guanfacine	Alpha-2 receptor agonist	Anxiety, panic, phobia	Dog: 1–3 mg/kg q8-12 h Cat: No established dose in cats. Anecdotal dose: 2–4 mg/cat q12 h	'As needed' or ongoing with TCAs and SSRIs. May be cost-prohibitive in some countries for ongoing use
Atenolol	Beta receptor antagonist	Anxiety, panic, phobia	Dog: 0.25–1 mg/kg q12 h Cat: 3.125–6.25 mg/cat q12 h	Reduce dose in cats with renal disease
Pindolol	Beta receptor antagonist	Anxiety, panic, phobia	Dog: 0.1–0.3 mg/kg q12 h Cat 1–2 mg/cat q12 h	May accelerate onset of SSRI effect
Propranolol	Beta receptor antagonist	Anxiety, panic, phobia	Dog: 0.5–2 mg/kg q12 h Cat: 1–5 mg/cat	Studies in humans show poor efficacy.

9.9.3.4 *Interactions with other medications*

Ergot alkaloids can be combined with SSRIs or TCAs when the effect of the latter appears insufficient. However, since ergot alkaloids also affect some 5HT receptors, caution should be exercised. Combinations with benzodiazepines, gabapentin, imepitoin or noradrenergic medications are considered safe.

9.10 Noradrenergic Medications

These medications augment the level of noradrenaline by either stimulating alpha-2 or blocking beta receptors (see Table 9.4).

9.10.1 Alpha-2 agonists

9.10.1.1 *Mode of action and metabolism*

These medications block noradrenaline release from the pre-synaptic neurons in the locus coeruleus. This pontine nucleus is an important modulator of the sympathetic nervous system (Tanaka *et al.*, 2000). Data show that locus coeruleus overactivity induces signs of fear and anxiety. By reducing the firing of these neurons, alpha-2 agonists block the physiological signs of anxiety and fear.

9.10.1.2 *Indications*

Dexmedetomidine oromucosal gel is licensed for dogs for the treatment of noise phobia (Korpivaara *et al.*, 2017a). Other indications include as-needed use for fears and anxieties, such as travel-related anxiety and fear during veterinary visits (Amat *et al.*, 2017; Korpivaara *et al.*, 2017b). One major advantage of dexmedetomidine oromucosal gel is that it can be given after signs of anxiety or panic appear (if the owner can apply it on the dog's gingiva), without the need to administer oral medication or when the patient will not take treats or food.

Clonidine is an alpha-2 agonist with similar indications to dexmedetomidine. It can also be used as an adjunct to SSRIs or TCAs for ongoing treatment of fears and anxieties such as separation-related distress, post-traumatic stress disorder and urine marking (Ogata and Dodman, 2011).

Guanfacine is another alpha-2 agonist with similar indications to dexmedetomidine and clonidine (Scholtysik, 1986). It may have a longer half-life in dogs than clonidine and dexmedetomidine and its bioavailability is higher (Kiechel, 1980). In addition, guanfacine showed less sedative effect and higher potency than other centrally acting alpha-2 agonists in reducing sympathetic activation, which may make it a preferable option for panic attacks and anxiety (Scholtysik, 1986).

9.10.1.3 Side effects and contraindications

Common side effects may include hypotension and sedation. Other possible side effects include sleep disturbances, paradoxical excitation, urinary incontinence and gastrointestinal upset. These medications should be used cautiously in geriatric or debilitated patients and those with cardiac disease and hypotension.

9.10.1.4 Interactions with other medications

Alpha-2 agonists can be combined with SSRIs or TCAs for the management of anxieties and fear (Ogata and Dodman, 2011). Further, these medications can be combined with gabapentin and benzodiazepines for acute panic attacks.

Care should be taken when combining alpha-2 agonists with other hypertensive medications, beta-adrenergic antagonists (see below) and other sedatives. Doses of anaesthesia should be adjusted, or alpha-2 agonists should be discontinued before anaesthesia.

TCAs can reduce the hypotensive effect of alpha-2 agonists, leading to hypertension. Combination of alpha-2 agonists with amitriptyline may lead to corneal ulcers.

9.10.2 Beta-adrenergic antagonists

9.10.2.1 Mode of action and metabolism

Medications from this class block beta-1, beta-2, beta-3, or all three receptors, thus preventing noradrenaline from binding and activating the sympathetic nervous system. The net effect is similar to alpha-2 agonists.

Propranolol is a beta-1 and beta-2 blocker that is used widely in human psychiatry for different conditions. However, a recent study evaluated its effect in humans and found poor results in reducing anxiety and panic (Steenen *et al.*, 2016). In addition, the bioavailability is highly variable and generally poor, and its half-life is short (Mills *et al.*, 2004).

Atenolol is a longer-acting, beta-1 selective blocker with a longer half-life and better availability (McAinsh and Holmes, 1983; Quiñones *et al.*, 1996). Pindolol is a partial beta-adrenoceptor/5-HT1A receptor antagonist that can augment the effect of SSRIs. It appears to accelerate the antidepressant response but does not increase the effectiveness of SSRIs in unresponsive human patients (Artigas *et al.*, 2006).

9.10.2.2 Indications

Beta-adrenergic receptor blockers may be beneficial for patients suffering from panic, phobia and anxieties. They are mostly used as adjuncts to SSRIs and TCAs but can also be combined with buspirone and benzodiazepines.

9.10.2.3 Side effects and contraindications

Side effects may include bradycardia, hypotension, dry mouth, nausea and ataxia. In some cases, urinary incontinence may appear. Beta-blockers are contraindicated in patients who suffer from a cardiac disease such as bradyarrhythmia or congestive heart failure, feline asthma and liver failure. They should be used cautiously in patients with diabetes mellitus and renal failure.

9.10.2.4 Interactions with other medications

Beta-blockers are metabolized by the CYP450 system (primarily CYP2D6). Strong inhibitors such as fluoxetine and paroxetine may increase serum levels of propranolol. Caution should be exercised when combining beta-blockers with medications with sedative effects such as gabapentin or benzodiazepines. Beta-blockers should not be combined with other hypotensive medications such as alpha-2 agonists.

9.11 Gamma-aminobutyric acid (GABAergic) Medications

These medications enhance the activity of GABA neurons, primarily in the limbic system (see Table 9.5).

Table 9.5. GABAergic medication doses and indications.

Medication	Class	Indications	Dose	Comments
Alprazolam	Benzodiazepine	Panic attacks, fear, anxiety	Dogs: 0.02–0.1 mg/kg q8–12 h Cat: 0.125–0.25 mg/cat q8–12 h	Excellent for panic attacks and 'as needed' use Can be given 30 minutes before an event and once more when the event starts
Clonazepam	Benzodiazepine	Anxiety, fear, hyperaesthesia, seizures, compulsive disorder, sleep disorders (hypnotic)	Dog: 0.2–1 m/kg q8–12 h Cat: 0.25–1 mg/cat q12–24 h	Long-acting Higher dose for seizures Do not exceed 8 mg in dogs
Diazepam	Benzodiazepine	Anxiety, fear, seizures, appetite stimulant	Dog: 0.5–2 mg/kg q8–12 h Cat: 1–2.5 mg/cat	Monitor closely in cats or avoid
Lorazepam	Benzodiazepine	Anxiety, fear, panic attacks	Dog: 0.02–0.1 mg/kg q8-12 h Cat: 0.5–1 mg/cat q8–12 h	
Oxazepam	Benzodiazepine	Anxiety, fear	Dog: 0.2–1 mg/kg q12–24 h Cat: 1–2.5 mg/cat q12–24 h	No anticonvulsant effect
Imepitoin	Partial GABA-A receptor agonist	Anxiety, fear, phobia, seizure	Dog: 10–30 mg/kg q12 h Cat: 50–100 mg/cat q12 h	Weak Ca channel blocker With lower doses, it may take 5–10 days to affect Use higher dose when using 'as needed'
Gabapentin	Ca channel blocker	Anxiety, fear, compulsive behaviours, seizures, pain	Dog: 10–30 mg/kg q8 h Cat: 5–25 mg/cat q8–12 h	Can be used 'as needed' 30–40 mg/kg dog, and 50-100 mg/cat
Pregabalin	Ca channel blocker	Anxiety, fear, compulsive behaviours, seizures, pain	Dog: 2.5–5 mg/kg q12 h Cat: 5–10 mg/cat q 12	Considered to have fewer side effects than gabapentin and more potent

9.11.1 Benzodiazepines

9.11.1.1 Mode of action and metabolism

These medications facilitate GABA activity by binding to GABA-A receptors in the CNS (Stahl, 2013). When the hypothalamic and limbic system receptors are activated, the effect is anxiolytic (Danneberg and Weber, 1983). The most commonly used benzodiazepines in veterinary psychiatry are alprazolam, clonazepam, lorazepam and oxazepam. Diazepam is less commonly used, given its effect on the liver, especially in cats (Center *et al.*, 1996). These medications have a rapid onset of action, and the effect lasts between two and 12 hours, depending on the medication (Crowell-Davis *et al.*, 2019).

Except for alprazolam, most benzodiazepines are metabolized by glucuronidation pathways in the liver (Center *et al.*, 1996). Benzodiazepines without intermediate metabolites (e.g. clonazepam, lorazepam and oxazepam) and alprazolam are considered safer for cats.

The choice between different benzodiazepine should be based on the desired duration. Alprazolam is a short-acting benzodiazepine with a duration of approximately two to three hours, while lorazepam lasts approximately four to six hours. Clonazepam and oxazepam are long-acting benzodiazepines with an average duration of eight to ten hours.

At the low end of the dose range, benzodiazepines act as muscle relaxants and appetite stimulants and have a mild calming effect. At the middle-dose range, benzodiazepines are anxiolytics and facilitate social interactions. At the high end of the dose range, benzodiazepines act as anticonvulsants and hypnotics.

Controversy exists regarding the effect of benzodiazepine on patients with fear-related presentations, especially where it is thought that the patient suppresses aggressive behaviours due to fear. This notion started in the 1960s in human psychiatry in patients taking diazepam and chlordiazepoxide (DiMascio, 1973). However, more recent data show that these claims are unsubstantiated (Rothschild, 1992; Joans and Hearron, 1996; Rothschild *et al.*, 2000). It is more likely that any possible disinhibition occurs as a result of side effects of benzodiazepines, including dysphoria and restlessness or paradoxical activation. It is also important to note that many patients with so-called 'disinhibition' were not inhibited at the start of the treatment. Finally, the beneficial effects of benzodiazepines and the emotional improvement of the patient are likely to outweigh any potential disinhibition.

Dependency is a concern that owners may have when discussing the possible use of benzodiazepines. This concept does not exist in veterinary patients as they do not take their own medications.

When discontinuing the use of benzodiazepines in patients who received it daily for an extended period (over several weeks), a gradual weaning process is necessary to avoid any withdrawal syndrome (development of anxiety and restlessness).

Given the wide dose range of benzodiazepines and their different effects at different doses, it is prudent to ask owners to test the dose before actual use. Owners should administer the test dose when they are present to evaluate the effect. The dose should be given when the daily routine is maintained and no unplanned or fear-evoking situation exists. The ideal dose in this scenario is the one where the patient is very calm to borderline lethargic. It is essential to remember that during the actual situation (e.g. the owner leaves the house and the dog stays alone), the effect will be counteracted by the patient's anxiety. Therefore, if, following an administration of a test dose, the owner sees no change, another test with a higher dose should take place.

9.11.1.2 Indications

Benzodiazepines can be used as an adjunct to SSRIs and TCAs for different presentations of anxiety, phobia and panic. Furthermore, benzodiazepines can be used as a single-agent treatment for many short-term or isolated situations such as noise phobia, veterinary visits, travel, grooming and owner departure. In low doses, benzodiazepines can be used as appetite stimulants.

9.11.1.3 Side effects and contraindications

Common side effects of benzodiazepines include sedation, ataxia, muscle relaxation, increased appetite and paradoxical excitation. In cats, diazepam was linked to cases of fatal hepatic necrosis (Center *et al.*, 1996).

9.11.1.4 Interactions with other medications

Benzodiazepines can be administered as an adjunct to SSRIs and TCAs, both on an ongoing or as-needed basis. Care should be taken to avoid additive effect when combining benzodiazepine with other sedatives, GABAergic medications or trazodone.

9.11.2 Imepitoin

9.11.2.1 Mode of action

Imepitoin is a low-affinity partial GABA-A receptor agonist and a weak Ca channel blocker that is licensed (in some countries) as an anti-epileptic for dogs. It has recently been shown to have anxiolytic properties in this species as well (McPeake and

Mills, 2017; Engel *et al.*, 2019). Imepitoin appears to be well tolerated in cats as well (Engel *et al.*, 2017).

9.11.2.2 Indications

Imepitoin is licensed as an anticonvulsant, and recently was also licensed for the treatment of noise phobia in dogs. Given its benzodiazepine-like effect, it may be beneficial for the treatment of the same indications (Engel *et al.*, 2018).

9.11.2.3 Side effects and contraindications

Side effects may include ataxia, vomiting, lethargy, increased appetite and hyperactivity.

9.11.2.4 Interactions with other medications

Imepitoin can be used as an adjunct to SSRIs and TCAs. Imepitoin should be used cautiously with other medications that may cause sedation such as GABAergic medications and trazodone.

9.11.3 Gabapentin and pregabalin

9.11.3.1 Mode of action and metabolism

Gabapentin and pregabalin block the voltage-sensitive calcium channel (VSCC) and are structurally related to GABA (Stahl, 2013). However, they do not mimic the effect of metabolism of GABA, but likely inhibit the release of excitatory neurotransmitters such as glutamate and noradrenaline (Graeme, 2006).

The bioavailability of gabapentin in cats reaches approximately 90%, and the peak effect is reached within ten days (Siao *et al.*, 2010). Excretion of gabapentin and pregabalin takes place via the kidneys.

9.11.3.2 Indications

Common indications include chronic pain, seizures and anxiety. These medications can be combined with SSRIs and TCAs as an adjunct for refractory anxiety and compulsive behaviours.

Gabapentin and pregabalin can be used for panic attacks and situational fears, such as travel-related problems or visits to the veterinarian, although a higher dose is necessary (van Haaften *et al.*, 2017; Pankratz *et al.*, 2018).

9.11.3.3 Side effects and contraindications

Since gabapentin and pregabalin have no active intermediate metabolites and minimal passage through the CYP450 metabolism, the likelihood of side effects is low. Common side effects include sedation, ataxia and gastrointestinal signs such as vomiting and diarrhoea. Owners should be advised to monitor for changes in animality.

Renal excretion is the main route of elimination. Therefore, care should be taken when prescribing these medications to patients with renal impairment.

9.11.3.4 Interactions with other medications

Both gabapentin and pregabalin can be combined with SSRIs, TCAs, trazodone, noradrenergic medications and other analgesics such as NSAIDs, amantadine, opioids and paracetamol.

9.12 Miscellaneous Medications

See Table 9.6 for doses and indications.

9.12.1 Carbamazepine

Carbamazepine is a tricyclic sodium channel blocker that has mood-stabilizing and antidepressant properties. It may also have serotonergic activity. The main indications of carbamazepine are seizures, neuropathic pain, impulsivity in dogs and head shaking in horses (Ambrósio *et al.*, 2002; Brooks, 2008; Haug, 2008).

9.12.2 Stimulants

These medications act on dopaminergic and noradrenergic pathways, enhancing the release of and blocking re-uptake of dopamine and noradrenaline. The main indications of methylphenidate are dextroamphetamine hyperkinesis. This diagnosis is controversial and might be related to other mental and emotional disorders (see Section 15.6.4 – Hyperkinesis).

Methylphenidate can be given twice daily (starting at a low dose and increasing every three days if necessary) to assess the patient for hyperkinesis. When effective, the patient's physiological parameters (e.g. pulse, respiration rate and temperature) and mental parameters (e.g. restlessness, pacing and repetitive behaviours) should decrease.

Table 9.6. Miscellaneous medications doses and indications.

Medication	Class	Indications	Dose	Comments
Carbamazepine	Na channel blocker	Anxiety, impulsivity, seizures, compulsive disorders	Dog: 5–10 mg/kg q12 h Cat: 15–25 mg/cat q12–24 h	Possible mild serotonergic effect
Amantadine	NMDA receptor antagonist	Pain, an adjunct to serotonergic medications for compulsive behaviours	Dog: 2–4 mg/kg q12 h Cat: 5–15 mg/cat q24 h	Can be combined with gabapentin, paracetamol and NSAIDs for pain control
Memantine	NMDA receptor antagonist	Pain, an adjunct to serotonergic medications for compulsive behaviours Adjunct for CDS	Dog: 0.5–1 mg/kg q24 h Cat: 1–5 mg/cat q24 h	
Methylphenidate	CNS stimulant	Hyperkinesis	Dog: 0.5–2 mg/kg q12 h	Start at low dose and increase 0.25 mg every 3 days if no response Do not exceed 2 mg/kg
Propentofylline	Xanthine derivative	CDS, apathy	Dog: 2.5–5 mg/kg q12 h Cat: 5–15 mg/cat q12–24 h	May improve interactions and mentation, but not memory
Haloperidol	Neuroleptic	Compulsive behaviour	Dog: 2–4 mg/kg Q12–24 h	
Risperidone	Neuroleptic	Impulsivity Dissociative disorder	Dog: 0.5–1 mg/m^2 q12–24 h	Can be combined with SSRIs for uncontrolled affective aggression
Topiramate	Na$^+$ channel blocker	Compulsive behaviour Anticonvulsant	Dog: 2–4 mg/kg q8–12 h Cat: 10–20 mg/cat q12 h	Can be combined with serotonergic medications

9.12.3 N-methyl-D-aspartate (NMDA) receptor antagonists

By blocking the NMDA receptors, medications such as memantine and amantadine reduce the effect of glutamate, the main excitatory neurotransmitter in the brain. These medications can produce dissociative anaesthesia in animals. Their main indications in veterinary medicine include analgesia, compulsive behaviours and, possibly, cognitive decline (Minkeviciene *et al.*, 2008; Schneider *et al.*, 2009; Wald *et al.*, 2009). These medications can cause ataxia and vomiting. Also, care should be taken when combining with other anticholinergic medications (e.g. clomipramine).

9.12.4 Propentofylline

This medication is a xanthine-derivative that selectively inhibits adenosine transport and phosphodiesterase enzyme. It may also improve hemodynamics in cerebral and peripheral compartments, thus reducing ischaemic damage to the brain and formation of free radical oxygen species and abnormal beta-amyloid proteins. Propentofylline stimulates the synthesis of nerve growth factor and inhibits inflammatory processes as well as excessive activation of microglia (Kapl and Rudolphi, 1998).

9.12.5 Antipsychotic/neuroleptic

These medications block dopamine receptors primarily in the limbic system and basal ganglia, producing chemical restraint and reducing stereotypic behaviours. Acepromazine, haloperidol and risperidone are among those that are used. Controversy exists about the use of these medications for mental and emotional disorders. Acepromazine was commonly used in the past for a variety of disorders. However, it is postulated that these medications produce chemical restraint, but not emotional calmness. Thus, the patient is likely to be physically inhibited while emotionally reactive. These medications should not be used as a single agent, or in cases of anxiety, fear, frustration or panic. They may be useful for compulsive behaviours, especially those where the patient may injure itself. Side effects are related to decreasing dopamine activity and blockade of alpha-adrenergic receptors. Side effects may include ataxia, akinesia, dystonia, bradycardia and hypotension. Chronic use may induce hyperprolactinaemia, which can lead to depression and anxiety. These medications should be used cautiously in geriatric patients or those with hepatic or renal dysfunction and seizures (Crowell-Davis *et al.*, 2019).

9.12.6 Topiramate

As a sodium-channel blocker, topiramate blocks the AMPA/Kainate receptors. It reduces the release of glutamate with the net result of increasing GABA release downstream of the glutamate pathways. Topiramate has an anticonvulsant effect but may be useful also for the treatment of abnormal and repetitive behaviours in dogs and cats (Podell, 2006).

Caution should be taken with patients suffering from hepatic or renal impairment. The most common side effects are anorexia, ataxia, vomiting and sedation. Topiramate can be combined with serotonergic medications.

References

Agnew, W. and Korman, R. (2014) Pharmacological appetite stimulation: rational choices in the inappetent cat. *Journal of Feline Medicine and Surgery* 16, 749–756.

Amat, M., Camps, T. and Manteca, X. (2016) Stress in owned cats: behavioural changes and welfare implications. *Journal of Feline Medicine and Surgery* 18(8), 577–586. DOI: 10.1177/1098612X15590867.

Amat, M., Le Brech, S., Garcia-Morato, C.T., Salichs, D., Pardes, B.M. *et al.* (2017) Preventing travel anxiety using dexmedetomidine hydrochloride oromucosal gel. In: Denenberg, S. (ed.) *Proceedings of the 11th International Veterinary Behaviour Meeting*. CAB International, Wallingford, UK, pp. 20–21.

Ambrósio, A.F., Soares-Da-Silva, P., Carvalho, C.M. and Carvalho, A.P. (2002) Mechanisms of action of carbamazepine and its derivatives, oxcarbazepine, BIA 2-093, and BIA 2-024. *Neurochemical research* 27(1-2), 121–130. DOI: 10.1023/A:1014814924965.

Argüelles, J., Enriquez, J., Bowen, J. and Fatjó, J. (2017) Mirtazapine as a potential drug to treat social fears in dogs: five case examples. In: Denenberg, S. (ed.) *Proceedings of the 11th International Veterinary Behaviour Meeting*. CAB International, Wallingford, UK, pp. 84–85.

Artigas, F., Adell, A. and Celada, P. (2006) Pindolol augmentation of antidepressant response. *Current Drug Targets* 7(2), 139–147. DOI: 10.2174/138945006775515446.

Björkholm, C. and Monteggia, L.M. (2016) BDNF – a key transducer of antidepressant effects. *Neuropharmacology* 102, 72–79. DOI: 10.1016/j.neuropharm.2015.10.034.

Black, K., Shea, C., Dursun, S. and Kutcher, S. (2000) Selective serotonin reuptake inhibitor discontinuation syndrome: proposed diagnostic criteria. *Journal of Psychiatry Neuroscience* 25, 255–261.

Brooks, D. (2008) Photic head shaking. In: Lavoie, J.P. and Hinchcliff, K.W. (eds) *Blackwell's Five-minute Veterinary Consult: Equine*, 2nd edn. Wiley-Blackwell, Ames, Iowa, pp. 590–591.

Bruyette, D., Ruhel, W.W. and Smidberg, T.L. (1995) Canine pituitary-dependent hyperadrenocorticism: a spontaneous animal model for neurodegenerative disorders and their improvement with l-deprenyl. *Progress in Brain Research* 106, 207–215.

Bueno, L., Fargeas, M.J., Fioramonti, J. and Honde, C. (1984) Effects of dopamine and bromocriptine on colonic motility in dog. *British Journal of Pharmacology* 82(1), 35–42. DOI: 10.1111/j.1476-5381.1984.tb16439.x.

Butz, R.F., Schroeder, D.H., Welch, R.M., Mehta, N.B., Phillips, A.P. *et al.* (1981) Radioimmunoassay and pharmacokinetic profile of bupropion in the dog. *The Journal of Pharmacology and Experimental Therapeutics* 217(3), 602–610.

Center, S.A., Elstonm, T.H., Rowland, P.H., Rosen, D.K., Reitz, B.L. *et al.* (1996) Fulminant hepatic failure associated with oral administration of diazepam in 11 cats. *Journal of the American Veterinary Medical Association* 209, 618–625.

Chávez, G., Pardo, P., Ubilla, M.J. and Marín, M.P. (2016) Effects on behavioural variables of oral versus transdermal buspirone administration in cats displaying urine marking. *Journal of Applied Animal Research* 44(1), 454–457. DOI: 10.1080/09712119.2015.1091335.

Ciribassi, J., Luescher, A., Pasloske, K.S., Robertson-Plouch, C., Zimmerman, A. *et al.* (2003) Comparative bioavailability of fluoxetine after transdermal and oral administration to healthy cats. *American Journal of Veterinary Research* 64(8), 994–998. DOI: 10.2460/ajvr.2003.64.994.

Cole, K.O. and Yonkers, K.A. (2004) Nonbenzodiazepines anxiolytics. In: Schatzberg, A.F. and Nemeroff, C.B. (eds) *Textbook of Psychopharmacology.* American Psychiatric Association Press, Washington DC, pp. 231–244.

Crowell-Davis, S.L., Seibert, L.M., Sung, W., Parthasarathy, V. and Curtis, T.M. (2003) Use of clomipramine, alprazolam, and behavior modification for treatment of storm phobia in dogs. *Journal of the American Veterinary Medical Association* 222(6), 744–748. DOI: 10.2460/javma.2003.222.744.

Crowell-Davis, S.L., Murray, T.F. and Mattos de Souza Dantas, L. (2019) *Veterinary Psychopharmacology*, 2nd edn. Wiley Blackwell, Hoboken, New Jersey.

Danneberg, P. and Weber, K.H. (1983) Chemical structure and biological activity of the diazepines. *British Journal of Clinical Pharmacology* 16(S2), 231S–244. DOI: 10.1111/j.1365-2125.1983.tb02295.x.

de Leeuw van Weenen, J.E., Parlevliet, E.T., Maechler, P., Havekes, L.M., Romijn, J.A. *et al.* (2010) The dopamine receptor D2 agonist bromocriptine inhibits glucose-stimulated insulin secretion by direct activation of the α2-adrenergic receptors in beta cells. *Biochemical Pharmacology* 79(12), 1827–1836. DOI: 10.1016/j.bcp.2010.01.029.

Dehasse, J. (1999) Retrospective study on the use of selegiline (Selgian®) in cats. *Proceedings of the American Veterinary Society of Animal Behavior*, Louisiana, New Orleans.

Dehasse, J. (2001) The use of sertraline in dog behaviour medicine. *Proceedings of the 3rd International Veterinary Behaviour Meeting*, British Columbia, Vancouver, pp. 195–196.

Delucchi, L., Martino, P., Baldovino, A., Pessina, P. and Rodrigues, A. (2010) Use of venlafaxine in the treatment of a canine narcolepsy-cataplexy case. *Journal of Small Animal Practice* 51(2), 132. DOI: 10.1111/j.1748-5827.2009.00908.x.

Denenberg, S. (2015) Animal behavior case of the month. *Journal of the American Veterinary Medical Association* 246(2), 194–196. DOI: 10.2460/javma.246.2.194.

Denenberg, S. and Landsberg, G. (2017) Current pharmacological and non-pharmacological approaches for therapy of feline and canine dementia. In: Landsberg, G., Madari, A. and Zilka, N. (eds) *Canine and Feline Dementia: Molecular Basic, Diagnostic, and Therapy*. Springer International Publishing AG, pp. 129–143.

DiMascio, A. (1973) The effects of benzodiazepines on aggression: reduced or increased? In: Garattini, E., Mussini, E. and Randall, L.O. (eds) *The Benzodiazepines*. Raven Press, New York, pp. 433–440.

Dodman, N.H. (1998) Pharmacologic treatment of aggression in veterinary patients. In: Dodman, N.H. and Shuster, L. (eds) *Psychopharmacology of Animal Behavior Disorders*. Blackwell Science, Malden, Massachusetts, pp. 41–63.

Dodman, N.H., Donnelly, R., Shuster, L., Mertens, P., Rand, W. *et al.* (1996) The use of fluoxetine to treat dominance aggression in dogs. *Journal of Veterinary Medical Association* 209, 1585–1587.

Duman, R.S. (1998) Novel therapeutic approaches beyond the serotonin receptor. *Biological Psychiatry* 44(5), 324–335. DOI: 10.1016/S0006-3223(98)00031-6.

Engel, O., von Klopmann, T., Maiolini, A., Freundt-Revilla, J. and Tipold, A. (2017) Imepitoin is well tolerated in healthy and epileptic cats. *BMC Veterinary Research* 13(1), 172. DOI: 10.1186/s12917-017-1087-3.

Engel, O., Masic, A., Landsberg, G., Brooks, M., Mills, D.S. *et al.* (2018) Imepitoin shows benzodiazepine-like effects in models of anxiety. *Frontiers in Pharmacology* 9, 1225. DOI: 10.3389/fphar.2018.01225.

Engel, O., Müller, H.W., Klee, R., Francke, B. and Mills, D.S. (2019) Effectiveness of imepitoin for the control of anxiety and fear associated with noise phobia in dogs. *Journal of Veterinary Internal Medicine* 33(6), 2675–2684. DOI: 10.1111/jvim.15608.

Ferguson, J.M. (2001) SSRI antidepressant medications: adverse effects and tolerability. *Primary Care Companion to the Journal of Clinical Psychiatry* 3(1), 22–27.

Ferguson, L.E., McLean, M.K., Bates, J.A. and Quimby, J.M. (2016) Mirtazapine toxicity in cats: retrospective study of 84 cases (2006–2011). *Journal of Feline Medicine and Surgery* 18(11), 868–874. DOI: 10.1177/1098612X15599026.

Fries, R.C., Kadotani, S., Vitt, J.P. and Schaeffer, D.J. (2018) Effects of oral trazodone on echocardiographic and hemodynamic variables in healthy cats. *Journal of Feline Medicine and Surgery*.

Graeme, J.S. (2006) The mechanisms of action of gabapentin and pregabalin. *Current Opinion in Pharmacology* 6, 108–113.

Gruen, M.E. and Sherman, B.L. (2008) Use of trazodone as an adjunctive agent in the treatment of canine anxiety disorders: 56 cases (1995–2007). *Journal of the American Veterinary Medical*

Association 233(12), 1902–1907. DOI: 10.2460/javma.233.12.1902.

Haberzettl, R., Bert, B., Fink, H. and Fox, M.A. (2013) Animal models of the serotonin syndrome: a systematic review. *Behavioural Brain Research* 256, 328–345. DOI: 10.1016/j.bbr.2013.08.045.

Hart, B.L., Eckstein, R.A., Powell, K.L. and Dodman, N.H. (1993) Effectiveness of buspirone on urine spraying and inappropriate urination in cats. *Journal of the American Veterinary Medical Association* 203(2), 254–258.

Hart, B.L., Cliff, K.D., Tynes, V.V. and Bergman, L. (2005) Control of urine marking by use of long-term treatment with fluoxetine or clomipramine in cats. *Journal of the American Veterinary Medical Association* 226(3), 378–382. DOI: 10.2460/javma.2005.226.378.

Haug, L. (2008) Canine aggression towards unfamiliar people and dogs. *Veterinary Clinics of North America: Small Animal Practice* 38, 1024–1041.

Heinonen, E.H., Anttila, M.I. and Lammintausta, R.A.S. (1994) Pharmacokinetic aspects of l-deprenyl (selegiline) and its metabolites. *Clinical Pharmacology and Therapeutics* 56(6), 742–749. DOI: 10.1038/clpt.1994.204.

Hewson, C.J., Luescher, U.A., Parent, J.M., Conlon, P.D. and Ball, R.O. (1998) Efficacy of clomipramine in the treatment of canine compulsive disorder. *Journal of the American Veterinary Medical Association* 213, 1760–1765.

Hopfensperger, M.J. (2016) Use of oral venlafaxine in cats with idiopathic cystitis or behavioral causes of periuria. *Proceedings of the American College of Veterinary Behaviorists Annual Symposium*, San Antonio, Texas, pp. 13–17.

Howell, S.R., Hicks, D.R., Scatina, J.A. and Sisenwine, S.F. (1994) Pharmacokinetics of venlafaxine and *O*-desmethylvenlafaxine in laboratory animals. *Xenobiotica* 24(4), 315–327. DOI: 10.3109/00498259409045895.

Ibáñez, M. and Anzola, B. (2009) Use of fluoxetine, diazepam, and behavior modification as therapy for treatment of anxiety-related disorders in dogs. *Journal of Veterinary Behavior* 4(6), 223–229. DOI: 10.1016/j.jveb.2009.04.001.

Irimajiri, M., Luescher, A.U., Douglass, G., Robertson-Plouch, C., Zimmermann, A. *et al.* (2009) Randomized, controlled clinical trial of the efficacy of fluoxetine for treatment of compulsive disorders in dogs. *Journal of the American Veterinary Medical Association* 235(6), 705–709. DOI: 10.2460/javma.235.6.705.

Joans, J.M. and Hearron, A.E. Jr. (1996) Alprazolam and suicidal ideation: a meta-analysis of controlled trials in the treatment of depression. *Journal of Clinical Psychopharmacology* 16, 208–211.

Kapl, D. and Rudolphi, K.A. (1998) New pharmacologic aspects in the neurologic profile of propentofylline. *Tierarztliche Praxis. Ausgabe K, Kleintiere/Heimtiere* 26(5), 317–321.

Kiechel, J.R. (1980) Pharmacokinetics and metabolism of guanfacine in man: a review. *British Journal of Clinical Pharmacology* 10(S1), 25S–32. DOI: 10.1111/j.1365-2125.1980.tb04901.x.

King, J.N., Simpson, B.S., Overall, K.L., Appleby, D., Pageat, P. *et al.* (2000) Treatment of separation anxiety in dogs with clomipramine: results from a prospective, randomized, double-blind, placebo-controlled, parallel-group, multicenter clinical trial. *Applied Animal Behaviour Science* 67(4), 255–275. DOI: 10.1016/S0168-1591(99)00127-6.

King, J.N., Overall, K.L., Appleby, D., Simpson, B.S., Beata, C. *et al.* (2004) Results of a follow-up investigation to a clinical trial testing the efficacy of clomipramine in the treatment of separation anxiety in dogs. *Applied Animal Behaviour Science* 89(3-4), 233–242. DOI: 10.1016/j.applanim.2004.06.003.

Knoll, J., Miklya, I., Knoll, B., Markó, R. and Kelemen, K. (1996) (–)Deprenyl and (–)1-phenyl-2-propylaminopentane, [(–) PPAP] act primarily as potent stimulants of action potential — transmitter release coupling in the catecholaminergic neurons. *Life Sciences* 58(10), 817–827. DOI: 10.1016/0024-3205(96)00014-8.

Korpivaara, M., Laapas, K., Huhtinen, M., Schöning, B. and Overall, K. (2017a) Dexmedetomidine oromucosal gel for noise-associated acute anxiety and fear in dogs – a randomised, double-blind, placebo-controlled clinical study. *Veterinary Record* 180(14), 356. DOI: 10.1136/vr.104045.

Korpivaara, M., Huhtinen, M., Aspergren, J. and Overall, K. (2017b) Oromucosal dexmedetomidine gel for alleviation of fear and anxiety in dogs during minor veterinary or husbandry procedures. In: Denenberg, S. (ed.) *Proceedings of the 11th International Veterinary Behaviour Meeting*. CAB International, Wallingford, UK, pp. 22–23.

KuKanich, B. (2013) Outpatient oral analgesics in dogs and cats beyond nonsteroidal antiinflammatory drugs. *Veterinary Clinics of North America: Small Animal Practice* 43(5), 1109–1125. DOI: 10.1016/j.cvsm.2013.04.007.

Landsberg, G.M. and Wilson, A.L. (2005) Effects of clomipramine on cats presented for urine marking. *Journal of the American Animal Hospital Association* 41(1), 3–11. DOI: 10.5326/0410003.

Landsberg, G.M., Melese, P., Sherman, B.L., Neilson, J.C., Zimmerman, A. *et al.* (2008) Effectiveness of fluoxetine chewable tablets in the treatment of canine separation anxiety. *Journal of Veterinary Behavior* 3(1), 12–19. DOI: 10.1016/j.jveb.2007.09.001.

Landsberg, G.M., Denenberg, S. and Araujo, J.A. (2010) Cognitive dysfunction in cats: a syndrome we used to dismiss as 'old age'. *Journal of Feline Medicine and Surgery* 12(11), 837–848. DOI: 10.1016/j.jfms.2010.09.004.

McAinsh, J. and Holmes, B.F. (1983) Pharmacokinetic studies with atenolol in the dog. *Biopharmaceutics & Drug Disposition* 4(3), 249–261. DOI: 10.1002/bdd.2510040306.

McPeake, K.J. and Mills, D.S. (2017) The use of imepitoin (Pexion™) on fear and anxiety related problems in dogs – a case series. *BMC Veterinary Research* 13(1), 173. DOI: 10.1186/s12917-017-1098-0.

Mealey, K.L., Peck, K.E., Bennett, B.S., Sellon, R.K., Swinney, G.R. *et al*. (2004) Systemic absorption of amitriptyline and buspirone after oral and transdermal administration to healthy cats. *Journal of Veterinary Internal Medicine* 18(1), 43–46. DOI: 10.1111/j.1939-1676.2004.tb00133.x.

Mengoli, M., Mendonça, T., Lee Oliva, J., Bienboire-Frosini, C., Chabaud, C. *et al*. (2017) Do assistance dogs show work overload? canine blood prolactin as a clinical parameter to detect chronic stress-related response. In: Denenberg, S. (ed.) *Proceedings of the 11th International Veterinary Behaviour Meeting*. CAB International, Wallingford, UK, pp. 112–114.

Milgram, N.W., Ivy, G.O., Head, E., Murphy, M.P., Wu, P.H. *et al*. (1993) The effect of l-deprenyl on behavior, cognitive function, and biogenic amines in the dog. *Neurochemical Research* 18(12), 1211–1219. DOI: 10.1007/BF00975038.

Mills, D. and Ledger, R. (2001) The effects of oral selegiline hydrochloride on learning and training in the dog: a psychobiological interpretation. *Progress in Neuro-Psychopharmacology and Biological Psychiatry* 25(8), 1597–1613. DOI: 10.1016/S0278-5846(01)00205-6.

Mills, P.C., Siebert, G.A. and Roberts, M.S. (2004) A model to study intestinal and hepatic metabolism of propranolol in the dog. *Journal of Veterinary Pharmacology and Therapeutics* 27(1), 45–48. DOI: 10.1111/j.1365-2885.2004.00547.x.

Minkeviciene, R., Banerjee, P. and Tanila, H. (2008) Cognition-enhancing and anxiolytic effects of memantine. *Neuropharmacology* 54(7), 1079–1085. DOI: 10.1016/j.neuropharm.2008.02.014.

Moon-Fanelli, A.A. and Dodman, N.H. (1998) Description and development of compulsive tail chasing in terriers and responses to clomipramine treatment. *Journal of the American Veterinary Medical Association* 212, 1252–1257.

Murphy, L.A., Barletta, M., Graham, L.F., Reichl, L.J., Duxbury, M.M. *et al*. (2017) Effects of acepromazine and trazodone on anesthetic induction dose of propofol and cardiovascular variables in dogs undergoing general anesthesia for orthopedic surgery. *Journal of the American Veterinary Medical Association* 250(4), 408–416. DOI: 10.2460/javma.250.4.408.

Nobukazu, K., Fumikazu, Y., Miki, Y., Koichi, K., Taiichiro, I. *et al*. (2009) Anxiolytic-like profile of mirtazapine in rat conditioned fear stress model. *Pharmacology, Biochemistry and Behavior* 92, 393–398.

Ogata, N. and Dodman, N.H. (2011) The use of clonidine in the treatment of fear-based behavior problems in dogs: an open trial. *Journal of Veterinary Behavior* 6(2), 130–137. DOI: 10.1016/j.jveb.2010.10.004.

Okkens, A.G. and Kooistra, H.S. (1997) Reproductive problems in the bitch and the queen. *Veterinary Quarterly* 19(sup1), 36–37. DOI: 10.1080/01652176.1997.9694798.

Ouslander, J.G. (2004) Management of overactive bladder. *New England Journal of Medicine* 350(8), 786–799. DOI: 10.1056/NEJMra032662.

Overall, K.L. and Dunham, A.E. (2002) Clinical features and outcome in dogs and cats with obsessive-compulsive disorder: 126 cases (1989–2000). *Journal of the American Veterinary Medical Association* 221(10), 1445–1452. DOI: 10.2460/javma.2002.221.1445.

Padala, P.R., Sadiq, H.J. and Padala, K.P. (2006) Urinary obstruction with citalopram and aripiprazole combination in an elderly patient. *Journal of Clinical Psychopharmacology* 26(6), 667–668. DOI: 10.1097/01.jcp.0000246219.35809.fd.

Pankratz, K.E., Ferris, K.K., Griffith, E.H. and Sherman, B.L. (2018) Use of single-dose oral gabapentin to attenuate fear responses in cage-trap confined community cats: a double-blind, placebo-controlled field trial. *Journal of Feline Medicine and Surgery* 20(6), 535–543. DOI: 10.1177/1098612X17719399.

Panksepp, J. (2016) The psycho-neurology of cross-species affective/social neuroscience: understanding animal affective states as a guide to development of novel psychiatric treatments. In: Wöhr, M. and Krach, S. (eds) *Social Behavior from Rodents to Humans. Current Topics in Behavioral Neurosciences*. Springer International Publishing AG, pp. 109–125.

Peroutka, S.J. (1985) Selective interaction of novel anxiolytics with 5-hydroxytryptamine1A receptors. *Biological Psychiatry* 20(9), 971–979. DOI: 10.1016/0006-3223(85)90194-5.

Pineda, S., Anzola, B., Olivares, A. and Ibáñez, M. (2014) Fluoxetine combined with clorazepate dipotassium and behaviour modification for treatment of anxiety-related disorders in dogs. *The Veterinary Journal* 199(3), 387–391. DOI: 10.1016/j.tvjl.2013.11.021.

Pobel, T., Caudrillier, M., Mills, D.S., Heath, S.E. and Harrington, L.J. (1997) Evaluation of the efficacy of selegiline hydrochloride in treating behavioural disorder of emotional origin in dogs. *Proceedings of the First International Conference on Veterinary Behavioural Medicine,* Birmingham, UK.

Podell, M.*et al*. (2006) New horizons in the treatment of epilepsy. *24th Annual Forum of the ACVIM Conference*, Louisville, Kentucky.

Pryor, P.A., Hart, B.L., Bain, M.J. and Cliff, K.D. (2001) Causes of urine marking in cats and effects of environmental management on frequency of marking. *Journal of the American Veterinary Medical*

Association 219(12), 1709–1713. DOI: 10.2460/javma.2001.219.1709.

Pugh, C.M., Sweeney, J.T., Bloch, C.P., Lee, J.A., Johnson, J.A. *et al.* (2013) Selective serotonin reuptake inhibitor (SSRI) toxicosis in cats: 33 cases (2004-2010). *Journal of Veterinary Emergency and Critical Care* 23(5), 565–570. DOI: 10.1111/vec.12091.

Quimby, J.M. and Lunn, K.F. (2013) Mirtazapine as an appetite stimulant and anti-emetic in cats with chronic kidney disease: a masked placebo-controlled crossover clinical trial. *The Veterinary Journal* 197(3), 651–655. DOI: 10.1016/j.tvjl.2013.05.048.

Quiñones, M., Dyer, D.C., Ware, W.A. and Mehvar, R. (1996) Pharmacokinetics of atenolol in clinically normal cats. *American Journal of Veterinary Research* 57, 1050–1053.

Rapoport, J.L., Ryland, D.H. and Kriete, M. (1992) Drug treatment of canine acral lick: an animal model of obsessive-compulsive disorder. *Archive of General Psychiatry* 49, 517–521.

Reisner, I. (2003) Diagnosis of canine generalized anxiety disorder and its management with behavioural modification and fluoxetine or paroxetine: a retrospective summary of clinical experience (2001-2003). *Journal of the American Animal Hospital Association* 39, 512.

Renoir, T. (2013) Selective serotonin reuptake inhibitor antidepressant treatment discontinuation syndrome: a review of the clinical evidence and the possible mechanisms involved. *Frontiers in Pharmacology* 4. DOI: 10.3389/fphar.2013.00045.

Robinson, R.T., Drafts, B.C. and Fisher, J.L. (2003) Fluoxetine increases GABAA receptor activity through a novel modulatory site. *Journal of Pharmacology and Experimental Therapeutics* 304(3), 978–984. DOI: 10.1124/jpet.102.044834.

Robinson, G.E., Fernald, R.D. and Clayton, D.F. (2008) Genes and social behavior. *Science* 322(5903), 896–900. DOI: 10.1126/science.1159277.

Rothschild, A.J. (1992) Disinhibition, amnesic reactions, and other adverse reaction secondary to triazolam: a review of the literature. *Journal of Clinical Psychiatry* 53, 69–79.

Rothschild, A.J., Shindul-Rothschild, J.A., Viguera, A., Murray, M. and Brewster, S. (2000) Comparison of the frequency of behavioral disinhibition on alprazolam, clonazepam, or no benzodiazepine in hospitalized psychiatric patients. *Journal of Clinical Psychopharmacology* 20(1), 7–11. DOI: 10.1097/00004714-200002000-00003.

Ruhel, W.W., Griffin, D., Bouchard, G. and Kitchen, D. (1996) Effects of l-deprenyl in cats in a one-month dose escalation study. *Veterinary pathology* 33(5), p 621.

Schneider, B.M., Dodman, N.H. and Maranda, L. (2009) Use of memantine in treatment of canine compulsive disorders. *Journal of Veterinary Behavior* 4(3), 118–126. DOI: 10.1016/j.jveb.2008.10.008.

Scholtysik, G. (1986) Animal pharmacology of guanfacine. *The American Journal of Cardiology* 57(9), E13–E17. DOI: 10.1016/0002-9149(86)90717-4.

Seksel, K. (2008) Behavior-modifying drugs. In: Maddison, J.E., Page, S.W. and Church, D.B. (eds) *Small Animal Clinical Pharmacology*. Saunders Elsevier, Philadelphia, Pennsylvania, pp. 126–147.

Seksel, K. and Lindeman, M.J. (1998) Use of clomipramine in the treatment of anxiety-related and obsessive-compulsive disorders in cats. *Australian Veterinary Journal* 76(5), 317–321. DOI: 10.1111/j.1751-0813.1998.tb12353.x.

Sherman, B.L. (2017) Use of psychopharmacology to reduce fear and anxiety in dogs and cats: a practical approach. In: Denenberg, S. (ed.) *Proceedings of the 11th International Veterinary Behaviour Meeting*. CAB International, Wallingford, UK, pp. 9–19.

Shirasaki, Y., Sugimura, M. and Sato, T. (2010) Bromocriptine, an ergot alkaloid, inhibits excitatory amino acid release mediated by glutamate transporter reversal. *European Journal of Pharmacology* 643(1), 48–57. DOI: 10.1016/j.ejphar.2010.06.007.

Siao, K.T., Pypendop, B.H. and Ilkiw, J.E. (2010) Pharmacokinetics of gabapentin in cats. *American Journal of Veterinary Research* 71(7), 817–821. DOI: 10.2460/ajvr.71.7.817.

Specchio, L.M., Iudice, A., Specchio, N., La Neve, A., Spinelli, A. *et al.* (2004) Citalopram as treatment of depression in patients with epilepsy. *Clinical Neuropharmacology* 27(3), 133–136. DOI: 10.1097/00002826-200405000-00009.

Spina, E., Santoro, V. and D'Arrigo, C. (2008) Clinically relevant pharmacokinetic drug interactions with second-generation antidepressants: an update. *Clinical Therapeutics* 30(7), 1206–1227. DOI: 10.1016/S0149-2918(08)80047-1.

Stahl, S.M. (2013) *Stahl's Essential Psychopharmacology*, 4th edn. Cambridge University Press, Cambridge, UK.

Steenen, S.A., van Wijk, A.J., van der Heijden, G.J.M.G., van Westrhenen, R., de Lange, J. *et al.* (2016) Propranolol for the treatment of anxiety disorders: systematic review and meta-analysis. *Journal of Psychopharmacology* 30(2), 128–139. DOI: 10.1177/0269881115612236.

Stein, D.J., Mendelsohn, I., Potocnik, F., Van Kradenberg, J. and Wessels, C. (1998) Use of the selective serotonin reuptake inhibitor citalopram in a possible animal analogue of obsessive-compulsive disorder. *Depression and Anxiety* 8(1), 39–42. DOI: 10.1002/(SICI)1520-6394(1998)8:1<39::AID-DA8>3.0.CO;2-0.

Stevens, B.J., Frantz, E.M., Orlando, J.M., Griffith, E., Harden, L.B. *et al.* (2016) Efficacy of a single dose of trazodone hydrochloride given to cats prior to veterinary visits to reduce signs of transport- and examination-related anxiety. *Journal of the American*

Veterinary Medical Association 249(2), 202–207. DOI: 10.2460/javma.249.2.202.

Tanaka, M., Yoshida, M., Emoto, H. and Ishii, H. (2000) Noradrenaline systems in the hypothalamus, amygdala and locus coeruleus are involved in the provocation of anxiety: basic studies. *European Journal of Pharmacology* 405(1-3), 397–406. DOI: 10.1016/S0014-2999(00)00569-0.

Thor, K.B. (2003) Serotonin and norepinephrine involvement in efferent pathways to the urethral rhabdosphincter: implications for treating stress urinary incontinence. *Urology* 62(4), 3–9. DOI: 10.1016/S0090-4295(03)00754-4.

van Haaften, K.A., Forsythe, L.R.E., Stelow, E.A. and Bain, M.J. (2017) Effects of a single preappointment dose of gabapentin on signs of stress in cats during transportation and veterinary examination. *Journal of the American Veterinary Medical Association* 251(10), 1175–1181. DOI: 10.2460/javma.251.10.1175.

Wald, R., Dodman, N. and Shuster, L. (2009) The combined effects of memantine and fluoxetine on an animal model of obsessive compulsive disorder. *Experimental and Clinical Psychopharmacology* 17(3), 191–197. DOI: 10.1037/a0016402.

Welch, R.M., Lai, A.A. and Schroeder, D.H. (1987) Pharmacological significance of the species differences in bupropion metabolism. *Xenobiotica* 17(3), 287–298. DOI: 10.3109/00498258709043939.

Wynchank, D. and Berk, M. (1998) Fluoxetine treatment of acral lick dermatitis in dogs: a placebo-controlled randomized double blind trial. *Depression and Anxiety* 8(1), 21–23. DOI: 10.1002/(SICI)1520-6394(1998)8:1<21::AID-DA4>3.0.CO;2-8.

Yalcin, E. (2010) Comparison of clomipramine and fluoxetine treatment of dogs with tail chasing. *Tierärztliche Praxis Ausgabe K: Kleintiere / Heimtiere* 38(05), 295–299. DOI: 10.1055/s-0038-1622860.

10 Problem Behaviours and Management in Cats and Dogs

Sagi Denenberg*

Langford Vets, University of Bristol, Langford, UK; North Toronto Veterinary Behaviour Specialty Clinic, Toronto, Canada

10.1 Introduction

The behaviours discussed in this chapter are all normal behaviours. Some may be intense or excessive, while others may be shown out of normal context. However, the common denominator for all is the owner's disapproval.

The most common reasons for presenting patients with problem behaviours are lack of stimulation or training, patients' and owners' frustration, inadvertent reinforcement or punishment, and unrealistic expectations.

It is important to address these problems even when they are not true pathology. Not only is owners' satisfaction critical for retaining the patient at home, but also some of these problem behaviours may develop into a true pathology later.

10.2 Addressing Problem Behaviours

10.2.1 Normal behaviour

When an owner presents a patient with problem behaviour, we must first determine if the behaviour is normal. Owners may consider the behaviour excessive or abnormal due to lack of knowledge or unrealistic expectations. For information about normal behaviours of cats and dogs see Chapters 4 and 5, respectively. For example, many owners may complain about 'counter-surfing' (see Section 10.4.2). Seeking food is one of the most basic and normal behaviours for animals. Once owners leave food on the counter, the animal will smell or see it and try reaching it. If the animal can reach and consume the food, it is reinforced and likely to repeat this behaviour.

10.2.2 Reviewing the problem

The next step is to define the behaviour. For this we must ask the owner to describe the behaviour and possibly observe it at the practice or using video. Ideally, owners can describe the situations, times and environments in which the behaviour takes place. Through this review we should be able to identify triggers and patterns for the behaviour. These would become useful when designing a management programme.

When reviewing the problem, it is essential to try to identify markers of normal or abnormal behaviours. For example, some dogs may bark 'excessively' when they hear or see another dog walking by the house. Other dogs may also vocalize when they see or hear a dog. However, their bark has a higher pitch and frequency, and lasts longer, which may indicate distress. Most owners can distinguish between different types of barking (Pongrácz *et al.*, 2005). Similarly, dogs may learn to jump on the owner for attention, while other dogs jump due to distress. The latter shows displacement behaviours, sympathetic activation and other distress-related behaviours.

10.2.3 The owner factor

We should also review the owner's involvement in the development and maintenance of the behaviour. While not always the owner's fault, there are areas where the owner contributed either by doing something that should not be done or did not do something that should have been done. At the same time, it is important not to blame the owner for these behaviours. Most owners feel guilty as it is,

*s.denenberg@bristol.ac.uk

 Small Animal Veterinary Psychiatry (ed. S. Denenberg)

DOI: 10.1079/9781786394552.0010

and further blaming or criticism is not helpful. Also, thinking that owners who feel guilty are more likely to engage with management is unsubstantiated. We should educate owners about normal behaviours, what to expect and how they can help their pets.

The first step when evaluating the owner's involvement is to examine their expectations. Many owners, for example, will inquire how to stop dogs from barking. The simplest answer is that dogs will always bark. It is, however, reasonable to expect dogs to stop barking when the owner gives the appropriate signal (where there are no pathologies).

Reviewing the animal's routines and care implemented by the owner help evaluate whether the patient's needs are met consistently. These needs include food and water, social interactions, exercise and elimination, and sleep and rest. Owners should provide their pets with outlets for normal behaviours (see Chapters 4, 5 and 6) to minimize the risk of problem behaviours. Routine veterinary care and feeding should also take place to reduce the risk of disease or nutritional deficits leading to problem behaviour (e.g. counter-surfing due to hunger).

Training should be evaluated as well. Untrained animals may show undesired behaviours. Some owners may assume that the pet knows what is expected of them and become frustrated when this is not the case. For example, cat owners may assume that cats know how to use the litter tray. While most cats need to be shown once or twice where the tray is, some cats may require more training and time. The latter may house-soil due to lack of training rather than to a true pathology. Using punishment in training may also lead to undesired behaviours, starting from avoidance to hiding and showing problem behaviour when the owner is not present.

10.2.4 Previous attempts to manage the problem

Often, before raising the problem with the veterinarian, owners have attempted to manage the situation, either alone or with someone else. It is important to review past attempts and identify what helped to a degree and what did not. It is equally important to review any past attempt that may have worsened the behaviour (e.g. punishment). As noted above, it is important not to criticize owners for punishing their pets. A simple discussion about the flaws of punishment and offering a different approach should suffice, in most cases, to stop using punishment.

Owners may have attempted techniques that would have worked. Possibly the owners did not persist or showed inconsistencies, leading to failure. Also, owners may inadvertently reinforce the problem or increase its severity. For example, many owners use extinction (see Sections 8.5.2.1 – Extinction, and 10.3.6). When used correctly, extinction should eliminate many problem behaviours such as jumping or barking at the owner for attention. However, if partway through the protocol of extinction, the owner gives attention, the dog may learn that a different (mostly higher) level of intensity is required to achieve its goal.

Owners may confront their pet when they show a problem behaviour; for example, try to remove a stolen object from the dog's mouth. Some dogs may think that the owner is playing with them and will start looking for more objects to steal and even present those to the owner as part of the play. Some dogs may develop aggression towards the owner when they try to remove the object.

10.3 Management Guidelines

Most problem behaviours have similar management guidelines in both cats and dogs. Following a careful assessment of the problem, its frequency and duration, possible triggers and past attempts to manage it, we can design an adequate management plan for the owner to follow. Ideally, the plan should be tailored for the individual patient rather than using a generic protocol.

10.3.1 Meeting needs

Animals spend long periods searching for food through hunting and scavenging. Therefore owners should use feeding toys instead of bowls. There are toys that owners can leave in one place and others that require more room for the patient to play in (see Handouts A9 and A10 – Feeding Toys and Stimulation for Cats and Dogs). Owners can use part of the food for training. Feeding toys provide mental stimulation and physical activity. They also keep the patient occupied in positive behaviour, leaving less time for undesired behaviours.

Most patients, including cats, will benefit from physical activity to reduce arousal and boredom. Taking dogs for walks or playing with them at home or in the garden is helpful. Similarly, owners should engage with cats using toys on wands, or soft toys they can throw for the cat to chase. Of course, the intensity and duration of the exercise should be matched to the individual patient's needs and health.

Owners should provide sufficient outlets for elimination, including walks, opening the door to the garden or using flap doors, and litter trays. Litter trays or the garden should be cleaned regularly to prevent the accumulation of excrement, vapours and smells that may deter the patient from returning to the area.

Social interaction is an important need for patients. Some owners assume that cats do not require socialization or need only minimal attention. This assumption, of course, is wrong. Some cats require or desire less attention than others, and less in comparison with dogs, but they do need attention. Ensuring that patients have sufficient social interactions with the owners is essential. Ideally, owners can set times throughout the day to interact with their pets (see Section 10.3.2). Social interactions can be met through training, play and affection.

Sleeping and resting occupy over 50% of the daily time budget (see Chapters 4 and 5). Ensuring that the patient has not only the time but also the appropriate location(s) is necessary. Many owners assume that their pets can sleep anywhere, anytime. This might be the case for some patients but not others. It would be best to educate owners to design a specific location for their pet to sleep. Owners may have daytime and night-time locations. Most pets will need to be trained to spend time there (see Handout C3 – Safe-haven). Pets follow their owners' routine and, as a result, are more active in the mornings and evenings when owners are active and around them. Most patients sleep through the night but not much through the day. Providing a calm and relatively dark place to sleep through the day is helpful. Many owners have several beds, or the patient can choose from a variety of locations. It may be that the patient has too many options.

10.3.2 Routine and predictability

Providing a consistent daily routine helps the patient anticipate what it is expected to do. It also ensures that the patient knows when each need is met. This predictability helps to reduce anxiety and arousal.

Routine and predictability also mean that owners should interact with the patient in the same manner each time. The patient learns to expect the same consequences from a particular interaction. For example, if the dog does not know what to expect when the owner returns home, it may try jumping, barking, running or mouthing the owner to get attention. However, if the owner trains the dog to sit each time the owner walks into the house, and only then gives attention to the dog, the owner provides a predictable and consistent outcome.

Part of the routine should include meeting all the patient's needs (see Section 10.3.1). It is helpful if owners introduce training several times daily (see below). Training helps expectations, increases consistency in interactions, and provides a predictable outcome.

10.3.3 Prevention

When we identify triggers for problem behaviours, we should attempt to remove or manage them. For example, if there are environmental triggers (e.g. food on the counter, noises or children's toys), owners should attempt to 'pet-proof' the environment. Using tools such as an indoor playpen, a separate room to leave the patient in when it is unsupervised and, in some cases, using a basket muzzle, can help to prevent stealing, chewing and mouthing. A white-noise machine may help to muffle sounds from other areas, which may be a trigger for the patient, leading to barking or jumping. Providing alternatives (e.g. feeding toys and chews, scratching posts and designated digging areas) may help to reduce the motivation to show problem behaviours.

When the owner is the trigger (e.g. rewarding attention seeking), we must teach the owner to stop inadvertently rewarding the behaviour they want to manage. Since habits are difficult to change, we should work on creating a gradual change through small changes and setting up a daily routine to support them. For example, owners may give attention when the dog is barking at them. We can teach the owner to use response substitution (see below) part of the time, ignoring the patient part of the time and preventing the behaviour by staying away (or keeping the patient away) for the rest of the time.

10.3.4 Training desired behaviours

Patients often show problem behaviours due to lack of knowledge of what is the desired behaviour. Further, owners often ask the wrong questions: 'How do I stop the behaviour?' When asking how to stop, in learning principles, owners are asking how to punish the patient. Punishment is administered to reduce the likelihood of repeating a particular behaviour (see Section 8.2 – Changing the Consequences of an Animal's Behaviour). Owners should ask: 'What should my pet do instead?'

Owners should focus not only on providing their pets' needs but also on teaching a set of behaviours to display in particular situations and rewarding these behaviours. Then, when the patient shows an undesired behaviour, the owner should ask it to perform the desired behaviour instead and then reward it. This approach is also known as *response substitution* (see Handout C7 – Response Substitution) and is based on *operant conditioning* (see Section 8.3.2.1 – Altering the motivation in the circumstances). For example, a dog may jump on the owner for attention. Instead of raising their voice, pushing the dog or even hitting it, owners should teach the dog to sit and only then provide a reward (attention in this case). Owners should start training the dog when it is calm and settled, and only later in more challenging situations. Initially, it might be difficult to change the behaviour as the dog may have learned to jump and was successful in getting attention in the past. Therefore owners should be patient, consistent and persistent with training. Moreover, using tools such as a head halter, lead and treats may be helpful.

10.3.5 Setting up to succeed

Owners require their pets to adjust to the their routine, environment and expectations. This task is difficult at times. Therefore, providing the patient with optimal conditions is paramount for success. Ideally, owners can start as soon as possible to prevent these behaviours from developing (see Chapter 6). When the problem already exists, owners should treat each encounter as a potential training session.

When owners anticipate a problem situation, they should plan on modifying it so that they can teach the pet the desired behaviour. For example, if the cat scratches the sofa regularly, the owner can manage the environment and interaction to teach the cat to use a scratching post. The first step is to ensure the cat has alternative scratching posts to use. Second, owners can prevent scratching by covering the area with a plastic sheet or using double-sided sticky tape. Next, the owner can teach the cat to use the designated scratching post using marker training (see Handout C6 – Marker Training).

If the problem has a consistent pattern, owners can modify the feeding schedule to either feed the animal as a distraction or keep the animal hungry before it starts with the behaviour so the owner can use food successfully to reward desired behaviours. For example, if the dog is pulling on-lead, owners should avoid feeding before walks, and take tasty treats with them on walks. The dog is then more motivated to focus on the owner and may learn faster for food.

10.3.6 Ignoring the behaviour

When the behaviour the patient is showing is a nuisance behaviour but not harmful to the patient or the environment, or disrupting the routine (e.g. a dog which is barking when a baby at home is sleeping), owners may ignore the behaviour. By ignoring the behaviour, owners remove all consequences, primarily reinforcement. The learning principle behind this option is known as *extinction* (see also Section 8.5.2.1 – Extinction). It is essential to rule out physical disorders and ensure the patient's needs are adequately met before ignoring the behaviours. It is unethical to ignore the patient's needs (e.g. pain, hunger or fear) even when interacting with the patient may reinforce the behaviour. Once the patient's needs are attended to, behaviour modification to reduce the motivation to show the behaviour can take place.

In many cases, the first response owners will see when ignoring the behaviour is an escalation. If the patient has learned that a particular level of the behaviour (e.g. barking for three minutes) means that the owner will give attention, the patient may start barking for longer periods to see if it gets attention. Also, the patient may show other attention-seeking behaviours, increased arousal and restlessness. Only if the owner is consistently ignoring the behaviour will the intensity and frequency slowly decrease. For more information see Section 8.5.2.1 – Extinction.

10.4 Undesired Behaviours – Cat

10.4.1 Chewing and sucking

Cats may chew or suck fabrics, plastics or wool (see Fig. 10.1). They may do so out of boredom or when trying to access food. Also, cats may chew as part of play behaviour. In some cases, the cat may learn that chewing is a functional tool to solicit the owner's

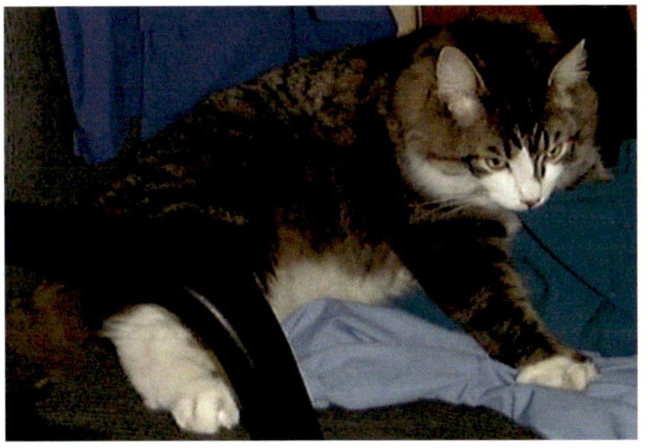

Fig. 10.1. Cats may enjoy chewing or sucking soft materials such as fabric, wool or plastic. It may be a form of play or attention seeking. Some cats may show this behaviour as a displacement behaviour when coping with boredom or anxiety. Cats may show this behaviour excessively, causing damage to themselves or the object (see Section 15.8 – Oral and Ingestive behaviours). (Photo courtesy of Sagi Denenberg.)

attention, and possibly even treats. Oriental breeds of cats seem to be overly represented in this group.

Owners should try providing alternatives such as toys the cat can chew, feeding toys or playing with the cat with toys on a wand (see Fig. 10.2A–C). Using catnip in toys may appeal to some cats. Eliminating access to objects the cat likes to chew might be helpful and possible at times. Punishment should not be part of the management.

We should rule out physical disorders such as dental pain, dietary deficiencies including hunger, and compulsive behaviours. If the object the cat is chewing is not valuable or one that may cause damage to the patient, it is possible to ignore the behaviour instead of reinforcing it with attention.

10.4.2 'Counter-surfing', climbing or jumping onto areas

Cats are very agile and flexible. They are also inquisitive and like to explore different areas. Also, cats like observing the area from high perching spaces. These three facts mean that, when possible, cats will jump onto high surfaces. Moreover, if the surface they are on provides reinforcements (e.g. food on the counter or a hiding place from a different animal), the cat will continue showing the behaviour.

Owners may feel that this behaviour is inappropriate; however, from the cat's point of view, the behaviour was successful and normal. Punishment is only likely to either stop the cat from jumping onto the surface when the owner is present or to learn to escape faster. In some cases, punishment may lead to aggression towards the owner.

When possible, avoiding reinforcement (e.g. leaving food on the counter) is helpful. Owners should provide alternatives such as cat towers or other spaces where the cat can perch and survey the area.

When the problem cannot be avoided, and providing alternatives is not helpful, the use of environmental deterrents might be useful. Air-spray canisters with motion sensors can be left in certain areas or using double-sided sticky tape might help to teach the cat that jumping onto a particular area might be aversive. It is important to weigh the benefit of such tools against the risk of developing anxiety and fear. The one advantage of such tools is the environmental aspect; the aversive outcome is not linked to the owner's presence. These tools should be used as the last option and only for a short period.

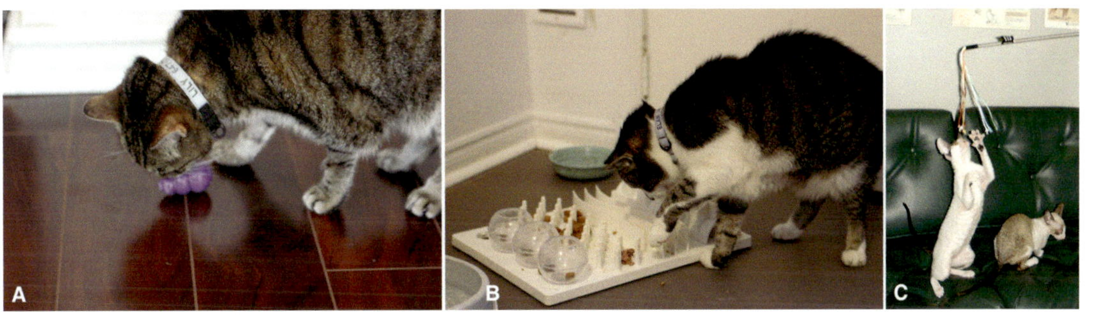

Fig. 10.2. Providing the cat with alternatives it can chew and play with alone (A, B) or with the owner (C) helps reduce undesired chewing and destroying of valuable belongings. (Photos courtesy of Sagi Denenberg)

10.4.3 Night-time activity

Cats are crepuscular animals; they are active at dusk and dawn. Often, cats are inactive through the day and have minimal to no interaction with the owners. As a result, the cat might be more active at night. Also, cats' natural prey, rodents, are more active at night. Hence a cat with hunting instincts and ability might be more active at night.

Physical disorders such as hyperthyroidism, pain, gastrointestinal diseases, cognitive dysfunction and hypertension may cause night-time activity. These must be ruled out first. The next step is to question the owner about the cat's routine and the environment to ensure that its needs are met.

Owners should implement a daily routine that includes ample stimulation before bedtime. Using toys and, possibly, training is helpful. If the cat is waking up as it is hungry, providing late-night meals, or automatic feeder (on a timer) may help. Owners should be instructed not to give the cat attention when it is seeking it at night. If necessary, owners should close the door to the bedroom to prevent the cat from coming inside or confining the cat to a different area of the house. Ignoring the cat might be difficult at times. When not possible, owners should try to ignore the cat and gradually prolong the time. All attention and reinforcement should be withheld. In some cases, using a medication (e.g. trazodone, or melatonin) may induce sleep and allow the owner to sleep as well. The medication may help to restore normal sleeping times.

10.4.4 Mounting

Mounting is a normal behaviour when displayed by a male towards a female in oestrus. In other contexts, the behaviour may not be pathological, but also not entirely normal. When cats mount each other, the owners or objects, physical disorders such as pain, testosterone production (in a neutered male), seizures, or spinal disorders should be considered. Also, the cat may show this behaviour as a displacement behaviour when trying to cope with a lack of stimulation, frustration or anxiety.

Once physical disorders have been ruled out, owners should address the environment and routine. If specific triggers were identified, they should be removed or managed. Based on observations, the owners should attempt to determine if a routine or schedule exists. Then play sessions, feeding toys and training should be implemented.

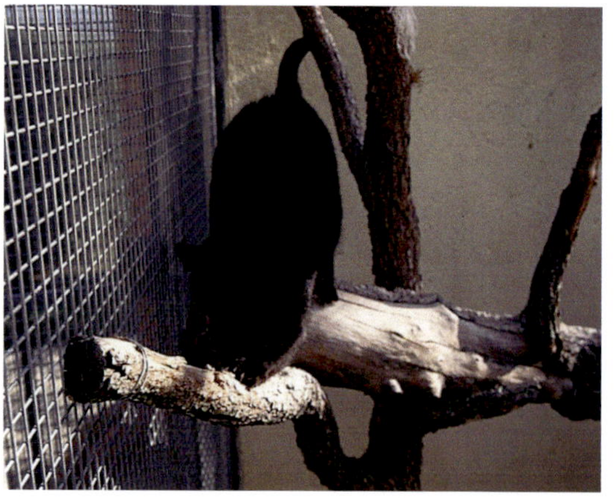

Fig. 10.3. Scratching is a normal behaviour that cats perform daily. Natural wood is one of the preferred surfaces to use. When possible, owners should provide cats with this material. When not possible, other textures such as cardboard, rope or carpet should be used. (Photo courtesy of Sagi Denenberg.)

If the behaviour is short, does not impair the cat's welfare or cause damage to objects, it is possible to ignore it while working to improve all other aspects including identification and removal of triggers. When the behaviour starts, owners should use response substitution to redirect the cat towards an alternative behaviour and then reward it.

10.4.5 Scratching

Cats scratch as part of their repertoire of normal behaviours. Scratching serves as communication (depositing scent and pheromones) and maintenance (e.g. claws and muscles) behaviours. Cats prefer scratching natural surfaces such as wood, and then synthetic surfaces such as carpets or commercial scratching posts (see Fig. 10.3). Cats may choose to scratch furniture or carpets at home instead of scratching posts. The behaviour is likely to be normal but redirected towards unacceptable (for the owner) objects.

Owners should provide the cat with several different scratching posts, including natural wood where possible. Rubbing catnip on the surface may help. A feline pheromone can be used to attract the cat to use a specific surface over others (Tynes *et al.*, 2017).

Regular nail trimming can help minimize the damage the cat may cause. Using tools such as

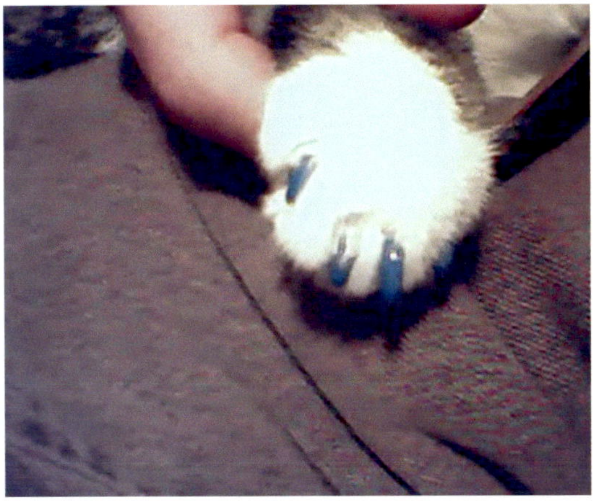

Fig. 10.4. Covering the claws with soft silicone might be an ideal solution. It allows the cat to continue performing the behaviour and prevents damage. These covers must be changed every several weeks or months as the claws grow and break if not trimmed. Many cats will accept these covers, but some will resist them. (Photo courtesy of Sagi Denenberg.)

silicone covers for the claws (see Fig. 10.4) is also helpful, though some cats will not tolerate it and will try removing it or show aggression towards the owners during the application process.

Direct punishment should be avoided; it only teaches the cat to avoid the behaviour when the owner is present. Also, it may lead to aggression towards the owner. Environmental deterrents such as double-sided sticky tape or a compressed-air canister with a motion sensor might be helpful. Also, these are not linked to the owner's presence or consistency. The use of such tools should be weighed against the possible development or increase of anxiety and fear. Amputation of the distal phalanx of the toes is still legally allowed and practised in some countries. The use of this horrific procedure should not be part of the management as there are better and more ethical tools available.

10.4.6 Vocalization

This section refers mainly to cats that, their owners feel, vocalize excessively. Most likely, the vocalization occurs through the night, probably interfering with the owner's sleep. Oriental breeds of cats appear to be more represented than other breeds.

Pain, metabolic and neurological disorders, and cognitive decline, are among the most likely physical disorders leading to excessive vocalization. Physical examination, laboratory tests and therapeutic trials should help to diagnose or rule out any physical disorder.

Cats may vocalize when anxious, fearful or frustrated. Also, a conflict between the cat and other cats or animals at home, or the owner, may lead to excessive vocalization. Hunger, attention seeking and oestrus are also likely to cause excessive vocalization.

We must review the owner's reaction to the cat's vocalization. Often, owners inadvertently reinforce this behaviour by providing attention or food in an attempt to stop the cat from vocalizing, especially at night.

Providing a predictable daily routine that includes all the cat's needs should help to minimize the problem. Owners should increase stimulation, especially before bedtime. Using feeding toys, timer feeders at night, training and affection may help to reduce the likelihood of vocalizing excessively.

Administering medications such as trazodone or clonazepam before bedtime may help both the patient and the owner to sleep better at night. It may also help to restore the normal sleep–wake cycle.

10.5 Undesired Behaviours – Dogs

10.5.1 Chewing

Dogs may spend long periods chewing objects such as bones, rawhides, sticks and plastic toys. When these are unavailable, dogs may chew other objects such as furniture or other possessions (e.g. shoes and children's toys). While owners find this behaviour inappropriate, most dogs appear to enjoy it.

Teething, dental pain, neurological and gastrointestinal disease, and pica can cause chewing. Similarly, boredom, frustration, anxiety and panic may lead to chewing. Therefore, the first step is to rule out these disorders.

Owners should provide acceptable outlets for chewing behaviours. Delivering meals inside a feed toy, and giving bones (real and plastic) or toys is helpful. It would also be helpful to implement play and training sessions, and exercise, as part of the daily routine.

When the dog is chewing an unacceptable object, the owners should distract them and then replace the object with an acceptable substitute. When possible, owners should 'dog-proof' the area to minimize both the options and rewarding the behaviour.

Using response substitution helps to teach the dog desired behaviours and reinforce them.

Punishment should not be part of the management. Also, confronting the dog over an object carries a risk of aggression. The dog may bite the owner to try to stop him from taking the object. Even if the owner is successful in removing the object, there is a higher likelihood of showing aggression the next time as the dog learned that it was not successful in keeping the object. Teaching the dog to drop objects on signal and rewarding it is a better and safer alternative to confrontation or punishment. When the dog does not drop the object (if it is well trained), the likelihood of aggression is even higher. Finding a more motivating treat may be necessary. Some dogs may learn that if they drop the object the owner will reward them. These dogs may look for more objects to chew and bring to the owner. At this point, owners should start ignoring the voluntary dropping of objects, and only reward the dog when they asked it to drop the object. Later, using an intermittent reward schedule (i.e. not rewarding each time, see Section 8.2.2.3 – Schedule of reinforcement) is helpful. The goal is to maintain the 'drop it' signal but not reward more chewing and stealing of objects.

When the owner cannot prevent the dog from chewing objects, the use of a basket muzzle should be considered. The muzzle should be used only when the owner cannot supervise the dog or secure the area. The muzzle should not be a substitute for training and optimizing the dog's routine and environment.

10.5.2 Counter-surfing and stealing objects

Dogs use their noses. If they can smell food on the counter or in the rubbish, they will try reaching it. Some dogs may jump on the counter or stand by it, barking and whining. Dogs may open cabinets searching for food. Often dogs will go into the bathroom to steal from the bins. This is a normal behaviour of scavenging and exploration.

Pica, boredom, nutritional deficits and hunger could lead to counter-surfing and stealing. When dogs find food or other objects they like, the behaviour is reinforced. Therefore, ruling out other underlying pathologies and ensuring the dog has sufficient stimulation, exercise and attention should help. Owners should train the dog to spend time in a different location (see Handout C3 – Safe-haven).

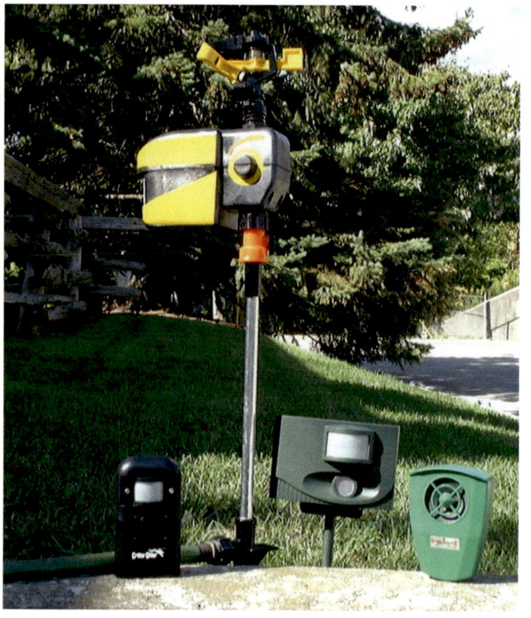

Fig. 10.5. Deterrent products such as motion-activated ultrasonic sounds or water spray may deter dogs from digging in certain areas. However, these products may cause anxiety and fear. Their main advantages over owner-applied punishment are consistency, timing and avoiding the environment rather than the owner. (Photo courtesy of Sagi Denenberg.)

Management is similar to undesired chewing (see above).

10.5.3 Digging

Digging is a normal behaviour of dogs. The three main motivations for digging are burying resources (e.g. bones and toys), scavenging for food, and hunting (e.g. rats, rabbits and vermin). This behaviour is unacceptable for owners when directed towards inappropriate surfaces (e.g. carpets and sofas) or causing damage to the garden. Given that digging is a normal behaviour, management is mostly aimed at providing the dog with appropriate outlets. Owners can allocate an area in the garden where the dog is allowed to dig, or a sandpit. Burying treats may help to attract the dog to this particular location rather than digging elsewhere. Providing other scavenging opportunities using feeding toys may reduce the motivation to dig for food. In some cases, placing deterrents such as a motion-activated water spray might help to reduce the behaviour (see Fig. 10.5). The benefits of such products should be weighed carefully against the potential for causing anxiety and fear.

It is essential to consider that some dogs may dig in an attempt to avoid or escape environmental threats such as other animals and noises, or confinement. These dogs will mostly dig around gates or fences and will exhibit other anxiety- and fear-related behaviours. Moreover, these dogs will attempt to escape these triggers in different environments (e.g. indoors). Finally, dogs with separation distress may also dig to try to follow the owner. The use of deterrent products in these cases is contraindicated as it will likely increase pre-existing anxiety and fear. Management of these dogs should focus on addressing the underlying triggers (see Section 13.2 – Separation-related Behaviour/Separation Distress).

10.5.4 Jumping on people or furniture

Jumping is a normal behaviour in dogs as part of their greeting or play behaviours. Jumping may be considered by some owners as inappropriate or unacceptable, especially with large dogs. Dogs may jump on their owners for attention. Owners should try avoiding reinforcing the behaviour by giving attention when the dog jumps on them. This is very difficult and may explain why the use of extinction (see Sections 8.5.2.1 – Extinction, and 10.3.6 - Ignoring the behaviour) is likely to fail. Therefore, management should focus on teaching alternative behaviours such as sit or paw instead of jumping. Training should start when the dog is calm and progress to more challenging situations. For example, when the owner walks into the room and gives the dog a signal to sit just before the dog is about to jump. Only once the dog sits should the owner give attention. Using a head halter is helpful to control the dog and direct it to sit instead of jumping. A lead attached to a collar or harness can be helpful as well; the owner can step on it to prevent the dog from jumping up. Punishment should be avoided. While it is likely to stop jumping, it is also likely to increase fear, anxiety and avoidance of contact with the owner.

10.5.5 Mounting

Mounting is a nuisance behaviour that many dogs show. It is normal when shown by a male mounting a receptive female. Puppies mount each other as part of play and practising adult behaviours. Also, dogs may mount each other while establishing social ranks. This behaviour is shown primarily by males; however, females may also show this behaviour. The patient may direct this behaviour towards other dogs or the owner. When mounting is directed towards the owner, it is not sexual behaviour. It is, in most cases, an attention-seeking behaviour. At times, especially following a high-intensity behaviour such as intense play, dogs that are highly aroused and have no appropriate outlet will direct mounting towards the owner. In these cases, mounting is a vacuum activity (see Section 7.3.3.1 – Vacuum activities). Physical disorders such as seizures, pain and abdominal pain may lead to thrusting movements.

Many owners feel embarrassed when their dogs mount. This is anthropomorphism. Punishment or trying to stop the patient without an appropriate alternative is likely to fail. Owners should focus on providing options to reduce high arousal following high-intensity behaviour. For example, following play, owners should provide the dog with a calm area and a chew toy. Also, disrupting play behaviour every two to three minutes to allow the dogs to settle down for a short period before playing again ensures that the patient's arousal level is not crossing the emotional threshold and the patient is able to control itself. Using a head halter to help to redirect the patient to sit is recommended, especially in cases where the dog is highly aroused. In some cases, neutering males may help to reduce mounting or its intensity.

10.5.6 Night-time activity

Most pets adapt to their owner's routine and are more active in the mornings and evenings. However, some dogs are more active at night when their owners are trying to sleep. The first step is to rule out physical disorders such as pain, gastrointestinal, neurological and other diseases (see Chapters 2 and 3). Pacing at night may also be a sign of cognitive dysfunction (see Chapter 16).

When the above conditions are ruled out or managed and the problem continues, owners should try to record more data on the behaviour. Details such as when, where, duration, environmental triggers and owners' responses are all helpful in identifying the cause of night-time activity. Psychiatric disorders such as anxiety, panic and phobia may account for this activity. If triggers are identified, we should attempt to remove or modify them. Environmental management (e.g. keeping the patient in an area where sounds of outdoor dogs or loud sounds are muffled, or placing a white-noise machine) should be part of the management (see Handout C3 – Safe -haven). Teaching the dog to settle down and rest is also helpful (see Handout C4 – Teaching a Pet how to Settle on Cue). When necessary, using medications such as trazodone, benzodiazepines and gabapentin may help these patients to sleep better at night (see Chapter 9).

When physical and psychiatric disorders are ruled out, owners should ensure that the patient's needs are met. A daily routine that includes daytime activities such as exercise, play and training should be implemented. Before bedtime, owners should ensure that the patient has eliminated and was fed. Using time-activated feeders at night helps in cases where hunger keeps the patient awake or leads to very early morning waking.

Owners should do their best to ignore the patient (once its needs are met, and no underlying pathology exists), although it may be very difficult. Giving the patient attention, even if it is in the form of punishment, may still reinforce the behaviour. Punishment is best avoided. Instead, owners may go to the patient to stop its activity using a lead and guide the patient to its night-time place and leave it there. Ideally, this is done without talking to the patient or providing any interactions other than taking it to its place.

10.5.7 Pulling on-lead

Walking dogs is a human concept. Owners like to walk a certain distance over a set time. Also, the timing of the walk depends on the owner's schedule not the dog. Dogs may want to walk at a different pace to the owner or are more curious about a particular smell or sight, while the owner may want to walk in a different direction. These are the most common reasons for dogs to pull while walking on-lead. Some dogs may pull in an attempt to avoid a particular area or trigger (e.g. other dogs, the veterinary practice or noises). While it may appear counterintuitive, pain may cause dogs to pull, especially back towards the home. Dogs in pain understand that once the walk is over, they may rest, and the pain reduces. Therefore, the faster they get back home, the sooner the pain will cease or reduce.

Owners should avoid punishing the patient for pulling. Instead, the focus should be on the owner teaching the patient to walk on a loose leash. Using treats and marker training to reinforce calm walking is helpful. Tools such as a head halter and front-attachment body harness are beneficial.

If the patient is pulling on-lead to avoid particular areas or triggers, the owner should first try to avoid these triggers and, later, design and implement a desensitization programme to teach the dog to accept these triggers.

10.5.8 Vocalization

Dogs have a wide range of vocalization, from barking to whimpering to growling and grunting. Most often, owners will complain about excessive barking. The term excessive denotes that, for the particular owner, barking in or at certain situations or times is unacceptable once it reaches a certain threshold. It may be that for a different owner, this level of barking might be acceptable. This complaint is subjective and depends on the owner's expectations and the context.

Dogs bark for many reasons, including warning, attention seeking, communication with other dogs or owners, or distress. It is important to first rule out physical disorders such as pain and neurological and cognitive decline. Next we must review the patient's routine and environment to ensure its needs are met. Owners may, inadvertently, reinforce the problem by giving the dog attention when it barks. Therefore, teaching the owner to ignore the behaviour when possible is helpful (see Section 10.3.6 - Ignoring the behaviour). It is only acceptable to ignore the behaviour once we rule out physical and psychiatric disorders (or manage them) and ensure that the patient's needs are met.

When excessive barking is the result of distress such as separation from the owner or panic during loud-noise events, a complete management programme including prevention, environmental management, behaviour modification and medications is necessary (see Chapter 13).

The focus of the management of nuisance barking is to teach the patient to stop barking and remain calm. Once the patient starts barking, the owner can distract it using a verbal signal or other sounds such as hand clapping. Once the patient stops barking, the owner should reward it. When the dog starts performing the task more rapidly and frequently, or even offers the behaviour (e.g. barks once and immediately stops and waits for a treat), the owners should start delaying the reward for increasing periods. Later, the owner can change from a consistent ratio to intermittent rewarding schedule (see Section 8.2.2.3 – Schedule of reinforcement). Continuing in this way, the owner is teaching the patient to be quiet rather than to stop barking. In other words, the patient learns that being quiet for increasing periods is the key to getting a treat.

The use of deterrent products such as a noise-activated spray or shock collar appeals to many owners. Using punishment may curb the behaviour rapidly; however, many patients will resume the behaviour when the product is no longer used or present. Some dogs may learn to modify the vocalization tone and pitch to avoid activation of the deterrent or to develop anxiety and fear (Juarbe-Diaz and Houpt, 1996; Wells, 2001; Moffat *et al.*, 2003).

References

Juarbe-Diaz, S.V. and Houpt, K.A. (1996) Comparison of two antibarking collars for treatment of nuisance barking. *Journal of the American Animal Hospital Association* 32(3), 231–235. DOI: 10.5326/15473317-32-3-231.

Moffat, K.S., Landsberg, G.M. and Beaudet, R. (2003) Effectiveness and comparison of citronella and scentless spray bark collars for the control of barking in a veterinary hospital setting. *Journal of the American Animal Hospital Association* 39(4), 343–348. DOI: 10.5326/0390343.

Pongrácz, P., Molnár, C., Miklósi, A. and Csányi, V. (2005) Human listeners are able to classify dog (*Canis familiaris*) barks recorded in different situations. *Journal of Comparative Psychology* 119(2), 136–144. DOI: 10.1037/0735-7036.119.2.136.

Tynes, V.V., Beck, A., Jeager, D.X. and Collin, J.F. (2017) Effect of synthetic feline pheromone on unwanted scratching in domestic cats. In: Denenberg, S. (ed.) *Proceedings of the 11th International Veterinary Behaviour Meeting*. CAB International, Wallingford, UK, pp. 45–47.

Wells, D.L. (2001) The effectiveness of a citronella spray collar in reducing certain forms of barking in dogs. *Applied Animal Behaviour Science* 73(4), 299–309. DOI: 10.1016/S0168-1591(01)00146-0.

11 Aggression – Cats

Jacqui Ley*

Melbourne Veterinary Specialist Centre, Glen Waverley, Victoria, Australia

11.1 Introduction

Aggression is a normal part of feline behaviour, like grooming and purring, and it serves many purposes for cats. Aggressive behaviour is used to retain territory, protect kittens and drive off threats from other cats or animals. Normal aggressive behaviour may be subtle or extreme. Aggressive behaviour may also be seen when cats are living with high levels of stress and as a sign of a psychiatric disorder. Diagnosing when aggression is a normal response to environmental change, a response to stress or a sign of mental health disease relies on understanding when cats are likely to be aggressive and how they show it.

11.2 Neurophysiology

The areas of the brain involved in aggressive behaviour are many. As more is discovered about the functioning of the brain, our understanding of how different areas integrate and modify the aggressive response is becoming more complex.

Two types of aggression can be distinguished: affective and predatory. Affective aggression (as a result of negative emotions such as fear, anxiety, frustration or pain) is characterized by a high degree of sympathetic up-regulation, with vocalizations and threat display, and its goal is to intimidate a potentially dangerous individual. Predatory behaviour is a normal behaviour and displayed with a lower degree of sympathetic up-regulation, fewer vocalizations and threats (as to not warn the prey), and the goal of the predator is to kill and eat prey. Affective and predatory aggressions are controlled by different neuronal pathways and are activated by different regions of the hypothalamus; medial for affective aggression and lateral for predatory aggression (Carlson and Birkett, 2017).

Areas identified as involving aggressive behaviour include the prefrontal cortex (dorsolateral prefrontal cortex, anterior cingulate cortex), amygdala, thalamus, hypothalamus and hippocampus. Other areas of interest are the bed nucleus of the stria terminalis (BNST), which plays a role in the generation of anxiety (Lebow and Chen, 2016). As the pathways for defensive aggression run from the medial amygdala through this area to the medial hypothalamus to the periaqueductal gray (PAG) (Panksepp and Biven, 2012), it is thought that the BNST may be of greater importance than previously supposed. Dysregulation of some areas may result in aggression with different characteristics. For example, more impulsive aggression may be seen when there is a lack of cortical regulation of the limbic system (Stahl, 2014).

The neurotransmitters identified as having a role in the generation and display of aggressive behaviour include the monoamines: serotonin, noradrenaline and dopamine as well as glutamate, gamma amino butyric acid (GABA) and acetylcholine (ACh). Relative levels of the neurotransmitters in different areas of the brain play a role in the expression of aggressive behaviour. With low levels of serotonin the prefrontal cortex increases the amount of dopamine and noradrenaline, increasing the probability of aggressive behaviour (Stahl, 2014).

11.3 Classifying Aggressive Behaviours

There are many ways to classify aggressive behaviours. While difficult, due to the complexity of aggressive behaviours, a definition of aggression is needed:

> Aggression includes all the species-specific behaviours that harm or threat to harm (not necessarily

*drjacquiley@msn.com

DOI: 10.1079/9781786394552.0011

to kill) another individual and, therefore, its display varies among species.

One of its primary functions is to distribute valuable but limited resources (e.g. food and safe spaces) among individuals and to protect oneself against injuries by others.

The reasons why a cat may be aggressive are many. Aggressive behaviours may occur between cats who share space, and may be directed at cats from other areas and individuals of other species. Cats vary on how likely they are to use aggressive behaviours, which can have serious consequences for them. Cats classed as proactive, that is outgoing and bold, were involved in more aggressive encounters and were at greater risk of being infected with feline immunodeficiency virus (Natoli *et al.*, 2005).

Aggressive behaviour is one part of a suite of behaviours considered to be agonistic. Scott (2015) defined agonistic behaviours as a 'system composed of behaviour patterns having the common function of adaptation to situations involving physical conflict between members of the same species'. This recognizes that aggressive behaviours include behaviours other than those that can cause physical injury. As such, it is not enough to only consider aggressive behaviours from the viewpoint of fighting behaviours but to also consider other behaviours such as threats, control of access and freezing when investigating aggressive behaviour between cats.

Aggressive behaviour can be the result of different motivations of the individual. Aggressive behaviour can be used in an instrumental manner (Manuck *et al.*, 2006), that is to achieve a goal. For example, a cat may use aggressive threats to drive away a cat that is invading the first cat's territory or removing other suitors from an in-season queen. Aggressive behaviours may also be classified as affective or impulsive aggression (Manuck *et al.*, 2006); that is, aggressive behaviour performed in response to the cat's internal emotional state. Aggression is often used to help manage and relieve a negative emotional state (such as from an affective disorder), such as being angry, fearful, anxious, painful or frustrated. So the cat who is frightened or frustrated by the intrusion of another cat into the first cat's territory uses aggression to manage or relieve this negative emotional state (affective aggression) and to drive away the perceived threat (instrumental aggression).

Aggression may also be considered offensive or defensive (Blanchard and Blanchard, 2006). Offensive aggression may occur because a resource, such as a territory or an oestrus female, is under dispute. If two cats are in an aggressive interaction, the offensively aggressive cat is the cat who initiates the aggressive encounter. The offensive threat may precede an attack and may end the encounter before any fighting occurs. If fighting occurs, areas targeted tend to be those that cause pain without permanently incapacitating the opponent. Cats may be bitten and scratched around the ears, legs and rump. When being offensively aggressive, the cat may be very confident in their behaviour and can be frightening to face.

Defensive aggression is aggression performed because the cat is forced to protect itself and escape is not seen as possible. Defensive attacks often target the vulnerable areas of the opponent such as the eyes and face and are often the last and most serious of the defensive pattern of the species (Blanchard and Blanchard, 2006). A cat may show defensive threats with the aim of preventing the need to fight. Defensive threats tend to emphasize the animal's size, weapons and readiness to use them. Generally, when possible, defensive behaviours that remove the need for fighting are utilized. Cats may leave an area, freeze or use defensive threat to avoid fighting. When defensive and offensive aggressive behaviours are compared, there are distinctive differences (see Table 11.1). When defensive, the cat keeps its body low and protected. The cat may twist its body so that its forelegs are free and can be used to react to the aggressor. In contrast, cats showing offensive behaviour stand tall and approach. Generally, the approach is very slow with low-pitched vocalizations. The victim is given the opportunity to leave the area by the slow threatening approach, although if they run they take the risk of being chased and attacked by the aggressor.

Predatory behaviour is also a type of aggressive behaviour. It is very different from affective aggression in that the cat is silent and secretive in preparing to be aggressive and waits to ambush suitable prey. The attack is fast, silent and aims to be lethal as quickly as possible. It is generally not considered with other aggressive behaviours (Wingfield *et al.*, 2006).

11.3.1 The body language of aggressive behaviours

Most aggressive behaviours by cats are silent and do not involve fighting at all. Aggressive behaviours tend to have a progression from threats through to

Table 11.1. Comparison of offensive and defensive aggressive behaviours in the cat.

	Offensive aggression	Defensive aggression
Motivation	A threat to resources – territory, food, mates	Threat to self
Threat behaviour	Block area, stare	Enlarge self – arch back, piloerection, weapons display, open-mouth hiss
Attack posture	Standing tall, charging	Body low, crouched so vulnerable areas are protected, may roll, forelegs are exposed, weapons displayed
Vocalization	'Mowl'	Scream
Attack directed at	Non-vulnerable areas – rump, ears	Vulnerable areas – eyes, head

more active and potentially injurious behaviours. The goal of threats is to prompt the other party into leaving without any actual fighting. This is very important as these threats may prevent injuries. If a cat can appear very large and very dangerous by puffing up its hair, arching its back and hissing, then it can avoid a potentially injurious or fatal interaction.

Aggressive behaviours have a progression from subtle but clear signals through to noisy attack and defensive behaviour. The metaphor of a ladder is often used to describe how the behaviours align with increasing arousal (see Fig. 11.1). This is not a perfect model but it is useful. At the lowest level of the ladder, a cat may start being threatening simply by positioning itself so that another cat or cats cannot access resources such as food, water, exits or litter trays. Some very confident cats will sprawl out on their sides or sit in a clearly visible place. Owners may interpret this behaviour as being 'playful' and 'friendly'.

The next level of aggressive behaviour may start with the parties staring at each other. The rungs of the ladder get progressively closer together as the aggressive encounter escalates. One cat may advance slowly on the other with its body raised and its tail down, with the tip twitching. This cat's head is held low with the ears forward and rotated outwards, and jaw clamped shut. It may give a deep growl. Sometimes the attacking cat will yowl (which might sound like they are chewing as they vocalize). Growling, yowling and snarling are used when the cat signals that it is threatening or actively attacking (Houpt, 2018).

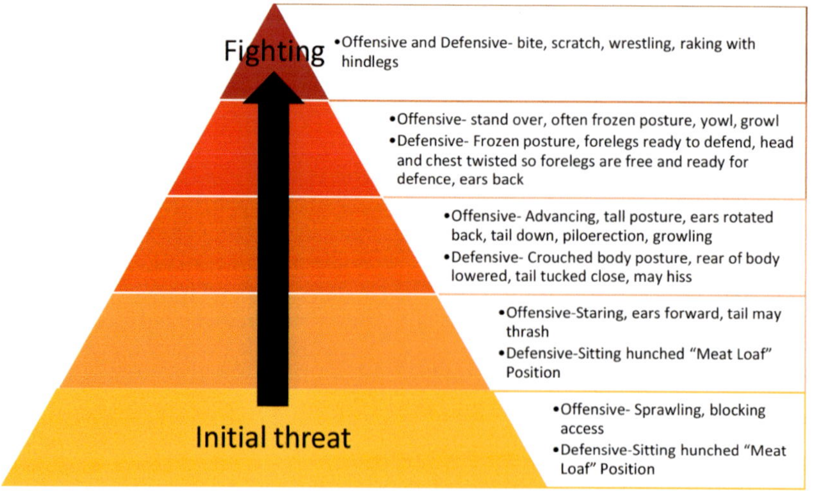

Fig. 11.1. Escalation of aggression. As the cat starts showing aggression, the initial behaviours are more subtle and diffuse. As aggression escalates, the behaviours become more intense, overt and directed towards the object of aggression.

As the offensive cat approaches, the other cat may pull back and may look for an escape. If it cannot or does not wish to leave, it tends to crouch and pull its head and neck in. The ears are held down and rotated back, and the cat may hiss or spit. The spit is generally made when a cat is defensive (Houpt, 2018). Usually, both cats will have dilated pupils and show piloerection, so they look bigger. There is often a stand-off with one cat threatening and the other seemingly frozen. If the threat does not resolve the problem, then fighting may occur with strikes by the forepaws, biting and grappling while raking with the hind paws.

It is essential to remember that while the ladder of escalation is an effective metaphor, some cats may escalate very fast (too fast for owners to evaluate) or might jump over several levels of the ladder. In addition, some cats may have dysfunctional communication skills and will not show all signs.

11.4 Development of Aggressive Behaviours

Aggressive behaviours are not seen until kittens have matured enough to be able to move around independently, to send and receive signals such as vocalizations and visual signals. Kittens show social play with pawing at each other, starting at two to three weeks of age as they develop the ability to walk and use their forepaws (Mendoza and Ramirez, 1987). Social play peaks at week 6 and stays high until it starts to decrease gradually between weeks 14 and 16. As social play waxes in preference for object-directed play, the kittens start to show more aggressive behaviours such as biting (Mendoza and Ramirez, 1987) and the defensive startle (arching their backs and piloerection) in response to stimuli they find threatening (Kolb and Nonneman, 1975). They also spit (Houpt, 2018).

Events and experiences during the kitten's development can have effects on its tendency to be aggressive as an adult. Early weaning, defined as permanent separation from the queen before 12 weeks of age, has been associated with higher levels of aggression, but not shyness, in cats (Ahola *et al.*, 2017). Early experiences have long-lasting effects on brain development and function that could easily be addressed by encouraging natural weaning of kittens by leaving them with their dam until greater than 12 weeks of age while providing contact with people.

11.5 Aggression and People

Aggressive behaviours by cats are among the most common reasons to relinquish cats to shelters or to present cats to veterinary behaviour clinics (Salman *et al.*, 2000; Denenberg *et al.*, 2005; Curtis, 2008). Amat *et al.* (2009) reported that 47% of feline presentations to the Animal Behaviour Clinic at the Barcelona School of Veterinary Medicine were for aggression. Most presentations were because of aggression directed towards people with play-related aggression and petting-related aggression. Aggression problems were more common in single-cat households than in multi-cat households. In many cases, the cats were defensively aggressive after being approached by people (Palacio *et al.*, 2007).

Aggressive behaviours by cats may occur as a part of normal feline behaviour, as a response to a stressful environment or as a manifestation of psychiatric disorder. Identifying the cause is important to help owners resolve the situation.

Many complaints about aggression in cats are about normal species-typical behaviour, highlighting the need for education of cat owners. Not having knowledge of cat behaviour and having high expectations of the cat were part of a group of risk factors considered modifiable for relinquishment of cats (Patronek *et al.*, 1996).

The goals of treating all aggression problems in cats should be safety for all concerned and quality of life (Beaver, 2004). Finding safe outlets of normal exploratory behaviour and providing suitable housing arrangements help reduce aggression between cats and people.

11.5.1 When normal cat aggressive behaviour is a problem for people

Sometimes the appropriate expression of aggressive behaviours by cats is a problem for the people they live with or live among. Feral and semi-owned cats fight and vocalize during the mating season and may keep people awake at night. More commonly, owners of companion cats find some of their cat's aggressive behaviours confusing.

11.5.1.1 Play aggression

Young cats are playful; it is part of what attracts people to keep cats. Play may include elements of predatory behaviour and agonistic behaviour, and it can be directed towards toys and other small objects. However, cats can direct their playful pouncing and biting to people and children and other cats if not provided with suitable outlets for their energy.

Opportunities for play directed to suitable objects needs to be provided for young cats (and playful older cats). Toys, such as food-dispensing toys and battery-operated toys, climbing posts, outside enclosures or time outside may all help to provide outlets for playful behaviour. The human targets of play aggression need to be prepared with suitable toys to which they can direct the cat's attention. All games should be with toys rather than hands or feet, so the cat does not associate these with play.

If ambushing is the cat's preferred game, it is also important that the owner does not run, which can provoke chasing. Instead, the owner should stand still and toss a toy or a treat ahead to encourage the cat to chase and play with it. Favourite ambush areas can also be removed or blocked where possible. Placing a collar with a bell on the cat might help to thwart the cat's sneak attack by alerting the victim.

When older or less playful cats are being pounced on by a playful cat, causing fighting, time apart and redirecting play to more suitable objects is recommended.

Punishment should not be used in managing play aggression – after all, the cat is playing. Water-spray bottles, yelling or admonishing the cat should be avoided. Owners should be encouraged to be pre-emptive and direct their cat to more acceptable play activities.

11.5.1.2 Fear-related aggression

When cats are frightened, some will use aggressive behaviours in an attempt to drive the threatening individual away. They may hiss, scratch and bite. Owners need to be aware of what induces fear in their cats and avoid it if possible (Beaver, 2004). If the cat must be exposed to a fear-inducing situation (such as a veterinary visit), then medication or nutraceuticals, such as alpha casozepine to help it be calmer, are indicated (Beata *et al.*, 2007; van Haaften *et al.*, 2017). If a cat has been frightened, owners need to resist the desire to comfort the cat. Many cats stay aroused and upset for a lengthy period after the event and to try to interact with them before they are ready may lead to redirected aggression (Beaver, 2004). Giving them a quiet, calm space until they are ready to instigate contact is required. Owners need to be told that their cat may stay aroused for a day (or more) after a very stressful event. The cat's arousal may not be obvious – this is probably due to it having evolved in a dangerous environment. Keeping one's emotional state quiet would have been an advantage for survival.

11.5.1.3 Petting induced aggression

Some cats, when petted for a while, suddenly show dilated pupils and a lashing tail (Wingfield *et al.*, 2006). If the person continues to pat the cat, they may be grabbed around the hand and arm and bitten and scratched. It is not clear why some cats react to petting like this; it may be that they find the repetitive stroking disturbing or overwhelming.

Management requires the owners to be aware of how much petting their cat likes and not to exceed this. Patting for a few seconds and then stopping and checking with the cat often allows the cat to feel comfortable and may extend patting sessions without leading to aggression. By checking in, the owner stops patting and allows the cat to indicate (it may look at the owner, nudge the hand or move under the owner's hand) that it would like more petting, or less, and gives it a chance to move away.

11.5.1.4 New cat introduction

A common event that causes unrest and disruption to a cat household is the introduction of a new cat. A survey of 252 households adopting a cat from a shelter found that of the 128 multi-cat households over half experienced fighting when new cats were introduced (Levine *et al.*, 2005). Many owners may get a new cat in the belief that their existing cat 'needs a playmate' or because a cat is ageing, and they may be surprised when the cats do not get along.

Household and neighbourhood cats may form a stable group. This group will have overlapping home territories where cats of the group will be tolerated. Stable groups of adult cats actively prevent new cats from joining their group (Turner, 2014).

When owners acquire a new cat, they need to mimic how a cat joins a stable group. The newcomer hangs around the edge of the group where it may be driven away. With persistence, it becomes tolerated and can claim an area for itself.

When a new cat is brought into a household, it needs to have controlled exposure to the household cats so that it and they can become familiar with each other with minimal fighting (Crowell-Davis *et al.*, 2004). The new cat should be confined to the area that will be its space or core territory. This space is defended against other cats (Bradshaw, 2013). The other cats should be able to smell the cat under the door, but visual exposure should be avoided. The main living area should be time-shared between the existing cats and the new cat, so they become familiar with each other's scents in the area.

The new cat can be given access to other rooms when the household cats are confined so that it can explore the house. This also puts its scent around the house, normalizing it for the other cats.

As the cats become familiar with each other, then they can be brought into the common area and fed as far apart as possible. Owners should use safety measures such as a carrier, stairgates, or lead and harness. The latter should be pre-trained, so the cat feels comfortable wearing it. If there is no aggressive behaviour, such as staring, hissing or growling, then they can stay in the space and gradually have longer supervised time together. If a cat is uncomfortable, escape to that cat's safe area should be available. If there is aggressive behaviour, the cats need to be separated and more time spent getting them familiar with each other.

Feline-appeasing pheromone, either sprayed or in a diffuser, may help the integration of a new cat into a household (DePorter *et al.*, 2019).

The time it takes to introduce a new cat may be longer than owners expect. Some cats may require several months to be habituated to each other. Owners need to be aware that considerable time may be needed to integrate new cats into a household.

11.6 Aggression as a Response to Stress

When cats are living in highly stressful situations, such as multi-cat households, some will attempt to cope with their stress by controlling interactions between themselves and other cats by using aggressive behaviour. The result is unsettled feline households and cats presenting to veterinary clinics with abscesses. Inter-cat aggressive behaviour may also be a factor in house-soiling and stress-related disease in other cats such as feline idiopathic cystitis, colitis and over-grooming (Mills *et al.*, 2014). When the stress is relieved, the cat's behaviour returns to within normal limits.

11.6.1 Multi-cat household

The most likely instigator is a male cat, but the victim cat may be male or female (Lindell *et al.*, 1997). Treatments that advise environmental management and medications are equally likely to be helpful in managing the situation.

It is easy to consider the important stressor in unsettled multi-cat households or colonies as simply being high cat density. However, cats can live in close proximity comfortably. In free-ranging colonies, the number of cats in an area reflects the nature and distribution of resources (Turner, 2014). In a household, the number of resources, such as feeding stations, water sources, resting and sleeping spaces, and toilet facilities, and the distribution of these, are probably more important than the number of cats with regard to inter-cat aggression. Cats in a household will have places where they can reliably be found at certain times of the day. They may time-share the spaces available to them to avoid cats with whom there is competition (Bernstein and Friedmann, 2014).

11.6.1.1 Management

Resources should be provided in sufficient numbers to allow cats to access what they need when they need it. This may mean many more toilet facilities, food stations, water stations and beds than owners and carers think. How the resources are distributed is also important. If all the feeders are in the same area, then it is one big feeder. Resources will need to be distributed around the space in clumps and be individualized to the cats in the household or colony. The owner or carer may need to experiment with how the resources are distributed to find the best combination for their cats.

Some general advice:

- Separate feeding stations. Cats have evolved to hunt small prey, so they tend to eat alone. Providing food bowls that are separated so the cats cannot see each other can reduce stress and fighting around food.
- Provide sufficient water bowls in different locations. Separate the water from feeding stations.
- Litter trays, resting areas and climbing towers all need two ways at least by which the cat can

access them. This prevents one cat from monopolizing access to resources. It also prevents cats from being trapped in the litter tray or a cat tower. Litter trays can be concealed behind a screen rather than covered over. This creates two access points.

- Provide a core territory and shared territory for the cats. Some cats may have to time-share the territory to avoid conflicts.
- Feline-appeasing pheromone in a diffuser may help settle aggressive cats.

11.6.2 Redirected aggression

Redirected aggression (sometimes known as displaced aggression) is a common form of aggressive behaviour seen in domestic cats and other animals (Chapman and Voith, 1990; Denenberg *et al.*, 2005). It is characterized by intense defensive arousal and aggression towards a target other than the inciting cause. One study found that redirected aggression was triggered most frequently by loud noises and other cats (Amat *et al.*, 2008). Cats with noise phobias were found to be over-represented compared to the control cats. Targets are commonly the owners or other cats in multi-cat households. Indoor cats were found to be more likely to show redirected aggression than cats that are allowed outside (Amat *et al.*, 2008). When triggered, the cats often display intense aggression attacks, which are hard to interrupt, exhibit uninhibited biting, and stay aroused long after the event.

Management of redirected aggression involves preventing the cat from seeing or otherwise experiencing its triggers. This may mean that owners keep the cat out of the rooms where it can see other cats. If keeping the cat away from the windows or trigger areas is not possible then blocking the view with curtains, blinds or with opaquing film applied over the windows or the areas where the cat can look outside, is advised.

It may also be necessary to prevent outside cats accessing private property by altering fences or other access points. Management may also involve minimizing sudden loud noises in the household.

11.6.3 Pain and physical diseases

Pain and physical disease (e.g. organ dysfunction, dermatological, gastrointestinal and neurological) are often overlooked causes of stress. Many low-grade chronic diseases may not be visible but can be a cause of a cat being irritable. Common diseases include arthritis, atopy, cystitis and large bowel disease (see Chapters 2 and 3). Cats, like many animals, do not display pain openly. If handled when painful, many cats will display defensive aggression. They may hiss when approached, patted or picked up. They may also strike with their forepaws to avoid being handled.

One study has identified chronic inflammation of the vomeronasal organ in cats and suggested that it may be a cause of inter-cat aggression (Asproni *et al.*, 2016).

Management requires diagnosis and treatment of painful conditions and other diseases. A full physical examination should be the first step if a cat is showing an increased tendency to be aggressive. Investigation of a change in behaviour in a cat should include full clinical evaluation and appropriate blood tests, laboratory tests and imaging to identify any disease. In some cases, a treatment trial for the suspected disease may be needed to identify if it is a cause of aggressive behaviours.

Moreover, getting older is not a reason to get aggressive. Older cats may have arthritis that makes being handled painful. This should be diagnosed and treated for the welfare of the cat (see Chapter 16).

11.7 Aggression as a Sign of Psychiatric Disorder

Some cats display aggressive behaviours as a sign of a psychiatric disorder. Most commonly, anxiety disorders, panic and impulsivity can lead to cats displaying out-of-context aggressive behaviours, using excessive levels of aggression, or being irritable, aroused and frequently aggressive. Aggressive behaviours can be difficult for owners to manage. Aggression due to a psychiatric disorder or due to stress is differentiated by the cat's response to environmental changes. If it does not abate after management strategies are implemented, then the cat needs to be examined for a psychiatric disorder that can cause aggressive behaviours.

11.7.1 History, assessment and diagnosis

Before any treatment and management plan can be implemented, it is vital to make a diagnosis so that appropriate treatment can be put in place. A diagnosis is made by collecting a thorough history, observation of the cat in their home environment without a stranger present (via video or pet camera), in the clinic or on a home visit, and a clinical examination. Medical problems are identified and quantified with appropriate laboratory tests, such as blood and urine, and further diagnostic tests as appropriate.

Aggressive behaviours do not need to be seen to be understood. The history allows the clinician to identify when the behaviour occurs, what triggers aggression and potential motivations for the behaviour. The description of the body language of the cat as well as its responses to changes in its environment and personality all help to identify the emotional state of the cat at the time of the aggressive incidents. Furthermore, how the cat manages stressors such as travel to the clinic or having a stranger in the house may help identify if the cat has a psychiatric disorder.

11.7.2 Diagnosis

As discussed previously, aggressive behaviours can be a normal behavioural response to environmental triggers; it can be a response to extreme environmental triggers, and it can be an abnormal response to normal environmental triggers due to the cat having a psychiatric disorder such as an anxiety disorder. Anxiety is an unpleasant emotional state that drives the individual to alter its behaviour to get some relief from unpleasant feelings. This may result in avoidant behaviour or aggressive behaviour. When the anxiety is excessive and has negative impacts on its day-to-day living, it can be classed as an anxiety disorder.

The diagnosis should consider that some types of aggression, such as fear aggression, may be seen in normal cats and cats with a psychiatric disorder. For example, a cat may demonstrate fear aggression because it encounters a large dog in the neighbourhood (normal response), because it is cornered by the bold, aggressive cat of the household (stress-related), or repeatedly whenever the owner approaches the cat where it is resting at home (aggression due to abnormal levels of fear).

While the diagnosis usually takes a descriptive form – identifying the targets of the aggressive behaviour (e.g. familiar cats, unfamiliar cats, familiar people, unfamiliar people and redirected aggression) – the clinician should identify the underlying mechanism. Knowing the pathology (e.g. anxiety, panic, frustration or impulsivity) directs the management and selection of medications (Denenberg and Dubé, 2018).

11.7.3 Treatment

Treatment of psychiatric disorders in cats requires attention to the environment of the cat, exercises to help the cat practise calm behaviour and medication to help manage the abnormal brain function.

11.7.3.1 Management of the environment

Providing a safe, reassuring and calm environment is essential for treating cases of aggression in cats. It may be necessary to separate cats that are fighting. This is done by creating safe areas for each cat or group of cats. Other areas of the house should be used as shared space that the cats (or group of cats) can use in a timeshare arrangement. This mimics how feral cats use space and provides a safe, threat-free environment for the anxious cat.

Scheduled time with the owner is also recommended. This does not have to be very long; approximately 15 minutes can be enough. It needs to happen at a regular point in the household routine to provide predictability for the cat. The owner is instructed to spend time doing what the cat likes. This may be playing, sitting quietly petting or grooming the cat, or just providing a lap.

The owner should be instructed to use a quiet, soothing voice with the cat rather than the high-pitched tone many people use. The owner should also keep their body language calm and steady to help their cat stay calm. If the cat is threatening, the owner should back away and leave the cat alone.

Some cats respond to food-dispensing toys but some may take time before they are calm enough to interact with the toys.

11.7.3.2 Settle exercises

Psychiatric disorders may prevent a cat from learning that normal events in its environment are not threatening, resulting in them using aggressive behaviour at inappropriate times. Exercises that reward calm behaviour and that encourage relaxation can be useful to encourage anxious cats to learn alternative ways of coping with stressors.

Owners should be asked to whisper 'good boy' or 'good girl' to their cat whenever they see a calm, relaxed behaviour such as lying in a relaxed fashion. By whispering, they are not arousing the cat, but they are rewarding calm behaviour. When the exercise is done correctly, the cat should not do anything beyond flicking an ear.

Many cats respond favourably to gentle and deep petting of the nape and shoulders area. This should be done only if there is no risk to the owner while petting the cat. If the owner notices that the cat keeps its head high, eyes open with a tense body, the owner should stop.

A settle exercise can be taught using treats. The cat is encouraged with treats to stay close to the owner. It is then asked or lured to make eye contact, and a treat is given. The cue 'stay' is given after the eye contact is rewarded, and the cat is given another treat for staying. The 'look' cue is given, and eye contact is rewarded again, and then the 'stay' cue is given. This sequence is repeated for about a minute. The cues are delivered in a calm and relaxed fashion. Through trial-and-error learning, the cat discovers the parameters of the exercise, and as it becomes familiar with it, the cat relaxes. Relaxed body language may include: relaxed eyes, ears rotated loosely forward, face relaxed, body muscles relaxed, breathing slowed and posture calm. With repetition, the exercise will induce a state of calm and relaxation on the cat. The exercise can then be introduced gradually into situations that have been stressful and aggression-provoking for the cat. Once the cat learns the exercise, treats should not be given as they may serve to keep the cat alert and waiting for more treats, which may be counterproductive. Also, owners should pay attention to the way the cat is taking the treat; some cats might become more aroused rather than calm.

11.7.3.3 Medication

Many cats with a psychiatric disorder that results in aggressive behaviours require medications to help them settle and be calm enough to learn more acceptable ways to manage their feelings of anxiety, panic or impulsivity. Typically, a baseline anxiolytic medication such as a selective serotonin re-uptake inhibitor (SSRI) or a tricyclic antidepressant (TCA) is used daily, and a situational medication, such as gabapentin, trazodone, mirtazapine or clonidine, is given when needed. Nutraceuticals may be added or used alone for some cats.

The SSRIs such as fluoxetine and TCAs such as clomipramine share common side effects due to their increasing serotonin in the synapse via their blockade of the serotonin transporter protein (see Section 9.8 – Serotonergic Medications). Lethargy was reported in four out of ten cats at doses higher than 0.4 mg/kg once a day; the lethargy resolved when the dose was lowered (Seksel and Lindeman, 1998). Urinary retention due to detrusor muscle paralysis caused by the medications is a rare but serious side effect. The paralysis is caused by the medication's anticholinergic effects and may appear in the first few days of treatment (Pfeiffer *et al.*, 1999; Verhamme *et al.*, 2008). Owners must monitor micturition and check that their cats are passing urine. If not, treatment is required and is supportive. The SSRI or TCA is stopped and the bladder emptied, either by catheterizing or by abdominocentesis. Bladder function may take up to a week to return to normal (Pfeiffer *et al.*, 1999) but if the problem is detected early, full recovery is expected.

References

Ahola, M.K., Vapalahti, K. and Lohi, H. (2017) Early weaning increases aggression and stereotypic behaviour in cats. *Scientific Reports* 7(1), 10412. DOI: 10.1038/s41598-017-11173-5.

Amat, M., Manteca, X., Brech, S.L., Ruiz de la Torre, J.L., Mariotti, V.M. *et al.* (2008) Evaluation of inciting causes, alternative targets, and risk factors associated with redirected aggression in cats. *Journal of the American Veterinary Medical Association* 233(4), 586–589. DOI: 10.2460/javma.233.4.586.

Amat, M., de la Torre, J.L.R., Fatjó, J., Mariotti, V.M., Van Wijk, S. *et al.* (2009) Potential risk factors associated with feline behaviour problems. *Applied Animal Behaviour Science* 121(2), 134–139. DOI: 10.1016/j.applanim.2009.09.012.

Asproni, P., Cozzi, A., Verin, R., Lafont-Lecuelle, C., Bienboire-Frosini, C. *et al.* (2016) Pathology and behaviour in feline medicine: investigating the link between vomeronasalitis and aggression. *Journal of Feline Medicine and Surgery* 18(12), 997–1002. DOI: 10.1177/1098612X15606493.

Beata, C., Beaumont-Graff, E., Coll, V., Cordel, J., Marion, M. *et al.* (2007) Effect of alpha-casozepine (Zylkene) on anxiety in cats. *Journal of Veterinary Behavior* 2(2), 40–46. DOI: 10.1016/j.jveb.2007.02.002.

Beaver, B.V. (2004) Fractious cats and feline aggression. *Journal of Feline Medicine and Surgery* 6(1), 13–18. DOI: 10.1016/j.jfms.2003.09.011.

Bernstein, P.L. and Friedmann, E. (2014) Social behaviour of domestic cats in the human home. In: Turner, D.C. and Bateson, P. (eds) *The Domestic Cat: The Biology of its Behaviour*. Cambridge University Press, Cambridge, UK, pp. 71–81.

Blanchard, D.C. and Blanchard, R.J. (2006) Stress and aggressive behaviors. In: Nelson, R.J. (ed.) *Biology of Aggression*. Oxford University Press, New York, pp. 275–291.

Bradshaw, J. (2013) *Cat Sense: the Feline Enigma Revealed*. Penguin, London.

Carlson, N.R. and Birkett, M.A. (2017) *Physiology of Behavior*, 12th edn. Pearson, Harlow, UK.

Chapman, B.L. and Voith, V.L. (1990) Cat aggression redirected to people: 14 cases (1981-1987). *Journal of the American Veterinary Medical Association* 196(6), 947–950.

Crowell-Davis, S.L., Curtis, T.M. and Knowles, R.J. (2004) Social organization in the cat: a modern understanding. *Journal of Feline Medicine and Surgery* 6(1), 19–28. DOI: 10.1016/j.jfms.2003.09.013.

Curtis, T.M. (2008) Human-directed aggression in the cat. *Veterinary Clinics of North America: Small Animal Practice* 38(5), 1131–1143. DOI: 10.1016/j.cvsm.2008.04.009.

Denenberg, S. and Dubé, M.B. (2018) Tools for managing feline problem behaviours: Psychoactive medications. *Journal of feline medicine and surgery* 20(11), 1034–1045. DOI: 10.1177/1098612X18806760.

Denenberg, S., Landsberg, G.M., Horwitz, D. and Seksel, K. *et al.* (2005) A comparison of cases referred to behaviorists in three different countries. In: Mills, D., Levine, E., Landsberg, G., Horwitz, D., Duxbury, M., *et al.* (eds) *Current Issues and Research in Veterinary Behavioural Medicine*. Purdue University Press, West Lafayette, Indiana, pp. 56–62.

DePorter, T.L., Bledsoe, D.L., Beck, A. and Ollivier, E. (2019) Evaluation of the efficacy of an appeasing pheromone diffuser product vs placebo for management of feline aggression in multi-cat households: a pilot study. *Journal of Feline Medicine and Surgery* 21(4), 293–305. DOI: 10.1177/1098612X18774437.

Houpt, K.A. (2018) *Domestic Animal Behavior*, 6th edn. Wiley Blackwell, Hoboken, New Jersey.

Kolb, B. and Nonneman, A.J. (1975) The development of social responsiveness in kittens. *Animal Behaviour* 23(2), 368–374. DOI: 10.1016/0003-3472(75)90085-8.

Lebow, M.A. and Chen, A. (2016) Overshadowed by the amygdala: the bed nucleus of the stria terminalis emerges as key to psychiatric disorders. *Molecular Psychiatry* 21(4), 450–463. DOI: 10.1038/mp.2016.1.

Levine, E., Perry, P., Scarlett, J. and Houpt, K.A. (2005) Intercat aggression in households following the introduction of a new cat. *Applied Animal Behaviour Science* 90(3-4), 325–336. DOI: 10.1016/j.applanim.2004.07.006.

Lindell, E.M., Erb, H.N. and Houpt, K.A. (1997) Intercat aggression: a retrospective study examining types of aggression, sexes of fighting pairs, and effectiveness of treatment. *Applied Animal Behaviour Science* 55(1-2), 153–162. DOI: 10.1016/S0168-1591(97)00032-4.

Manuck, S.B., Kaplan, J.R. and Lotrich, F.E. (2006) Brain serotonin and aggressive disposition in humans and nonhuman primates. In: Nelson, R.J. (ed.) *Biology of Aggression*. Oxford University Press, New York, pp. 65–113.

Mendoza, D.L. and Ramirez, J.M. (1987) Play in kittens (*Felis domesticus*) and its association with cohesion and aggression. *Bulletin of the Psychonomic Society* 25(1), 27–30. DOI: 10.3758/BF03330067.

Mills, D., Karagiannis, C. and Zulch, H. (2014) Stress—its effects on health and behavior. *Veterinary Clinics of North America: Small Animal Practice* 44(3), 525–541. DOI: 10.1016/j.cvsm.2014.01.005.

Natoli, E., Say, L., Cafazzo, S., Bonanni, R., Schmid, M. *et al.* (2005) Bold attitude makes male urban feral domestic cats more vulnerable to feline immunodeficiency virus. *Neuroscience & Biobehavioral Reviews* 29(1), 151–157. DOI: 10.1016/j.neubiorev.2004.06.011.

Palacio, J., León-Artozqui, M., Pastor-Villalba, E., Carrera-Martín, F. and García-Belenguer, S. (2007) Incidence of and risk factors for cat bites: a first step in prevention and treatment of feline aggression. *Journal of Feline Medicine & Surgery* 9(3), 188–195. DOI: 10.1016/j.jfms.2006.11.001.

Panksepp, J. and Biven, L. (2012) *Archeology of the Mind: Neuroevolutionary Origins of the Human Emotions*. N.W. Norton and Co, New York.

Patronek, G.J., Glickman, L.T., Beck, A.M., McCabe, G.P. and Ecker, C. (1996) Risk factors for relinquishment of cats to an animal shelter. *Journal of the American Veterinary Medical Association* 209(3), 582–588.

Pfeiffer, E., Guy, N. and Cribb, A. (1999) Clomipramine-induced urinary retention in a cat. *The Canadian Veterinary Journal* 40(4), 265–267.

Salman, M.D., Hutchison, J., Ruch-Gallie, R., Kogan, L., New, J.C. *et al.* (2000) Behavioral reasons for relinquishment of dogs and cats to 12 shelters. *Journal of Applied Animal Welfare Science* 3(2), 93–106. DOI: 10.1207/S15327604JAWS0302_2.

Scott, J.P. (2015) Agonistic behavior of mice and rats: a review. *Integrative and Comparative Biology* 6(4), 683–701.

Seksel, K. and Lindeman, M.J. (1998) Use of clomipramine in the treatment of anxiety-related and obsessive-compulsive disorders in cats. *Australian Veterinary Journal* 76(5), 317–321. DOI: 10.1111/j.1751-0813.1998.tb12353.x.

Stahl, S. (2014) *Stahl's illustrated Violence: Neural Circuits, Genetics and Treatment*. Cambridge University Press, New York.

Turner, D.C. (2014) Social organisation and behavioural ecology of free-ranging domestic cats. In: Turner, D.C. and Bateson, P. (eds) *The Domestic Cat: The Biology of its Behaviour*. Cambridge University Press, Cambridge, UK.

van Haaften, K.A., Forsythe, L.R.E., Stelow, E.A. and Bain, M.J. (2017) Effects of a single preappointment dose of gabapentin on signs of stress in cats during transportation and veterinary examination. *Journal of*

the American Veterinary Medical Association 251(10), 1175–1181. DOI: 10.2460/javma.251.10.1175.
Verhamme, K.M.C., Sturkenboom, M.C.J.M., Stricker, B.H.C. and Bosch, R. (2008) Drug-Induced urinary retention. *Drug Safety* 31(5), 373–388. DOI: 10.2165/00002018-200831050-00002.
Wingfield, J.C., Moore, I.T., Goymann, F., Wacker, D.W. and Sperry, T. (2006) Contexts and ethology of vertebrate aggression: implications for the evolution of Hormone-Behaviour interactions. In: Nelson, R.J. (ed.) *Biology of Aggression.* Oxford University Press, New York, pp. 179–210.

12 Aggression – Dogs

Carlo Siracusa*

Department of Clinical Sciences and Advanced Medicine, School of Veterinary Medicine, University of Pennsylvania, Philadelphia, Pennsylvania, USA

12.1 Introduction

Dog aggression is a prominent topic in veterinary psychiatry and a relevant public health problem. Dog aggression directed to people or other animals has been consistently reported to be among the most frequent problems referred to veterinary psychiatrists (Denenberg *et al.*, 2005; Bamberger and Houpt, 2006; Fatjo *et al.*, 2007; Siracusa *et al.*, 2017). Dogs bite an estimated 1.5% of the US population (Gilchrist *et al.*, 2008) and 1.9% of the UK population (Westgarth *et al.*, 2018) each year. Nevertheless, primary care veterinarians often feel that is not their responsibility to initiate a conversation about behaviour problems, including aggression, with their clients (Patronek and Dodman, 1999) and inaccurate information about dog aggression and its treatment is readily available in the media (Herron *et al.*, 2009).

12.2 Neurophysiology of Aggression

From a neurophysiological standpoint, two types of aggression can be distinguished: affective and predatory. Affective aggression is characterized by a high degree of sympathetic up-regulation, with vocalizations and threat display, and its goal is to intimidate a potentially dangerous individual. Predatory behaviour is displayed with a lower degree of sympathetic up-regulation, fewer vocalizations and threats (predators do not want to be discovered early by their prey), and the goal of the predator is to kill and eat prey. Affective and predatory aggression are controlled by different neuronal pathways and are activated by different regions of the hypothalamus (medial for affective aggression, and lateral for predatory aggression) (Carlson and Birkett, 2017). In this chapter, affective aggression is referred to as aggression, and predatory aggression as predatory behaviour.

Different regions of the brain hierarchically control aggression. The periaqueductal gray nucleus (PAG) in the brainstem programmes the actions of an animal displaying aggressive behaviour. The PAG is activated or inhibited by the hypothalamus and the amygdala, which control the response to a perceived threat by activating the stress response. The stress response is the biological response activated when an animal perceives a threat or challenge. The activation of this response can result, among other biological processes, in four different behaviour displays: aggression (fight), escape (flight), tonic immobility (freeze), displacement (fidget) (Carlson and Birkett, 2017). Based on their animality, dogs tend to respond to threats with consistent behaviour responses in similar contexts (coping strategy). The dog's reaction (e.g. aggression or escape) is determined by analysis of the perceived stimuli, environmental options, physical abilities and past experiences. This last process is mainly regulated by superior brain areas like the sensory cortex and the ventromedial prefrontal cortex; the latter has an inhibitory role on the emotions controlled by the amygdala.

The neurotransmitters identified as having a role in the generation and display of aggressive behaviour include the monoamines: serotonin, noradrenaline and dopamine as well as glutamate, gamma amino butyric acid (GABA) and acetylcholine (ACh). Relative levels of the neurotransmitters in different areas of the brain play a role in the expression of aggressive behaviour. Low levels of serotonin in the prefrontal cortex increase the amount of dopamine and noradrenaline, increasing the probability of aggressive behaviour (Stahl, 2014). Furthermore, serotonin (5-HT) is known to

*carlosiracusa@gmail.com

 Small Animal Veterinary Psychiatry (ed. S. Denenberg)
DOI: 10.1079/9781786394552.0012

modulate the emotional response and the display of aggressive behaviour, with lower levels of serotonin promoting a more risky and impulsive reaction to a perceived threat (Reisner *et al.*, 1996; León *et al.*, 2012; Bear *et al.*, 2016; Carlson and Birkett, 2017).

12.3 Aggression as a Normal Social Behaviour

From an ecological and ethological perspective, aggression is a normal behaviour that can be observed across the entire animal kingdom. Aggression includes all the species-specific behaviours that harm or threat to harm (not necessarily to kill) another individual and, therefore, its display varies among species. One of its primary functions is to distribute valuable but limited resources (e.g. food and safe spaces) among individuals and to protect oneself against injuries by others. Indeed, aggressive behaviour is triggered by the perception of a potential threat. Aggression, together with affiliative behaviours, helps to maintain stability within a social group by dividing resources and assigning each individual a position in the social network. While affiliative behaviours are used to increase proximity among individuals of a social group, aggressive behaviours are used to keep or increase the distance between individuals of a group. Outside of a social group, aggression helps to defend the territory and the resources in it (Miklosi, 2015; Bradshaw and Rooney, 2016; Nelson and Kriegsfeld, 2018). Many of the aggressive behaviours that an animal performs are threats rather than harmful behaviours, and their goal is to avoid a direct physical confrontation that may result in fatal injuries. Fighting is rarely the first choice for a healthy animal because it is dangerous and highly energy-consuming. Functionally, predation is not an aggressive behaviour since its goal is destroying and eating an individual and not defending resources or responding to threats (Miklosi, 2015; Bradshaw and Rooney, 2016).

This definition of aggression applies very well to non-captive wolves that use species-specific affiliative and aggressive behaviours to increase or decrease their distance, leave or join a group. Through these behavioural repertoires, wolves can keep stability in their social unit, a family of genetically related individuals, minimizing fights and injuries (Mech and Boitani, 2003; Miklosi, 2015). A stable hierarchy in wolves is maintained through affiliative behaviours, ritualized aggressive displays (threats) and deferential behaviours. Actual fights are infrequent. When severe conflicts arise between two individuals, such as a mature breeder and its male yearling offspring, the young usually disperses to form its own family (Mech and Boitani, 2003).

Although the wolf is the ancestor of the domestic dog and the two species are closely related from a genetic standpoint, it is essential to keep in mind that the domestic dog has experienced an extensive artificial selection that has profoundly altered its physical and behavioural phenotype. It suffices to compare the picture of a pug dog to the image of a grey wolf to understand how profound the effect of the artificial selection on the domestic dog is. Multiple cognitive studies confirm that the same effect is visible in the behaviour of the domestic dog (Miklosi, 2015). The social behaviour of grey wolves, including their affiliative and aggressive behaviour, has been modified via artificial selection to create an animal, the domestic dog, whose social behaviour is oriented primarily towards humans. The domestic dog is a species that is highly dependent on humans and therefore is continually trying to adapt its affiliative and aggressive behaviour to the environment that it shares with them. Contrary to the natural environment of wild species, the environment in which humans and dogs live is highly variable. The domestic dog can live in a small apartment in Toronto or London as well as on a farm in Maine or Wales. This adaptability to extremely different environments is behind the success of the dog as a domestic species, and it is related to great plasticity of the dog's social behaviour (Bonanni and Cafazzo, 2014; Boitani *et al.*, 2016; Macdonald and Carr, 2016).

Dogs can form wolf-like societies with conspecifics under appropriate conditions, with a defined social structure and hierarchy, or can congregate in dynamic groups around resources and proximity to humans, without forming a clear social structure and hierarchy. For this reason, affiliative and aggressive interactions among dogs, and between dogs and humans, should be interpreted within the specific context in which they happen. Using a rigid paradigm about hierarchy extrapolated from the wolf social behaviour (the pack model or dominance theory) to interpret the dog social behaviour is flawed and may lead to dangerous outcomes in a clinical and training setting. Although the dominance theory is frequently used to explain the aggressive behaviour of domestic dogs by the popular media, the scientific community rejected this theory more than a decade ago (Mech, 2008; Welfare in Dog Training, 2019). Since then, scientists have shifted their focus to studying and interpreting dog cognition and communication. This knowledge is now applied to understanding how dogs interact with different individuals in the diversified contexts that they can encounter in their lives. These tools have allowed us to understand that dogs communicate differently with humans and animals, often relying more on information coming from humans than from other dogs.

Domestication has created a new canine species that is highly dependent on humans and that struggles to understand how to navigate safely a world created by humans for humans, where the social rules are continuously changing across places and societies. Cognitive studies show that dogs are constantly trying to read the body language of humans and are more likely to follow their directions when humans show a friendly attitude (Miklosi, 2015). Dogs are captive animals and do not have the freedom to leave or join a group as wolves do; they are forced by humans to live in an environment and with individuals that they may not find safe. Aggressive interactions result from a dog feeling threatened in an environment that it does not control and in which it often feels unsafe.

12.4 The Relevance of Individual Interactions in Social Behaviour

Due to the behavioural plasticity favoured by domestication, dogs can successfully adapt to different environmental conditions. This high adaptability makes it impossible to define a social structure that fits all interactions involving dogs. In this ever-changing environment, we have to observe the individual dog and its interactions in a specific context to understand its social behaviour and emotions. Observing the communication signals that a dog sends to another dog or a human is the most effective way to understand a specific social interaction, in the absence of a stable social paradigm to use. Genes, past experiences and epigenetics (e.g. experiential and environmental effects on gene translation) influence the dog's behaviour. These factors will determine the animality of an individual dog and its propensity to respond aggressively (fight response) to a perceived stressor. The role of genetics and epigenetics in dog aggression has not been accurately quantified. Although an aggressive and impulsive temperament (i.e. characterized by a lack of inhibitory control (see Section 7.4.1 – Impulsivity)) has been associated with genes encoding serotonergic and dopaminergic receptors, the effect of early experience on the same genes makes it difficult to quantify the heritability of these traits (Van Der Berg, 2016). The relative contribution of genes on dog behaviour is substantial enough to allow the selection of different phenotypes (Lewis, 2016), and different behaviour profiles have been identified for several breeds (Duffy *et al.*, 2008). However, the effect of experience, in particular perinatal, is thought to outweigh the effect of genes in the development of a dog's behaviour (Wilsson, 2016).

The best tool to decode the emotions of a dog is observing and understanding its communication, including body language and vocalizations. Recognizing early signs of increasing arousal (e.g. yawning, lip licking, mydriasis, piloerection, stiffness and averted gaze) is essential to prevent the escalation of an antagonistic interaction into overt aggression (e.g. barking, growling, snarling, lunging, snapping and biting). How quickly a dog will escalate from early or subtle signs of mounting arousal to overt aggression can significantly vary among individuals. Impulsive dogs will show subtle signs of early stress that will last for a short time (De Keuster and Jung, 2010). Dogs may also shift from one coping strategy to another as the context of the interaction evolves; for example, a dog may show subtle signs when a stranger approaches, run away when the person gets closer, and then become aggressive if the person tries touching it. Although the animality of a dog determines its common coping response, this context-related variability of coping strategies must be accounted for when evaluating the risks related to dog aggression. From here derives, in fact, one of the most important assumptions regarding dog aggression: ALL dogs can bite if the appropriate situation presents.

The display of affective aggression can vary from an overtly fearful, defensive body language (e.g. ears back, low body posture, tail down and averted gaze) to a more proactive offensive body language (e.g. staring, lunging at, running after and high body posture). Many dogs will show an ambivalent body language (conflict-related behaviour) with both defensive and offensive signs (e.g. rolling over and growling with teeth showing), which has been associated with a high level of arousal experienced by these individuals (Horváth *et al.*, 2007). These differences are determined by the different animality of dogs (genetics, epigenetics and early experience); the specific context in which the interaction happens, including the presence of barriers that may interfere with a dog's ability to communicate appropriately, and the value of a resource; and the learning that has occurred in previous similar experiences. Even when the body language displayed is offensive, the origin of this aggressive behaviour is still rooted in the perception of a threat or challenge perceived by the animal that activates the response.

12.5 When Dog Aggression Becomes a Behaviour Problem

All dogs use antagonistic interactions (e.g. staring at or pushing away another individual) to protect valuable resources and individual safety. Overtly aggressive behaviour can be a part of these normal interactions. These conflicts often resolve with a short and safe interaction and do not escalate to a bite. For example, if a dog growls at another over a resource, and the receiver ceases his threatening behaviour, this interaction will be brief and uneventful.

However, aggression can lead to a dangerous interaction and become a problem when a dog sends appropriate antagonistic signals, but the receiver does not respond appropriately. This can happen accidentally in specific contexts in which none of the two individuals interacting is displaying abnormal behaviour. For example, a dog may bite a child that inflicts pain to the animal and does not stop when the dog growls in response. Another example is a dog barking at another dog that is entering its safe personal space, but the receiver cannot walk away because it is walked on a lead by the owner. In these cases, dogs that are barking and growling at first do not show abnormal behaviour, but the inappropriate response to their signals (i.e. the receiver continues the unsafe interaction) amplifies their perception of threat and triggers a quick escalation of their aggression. This aggression can usually be addressed with changes in the environment and behaviour modification, such as making sure that two unfamiliar dogs that are allowed to interact for the first time are not forcibly restrained or held on a tight lead.

Selective breeding and human intervention (surgeries and grooming) have led to the development of different appearances in dogs. Certain breeds are incapable of using a full repertoire of behavioural signals. For example, French bulldogs cannot use their tail effectively, while the eyes of English sheepdogs may be covered by hair.

In other cases, either the dog that is showing aggressive behaviour or the receiver (or both) have inappropriate social skills. This happens when a dog responds to a mild antagonistic sign, such as an incidental short stare, with very intensive aggression, or when a dog bites another dog that is showing affiliative behaviour like a play bow. Such behaviour is usually the result of an underlying dysregulation in the emotional response of the animal with excessive arousal that causes excessively aggressive responses to benign interactions or threats of mild-to-moderate intensity. Abnormalities or lesions in the brain areas that control aggressive behaviour, lower concentrations of central 5HT, or higher of noradrenaline or dopamine have been associated with increased aggression (Reisner *et al.*, 1996; Amat *et al.*, 2013; Bear *et al.*, 2016; Gerken *et al.*, 2016; Carlson and Birkett, 2017). This dysregulation usually requires professional help from a veterinary psychiatrist who should determine the source of the abnormal behaviour (primary problem behaviour versus medical problem) and determine appropriate treatment, including psychotropic medication if indicated.

Based on these premises, we propose to define dog pathological aggression as:

> A display of aggressive behaviour characterized by a disproportionately intense response to a benign interaction or to a mild-to-moderate trigger, or by the inability of the dog to quickly return to a basal level of arousal once the threatening stimulus is removed, and by its failure to respond appropriately to environmental cues (including training via operant conditioning) secondary to the excessive arousal.

Because all affective aggression is invariably caused by an activation of the stress response, whether adaptive or pathological (Bear *et al.*, 2016), all proposed classifications of dog aggression are subjective and not based on a well differentiated underlying neurophysiology/pathology. The goal of this chapter is to provide the reader with a general knowledge of the mechanisms, signs and treatment of affective aggression applicable to multiple contexts, rather than proposing a fictitious classification. We will only differentiate two contexts based on the target of dog aggression: affective aggression directed to people, and affective aggression directed to other dogs. We will briefly review predatory behaviour and inappropriate play that, even if they are not forms of affective aggression, can cause significant injuries and carry liability.

12.6 General Guidelines for the Management of Aggression

The first step in managing aggression problems in dogs is to rule out or manage medical abnormalities. A full physical examination and any necessary imaging and laboratory tests should take place before establishing a diagnosis and treatment. Sensory decline, metabolic and inflammatory diseases, and painful conditions are among the most common causes of aggression in dogs. For more information see Chapters 2 and 3.

The treatment of affective aggression includes three components, regardless of the specific target and context:

- establishing a safe environment through strict preventive measures;
- modifying the environment to minimize as much as possible the perception of threats and challenges that would activate the stress response; and
- using behaviour modification to enhance the communication between the dog and its owner, so that the latter will be able to direct the dog's behaviour predictably in situations at risk for aggression.

These interventions will ultimately result in increased control over the environment by the dog and, therefore, in reduced activation of the stress response (Notari, 2009). Dogs that perceive the situation as stable and predictable feel safer in it and are less likely to show aggression (Lindell, 2018a, b, c, d).

12.6.1 Safety

Establishing a safe environment must always be the first step in the treatment of affective aggression. Other components of the treatment take time to implement and yield noticeable results, while safety can be enacted immediately by establishing and following clear and specific safety rules. Once the owner can operate in safety, environmental and behaviour modification can be implemented. For example, if a dog is presented for a history of biting unfamiliar children, our first step must be recommending the owner avoids any interaction between the dog and unfamiliar children. Within this safe context, we can then work on setting the right environment and implementing the training for a successful introduction to children. Creating a safe environment will drastically minimize the exposure of the dog to the stimuli that are perceived to be a threat or challenge and will consequently promote desensitization to these stimuli. The environmental and behaviour modification will then provide the owner and the dog with the tools to implement a controlled exposure to the threatening stimuli. This will, in turn, increase the dog's perception of safety and will promote a less aroused and aggressive behaviour. At this point, the safety rules can be adjusted according to the modified environment and the trained behaviour and, if appropriate, less strict rules can be put in place.

12.6.2 Environmental modification

Changes in the environment should be implemented with two main goals in mind: first, facilitating the enforcement of the safety rules established; and second, increasing the control that the dog has on its environment to reduce its distress and arousal.

When enforcing safety, the use of physical barriers is often necessary to prevent interactions that may potentially lead to aggression. For example, the use of a physical barrier (e.g. a gate, crate or closed door) to separate a dog from home visitors must be considered for dogs showing affective aggression towards unfamiliar people.

All dogs must be provided with safe spaces at home and outside. Dogs must always be given the possibility of retreating to safety where they can stay undisturbed when they feel unsafe or overstimulated. This will allow them the potential to respond to the increased arousal and distress by enacting an escape-type response rather than an aggression-type response. Aside from necessary and structured interactions (e.g. a veterinary visit), no dog should be forced to have interactions that are not safe and enjoyable (to the animal itself) since this may escalate to aggression. This is particularly important for dogs with a history of aggression and for interactions between dogs and small children.

Choosing the right tools to handle and contain a dog is extremely important. Simple collars, head collars, and harnesses must always be preferred to prong collars and choke chains (Herron *et al.*,

2009; Grohmann *et al.*, 2013). Leads should be robust and of fixed length. Retractable leads should be avoided for aggressive dogs since they don't give adequate control during walks. Training the dog to wear a basket muzzle can be very helpful in specific situations but should not be considered a safe choice as they will indiscriminately expose dogs to situations that are known to trigger their aggression (Corridan, 2009; Hunthausen, 2009).

12.6.3 Behaviour modification

The primary goal of behaviour modification is improving the communication between dogs and people (usually their owners) and other dogs (see Chapter 8). Because dogs are highly dependent on their owners to gain control over their environment (Miklosi, 2015), the use of behaviour modification will help them to feel safer in their environment and decrease the likelihood of resorting to aggression secondary to activation of the stress response.

To accomplish this goal, behaviour modification should be focused first on establishing consistent and predictable channels of communication between the dog and the owner and, second, on providing the dog with directions to increase its control over the environment. When excessive arousal does not allow the dog to 'think' of a safe coping strategy, it is the owner's responsibility to 'explain' to the dog how to safely handle a potentially challenging situation. For example, during walks on a lead, a dog might become increasingly distressed by the presence of another dog. The owner must redirect the dog's behaviour towards the desired behaviour (e.g. 'watch' or 'touch' the owner's hand) using operant conditioning while moving the dog away from the second dog.

When using behaviour modification with an aggressive or overly aroused dog, it is essential to keep in mind that the level of distress that the dog is experiencing will influence its ability to respond to cues. In general, highly aroused and distressed dogs encounter difficulties in reacting appropriately to operant conditioning since their ability to perform voluntarily may be impaired (Mills, 2009; Notari, 2009). The use of classical conditioning may be granted in cases when the dog is not responding due to its excessive arousal or distress. In these cases, exposing the dog to a 'positive opposite' (e.g. a high-value treat), without asking it to perform an operant behaviour, may help to change the dog's emotional state to a more positive one and to improve the association with the distressing context. If the dog is too aroused to perform on operant conditioning, the owner should not be worried about using a high-value positive stimulus since the latter will not act as a reinforcer of the fearful and aggressive behaviour of the dog, which is, at that point, not operant (voluntary). For more information on learning principles and behaviour modification, see Chapter 8.

12.6.4 Using psychoactive medication to treat dog affective aggression

Many cases of dog affective aggression can be treated and managed using the three-component approach described above. Some cases, however, may benefit from the use of psychoactive medication. When the aggression is recurrent, characterized by a high degree of emotional arousal and impulsivity, and does not respond well to environmental and behaviour modification, the use of medication may help. The goal of medication treatment is to reduce excessive arousal and impulsivity and, therefore to facilitate the behaviour modification (see Chapter 9).

No psychoactive medication is licensed for use in dog aggression. These medications are used off-label to address the underlying affective disorder and arousal level. Because of the role played by serotonin in regulating anxiety and aggression (Reisner *et al.*, 1996; Amat *et al.*, 2013; Bear *et al.*, 2016; Carlson and Birkett, 2017), serotonergic medications, in particular SSRIs and TCAs (see Section 9.8 – Serotonergic Medications) are used in the treatment of dog aggression (Crowell-Davis and Landsberg, 2009; Landsberg *et al.*, 2013; Overall, 2013). There is no specific dosage or frequency of administration used for aggression problems, and the general indications about the use of these medications should be followed. It is essential to make the client aware that the use of medication does not eliminate aggression and the risk that a bite may occur.

For this reason, psychoactive medications must be considered a complement to the treatment for aggression. Strict safety strategies, environmental and behaviour modification will still represent the core components of the treatment for dog aggression. SSRIs and TCAs, as well as many other psychoactive medications, can cause a paradoxical increase in arousal and aggression. The treatment should be immediately discontinued if aggression worsens and a different medication should be chosen.

12.7 Dog Aggression Directed to People

Aggression towards people is a common problem; approximately 68% of dogs are referred for aggression problems in urban areas (Siracusa *et al.*, 2017). Between 2001 and 2003, an estimated 4.5 million people in the USA (1.5% of the population) were bitten each year. Of these, 19% required medical attention. Children were more likely than adults to receive medical attention for a dog bite. Among adults, bite rates decreased with increasing age (Gilchrist *et al.*, 2008). These statistics do not include people that have been a victim of dog aggression not resulting in a bite injury. Also, there are unreported dog bites. Therefore, the real magnitude of dog aggression directed to people is likely to be much higher.

In a study conducted in the UK (Westgarth *et al.*, 2018), 25% of 694 people surveyed reported having been bitten by a dog during their lifetime, with only a third of bites described requiring further medical treatment and 0.6% hospital admission. The yearly incidence of dog bites was 1.9%. Males were twice as likely to have been bitten in their lifetime than females. Regarding all bites described, most commonly, people were bitten by a dog that they had never met before the incident (54.7%).

These numbers clearly show that dog aggression is a public health problem and not just a dog behaviour problem. Bite prevention relies on public education about dog behaviour and early detection of situations at risk, and veterinarians have a pivotal role in both processes.

Although dog bites can happen in any context in which dogs and people are present together, there are situations in which bites tend to occur with a frequency higher than average. In many cases, the triggers for bites are interactions that the dog perceives as threatening. Interactions that are safe among humans may not be perceived as safe by dogs. Interactions between dogs and children are a typical example. Owners consider their interactions with children to be safe and, therefore, think the dog sees the situation as safe. However, dogs might find interactions with children threatening and are more likely to inflict a severe bite on children than on adults. Most dogs (66%) that bite a child have never done so in the past, and 19% of them have never bitten a human before (Reisner *et al.*, 2007). Food guarding is the most frequent cause of bites (43%) directed to children in the household, while entering the dog's territory (i.e. the house, garden and area surrounding the house) represents the most common trigger (53%) for bites directed to unfamiliar children (Reisner *et al.*, 2007).

In a study conducted in the UK (Oxley *et al.*, 2018), most bites (35%) happened when people interacted or tried to interact with dogs. In another study (Rezac *et al.*, 2015), bending over the dog preceded 76% of bites to the face, and gazing between victim and dog preceded 19% of bites to the face. Dogs can find both behaviours extremely threatening.

12.7.1 Aggression directed to unfamiliar people

In this chapter, we define unfamiliar people as individuals that do not live in the same household as the dog. These people do not belong to the stable social group of the dog. The group of unfamiliar people is not homogeneous and may include people that are strangers to a dog and people with which a dog has regular interactions. This difference in the frequency of contact can influence the affiliative and antagonistic interactions that a dog shows towards specific unfamiliar individuals. However, the lack of a stable, frequent and consistent contact happening within the dog's territory (with its resources) characterizes all these interactions to different degrees. The lack of a bond within a stable social group increases the probability that a dog may perceive the interaction with an unfamiliar person as potentially threatening and unsafe. Whether a dog fears for its personal safety (fear-related aggression), for its resources (resource guarding) or for the invasion of the space that it actively patrols and defends (territorial aggression), the perception of a potential threat and the activation of the stress response are behind the display of affective aggression to strangers.

The perception of a specific stimulus as a threat can vary significantly among individual dogs. Some dogs interact with strangers with minimal or no distress; others will tolerate interaction without direct physical contact. Some dogs will react aggressively to a stranger just entering their safe inter-individual space. The perception of a potential threat is determined by the genetics and epigenetics of the dog, its experience and the environment.

In dogs with known aggression problems, 63% showed aggression towards unfamiliar people in a non-aversive situation, 45% when interacting outdoors, 35% during veterinary examination or grooming, and 44% showed aggression towards unfamiliar children (Siracusa *et al.*, 2017).

In clinics, aggression towards unfamiliar people is often categorized based on its motivation and context:

- fear-related aggression: barking and/or growling and/or baring teeth and/or lunging and/or snapping and/or biting or attempting to bite in response to a perceived threat from an unfamiliar person;
- resource guarding: barking and/or growling and/or baring teeth and/or lunging and/or snapping and/or biting or attempting to bite an unfamiliar person in the presence of a high-value item, typically food, toys, or resting places;
- territorial aggression: barking and/or growling and/or baring teeth and/or lunging and/or snapping and/or biting or attempting to bite in response to an unfamiliar person entering the space that a dog actively defends; and
- affective aggression can be exacerbated by frustration when an animal is prevented by a physical barrier (e.g. lead, crate or fence) to interact freely with an individual. This behaviour is sometimes referred to as 'barrier frustration' and 'lead-related aggression'.

As for all the other diagnoses mentioned in this section and the following section, these diagnoses help the clinician to convey more information about the motivation and context in which a dog displays aggression. However, they do not correspond to different underlying neurophysiological/pathological mechanisms. These diagnostic categories are all, in fact, displays of affective aggression with activation and, sometimes, dysregulation of the emotional response and corresponding arousal.

12.7.1.1 Specific treatment recommendations

Risk management is the first step; all unnecessary interactions should be avoided even when the risk that a bite occurs is low. The dog must always be under the owner's direct control and supervision when around unfamiliar people. A dog that is fearful of unfamiliar people does not need to be exposed to people indiscriminately for socialization.

In public areas, the dog must always be on a fixed-length lead. The use of coercive methods (e.g. prong collars, choke chains, electronic collars) must be avoided to prevent further increase of distress, emotional arousal and fear that may result in an increased risk of bites to people and physical injuries to the dog (e.g. damage to the trachea or brain) (Herron *et al.*, 2009; Grohmann *et al.*, 2013). Martingale collars, front-clipped harnesses and head halters are safe and effective tools. Head halters require prior desensitization and should be used with caution in dogs that become very aroused and jump in the air because of increased risk of a neck injury. A basket muzzle may be used to prevent aggression but the dog should never be left unsupervised, and unfamiliar people should not be allowed to reach for it. Response substitution (e.g. teaching the dog to 'look' on cue) can be used to redirect the dog's attention on the owner during walks (Mills, 2009).

Dogs with a history of aggression towards unfamiliar people should never be left unsupervised in a garden without a solid fence tall enough to prevent the dog from jumping out. Electric fences are not able to reliably prevent a dog from escaping the garden (Starinsky *et al.*, 2017).

If a dog shows aggression to unfamiliar people visiting at home, safety measures should be adopted to prevent injuries. Often dogs get very aroused whenever there is a change in the environment caused by an unfamiliar person entering or exiting a room, standing up from a sitting position, or moving from one place to another. In these circumstances, the owner should supervise the dog and may need to keep the dog on a lead or confined behind a physical barrier. Interactions between the visitor and the dog should be kept at the minimum level tolerated by the dog (as shown by its body language), and contact between the two of them should never be forced. Caution should be exercised around children that are less likely to follow safety rules. Dogs should never be left unsupervised with children, and dogs with a history of aggression to unfamiliar children should be restrained or confined in their presence.

Following risk management, behaviour modification can be used to introduce the dog to unfamiliar people in a gradual manner under controlled settings. A desensitization programme provides the owners with an effective tool to teach the dog how to react appropriately to the presence of an unfamiliar person. Dogs should be under their owner's control using leads, harness and head halter or a muzzle. Once the threshold (the distance at which the dog starts reacting towards the unfamiliar person) is identified, owners can begin working with the dog under the threshold. Only when the dog is calm (shows no signs of emotional distress), focuses on the owner and responds to signals, can the owner gradually decrease the distance from the other person while associating their presence with a positive outcome (See Chapter 8).

The result of the introduction protocol can be highly variable and often will not culminate in safe physical contact between the dog and the person involved. Some dogs will learn to be comfortable around a specific unfamiliar individual, while others will tolerate this person only at a distance and with minimal interactions (Lindell, 2018a).

Unfamiliar people should not approach dogs in possession of high-value resources (e.g. toys, bones or food-filled toys). Similarly, dogs resting or sleeping, especially in their preferred places, should not be disturbed by unfamiliar people.

Pain is a frequent cause of aggression directed to veterinarians and groomers. Once the cause of pain is removed, it may be necessary to desensitize the animal who now associates being handled by the veterinarian or groomer with the feeling of pain.

A few dogs with high emotional dysregulation, which experience excessive fear and show severe aggression around unfamiliar people, may not tolerate any degree of exposure to and interaction with unfamiliar people. Medication treatment is indicated when the aggression is associated with excessive emotional dysregulation.

12.7.2 Aggression directed to familiar people

In this chapter, we define familiar people as individuals that consistently live in the same household with the dog. These people belong to the stable social group of the dog, on which the dog is dependent. This dependence is at the base of the affiliative relationship between human and dog and defined as 'attachment' (Miklosi, 2015). Developing a social bond and an affiliative relationship does not entirely protect from the occurrence of antagonistic interactions (conflict-related behaviour) when at least one of the two individuals perceives the interaction as potentially threatening or challenging. Antagonistic interactions have been observed in families of wolves (Packard, 2003) and feral dogs (Bonanni and Cafazzo, 2014) and are considered normal in cohesive and stable groups. These conflicts do not usually escalate to severe aggression with injuries and are characterized by an association of aggressive (e.g. snarling), deferential (e.g. lowering the body) and appeasing behaviours (e.g. pawing). Therefore, the existence of conflict and aggression in a cohesive social group does not have to be considered abnormal, and it should not be assumed that it is an attempt to initiate an escalating fight to gain unchallenged leadership. Conflicts may be observed to gain or retain access to a specific valuable resource and may remain limited to this specific context.

Similarly, expected aggressive behaviours like snarling or growling directed to familiar people could also be observed in dogs that have developed a strong and stable social bond with their human companions. For example, a dog may snarl when the owner attempts to remove a high-value item from its mouth while showing at the same time deferential behaviours like lowering the body and pointing the ears back. These restricted episodes are unlikely to escalate into more generalized aggression (depending on the owner's reaction) and are not an attempt by the dog to conquer a higher hierarchy level. A dog in this situation is just asking to be left undisturbed with its resource (which, paradoxically, was probably provided by the same human companion that is now challenging it). Therefore, the most sensible response to this aggressive behaviour is to allow the dog to retain access to its resource without engaging in an escalating conflict that may result in injury.

Although some parallels exist between the communication used within a group of wolves or dogs and the body language that dogs use with humans, it should always be remembered that the bond between dogs and humans is different in nature from the intra-species bond, and the domestication process has shaped it. This is also confirmed by the fact that many dogs show remarkably different behaviour when interacting with other dogs and when interacting with humans. Moreover, domesticated dogs living in a household are captive and kept in a, more or less, strict, confined state. This can significantly influence their ability to show appropriate social interactions. For example, a dog that is approached while in possession of a high-value resource may snarl and walk away to a different room or the garden, if accessible, but may proceed to growl if confined to a crate or tethered because it is deprived of the possibility to remove itself from the context. If conflicts repeatedly happen in the household, the behaviour response of the dog can also escalate as a result of sensitization (i.e. continuous exposure leading to more immediate and intense reaction) or classical conditioning (i.e. associating the person approaching with a negative outcome). In this way, an expected mild-to-moderate aggressive interaction that can be considered part of a dog's normal behaviour repertoire can escalate into a severe and dangerous interaction, even in dogs that do not have a pathological dysregulation of their emotional response.

In dogs presented for aggression problems, 46% showed aggression towards familiar people over resources, 34% when disturbed while resting or sleeping, 34% during non-aversive situations, 27% when groomed or medicated, 27% during painful or aversive interactions, and 15% during aversive, but not painful, interactions. Of these dogs, 19% showed aggression towards children (Siracusa *et al.*, 2017).

Some dogs which show aggression towards unfamiliar people may suffer from emotional dysregulation and high arousal level. These dogs are likely to show a pathological form of affective aggression. These cases are extremely dangerous due to the inability to avoid some of the contexts that would trigger aggression in the home.

In clinics, aggression towards familiar people is often categorized based on its motivation or context:

- conflict-related aggression: barking at and/or growling at and/or baring teeth at and/or lunging at and/or snapping and/or biting or attempting to bite people living in the same household;
- resource guarding: barking and/or growling and/or baring teeth and/or lunging and/or snapping and/or biting or attempting to bite a familiar person in the presence of a high-value item, typically food, toys or resting places – this diagnosis can be used when this specific aggressive interaction is the only sign observed and is not included in a broader diagnosis of conflict-related aggression; and
- affective aggression can also be exacerbated by frustration when the dog is prevented from obtaining a specific goal or object. In some cases the dog may redirect its behaviour towards a familiar person, a behaviour sometimes called 'redirected aggression'.

12.7.2.1 Specific treatment recommendations

All the situations that the dog perceives as an actual or potential threat in the interactions with familiar people should be identified and avoided when possible. For example, if aggression is associated with the dog being disturbed while resting or sleeping, the animal should be given a safe spot in which it can rest and sleep undisturbed. If someone needs to interact with the dog, he/she should call the dog away from the resting spot. Similarly, a dog that shows aggression over resources can be left undisturbed or even confined when in their possession (if this is not dangerous to the dog's health).

Unfortunately, not all situations can be easily avoided and aggression may become very difficult to prevent and control. Dogs that show severe aggression when handled or medicated by familiar people are at increased risk of being rehomed and euthanized even after having received treatment from a veterinary psychiatrist (Siracusa *et al.*, 2017).

Once a safe environment has been established through avoidance of triggers, behaviour modification can help to manage some conflicts safely and successfully. First, the intensity of a stimulus that would trigger aggression should be determined. Once this threshold is identified, a similar stimulus, but at a below-threshold intensity, should be repeatedly presented together with a high-value treat. The intensity can then be progressively increased as long as the dog is calm and does not show signs of increased arousal or emotional distress. For example, if wiping the paws of a dog triggers growling and attempting to bite, the owner should at first not wipe the paws. The owner then starts presenting the towel used to wipe paired with high-value treats and progressively decreasing the distance from the paws. If the dog is comfortable with this process, the owner may then attempt to touch the paws gently while offering treats. Following the same rules, the intensity of the interaction can be progressively increased but keeping it always below the threshold that would cause aggression (Lindell, 2018b).

Due to the difference in social communication and interaction between the two species, some human body language can be perceived as threatening by dogs. For example, staring at and bending over, as well as hugging or kissing, are not normal behaviours in the dog social repertoire (Rezac *et al.*, 2015; Oxley *et al.*, 2018). Therefore, these postures and interactions may be perceived as threatening by fearful dogs and may trigger a defensive response displayed as aggression. Owners should attempt to establish effective communication with their dogs. A simple way is pairing a discriminative signal with each interaction. The signal might be a word or hand signal. For example, before brushing the dog, the owner might say 'brushing time', and then proceed to brush the dog gently while offering treats. With multiple repetitions, the dog learns the pattern of the interaction and expects a positive outcome.

Young children are at risk of being bitten even during positive interactions (Reisner *et al.*, 2011). Children should never be left unsupervised with dogs and should be separated from them using a physical barrier if the dog has a history of aggression towards familiar people. The presence of adolescent children has been identified as a risk factor for rehoming and euthanasia (Siracusa *et al.*, 2017).

Highly fearful and anxious dogs, whose arousal level is very high, may have severe limitations in forming an appropriate bond with one or more individuals living in their household and may not be able to accept any close interaction with these people. In these cases, the use of psychoactive medications is indicated to facilitate behaviour modification.

12.8 Aggression between Dogs

Aggression between dogs is very commonly observed in veterinary practices (Fatjo *et al.*, 2006). The incidence of cases appears to be related to the density of dogs in the area, ranging from 11% in rural areas (Denenberg, unpublished data), 16% in suburban areas (Bamberger and Houpt, 2006) to 51% in urban areas (Siracusa *et al.*, 2017).

12.8.1 Aggression directed to unfamiliar dogs

Unfamiliar dogs are defined here as dogs that do not live in the same household. Although some dogs that do not live in the same house develop a social bond if they meet frequently, their bond should be considered different in quality and intensity from the bond that household dogs develop. Unfamiliar dogs that meet outside the house rarely compete for the same valuable resources and, due to their short interactions, do not undergo the same learning processes that dogs living together in a confined space experience. For this reason, the behaviour that a dog shows towards familiar and unfamiliar dogs can be very different. A dog may experience fear leading to aggression around unfamiliar dogs and may trust familiar dogs without showing any aggression. Conversely, a dog may enjoy short interactions in an open space with unfamiliar dogs but may develop aggression towards household dogs with which it consistently competes for resources and spaces.

In clinics, aggression to unfamiliar dogs is often categorized based on its motivation and context:

- fear-related aggression: barking and/or growling and/or baring teeth and/or lunging and/or snapping and/or biting or attempting to bite in response to a perceived threat from an unfamiliar dog;
- resource guarding: barking and/or growling and/or baring teeth and/or lunging and/or snapping and/or biting or attempting to bite an unfamiliar dog in the presence of a high-value item, typically food, toys or resting places;
- territorial aggression: barking and/or growling and/or baring teeth and/or lunging and/or snapping and/or biting or attempting to bite in response to an unfamiliar dog approaching or entering the space that a dog actively defends; and
- frustration: aggression can be exacerbated when an animal is prevented, using a physical barrier, from interacting freely with an individual. The physical barrier can be a gate or lead (sometimes referred to as 'barrier frustration' and 'lead-related aggression'). Repeated frustration experienced while meeting unfamiliar dogs on a lead may also cause sensitization and result in aggression progressively exacerbating over time.

12.8.1.1 Specific treatment recommendations

Avoidance is the most effective strategy to prevent aggression directed to unfamiliar dogs and decrease the related liability. Always when possible, unnecessary interactions involving a dog with a history of aggression to unfamiliar dogs should be avoided, even when the risk that a bite occurs is low. Owners should avoid uncontrolled exposure for unfamiliar dogs to socialize an aggressive dog. Indiscriminate exposure to dogs will likely result in further sensitization and increased emotional arousal and aggression.

A basket muzzle may be used to prevent aggression, but the dog should never be left unsupervised, and unfamiliar dogs should not be allowed to approach. Response substitution (e.g. teaching the dog to 'look' on cue) can be used to redirect the dog's attention on the owner during walks. Electric fences are not a suitable substitute for solid fences and cannot reliably prevent a dog from leaving the garden and attacking an unfamiliar dog.

In public, the dog must always be on a fixed-length lead connected to a safe collar, harness or head halter. The use of coercive tools (e.g. prong collars, choke chains, electronic collars) must be avoided to prevent further increase of distress, emotional arousal and fear that may result in an increased risk of bites to people and physical injuries to the dog (e.g. damage to the trachea or brain) (Herron *et al.*, 2009; Grohmann *et al.*, 2013).

Behaviour modification can be used to introduce unfamiliar dogs with a history of aggression. Calm dogs with appropriate social skills are an ideal match for reactive dogs, while introducing two highly reactive dogs may be an operation destined to fail. At the beginning of the training protocol, each of the two dogs should be trained with a cue to redirect their attention towards the owner (e.g. 'watch me') via operant conditioning. This skill can be used to walk the dogs at a long distance while asking them to stay focused on the owner. Rewarding the dogs for complying with this request will also create a positive association with the presence of the other dog. The owner then gradually decreases the distance between the two dogs if the dogs appear calm. Finally, the two dogs can be allowed to interact on a loose lead in a large fenced area, possibly wearing a muzzle. Depending on the dog's animality, an introduction protocol may culminate in full safe interaction with physical contact between the two dogs, or may have limited results with the dogs only being able to walk safely at a distance. Close interaction or physical contact between dogs that are uncomfortable with each other (as shown by their body language) should never be forced.

Dogs experiencing excessive arousal in response to meeting unfamiliar dogs, sometimes even from a long distance, can be difficult to control during walks. In this case, the use of psychoactive medications is indicated to decrease the arousal and facilitate learning and training to improve the safety and quality of walks outdoors.

12.8.2 Aggression between household dogs

Dogs living in the same household can form a strong social bond but will also experience social conflicts. As discussed above, conflict is also expected in very cohesive groups, and it is usually mitigated and resolved by affiliative and appeasing behaviour. Aggression towards a familiar dog over resources appears to be one of the most common presentations in referral centres, reaching approximately 65% of the cases (Siracusa *et al.*, 2017). Unfortunately, not all aggressive interaction within a group of dogs can be resolved, and some of these escalate into severe and dangerous fights (Siracusa, 2016). Inappropriate social and communication skills, temperamental reactivity and excitability, poor environmental control because of human interference, space distribution and availability, and confinement should be considered in cases of aggression between household dogs (De Keuster and Jung, 2010; Landsberg *et al.*, 2013).

Aggression between household dogs is more frequent among same-sex than among mixed-sex, with female–female aggression carrying the worst prognosis (Sherman *et al.*, 1996; Bamberger and Houpt, 2006; Wrubel *et al.*, 2011; Overall, 2013). The aggressor will initiate an aggressive interaction by sending a threatening signal (e.g. staring, growling, snarling or biting). The aggressor tends to be younger than the victim and to have arrived in the home more recently in more than 50% of reported cases (Sherman *et al.*, 1996; Wrubel *et al.*, 2011). Among the most frequently reported triggers for aggression between household dogs are resource guarding, excitement, interacting with the owner, and approaching the dog over a resting spot (Sherman *et al.*, 1996; Wrubel *et al.*, 2011).

In clinics, aggression towards familiar dogs is often categorized based on its motivation and context:

- Intra-species affective aggression: barking at and/or growling at and/or baring teeth at and/or lunging at and/or snapping and/or biting or attempting to bite dogs living in the same household. Because of the complex nature of aggression between household dogs and its multiple causes, this diagnosis based on the underlying neurophysiology of the aggressive response observed is preferred to other diagnoses like 'status-related aggression' and 'fear-related aggression' (Siracusa, 2016).
- Resource guarding: barking and/or growling and/or baring teeth and/or lunging and/or

snapping and/or biting or attempting to bite a familiar dog in the presence of a high-value item, typically food, toys or resting places. This diagnosis can be used when this specific aggressive interaction is the only sign observed and is not included in a broader diagnosis of intra-species affective aggression. A possible motivation to show this type of aggression may be the desire to keep the other dog away, not due to fear of losing a resource, but due to frustration (see Section 7.4.2.2 – Frustration).

12.8.2.1 Specific treatment recommendations

In cases of mild-to-moderate aggression (e.g. snarling or growling) between two household dogs limited to one or a few specific contexts, such as protection of resources, avoidance of these contexts, supervision and environmental changes by the owners may be effective in preventing escalating aggression and injuries.

If there is a severe history of aggression between household dogs, separation using physical barriers is often a necessary first step. In some cases, it may suffice to separate the dogs only when the owner cannot directly supervise them. In the case of repeated severe aggression that has led to sensitization and high anticipatory anxiety when the dogs are together, complete separation at all times is indicated. This will be the first step of a process of desensitization of the dogs to the presence of each other.

Following separation, the emotional arousal and chronic distress previously experienced by the dogs will decrease, and the dogs will look more comfortable (this may take several weeks or more and may require the use of psychoactive medications). At this point, behaviour modification can be used to facilitate reintroduction. Two owners should keep the dogs on a loose lead at a safe distance (i.e. a distance that does not trigger behaviours and signs of increasing arousal, and from which the dogs cannot make physical contact even when the lead is fully extended). If only one owner is available, then the dogs should be separated with a physical barrier (e.g. gate or tether) and the owner should control the aggressor. The sight of the other dog should be associated with a positive stimulus, e.g. receiving a high-value treat. Response to verbal cues trained by operant conditioning, such as 'watch me' or 'touch', can be beneficial to redirect the attention of a dog that shows signs of discomfort during the reintroduction process (e.g. gazing at the other dog, stiffening his body, showing repeated yawning and lip licking). Progressively, the owner can attempt to increase the length of the interaction and decrease the distance between the two dogs. The lead should be dropped only if the dogs appear to be completely comfortable around each other. A successful reintroduction would allow the dogs to be together without supervision or use of physical containment. While a noticeable improvement was observed in most cases, a full resolution is difficult to attain (Sherman *et al.*, 1996; Wrubel *et al.*, 2011).

For safety, the owners must never use their arms or legs to separate their household dogs during a fight. Instead, they should use loud noises, heavy blankets or indoor leads on each dog.

Psychoactive medications are indicated when the excessive emotional dysregulation and arousal of a dog increases the probability that a severe fight may occur and interfere with the behaviour modification.

12.9 A Note on Predatory Behaviour and Misdirected Play

Aggressive behaviour due to predatory behaviour (i.e. non-affective) has far less clinical relevance than affective aggression (Bamberger and Houpt, 2006; Siracusa *et al.*, 2017). Dog predatory behaviour is usually directed towards non-human animals and, as discussed at the beginning of this chapter, is characterized by a specific body language (e.g. lowering the body posture, pointing at the prey, and absence of vocalization) (Miklosi, 2015; Lord *et al.*, 2017). Contrary to popular belief, dogs' aggression towards children is an affective disorder, not predatory (Reisner *et al.*, 2007, Reisner *et al.*, 2011). Because the primary goal of a dog displaying predatory behaviour is killing the prey, this is very dangerous and pathological behaviour. When predatory behaviour towards a target is confirmed, the latter should be permanently separated using a physical barrier. Welfare-friendly behaviour modification is unlikely to eliminate or significantly reduce the behaviour since predation is a strongly motivated normal behaviour and essential to the survival of an animal.

Playful behaviour by a dog can cause injuries when the animal is excessively aroused and does not control its fine movements well. Small children are particularly exposed and should always be supervised when playing with dogs. Rough play should always be avoided, and play that minimizes physical contact should be preferred. Playing with toys, the dog can grab and pull, or playing fetch is an appropriate play. If a dog becomes overly aroused and starts mouthing when playing, play sessions should be kept at a length that prevents this over-arousal. Stuffed and squeaky toys, and food-filled toys, are very useful to redirect and displace a dog's arousal and should be readily offered to dogs that become overly aroused (Sung, 2018).

References

Amat, M., Le Brech, S., Camps, T., Torrente, C., Mariotti, V.M. *et al.* (2013) Differences in serotonin serum concentration between aggressive English cocker spaniels and aggressive dogs of other breeds. *Journal of Veterinary Behavior* 8(1), 19–25. DOI: 10.1016/j.jveb.2012.04.003.

Bamberger, M. and Houpt, K.A. (2006) Signalment factors, comorbidity, and trends in behavior diagnoses in dogs: 1,644 cases (1991-2001). *Journal of the American Veterinary Medical Association* 229(10), 1591–1601. DOI: 10.2460/javma.229.10.1591.

Bear, M.F., Connors, B.W. and Paradiso, M.A. (2016) *Neuroscience, Exploring the Brain*, 4th edn. Wolters Kluwer, Philadelphia, Pennsylvania.

Boitani, L., Francisci, F., Ciucci, P. and Andreoli, G. (2016) The ecology and behavior of feral dogs: a case study from central Italy. In: Serpell, J. (ed.) *The Domestic Dog: Its Evolution, Behavior And Interactions with People*, 2nd edn. Cambridge University Press, Cambridge, UK, pp. 342–368.

Bonanni, R. and Cafazzo, S. (2014) The social organization of a population of free-ranging dogs in a suburban area of Rome: a reassessment of the effects of domestication on dogs' behavior. In: Kaminski, J. and Marshall-Pescini, S. (eds) *The Social Dog; Behavior and Cognition*. Academic Press, San Diego, California, pp. 63–104.

Bradshaw, J. and Rooney, N. (2016) Dog social behavior and communication. In: Serpell, J. (ed.) *The Domestic Dog: Its Evolution, Behavior and Interactions with People*, 2nd edn. Cambridge University Press, Cambridge, UK, pp. 133–159.

Carlson, N.R. and Birkett, M.A. (2017) *Physiology of Behavior*, 12th edn. Pearson, Essex, UK.

Corridan, C. (2009) Basic requirements for good behavioural health and welfare in dogs. In: Horwitz, D.F. and Mills, D.S. (eds) *BSAVA Manual of Canine and Feline Behavioural Medicine*, 2nd edn. BSAVA, Gloucester, UK, pp. 24–34.

Crowell-Davis, S. and Landsberg, G. (2009) Pharmacology and pheromone therapy. In: Horwitz, D.F. and Mills, D.S. (eds) *BSAVA Manual of Canine and Feline Behavioural Medicine*, 2nd edn. BSAVA, Gloucester, UK, pp. 245–258.

De Keuster, T. and Jung, H. (2010) Aggression towards familiar people and animals. In: Horwitz, D. and Mills, D.S. (eds) *BSAVA Manual of Canine and Feline Behavioural Medicine*, 2nd edn. BSAVA, Gloucester, UK, pp. 182–210.

Denenberg, S., Landsberg, G.M., Horwitz, D. and Seksel, K. *et al.* (2005) A comparison of cases referred to behaviorists in three different countries. In: Mills, D., Levine, E., Landsberg, G., Horwitz, D., Duxbury, M., *et al.* (eds) *Current Issues and Research in Veterinary Behavioural Medicine*. Purdue University Press, West Lafayette, Indiana, pp. 56–62.

Duffy, D.L., Hsu, Y. and Serpell, J.A. (2008) Breed differences in canine aggression. *Applied Animal Behaviour Science* 114(3-4), 441–460. DOI: 10.1016/j.applanim.2008.04.006.

Fatjo, J., Ruiz de la Torre, J.S. and Manteca, X. (2006) The epidemiology of behavioural problems in dogs and cats: a survey of veterinary practitioners. *Animal Welfare* 15, 179–185.

Fatjo, J., Amat, M., Mariotti, V.M., de la Torre, J.L.R., Manteca, X. *et al.* (2007) Analysis of 1040 cases of canine aggression in a referral practice in Spain. *Journal of Veterinary Behavior* 2(5), 158–165. DOI: 10.1016/j.jveb.2007.07.008.

Gerken, A.T., Gross, A.F. and Sandrs, K.K. (2016) Aggression and violence. In: Stern, T.A., Fava, M., Wilens, T.E. and Rosenbaum, J.F. (eds) *Massachusetts General Hospital Comprehensive Clinical Psychiatry*, 2nd edn. Elsevier, Philadelphia, Pennsylvania, pp. 709–717.

Gilchrist, J., Sacks, J.J., White, D. and Kresnow, M.-J. (2008) Dog bites: still a problem? *Injury Prevention* 14(5), 296–301. DOI: 10.1136/ip.2007.016220.

Grohmann, K., Dickomeit, M.J., Schmidt, M.J. and Kramer, M. (2013) Severe brain damage after punitive training technique with a choke chain collar in a German Shepherd dog. *Journal of Veterinary Behavior* 8(3), 180–184. DOI: 10.1016/j.jveb.2013.01.002.

Herron, M.E., Shofer, F.S. and Reisner, I.R. (2009) Survey of the use and outcome of confrontational and non-confrontational training methods in client-owned dogs showing undesired behaviors. *Applied Animal Behaviour Science* 117(1-2), 47–54. DOI: 10.1016/j.applanim.2008.12.011.

Horváth, Z., Igyártó, B.-Z., Magyar, A. and Miklósi, A. (2007) Three different coping styles in police dogs exposed to a short-term challenge. *Hormones and Behavior* 52(5), 621–630. DOI: 10.1016/j.yhbeh.2007.08.001.

Hunthausen, W. (2009) Preventive behavioural medicine for dogs. In: Horwitz, D.F. and Mills, D.S. (eds) *BSAVA Manual of Canine and Feline Behavioural Medicine*, 2nd edn. BSAVA, Gloucester, UK, pp. 65–74.

León, M., Rosado, B., García-Belenguer, S., Chacón, G., Villegas, A. *et al*. (2012) Assessment of serotonin in serum, plasma, and platelets of aggressive dogs. *Journal of Veterinary Behavior* 7(6), 348–352. DOI: 10.1016/j.jveb.2012.01.005.

Lewis, T.W. (2016) Improving the efficacy of selection on complex traits—A brief review of quantitative genetic methods and considerations for measurement of phenotypes. *Journal of Veterinary Behavior* 16, 76–80. DOI: 10.1016/j.jveb.2016.06.003.

Lindell, E.M. (2018a) Aggression/Canine: human directed/Unfamiliar people. In: Horwitz, D. (ed.) *Blackwell's Five-Minute Veterinary Consult Clinical Companion, Canine and Feline Behavior*, 2nd edn. Wiley Blackwell, Hoboken, New Jersey, pp. 58–69.

Lindell, E.M. (2018b) Aggression/Canine: human directed/Familiar people. In: Horwitz, D. (ed.) *Blackwell's Five-Minute Veterinary Consult Clinical Companion, Canine and Feline Behavior*, 2nd edn. Wiley Blackwell, Hoboken, New Jersey, pp. 45–57.

Lindell, E.M. (2018c) Aggression/Canine: Interdog/Unfamiliar dogs. In: Horwitz, D. (ed.) *Blackwell's Five-Minute Veterinary Consult Clinical Companion, Canine and Feline Behavior*, 2nd edn. Wiley Blackwell, Hoboken, New Jersey, pp. 89–99.

Lindell, E.M. (2018d) Aggression/Canine: Interdog/Familiar dogs. In: Horwitz, D. (ed.) *Blackwell's Five-Minute Veterinary Consult Clinical Companion, Canine and Feline Behavior*, 2nd edn. Wiley Blackwell, Hoboken, New Jersey, pp. 79–88.

Landsberg, G., Hunthausen, W. and Ackerman, L.F. (eds) (2013) *Behavior Problems of the Dog and Cat*, 3rd edn. Saunders Elsevier, London.

Lord, K., Schneider, R.A. and Coppinger, R. (2017) Evolution of working dogs. In: Serpell, J. (ed.) *The Domestic Dog: Its Evolution, Behavior and Interactions with People*, 2nd edn. Cambridge University Press, Cambridge, UK, pp. 42–66.

Macdonald, D.W. and Carr, G.M. (2016) Variation in dog society: between resource dispersion and social flux. In: Serpell, J. (ed.) *The Domestic Dog: Its Evolution, Behavior and Interactions with People*, 2nd edn. Cambridge University Press, Cambridge, UK, pp. 319–341.

Mech, D. (2008) Whatever Happened to the Term "Alpha Wolf"? *International Wolf* 18, 4–8.

Mech, L.D. and Boitani, L. (2003) Wolf social ecology. In: Mech, L.D. and Boitani, L. (eds) *Wolves: Behavior, Ecology and Conservation.The University of Chicago Press*. Chicago, Illinois, pp. 1–34.

Miklosi, A. (2015) *Dog Behavior, Evolution and Cognition*, 2nd edn. Oxford University Press, Oxford, UK.

Mills, D.S. (2009) Training and learning protocols. In: Horwitz, D.F. and Mills, D.S. (eds) *BSAVA Manual of Canine and Feline Behavioural Medicine*, 2nd edn.. BSAVA, Gloucester, UK, pp. 49–64.

Nelson, J.R. and Kriegsfeld, L.J. (2018) *An Introduction to Behavioral Endocrinology*, 5th edn. Oxford University Press, New York.

Notari, L. (2009) Stress in veterinary behavioural medicine. In: Horwitz, D.F. and Mills, D.S. (eds) *BSAVA Manual of Canine and Feline Behavioural Medicine*, 2nd edn. BSAVA, Gloucester, UK, pp. 136–145.

Overall, K.L. (2013) *Manual of Clinical Behavior Medicine for Dogs and Cats*. Elsevier Mosby, St. Louis, Missouri.

Oxley, J.A., Christley, R. and Westgarth, C. (2018) Contexts and consequences of dog bite incidents. *Journal of Veterinary Behavior* 23, 33–39. DOI: 10.1016/j.jveb.2017.10.005.

Packard, J.M. (2003) Wolf behavior: reproductive, social, and intelligent. In: Mech, L.D. and Boitani, L. (eds) *Wolves: Behavior, Ecology and Conservation*. The University of Chicago Press, Chicago, Illinois, pp. 35–65.

Patronek, G.J. and Dodman, N.H. (1999) Attitudes, procedures, and delivery of behavior services by veterinarians in small animal practice. *Journal of the American Veterinary Medical Association* 215(11), 1606–1611.

Reisner, I.R., Mann, J.J., Stanley, M., Huang, Y.Y. and Houpt, K.A. (1996) Comparison of cerebrospinal fluid monoamine metabolite levels in dominant-aggressive and non-aggressive dogs. *Brain Research* 714(1-2), 57–64. DOI: 10.1016/0006-8993(95)01464-0.

Reisner, I.R., Shofer, F.S. and Nance, M.L. (2007) Behavioral assessment of child-directed canine aggression. *Injury Prevention* 13(5), 348–351. DOI: 10.1136/ip.2007.015396.

Reisner, I.R., Nance, M.L., Zeller, J.S., Houseknecht, E.M., Kassam-Adams, N. *et al*. (2011) Behavioural characteristics associated with dog bites to children presenting to an urban trauma centre. *Injury Prevention* 17(5), 348–353. DOI: 10.1136/ip.2010.029868.

Rezac, P., Rezac, K. and Slama, P. (2015) Human behavior preceding dog bites to the face. *The Veterinary Journal* 206(3), 284–288. DOI: 10.1016/j.tvjl.2015.10.021.

Sherman, C.K., Reisner, I.R., Taliaferro, L.A. and Houpt, K.A. (1996) Characteristics, treatment, and outcome of 99 cases of aggression between dogs. *Applied Animal Behaviour Science* 47(1-2), 91–108. DOI: 10.1016/0168-1591(95)01013-0.

Siracusa, C. (2016) Status-related aggression, resource guarding, and fear-related aggression in 2 female mixed breed dogs. *Journal of Veterinary Behavior* 12, 85–91. DOI: 10.1016/j.jveb.2015.12.001.

Siracusa, C., Provoost, L. and Reisner, I.R. (2017) Dog- and owner-related risk factors for consideration of euthanasia or rehoming before a referral behavioral consultation and for euthanizing or rehoming the dog after the consultation. *Journal of Veterinary Behavior* 22, 46–56. DOI: 10.1016/j.jveb.2017.09.007.

Stahl, S. (2014) *Stahl's Illustrated Violence: Neural Circuits, Genetics and Treatment*. Cambridge University Press, New York.

Starinsky, N.S., Lord, L.K. and Herron, M.E. (2017) Escape rates and biting histories of dogs confined to their owner's property through the use of various containment methods. *Journal of the American Veterinary Medical Association* 250(3), 297–302. DOI: 10.2460/javma.250.3.297.

Sung, W. (2018) Mouthing/play biting and aggressive play: canine. In: Horwitz, D. (ed.) *Blackwell's Five-Minute Veterinary Consult Clinical Companion, Canine and Feline Behavior*, 2nd edn. Wiley Blackwell, Hoboken, New Jersey, pp. 805–814.

Van Der Berg, L. (2016) Genetics of dog behavior. In: Serpell, J. (ed.) *The Domestic Dog: Its Evolution, Behavior and Interactions with People*, 2nd edn. Cambridge University Press, Cambridge, UK, pp. 70–92.

Welfare in Dog Training (2019) What's Wrong with Using 'Dominance' to Explain the Behaviour of Dogs? Available at: https://www.dogwelfarecampaign.org/why-not-dominance.php (accessed 31 August 2019).

Westgarth, C., Brooke, M. and Christley, R.M. (2018) How many people have been bitten by dogs? A cross-sectional survey of prevalence, incidence and factors associated with dog bites in a UK community. *Journal of Epidemiology and Community Health* 72(4), 331–336. DOI: 10.1136/jech-2017-209330.

Wilsson, E. (2016) Nature and nurture: how different conditions affect the behavior of dogs. *Journal of Veterinary Behavior* 16, 45–52. DOI: 10.1016/j.jveb.2016.10.002.

Wrubel, K.M., Moon-Fanelli, A.A., Maranda, L.S. and Dodman, N.H. (2011) Interdog household aggression: 38 cases (2006-2007). *Journal of the American Veterinary Medical Association* 238(6), 731–740. DOI: 10.2460/javma.238.6.731.

13 Affective Disorders in Cats and Dogs

Sagi Denenberg*

Langford Vets, University of Bristol, Langford, UK; North Toronto Veterinary Behaviour Specialty Clinic, Toronto, Canada

13.1 Introduction

While aggression in both cats at dogs is a major problem and a reason for presentation to veterinary surgeries, and of public health concern, there are numerous other reasons for presentation. The following chapters will detail elimination problems (14), abnormal and repetitive behaviours (15) and ageing-related problems (16). This chapter will focus on presentations related to anxiety disorders, panic disorders, frustration-related presentations and some miscellaneous problems. Presentations that include aggression as a result of affective disorders are discussed in Chapters 11 (cats) and 12 (dogs).

The presentation is why owners come to see us. Our goal is to find the underlying emotional and mental disorders that lead to the presentation (see Chapter 7). Many patients may have more than one existing disorder – the diagnosis may be complicated at times. In this chapter, we review the most common presentations (and some less common). Using a phenomenological approach, we will describe the disorder, consider the context (including environment, routine and peripheral behaviours) and the patient's physical health and needs, and reach a diagnosis. Management of these disorders requires a combination of environmental management, behaviour modification (see Chapter 8) and, at times, psychoactive medications (see Chapter 9).

13.1.1 Anxiety

Anxiety disorders are among the most prevalent causes for presentations of cats and dogs to veterinarians. Anxiety and fear are commonly used interchangeably, though they are different. Anxiety is the anticipation of future threat, whereas fear is an emotional response to present or perceived imminent threat. These emotions overlap in both the neuroanatomical and the neurochemistry, and in behaviours. However, anxiety-related behaviours are focused on vigilance and monitoring the situation in preparation for future danger, whereas fear-related behaviours are focused more on repulsion of or escaping the threat. Both anxiety and fear lead to increased arousal. Anxiety primarily leads to cortical arousal seen as muscle tension, scanning of the area and restlessness. Fear is associated with strong activation of the autonomic nervous system leading to physiological changes such as tachycardia, tachypnea, muscle tremors and dilated pupils.

Contrary to common beliefs, in both fear and anxiety the patient will attempt to avoid first when possible. When the patient cannot avoid, it will confront the threat. These emotions are adaptive; they are meant to help the animal avoid dangerous situations (present or future) and thus survive. Anxiety and fear become maladaptive when they are chronic (i.e. several months, though no timeframe is agreed upon), limit the patient's ability to learn, are excessive in reaction in relation to the trigger and context (which is subjectively assessed by the clinician) and when they impair the welfare of the patient. For example, it is adaptive for a kitten to show apprehension and fear when encountering new animals or people. However, with sufficient introductions that are calm and positive, the kitten will habituate to the presence of people and animals and will be able to generalize this to new people in the future. However, some kittens show excessive avoidance and even aggression when encountering new people as a result of maladaptive fear and anxiety. These kittens will not habituate or only habituate to several people (e.g. the immediate family) but will not be able to generalize it to other people. This kitten

*s.denenberg@bristol.ac.uk

DOI: 10.1079/9781786394552.0013

will continue to show anxiety- and fear-related problems in the future.

Learning and memory are affected by chronic fear and anxiety due to the level of corticosteroid hormones such as cortisol, which in turn reduce the level of brain-derived neurotrophic factor (BDNF) (Chen *et al.*, 2001; Kuma *et al.*, 2004). As a neurotrophin, BDNF plays a role in neuronal genesis, proliferation and plasticity (Mahar *et al.*, 2014). It is an important part of memory formation and consolidation.

13.1.1.1 Phobia

Phobia is an exaggerated and persistent fear reaction that is out of proportion to the trigger. The physiological and emotional response can cripple the patient and is maladaptive. Phobias are specific to the trigger. The focus of the patient is the avoidance of the situation. The reaction can be so intense that the patient will shut down in terror (tonic immobility). Some patients may react in the opposite way; a manic behaviour that is aimed at avoiding the situation or trigger. In some cases, a phobia may be accompanied by a panic attack (see below).

13.1.1.2 Panic

Panic is a sudden development of intense fear response accompanied by robust activation of the sympathoadrenomedullary (SAM) and the hypothalamic-pituitary-adrenal (HPA) systems. Within seconds to minutes, the patient experiences physical and cognitive changes, including very high emotional and physiological arousal (see Section 7.4.3 – Arousal). The reaction is maladaptive and limits the patient from using full cognitive abilities.

Panic can be seen as part of anxiety disorders; however, it can be seen in other disorders, such as depression, post-traumatic stress disorder, and hypersensitivity-hyperactivity disorder. Panic can serve as a prognostic marker, indicating the severity of the problem.

13.1.2 Frustration

Frustration is probably one of the most underdiagnosed or disregarded emotions that play a vital role in problem behaviours in dogs and cats. The tendency to focus on fear and anxiety as the main (or sole) cause of many undesired behaviours is wrong and leads to not only lower success rates when treating psychiatric disorders but also to reduced welfare of the patient.

Frustration can be broadly defined as the inability to access or achieve resources which were previously available to the animal. For example, a cat may show frustration-related behaviours when the flap door is locked, and it cannot go out as before, or a dog may show frustration when an owner is withholding a treat or a toy. Fig. 13.1 describes the activation of the frustration pathway. It is important to note that the animal will not show frustration in a situation where a novel trigger is presented unless fear is also present. That is, the animal might show frustration due to its inability to avoid the threatening trigger. Frustration may also lead to more intense behaviours including activation of the rage component of the network (see Section 7.4.2.2 – Frustration). This activation is likely to cause aggression when the patient is frustrated (see Chapters 11 for cats, and 12 for dogs). Further, due to increased cortical arousal as a result of repeated or chronic frustration, the patient may exhibit displacement behaviours (see Sections 7.3.3.2 – Displacement behaviours, and 7.4.3 Arousal) and abnormal and repetitive behaviours (see Chapter 15).

Unlike anxiety and fear, where the animal's first choice is to avoid the trigger, a frustrated animal is more likely to confront the trigger in an attempt to achieve its goal. For example, a dog that is afraid of other dogs is likely to try avoiding, whereas a dog frustrated by another invading its personal space is more likely to show aggression.

Like anxiety and fear, frustration is an adaptive emotion that is meant to help the animal gain access to and control resources vital for survival. Therefore, increased or unsolved frustration should not only be seen as an undesired behaviour but also as a welfare concern (Stephen and Ledger, 2005; Jakovcevic *et al.*, 2013).

While frustration is an affective state (emotional reaction to a trigger), it may also be a temperament trait lasting over a long period or in many situations. Clinically speaking, frustration-related situations can be divided into five domains based on the presentation and context (McPeake *et al.*, 2019). The work described below investigated frustration in dogs; however, cats are likely to show similar characteristics. More information on the identification of frustration can be found in McPeake *et al.*, 2019 and https://ipstore.lincoln.ac.uk/. It is essential to note that patients are not limited to one category of frustration (see below).

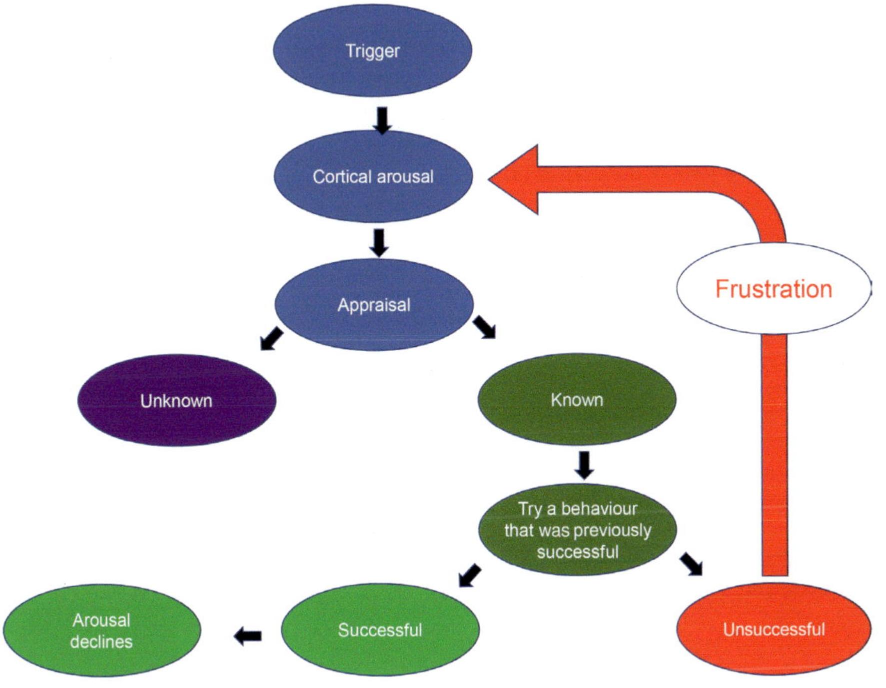

Fig. 13.1. Development of frustration .

Once the animal encounters a trigger, cortical arousal (perception and assessment) takes place. If the trigger is familiar (i.e. the animal encountered it before), the animal will try mounting a reaction that led to a successful outcome in the past. If this reaction, or similar, is unsuccessful, like in the past, the frustration network is activated, leading to increased arousal and repeated cycles. It is important to note that a novel trigger will not elicit frustration.

13.1.2.1 Frustration due to lack of autonomous control

This might be the most important presentation of frustration – when the animal cannot control its environment and is not free to express the behaviour it wants. These patients may show frustration when they are confined (e.g. on a lead or with a closed window) or restrained, or when they perceive a threat to their direct resources such as food, toys or environment. This frustration may lead to aggression over resources or redirected when the patient cannot access the inciting trigger.

13.1.2.2 Frustration due to barriers

The patient is limited from achieving its goal due to a physical barrier. The patient may persevere in its attempt to achieve its goal. It may present behaviour such as digging, scratching, jumping and pacing. It may also vocalize including barking, whimpering and howling.

13.1.2.3 Frustration due to unmet expectations

Patients learn from past behaviours and situations. Any change of predictable routines or environments will lead the patient to attempt to restore the previous situation or avoid the new one. When the patient fails to do so, frustration will develop. These patients will show frustration in situations such as schedule changes (e.g. the owner is late to return and feed the dog), and when the owner withholds a reward. A common example is when the owner attempts to change the patient behaviour using extinction; frustration will lead to an initial increase of the behaviour, and later to extinction burst.

13.1.2.4 *Frustration when attempting to cope with changes*

These patients will show frustration when they cannot achieve a specific goal. The patient may show restlessness and irritability. Examples include owners who decide to no longer allow the patient on the bed (when it used to sleep there), or when owners stop a dog from reaching other dogs it wants to play with.

13.1.2.5 *General frustration*

Patients in this group are likely to show frustration as part of their temperament. It is also possible that their frustration level is a result of the summation of triggers. These patients are likely to show frustration daily in what would be considered benign situations such as lateness to take the dog for a walk or provide its meal. Furthermore, other factors such as pain, other diseases, and fear and anxiety are likely to increase frustration.

13.2 Separation-related Behaviour/ Separation Distress

Separation-related behaviour (SRB) is a general term that encompasses a group of undesired behaviours that are seen when the patient is separated from the owner. The older (and more common) term 'separation anxiety' is inaccurate at best. These patients are likely to be distressed; however, the underlying causes may be different. Another common error is to assume that all SRBs are due to anxiety.

Not much is known about separation-related behaviours in cats compared to dogs. For many years, and still now, cats were thought to be less social than dogs, and a species that does not require much attention or care. It is likely that many cat owners miss signs of SRB, so less information is available. While attachment between the cats and their owners is less clear than the one in dogs, it is likely to be similar given that both species are captive, dependent on the owners for needs, and domesticated for thousands of years (Driscoll *et al.*, 2007; Vitale *et al.*, 2019).

Separation-related behaviours are among the most difficult problems to manage. Patients are dependent on owners for their needs (both social and physical) and cannot cope well with the owner's absence. Also, chronic cases of SRB are likely to increase the HPA and SAM activation leading to a reduced level of BDNF (Moesta *et al.*, 2019). In turn, a low BDNF level may reduce the patient's ability to learn. Further, it is unlikely that owners can completely avoid the trigger (i.e. leaving the patient alone). Finally, when the problem occurs, owners are not present, by definition, and therefore cannot be there to help the patient as they would in many other situations.

13.2.1 Diagnosis

The first step is to rule out physical disorders leading to signs of SRB. Patients may be in pain or have gastrointestinal disorders, hyperthyroid (in cats) or neurological diseases. Moreover, physical disorders may lead to anxiety and frustration if the patient depends on the owner for help or comfort in alleviating those. Some examples include a dog with colitis who depends on the owner to go outside to eliminate or a cat with arthritis who depends on the owner to be picked up to its perch. Next, we must evaluate the patient routine and environment. Patients who show SRB are possibly under-stimulated or under-exercised.

Several emotions are likely to play a role in the development and maintenance of SRB. It is important to differentiate or identify those so that we can institute effective management. Equally, it is essential to remember that these emotions are not mutually exclusive.

Patients may experience anxiety around times that the owner is likely to leave the house, and when the owner is absent. The anxiety is about abandonment. Signs may include restlessness, pacing, following the owner around the house, lack of sleep, excessive reactivity to noises and movements, and intense greeting behaviours. The patient may attempt to sit on window sills or watch out of the window and wait for the owner by the door. House soiling, vocalization and damage to property are among the most common complaints (see Fig. 13.2).

When the owner is leaving or shortly after, the patient may show signs of a panic attack (see Section 13.7), indicating a more severe problem. These signs may include distressed vocalization (howling, barking and whimpering), muscle tremors, dilated pupils, urination and defecation, panting and excessive salivation, anorexia, or the patient may shut down and become immobilized until the owner's return (see Figs. 13.3 and 13.4).

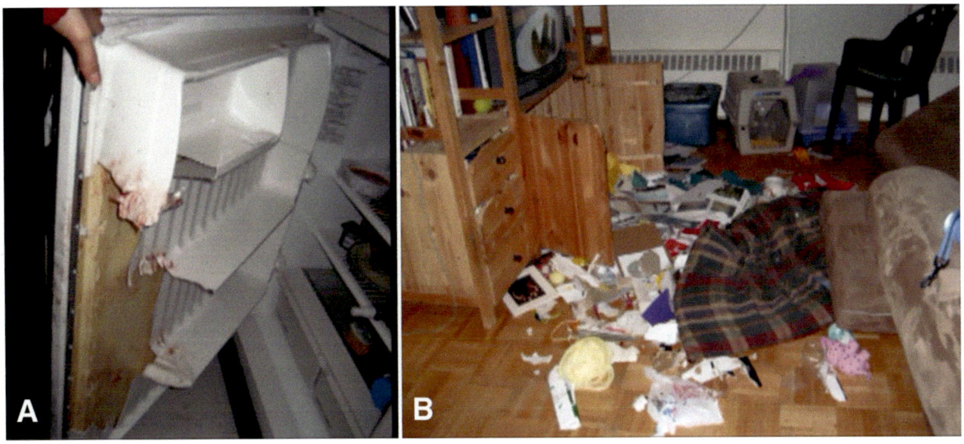

Fig. 13.2. Separation distress due to anxiety. The patient may cause damage to property or personal objects. Most damage is done as a displacement behaviour rather than intentional. The targets (e.g., furniture, doors, or a personal belonging) are not specific. (Photos courtesy of Sagi Denenberg.)

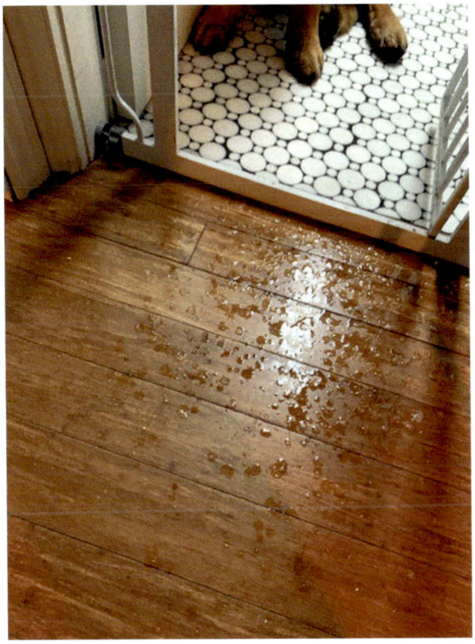

Fig. 13.3. Panic attack. The dog in this case was drooling excessively while standing by the stairgate the entire time it was left alone. (Photo courtesy of Sagi Denenberg.)

Grief (loss of attachment figure) may be part of SRB in dogs and cats. It can lead to signs of withdrawal, apathy, anorexia when left alone, and mournful vocalization.

Patients with SRB are likely to have reduced ability to learn in the context of separation. It would be expected that pets will adjust to the owner's routine, especially young and healthy animals, or, in other words, habituate to the owner's absence. These patients are likely to go through the opposite process; they become sensitized to the owner's absence. As a result, a phobia may develop; the patient's emotional reaction to the owner's absence, even a very brief absence or leaving the room, is intense and coupled with a strong physical reaction.

Frustration also plays a role. These patients are not always anxious, and their behaviours are meant to solve the current situation and reunite with the owner or escape their confinement. These patients may cause destruction or damage towards exits when trying to leave the area (see Fig. 13.5). They may also destroy objects as redirected behaviour. A frustrated animal is less likely to follow the owner around the house, show hypervigilance, house soil or show anorexia when left alone. Also, the patient may show aggression in an attempt to stop the owner from leaving.

Owners are more likely to miss covert signs of SRB. The most common complaints are intense vocalization, damage to property or objects, and house soiling. Unless carefully observed (possibly using a video camera), owners are likely to miss the patient who is lying by the door without movement but is not sleeping, or the one who is pacing the entire time the owner is away.

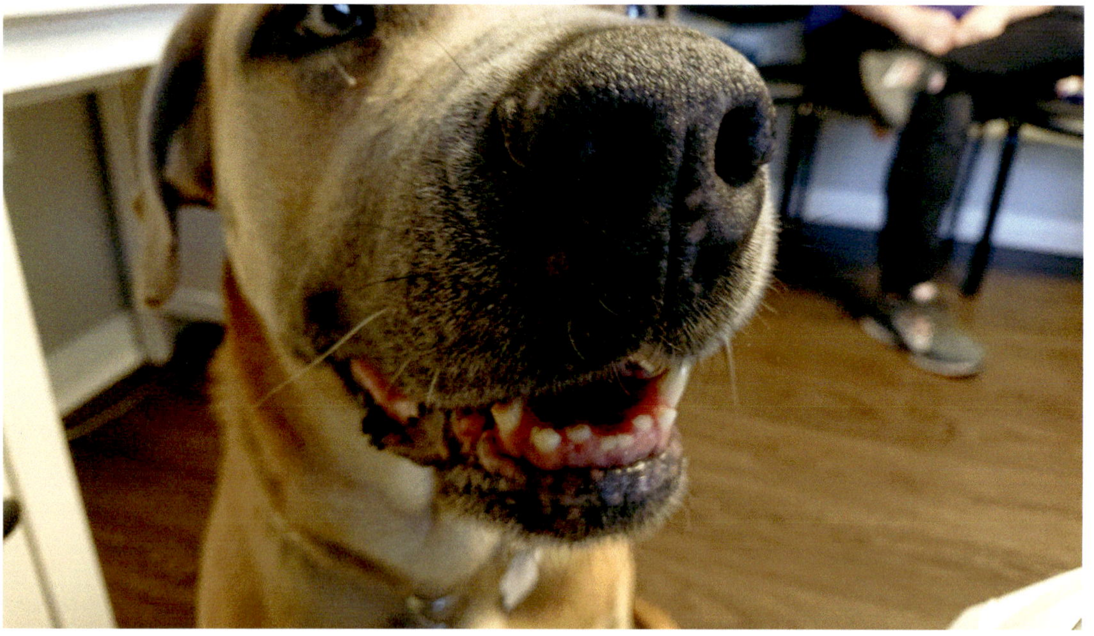

Fig. 13.4. Panic attack. When suffering a panic attack, pain sensation is muted. The patient may injure itself during its attempt to follow the owner or escape the situation. This dog broke its teeth while trying to escape. (Photo courtesy of Sagi Denenberg.)

When owners report that the patient is following them all over the home, seems to have light sleep (i.e. wakes up to each minor sound or movement), or seems to shut down when the owner prepares to leave home, we must be proactive and ask more questions. These questions include asking about the patient's behaviour when the owners prepare to leave and return, eating when left alone (a common description is a pet who will not eat treats or food when left alone, and will eat immediately following the owner's return), or sleep quality and duration. Leaving a video camera is a useful tool. However, we must keep in mind that assessing whether the patient is sleeping when left alone may be difficult as it may lie down and even close its eyes, but not necessarily sleep. Activity collars may be used; however, the data rendered are processed, and the software is not likely to differentiate between sleeping to tonic immobility.

Additional questions should include asking about the patient behaviour when left with someone who is not the main attachment figure, environmental events (e.g. waste collection, construction nearby or people arriving at the door) and other psychiatric disorders. SRB is likely to show comorbidity with other disorders involving anxiety, phobias or frustration.

The patient may cause damage to property or personal objects. Most damage is done as a displacement behaviour rather than intentional. The targets (e.g. furniture, doors or personal belongings) is not specific.

13.2.2 Management

The first step is to address any underlying physical disorder that may cause similar clinical signs (see Chapters 2 and 3) or leads to anxiety, given the patient's inability to manage the situation alone.

Next we need to address the patient's routine and environment. Owners should implement a predictable and consistent daily routine that meets the patient's need for exercise and stimulation, social interactions, elimination, feeding and sleep. The routine should be designed in such a way that the patient is exercised (including play sessions with cats) and eliminates before departure. Owners

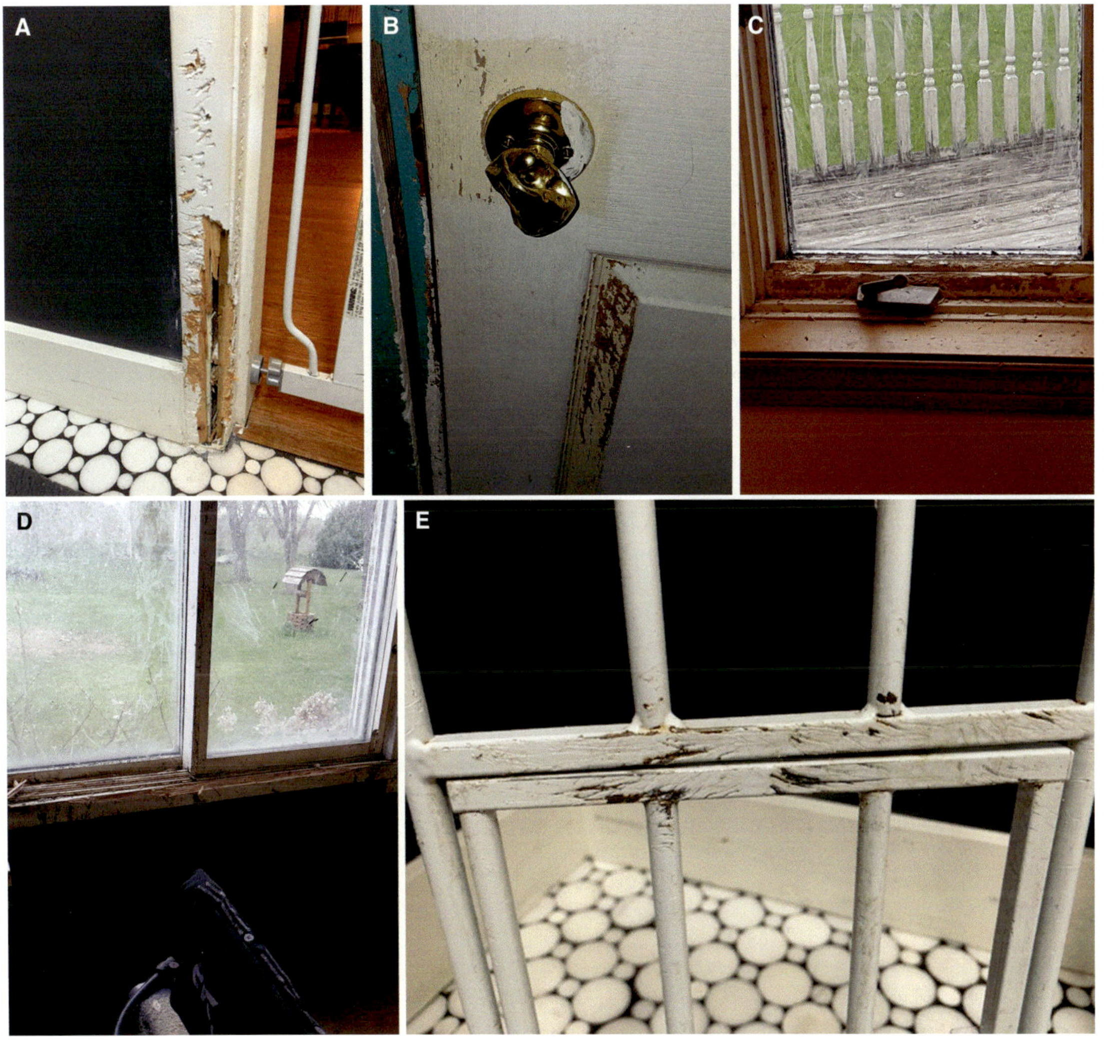

Fig. 13.5. Separation distress due to frustration. The patient may cause damage, similar to SRB as a result of anxiety. In the case of frustration, the damage is targeted primarily at exits. In this case, the damage is more deliberate as the patient is trying to break its confinement. (Photos courtesy of Sagi Denenberg.)

should meet the patient's social needs through training, play and affection before leaving. Then, when leaving, the owner should leave the patient with food and treats, ideally inside feeding toys. Many patients will not eat when left alone; providing less food when the owner is at home and more food (ideally, a higher-value food) when the owner is absent may stimulate the patient to eat when alone. Once the patient is eating, it is likely to be slightly more settled, though it is not clear if the patient was calmer and therefore ate, or ate and therefore was calmed. In any event, once the patient eats when left alone, the situation is better than before.

Ideally, owners can design a safe space for the patient to stay when left alone (see Handout C3 – Safe Haven). Training should only be done when the owner is at home to allow the patient out before it becomes distressed. Only once the patient is voluntarily spending time in this location when the owner is at home (or possibly when left alone) can the owner start using this place when they leave the patient alone. Working with the patient on calming down on a signal (see Handout C4 – Teaching a Pet How to Settle on Cue) is useful; in future departures, owners can use this exercise to calm the patient before leaving it alone.

If the patient's arousal level is not limiting the patient from learning (as it usually is) before the owner is leaving, we can attempt to start desensitizing the patient to departure signals and later to the owner's absence (see Handout D14 – Desensitization – Separation-related Problems). In many cases, this part of the management can only be implemented following the use of medications that help the patient to calm down first (see below).

Upon returning home, the patient may show an exaggerated greeting behaviour, including jumping on the owners, mouthing, pacing and barking. Owners can ignore this behaviour until the patient stops and only then give attention (see Section 8.5.2.1 – Extinction). However, a preferred option is to guide the patient to show the desired behaviour (e.g. sitting by the door when the owner enters the home). The latter option requires the owners to be more proactive, including preparing treats by the door, have a lead ready, or practise it several times daily (i.e. leaving and coming back inside). The owner should choose a behaviour they prefer the patient to show. The behaviour must be simple enough and tangible so the patient can learn; for example, sitting by the door. Training should take place when the patient is not expecting the owner to leave; the owner has several minutes to train the patient and has treats ready (see Handout C1 – Set Up to Succeed). The owner can step outside and return almost immediately and ask the patient to sit. The owner may need to use a lead or head halter, or lure the patient. Once it sits, the owner should reward it. This exercise should continue until the patient sits immediately, without a verbal signal, when the owner comes back inside. This option, response substitution (see Handout C7 – Response Substitution), is likely to work faster than extinction and reduce the patient's frustration when the owner is standing and ignoring it.

Adding a pet to serve as a companion is not likely to help. Although the patient and the new animal may form a positive relationship, it may not help the patient as the attachment is to the owner. In some cases, adding an additional pet may worsen the situation or create new problems (in both the existing and new animal in the home). The desire to add a 'friend' is anthropomorphic.

Many cases of SRB (less likely when frustration is the sole cause) require the use of medications to reduce the patient's negative affective state. Since the problem revolves mostly around anxiety and high arousal level, the use of serotonergic medications such as clomipramine and fluoxetine is the mainstay approach. When the patient shows SRB coupled with panic attacks, the use of noradrenergic medications such as clonidine or dexmedetomidine may be helpful to reduce signs related to an intense activation of the SAM and HPA systems. The use of medications to allow the patient to calm down when they struggle with the owner's departure is useful. Benzodiazepines (e.g. alprazolam, lorazepam or clonazepam), high-dose gabapentin or trazodone can help reduce intense fear or phobia signs by increasing the threshold for reactivity.

13.3 Travel Anxiety

Travelling is not an innate behaviour or situation for animals. They must learn to spend time in a moving vehicle. The process of habituating to travel is best done when the animal is young and has no negative bias (e.g. the socialization period). When done gradually and coupled with a positive outcome, most animals habituate (see Chapter 6 for more information).

There are three likely reasons for patients to show high arousal, agitation, restlessness and somatic signs (e.g. trembling, drooling, dilated pupils and panting) (see Fig. 13.6). Some patients are anxious about the travel itself, including the motion and vibration, sounds and moving objects. The second group of patients who show anxiety during travel are likely to be anxious about the destination or purpose of the travel, not the travel itself. The third group is likely to be patients who suffer from motion sickness rather than anxiety.

13.3.1 Diagnosis

These patients show hesitation or even avoidance of the vehicle. When walking from the home towards the vehicle, they may try to avoid it. Often owners must put dogs into the vehicle even when they are able to jump inside. These patients may become hypervigilant when they hear the owner

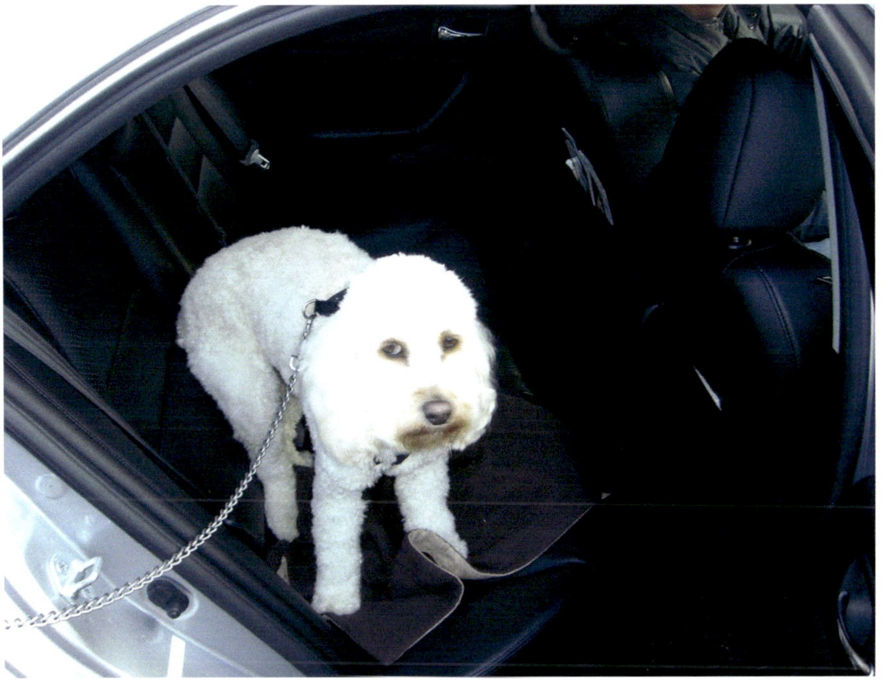

Fig. 13.6. This patient shows typical signs of distress in the car. The body language is low and inhibited, the tail is low, the ears are back, and the patient holds its head low. This patient must be picked up and put into the car; it will not jump inside.(Photo courtesy of Sagi Denenberg.)

taking the keys or giving any other signal that predicts travelling.

Once inside the vehicle, they are restless, pacing and panting, barking, and have difficulty concentrating on the owner. Some patients may also suffer from panic attacks, including robust activation of the SAM and HPA systems (see Section 13.7).

The use of antiemetics or medications that counteract nausea can help to differentiate between motion sickness and anxiety. Using medications such as an antihistamine or similar that may lead to drowsiness may help to alleviate the signs but not differentiate the cause. Moving small dogs and cats to a higher position where they can see the road may also help to alleviate some of the signs (motion sickness is often the result of lack of synchronization between the movements felt by the vestibular apparatus and static image (e.g. crate or foot well) seen by the visual cortex).

Patients who are anxious due to the unknown destination often show signs of anxiety on the way from the home to the destination. However, on the way back home, these patients are likely to be calmer as they anticipate that the destination is the home.

13.3.2 Management

Using antiemetic or medications for nausea such as maropitant, non-drowsy antihistamines or low-dose acepromazine can be useful for those patients who suffer from motion sickness. Keeping the patient high so it can see the road, providing fresh air during the ride, and possibly a small meal before the travel, can help.

When the patient suffers from anxiety that is limited to vehicle travel, the use of as-needed medications such as trazodone, benzodiazepines, gabapentin or alpha-2 agonist can help. Owners should give a test dose at home before taking the patient for a car ride. An optimal response at home is mild lethargy. The travel effect will counteract some of the effects of the medication; therefore the response will be more limited during the travel.

Working on desensitization to car rides (see Handout D11 – Desensitization – Car Rides) may be helpful. Owners should be slow and patient and try avoiding unnecessary travels with the patients while working on desensitization.

When the patient is anxious about the destination, giving a predictable and consistent signal may help. Owners should choose a signal and give it before each travel to a specific destination. For example, when taking the dog to the park, the owner should first say 'going to the park' and then take the dog to the car and drive to the park. When going to the vet, the owner should say 'going to the vet' and then travel to the vet. This exercise is difficult due to time constraints. However, the owner can set this up and try frequently travelling after giving the signal.

In many cases, the problem is combined (e.g. travel anxiety and motion sickness), and combined management is necessary.

13.4 Generalized Anxiety

Excessive and long-term anxiety in more than three situations. This anxiety is maladaptive; the patient is showing more intense signs than non-pathological anxiety and will not settle once the situation is finished. Owners are often confused by generalized anxiety as no tangible triggers exist. There are no specific triggers since the patient is anxious about everything from interactions with the owner and other people and animals, walks and exercise, handling, noises, or changes in routine and environment. In other words, the patient is showing signs of anxiety consistently through the day, not limited to specific contexts. The patient is likely to displace these behaviours regardless of the owner's presence.

13.4.1 Diagnosis

The patient displays multiple displacement behaviours, restlessness, hypervigilance, difficulties to settle down and rest, hyposomnia and attention-seeking behaviours. The patient may withdraw from multiple situations and become inhibited in its interactions. Changes in feeding behaviours such as anorexia or ravenous and indiscriminate eating may be noted.

Patients may show excessive attention-seeking behaviours. These behaviours are likely to be more intense than those shown when the patient presents learnt attention-seeking. Also, providing attention is likely to be insufficient to calm the patient.

In some cases, panic attacks may accompany generalized anxiety. In this case, the patient may disconnect from the owner, ignore food or toys, and exhibit somatic signs indicated by robust activation of the SAM and HPA systems (see Section 13.7).

Physical disorders such as pain, hyperadrenocorticism, hyperthyroid (cats) and diabetes should be ruled out. In cases where the patient is withdrawn and inhibited, hypoadrenocorticism should be ruled out. Often these patients also present signs of allergies and gastrointestinal diseases such as colitis. (See Chapters 2 and 3 for more information.)

13.4.2 Management

Since there are no patterns or specific triggers, the aim of management is focused on optimizing the patient's environment and routine. Owners should attempt to teach the patient to go to its safe space when it is anxious (see Handout C3 – Safe Haven) by providing a calm and quiet area where they can give food, water, and affection. It would be best if owners can implement a daily routine that includes set times the patient is in its safe place for rest and sleep. Providing cats with a high perching space is beneficial.

Meeting the patient's need to exercise (indoor and outdoor), including play, is essential. When the patient is afraid to walk outside, indoor or garden only walks (when possible) should substitute walks on streets or roads. Using feeding toys provides mental stimulation. Moreover, it may keep the patient engaged in desired behaviours at times when it is likely to show anxiety (see Handouts A9 and A10 – Feeding Toys and Stimulation for Cats and Dogs).

Training the patient (cats included) is useful to engage the patient in calm, predictable and consistent interactions. The goal is not better performance in training; it is to help the patient focus on desired behaviours.

Teaching the patient to settle on a signal (see Handout C4 – Teaching a Pet How to Settle on Cue) may become useful when the patient exhibits intense signs of anxiety and possible panic attacks. Owners should be aware that this exercise is difficult in calm pets, let alone in a highly anxious patient.

The use of medications is necessary to alleviate anxiety. Long-term daily use of serotonergic medications such as SSRI or TCA is the first choice.

When the signs are intense, adding a secondary medication, primarily GABAergic medication, such as benzodiazepines, gabapentin or pregabalin, and imepitoin may be beneficial to increase the patient's reactivity threshold.

For patients who are inhibited and withdrawn, using selegiline may provide better control of their anxiety. Another option is using other dopaminergic medications such as bupropion. When the patient experiences panic attacks, using alpha-2 agonists such as clonidine or a beta-blocker such as propranolol or pindolol may be beneficial.

13.5 Fear

As mentioned above (see Section 13.1.1), fear is an adaptive emotion that helps the animal to survive by avoiding dangerous or threatening triggers. Non-pathological fear is accompanied by activation of the sympathetic nervous system and the HPA axis. The animal will have an appropriate appraisal process and mount the appropriate response (which is not synonymous with acceptable response).

However, when the patient is consistently encountering the trigger or triggers that lead to fear, or the intensity of the trigger(s) increase(s), or the patient cannot mount an appropriate response, the level of fear may become pathological. Once fear becomes pathological, the involved behaviours are more intense and may lead to the development of other maladaptive disorders such as phobia and panic (see below). Unlike phobia or panic, fearful animals show behaviours that are within normal proportion to the trigger.

13.5.1 Fearful behaviour

These behaviours are seen when the trigger is present; there is a clear pattern. Fearful behaviours are focused on avoiding the trigger and survival. There are three groups of fearful behaviours, and the patient may exhibit some or all of them (though not at the same time). The patient may exhibit active or passive avoidance or active repulsion (see Chapters 11 and 12 for more details about active repulsion). The selection between these depends on the patient's experience, options, physical health and genetics. For example, a cat may decide to run away from another cat if it is healthy and has an option to run away. However, if the cat is in pain or confined, it may choose passive avoidance.

Active avoidance behaviours include running away and hiding. Passive avoidance behaviours include cowering, low ears and tail, turning the head away, and tonic immobility (see Figs. 13.7 and 13.8A–C). Active repulsion is aggression (see Fig. 13.9). In all cases, signs linked to activation of the sympathetic and HPA systems (e.g. trembling, mydriasis, panting and tachycardia) will appear.

13.5.2 Management

The first step is to rule out or treat physical disorders such as hyperadrenocorticism, hyperthyroid, pain, and neurological and musculoskeletal disorder. Once these are ruled out or managed, owners can focus on identifying triggers and patterns. Maintaining a diary is helpful in gathering the necessary information (see Handout A7 – Behaviour Diary Template).

Based on the information gathered through the owner's history and diary, triggers and patterns should be identified and prioritized. There are several options to prioritize triggers, including the owner's preference, intensity or risk, and the ability to avoid triggers. When possible, we must attempt to desensitize the patient to those triggers that are unavoidable or pose a higher risk (to the patient or surrounding people and animals). This prioritization may not always be similar to that of the owner's. Owners tend to focus on the more salient features rather than the ability to manage the situation. For example, owners often will prioritize the dog's fear of people on walks or traffic sounds over fear of noises inside the home or family members. However, it is easier (though not easy) to avoid people and traffic sounds, by altering the routine and environment, than it is to avoid sudden sounds at home.

The first step should be to design a routine or time-management and environmental plan to avoid as many triggers as possible. At times, we want to avoid triggers that will be reintroduced later through a desensitization programme. Depending on the specific fear, owners should attempt to control the environment or the patient's exposure to the trigger(s). For example, altering the time of the day the dog is walked, or preventing the cat from accessing an area when visitors arrive, help minimize exposure to the trigger. At home, allocating a secure place to keep the patient when triggers might be present (e.g. visitors, noise or other animals) is helpful. Teaching the patient to spend time in this

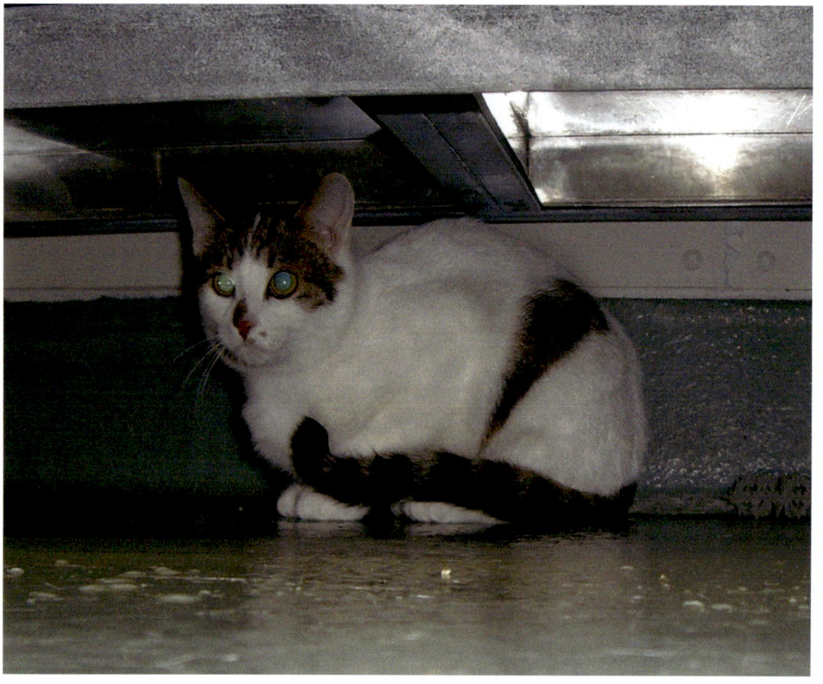

Fig. 13.7. Active avoidance. This patient is showing active avoidance. Note the dilated pupils, cowered body, and location of the patient. (Photo courtesy of Sagi Denenberg.)

area may be complicated and require patience and persistence (see Handout C3 – Safe Haven).

At the same time that we attempt to avoid triggers, we can start working with the patient on basic training such as 'watch me' and 'touch' and loose-leash walks (see Handouts C2 – How to Teach a 'Watch Me' and 'Touch' Cue and C10 – Training Loose-leash Walks), and settle exercises (see Handout C4 – Teaching a Pet How to Settle on Cue). These exercises help us to manage the patient during the desensitization programme.

Once the patient is calmer, we can tailor a desensitization programme to help modify the patient's behaviour when encountering the threatening trigger(s). The programme must be designed for each trigger separately based on the priority list (for more information see Section 8.5.3 – Specific considerations concerning the use of desensitization

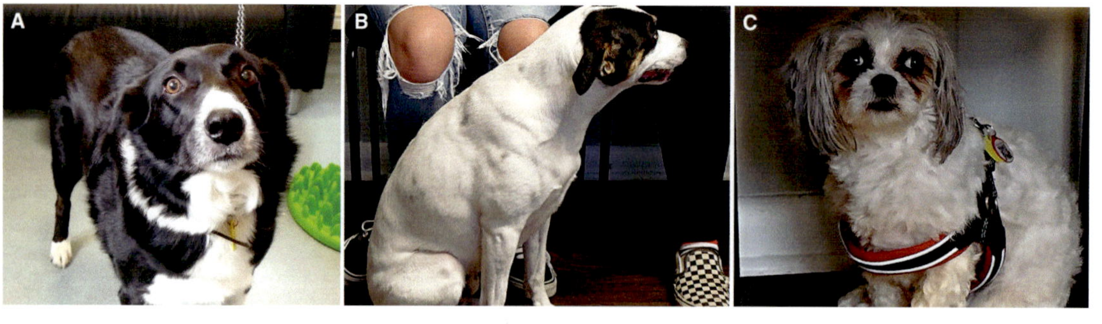

Fig. 13.8. A-C. Fearful body language. The dogs in these images are fearful and show short-term tonic immobility (A and B) or avoidance (C). Note the ears and tail position, low body and dilated pupils. (Photos courtesy of Sagi Denenberg.)

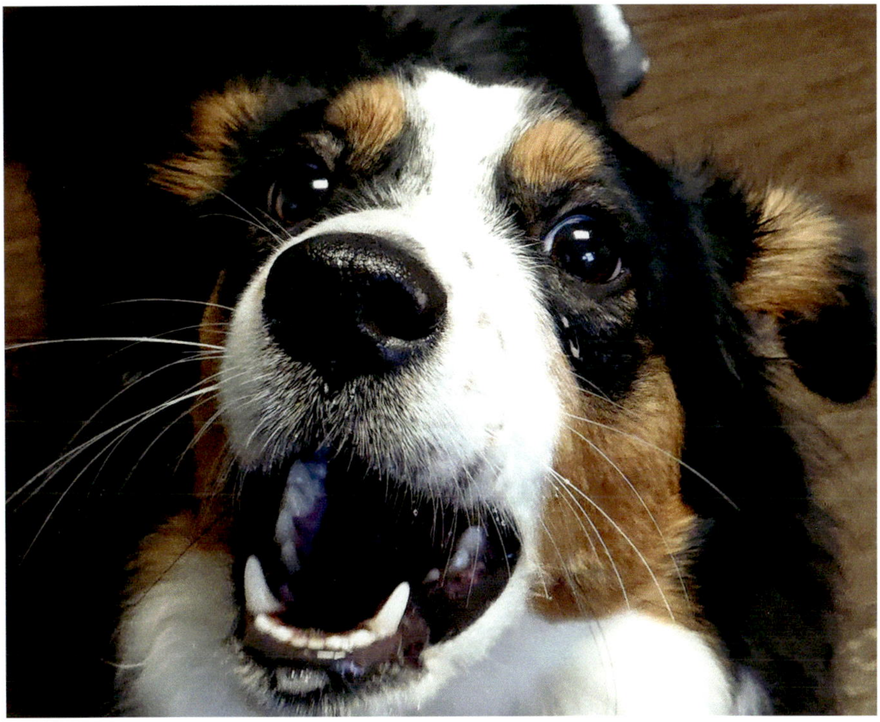

Fig. 13.9. Active repulsion. The dog in this image is fearful and is showing aggression to repulse the trigger. Note the ears position, open mouth in V shape, dilated pupils, and low body. (Photo courtesy of Sagi Denenberg.)

and counter-conditioning). The process is similar in all cases; however, the patient's response might vary. It is essential to maintain low-level exposures and keep the patient under the threshold for reactivity. Further, once the patient becomes aroused by one exercise, it may remain aroused for quite some time. Therefore, owners should follow closely for signs of high arousal (see Section 7.4.3 – Arousal) and allow the patient sufficient time to settle down between sessions. Appendix D contains specific desensitization protocols for different triggers.

When fear and arousal levels are pathological (see Section 7.4.3 – Arousal) and limit the patient's ability to process the information given by the owners and the environment, the use of medications is helpful. Medications can be given as needed through desensitization exercises or when the owner cannot avoid the trigger. When owners cannot avoid or predict different triggers, the ongoing use of medications may be necessary.

GABAergic medications such as gabapentin or pregabalin, or benzodiazepines (e.g. alprazolam, lorazepam or clonazepam) are among the best first-choice medications for as-needed use. They can also be used ongoing. When the problem is intense and includes many signs of high arousal, the use of serotonergic medications such as SSRI or TCA, or trazodone, might be indicated.

13.5.3 Phobia

A phobia is an exaggerated fear or anxiety about a specific trigger or situation. The patient will experience this response, within seconds, each time the trigger or situation is presented. The primary goal of the patient is to avoid the situation whenever possible. When impossible, the patient may show tonic immobility or even catatonia. In cases of true phobia, the reaction is out of proportion to the actual trigger or situation. The patient is distressed and dysfunctional.

Another key diagnostic criterion is that the reaction is specific to a trigger or situation. However, it is essential to remember that the patient may suffer from several phobias. The degree of reaction may vary from intense anticipatory behaviour (anxiety) to a full panic attack, including a robust activation of the SAM and HPA systems.

Owners tend to look for rationale or a cause; this may be a frustrating situation. Phobias are irrational in their intensity and accompanied behaviours. Further, there may not be a tangible cause for owners to identify. For example, fear of loud noises, such as thunder, is an adaptive fear (e.g. avoidance of lightning storms, which may kill the animal). However, some patients exhibit noise phobia where the reaction is either unnecessary, as the patient is protected at home, or the patient becomes immobilized and therefore more likely to be vulnerable.

During a phobic event, the patient becomes highly aroused, distressed and dysfunctional. Often the patient will disconnect from the owners and the environment; they will not listen, they ignore food or toys, and even punishment and pain.

Many somatic signs such as trembling, mydriasis, tachycardia, tachypnea, excessive salivation and panting can be seen. Once the phobic stimulus has ended, the patient starts to recover. However, the recovery period may last several hours or more. The patient may be very vigilant and aroused for long periods, or sleep for long periods.

Management of phobia requires owners to try to minimize the impact of phobic stimuli on the patient by modifying the environment and routine, and medications. First-choice medications include gabapentin or pregabalin, or benzodiazepines. If the phobic stimuli are present often or unavoidable, then adding SSRI, TCA or SNRI is necessary.

13.5.3.1 Agoraphobia

In human psychiatry, agoraphobia refers to marked fear or anxiety in public or open spaces, when interacting with a large number of people and being outside of the home alone. While it is difficult to assess these emotional parameters and thoughts in veterinary patients, those patients who show marked fear and anxiety before leaving, or having left, the home may have agoraphobia.

Diagnostic criteria include increased vigilance when the owner prepares to take the patient for a walk or out of the house, trying to avoid being taken out (e.g. running away from the lead or harness, hiding or even showing aggression towards the owner), and once outside the patient shows marked fear including freezing, refusal to move and panic attack.

Differential diagnosis includes pain, other phobias or anxieties, or aggression towards the owner while handling the patient. Patients should be screened for any physical disorder, including vision impairment, pain and neurological disorders.

The first goal is to avoid the phobic stimulus when possible. Owners should not force the patient out of the house. Instead, an indoor elimination area (e.g. litter trays or pads) should be placed. Some patients will go out to the garden but not to the street. Owners can exercise and stimulate the patient indoors. In some cases, social learning may facilitate walks. Trying to take the dog for a walk with other dogs might be helpful.

The use of gabapentin, pregabalin or benzodiazepine is indicated to alleviate the signs or reduce the intensity of the phobia. Adding SSRI or SNRI is helpful. When the patient experiences panic attacks, before or during outings, adding clonidine or dexmedetomidine or beta-blocker may be beneficial.

A desensitization programme should follow, once the patient's arousal level is sufficiently low to allow it to learn. Owners should start with brief outings by the house during calm times (e.g. minimal traffic, pedestrians and noise) and reward the patient for calm behaviour (see Handout D9 – Desensitization – Walks).

13.5.3.2 Neophobia

Neophobia is intense fear or anxiety when encountering anything new in the environment or routine. The patient shows marked reaction each time it encounters the trigger. It is common and acceptable for animals, especially young ones, to show fear of novel objects or circumstances they eventually habituate, whereas the neophobic patient does not – it may become sensitized.

The main goal of the patient is to avoid the phobic stimulus (e.g. waste bin on the road, a new person in the environment, or change in routine) and restore previous routine or environment.

Differential diagnosis includes pain, sensory impairment, neurological disease, other phobias and anxieties, and panic attacks. True neophobia means that the patient consistently shows the reaction over a prolonged period (e.g. several months) and the intensity remains very high. This is not the same situation that occurs when young animals (e.g. kittens or puppies) first encounter new situations or people and may show anxiety or panic attack. Many of those young animals, even those deprived of appropriate socialization (see Chapter 6), eventually habituate. Those who do not may develop neophobia.

Patients with neophobia are not selective; they will react to each new stimulus. This is in contrast to patients that have specific fear or anxieties and will respond only to those triggers. We must keep in mind that the patient may have several fears or anxieties and therefore may respond to many triggers.

Owners should attempt to maintain the environment and routine as predictable and consistent as possible to avoid phobic events. When the need arises to introduce a new stimulus, a gradual introduction is the best approach. The environment should remain similar other than the stimulus. Owners should teach the patient to settle down first (see Handout C4 – Teaching a Pet How to Settle on Cue). Once the patient is calm, the trigger can be introduced with low intensity (e.g. from a distance or low-volume) while providing the patient with positive reinforcement. Only once the patient appears to habituate can the owner move the patient closer to the trigger or increase the intensity of the situation.

Often, the use of serotonergic medications, coupled with GABAergic medications, is necessary. When the patient also exhibits signs of panic attacks, alpha-2 agonists or beta-blockers can be added.

13.5.3.3 Phonophobia

Phonphobia is intense fear or anxiety when encountering sounds. The patient will aim to avoid the sound by escaping or hiding. When the patient fails to do so, it may show tonic immobility or catatonia. Often, phonophobia is accompanied by a panic attack that leads to robust activation of the SAM and HPA systems (see Section 13.7).

Fear of loud noises is innate and adaptive. However, when it escalates or when the patient does not seem to habituate, a true phobia may develop. The reaction becomes maladaptive and a serious welfare concern. Approximately 40–50% of owners report noise sensitivities in their pets, and the age of onset is between one and two years (Blackwell *et al.*, 2005; Tiira *et al.*, 2016). In contrast, less than 20% of owners are likely to seek help (Dale *et al.*, 2010). The degree of phobia seems to escalate with age, and females are more likely to develop this phobia (Storengen and Lingaas, 2015).

Phonophobia (also known as sonophobia or ligyrophobia) appears to divide into two sub-categories based on the saliency of the sound (Blackwell *et al.*, 2013; Bowen *et al.*, 2013). The first sub-category includes more salient sounds such as thunder, fireworks and gunshot. The second sub-category includes less salient sounds such as traffic and domestic sounds (e.g. vacuum cleaner, lawnmower or electronic sounds).

Patients who showed a phobia when experiencing a more salient sound (e.g. thunder) were more likely to show a phobia to a different salient sound (e.g. fireworks), but not to less salient sounds (e.g. traffic). This characteristic may indicate that the patient generalizes the phobia (Blackwell *et al.*, 2013). Patients who exhibit a phobia to less salient sounds (e.g. traffic, voices or sneezing) were more likely to have other comorbidities (e.g. separation-related distress or generalized anxiety) than patients with a phobia to more salient sounds, possibly indicating a genetic trait of overall fearfulness.

Some patients may show a variant of phonophobia to thunder. These patients may also respond to other indicators of thunderstorms than just the sound. Other factors may include changes in barometric pressure, static electricity, wind, heavy rain and changes in ambient light.

Differential diagnoses include other phobias and anxieties, panic attacks due to other causes, neurological disorders, sensory deficits and gastrointestinal disorder. Pain is likely to play a major role, both as a differential diagnosis and as a contributor to the development and maintenance of phobia (Lopes Fagundes *et al.*, 2018). Further, some sounds such as gunshot and fireworks are above 100 decibels and may cause pain to those animals who are in proximity to the source (see Table 13.1).

In human medicine, hyperacusis (increased sensitivity to different sounds or frequencies) and

Table 13.1. Sound intensity.

Source	Decibel (dB)
Conversation, TV	50–70
Loud voices, vacuum, engines, door shutting	80–100
Fireworks (50–100 m away), motorcycles, heavy machinery	100–120
Thunder	110–130
Gunshot (50–100 m away)	130–160

misophonia (an intense negative emotional reaction to different sounds) affect people's behaviour when they hear the sounds they are sensitive to. It is unclear if animals suffer from similar conditions or show phobic reactions.

While it may be very difficult or near impossible at times, the first and most important aspect of the management of phobophobia is prevention. Owners should attempt to avoid any phobic trigger when possible (e.g. avoiding areas with traffic, muting electronic devices at home and speaking softly). When the owners cannot avoid environmental sounds (e.g. thunder or fireworks), a combination of environmental and routine modification and medications is necessary.

Owners should attempt to teach the patient to spend time in a calm and relatively sound-isolated area (see Handout C3 – Safe Haven). Using a white noise such as a dedicated machine, online sounds, humidifier or a fan can help to muffle sounds from the outside. Placing soundproofing in walls or using a room with no exposure to the outside (e.g. basement, bathroom or a utility room) may help to minimize the impact of the sound. Playing music is also possible. Owners should teach the patient to go to its area several times daily for rest, food, affection and chews. Ideally, the patient learns to associate the area with a positive outcome.

When owners are aware of a noise event (e.g. thunderstorm or fireworks), they should take the patient to its safe haven ahead of time. Before placing the patient there, owners should ensure the patient's needs are met. Dogs should be walked or let out to the garden. Cats can go out but placed back inside before the start of the event. Owners should place litter trays and elimination pads in the room. Owners should attempt to engage with the patient using training and treats to distract it from the noise.

For acute and severe phobias, using GABAergic medications such as imepitoin, gabapentin, pregabalin or benzodiazepine is helpful. If the patient also shows a panic attack, the use of alpha-2 agonists such as dexmedetomidine or clonidine is helpful. When the patient exhibits long-term phobia or has multiple triggers, adding ongoing serotonergic medications (e.g. TCA, SSRI or SNRI) is indicated.

When the patient is calm, ideally when there are no noise events (e.g. not during thunderstorm season), a desensitization programme should be implemented. Owners can start using recorded sounds on computers or mobile phones with low volume and later increase (see Handout D13 – Desensitization – Noises). Some patients may not respond to recorded sounds (especially patients with storm phobia). In these cases, desensitization should take place during 'live' events when owners attempt to muffle the sounds.

Using tools such as ear covers, head covers, body wraps or eye covers has been advocated for both dogs and cats. However, their efficacy is not proven. Also, owners should closely observe the patient to ensure that these products do not cause more problems or possibly distract the patient by being a problem themselves. When deciding to use such a product, owners should attempt to introduce it slowly and gradually, while associating it with a positive outcome.

Early exposure through socialization may have a protective effect; puppies who were born through shooting season were less likely to develop phonophobia (Blackwell *et al.*, 2005). Owners of young kittens and puppies, and breeders, should attempt to start exposing these animals to different noises at a very young age. Screening of young animals should take place early on by asking questions and addressing owners' concerns. All animals show a startle reflex when they encounter sudden and loud noises. This is not an indication of phobia. However, when a young animal shows intense startle, which is followed by somatic changes such as prolonged tachycardia, panting or mydriasis, and behavioural avoidance, we should not only monitor it but also start basic desensitization. Monitoring alone is insufficient; being proactive is more important.

Sound volumes are measured in decibels. Any noise over 80–85 dB will cause irritation, and over the long term may cause hearing impairment. Noise over 130–140 dB can also cause pain.

13.5.3.4 Social phobia

This disorder is not well defined in veterinary psychiatry. In human psychiatry, social phobia refers to marked fear or anxiety in social situations, including interactions with other people. It is likely that veterinary patients who show intense fear and anxiety near other animals or people may have a variant of this disorder.

The patient aims to avoid any interaction with other animals (usually conspecies) or people. If it cannot avoid this, it may show tonic immobility or even catatonia. Multiple exposures to the same phobic stimulus do not help the patient to habituate. Some patients may also show a panic attack.

Management of social phobia is similar to other phobias. The starting point is avoidance, through environmental and routine modifications, and the use of medications to reduce the intensity of the response. Then a desensitization programme can follow.

13.6 Post-traumatic Stress Disorder (PTSD)

This diagnosis is controversial in veterinary psychiatry as we cannot assess the cognitive involvement in this disorder. The behaviour we see may be attributed to other phobic or anxiety disorders, especially those involving panic attacks. A key diagnostic criterion is the immediate, intense and out-of-proportion reaction following a traumatic event. A traumatic event may be rehoming, a veterinary visit, a noise event or an attack by another animal.

Unlike phobia, the patient may exhibit signs of intense fear or panic, even when the trigger is not present. This is due to endogenous factors such as memories from the event. Moreover, it is likely that during the traumatic event the patient created a memory of predicting signals (e.g. noise, sight or smell). In many cases, one predicting signal is sufficient to elicit a full reaction.

Signs of PTSD may not appear immediately following the traumatic event. It may take several weeks or longer for signs to appear. Further, the number of signs and the severity may change with time. Some patients may experience spontaneous recovery, whereas others will require life-long management. Like many other emotional disorders, some individuals are likely genetically prone to the development of PTSD.

The main goal of the patient, as evidenced by its behaviour, is to avoid the trigger. The patient may try escaping or hiding, and when it cannot, the patient may show tonic immobility. In other cases, the patient may show increased irritability and even aggression towards the trigger (when present). Commonly seen signs include displacement behaviours (see Section 7.3.3.2 – Displacement behaviours), hypervigilance, restlessness, dissociative clinical signs (e.g. disconnect from the owner and hypoaesthesia) and anorexia. When a panic attack is part of PTSD, signs such as mydriasis, tachycardia and tachypnea, trembling, salivation, diarrhoea and emesis may be seen.

13.6.1 Management

The first step is to try to avoid triggers. This is not always possible since some of the triggers are endogenous. Owners should maintain a diary, which may help to identify triggers such as locations, times, sights or sounds.

In-between episodes, owners should work with the patient on basic training and calming techniques (see Handouts C1 – Set Up to Succeed; C2 – How to Teach a 'Watch Me' and 'Touch' Cue; and C4 – Teaching a Pet How to Settle on Cue). Later, a desensitization programme should be implemented, starting with the predicting triggers.

Medications such as benzodiazepines and gabapentin are useful prior to or during an event. When PTSD is accompanied by a panic attack, adding clonidine or dexmedetomidine is beneficial. For frequent or unpredictable incidents, or for those patients who exhibit increased arousal between episodes, the use of serotonergic medications such as SSRI or TCA is indicated.

13.7 Panic

Panic is an emotional and physiological response involving intense fear and robust activation of the SAM and HPA systems. Peak effect is reached within minutes of activation. Panic in veterinary patients mostly occurs as part of anxiety disorder but can be seen in other disorders such as abnormal and repetitive behaviours (see Chapter 15), post-traumatic stress disorder (see above) and cognitive dysfunction (see Chapter 16). In these contexts, panic attacks serve as an indicator of severity and as a (poorer) prognostic factor.

It is unclear if veterinary patients have panic disorder. In human psychiatry, panic disorder is defined as 'recurrent unexpected panic attacks' and a key diagnostic is the unpredictability of attacks. It appears that in the veterinary patient, panic is mostly linked to a specific trigger (e.g. phobia or anxiety). Also, we cannot determine if the patient truly has no trigger.

Clinical signs of panic include tachycardia, tachypnea and sometimes dyspnea, mydriasis, trembling, excessive salivation (although some patients may have a dry mouth) and sweating. Some patients may have other psychosomatic signs such as diarrhoea, nausea (which may lead to vomiting), restlessness and irritability, and loss of control over bodily sphincters leading to the evacuation of the bladder or colon. The patient will attempt to escape from the situation, and when it cannot, it will show tonic immobility (freeze). Panic may also lead to hypoaesthesia (reduced pain sensation), disconnect from the owner and vocalization such as whimpering, howling or whining.

Whereas panic disorder is unpredictable, most panic attacks can be predicted based on the past responses of the patient in similar situations. When predicted, owners should attempt to avoid situations that lead to panic attacks. Administering medications at the time of a panic attack is necessary. However, administering medications pre-emptively may have a greater effect and help to facilitate learning during these situations (see below).

Differential diagnoses include physical disorders such as seizures and other neurological disorders, pain and gastrointestinal and endocrine diseases. Emotional differential diagnoses include other fears and anxieties.

13.7.1 Management

Management of panic always involves medications. The reaction is intense and limits the patient's ability to learn and execute appropriate cognitive functions. Panic leads to strong discharge of noradrenaline from the locus coeruleus and activation of noradrenergic neurons in the median raphe, periaqueductal gray, amygdala, hippocampus, anterior cingulate cortex and medial prefrontal cortex (Sobanski and Wagner, 2017). The net result is an intense activation leading to inhibition of serotonergic and GABAergic neurons. Therefore, medications that inhibit the locus coeruleus or increase the net GABA effect are the first choice to manage panic attacks.

Alpha-2 agonists such as dexmedetomidine or clonidine, or beta-blockers such as pindolol or propranolol, may be beneficial in counteracting the effect of noradrenaline. These medications can reduce the intensity of the panic the patient experiences during the event. It is best to give the medication before a known situation that may lead to a panic attack (e.g. prior to a thunderstorm or fireworks, or a veterinary visit). However, giving those once the first sign of panic is noted may be beneficial, though a higher dose is likely to be necessary.

Benzodiazepines such as alprazolam are also indicated in panic attacks. They elevate the reactivity threshold and reduce the likelihood of experiencing panic. Other GABAergic medications such as gabapentin, pregabalin or imepitoin can be used as well. When panic attacks occur frequently, serotonergic medications such as SSRI or TCA should be added.

13.8 Depression and Dysthymia

This diagnosis is controversial in veterinary psychiatry; we lack evidence about the cognitive aspect of this disorder. We do not know if our patients think about stressors and long-term prospects as humans do. We can only evaluate the behaviour we see.

Signs of depression include changes in appetite (anorexia or ravenous appetite) leading to weight changes (loss or gain), changes in sleep (insomnia or hypersomnia), withdrawal from interactions with the owners or other animals, inactivity and overall low energy. It is critical to compare the patient to its past behaviour and the normal (biological) behaviours of the species (and to a lesser degree the breed). When these signs appear most of the day and most days, over a prolonged period (e.g. months), the term dysthymia is used.

Possible causes for depression include changes in the routine or environment such as loss of a companion (animal or person), changes in routine (e.g. the owner is going back to work) and rehoming. These causes may trigger a negative emotional state, which in human psychiatry would be referred to as 'feelings of hopelessness'.

Differential diagnoses include any physical disorder that may lead to lethargy and low energy levels, for example hypothyroid, diabetes, hypoadrenocorticism, neurological and gastrointestinal disorders, and painful conditions. Anxiety disorders and cognitive decline are also among possible differential diagnoses.

13.8.1 Management

Given that patients with depression are withdrawn and tend to avoid interactions, the first step is not to force them to interact. It is a common mistake; owners want to encourage the patient to interact but do so with higher intensity or frequency than the patient can manage. Therefore, a slow and gradual approach is necessary. Using marker training (see Handout C6 – Marker Training) can be beneficial in encouraging the patient to continue showing desired behaviours and shaping the response as the patient starts showing these behaviours more frequently. For example, the owner may mark the desired behaviour each time the cat walks into the room. Once the cat walks into the room more frequently, possibly in anticipation of a treat, the owner stops marking as soon as the cat enters the room and starts marking when the cat stays in the room for a short period. Later, the owner marks only when the cat approaches the owner. To increase the likelihood of the patient showing the desired behaviour, owners can set up these sessions (see Handout C1 – Set Up to Succeed).

Owners may try to train and play with the patient. High obedience level is not the goal; it is the interaction and engagement with the patient. Owners may feed through training and play instead of meals, and use high-value treats to maintain the patient's engagement level. Providing a consistent daily routine and environment helps the patient to gain more control over its life, for example by approaching the owner at designated meal- or playtimes or going to the door when it is time for a walk. This may reduce the 'feeling of hopelessness'.

When signs of depression last several weeks and environmental and behaviour modification techniques are not successful in ameliorating the signs, medications are indicated. Similar to most other emotional disorders, serotonin plays a crucial role in depressive disorder. Unlike anxiety disorders, the level of noradrenalin may be low in depression, leading to apathy and withdrawal. The use of SSRI or SNRI is considered the first line of medications. TCA and other serotonergic medications may be useful as well.

Since the level of prolactin increases in chronic depression (dysthymia), the use of MAOIs such as selegiline or DRI such as bupropion may be useful (Pageat *et al.*, 2007). The use of mirtazapine is indicated in patients with anorexia. It can be added to other serotonergic medications (Argüelles *et al.*, 2017).

References

Argüelles, J., Enriquez, J., Bowen, J. and Fatjó, J. (2017) Mirtazapine as a potential drug to treat social fears in dogs: five case examples. In: Denenberg, S. (ed.) *Proceedings of the 11th International Veterinary Behaviour Meeting*. CAB International, Wallingford, UK, pp. 84–85.

Blackwell, E., Casey, R. and Bradshaw, J. (2005) *Firework Fears and Phobias in the Domestic Dog*. RSPCA, Horsham, UK.

Blackwell, E.J., Bradshaw, J.W.S. and Casey, R.A. (2013) Fear responses to noises in domestic dogs: prevalence, risk factors and co-occurrence with other fear related behaviour. *Applied Animal Behaviour Science* 145(1-2), 15–25. DOI: 10.1016/j.applanim.2012.12.004.

Bowen, J., Calvo, P., Bulbena, A. and Fatjó, J. (2013) Clinical characterisation of noise sensitivity in dogs. *Journal of Veterinary Behavior* 8(4), e44. DOI: 10.1016/j.jveb.2013.04.058.

Chen, B., Dowlatshahi, D., MacQueen, G.M., Wang, J.F. and Young, L.T. (2001) Increased hippocampal BDNF immunoreactivity in subjects treated with antidepressant medication. *Biological Psychiatry* 50(4), 260–265. DOI: 10.1016/S0006-3223(01)01083-6.

Dale, A.R., Walker, J.K., Farnworth, M.J., Morrissey, S.V. and Waran, N.K. (2010) A survey of owners' perceptions of fear of fireworks in a sample of dogs and cats in New Zealand. *New Zealand Veterinary Journal* 58(6), 286–291. DOI: 10.1080/00480169.2010.69403.

Driscoll, C.A., Menotti-Raymond, M., Roca, A.L., Hupe, K., Johnson, W.E. *et al.* (2007) The near eastern origin of cat domestication. *Science* 317(5837), 519–523. DOI: 10.1126/science.1139518.

Jakovcevic, A., Elgier, A.M., Mustaca, A.E. and Bentosela, M. (2013) Frustration behaviors in domestic dogs. *Journal of Applied Animal Welfare Science* 16(1), 19–34. DOI: 10.1080/10888705.2013.740974.

Kuma, H., Miki, T., Matsumoto, Y., Gu, H., Li, H.-P. *et al.* (2004) Early maternal deprivation induces alterations in brain-derived neurotrophic factor expression in the developing rat hippocampus. *Neuroscience Letters* 372(1-2), 68–73. DOI: 10.1016/j.neulet.2004.09.012.

Lopes Fagundes, A.L., Hewison, L., McPeake, K.J., Zulch, H. and Mills, D.S. (2018) Noise sensitivities in dogs: an exploration of signs in dogs with and without musculoskeletal pain using qualitative content analysis. *Frontiers in Veterinary Science* 5, 17. DOI: 10.3389/fvets.2018.00017.

Mahar, I., Bambico, F.R., Mechawar, N. and Nobrega, J.N. (2014) Stress, serotonin, and hippocampal neurogenesis in relation to depression and antidepressant effects. *Neuroscience & Biobehavioral Reviews* 38, 173–192. DOI: 10.1016/j.neubiorev.2013.11.009.

McPeake, K.J., Collins, L.M., Zulch, H. and Mills, D.S. (2019) The canine frustration questionnaire: development of a new psychometric tool for measuring frustration in domestic dogs (*Canis familiaris*). *Frontiers in veterinary science* 6(152). DOI: 10.3389/fvets.2019.00152.

Moesta, A., Kim, G., Wilson-Frank, C.R., Weng, H.Y. and Ogata, N. (2019) Comparison of serum brain-derived neurotrophic factor in dogs with or without separation anxiety. *Journal of Veterinary Behavior; Clinical Applications and Research* 35, 14–18.

Pageat, P., Lafont, C., Falewée, C., Bonnafous, L., Gaultier, E. *et al*. (2007) An evaluation of serum prolactin in anxious dogs and response to treatment with selegiline or fluoxetine. *Applied Animal Behaviour Science* 105(4), 342–350. DOI: 10.1016/j.applanim.2006.11.004.

Sobanksi, T. and Wagner, G. (2017) Functional neuroanatomy in panic disorder: status quo of the research. *World Journal of Psychiatry* 7(10), 12–33. DOI: 10.5498/wjp.v7.i1.12.

Stephen, J.M. and Ledger, R.A. (2005) An audit of behavioral indicators of poor welfare in kenneled dogs in the United Kingdom. *Journal of Applied Animal Welfare Science* 8(2), 79–95. DOI: 10.1207/s15327604jaws0802_1.

Storengen, L.M. and Lingaas, F. (2015) Noise sensitivity in 17 dog breeds: prevalence, breed risk and correlation with fear in other situations. *Applied Animal Behaviour Science* 171, 152–160. DOI: 10.1016/j.applanim.2015.08.020.

Tiira, K., Sulkama, S. and Lohi, H. (2016) Prevalence, comorbidity, and behavioral variation in canine anxiety. *Journal of Veterinary Behavior* 16, 36–44. DOI: 10.1016/j.jveb.2016.06.008.

Vitale, K.R., Behnke, A.C. and Udell, M.A.R. (2019) Attachment bonds between domestic cats and humans. *Current Biology* 29(18), R864–R865. DOI: 10.1016/j.cub.2019.08.036.

14 Elimination Problems in Cats and Dogs

Sagi Denenberg*

Langford Vets, University of Bristol, Langford, UK; North Toronto Veterinary Behaviour Specialty Clinic, Toronto, Canada

14.1 Introduction

Inappropriate elimination (also referred to as house soiling by different sources) in cats and dogs is a common presentation in veterinary surgeries and referral centres and may lead to relinquishment or euthanasia (Salman *et al.*, 2000; Denenberg *et al.*, 2005). Elimination is a normal physiological function of disposing of waste products, and part of communication behaviour in cats and dogs (Carney *et al.*, 2014; Lisberg and Snowdon, 2014).

Elimination in 'inappropriate' locations should be divided into normal but unacceptable (for the owner), and pathological elimination. The former requires training and providing optimal routine and environment while the latter requires behaviour modification, medications and, possibly, surgical intervention.

There are different terms used to describe the different presentations, with no agreement between sources. To avoid confusion, in this text we use the term inappropriate elimination to describe both urine and faecal elimination (regardless of the underlying reason) in undesired locations. Further, we use the terms *periuria* and *perichezia* to describe urine and faeces elimination, respectively, for any reason in undesired locations. Both periuria and perichezia can be further divided into marking behaviour (communication) and inappropriate latrine behaviour (eliminating waste products).

14.1.1 Training

Young animals or animals in new environments (e.g. following a move to a new house) must learn where to eliminate. From the animal's point of view, elimination is appropriate in any location that is not its feeding or sleeping area. Therefore, unless the owner provides the animal with ideal conditions (routine and location), it may eliminate in areas the owner considers inappropriate. (See also Sections 6.5.1 – Litter trays; and 6.6.1 – House training.)

14.1.1.1 Training cats

Many owners assume that cats naturally know to use litter trays. While the cat's normal behaviour is to look for surfaces to dig and later bury their urine or faeces, and in most cases very little intervention is required, the owner must still condition the cat to the tray or area. Owners should take kittens to the litter tray and place them there several times daily. The tray should be in an easily accessible area, especially for kittens, and they should be able to walk into the tray. If the kitten soils outside the tray, the owner can transfer the faeces or urine-soaked paper towel into the litter tray to draw the kitten to use it in the future. The kitten should be rewarded once it has soiled in the tray. The litter should be scooped and refreshed daily, and the tray cleaned weekly. For more information on litter tray training, see Handout C8 – Litter Tray Training.

Owners should attempt to reward the kitten when it uses the litter tray. A marker is an excellent tool for this purpose (see Handout C6 – Marker Training). Punishment should be avoided; it is only likely to teach the kitten to eliminate when the owner is not present. If the kitten is consistently eliminating outside the tray, owners should consider confinement in a small area with food and water, bed and litter tray. It may help the kitten to learn to

*s.denenberg@bristol.ac.uk

DOI: 10.1079/9781786394552.0014

use the tray rather than other areas. Confinement should not be used instead of supervision and meeting the kitten's needs.

Providing several options (e.g. different boxes, locations or litters) can help to promote the kitten to choose its preferred location and use the tray more frequently. Allowing kittens outdoors (supervised initially) is helpful – most cats with outdoor access will eliminate outside almost exclusively. Finally, owners should ensure that no other animal in the home is blocking the way or limiting the access of the kitten to the tray.

14.1.1.2 Training dogs

Training in dogs should follow similar guidelines. Most dog owners prefer their dogs to eliminate outdoors, and dogs do not have the same preferences as cats; hence the initial training might be more time- and effort-consuming. Like cats, dogs prefer not to eliminate near their feeding or sleeping area.

The key to successful training is guiding the dog to appropriate elimination areas and rewarding it when it soils there. Unfortunately, many owners still use punishment (e.g. reprimanding or pushing the dog's nose into the excrement). While punishment may teach the dog not to eliminate in specific areas it may increase anxiety and fear and avoidance of the owner, teach the dog to eliminate while the owner is not present, and possibly lead to aggression towards the owner. Below are some simple guidelines to train dogs to eliminate in appropriate locations (see Handout C9 – Housetraining Your Puppy). These guidelines apply to puppies and adults alike, keeping in mind that puppies have a lower ability to hold the urine and faeces and may need to eliminate more frequently.

- Crate/room: when owners cannot supervise the puppy, they should confine it in a small area with food and water and a bed – dogs prefer not to eliminate close to their resources. Confinement is not a replacement for training and supervision (see below) and should be used sparingly. The area should be large enough for the puppy to walk inside, stand, turn around, and lie comfortably. Also, it should have sufficient space for food and water and toys. Placing an appeasing pheromone diffuser in the area might be helpful to create a calm and positive environment. It is important to note that puppies that were confined for extended periods (e.g. puppy mill, shelters or pet shop) before adoption may soil in their crate and even lie in it. This is a pathology forced on the puppy due to poor environmental conditions and routine. These puppies should not be confined, or confined only for short periods each time.
- Routine: owners should design a daily routine that meets the puppy's needs (e.g. feeding, play and exercise, sleep and rest, social interactions and elimination). The routine should include ample opportunities to eliminate in appropriate locations. Only once the owner ensures that the puppy's needs, except sleep and food, are met, can they confine the puppy. Feeding and sleep times help in the regulation of the gastrointestinal and urinary systems so the owners can predict when the puppy will need to eliminate. Puppies will need to eliminate approximately five to ten minutes after playing or training, and less than that after waking up. Owners should be ready to take the puppy to their preferred location (e.g. garden or indoor toilet area) based on these timeframes. The average transition time of solid diets, in a puppy, is two hours. Therefore, owners should take the puppy out approximately two hours after a solid meal.
- Supervision: when the puppy is allowed out of its crate or room, as part of the daily routine, owners should supervise it. Owners must keep in mind that it only takes a few seconds for the puppy to eliminate. Therefore, supervision means that owners must keep their eye on the puppy. Owners can attach a long leash from their belt or waist to the puppy so that they can ensure the puppy comes with them wherever they go. Most puppies will show signs of impending elimination; they will become restless, sniff the floor or along the walls, circle, try leaving the area, and squat. As soon as the owners recognize these signs, they should distract the puppy (e.g. calling its name or clapping hands), and then take the puppy outside. Ideally, owners should follow the puppy outside to ensure it eliminates. If the puppy did not eliminate and then is brought back inside, the owners should supervise it or place it back in its area. However, within 10–15 minutes, they should take the puppy back out again. Once the puppy eliminates, owners can allow it to be free around the house until the next anticipated elimination time. Owners can also allow the puppy to be free for a while, and then place it back in its space for rest, food or chew.

- Teach desired location: elimination is a normal behaviour and a physiological need. Punishing a puppy when it eliminates is likely to cause more problems than solve them. If the puppy has eliminated at home, it would be best if the owner ignored it. It should serve as a learning experience to the owner to supervise the puppy at those times or areas or use confinement. Owners should clean the area thoroughly using biological cleaners and possibly spraying it with a pheromone product. Instead of punishment, owners should reward the puppy when it eliminates in the desired location. A marker is an excellent tool to signal the desired behaviour and provide a reward (see Handout C6 – Marker Training). It is possible to train puppies to eliminate on a signal. Timing is important for a successful outcome. The owner should follow the puppy to the elimination area. As soon as the puppy is about to eliminate, the owner should give a verbal signal, and provide a reward once the puppy has finished. With sufficient repetitions, the puppy may learn the signal. Then owners can take the puppy out before confinement, car travel or sleep and give the puppy the signal. Also, owners can reinforce requests to go outside to eliminate. Many puppies and dogs learn after some time to go to the exits or the owner when they need to eliminate. Owners can reinforce these behaviours by taking the puppy outside and even providing a treat once the puppy eliminates. These consequences will reinforce the 'asking' behaviour the puppy shows. Placing a bell on the door, especially if the puppy scratches it, may help in training the puppy to alert the owners when it needs to go outside to eliminate. Owners should note that some puppies learn that these are signals to go outside, not necessarily to eliminate. If this behaviour is problematic for the owner, they can ignore the puppy at times when they are certain the puppy does not need to eliminate (e.g. shortly after elimination). Placing a flap door to allow puppies to go outside independently from the owner may be helpful.

14.1.2 Ruling out physical disorder

When presented with a patient with a complaint of inappropriate elimination, especially if the patient was well trained prior to presentation, the possibility of physical pathology must be investigated. Many painful, neurological, gastrointestinal and urological diseases can cause inappropriate elimination. For more information, see Chapters 2 and 3. Puppies and kittens that appear refractory to house training should be investigated as well. The underlying cause might be a physical pathology. Tables 14.1 and 14.2 show the most common causes of inappropriate elimination in cats and dogs, respectively.

A full physical examination, urinalysis, blood analysis and stool sample should be performed on each patient presenting with inappropriate elimination. Since physical pathologies could be intermittent, it is important to remember that normal results of physical examination or laboratory tests do not completely exclude underlying physical pathology. Therefore, owners should be encouraged to proceed with these steps as soon as the pet starts eliminating in inappropriate locations.

Physical pathology might be an inciting factor, but not necessarily a maintaining factor. For example, transient pain or infection may lead to elimination outside the litter tray. The cat may be treated for this pathology but persist in eliminating outside the tray due to learning (e.g. the litter tray might be conditioned with pain or discomfort). Moreover, physical pathologies might be both the inciting and maintaining factors, and continuous treatment may be required alongside environmental and behavioural management. For example, a dog may develop diabetes mellitus and start eliminating inside the house. The dog will require life-long care for diabetes. The dog still might eliminate inappropriately while the disease is not well regulated. Also, the dog may learn to soil at home as emptying a full bladder provides a relief (reward feeling).

14.1.3 Hygiene

It is essential to remember that at the root of the problem (after ruling out physical and psychiatric disorders) is the word 'inappropriate'. What is appropriate for the animal may not be appropriate for the owner and vice versa. When owners decide where it is appropriate for their pet to eliminate, they must take into account the animal's needs.

Like us, animals prefer a clean latrine and, ideally (unless it is a form of communication), a quiet area. Owners should place litter trays in areas with minimal traffic or behind a visual barrier. Similarly, elimination areas for dogs should be easily accessed.

Possibly, animals avoid the heavily soiled area due to parasites and disease spreading. Cleaning the

Table 14.1. Examples of physical pathologies leading to inappropriate elimination in cats. These diseases are often accompanied by signs other than elimination. It is important to rule these out before addressing a possible mental or emotional disorder. Some of these diseases may need to be managed life-long alongside psychiatric disorder. These diseases may be the inciting cause, but not always a maintaining factor.

Pathology	Elimination	Other signs
Pain: Dermatological (e.g. pododermatitis, anal sacculitis) Gastrointestinal Musculoskeletal Neuropathic Urological	Urine and faeces	Vocalization, inactivity, licking excessively, anorexia, aggression, pain when squatting
Neurological: Cognitive dysfunction Degenerative CNS disease Infections Neuromuscular (e.g. incontinence) Sensory decline Tumours	Urine and faeces	Related to the specific pathology Aimless walking, circling, head tilt, vocalization, anorexia, urination and defecation where resting
Gastrointestinal: Colitis Constipation Pathologies leading to polyphagia Pancreatitis	Faeces	Diarrhoea, increased frequency and volume, haematochezia, steatorrhoea, urgency, polyphagia, pain when passing faeces
Urological: Feline interstitial cystitis Incontinence Infections Renal insufficiency Urinary calculi	Urine	Pain when urinating, urgency, urinating when sleeping, haematuria, vocalization, excessive licking of genitals Polyuria and polydipsia
Metabolic: Diabetes Insipidus Diabetes Mellitus Hyperthyroidism Hepatic disease	Urine and faeces	Polyuria and polyphagia, weight loss, vocalization, restlessness and increased activity, dull coat

area regularly by scooping the litter or picking up and removing excrement is necessary to maintain cleanliness. If using litter trays, changing the litter and washing the tray should be done regularly. The frequency depends on the number of animals using the tray or area. Covered litter trays may appeal to owners; however, ammonia vapours may remain inside and even adhere to the cover. This may decrease the appeal of the tray. Boxes should be opened regularly to ventilate.

14.2 Elimination Problems in Cats

Cats are fastidious about their elimination routines and locations. Cats may soil outside these locations due to physical pathologies, changes in preferences or development of aversions, and anxiety disorders.

It is important to note that elimination, primarily urine, is also a form of communication, and therefore may be normal but unacceptable (Carney *et al.*, 2014). The prevalence of inappropriate elimination appears to be higher in urban areas than in rural communities or where cats are allowed to go outdoors (Denenberg, 2019, unpublished data). When cats have free access outdoors, they may mark their territory using urine; however, owners may miss this behaviour as it is not causing an indoor problem. In large urban areas, the prevalence reaches nearly 60% and involves primarily aversion to the owner's designated

Table 14.2. Examples of physical pathologies leading to inappropriate elimination in dogs. These diseases are often accompanied by signs other than elimination. It is important to rule these out before addressing a possible mental or emotional disorder. Some of these diseases may need to be managed life-long alongside psychiatric disorder. These diseases may be the inciting cause, but not always a maintaining factor.

Pathology	Elimination	Other signs
Pain: Dermatological (e.g. pododermatitis, discoid lupus, anal sacculitis) Gastrointestinal (e.g. inflammatory bowel disease, acid reflux) Musculoskeletal Neuropathic Urological	Urine and faeces	Vocalization, anorexia, insomnia, limping, licking excessively, attention-seeking, aggression Signs related to the specific disease
Neurological: Cognitive dysfunction Degenerative disease Encephalitis hepatoencephalopathy Infections neuromuscular Tumour	Urine and faeces	Circling, pacing, head tilt, vocalization, aimless walking, vomiting, head pressing Signs related to the specific pathology
Gastrointestinal: Colitis Constipation Exocrine pancreatic insufficiency Infections Inflammatory bowel disease Pancreatitis	Faeces	Increased frequency and volume, diarrhoea, steatorrhoea, haematochezia, urgency, vomiting
Urological: Calculi Cystitis Incontinence Infections (e.g. pyelonephritis, UTI) Renal disease	Urine	Vocalization, increased frequency and urgency, changes in volume, polyuria and polydipsia, changes related to the specific pathology
Metabolic: Diabetes Insipidus Diabetes Mellitus Hyperadrenocorticism Hepatic dysfunction	Urine and faeces	Aggression, anxiety, apathy, polydipsia and polyuria, polyphagia, changes specific to the pathology

location or substrate (Denenberg *et al.*, 2005; Amat *et al.*, 2009).

14.2.1 Diagnosis

Considering how prevalent and important this presentation is, and the potentially dire consequences (relinquishment or euthanasia), it is surprising that no clear algorithm exists to diagnose the underlying pathology. Fig. 14.1 attempts to give such an algorithm. It is important to remember that this algorithm offers help in approaching a patient with inappropriate elimination. However, other factors, such as other coexisting psychiatric disorders, social interactions, environment and litter tray hygiene, should be considered. There are many reported signs and risk factors; however, many have only weak evidence to support them (Barcelos *et al.*, 2018). Moreover, about a third of veterinarians in first-opinion practices are not able to make a diagnosis based on these signs (Bergman *et al.*, 2002).

While it is accepted by many that physical disorders such as urinary tract diseases are closely linked to inappropriate elimination, it is prudent to remember that any such link might be anecdotal. Several studies have pointed to physical disorders as risk factors, while others did not find any such

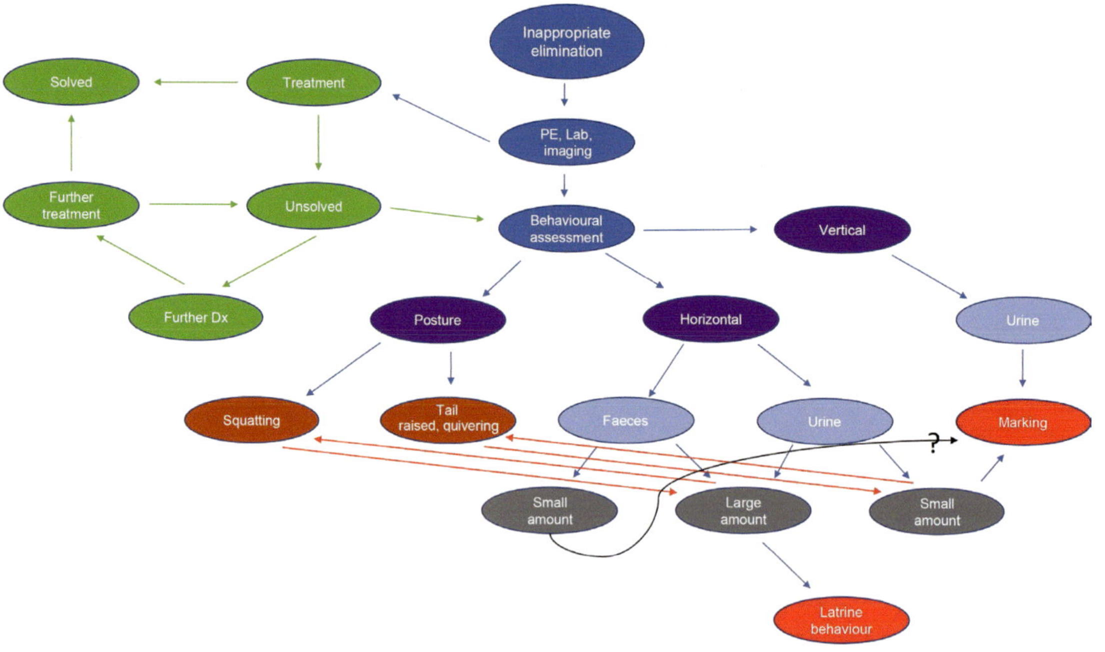

Fig. 14.1. A suggested algorithm for the diagnosis of inappropriate elimination in cats. This algorithm focuses only on the behaviour of the patient, the surface and deposits. It does not take into account other psychiatric pathologies, social interactions and owners' responses. Following this algorithm helps guide the clinician. However, the final diagnosis should be established when considering all factors.

relationship (Horwitz, 1997; Frank *et al.*, 1999; Tynes *et al.*, 2003; Barcelos *et al.*, 2018). Therefore, each patient presented for inappropriate elimination should be thoroughly screened for possible physical pathologies. At the same time, when physical pathologies exist, they may be unrelated to inappropriate elimination, and their treatment may not solve the problem.

14.2.1.1 Physical pathologies

When presented with a patient that is eliminating in the home, we first must rule out physical disease. A full physical examination and laboratory tests such as urinalysis or imaging, such as abdominal radiographs, are the first steps to take. The owner's history and, possibly, video of the patient eliminating may help as well. We must look for indications of pain leading to house soiling; chronic pain may not be evident during physical examination (see Chapter 3). Patients in pain will not only avoid the litter tray but also avoid other situations or behaviours. They may not jump onto perches, avoid contact, hide and show aggression. When not sure, we can ask the owners to capture footage of the patient during regular activities (see Handout A8 – Pain Assessment).

14.2.1.2 Behavioural analysis

Once we rule out physical disorders, we should focus on the behaviour of the patient in order to establish a diagnosis. If not already available at the time of presentation, owners should maintain a diary of the patient's elimination. Try recording details such as posture, elimination behaviour, surfaces and location, type of and quantity of elimination, frequency and the owner's reaction. The diary is valuable for both diagnosis and designing a management plan. Maintaining the diary long term may also help to assess progress.

- Posture: a description of the patient when it eliminates could be helpful. Other than possible pain, posture can help in identifying the underlying pathology. For example, a patient that is squatting with a slightly raised tail may show preferences of aversions leading to inappropriate

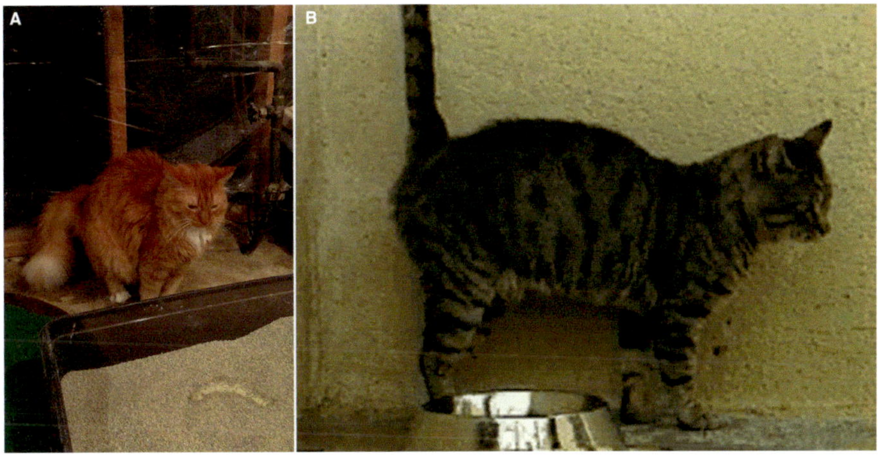

Fig. 14.2. A cat who is presented with inappropriate latrine behaviour is likely to show normal elimination posture including squatting with semi-raised tail and depositing urine or faeces on horizontal surfaces (A). A cat who is marking is likely to back onto a vertical surface and spray small amounts of urine (B). It is important to remember that these descriptions are suggestive but not an absolute diagnosis. (Photos courtesy of Sagi Denenberg.)

latrine behaviour (see Fig. 14.2A), whereas a cat that backs onto a wall and raises its tail may be marking (see Fig. 14.2B).

- Elimination behaviour: when possible, owners should attempt to describe the patient eliminating. Paying attention to signs such as attempts to bury faeces, sniffing the area before and after elimination, circling, running away, or depositing other scents (e.g. kneading or bunting) is helpful. Marking patients are likely to back onto a vertical surface, deposit a small amount of urine (and rarely faeces) and then possibly also knead. Their tail is likely to quiver. Patients with inappropriate latrine behaviour are likely to circle the area, sniff it, attempt to bury it and walk away from the area.
- The surface on which the patient eliminates may indicate the underlying cause. Deposits on a vertical surface are likely to indicate marking, while horizontal surfaces are more likely to indicate inappropriate latrine behaviour. As mentioned before, these signs are suggestive but not diagnostic on their own. The patient may attempt to deposit urine on a wall and miss. Similarly, the patient may mark new scents or the owner's personal belongings (e.g. shoes, bag or bed), and deposit urine on horizontal surfaces.
- Type and quantity: latrine behaviour includes both urine and faeces, and the amount is usually large (e.g. a full bladder or colon evacuation). Marking is primarily urine (rarely faeces, also known as *middening*). Marking behaviour is mostly small amounts of urine.
- Social interactions: questions should include interactions with the owners and other animals in the home (if applicable). Again, video of the cat interacting with other animals in the house is useful. One of the risk factors, leading to inappropriate elimination in cats, is a multi-cat household (Pryor *et al.*, 2001). However, the number of cats in the house (apart from the patient) appears to be irrelevant as long as there is at least one more (Barcelos *et al.*, 2018). Any disruption of a solitary lifestyle may be a trigger. Multi-cat households were over-represented in both cases of periuria and perichezia, possibly indicating that it is not only anxiety but also competition over resources that contributes to inappropriate elimination. Owners may miss subtle signs of conflict or even covert aggression. Similarly, a cat may avoid its litter tray (or outdoor elimination area) due to a dog or children in the house. If there are other cats in the home, we should inquire about their toileting routine. For example, some cats use a specific litter tray exclusively, while leaving the others.
- Environment: gathering details about the patient's environment can help in making a diagnosis. When a house visit or videos and photos of the environment are not an option, a

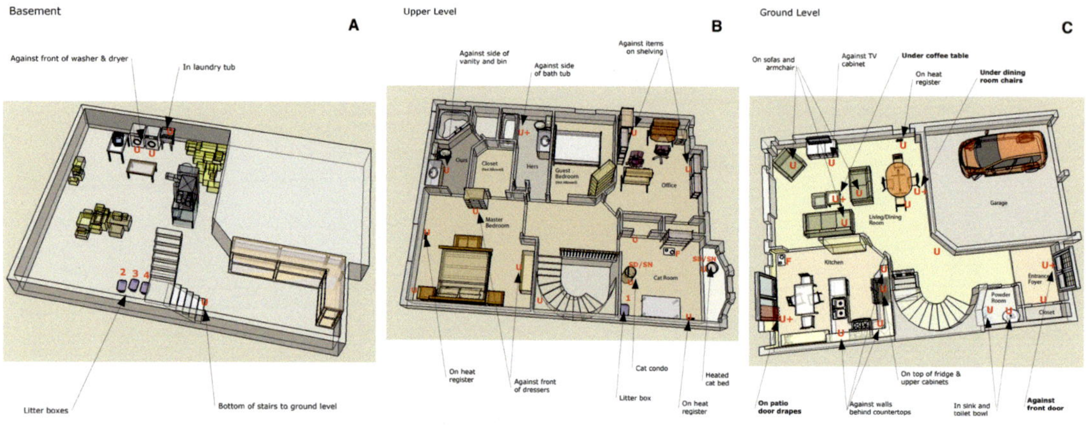

Fig. 14.3. Owners can bring a plan of their home to show where the cat is soiling. It is helpful if owners also indicate where the patient sleeps, plays, eats, perches or hides. All levels of the home should be mapped. Owners can use the following key: F – food, P –perching, R – resting place, S – stools, SD – sleeps during the day, SN – sleeps during the night, U – urine, W – water. (Photos courtesy of Sagi Denenberg.)

description of the patient's environment including litter tray, where it soils, sleeping and eating area, perches, and outdoors (if it has access or watches the garden) helps in differentiating between the different diagnoses (see Fig. 14.3). As part of the physical environment review, we should ask about resources such as food, water, sleeping area and toys.

- Litter trays: we should gather details about the number, locations, types of tray and litter, and cleaning routines. The number of litter trays and their type does not appear to be a contributing risk factor. However, cleanliness is a major factor; cats appear to avoid litters that are contaminated with urine or faeces (Ellis *et al.*, 2017).
- Changes: any changes (before and after the problem started) to the household, including environment, people and other animals, should be noted. In addition, changes in routine, feeding, litter tray (number, locations, shape and size, and litter) should be noted.

14.2.1.3 Development

Like many other problems, inappropriate elimination tends to follow a development curve. It is important to ask the owner about possible inciting factors and maintaining factors. Owners will not always know the answers; however, any information may be helpful. We should try to identify any events, changes or diseases that occurred before the patient started eliminating in inappropriate locations. Next, we should inquire about any changes that occurred since the problem first appeared. For example, has the patient developed a new elimination pattern? Is it more frequent? Has the volume of urine or stool changed? Are there new locations? Reviewing any factors that may maintain the problem helps in designing a management programme that may eliminate those. Among these factors, the owner's response (e.g. reaction to the patient, cleaning soiled areas, and past efforts to correct the situation) are among the most common maintaining factors.

14.2.1.4 Identifying the soiling patient

In a multi-cat household, the diagnosis might be complicated. At times, the owners do not know which the soiling cat is, or more than one cat may soil. In this case, there are several options to identify the soiling cat. If the owners still are unable to identify the soiling cat, or there are more than one that soils, treatment should apply to all. Identifying the soiling cat can be done in several ways; however, the best way is observation (direct or using cameras).

The owners can separate the cats, primarily confining the one they suspect is inappropriately eliminating. The length of separation depends on the frequency of soiling. For example, if the owners find evidence of inappropriate elimination only once a week, then at least two weeks of separation are necessary. Separation may not help as changing the routine, environment and dynamic in the household may change the patient's behaviour. If the reason for the problem is negative social interactions between the cats in the house, separation might benefit the cats, reducing the likelihood of inappropriate elimination (which may resume upon reintroducing the cats). Also, separation may cause the opposite effect, leading to increased anxiety and fear-related problems. This, in turn, may lead to a higher chance of inappropriate elimination by other cats in the home.

Owners can administer fluorescein orally (2.5–5 ml of the ocular drops or mix 4–6 strips with soft food). Fluorescein passes through the kidneys and is eliminated in the urine. Owners should follow the patient's urination for 24 hours, using an ultraviolet lamp to detect fluorescence residue in the urine. This method is not 'bulletproof' as the fluorescein concentration in the urine may be low, or it may be neutralized by acidic urine (Neilson, 2004). In both cases, it will not fluorescence. Non-toxic shavings from children's paints may be detected in the patient's faeces.

14.2.2 Marking behaviour

Marking is a way of communication. Cats mark using urine, and secrete from different glands such as anal, cheek and interdigital glands (Borchelt and Voith, 1996). It is used by both male and female, mostly intact. Cats mark their territory to avoid conflicts between different individuals, inform about reproductive status (e.g. female in oestrus), and during a conflict. Cats use both urine and faeces to mark, although the latter is very infrequent.

When a patient is presented with periuria or perichezia, the first step is to rule out physical disorders. Once these are ruled out or managed, the next step is to differentiate marking from inappropriate latrine behaviour. We should look for signs beyond the urination (and, rarely, defecation) behaviours. Noting other signs of psychiatric disorders such as anxiety, phobia or conflicts may help in diagnosing the correct underlying disorder. Emotional urination and defecation as a result of anxiety, chronic distress or phobias are also known as *enuresis* and *encopresis*, respectively. Cats who are described as relaxed by their owners are about one third less likely to urine-mark (Barcelos *et al.*, 2018). The exact purpose of marking is unclear. Possible reasons include self-assuring or comforting behaviour, attempts to deter rivals and threats, or displacement behaviour.

The term 'urine spraying' is sometimes used to describe urine marking behaviour. However, the pathognomonic behaviour (i.e. backing onto a vertical surface with raised and quivering tail while spraying a small amount of urine) may not be present in all urine-marking situations. The marking cat may deposit larger amounts of urine onto a horizontal surface such as visitors' shoes, or its owner's bed or clothing, and other animals' beds. Similarly, when we find small amounts of faeces in similar locations, the possibility of middening (faeces marking) should be considered. It is important to note that the correlation between urine marking and faeces marking is poor. In other words, a patient who is urine marking, unlike latrine behaviour, is not more likely to also faeces mark.

Unlike latrine behaviours (see Section 14.2.3), marking behaviour may appear disorganized. The frequency, location and amounts vary depending on the underlying psychiatric disorder. One clue is the location and its significance to the cat. Marking behaviour tends to occur around windows and doors, personal belongings (the owner's), other animals or the patient itself. The patient is likely to continue using the litter tray alongside marking.

Marking may be a sexually dimorphic behaviour (that is, gender related); data suggest that males are more commonly represented in this category. However, more recent data did not show any such connection (Barcelos *et al.*, 2018). Also, the behaviour might be influenced by gonadal hormones as intact patients (both male and female) are over-represented (Bradshaw and Cameron-Beaumont, 2000). Male patients living with females are more likely to show marking behaviour compared to male patients living with other males (Hart and Cooper, 1984).

14.2.2.1 Management

Management is aimed at eliminating or controlling the underlying psychiatric disorder leading to marking behaviour. Owners must be advised that a combined (behavioural, environmental and routine) approach is necessary.

The first step is to address any conflict between the patient and other animals or people in the home (or outside). A common observation by many owners is that an outdoor cat is a trigger (Pryor *et al.*, 2001). Owners should attempt to manage such conflict. When the conflict is with a different cat in the home, the owners should start by separating the cats. Ideally, the patient and the other cat each have their own separate area (e.g. different rooms). The owners should provide all their needs (e.g. food, water, litter, toys and affection) in those rooms. The rest of the house should be used as a timeshare area; that is, owners should confine one cat and allow the other to roam the house. When they want to allow the second cat out, they must confine the first cat and only then allow the second one out. Once the owners establish safety and can reduce the conflict between the cats (by using prevention), a desensitization programme can be designed. The goal is to re-establish positive interactions between the cats in question. For more information on the management of conflicts in a multi-cat household, see Section 11.7 – Aggression as a Sign of Psychiatric Disorder.

When the conflict is with an outdoor animal, owners should try to avoid the situation. When possible, owners should prevent access of outdoor animals into their garden. Using higher fences is helpful but not always possible. The use of booby traps might be beneficial; however, the risk versus the benefits should be carefully considered. If the patient is going outdoors freely (e.g. using a cat flap), it may be affected by these traps as well, and possibly develop more anxiety or phobias. If blocking outdoor animals' access is not possible, then attempts should be made to prevent the patient from seeing those animals. Owners should try to limit the access of the patient to areas where it can watch the garden, close the curtains or blinds, and even frost part of the window. Allowing the patient freely outdoors may increase stimulation and opportunities to eliminate outside. However, free access (e.g. using a cat flap) is also associated with an increased risk of marking behaviour (Barcelos *et al.*, 2018). A good (although more time-consuming) compromise is to allow the patient outdoors under supervision.

When the trigger of enuresis and encopresis is the owners or other people, an approach of prevention and behaviour modification should be implemented. Owners should ensure that they meet the patient's needs. These needs include not only food, water, litter tray, toys and sleeping area, but also stimulation and attention. A daily routine should be set, including times that owners interact with their cats, ideally using toys and affection, and times when the patient is left alone to rest and sleep. The patient should have designated sleeping areas where it can be left alone in a calm, quiet and relatively dark environment that promotes sleep. Owners should not 'force' the patient to have attention. When the patient appears aroused (e.g. dilated pupils, swatting tail, piloerection, or tense body) it should be left alone.

Many owners provide indoor cats with access to view outdoor birdfeeders. Unfortunately, this is more likely to cause frustration in a predator that is unable to exercise its genetics. This frustration may translate to more disorders and should be avoided. Instead, owners should use feeding toys, chase toys and three-dimensional spaces (e.g. shelves or closets) to stimulate the patient. The patient should also have hiding places with two accesses so it can avoid oncoming people or other animals in the home.

When visitors to the patient's environment are the trigger, owners should manage the patient's routine and environment. The patient should have its safe space and should be placed there before visitors arrive.

If the patient is marking the same areas frequently, owners can try to prevent access or change the function of the area. First, they should clean the area thoroughly using biological cleaners or diluted bleach products. Preventing access using a booby trap, a closing door, double-sided sticky tape, or other deterrents should be considered carefully. This approach may not only increase anxiety in an already anxious patient, but also it may only teach the patient to use different locations. Using the area as a feeding station or sleeping area might be helpful, and less likely to increase anxiety. The use of pheromone products, although controversial by some authors, was found to be effective in the management of marking behaviours (Mills *et al.*, 2013). Spraying the area with feline facial pheromone or placing a nearby diffuser may reduce the patient's anxiety and promote more calmness. Providing a litter tray in the area may encourage the patient to use it. While many owners dislike having a litter tray in many of those areas, a simple reminder that a litter tray is easier to clean than a carpet or windowsill should suffice in most cases. Ideally, these measures are not life-long but short-term. If the cat is spraying urine onto vertical spaces, two litter trays can be used; one horizontally and the other placed inside the first one in a vertical position protecting the wall (see Fig. 14.4).

Litter trays should be placed in areas acceptable to both the owner and the patient. The litter should

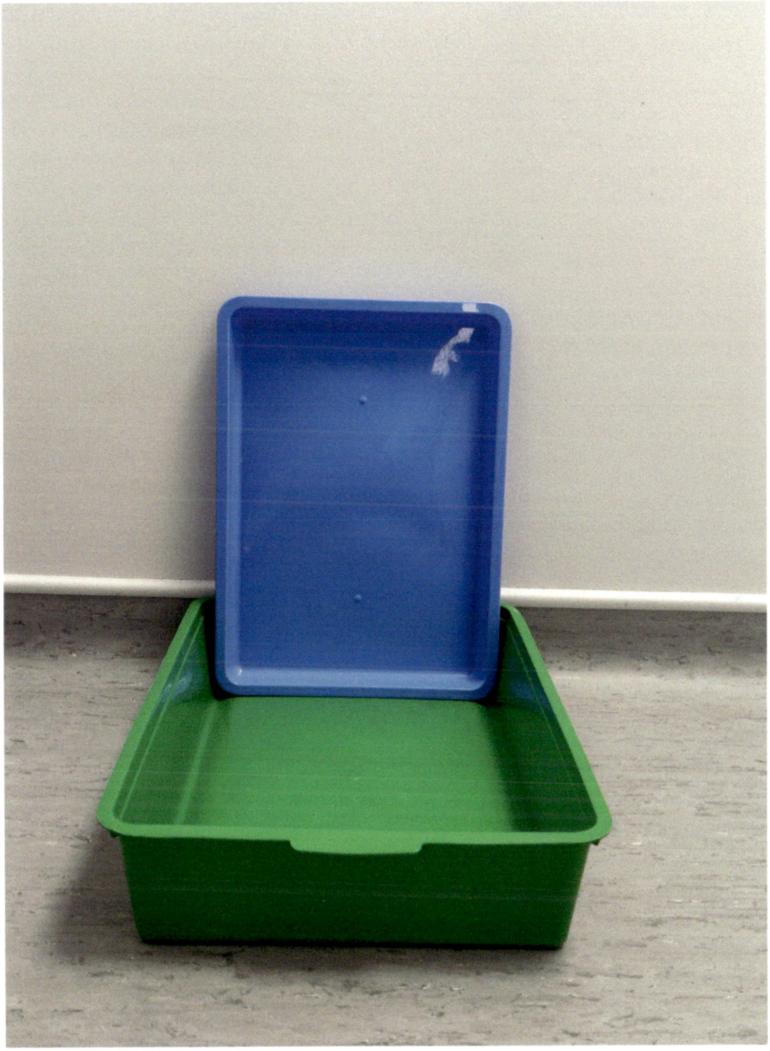

Fig. 14.4. Using two litter trays against a vertical surface may help to clean the area and encourage the patient to use a litter tray instead of marking. The trays can be gradually moved away as the management starts creating a change. (Photo courtesy of Sagi Denenberg.)

be cleaned regularly (ideally several times daily) and changed frequently (ideally weekly) to avoid any physical remnants (Ellis *et al.*, 2017) or odours. For more information on litter tray management, see Section 14.2.3.1.

Punishment should never be part of the management. Punishment, at best, may stop the patient from marking when the owner is present or in specific locations. However, punishment is likely to increase anxiety and fear, and avoidance of or aggression towards the owner.

14.2.2.2 Surgery

While it is important to remember that the evidence to support marking behaviour as a sexually dimorphic behaviour and hormonally related is weak, neutering might be helpful. Neutering cats at a prepubertal age seems to have a protective effect, and neutering adults who already mark may also help (Hart and Barrett, 1973; Hart and Cooper, 1984). However, approximately 10% of males and 5% of females will continue marking following neutering.

14.2.2.3 Psychopharmacology

Almost all cases of enuresis and encopresis will require the use of medications to manage the underlying pathology. First-choice medications mostly include serotonergic medications such as SSRIs, TCAs or buspirone. Currently, only clomipramine is licensed (in Australia) for urine marking in cats.

The goal of using medications is not to directly stop the patient from marking but to reduce arousal, anxiety and other underlying pathologies. Only once these are resolved or managed will the patient cease (or reduce) marking. Owners must be advised that the use of medications is only part of the management, not the entire management.

A notable (yet infrequent) side effect of several serotonergic medications or medications with a strong antihistaminic effect (e.g. amitriptyline) is urethral spasms. We should caution owners to monitor the patient's urine output to ensure that marking stops, not urination overall.

14.2.3 Inappropriate latrine behaviour

This presentation includes patients who eliminate in areas that owners consider unacceptable. Anxieties, fears or other psychiatric disorders are less likely to play a role in this presentation, compared to marking behaviour. Inappropriate latrine behaviour involves both urine and faeces and appears to be equally prevalent in males and females. Unlike marking behaviour, there is a strong correlation between urine elimination and faeces elimination in unacceptable locations (Barcelos *et al.*, 2018). It is likely that when the patient is not using the litter tray due to aversions, or it prefers a different area, it will use the area for all types of elimination.

Inappropriate latrine behaviour is divided into aversion and preference. The patient may develop an aversion to the litter, tray or location. Possible risk factors include the type of litter, cleanliness of the litter, location, previous disease or pain associated with elimination, and conflict between the patient and other animals at home. Older data suggest different litter tray factors such as size, number of trays, type of litter and the chemical properties of the litter (e.g. clumping versus non-clumping, scented versus non-scented, and odour neutralizers); however, newer data found no evidence to these claims (Horwitz, 1997; Grigg *et al.*, 2013; Hart and Hart, 2014; Barcelos *et al.*, 2018). Of all risk factors suggested, it appears that the main two are the cleanliness of the litter and possible competition over resources with another cat at home (Ellis *et al.*, 2017; Barcelos *et al.*, 2018). The patient may also develop a preference for a different location or surface. It is likely that when the patient eliminates in an area that owners find unacceptable, the owners are more likely to clean the area faster and better than cleaning the litter tray; hence providing a more desired (by the patient) elimination area.

As noted above, the presence of another cat at home may increase the risk of inappropriate behaviour. Even when there is no conflict between the cats, it is possible that the second cat is a competitor over or blocks the access to the litter tray, leading to inappropriate latrine behaviour. The effect of a second cat, in this case, is not as strong as in the case of marking behaviour.

The typical presentation of inappropriate latrine behaviour includes the patient walking to the area, possibly attempting to dig, squatting to eliminate (urine or faeces) and then attempting to cover the area. Variations may exist in this behaviour; however, it is almost invariably on horizontal surfaces, a full bladder or colon evacuation, and the patient shows no other marking behaviours in the area. Cats which never attempted to dig in the litter may be at a higher risk of developing inappropriate latrine behaviour (Horwitz, 1997). The patient may still use the owner-designated area (e.g. litter tray) for part of its elimination.

In many cases, inappropriate latrine behaviour is very organized; that is, the patient will return to the same specific location or locations, have a routine, and will use it daily. The latter may change based on the litter tray cleanliness. Some patients may use one area (or litter tray) for urine and a second for faeces.

14.2.3.1 Management

As with any presentation of inappropriate elimination, the first step is to rule out any physical abnormality that may cause or contribute to this problem. If the patient continues to eliminate in inappropriate locations after physical conditions have been ruled out or treated, a behavioural approach should take place. It is essential to remember that in some cases, both medical and behavioural factors coexist.

Since inappropriate latrine behaviour mostly involves learning and environmental factors, management should focus on environmental modification, routine, meeting the patient's needs and training.

Owners should maintain a diary of the patient's behaviours. The diary should include details such as locations and surfaces, frequency, time of day, type of elimination, the patient's behaviour, and presence of other animals and people. The diary helps to identify patterns and establish a management plan.

Litter cleanliness is one of the main risk factors; owners should address litter tray hygiene first. The frequency of cleaning and completely changing the litter should increase from its presence. The actual frequency depends on the patient and the presence of other cats at home. Cats will urinate between two and four times daily, and defecate at least once daily (depending on diet). Therefore, the litter should be scooped at least once daily, if not more frequently. Using an automatic litter tray (self-cleaning) may help the owner. However, some of these trays may scare the patient as they work. Also, in the author's opinion, these trays do not clean the litter adequately, especially when considering a patient who is already avoiding the tray.

Adding more trays in different locations may help in litter management as it gives the patient more options. However, there is no evidence that the 'rule of thumb' suggesting that the number of trays should be the number of cats plus one is valid. Nearly 70% of owners of all cats (appropriately and inappropriately eliminating) do not follow this rule (Barcelos *et al.*, 2018).

Next, owners should offer the patient several options. If the patient is still using the litter tray, even partially, it should serve as a 'control' when conducting a preference trial. Since owners often resist placing the tray in different locations and trays are more expensive, the first step is to test different litters. The duration of each phase depends on how frequently the patient eliminates. Also, owners should be aware of a 'novelty' factor; the patient is likely to use the new litter at first, but it may not continue using it in the future. Therefore, approximately two weeks is an appropriate period to test each litter. We should leave the existing litter tray unchanged and add a second tray, existing or new (but identical), near it with a new type of litter. After testing several litters, owners can test different boxes or locations using the same approach. This approach is time-consuming and may take many weeks to find the patient's preference. Giving more than one new option each time (e.g. trying several litters simultaneously) may accelerate the process. Following the patient's preference may also help; that is, owners should consider placing a litter tray where the cat eliminates, or use the same surface (e.g. carpet) that the patient is preferring.

When owners identify (based on the diary) the patient's preferred location, they may try preventing access to it or changing the function. Using booby traps to prevent access may stop the patient from going to those areas; however, it may only teach the patient to use different locations or lead to anxiety and fear. Owners might be able to block the patient's access to the room or area by closing doors or confining the patient. If the diary shows a routine, owners can use prevention, supervision or confinement at times when the patient is most likely to eliminate. Placing food, water or a bed in the area may stop the patient from eliminating in those areas. Soiled areas should be cleaned thoroughly using biological cleaners or mild bleach.

While owners try to reduce the appeal of the area the patient is using, they should attempt to improve the appeal of the place they wish the patient to use. Any deterrents in the area (e.g. noise, traffic, competition or odours) should be removed or managed. The location should be easily accessed, especially if the patient is painful or visually impaired.

The patient may need to be retrained to use the litter. Owners should follow the same general approach used in kittens (see Section 14.1.1.1). However, more care and effort are usually required. Training should focus on rewarding elimination in desired locations rather than punishing inappropriate elimination. The patient may need to be confined in a small area with food, water, a bed and a litter tray, so it is encouraged to use the tray to avoid elimination where food and water are. Confinement should take place at times when the patient is likely to eliminate. If the owner is present when the patient uses the tray, they should reward the patient. Then the patient should be allowed freely in the home until the next elimination time approaches. If the patient does not have a set routine or the owner cannot predict when it is about to eliminate, the patient should always be confined unless supervised by the owners. Confinement is not instead of supervision and providing the patient's needs.

Another option that may help to manage the problem is placing a litter tray where the patient is currently eliminating. Once the patient starts using the tray regularly, the owners should gradually (every several days) move it towards the desired location.

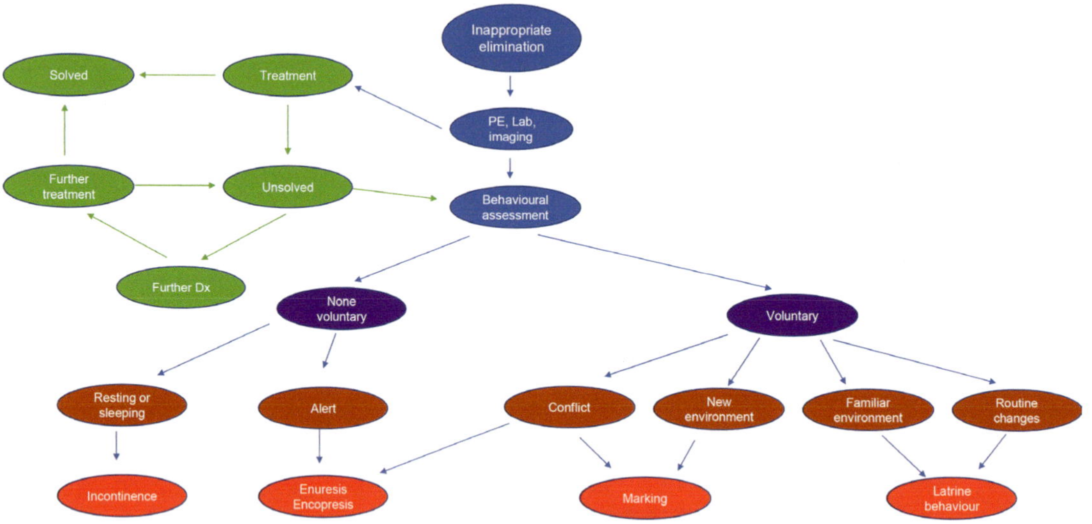

Fig. 14.5. A suggested algorithm for the diagnosis of inappropriate elimination in dogs. This algorithm focuses only on the behaviour of thepatient, and the patients ability to control the behaviour. It does not takeinto account other psychiatric pathologies, social interactions, and owners'responses. Following this algorithm helps guide the clinician. However, thefinal diagnosis should be established when considering all factors.

14.3 Elimination Problems in Dogs

Inappropriate elimination problems in dogs are similar to those in cats; however, the presentation is less prevalent in dogs. Nearly 10% of dogs presented to referral centres perform inappropriate elimination (Denenberg *et al.*, 2005), which is one of the risk factors for relinquishment or euthanasia (Salman *et al.*, 2000). Dogs may use urine and faeces to mark their environment and may also show enuresis and encopresis.

14.3.1 Diagnosis

Diagnosis of patients presented with inappropriate elimination follows the same rules as in cats. Physical disorders, training and psychiatric disorders can all contribute. One of the first questions should be about the patient's past training; whether it was fully trained before. Fig. 14.5 provides an algorithm to diagnosing the underlying cause of inappropriate elimination in dogs. It is important to note that this algorithm is not taking into account the patient's past training, the owner's responses, and other comorbidities, and therefore should be used as a suggestive diagnostic tool.

14.3.1.1 Physical disorders

Like cats, the first step is to rule out any physical disorder that may lead to increased soiling frequency, volume, urgency or in inappropriate locations. Hormonal disorders, painful conditions, sensory decline, cognitive dysfunction, and urinary and gastrointestinal diseases can all lead to inappropriate elimination. Table 14.2 illustrates the most common physical disorders. For more information, see Chapters 2 and 3.

14.3.1.2 Behavioural analysis

Following management of physical disorders, we should focus on the patient's behaviour, environment and emotional health. Maintaining a diary may help to identify patterns, triggers, routines and locations.

The first question should be about the patient's past elimination behaviours. We must verify that the patient was fully trained to eliminate in desired locations, and this has changed. If the patient was not fully trained, then repeating the training process with more care and patience, ensuring consistency and providing an optimal learning environment, should help (see Section 14.1.1.2).

An important question to ask is about the patient's ability to control its elimination. Some forms of elimination occur involuntarily. When the patient cannot control its elimination and is resting or sleeping, the likely diagnosis is incontinence. When the patient is unable to control its elimination but is alert, the likely diagnoses are enuresis and encopresis. When the patient is in full control of its elimination, the underlying causes are most likely marking, inappropriate latrine behaviour or conflict. However, some patients who control their elimination may still show enuresis or encopresis. Furthermore, description or observation of the patient's body postures before, during and following elimination is helpful. Observing the patient's environment may help to identify possible triggers.

14.3.2 Marking behaviour

Both males and females will mark their environment, although it is seen mostly in intact males. Dogs will mark new environments and scents (e.g. visitors' possessions, new homes, and even new family members). Oestrus females are likely to increase marking in intact males. When countermarking, dogs tend to urinate over existing scents. The presentation mostly involves urination and, infrequently, defecation. The typical body posture includes raising one hind foot to aim the urine stream over the existing scent. The patient may show additional marking behaviours such as scratching the ground with its hind feet. The patient will usually void small amounts of urine in different locations.

14.3.2.1 Management

Neutering appears to be helpful; approximately 80% of male dogs stop marking (Neilson *et al.*, 1997). Introducing new environmental triggers (e.g. people and other animals, or new environments) gradually and under supervision may help. Owners may teach the patient to eliminate on signal and then take it to eliminate before exposing to a trigger. Separating the patient and confining it in a safe area when visitors arrive may help.

When introducing the patient to a new environment, the use of appeasing pheromones (either a spray or a diffuser) may reduce arousal and promote calmness. Similarly, placing toys, food and water, or a bed may help reduce marking by changing the function of the area and providing familiar items. The areas where the patient marked should be cleaned thoroughly using biological cleaners or diluted bleach. Pheromones can be sprayed on the area.

When marking is due to anxiety or high arousal, the use of medications is helpful. The first choice is serotonergic medications such as SSRI or TCAs. For more information, see Section 9.8 – Serotonergic Medications.

14.3.3 Inappropriate latrine behaviour

Changes in routine (e.g. new job, school year starting or sickness) or the environment (e.g. a new home) may lead a well trained patient to eliminate in inappropriate locations until it learns where the new appropriate location is. It can take a long time for the patient to adjust to a new routine, and owners must be aware of these changes.

Changes in diets may also cause inappropriate latrine behaviours. Diets that are high in fibre may cause more faeces production and a higher urgency to eliminate. Also, rapid changes in diet that the patient might be sensitive to may lead to inappropriate elimination.

14.3.3.1 Management

Any changes to the environment or routine must be considered carefully. Owners should attempt to make those changes gradually to allow the patient to adjust. Also, changes in feeding schedule should take place. Often, owners continue feeding the patient at the same time as before, even when the routine has changed.

When moving to a new home, owners should take the patient out more frequently to their desired elimination area. Once the patient eliminates there, a reward should be given. If the patient comes back inside but did not eliminate, the owner should supervise or confine the patient and allow it outside again shortly after. For more information on training, see Section 14.1.1.2.

14.3.4 Enuresis and encopresis

The patient is often distressed or highly aroused when eliminating. Often this behaviour is involuntary; however, the patient is alert and reactive. The underlying mechanism is excessive arousal (see Section 7.4.3 – Arousal) triggered by conditions such as anxiety, phobias, panic and excitement. Common triggers include people approaching the patient, separation distress, noise aversions and other phobias.

The patient's body language is often the best indication alongside the context. During panic attacks, the patient often will present multiple displacement behaviours, roll on its side or back with ears pinned back while attempting to avoid eye contact, freeze and void urine (and sometimes stools). The amount of urine is often a full bladder. When the patient is highly excited, it usually stands with a cowering or arched back, wagging its tail and attempting to establish physical contact with the person or dog it sees while dribbling small amounts of urine.

Patients with separation distress can hold their urine and faeces for extended periods when the owners are present (for more information, see Section 13.2 – Separation-related Behaviour/Separation Distress). However, once left alone, the patient may eliminate even if it eliminated shortly before the owners left home. Often, urination is aimed at exits (windows and doors).

14.3.4.1 Management

Management aims to reduce the underlying arousal level. Doing so helps the patient to gain control over its bodily functions and assess the situation differently. This is achieved via prevention of known triggers, minimizing when prevention is not possible, and behaviour modification.

Owners should take patients outside who show enuresis or encopresis when meeting people and dogs. Introductions should be done gradually to allow the patient to adjust. A desensitization programme helps to teach the patient how to respond calmly. Before each training session, the patient should be taken outside to eliminate. Then owners must ensure that the trigger (dog or person) is calm and under control, i.e. does not approach too fast or in excitable/threatening manner. Once the patient starts showing signs of increased arousal, the other person or dog stops, and the owners should work with the patient on calming down before continuing. For more information on desensitization, see Appendix D for desensitization protocols.

People who greet the patient must avoid direct contact, reaching too fast, talking loudly, or attempting to pet a patient that is visibly avoiding them or shows signs of distress. If the patient shows signs of conflict and displacement behaviours when the other dog or person approaches, owners should stop the interaction and remove the patient to a different area to allow it to settle down.

Punishment is never part of the management. These patients are distressed already, and punishment will only increase it. These patients are not soiling purposely (for spite). They are merely expressing their negative (except for excessive excitement) emotional state.

14.3.4.2 Psychopharmacology

Medications are an integral part of most cases of enuresis and encopresis. These patients are unable to control their emotions and, as a result, their physiological functions. The first choice is usually serotonergic medications such as SSRIs or TCAs. In situational cases or when the trigger is a panic attack, medications such as benzodiazepines (e.g. alprazolam or lorazepam) or alpha-2 agonists such as clonidine and dexmedetomidine are helpful. For more information, see Chapter 9.

References

Amat, M., de la Torre, J.L.R., Fatjó, J., Mariotti, V.M., Van Wijk, S. *et al.* (2009) Potential risk factors associated with feline behaviour problems. *Applied Animal Behaviour Science* 121(2), 134–139. DOI: 10.1016/j.applanim.2009.09.012.

Barcelos, A.M., McPeake, K., Affenzeller, N. and Mills, D.S. (2018) Common risk factors for urinary house soiling (periuria) in cats and its differentiation: the sensitivity and specificity of common diagnostic signs. *Frontiers in Veterinary Science* 5, 108. DOI: 10.3389/fvets.2018.00108.

Bergman, L., Hart, B.L., Bain, M. and Cliff, K. (2002) Evaluation of urine marking by cats as a model for understanding veterinary diagnostic and treatment approaches and client attitudes. *Journal of the American Veterinary Medical Association* 221(9), 1282–1286. DOI: 10.2460/javma.2002.221.1282.

Borchelt, P.L. and Voith, V.L. (1996) Elimination behavior problems in cats. In: Voith, V.L. and Borchelt, P.L. (eds) *Readings in Companion Animal Behavior*. Veterinary Learning Systems, Yardley, Pennsylvania, pp. 179–190.

Bradshaw, J. and Cameron-Beaumont, C. (2000) The signalling repertoire of the domestic cat and its unrelated relatives. In: Turner, D.C. and Bateson, P. (eds) *The Domestic Cat: The Biology of Its Behaviour,* 2nd edn. Cambridge University Press, Cambridge, UK, pp. 67–93.

Carney, H.C., Sadek, T.P., Curtis, T.M., Halls, V., Heath, S. *et al.* (2014) AAFP and ISFM guidelines for diagnosing and solving house-soiling behavior in cats. *Journal of Feline Medicine and Surgery* 16(7), 579–598. DOI: 10.1177/1098612X14539092.

Denenberg, S., Landsberg, G.M., Horwitz, D. and Seksel, S. *et al.* (2005) A comparison of cases referred to behaviorists in three different countries. In: Mills, D.S., Levine, E., Landsberg, G., Horwitz, D., Duxbury, M., *et al.* (eds) *Current Issue and Research in Veterinary Behavioral Medicine*. Purdue University Press, West Lafayette, Indiana, pp. 56–62.

Ellis, J.J., McGowan, R.T.S. and Martin, F. (2017) Does previous use affect litter box appeal in multi-cat households? *Behavioural Processes* 141(Pt 3), 284–290. DOI: 10.1016/j.beproc.2017.02.008.

Frank, D.F., Erb, H.N. and Houpt, K.A. (1999) Urine spraying in cats: presence of concurrent disease and effects of a pheromone treatment. *Applied Animal Behaviour Science* 61(3), 263–272. DOI: 10.1016/S0168-1591(98)00195-6.

Grigg, E.K., Pick, L. and Nibblett, B. (2013) Litter box preference in domestic cats: covered versus uncovered. *Journal of Feline Medicine and Surgery* 15(4), 280–284. DOI: 10.1177/1098612X12465606.

Hart, B.L. and Barrett, R.E. (1973) Effects of castration on fighting, roaming, and urine spraying in adult male cats. *Journal of the American Veterinary Medical Association* 163(3), 290–292.

Hart, B.L. and Cooper, L. (1984) Factors relating to urine spraying and fighting in prepubertally gonadectomized cats. *Journal of the American Veterinary Medical Association* 184(10), 1255–1258.

Hart, B.L. and Hart, L.A. (2014) Feline behavioural problems and solutions. In: . Turner, D.C. and Bateson, P. (eds) *The Domestic Cat: The Biology of its Behaviour*. Cambridge University Press, Cambridge, UK, pp. 201–212.

Horwitz, D.F. (1997) Behavioral and environmental factors associated with elimination behavior problems in cats: a retrospective study. *Applied Animal Behaviour Science* 52(1–2), 129–137. DOI: 10.1016/S0168-1591(96)01073-8.

Lisberg, A.E. and Snowdon, C.T. (2014) Effects of sex, social status and gonadectomy on countermarking by domestic dogs, *Canis familiaris*. *Animal behaviour* 77, 1147–1154.

Mills, D.S., Dube, M.B. and Zulch, H. (2013) *Stress and Pheromonatherapy in Small Animal Clinical Behaviour*. Wiley-Blackwell, Chichester, UK.

Neilson, J. (2004) The use of fluorescein in cats to identify participants in housesoiling. *Proceedings of the American College of Veterinary Behaviorists*, Philadelphia, Pennsylvania.

Neilson, J.C., Eckstein, R.A. and Hart, B.L. (1997) Effects of castration on problem behaviors in male dogs with reference to age and duration of behavior. *Journal of the American Veterinary Medical Association* 211(2), 180–182.

Pryor, P.A., Hart, B.L., Bain, M.J. and Cliff, K.D. (2001) Causes of urine marking in cats and effects of environmental management on frequency of marking. *Journal of the American Veterinary Medical Association* 219(12), 1709–1713. DOI: 10.2460/javma.2001.219.1709.

Salman, M.D., Hutchison, J., Ruch-Gallie, R., Kogan, L., New, J.C. *et al.* (2000) Behavioral reasons for relinquishment of dogs and cats to 12 shelters. *Journal of Applied Animal Welfare Science* 3(2), 93–106. DOI: 10.1207/S15327604JAWS0302_2.

Tynes, V.V., Hart, B.L., Pryor, P.A., Bain, M.J. and Messam, L.L.M. (2003) Evaluation of the role of lower urinary tract disease in cats with urine-marking behavior. *Journal of the American Veterinary Medical Association* 223(4), 457–461. DOI: 10.2460/javma.2003.223.457.

15 Abnormal and Repetitive Behaviours in Cats and Dogs

Sagi Denenberg*

Langford Vets, University of Bristol, Langford, UK; North Toronto Veterinary Behaviour Specialty Clinic, Toronto, Canada

15.1 Introduction

Abnormal and repetitive behaviours (ARBs) are groups of pathological movements and sequences arising from normal maintenance behaviour. These behaviours are excessive in nature, ritualistic, do not serve a biological or functional purpose, and impair the quality of life of the animal (Mason, 2006).

These behaviours may be the consequence of an impoverished environment, boredom, conflict and frustration, anxieties and fear, and brain pathologies. Often, ARBs are divided into several groups based on their common presentations. These groups include hallucinations, activity patterns, self-injuries, and oral behaviours. Other abnormal behaviours include sleep and dissociative disorders.

15.1.1 Stereotypic behaviours

These behaviours are mostly seen when the patient is unable to or prevented from pursuing normal, species-specific behaviours. Stereotypic behaviours are more commonly seen in zoo and production animals, and horses. Stereotypic behaviours are repetitive in a rigid pattern (fixed-action), serve no function, and are mostly motoric (i.e. movement-related behaviours).

15.1.2 Compulsive behaviours

Similar to stereotypic behaviours, compulsive behaviours are repetitive and excessive. However, unlike stereotypic behaviours, compulsive behaviour is less rigid (that is the pattern may change) and appears to be goal-orientated. For example, spinning is a stereotypic behaviour, usually rigid in nature, and serves no purpose. Tail chasing is a compulsive behaviour; the patient is trying to catch its tail. At times, the patient will try circling to one side or the other to grab the tail, or it may then lie on the ground and try reaching its tail. Once the tail is caught, the behaviour ceases (even if only for a short period). Stereotypic behaviour continues for a fixed number of repetitions and then stops (even if only for a short period).

Compulsive behaviours might be self-rewarding. Once the goal is achieved, dopamine is released, providing strong reinforcement. Equally, beta-endorphins and endogenous opioids, which are released during and following the behaviour, serve to reinforce the behaviour.

15.1.3 What about obsession?

While most owners would answer that their pets are able to obsess, this question is difficult to answer. In human psychiatry, there is ample evidence to support a cognitive and deliberate intention behind many compulsive behaviours. Take, for example, people who wash their hands excessively numerous times daily. Once this person starts washing his or her hands, they will do so an excessive number of times over a short period (compulsive behaviour). However, this person can explain and justify the behaviour as fear of bacteria (obsession). We cannot have the same level of interactions with our patient; hence, the question remains open.

To assume that animals can obsess, we must first assume that they have the required level of cognition and emotions. Since our patients possess the same brain structures and neurotransmitters, it is

*s.denenberg@bristol.ac.uk

DOI: 10.1079/9781786394552.0015

reasonable to assume that their ability is similar to ours. Moreover, a growing body of evidence suggests that dogs and cats show similar results on assays as people, when considering their inability to communicate with us verbally.

Direct observation of our patient can confirm their cognitive abilities. For example, a dog may have seen a rat in the garden but was unable to catch it, or its owner hid a ball behind a piece of furniture. These dogs may return to the same location time and again, and might even show intense focus and agitation or distress when they cannot access their goal. This reaction, which is likely coupled with frustration, may indicate obsession.

15.2 Pathophysiology

While all ARBs may have a similar underlying pathology, differences exist in their presentation. ARBs might be on a spectrum, and their expression depends on the individual's animality and neuro-evolutionary composition (McElroy *et al.*, 1994; Stein, 2000). For example, some ARBs, such as spinning, circling, barking and tail chasing, are likely to develop subsequent to situations of high arousal. Conversely, self-injurious or oral ARBs such as hyperaesthesia, psychogenic alopecia, flank sucking or acral lick dermatitis may develop as a result of deprivation and inactivity. In species where locomotion is essential (e.g. equine) some of the most common ARBs include pacing and stall kicking, whereas in species such as ruminants who graze and masticate for long hours, most common ARBs include tongue rolling and preputial suckling. Primates and cats spend long hours grooming, and their most common ARBs include excessive grooming-like behaviours.

15.2.1 Neurochemistry

It is likely that most neurotransmitters play a role in the development and maintenance of ARBs. Not only their absolute level but also their relative level and interactions with other neurotransmitters are responsible.

15.2.1.1 Serotonin

The study of ARBs received most of its momentum following the discovery of the effect serotonergic medications have on what was considered a refractory condition. Early studies with clomipramine proved its efficacy when compared to desipramine (noradrenergic) (Zohar and Insel, 1987). These results suggest that serotonin plays a significant role in ARBs compared to noradrenaline, which plays a minimal role. This is in contrast to anxiety and panic disorders (see Chapter 13) where both serotonin and noradrenaline play an equal role.

Since then, more studies have proved the efficacy of serotonin re-uptake inhibitors such as citalopram (Stein *et al.*, 1998), clomipramine (Goldberger and Rapoport, 1990; Rapoport *et al.*, 1992; Hewson *et al.*, 1998; Moon-Fanelli and Dodman, 1998) and fluoxetine (Wynchank and Berk, 1998; Irimajiri *et al.*, 2009).

15.2.1.2 Dopamine

Dopamine levels in the brain influence both the increase and decrease of ARBs (Goodman *et al.*, 1990). Dopamine agonists such as amphetamines may induce stereotypic behaviours such as overgrooming and self-injurious behaviours (Hartgraves and Randall, 1986; Martin *et al.*, 1998). Conversely, dopamine antagonists (e.g. haloperidol) appear effective in the management of ARBs (Iglauer and Rasim, 1993). Dopaminergic augmentation of serotonergic medications may provide better results in the management of refractory ARBs (McDougle *et al.*, 1994).

15.2.1.3 Glutamate and Gama aminobutyric Acid (GABA)

As the main excitatory neurotransmitter, glutamate is the most ubiquitous neurotransmitter in the cortex. Glutamatergic neurons are extensively distributed across various brain regions, including basal ganglia, cerebellum, brainstem circuits and various intracortical and cortico-subcortical connections (Pittenger *et al.*, 2011). Among other circuits, glutamate acts on the cortico-striato-thalamo-cortical (CSTC) circuit.

GABA is the main inhibitory neurotransmitter in the cortex. Increased activity of the GABAergic pathway reduces the activity of neurons and is likely to help in the management of ARBs.

The use of glutaminergic medications such as NMDA receptor antagonists (e.g. memantine) or sodium channel blockers (e.g. topiramate) help to augment the CSTC circuit and reduce compulsive behaviours. These medications help to augment the effect of serotonergic medications (see Chapter 9).

15.2.1.4 Other neurotransmitters

Research into the role of other neurotransmitters is ongoing. Beta-endorphins, neuropeptide Y, substance P, and others are likely playing a role and medications that augment their effects might be useful (Korff and Harvey, 2006).

15.2.2 Neuroanatomy

Most recent data implicate the CSTC circuit as the main circuit involved in the development of ARBs. A glutaminergic dysfunction in this circuit is implicated in many compulsive disorders. Through the direct CSTC pathway, glutamate excitatory signals from the orbitofrontal cortex and the anterior cingulate cortex increase GABAergic (inhibitory) signalling to downstream inhibitory nuclei such as substantia nigra and globus pallidus interna (Pauls *et al.*, 2014). This is a rather simplistic view as there are four circuits involved (Lochner and Stein, 2003):

1. circuit involving projections from sensorimotor cortex via putamen;
2. circuit involving projections from paralimbic cortex via the nucleus accumbens;
3. projections from orbitofrontal cortex to the ventromedial caudate nucleus; and
4. projections from the dorsolateral prefrontal cortex via dorsolateral caudate nucleus.

Other centres such as the amygdala and the hippocampus, likely play a role in the development and maintenance of ARBs (Adler *et al.*, 2000).

15.3 Diagnosis

The approach to diagnosing ARBs should consist of an evaluation of physical and mental parameters, and environmental factors such as the patient's routine, household and welfare.

15.3.1 Physical disorders

The first step in approaching cases of ARBs is to rule out any physical disorder. Many diseases such as neurological, dermatological, metabolic and organ disorders can lead to ARBs. A full physical examination and laboratory tests (e.g. blood, urine, cerebrospinal fluid [CSF] analysis or biopsy) should take place. If a disease was detected, then suitable management should follow. If no disease was detected, a medication trial might be warranted in certain situations. The latter is most commonly the situation in cases of chronic pain. For a more in-depth discussion about physical conditions that may lead to ARBs, see Chapters 2 and 3.

15.3.2 Psychiatric disorder

ARBs may be the consequence of poor mental and emotional health. Reviewing not only the immediate presentation but also the entire spectrum of mental and emotional health is necessary when attempting to diagnose, and later manage, ARBs.

ARBs might arise as a result of chronic anxieties, panic attacks, frustration and poor welfare. A thorough review of the patient's behaviour, routine and environment is essential. Questions regarding specific behaviour should help to differentiate between physical and psychiatric disorders:

- What are the presenting signs? ARBs divide into several groups (e.g. hallucinations, activity patterns, self-injurious, and oral and ingestive behaviours).
- When did the behaviour start and did it develop since first noted? ARB with an acute onset and high intensity without progress is more likely to indicate a physical disorder. More gradual and prolonged development is likely to indicate a psychiatric disorder.
- What are the frequency and patterns of the behaviour? When ARBs occur without any known frequency or pattern, the likely underlying cause is physical disorders such as seizures. Most psychiatric disorders will show a certain pattern and frequency. It is, however, essential to remember that certain physical disorders such as pain may have frequency and pattern (e.g. occurs only following exercise).
- Is there any trigger? Lack of triggers, after a careful review of the problem, is more likely to indicate a physical disorder. However, when ARBs reach a high intensity and frequency, true compulsive behaviour might be 'emancipated' from any trigger. Thus, it may appear without clear triggers, patterns or frequency.
- Can the patient be interrupted, and will it continue? Seizures cannot be interrupted. Many

other physical conditions cannot be interrupted (although when owners use punishment, some patients will stop showing the behaviour when the owner is present). Most ARBs can be interrupted. However, many patients will resume the activity shortly later. Moreover, some patients will respond with aggression if the owner tries stopping them.

- Do any siblings show similar behaviours? There are likely to be genetic predispositions for certain ARBs in dogs and cats (Dodman *et al.*, 2010). When possible, owners should inquire about their pet's siblings.
- What were the owners' attempts to manage the behaviour so far? Owners may inadvertently reinforce behaviours, especially in puppies and kittens, and contribute to the development of the problem. In some cases, owners will contribute to frustration, conflict and anxiety by using punishment-based training, not providing for the patient's needs, or neglect. The environment where the patient lives may contribute by containing many triggers and no outlets.

15.3.2.1 Diary

Owners will not always have the answers to the above questions. In this case, more data is necessary. We can ask owners to maintain a diary to gather more information. The diary should include specific information about the presentation itself, such as:

- When is the behaviour likely to occur? Times and triggers should be noted.
- How long does each episode last?
- Does it occur in specific environments or situations?
- Who else is present at the time?
- Can you interrupt the behaviour? If yes, will the patient resume it immediately?
- Is the patient coherent and responsive while performing the behaviour?
- Are there more ARBs?
- Is the behaviour escalating? More frequent and more intense?
- What are the owner's reactions?

15.3.2.2 Observation

It is helpful to observe the behaviour either directly or via video. Observations help to identify underlying motivations such as anxiety, panic, frustration and conflict. In addition, video can be helpful to assess future progress by comparison to the baseline videos.

15.4 Management

Managing ARBs may be complicated at times. Not only is the psychiatric approach likely to require complex behavioural and environmental management and medications, but also, at times, there are complicating factors such as emotional and physical disorders.

It is important to remember that whether the inciting cause was psychiatric or a physical disorder, the maintaining factors may be both. For example, a dog may lick its carpal area, causing injuries as a result of pain. If undiagnosed or untreated, pain may continue to lead to more licking and biting the area. At the same time, a compulsive component may develop due to dopaminergic self-rewarding sensation and the release of local opioids and cytokines that numb the pain. Therefore, the management of both physical and psychiatric disorders may be required in many cases. The latter is especially true in ARBs that include self-injurious behaviours, but also in many gastrointestinal conditions and others.

15.4.1 Triggers

In some cases, triggers can be detected. However, when possible, triggers should be removed or managed. Even removing only a few may help reduce summation of effects. When we cannot remove the trigger, we might be able to implement a behaviour modification programme to change the patient's motivation to repeat the behaviour (see Chapter 8). By changing the patient's motivation, we can decrease the severity of the presentation, and later teach the patient an alternative response (see 'Response substitution' below).

15.4.2 Optimizing the environment and routine

Many ARBs may result from a suboptimal routine and environment. Many cats' and dogs' needs are unmet by their owners. Therefore, optimizing the routine and environment is helpful. Owners should attempt to introduce a predictable daily routine that meets the patient's needs. There are five essential needs to meet several times daily. These include feeding, elimination, rest and sleep, social interactions and physical activity. Based on the diary (see Section 15.3.2.1), owners should try to ascertain when the patient is most likely to engage in ARBs. Then, implementing training and play sessions, feeding or exercise at those times is likely to reduce ARBs. Ideally, the daily routine should be consistent each day. Predictability reduces anxiety as the patient learns to expect certain interactions at different times.

Feeding patients is more than nutrients and calories; it is also an important behaviour that wild and feral animals spend a long time performing. Therefore, owners should feed the patient in meals, several times daily, and use feeding toys (see Handouts A9 and A10 – Feeding Toys and Stimulation for Cats and Dogs). When possible, feeding should take place at times when the patient is most likely to engage in ARBs.

As part of the daily routine, owners should attempt to work on training with the patient. This approach includes cats as well. While it is more difficult to train a cat compared to a dog, it is possible and rewarding. Success in training is not the main parameter. In this case, training is mostly done to provide a distraction at times when the patient is likely to engage in ARBs and provide a positive and structured interaction with the owner. Owners should initiate the training using a signal, provide positive outcomes, and end the training using a signal (e.g. open hands and saying 'done').

15.4.3 Response substitution

It would be helpful if owners could stop the patient from engaging in ARBs positively and calmly. To do so, the owner must first train the patient several signals that later can be used. For example, owners can train their pet signals such as 'watch me' and 'touch' (see Handout C2 – How to Teach a 'Watch Me' and 'Touch' Cue). These are simple signals for patients to follow, even when they are highly aroused. Once the patient is trained well in these behaviours, owners can attempt to give the signal during times when the patient is likely to engage in ARBs. Ideally, owners can prevent the patient from starting by engaging with it when it is likely to start. Also, the sooner the owner can give the signal, the more likely they are to succeed.

When the patient is not well trained, or is too intense, using tools such as a head halter, lead, or even using hands (when there is no risk of biting) to stop the behaviour and redirect the patient's attention towards the owner, might be necessary.

Once the patient stops the behaviour, the owner should try reinforcing it using treats, toys, affection or praise. The next step is to try to maintain the length of time between episodes. Once the patient stops the behaviour more consistently following the signal, owners should start delaying the reward they give. Slowly and gradually, the time is prolonged, maintaining the same response. For example, if a dog is spinning, the owner should stop the dog using a signal such as 'sit'. Once the dog stops, the owner should reward the dog. Initially, the reward is given immediately as the dog stops; later, the reward should be given 15 seconds after the dog stops, and then 30 seconds later. The goal is to teach the patient that the longer it is not engaging in ARBs the more rewards it will receive.

15.4.4 Settle exercise

Owners should teach their pet to settle and relax (see Handout C4 – Teaching a Pet How to Settle on Cue). Training starts when the patient is about to sleep. This is when it is most calm. We cannot 'force' patients to calm down; we can take advantage of the opportunities presented to us. Owners should attempt to identify the best time and place; that is when and where the patient consistently goes to sleep. Several signals can be associated with falling asleep, which later can be used elsewhere:

- Visual/environmental signal: a mat, towel or blanket; owners should place the mat where the pet is likely to sleep.
- Tactile/touch: owners should slowly and gently pet the patient. Petting should focus on the dorsal neck, shoulders, ventral torso and ears. These areas appear to help patients to calm down. If the patient is aggressive or appears aroused as a result of the touch, the owner should either hold their hand on the same area or avoid touching altogether.
- Verbal signal: the owner should choose a word or a phrase such as 'calm down' or 'relax' to use at these times.
- The tone of voice: owners should use a calm, low and soft voice – a whisper.

As the patient lies on the mat, the owner should gently pet it and whisper the signal. Over several minutes, the patient is likely to fall asleep as it is part of their routine. In most cases, this phase is easily achieved. The challenge is to transfer the signal and feeling to other times and situations. Owners should first practise where they achieve success, and later attempt it during other times.

The expectation is reduced arousal, not sleeping. Owners should be instructed to watch for changes in the patient's body language and look for so-called 'biofeedbacks' or changes in the patient's physiology. For example, if the dog was spinning, and then stopped, the owner should attempt using this calming protocol by first asking the dog to sit on the mat (response substitution). Then the owner can gently pet the dog and whisper the signal. If the dog becomes more relaxed sitting or lying down, and instead of panting takes a deep breath, the exercise is successful. The more owners practise it, the better the result will be. Owners should be advised that this exercise is challenging and may require weeks or months to complete.

15.4.5 Prevention

In cases of self-injurious behaviours or when the patient might show aggression towards people or other animals in its vicinity, owners should implement prevention. Tools such as Elizabethan collar, head halter, crate or a basket muzzle may be used. If the trigger is environmental, such as lights or shadows, keeping the patient inside a dark room with little light may help it rest instead of performing ARBs.

Owners can teach the patient to spend time in a safe haven, an area that is associated with calmness, positive outcome and rest (see Handout C3 – Safe Haven). Not all patients will find this place calming, especially at first; therefore, it will require training and routine management. First, owners should try to identify the appropriate location. A bedroom, utility room or crate might be the ideal location. Second, when placing the patient in its safe haven, owners should consider leaving chews, feeding toys and water (except for psychogenic polydipsia – see Section 15.8.2). Turning off the lights in the area, except for a small light, or covering the crate, and placing a white-noise machine can minimize environmental stimuli. The use of pheromone diffusers might be helpful to calm the patient in the area.

Next, the owners should design a daily routine that includes times when the patient is left in its safe haven. The patient should be taken there several times daily, only after its needs are met. In the beginning, owners should leave the patient inside its safe haven only for short periods, and only once it is more accustomed to it can the patient be left for longer periods. The ideal result of this exercise is to teach the patient to choose to go to this place to settle and rest. Owners should be advised that this exercise is challenging and may require weeks or months to complete.

15.4.5.1 Is prevention making it worse?

There is a controversy about attempting to stop the patient from performing ARBs. In some cases, it is thought that ARBs arise as a coping mechanism for low welfare, frustration or boredom. ARBs might be the only way the patient can manage its daily life successfully.

Therefore, stopping ARBs without addressing the underlying motivation, might eliminate the patient's coping mechanism without providing alternatives. We must decide on the best approach. If the patient injures itself, then we must stop the behaviour. However, if the patient is not injuring itself or posing a risk to people and animals around it, or causing damage to the household, then we may allow it to continue. By changing the underlying motivation, we will reduce the likelihood of repeating the behaviour. In most cases, the approach is a combination of prevention and management while attempting to reduce or change the motivation.

15.4.6 Medications

15.4.6.1 Psychiatric medications

Many ARBs require the use of psychiatric medications as part of the management given the complexity and the likelihood of neurotransmitters pathology. For a more in-depth discussion of these medications, see Chapter 9.

The first choice is usually a serotonergic medication. SSRIs and TCAs have proven efficacy in both human and animal models of obsessive-compulsive disorder. It is important to note that some TCAs (e.g. amitriptyline and doxepin) also have a strong antihistaminic effect and might be useful for ARBs that may have a pruritic presentation (e.g. paw licking, and acral lick dermatitis (see Section 15.7.1).

Benzodiazepines are also useful in the management of ARBs. These are usually given as an adjunct to serotonergic medications, although they can be used individually. Other GABAergic medications, such as gabapentin, pregabalin and imepitoin, might be beneficial as well.

Since glutamate is implicated in the pathology of ARBs, given its role in the CSTC circuit, the use of glutaminergic medications may be beneficial. Memantine and amantadine might be beneficial as an adjunct to serotonergic medications in alleviating the signs of ARBs. Topiramate reduces the release of glutamate and increases the release of GABA, and might be beneficial as an adjunct to serotonergic medications.

15.4.6.2 Medications for physical conditions

When ARBs are possibly related to a neurological condition, the use of anticonvulsants such as levetiracetam (dog: 10–30 mg/kg q8 h; cat: 10–50 mg q8 h), phenobarbital (dog: 2–4 mg/kg q12 h; cat: 5–15 mg q12 h), or gabapentin (dog: 10–40 mg/kg q8 h; cat 25–50 mg q12 h) might be useful. It is important to note that these medications may also have a sedative effect and, therefore, stop the behaviour but not the cause.

Analgesic medications should be used as part of the trial for diagnosis, and the management. Analgesics should be used for at least six weeks after all signs have disappeared. The use of opioids is controversial. Some data suggest that the use of opioid antagonists such as naltrexone (dog: 1–2 mg/kg q12 h; cat 25–50 mg q24 h) might be beneficial. The effect of the latter is lower compared to other options and might only be successful in the early stages before the behaviour is 'emancipated'.

Where tissue damage exists, antibiotics should be given. The use of antibiotic should be based on culture and sensitivity. It is essential to note that superficial culture may be different from deep tissue culture. In one study, only about a third of dogs have similar cultures from both superficial and deep tissue (Shumaker *et al.*, 2008). Antibiotic treatment should continue for at least six weeks after all signs have resolved, and possibly a negative culture.

Anti-pruritic medications may also be necessary for ARBs where pruritus might be the inciting or maintaining factor. Antihistamines such as diphenhydramine, loratadine or cetirizine might be useful. More recently, oclacitinib was approved for use in dogs and can be used for cats as well. More advanced, or intense, cases may require the use of steroids; however, their benefits should be weighed against possible side effects. TCAs such as amitriptyline and doxepin have a strong antihistaminic effect and might be useful as well.

15.5 Hallucinatory Behaviours

15.5.1 Fly-snapping

This disorder is more common in the dog (primarily Cavalier King Charles spaniel) than the cat. The patient will sit or stand and appear calm. Then it would display a normal behaviour pattern that is meant to catch flies. The patient will start staring towards the ceiling or walls, look around the area and then snap and attempt to bite the air. However, the behaviour is aimless as no flies are present. The patient may present an isolated episode or a sequence of several episodes. The most common physical disorders leading to fly-snapping are seizures, syringomyelia, hepatoencephalopathy, pain and, possibly, ocular disorders.

15.5.2 Shadow/light reflection chasing and pouncing

Patients presented with this presentation appear to follow shadows with the sight, and then attempt to jump on the shadow. Pouncing resembles hunting or scavenging behaviour. The patient will stare towards a specific focal point, and then prepare to pounce. Mostly, the patient will be focused on the point for several seconds or minutes as if observing prey. Then it may cower and lunge towards the focal point. The patient tends to have dilated eyelids and pupils. Cats may be rigid, with tail wagging tensely, and low body posture. Often, after pouncing, the patient stops and looks down to see if it caught the shadow. Seizures, vision impairment, abdominal pain and spinal pain should be ruled out.

15.5.3 Staring

The patient is presented for prolonged staring towards an imaginary object (see Fig. 15.1). At times, owners will describe it as if the patient is staring at the stars (stargazing). This behaviour can take place in any environment (both indoors and outdoors) and continue for long periods. Sometimes the patient can be distracted by calling it or waving a hand in its line of vision. However, most often, the patient will resume the behaviour immediately. When patients sit and stretch their necks upwards, staring at the ceiling or sky, they should

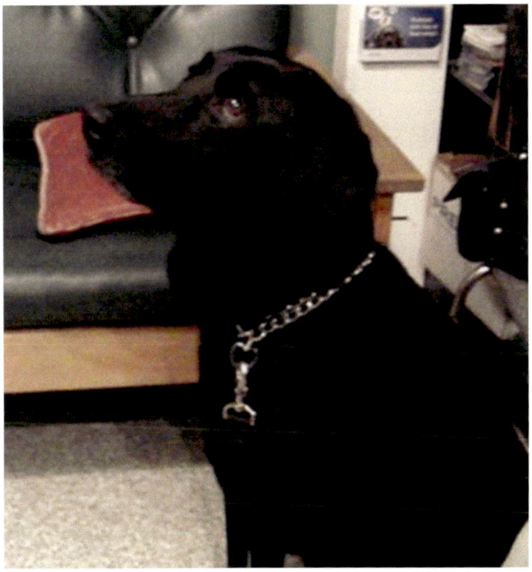

Fig. 15.1. Staring. This dog spends long periods sitting or standing and staring upwards. It is not looking at any particular object or towards a specific location. This dog will show this behaviour both indoors and outdoors, and at any time of the day or night. (Photo courtesy of Sagi Denenberg.)

be evaluated for possible neck pain, acid reflux disease or spinal injuries. Other possibilities include vision impairment, glaucoma, dental disease or seizures.

15.6 Activity Patterns

15.6.1 Circling and spinning

The patient is presented for spinning around its body axis or circling around an area or object (e.g. garden, tree, furniture or room). The behaviour is very stereotypic (see Figs. 15.2 and 15.3); that is, the patient is likely to run or spin at the same speed, number of times, and pattern each episode. No particular aim can be identified; the patient is not trying to catch its tail or reach a certain area. Some patients may grab their tail while spinning, accidentally at times, but this will not end the episode. Most patients will continue showing this behaviour until the point of exhaustion. In many cases, marks on the surface (e.g. tracks on the grass or carpet) can be seen. Some patients may show aggression if the owner is physically trying to stop it. Seizures and other neurological diseases, pain and

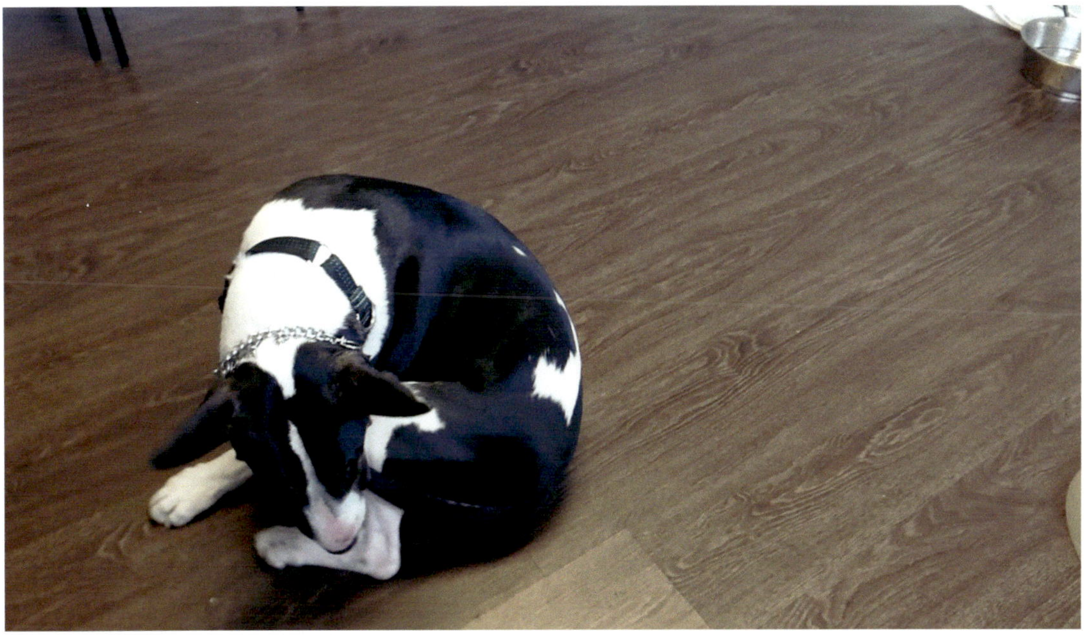

Fig. 15.2. Spinning. This English bull terrier is showing spinning behaviours. While it has its tail in its mouth, it is not the goal of the behaviour. This dog would spin using the same pattern and speed seven times and then stop and sit, and then start again. During most episodes, the dog spins to its left. (Photo courtesy of Sagi Denenberg.)

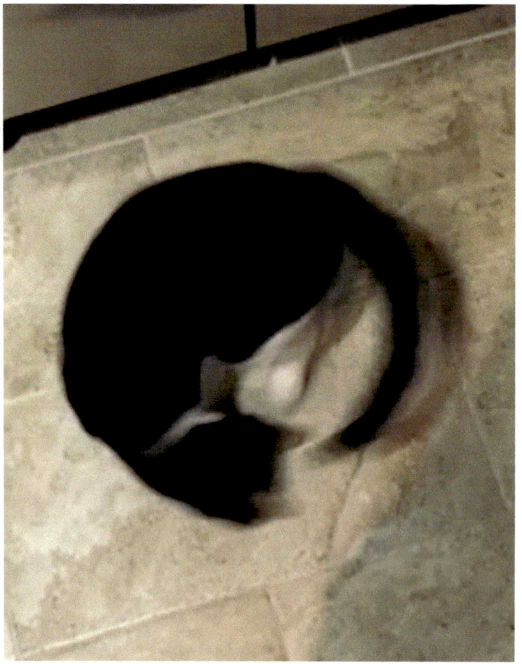

Fig. 15.3. Spinning cats. Similar to dogs, cats may show spinning behaviour. This cat would spin to both sides (not during the same episode). The behaviour is very rigid; the cat would spin with the same speed and pattern for five circles before stopping for a short period. This cat has lost weight despite a ravenous appetite. (Photo courtesy of Sagi Denenberg.)

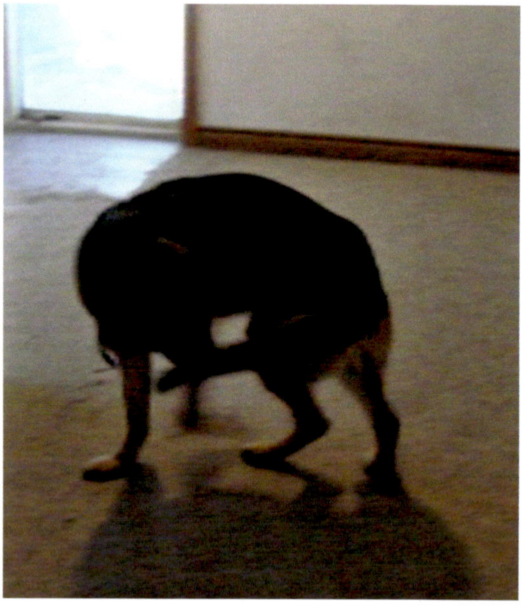

Fig. 15.4. Tail chasing. This dog is chasing its tail. It will attempt to grab the tail in different ways. The dog would spin to either the left or right, fall on its side and turn backwards, or even try reaching its tail between its hind feet. Once the tail is caught, the behaviour ceases (even if only for a short period). (Photo courtesy of Sagi Denenberg.)

vestibular disease are all possible causes of spinning and circling.

Spinning is reported to have a high incidence in English bull terriers and was associated with increased aggression and trance-like behaviour (mostly evident as walking a short distance very slowly, lifting one foot at a time, and appearing incoherent) (Moon-Fanelli *et al.*, 2011). Males seem more likely to show this behaviour than females.

15.6.2 Tail chasing

The patient is trying to catch its tail. This behaviour is different from spinning, as the goal is the tail. Once the patient grabs hold of its tail, it will stop (even for a short period). Unlike the spinning, the patient may spin in either direction, at different speeds and number of times. Also, it may lie on its side trying to grab the tail without any spinning. The behaviour may be highly intense, leading to injuries of the tail. Some patients may show aggression if the owner is trying to stop them. Amputating the tail is not likely to stop the behaviour and may increase it, as physical conditions such as inflammation and pain following amputation may increase the desire to bite the area. Common physical conditions that underlie this condition include local inflammation and pain, pruritus, anal sacs disease, spinal pain, parasites and seizures. German shepherd dogs appear to be more likely to develop this condition (see Fig. 15.4).

15.6.3 Turning and checking

The most common presentation includes a patient who turns its head around towards its flanks or hips and looks. The patient may turn its head to either direction and stare for several seconds or longer, then it would resume its previous activity. Abdominal and spinal pain, parasites and gastrointestinal diseases are among the most likely causes.

15.6.4 Hyperkinesis

Patients are usually presented for excessive restlessness, and often agitation. Most patients are lean or underweight, may have a dull coat and pronounced muscle definition. In cases of 'true' hyperkinesis, the sympathetic tone is high as evidenced by tachycardia, tachypnea, hypertension, dilated pupils, and often higher body temperature, including during resting. These patients often suffer from lack of sleep. They have a normal appetite, or even higher-than-normal to support their high metabolic rate. Many patients will present ARBs such as pacing, jumping, circling or other frantic random activity patterns.

Unlike increased restlessness in anxiety disorder, these patients do not appear distressed. Also, the patient is less likely to respond to behaviour modification exercises, and no specific triggers (e.g. times, environment or situations) can be identified. Possible differential diagnoses include boredom, frustration, anxiety, pain, seizures, pituitary tumours and hyperthyroidism.

Diagnosis is based on clinical signs, documenting a strong sympathetic tone and response to medication. The most commonly used medications are stimulants, such as methylphenidate. These can be used alone or in combination with SSRIs, TCA and gabapentin. Another option is alpha-2 agonists such as clonidine.

It is worth noting that while this presentation might be common based on owners' assessment, true hyperkinesis is very infrequent. Often these patients are anxious or lack mental and physical stimulation, and their needs are unmet by their owners.

15.7 Self-injurious Behaviours

15.7.1 Acral lick dermatitis, nail-biting and paw-licking

Acral lick dermatitis is more common in dogs than cats. The patient will lick an area on its feet (front primarily) and may cause tissue damage (see Fig. 15.5). The area is usually discrete, at least at first, but may progress later to cover most of the foot. Often discolouration of the fur can be seen due to licking. The disorder could be self-rewarding as tissue damage leads to release of local cytokine and opioids that provide a local anaesthetic effect and activate a reward loop, including dopamine release. The pet can often be disrupted but will resume the activity immediately following the owner

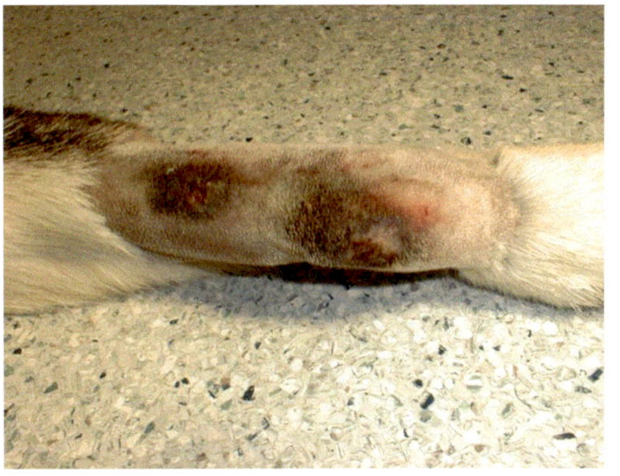

Fig. 15.5. Acral lick dermatitis. This dog is licking its foreleg excessively until a lesion develops. Once the lesion exists, it creates further irritation and more reason to lick the area, thus initiating a vicious cycle. Treatment is likely to require both mental and physical health approaches. (Photo courtesy of Sagi Denenberg.)

leaving it alone again. Boredom, frustration, anxiety and panic may lead to this disorder. However, the most likely causes are physical disorders including pain, mast cell tumours, fungal and bacterial infections, and allergies (Denerolle *et al.*, 2007). Nail-biting might be the result of allergies, fungal infections and immune-mediated diseases such as discoid lupus erythematosus

The distribution of the lesions might be useful in determining whether a physical or psychiatric disorder is more likely. Lesions in areas hard to reach by licking are less likely to be psychogenic. Similarly, several lesions in different locations are more likely to be a physical disorder in origin.

Patients may also lick and bite other accessible areas of the body (e.g. paws and tail). The severity can range from mild discolouration of the coat to extensive damage of the tissue (see Figs. 15.6 and 15.7).

15.7.2 Flank-sucking

The patient will often lie on its side and turn towards its flank and hold it in its mouth. Occasionally, the patient will bite the area, but more often it will hold it while performing sucking motions. Infrequently, the flank is damaged above a minor inflammation. This disorder is most likely seen in Doberman pinschers and Dalmatians. Pain, gastrointestinal disease, allergies and parasites are the most likely

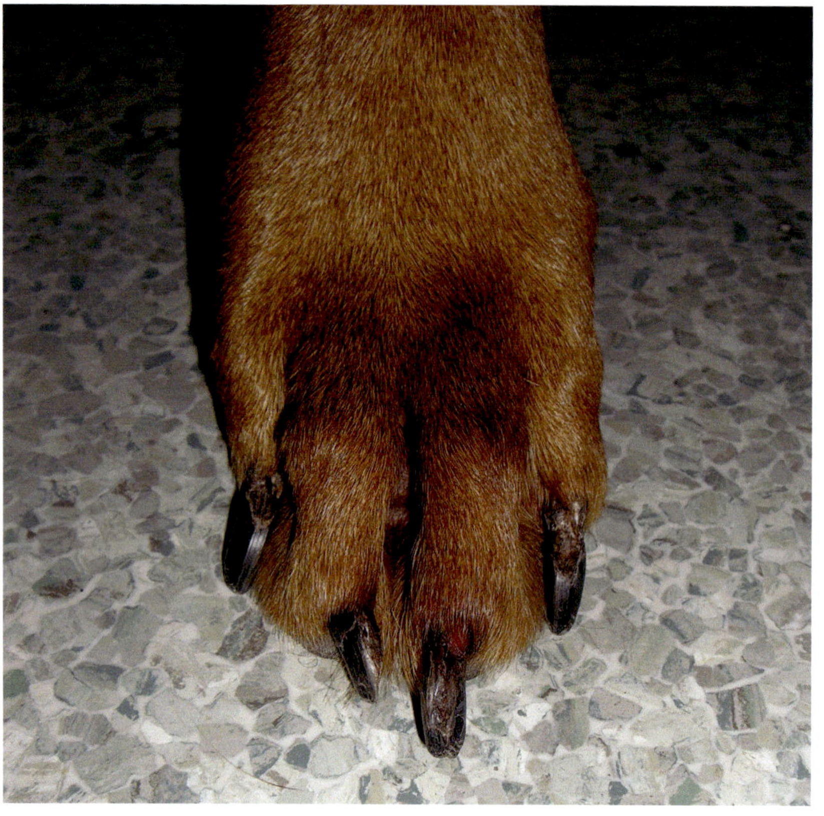

Fig. 15.6. Paw-licking. A minor case of paw-licking leading to discolouration of the skin and minor lesions of the skin and nails. Only once physical disorders such as allergies, lupus or fungal infections are ruled out can a mental disorder be diagnosed. (Photo courtesy of Sagi Denenberg.)

physical conditions to cause this behaviour. Anxiety, boredom and panic are the most likely psychiatric disorders leading to flank-sucking.

15.7.3 Hyperaesthesia

A poorly understood syndrome in both cats and dogs (less likely), leading to a range of abnormal behaviours. Owners often describe their cat as if it has 'seen a ghost'. The hallmark of this condition is the rippling or twitching of the skin on the back (thoracolumbar spinal area). Often, touching the area may elicit the behaviour. A typical episode starts with the skin rippling, while the cat is sitting and looking at it. Then the tail usually starts wagging in an intense and erratic pattern. The cat's pupils are dilated, and it may vocalize (crying and hissing). Next, the cat may turn and attempt to bite or bite the thoracolumbar area, flanks, thighs or tail. Some cats lie on their side while screaming and biting the area and kicking with their hind feet. In most cases the cat will then jump and run away from the area, defecating at times. This syndrome is often associated with urine marking and aggression when touched in the area.

Hyperaesthesia is a complex syndrome that may have neurological, dermatological, pain and gastrointestinal causes. A complete physical examination, coupled with laboratory tests, is the first step. Advanced imaging, including MRI or the spine, is recommended. Skin biopsies and scraping for parasitology and culture should be collected. Trials with analgesics, anti-pruritis, anticonvulsants and parasite control should follow. If physical disorders are ruled out, evaluation of the patient's environment, routines and welfare should take place. Among

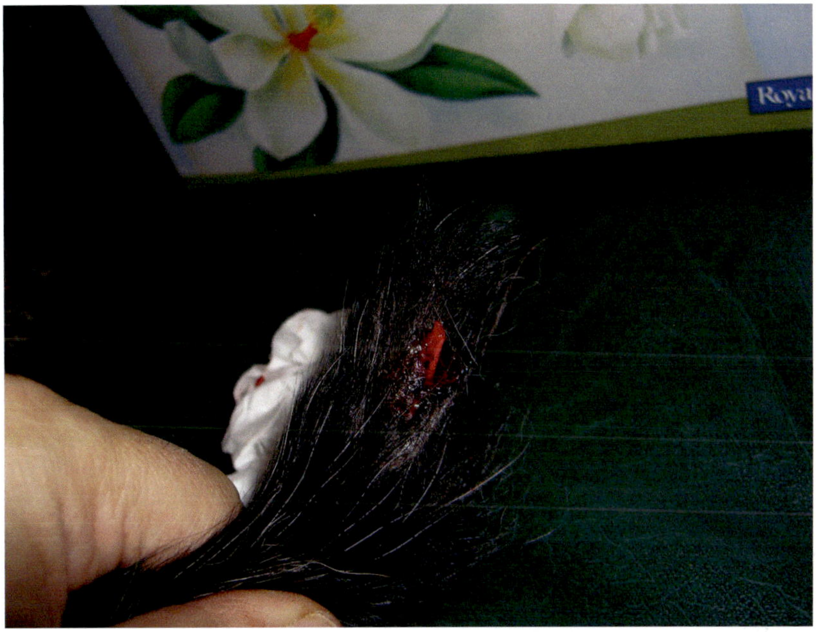

Fig. 15.7. Tail-biting. This cat bit the tip of its tail several times leading to severe injuries. Physical disorders such as allergies, pain, neuropathies and trauma must be considered first. Treatment of this disorder requires both addressing the existing wound and the underlying cause. (Photo courtesy of Sagi Denenberg.)

the most successful medications are SSRIs and anticonvulsants.

15.7.4 Psychogenic alopecia

The patient licks itself, barbering the fur (see Fig. 15.8). This condition is more common in cats than dogs, and mostly around the ventral abdomen or flanks. In true psychogenic alopecia, the damage is self-inflicted, including local inflammation, broken hair shafts (while the follicles are healthy), and no pruritus is present. Therefore, a full range of dermatological evaluation including skin scraping for parasite evaluation, fungal and bacterial cultures, anti-pruritic and parasite control medications, allergy testing, including a food trial, and biopsies should take place (Waisglass *et al.*, 2006).

15.8 Oral and Ingestive Behaviours

15.8.1 Pica

Pica (a depraved appetite) is sometimes seen in dogs and cats, and the most common presentation is coprophagia in dogs or chewing strings and plastic in cats. The patient may harm itself by eating poisonous, toxic or contaminated objects. Of course, the risk of a gastric or intestinal foreign body obstruction exists (see Fig. 15.9).

Pica might be a subjective problem, that is, the owner may dislike what the patient is eating (as in the case of coprophagia) or feel that the behaviour is excessive, whereas it may be normal.

Pica might be the result of gastrointestinal diseases, including pancreatic disease. Oral, gastrointestinal and abdominal pain may also lead to pica. It is less likely that nutritional deficits will be the underlying cause of pica.

Lack of oral stimulation or boredom may lead to pica as a coping mechanism. Similarly, anxieties may lead to pica as the behaviour may start as a displacement behaviour and later progress into a compulsive disorder. Also, some owners may inadvertently reinforce the problem by giving attention when the dog or cat presents the problem (e.g. chasing the pet or confronting it).

15.8.2 Psychogenic polydipsia

Average water intake in dogs and cats is 20–30 ml/kg/day depending on the diet, temperature and

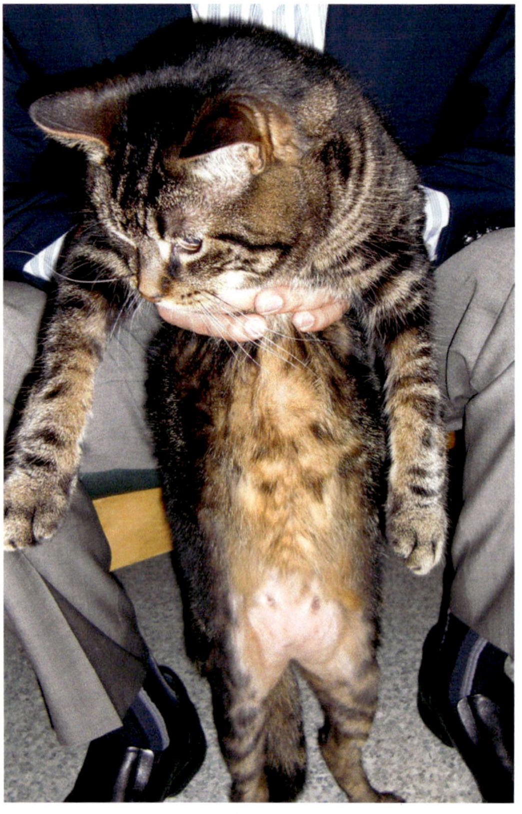

Fig. 15.8. Psychogenic alopecia in cats. This cat was presented for psychiatric assessment. Once all physical disorders were ruled out, management using environmental and behaviour modification and medications were used. The cat's coat started improving, reaching full resolution (with infrequent and minor flare-ups during routine changes). Note the distribution of the lesions; mostly lower abdomen. (Photo courtesy of Sagi Denenberg.)

activity. Once the patient consistently drinks over 90 ml/kg/day, we can consider polydipsia. The most common owner's complaint is about excessive urination possibly leading to house-soiling problems. Some of the most likely causes of this presentation are physical, not psychiatric. These include hormonal imbalances such as diabetes mellitus and insipidus, renal disorders, pituitary adenoma and metabolic diseases.

Diagnostic tests such as blood and urine analyses, abdominal imaging and scanning of the pituitary gland help make a diagnosis. When laboratory tests yield no answer, a water deprivation test or a desmopressin (DDAVP) trial may be considered; the latter two should take place under veterinarian supervision to prevent dehydration.

Owners should provide the patient with measured amounts of water divided into several portions throughout the day. Low-sodium diet and treats should be used. Providing ice cubes as part of the daily water intake helps increase stimulation and occupy the patient in a positive interaction.

15.8.3 Licking and chewing behaviours

Oral behaviours such chewing or sucking fabrics (see Fig. 15.10) and other materials, gulping, lip-smacking and licking of surfaces or people may be compulsive. Often causes such as boredom, anxiety or frustration may underlie these conditions. However, physical conditions such as gastric oesophageal reflux disease, inflammatory conditions, parasites or motility disorders may account for these behaviours (Bécuwe-Bonnet *et al.*, 2012).

15.9 Sleep Disorders

Sleep is a normal behaviour; it is part of the restorative (physical and cognitive) process of the brain and body, and it is critical for survival. External and internal factors influence sleep. External factors include daylight, owners' routine, other animals, noise and temperature. Internal factors include emotions, pain, hunger, diseases and biological rhythms. Sleep disorders are secondary to different pathologies such as anxiety, pain or neurodegenerative disorders. Sleep disorders infrequently occur in cats and dogs and range from mild to severe (Zanghi, 2017).

The first step in the diagnosis of sleep disorders is to rule out underlying physical pathologies such as painful conditions, neurodegenerative disorders and seizures, hormonal disorders or gastrointestinal disease. A full physical examination, blood analysis and imaging (such as MRI) are necessary. CSF analysis might help to identify a deficiency in hypocretin-1 leading to sporadic narcolepsy in dogs (Ripley *et al.*, 2001). Familial narcolepsy (in Doberman pinschers or labrador retrievers) is due to mutation in hypocretin-2 receptor gene. Thus, dogs with this type of narcolepsy will have normal hypocretin level in the CSF. Cognitive decline in dogs and cats (see Chapter 16) may lead to altered sleep–wake cycle and hyposomnia.

Next, we must rule out emotional disorders such as anxiety, panic attacks or disorders, and

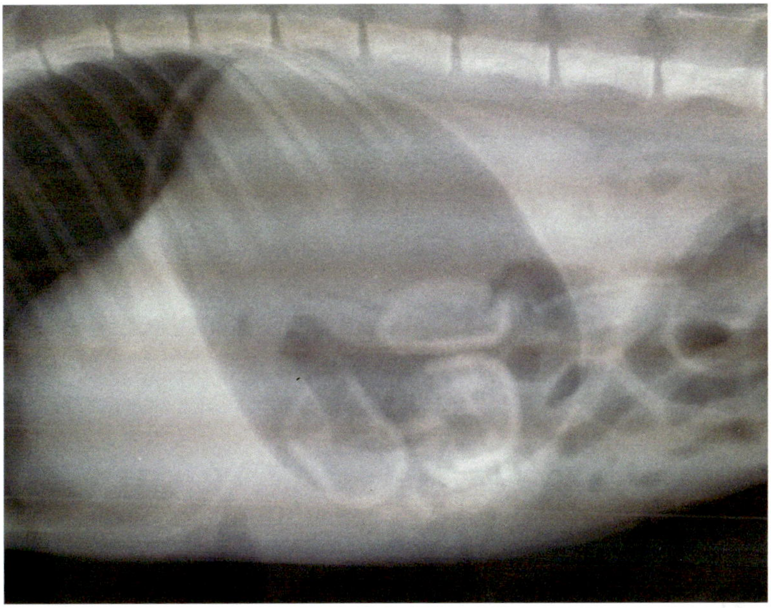

Fig. 15.9. Pica in cats. This cat ingested the rubber from a baby's dummy (pacifier), leading to a gastric foreign body. This was not accidental ingestion; the cat chewed and swallowed several of these, and continued doing so after the surgery. (Photo courtesy of Sagi Denenberg.)

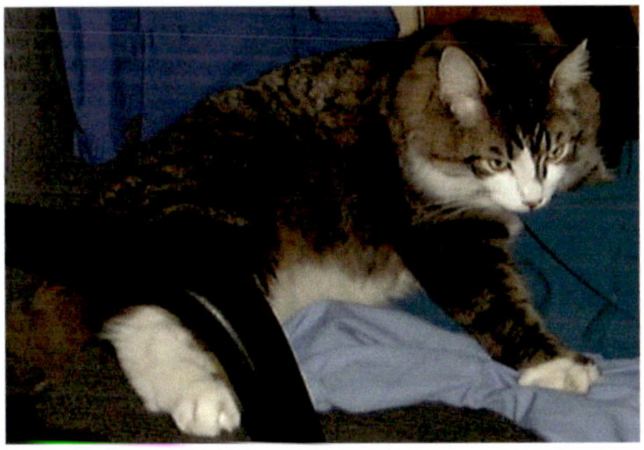

Fig. 15.10. Fabric sucking. This cat shows fabric sucking behaviour, which was likely to have started as a coping mechanism or vacuum activity as a result of lack of stimulation. It has developed into a compulsive behaviour where the cat would frequently engage in this behaviour during different times and environments. This behaviour has not escalated beyond sucking; the cat never caused damage to the garment or ingested pieces of it. (Photo courtesy of Sagi Denenberg.)

phobias (see Chapter 13). These disorders may lead to insomnia and altered sleep–wake cycle and signs similar to sleep disorders. Depression may lead to hypersomnia in cats and dogs. Daily schedule, lack of stimulation (physical and mental) and unpredictable owners' routines may also lead to changes in the sleep–wake cycle.

15.9.1 Hyposomnia and insomnia

Dogs and cats spend approximately 60% of the day in resting and sleeping behaviour. Many acute and chronic conditions cause lack of appropriate sleep (quality and quantity). These patients cannot fall asleep, and when they do sleep, their sleep is shallow and they wake up easily. Sleep deprivation for any reason, ultimately, will lead to more irritability, arousal and even aggression.

15.9.1.1 Diagnosis

Since hyposomnia and insomnia are secondary to physical and emotional pathologies, the diagnosis is aimed at finding the underlying causes. A full physical examination, laboratory testing and imaging should be the first step. When necessary, a medication trial (e.g. analgesia) should follow.

When talking to owners, we should note the daily routine, level of exercise and stimulation, and any indication of emotional disorders. Owners should maintain a diary (see Handout A6 – Diary), which may help to identify patterns and triggers (both internal and external).

15.9.1.2 Management

Once physical and emotional disorders are either ruled out or managed, we can address hyposomnia or insomnia if they still exist. The first step is to design a strict daily routine. Owners should ensure that the patient receives ample daytime stimulation and allow sufficient night-time (and some daytime) sleep times. The patient should have a designated sleep area in the home. The place should be comfortable, accessible, relatively dark and calm (see Handout C3 – Safe Haven). Owners should train the patient to go there as part of its daily routine. At the same time, owners should try avoiding any disturbances to allow the patient to sleep.

Before the patient is in its place, owners should ensure the patient's needs (e.g. elimination, exercise, interactions and play, and food) were met. The use of feeding toys, play and exercise helps to stimulate the patient. Intense activities should be followed by calmer activities such as chewing a bone or licking soft food from a Kong toy.

In many cases of chronic hyposomnia and insomnia, the circadian rhythm and the patient's sleep–wake cycle have been altered and fixed to a new rhythm. Even after managing the underlying cause, the patient may not revert to the previous rhythm. In these cases, the use of medication is necessary if routine and environmental management failed. Owners can try using melatonin to regulate the sleep–wake cycle, though good evidence is lacking. Clonazepam, a long-acting benzodiazepine, is a useful hypnotic that may help to regulate the sleep–wake cycle. Other options include trazodone or gabapentin.

15.9.2 Rapid eye movement behaviour disorder

Rapid eye movement (REM) sleep is not a passive or inhibited function of the brain; it is an active process of an intense brain function. Electroencephalogram (EEG) waves during REM sleep are similar to EEG waves during wakefulness; they are fast and desynchronized. As a result, autonomic physiological activities such as breathing, pulse, blood pressure change, usually increase. The animal is likely dreaming during this phase. During REM sleep, muscle hypotonia (or complete atonia of some muscles) develops. This disconnect ensures that the animal is not active while dreaming. The diaphragm and the laryngeal, facial, distal limbs and tail muscles are not fully affected by hypotonia (Hendricks *et al.*, 1989). Therefore, during the REM sleep phase, the animal may vocalize, paddle its limbs (dogs only) and have facial twitches.

REM behaviour disorder (RBD) accounts for most parasomnia (altered or abnormal sleep behaviours) in cats and dogs. In human medicine, parasomnias are closely linked to neurodegenerative disorders later in life. Therefore, scanning patients is helpful; however, if no lesions are found, it is important to consider repeating the scan several months later.

RBD can occur during both day- and night-time sleep and may last from a few seconds to several minutes. There is no breed or sex predilection and most patients start exhibiting this disorder at a young age (less than a year in dogs) (Schubert *et al.*, 2011).

15.9.2.1 Diagnosis

The diagnosis of RBD in veterinary patients is primarily based on clinical signs (observation) and ruling out other possible causes. Differential diagnoses include seizures, neurodegenerative disorders, infectious diseases of the CNS, gastroesophageal reflux disease, and non-REM parasomnias.

The use of polysomnography is the best tool to diagnose different parasomnias. However, given the cost involved and the difficulties in fitting (and keeping) the electrode on the patient, this method is reserved for research.

Patients with RBD are likely to become very active since the muscular hypotonia is not present. The patient may walk or run, show aggression, bark and eliminate. During this time, the patient is incoherent and non-responsive to the owner's signals. One of the main differences between RBD and non-REM parasomnia is the patient's wakefulness. If the owner can easily wake the patient up from this episode (e.g. clapping their hands so that the patient immediately stops and focuses on them), it is most likely REM parasomnia. However, if the patient is difficult to arouse and appears agitated or confused, it is likely to be a non-REM parasomnia.

15.9.2.2 Management

Treatment of parasomnia invariably requires the use of medications. The use of hypnotics, such as clonazepam, or anticonvulsants, such as potassium bromide (KBr), is helpful. Other options include oxazepam, gabapentin and melatonin. A recent survey found Kbr to be more effective than the other options (Schubert *et al.*, 2011). However, the author's experience is that the combination of clonazepam and melatonin was effective in 13 out of 14 cases (Denenberg, unpublished data). In human medicine, serotonergic medication use in RBD is controversial. Serotonergic medications reduce REM sleep and may affect the transition between non-REM to REM sleep. Trazodone is an exception and can be used. Bupropion, a dopaminergic medication, enhances REM sleep and may offer a beneficial effect.

Owners should ensure that the patient is sleeping in a secure area where it cannot injure itself or come out and show aggression (see Handout C3 – Safe Haven). Further, owners should ensure that the patient is well stimulated (both physically and mentally) and has its needs met.

When the patient is showing RBD, owners should attempt to wake it up in a safe manner. Instead of touching the patient or being next to it, owners should call its name, clap their hands or make a different sound. Once the patient is awake, owners should call it and try refocusing its attention on the owner. It is essential to differentiate RBD from non-REM parasomnia. Waking a patient with non-REM parasomnia may lead to aggression, confusion and erratic behaviours.

Treatment with medications and a safe sleeping location is likely to be a lifelong management. However, the long-term prognosis tends to be favourable.

15.9.3 Non-REM parasomnia

Non-REM (NREM) is the first phase of sleep. As the patient calms down and prepares to sleep, the brain activity slows down (Alpha waves on EEG). Soon after this, the patient enters the first phase (N1) of NERM sleep. It becomes drowsy, and a process of physiological inhibition starts (slower breathing rate, lower pulse and blood pressure). At the same time, a full muscle atonia is not present; the patient may show jerking motion of limbs or head.

Next, the patient enters the second phase, N2 or light sleep. The EEG wave is theta and includes sleep spindles (a short burst of rapid waves among the slower waves). These spindles are coupled with a short exchange of muscle tone and relaxation. The process of physiological inhibition continues. The last phase is N3, also known as slow-wave sleep (SWS). EEG measurements show delta waves. In this phase, the patient is in a deep sleep, coupled with full muscle atonia. This stage is followed by REM sleep.

There are several types of non-REM parasomnia, including nightmare, night terrors and sleepwalking; however, it is difficult to assess whether veterinary patients experience these. NREM parasomnia appears during SWS sleep (N3) when it is the most difficult to wake the patient.

15.9.3.1 Diagnosis

NREM parasomnia infrequently occurs in patients. The patient may show intense aggression with minimal inhibition. Unlike RBD, it is difficult to wake these patients, and when they wake up during SWS, they appear disorientated, unco-ordinated, and may not recognize their owners. The patient may vocalize, open its eyes, move around the room and eliminate. However, they are not awake – they may fall and hit furniture or walls.

A complete physical examination, laboratory tests and brain imaging are necessary to rule out differential diagnoses such as seizures, RBD, neurodegenerative disorders and toxins. Emotional differentials include panic attacks, affective aggression and other abnormal and repetitive behaviours. Paradoxical drug reaction (e.g. benzodiazepines) may induce similar signs to NREM parasomnias.

Owners may change the layout of the area (e.g. place a stairgate or pillows around) where the patient sleeps, once it has fallen asleep. If the patient presents an NERM parasomnia, it is likely to hit the object as it walks. Patients that are awake will avoid these objects when walking.

15.9.3.2 Management

Similar to RBD, treatment requires medications and safe environment to confine the patient. However, unlike RBD, owners should not attempt to wake the patient. Instead, the patient should be left alone as it will go back to sleep. Most NREM parasomnias are likely to last only several minutes.

15.10 Hypersensitivity-hyperactivity Syndrome

Hypersensitivity-hyperactivity (HSHA) occurs mostly in very young patients (average age of onset is two months). These patients show increased motor activity and inability to settle down, more than expected in normal kittens or puppies. The behaviour is usually very disorganized, and the patient lacks many normal behaviour patterns. For example, dogs do not show appeasement behaviour following an episode of aggression, or they lack bite inhibition during a play fight. Patients with HSHA are sleep-deprived (average 7 hours daily), underweight (although they may have a voracious appetite) and irritable. One of the hallmarks of this syndrome is an extremely low reactive threshold to environmental stimuli.

There are two stages to HSHA, defined by the signs and the differences in sleep and appetite. In stage one, patients lack bite inhibition, play and explore excessively, and show anticipatory behaviours (hypervigilance; reacting to each stimulus in the environment). Their appetite and sleep patterns are normal. Stage two includes all the signs seen in stage one and includes hyposomnia and lack of satiety (including nondiscriminatory appetite).

Patients may show aggression towards people or other animals. However, the aggression is not directed towards a specific stimulus and can be random. That is, the patient may bite the owner who is playing with it at one time but not others. Also, the bite is uninhibited, and there are no warning signs. The aggression is not a result of an underlying affective disorder (see Chapters 11 and 12) but a consequence of the excessive motoric activity. For example, a puppy with HSHA will mouth the owners, possibly forcefully, when they are highly aroused. The bite is not meant to achieve a goal (e.g. distance increasing or maintaining resources) as it might be in different situations.

HSHA is a life-long disorder that may have genetic and pre- and postnatal factors. The prognosis for successful management is favourable with early intervention. Adult patients who are presented with HSHA that has been present since a young age carry a poorer prognosis.

15.10.1 Management

Treatment requires the use of psychoactive medications that aim to reduce the overactivity and arousal while increasing the reactivity threshold. Currently, the preferred medication is selegiline (0.5–1 mg/kg, in the morning). Other options include SSRI or TCA. Treatment with psychoactive medications is usually lifelong.

Using behaviour techniques such as structured play, settle exercises and training focus on managing the behaviour. The success of these techniques is based on the success of the medications. Owners are instructed to have a predictable and strict daily routine and create a calm environment for the patient. The environment should be dark, quiet and relatively barren. The owners establish play sessions with clear signals for the start and end of the session. Early sessions include minimal play with many breaks to settle and breathe deeply. With success, the session might include more play, fewer breaks and more stimulating play.

We should inform owners that this condition can only be managed but not cured. Early stages require more time and effort; however, with improvement, these patients can have a long and successful life.

15.11 Dissociative Syndrome

A progressive loss of connection to reality and the increase of hallucinations, a dissociative disorder can be interpreted as a partial seizure or a true psychiatric pathology. During the phase of hallucinations, the patient might show severe and dangerous aggression towards people and animals. The human parallel to this disorder is schizophrenia.

The disorder usually appears in patients between the ages of 12 and 20 months. While it may appear later in life, it has likely been present but was not diagnosed. Owners are likely to complain about abnormal and repetitive behaviours and aggression.

In dogs, there might be a genetic component to this disorder; it appears more prevalent in German shepherd dogs and bull terriers. Careful examination of the dog's past may show the first clinical signs starting at four to seven months of age, especially in German shepherd dogs. This is known as the premorbid phase. The main characteristic of this phase is social behaviour changes. The patient becomes more withdrawn from its social group, may start showing aggression, and there are no clear signs or reasons for these changes.

Moreover, owners may notice changes in normal behaviour sequences without apparent reason. The patient might start playing and then stop and withdraw or attack. Females are more likely to withdraw, while males are more likely to attack.

Diagnosis is made based on clinical signs and a description of the patient's behaviour. Patients might be underweight or even reach cachexia as a result of increased activity, although their appetite might be normal. Later, the owners may notice changes to the patient's consciousness level.

There are two groups of clinical signs of this disease. For diagnosis, at least three signs of group one and one sign from group two are needed. Clinical signs in group one include onset around puberty and under five years of age, evidence of hallucinations, stereotypic behaviour during hallucinations, stupor phases that might be accompanied by self-injurious behaviours, and a premorbid phase. Group-two clinical signs include dilation of the third ventricles of the brain and occipital region peaks isolated on an electroencephalogram. Primary hormonal disorders, partial seizures, iatrogenic (medication-related) and brain tumours can mimic signs of dissociative disorders and must be ruled out.

The prognosis is generally poor. Early diagnosis and aggressive treatment can bring partial relief. Late-stage diagnosis is usually unsuccessful. It is estimated that under a third of patients respond to treatment overall. The treatment is mainly pharmacological. Early or mild cases may benefit from fluoxetine 1–4 mg/kg sid, while more advanced cases may benefit from neuroleptics such as risperidone (0.5–1 mg/m2 sid).

Owners should be made aware of the success rate and the risk of aggression. Environmental modification and routine changes should help to manage patients. When the dogs are near their owners, they should be tethered or muzzled. It is more difficult to limit cats unless confinement is used frequently. When left unsupervised the patient should be confined, and the owner should provide stimulation. The environment should be calm, quiet and relatively dark. Aggressive episodes may occur without any reason or provocation and might be very violent. In addition, the patient cannot be disrupted or redirected using signals or treats.

References

Adler, C.M., McDonough-Ryan, P., Sax, K.W., Holland, S.K., Arndt, S. *et al.* (2000) fMRI of neuronal activation with symptom provocation in unmedicated patients with obsessive compulsive disorder. *Journal of Psychiatric Research* 34(4-5), 317–324. DOI: 10.1016/S0022-3956(00)00022-4.

Bécuwe-Bonnet, V., Bélanger, M.-C., Frank, D., Parent, J. and Hélie, P. (2012) Gastrointestinal disorders in dogs with excessive licking of surfaces. *Journal of Veterinary Behavior* 7(4), 194–204. DOI: 10.1016/j.jveb.2011.07.003.

Denerolle, P., White, S.D., Taylor, T.S. and Vandenabeele, S.I.J. (2007) Organic diseases mimicking acral lick dermatitis in six dogs. *Journal of the American Animal Hospital Association* 43(4), 215–220. DOI: 10.5326/0430215.

Dodman, N.H., Karlsson, E.K., Moon-Fanelli, A., Galdzicka, M., Perloski, M. *et al.* (2010) A canine chromosome 7 locus confers compulsive disorder susceptibility. *Molecular Psychiatry* 15(1), 8–10. DOI: 10.1038/mp.2009.111.

Goldberger, E. and Rapoport, J.L. (1990) Canine acral lick dermatitis: response to the antiobsessional drug clomipramine. *Journal of the American Hospital Association* 27, 179–182.

Goodman, W.K., McDougle, C.J., Price, L.H., Riddle, M.A., Pauls, D.L. *et al.* (1990) Beyond the serotonin hypothesis: a role for dopamine in some forms of obsessive compulsive disorder? *The Journal of Clinical Psychiatry* 51 Suppl, S36–43.

Hartgraves, S.L. and Randall, P.K. (1986) Dopamine agonist-induced stereotypic grooming and self-mutilation following striatal dopamine depletion. *Psychopharmacology* 90(3), 358–363. DOI: 10.1007/BF00179191.

Hendricks, J.C., Lager, A., O'Brien, D. and Morrison, A.R. (1989) Movement disorders during sleep in cats and dogs. *Journal of the American Veterinary Medical Association* 194(5), 686–689.

Hewson, C.J., Luescher, U.A., Parent, J.M., Conlon, P.D. and Ball, R.O. (1998) Efficacy of clomipramine in the treatment of canine compulsive disorder. *Journal of the American Veterinary Medical Association* 213(12), 1760–1765.

Iglauer, F. and Rasim, R. (1993) Treatment of psychogenic leather picking in psittacine birds with a dopamine antagonist. *Journal of Small Animal Practice* 34(11), 564–566. DOI: 10.1111/j.1748-5827.1993.tb03550.x.

Irimajiri, M., Luescher, A.U., Douglass, G., Robertson-Plouch, C., Zimmermann, A. *et al.* (2009) Randomized, controlled clinical trial of the efficacy of fluoxetine for treatment of compulsive disorders in dogs. *Journal of the American Veterinary Medical Association* 235(6), 705–709. DOI: 10.2460/javma.235.6.705.

Korff, S. and Harvey, B.H. (2006) Animal models of obsessive-compulsive disorder: rationale to understanding psychobiology and pharmacology. *Psychiatric Clinics of North America* 29(2), 371–390. DOI: 10.1016/j.psc.2006.02.007.

Lochner, C. and Stein, D.J. (2003) Heterogeneity of obsessive-compulsive disorder: a literature review.

Harvard Review of Psychiatry 11(3), 113–132. DOI: 10.1080/10673220303949.

Martin, A., Scahill, L., Vitulano, L. and King, R.A. (1998) Stimulant use and trichotillomania. *Journal of the American Academy of Child & Adolescent Psychiatry* 37(4), 349–350. DOI: 10.1097/00004583-199804000-00009.

Mason, G.J. (2006) Stereotypic behaviour in captive animals; fundamentals and implications for welfare and beyond. In: Mason, G.J. and Rushen, J. (eds) *Stereotypic Animal Behavior: Fundamentals and Applications to Welfare*. CAB International, Wallingford, UK, pp. 325–356.

McDougle, C.J., Goodman, W.K., Leckman, J.F., Lee, N.C., Heninger, G.R. *et al.* (1994) Haloperidol addition in fluvoxamine-refractory obsessive-compulsive disorder. A double-blind, placebo-controlled study in patients with and without tics. *Archives of General Psychiatry* 51(4), 302–308. DOI: 10.1001/archpsyc.1994.03950040046006.

McElroy, S.L., Phillips, K.A. and Keck, P.E. (1994) Obsessive compulsive spectrum disorder. *The Journal of Clinical Psychiatry* 55 Suppl, 33–51.

Moon-Fanelli, A.A. and Dodman, N.H. (1998) Description and development of compulsive tail chasing in terriers and response to clomipramine treatment. *Journal of the American Veterinary Medical Association* 212(8), 1252–1257.

Moon-Fanelli, A.A., Dodman, N.H., Famula, T.R. and Cottam, N. (2011) Characteristics of compulsive tail chasing and associated risk factors in bull terriers. *Journal of the American Veterinary Medical Association* 238(7), 883–889. DOI: 10.2460/javma.238.7.883.

Pauls, D.L., Abramovitch, A., Rauch, S.L. and Geller, D.A. (2014) Obsessive-compulsive disorder: an integrative genetic and neurobiological perspective. *Nature Reviews Neuroscience* 15(6), 410–424. DOI: 10.1038/nrn3746.

Pittenger, C., Bloch, M.H. and Williams, K. (2011) Glutamate abnormalities in obsessive compulsive disorder: neurobiology, pathophysiology, and treatment. *Pharmacology & Therapeutics* 132(3), 314–332. DOI: 10.1016/j.pharmthera.2011.09.006.

Rapoport, J.L., Ryland, D.H. and Kriete, M. (1992) Drug treatment of canine acral lick. an animal model of obsessive-compulsive disorder. *Archives of General Psychiatry* 49(7), 517–521. DOI: 10.1001/archpsyc.1992.01820070011002.

Ripley, B., Fujiki, N., Okura, M., Mignot, E. and Nishino, S. (2001) Hypocretin levels in sporadic and familial cases of canine narcolepsy. *Neurobiology of Disease* 8(3), 525–534. DOI: 10.1006/nbdi.2001.0389.

Schubert, T.A., Chidester, R.M. and Chrisman, C.L. (2011) Clinical characteristics, management and long-term outcome of suspected rapid eye movement sleep behaviour disorder in 14 dogs. *Journal of Small Animal Practice* 52(2), 93–100. DOI: 10.1111/j.1748-5827.2010.01026.x.

Shumaker, A.K., Angus, J.C., Coyner, K.S., Loeffler, D.G., Rankin, S.C. *et al.* (2008) Microbiological and histopathological features of canine acral lick dermatitis. *Veterinary Dermatology* 19(5), 288–298. DOI: 10.1111/j.1365-3164.2008.00693.x.

Stein, D.J. (2000) Neurobiology of the obsessive-compulsive spectrum disorders. *Biological Psychiatry* 47(4), 296–304. DOI: 10.1016/S0006-3223(99)00271-1.

Stein, D.J., Mendelsohn, I., Potocnik, F., Van Kradenberg, J. and Wessels, C. (1998) Use of the selective serotonin reuptake inhibitor citalopram in a possible animal analogue of obsessive-compulsive disorder. *Depression and Anxiety* 8(1), 39–42. DOI: 10.1002/(SICI)1520-6394(1998)8:1<39::AID-DA8>3.0.CO;2-0.

Waisglass, S.E., Landsberg, G.M., Yager, J.A. and Hall, J.A. (2006) Underlying medical conditions in cats with presumptive psychogenic alopecia. *Journal of the American Veterinary Medical Association* 228(11), 1705–1709. DOI: 10.2460/javma.228.11.1705.

Wynchank, D. and Berk, M. (1998) Fluoxetine treatment of acral lick dermatitis in dogs: a placebo-controlled randomized double blind trial. *Depression and Anxiety* 8(1), 21–23. DOI: 10.1002/(SICI)1520-6394(1998)8:1<21::AID-DA4>3.0.CO;2-8.

Zanghi, B.M. (2017) Sleep disorders. In: Ettinger, S.J., Feldman, E.C. and Cote, E. (eds) *Textbook of Veterinary Internal Medicine: Diseases of the Dog and Cat*. Elsevier, St. Louis, Missouri, pp. 1410–1413.

Zohar, J. and Insel, T.R. (1987) Obsessive-compulsive disorder: psychobiological approaches to diagnosis, treatment, and pathophysiology. *Biological Psychiatry* 22(6), 667–687. DOI: 10.1016/0006-3223(87)90199-5.

16 Ageing-related Problems in Cats and Dogs

Sagi Denenberg*

Langford Vets, University of Bristol, Langford, UK; North Toronto Veterinary Behaviour Specialty Clinic, Toronto, Canada

16.1 Introduction

In the past two decades, advances in veterinary medicine and nutrition, and ownership, have led to increases in the average lifespan of dogs and cats. However, it also means that now we see more age-related diseases. A senior pet is the one who has reached 75% of its estimated lifespan. While it is somewhat easier to determine this average in pure-bred animals, mixed breeds are more challenging to estimate. The author uses a simple rule-of-thumb to estimate lifespan in crossbred dogs: small dogs are considered seniors when they reach 12 years of age, medium-sizes dogs over 10, large dogs over 9, and giant dogs are considered senior when they are over 7 years of age. Cats are considered senior over 12 years of age.

The process of ageing contributes to the development of two groups of diseases: physical and mental. As the body ages, different systems become less efficient and more susceptible to changes in the body equilibrium. As a result, systems' dysfunction, mutation and deterioration take place. Abnormal products such as toxic proteins (e.g. beta-amyloid) or toxic free radicals are formed and can damage different tissues. Further, often the changes are occurring in several systems at the same time. The immune, cardiac and skeletal systems also degenerate, leading to a reduced ability of the animal to cope with daily triggers. The pet sensory system declines as well. With reduced sight, hearing, olfaction and tactile abilities, the pet may feel less competent to interact with its environment. As a result, anxieties and fear may develop or worsen in senior pets as compared to young adults.

In many, if not most, senior pets, the first, and sometimes the only, change that might indicate the development of different abnormalities is a behavioural change (see Table 16.1). Senior pets may avoid many interactions, become more withdrawn and apathetic, or irritable and even aggressive. Moreover, senior pets may develop cognitive changes leading to confusion, disorientation and memory loss.

16.2 Addressing Behavioural Problems in Senior Pets

Senior pets should be evaluated at least twice yearly if no health concerns are present. The frequency may increase if the pet is presenting chronic health concerns. Aside from a complete physical examination, and laboratory tests, a full behavioural screen should take place. The author is using a simple questionnaire (see Handouts A5 – Cat Cognitive Dysfunction Questionnaire, and A6 – Dog Cognitive Dysfunction Questionnaire) to help to detect any behavioural change that may not be apparent during the visit to the surgery. The questionnaire can be given to the owner to fill in prior to the visit. Based on the owner's answers, further discussion can take place.

Early identification of behavioural clinical signs allows for most optimal care to be given. Unfortunately, unless we ask specific and direct questions, most owners do not report these clinical signs. Among other reasons, owners might not be aware that the veterinary surgeon can provide care and help for their pet, they may be concerned about the recommendation of euthanasia, and perhaps believe that the clinical signs are part of

*s.denenberg@bristol.ac.uk

DOI: 10.1079/9781786394552.0016

Table 16.1. Possible behavioural clinical signs of physical diseases.

Possible behavioural signs	Possible causes
Changes in appetite Disorientation Fear/anxiety Irritability Lethargy/apathy Reduced interest in play and activity Vocalization Withdrawal/avoidance	Cardiovascular: cardiomyopathy, hypertension hypoxia ischaemia mitral insufficiency
Aggression/irritability Hyperaesthesia Reduced interest in exercise or play Reduced self-hygiene Restlessness – pacing Sleep–wake cycle changes/restlessness Stereotypic – licking/self-trauma	Dermatologic: allergies atopy autoimmune diseases dermatitis fungal diseases parasites
Aggression Avoidance/withdrawal House soiling Night-time waking Pica/coprophagia Reduced appetite Stereotypic – licking Stereotypic – pacing	Digestive: constipation dental/oral diseases hepatic diseases infectious/inflammatory nutritional imbalances pain
Aggression (over food/water) Activity – increased/decreased/apathy Appetite – increased/decreased House soiling/urine marking Irritability Restlessness – pacing Sleep–wake cycle Stereotypic – licking Vocalization	Endocrine: diabetes insipidus diabetes mellitus hyperadrenocorticism hyperthyroidism hypoadrenocorticism hypothyroidism insulinoma
Aggression Avoidance Reduced interest in exercise or play Reduced self-hygiene Sleep–wake cycle changes/restlessness Vocalization	Musculoskeletal: arthritis degenerative diseases muscular dystrophy pain
Aggression Avoidance Decreased response to stimuli Disorientation Fear/anxiety Reduced learning ability Vocalization	Sensory: cataracts/lenticular sclerosis loss of hearing loss of vision
Aggression House soiling/marking Pacing Sleep–wake changes Withdrawal/avoidance	Urinary tract: idiopathic cystitis renal diseases urinary incontinence urinary tract infection urolithiasis

normal ageing. Being proactive and educating owners about senior pet care and management options is the best tool we have to address the appropriate level of care for these pets.

When a senior pet is presented due to behaviour problems, the first task is to rule out or treat a physical disease. Only once those are addressed, can we move towards managing behaviour problems. Frequently, we must manage both physical and behavioural diseases simultaneously.

Management of behaviour problems in senior pets is more challenging and limited compared to younger animals. This is due to deteriorated physical health, including sensory decline, pain and reduced cognition in some cases. Moreover, many senior pets are being treated for other physical conditions with medications that may contradict the use of psychoactive medications. Owners must be patient when managing senior pets and have realistic expectations.

Most behavioural problems in senior pets are similar to those in younger pets, and so is the management. Therefore, this chapter will focus on those problems that have more specific concerns for senior pets. For a complete discussion of other problems, see the relevant chapters.

16.2.1 Aggression

Aggression in senior dogs and cats may have similar underlying causes to those in younger pets. Once physical changes that can lead to aggression (e.g. pain, central nervous system [CNS] disease or diabetes mellitus) are ruled out, the focus is on the animal's internal or external behavioural causes. For more details, see Chapter 11 (for cats) or Chapter 12 (for dogs).

Several age-related changes may account for differences in, or possibly increased, aggression in senior pets. Senior dogs and cats may have reduced mobility due to degenerative joint disease, and their ability to avoid specific triggers or situations is reduced. As a result, the pet might be more likely to respond with aggression rather than avoiding. Similarly, with reduced sensory capacity (e.g. reduced vision or hearing), the animal might be surprised by triggers and is forced to react with aggression. Finally, the ability of the senior pet to communicate (both transmitting and receiving the message) might be impaired due to different physical diseases, leading to increased aggression.

16.2.1.1 Treatment

In many cases of aggression in senior pets, we are limited in our ability to implement a behaviour modification plan that is based on learning and memory due to the animal's physical and mental conditions. Therefore, safety through environmental management is the first goal. Owners should be taught to identify triggers and situations that lead to aggression and try preventing or avoiding them. The animal should have a safe environment in the home, where it can stay, rest and sleep. The owners should manage the animal's routine so that it is predictable and creates separation when necessary. The safe environment should include easily accessible perches and hiding areas for cats, and possibly covered crates for dogs.

When possible, desensitization and counter-conditioning exercises should take place. Owners should have realistic expectations of what can be achieved. Also, the implementation of such programmes is likely to require more time and effort than for younger animals. For more details on the management of aggression, see the relevant chapters.

16.2.2 Anxiety disorders

With reduced physical and mental capacities, senior pets' ability to cope with changes (e.g. routine, household or environment) is reduced. As a result, anxiety may develop or worsen. Further, anxieties that existed through the years may exacerbate through learning (e.g. sensitization). Senior pets may develop similar disorders (e.g. phobias, panic attacks, noise sensitivities, or separation-related) to younger animals. Finally, due to physical changes, senior pets may develop new anxieties or frustration-related disorders. For example, a senior cat may not be able to reach its favourite perch on a tower due to degenerative joint disease. The cat may become more anxious about its inability to avoid different situations, or frustrated that it cannot reach its favourite spot. Owners, too, may cause more anxiety by expecting senior pets to behave as they did in the past or not addressing age-related changes.

16.2.2.1 Treatment

Anxiety disorders in senior dogs and cats require similar management to younger cats. For more details, see Chapter 13. The management requires more patience, consistency and persistence than the management of similar disorders in younger animals. Owners should strive to match the needs of the senior pet and provide predictability and safety. To reduce frustration, owners should attempt to provide easy access to resources or preferred locations (e.g. provide a ramp to climb onto the windowsill), and avoid rapid or unnecessary changes.

The use of psychoactive medications might be useful and necessary. However, it might be limited due to concurrent physical diseases. Therefore, careful selection or dose adjustments are required. Also, the use of nutraceuticals might be beneficial and safer in some cases.

16.2.3 Excessive vocalization

This is a subjective problem based on owners' perceptions, and the main objectives are to determine the cause and try to reduce it. There are many physical disorders (e.g. hyperthyroid, pain or CNS disease) that may lead to increased vocalization at different times of the day. Increased anxieties or fear-related conditions might also lead to increased vocalization. For more information on cats and dogs, see Chapter 10.

The first step is to collect information about this behaviour. Owners should record data on when, where, how long, possible triggers (e.g. food, attention, outdoor animals or noises), and the reactions of the pet. Also, owners should view recent history before the problem started. For example, recent changes to the household or environment may trigger excessive vocalization.

16.2.3.1 Treatment

Once we identify the cause, we may implement appropriate management. Physical disorders must be ruled out or addressed first, and then we can approach behavioural management. Owners should ensure the animal's needs are met regularly through a predictable daily routine. For example, a dog who vocalizes at night might be hungry. Therefore, providing a late-night meal might reduce vocalization (see also 16.2.5 – Night waking). Owners should remember that giving attention may reinforce attention-seeking behaviours. Only when different diseases (e.g. pain or nausea) are ruled out, and the animal's needs are met, should owners be instructed to ignore the animal.

The focus should be on reinforcing calm and desired behaviours rather than trying to stop (punish) undesired behaviours. The animal can be taught a calm or quiet signal at times when it is not vocalizing, using reward-based training. Then, when the cat or dog starts vocalizing, the owner may give the signal and reward the animal if it stops. With sufficient repetitions, once the animal learns to stop vocalizing more rapidly and consistently, the owner can shape the behaviour. That is, instead of providing the reward immediately, as the animal stops vocalizing, the owner will start delaying the reward, gradually increasing the time that the animal is quiet. Later, the owner may change from a constant reinforcement ratio (e.g. reward after each repetition) to a variable reinforcement ratio (rewarding the behaviour randomly).

Marker training (see Handout C6 – Marker Training) might be beneficial in managing excessive vocalization. First, the owner must condition the cat or dog to the marker. For example, pairing finger-snapping with a tasty treat. Then, when the animal is conditioned (that is getting excited when it hears the marker), the owner can start using the marker to signal calm behaviours. The owner is instructed to ignore the cat or dog when it vocalizes, and mark quiet behaviour once the pet stops. As noted above, the objective is to move towards a variable reinforcement ratio of calm behaviours.

16.2.4 House soiling

House soiling is a commonly reported behaviour problem in senior pets. There are numerous physical disorders that may lead to this presentation including those that are more widely seen in senior pets (e.g. renal disease, urinary incontinence, cognitive decline or degenerative joint diseases), or those that can be found in any age, such as diabetes mellitus, Cushing's disease or inflammatory bowel disease. There are also behavioural reasons such as enuresis, encopresis, substrate/location aversion or preferences, and marking behaviour.

The first step is to rule out any physical disorder or to manage these. A full physical examination and relevant laboratory tests are always indicated. Owners should keep a diary of the soiling behaviours, including, if possible, video of the animal. These data might help to identify patterns, routines or indications of physical disorders.

It is essential to ascertain that the animal in question was appropriately house-trained in the past, and this is truly a new problem rather than lack of training. The household routine and environment should be evaluated for any recent changes prior to the start of the problem.

16.2.4.1 Treatment

Owners of senior cats and dogs with physical or sensorial impairment should provide easier access to elimination areas. For example, providing a litter tray in a dark or difficult-to-access location (e.g. basement) may limit the cat's ability to access it. Similarly, going down many stairs or walking a long distance to reach the field may restrict the dog's ability to eliminate in appropriate locations.

Once physical disorders are ruled out or addressed, owners should ensure the animal has a consistent daily routine that allows ample opportunities for appropriate soiling. For example, dogs should have enough access to the garden or walks. Similarly, cats that depend on their owners to be let out should have sufficient access to the garden. For more information about routine management of house soiling in cats and dogs, see Chapter 14. Underlying causes of marking behaviours should be identified, and a behaviour modification programme should be prescribed.

The animal's environment should be modified as well. If the animal returns to the same location each time, the function of the location might be changed from latrine to a feeding station or sleeping area. The owner should clean the area thoroughly using biological cleaners. Once the area is cleaned, food or beds can be placed there. In addition, using pheromone products might help.

16.2.5 Night waking

Most cats and dogs adapt to their owner's routine and spend most of the night sleeping. Cats, in particular, are crepuscular (dusk and dawn activity) creatures (Fitzgerald and Turner, 2000). An altered sleep–wake cycle may lead to cats and dogs becoming more active at night. While this behaviour can occur in all ages, it tends to be more common in senior cats and dogs.

Any disease that causes pain or altered metabolism can lead to night waking. Pain as a result of arthritis or gastrointestinal conditions is one of the leading causes of restlessness and inability to sleep. Pets may pace, circle, lie down and get up, and stand in one place. Any disease that leads to increased urination, thirst or appetite (e.g. diabetes mellitus, diabetes insipidus or hyperadrenocorticism) may lead to restlessness, frequent need to go out, and agitation. Hypertension and hyperthyroidism are among the leading causes in senior cats. Cognitive dysfunction might also lead to an altered sleep–wake cycle in senior pets.

Primary behavioural causes include anxiety disorders, compulsive behaviours (e.g. circling, pacing or hallucinations) and conflict with other pets in the home. Boredom and lack of daytime stimulation may contribute to night waking in pets. Night waking could be part of attention-seeking behaviour in senior pets, especially if the pet feels more insecure at night. Often, excessive vocalization is also part of the clinical picture.

Owners may reinforce, inadvertently, this problem by giving attention to the animal. Changes in household routine or the environment may also contribute. Finally, in some cases, the inciting causes may not be the maintaining factors. Therefore, addressing both is necessary at times.

16.2.5.1 Treatment

As with any other behaviour problem, the first step is to rule out or manage any physical disease causing night waking. However, some conditions cannot be managed effectively (e.g. sensory or cognitive decline, or degenerative joint disease), reducing the success rate of managing night-time waking. Long-term, or possibly life-long, medications and management may be required (Landsberg *et al.*, 2011).

The next step is to try to identify both inciting and maintaining factors. Ideally, these factors can be removed by addressing the pet's daily routine and environment, and meeting its needs throughout the day. Owners should attempt to increase daytime stimulation, both physical and mental, based on the pet's ability. Also, any reinforcement (maintaining factor) should be removed.

Rewarding calm behaviours, rather than trying to stop undesired behaviours, should reflect the primary approach that owners should take. Owners can use marker training to signal calm behaviours as they take place.

Owners should maintain a predictable and consistent daily routine. If the pet is hungry overnight, providing a late-night meal might reduce restless behaviours overnight. Also, providing food in timed (automatic) feeders might help.

Where a conflict between pets in the home is the problem, the pets should be separated overnight, each in their respective places. Owners should slowly establish these locations by providing positive outcomes for spending time there. The use of pheromones might be beneficial to help pets settling down in those places.

In some cases, the use of psychoactive medications or hypnotics is necessary. Trazodone or clonazepam are two useful medications for hyposomnia or insomnia in pets. For anxiety-related night-time waking, the use of a serotonergic medication might be beneficial. Finally, for night-time waking as a result of cognitive decline, selegiline might be indicated.

16.2.6 Abnormal and repetitive behaviours

Senior pets may show similar abnormal and repetitive behaviours (ARBs) to younger animals. With the increased risk of physical disease, so is the risk of ARB as a result of physical changes increasing. Conditions such as pain, sensory decline, CNS diseases including tumours, organ dysfunctions and metabolic diseases might lead to the development of ARB. Cognitive decline may lead to behaviours that are abnormal and repetitive such as excessive pacing.

Primary behavioural conditions such as anxiety disorders, frustration and boredom might also contribute to the development of ARB in senior pets. For more information on different abnormal and repetitive behaviours in dogs and cats, including diagnosis and management, see Chapter 15.

16.2.6.1 *Treatment*

Behavioural management can follow if primary physical diseases are ruled out or treated. Often, both physical and behavioural treatments must be applied at the same time. Medications to control pain, cognitive decline or other diseases may be used.

Owners should be advised to maintain a diary of the behaviour, including information such as when, where, how long, can the animal be distracted, possible triggers, and the animal's mentation. These data help to identify the inciting and maintaining factors and differentiate physical from mental causes.

Owners should remove any reinforcement they may provide to the animal. Next, addressing the animal's routine and environment must take place. The animal should be free to express normal behaviours within its environment — increasing stimulation where adequate and providing a consistent and predictable daily routine should help. Owners can work with their pet on basic training, play with toys, and use feeding toys instead of bowls for feeding.

Focusing on calm behaviours rather than punishing the animal in an attempt to stop the behaviour is necessary. Owners can try stopping the behaviour using redirection signals (e.g. response substitution – see Chapter 8) and then reward an alternative behaviour. Using tools such as a lead and head halter might be beneficial.

When ARB leads to reducing the quality of life, the use of medications is beneficial. The most commonly used medications are serotonergic. Other options may include buspirone, benzodiazepines and gabapentin. For more information, see Chapter 9. We may have to adjust the dose or medication depending on the animal's health and other medication it might be taking.

16.3 Cognitive Dysfunction

Cognitive dysfunction syndrome (CDS) is a progressive and degenerative disease of the brain. The clinical hallmarks of CDS are memory loss, reduced cognitive abilities and confusion (Landsberg *et al.*, 2010, 2011) The underlying pathology involves continuous damage to neurons leading to cerebral atrophy, particularly around the third ventricles and hippocampus (Colle, *et al.*, 2000; Tapp *et al.*, 2004; Gunn-Moore *et al.*, 2006). There are many parallels between the pathology of CDS in pets, dogs in particular, and people with Alzheimer's disease (Takeuchi *et al.*, 2008).

There are several likely causes for this pathology. With ageing, the circulatory system becomes less efficient, leading to micro-haemorrhages and infarcts formation (Cummings *et al.*, 1996; Gunn-Moore *et al.*, 2006). As a result, oxygen perfusion to tissues is compromised, leading to reduced mitochondrial function in neurons and higher production of toxic oxygen-free radicals (TFR). These TFRs destroy or change different cell metabolites, such as proteins, and damage the cell membrane (Head *et al.*, 2002; Sullivan and Brown, 2005). The formation of beta-amyloid protein oligomers creates extracellular plaques that possibly affect the ion channels (primarily Ca^{+2}), leading to apoptosis (Takeuchi *et al.*, 2008). The distribution of beta-amyloid is somewhat different between dogs and cats. In dogs, the distribution is more discrete, while in cats, it is more diffuse (Landsberg *et al.*, 2010, 2011). The amount of beta-amyloid deposition in neurons and perivascular correlates with the age of the cat or dog (Nakamura *et al.*, 1996; Head *et al.*, 2005).

Why do many owners avoid reporting the clinical signs of cognitive dysfunction to their vets? There are several likely explanations. Owners may not be aware of early clinical signs, especially if they are minimal. Also, unless the owner pays close attention, clinical signs may go unnoticed. Clinical signs might be easier to diagnose in working dogs (e.g. guide dogs and police dogs) whose behaviour is stricter and more dependent on trained behaviours. Many pet dogs and most cats do not perform to the same level; therefore, owners might miss mild signs such as wandering into a room or environment or forgetting to eat a meal or two. Further, owners may not know that management of cognitive decline exists (see Section 16.3.5) or believe that the veterinary surgeon may recommend euthanasia. Finally, owners may feel that this is part of normal ageing and that no management is warranted.

We must be proactive and ask specific questions during each routine visit of ageing cats and dogs. Moreover, discussing the likelihood of CDS with owners of adult cats and dogs, and informing them about the possibility of this disease and management options, may encourage owners to pay close attention to clinical signs and report them. The use of screening questionnaires (see Handouts A5 – Cat Cognitive Dysfunction Questionnaire, and A6 - Dog Cognitive Dysfunction Questionnaire) may be helpful to identify potential patients and offer early intervention.

16.3.1 Diagnosis

The primary clinical signs of CDS in dogs and cats are divided into five groups: disorientation and confusion; changes in normal routines and behavioural patterns; changes in interactions with people and other animals; activity changes; and memory loss. A cat or a dog with cognitive dysfunction may forget to eat, forget where it usually soils or forget when it is time for a walk. Similarly, the animal may forget past training and people it associated with in the past. Owners may complain about house soiling, changes in interactions and weight loss.

Natural biological rhythms may change as well. Cats and dogs with CDS may become more active, especially at times when they used to sleep, or sleep more than before. They may need to soil at different times than they did previously. The animal might walk into an environment, even a familiar one, and wander or stand and appear confused. It might wander into a corner without the ability to back out of it. Finally, the pet may seem more anxious.

To date, there are no definitive tools to diagnose CDS in cats and dogs (Denenberg *et al.*, 2017). The diagnosis is based on the exclusion of other possible causes. A full physical examination, including appropriate laboratory tests and imaging, should precede behavioural assessment. At times, a medication trial may be warranted, especially if pain is suspected. Any current physical disease must be addressed first. On the other hand, finding a physical or behavioural disease in senior pets does not exclude the possibility of concurrent cognitive dysfunction syndrome.

16.3.2 Medical differentials of cognitive dysfunction in cats and dogs

Central nervous system diseases may directly alter the pet's consciousness and responsiveness. In addition, extra-cranial diseases may also affect the CNS and indirectly affect its function, and lead to CDS-like clinical signs. Chronic exposure to CNS toxins might lead to the development of clinical signs similar to CDS. Any debilitating or chronic disease may lead to increased anxiety, irritability, changes in sleep–wake cycles, and avoidance.

16.3.2.1 Cardiovascular diseases

Cerebral hypoxia might be the result of ischemia, hypotension or other compromised circulation within the CNS or extra-cranially. The pet may appear withdrawn, lethargic or confused. Moreover, the cat or dog might present reduced social interactions, awareness and activity levels.

Cardiovascular diseases in cats and dogs may lead to exercise intolerance, increased irritability and reduced appetite. The pet may start pacing at night, showing altered sleep–wake cycles. Hypertension and congestive heart failure may lead to the development, or increase, of anxiety as a result of dyspnoea at times, cardiac palpitations and arrhythmias, and cerebral hypoxia.

16.3.2.2 Endocrine diseases

House soiling in senior dogs may be the result of diabetes insipidus rather than cognitive dysfunction. Also, the animal may show night-time restlessness and pacing due to the need to be let out to eliminate.

Night-time waking, house soiling and lethargy may be the result of hyperglycaemia in diabetes mellitus in cats and dogs. Increased drinking and appetite may lead to aggression over resources. Advanced stages of diabetes mellitus may lead to the development of hyperkalaemia, leading to lethargy, withdrawn behaviour with reduced interactions, and disorientation.

Hyperadrenocorticism might lead to increased anxiety-like clinical signs as a result of chronic over-activation of the hypothalamic-pituitary-adrenal axis with the excessive production of cortisol. Dogs may become more irritable, aggressive and restless. With polyphagia, polydipsia and polyuria, the dog might show aggression over resources, house soiling, night-time pacing and exercise intolerance.

Hypoadrenocorticism might result in lethargy and apathy, and the dog may appear withdrawn. Increased levels of potassium and, in some cases, hypoglycemia are responsible for these signs. Some pets are presented for exercise intolerance and disorientation.

Hyperthyroidism in cats (and possibly iatrogenic in dogs) may lead to increased restlessness, agitation, aggression, night-time pacing and vocalization. Some cats might display abnormal and repetitive behaviours.

Hypothyroidism in dogs (and possibly iatrogenic in cats) might lead to lower-rate metabolism. Clinical signs may include lethargy, exercise intolerance, changes in sleep–wake cycle and reduced interactions.

Insulinomas are rare in cats and dogs (Meleo and Peterson, 2014). Oversecretion of insulin will lead to hypoglycemia. The animal may appear withdrawn, disoriented, confused and fearful. Other clinical signs may include sleep–wake cycle alterations and increased vocalization.

16.3.2.3 Gastrointestinal and hepatic diseases

Diseases that lead to abdominal pain, discomfort, acid reflux and nausea may cause cats and dogs to wake up at night, vocalize and become irritable. Further, these diseases may cause lip-licking, lip-smacking, licking surfaces and owners, and other anxiety-related signs.

Bowel diseases such as inflammatory bowel syndrome and infections that affect motility can lead to diarrhoea and house soiling. Dogs that are well trained not to soil at home might develop anxiety as a result of house soiling. In contrast, constipation may lead to pain and signs of withdrawal, night-time pacing, avoidance of interactions, reduced appetite and aggression.

Exocrine pancreatic insufficiency might lead to indigestion, pain, reduce activity, and eating non-food items (pica) in pets. Pancreatitis may cause pain, nausea and vomiting. Pets with pancreatic diseases might be restless, irritable and more aggressive.

Hepatic dysfunction may lead to reduced absorption of nutrients that are essential for proper nerve cell function, indigestion and pain. Moreover, hepatic encephalopathy may be the result of hepatic shunts and microvascular dysplasia (portal atresia). The result is toxaemia, an increased level of ammonia that may lead to an adverse effect on the CNS. The pet might appear disorientated, confused, irritable and more aggressive. Also, abnormal and repetitive behaviours may emerge.

16.3.2.4 Pain

Pain may be the result of almost all diseases. Pain may be acute or chronic, localized or generalized, and lead to increased irritability, aggression and exploration, or reduced activity, apathy and withdrawal (see Chapter 3). Pain is expressed through species-specific behaviours. Dogs are more likely to show overt signs of pain, including vocalization, limping, licking and aggression. Cats, on the other hand, are more likely to avoid performing certain behaviours such as jumping onto counters, hunting or seeking affection. These behavioural signs might be considered changes in interactions, sleep–wake cycle changes, and confusion.

Pain may also alter specific behavioural patterns. For example, cats with urinary tract pain may avoid the litter tray if it becomes associated with pain. Similarly, if the pet learns that it cannot avoid pain (e.g. move away when in pain from arthritis), it might become more aggressive. Dental pain may lead to reduced appetite.

Localized pain may lead to the development of abnormal and repetitive behaviour such as excessive licking and self-injury of a particular joint or area on the body. The release of opioids, endorphins and enkephalins serve as local analgesia and reinforce the licking behaviour.

Pets with chronic pain eventually alter their behaviour in an attempt to ease or avoid pain. They may eat less, sleep less and become lethargic or more anxious.

16.3.2.5 Sensory decline

Ageing may lead to reduced vision and hearing, and possibly olfaction abilities. Lenticular sclerosis is an ageing of the lens, leading to impaired vision, especially in low light. Pathological conditions, such as cataracts, might lead to partial or complete blindness. Any disease along the auditory pathways may affect the pet's hearing.

Reduced sensory capabilities affect the pet's ability to perceive information, including threats, and communicate with the environment. Cats and dogs may become more anxious, aggressive and irritable. They might also exhibit night-time waking and vocalization, reduced appetite and house soiling. Owners may complain about changes in interactions, restlessness, sleep–wake cycle changes, disorientation and confusion.

16.3.2.6 Urinary tract diseases

Chronic kidney disease (CKD) is a common disease in senior pets that leads to increased urination and drinking. Owners may complain about house soiling and aggression over resources (water).

Furthermore, CKD may lead to nausea and reduced appetite and abdominal pain. Owners may report that the pet forgets to eat, and is licking excessively. In more advanced stages, with increasing azotaemia and hyperkalaemia, signs of confusion, disorientation and lethargy may appear.

Lower urinary tract diseases, such as idiopathic cystitis or feline urinary syndrome, may lead to house soiling in pets. Typical accompanying signs include increased anxiety, pain, irritability and aggression. Pets may vocalize, pace and have altered sleep–wake cycle.

Urinary incontinence may develop, particularly in ageing bitches. Owners might complain about house soiling and forgetting to go outside to soil.

16.3.3 Behavioural differentials of cognitive dysfunction in dogs and cats

Many primary behavioural diseases may lead to similar signs of cognitive decline. See Section 16.2 and other relevant chapters for more information. A thorough evaluation of the cat or dog history, observation of current behaviours and identifying the clinical signs of CDS during situations in which the primary behavioural differential does not occur can help in diagnosis. Primary behavioural diseases can take place concurrently with CDS in cats and dogs and may complicate the diagnosis.

16.3.4 Standardized laboratory tests

Cognitive dysfunction syndrome is challenging to assess in owned cats and dogs due to the lack of clinical diagnostic tests, owners and household variability, and different training levels of cats and dogs at home.

However, in a standardized setting in laboratories, where all animals receive the same care, training, diets and medical care, it is possible to detect signs of cognitive decline at an earlier age, based on an accurate battery of tests (Levine *et al.*, 1987; Cotman and Head, 2008). These tests involve teaching the cat or dog a specific behaviour, and after reaching the desired success rate the task is changed. The tests measure the animal error or success rate in comparison to a younger, cognitively intact cat or dog (Head *et al.*, 1995; Christie *et al.*, 2005; Milgram, 2010). In one test, the cat or dog is presented with a tray, and on it there are different objects. Underneath one of the objects, the well is filled with canned food, while the other wells, under the other objects are empty. All objects are baited with canned food to eliminate olfactory bias. During the first phase of the test, the cat or dog must learn that the food is always under the same object (discrimination test). Once the cat or dog learns that the food is always under a specific object (reach the success criterion), the tester then switches the food to a different well underneath a different object (reversal phase). The cat or dog then must learn the new protocol. The number of errors made is the measurement of the animal's cognitive ability. A similar test involves identical objects and food placed underneath one of them. In this test, the cat or dog must learn that a marker (a different object) is placed near the correct well (landmark test). This time, the marker is slowly moved along the tray in increasing distance from the correct object. Two other tests investigate the spatial memory of the animal by presenting the tray with food baited well under objects, and using an increasing time delay the cat or dog has to identify where the food is.

Later, the position of the food is reversed (delayed non-matching to position, and egocentric tests, respectively). For more details of these tests and applications see other sources (Christie *et al.*, 2005; Landsberg *et al.*, 2010, 2011; Milgram, 2010; Landsberg and Malamed, 2017).

16.3.5 Treatment of cognitive dysfunction in dogs and cats

The approach to the treatment of CDS in cats and dogs should be multimodal. There are four modalities of treatment: medications, supplements, diets, and behavioural approach. A combination of some or all of these modalities yields the best result. The main aims of treatment are enhancing neuronal function and transmission, reducing the production and elimination of toxic free radicals, strengthening the integrity of neurones, and overall improvement of brain metabolism. While not available at this time, using stem cells therapy for CDS is currently under research.

Like any other disease, early intervention and tailored management is optimal. Currently, there are a few medications, supplements and diets licensed for dogs. The options for cats are more limited and extrapolated from dogs.

Still, owners should be made aware that there is no cure for CDS in cats and dogs. Treatment aims to minimize the signs, slow the deterioration and improve the cat's or dog's quality of life.

16.3.5.1 *Medications*

Selegiline is classified as a preferential and irreversible inhibitor of the enzyme monoamine oxidase type B (MAOB), although the mode of action is not entirely understood. In high doses, it might also have a minor effect on MAO type A. The enzyme MAOB degrades catecholamines (dopamine, noradrenaline and serotonin) in the brain. The main impact of selegiline is thought to be due to the increase in dopamine, leading to an improvement in clinical signs of CDS (Head *et al.*, 1996; Ruehl *et al.*, 1997).

Among other effects, selegiline also enhances the activity enzyme superoxide dismutase, leading to an increased rate of toxic free radicals removal, stimulating the release of catecholamines and inhibiting the re-uptake of catecholamines (Carrillo *et al.*, 1994; Denenberg *et al.*, 2018).

Selegiline is licensed for dogs (in North America) for the treatment of CDS, but not in cats. However, there is a growing body of evidence of its usefulness in cats as well (Landsberg *et al.*, 2010). Selegiline, as other MAO inhibitors, should not be given concurrently with other medications that enhance catecholamines, in particular serotonin. In human medicine, people who take MAO inhibitors are cautioned not to eat foods that contain tyramine, as it may lead to a fatal reaction. While no such warning exists in veterinary psychiatry, it is prudent to caution pet owners as well.

The xanthine derivative, propentofylline, is licensed to improve dullness and lethargy in dogs. It may prevent platelets aggregation, thereby reducing the risk of thrombus formation, leading to improved microcirculation in the brain (Parkinson *et al.*, 1994). The result is enhanced oxygenation of the brain. While it is not licensed for cats, there is anecdotal evidence to support its use in this species (Gunn-Moore *et al.*, 2007; Landsberg *et al.*, 2010).

Nicergoline is an ergot alkaloid derivative that may be beneficial in CDS (Siwak *et al.*, 2000b). As an I1-adrenoceptor antagonist, it induces vasodilation and increases arterial blood flow; enhances cholinergic and catecholaminergic neurotransmitter function; inhibits platelet aggregation; promotes metabolic activity, resulting in increased utilization of oxygen and glucose; and has neurotrophic and antioxidant properties (Winblad *et al.*, 2008).

Adrafinil and modafinil are both eugeroic substances that improve alertness, stabilize the sleep–wake cycle and have weak dopamine transporter blocker effect (Siwak *et al.*, 2000a). Adrafinil is converted slowly to modafinil *in vivo*, and the postulated mechanism is likely related to the enhanced noradrenergic activity. Adrafinil was shown to have a stronger effect on activity level compared to nicergoline or propentofylline (Siwak *et al.*, 2000b). One study found that adrafinil improved alertness and learning (discrimination task); however, it impaired memory development (Siwak *et al.*, 2003).

Given that anticholinergic medications may worsen the pathology of CDS, the opposite may apply; the use of cholinesterase inhibitors such as donepezil and phenserine was found to improve memory and learning in senior dogs (Pugliese *et al.*, 2007; Araujo *et al.*, 2011; Cross *et al.*, 2016). However, further research is required to establish the appropriate dose range and safety.

16.3.5.2 Natural supplements

Natural supplements offer another option for the management of CDS in pets. These supplements are considered to be safer and can be combined with medications. Furthermore, many cats and dogs suffering from CDS also suffer from other diseases (e.g. renal or cardiac disease), which may exclude the possibility of using medications for CDS.

Many of these supplements contain similar ingredients, and they aim to reduce the risk of toxic free radical damage, strengthen the neuron integrity and enhance neuronal function.

Senilife® (Ceva Animal Health) contains phosphatidylserine, ginkgo biloba, vitamins B6 and E and resveratrol and was found to help improve cognition in dogs with CDS (Osella *et al.*, 2007; Araujo *et al.*, 2008). No information has been published for cats.

Aktivait® (VetPlus Ltd) contains phosphatidylserine, vitamins C and E, selenium, omega-3 fatty acids, alpha-lipoic acid (dog product only), coenzyme Q and L-carnitine. The cat product does not contain alpha-lipoic acid due to possible toxicity. The dog product was shown to lead to an improvement in social interactions and reduce disorientation and house soiling (Heath *et al.*, 2007).

Cholodin®-Fel (MVP Laboratories Inc.) is a product containing choline, phosphatidylcholine, methionine, inositol, vitamins B and E, zinc, selenium and taurine. A small study of 21 cats showed some improvement in signs of disorientation (Messonier, 2001).

As an essential part of the cell membrane, the phospholipid phosphatidylserine helps to facilitate the signal transduction in neurons, maintain the membrane fluidity and structure, and facilitates cholinergic transmission (Tsakiris and Deliconstantinos, 1985).

Ginkgo biloba is a plant extract that contains high levels of terpenoids and flavonoids, both of which are antioxidants. Ginkgo biloba is used today in both human and animal medicine for a variety of purposes including cognitive dysfunction, cancer treatment, eye problems and more. However, to date, there is no conclusive evidence of its positive effect on the treatment of cognitive dysfunction (DeKosky *et al.*, 2008; Vellas *et al.*, 2012). Other antioxidants found in these supplements include resveratrol, vitamins B6 (pyridoxine), C and E.

Novifit® (Virbac Animal Health) contains S-Adenosyl-L-methionine (SAMe), a naturally produced substance from the amino acid methionine and adenosine triphosphate (ATP). SAMe is a co-substrate in many different metabolic processes in the body, including methyl transfer, enzyme enhancer, upregulate monoamine metabolism, and plays a role in cell membrane fluidity (Bottiglieri, 2013). Compared to placebo, SAMe was shown to improve the clinical sign of CDS in dogs (Rème *et al.*, 2008). Further, in a laboratory setting, SAMe was found to reduce the number of errors that ageing cats and dogs perform when learning new tasks (Araujo *et al.*, 2012).

Neutricks™ (Neutricks LLC) contains apoaequorin, a calcium-binding protein found in jellyfish (*Aequorea Victoria*). This protein might play a role in nerve cells transduction by enhancing the calcium channels. Apoaequorin was found to improve learning and attention in a small study of dogs in a laboratory setting (Milgram *et al.*, 2015).

16.3.5.3 Dietary management

In recent decades, a growing understanding of how different supplements affect metabolism in the body and brain has led to the development of diets to aid in the management of cognitive dysfunction in cats and dogs. These diets contain various ingredients that aim to reduce the risk of damage created by toxic free radicals, enhance metabolism (particularly the neuronal membrane and the mitochondria) and facilitate nerves transduction.

Hill's Prescription Diet contains a high level of antioxidants such as vitamins C and E, selenium, beta-carotene and other carotenoids, and flavonoids. It also contains mitochondrial C-factors such as alpha-lipoic acid and L-carnitine. Studies in dogs have shown improvement in learning and clinical signs of CDS when compared to placebo (Araujo *et al.*, 2005; Head, 2007).

Purina Pro Plan Veterinary Diet NC NeuroCare is a diet for senior dogs that is supplemented with medium-chain triglycerides (MCT). With poor oxygen perfusion, the ageing brain is struggling to metabolize glucose as its energy source (London *et al.*, 1983). Medium-chain triglyceride can provide a higher level of ketones, which are a more readily available source of energy than glucose in hypoxic metabolism (Taha *et al.*, 2009). A recent double-blinded, placebo-controlled clinical study of dogs with signs of CDS found a significant improvement in the clinical signs of cognitive dysfunction in dogs (Pan *et al.*, 2018).

A senior cat and dog diet from Royal Canin (Mature Consult) contains a blend of antioxidants, L-tryptophan and phosphatidylserine and aims to help cognitive function.

16.3.5.4 Behavioural management

Behavioural and environmental management is likely to be the most critical aspect of managing cats and dogs with CDS. Many senior pets have concurrent physical or mental diseases that may contradict the use of medications. While supplements and diets might be beneficial in the management of CDS, the effect of behavioural management was found to be more profound (Milgram *et al.*, 2004; Head, 2007).

Management of senior pets must be tailored to the individual animal's needs and abilities. Many senior pets suffer from sensory decline, degenerative joint diseases, muscular dystrophy, cardiac diseases, or other metabolic diseases that limit their ability to exercise, play and interact with their environment. Also, the management must be species-specific. That is, cats' and dogs' needs are not always the same. While both species need food and water, exercise, social interactions with their owners and opportunities to eliminate, cats require perching and climbing spaces, hiding areas and scratching posts, whereas dogs require walks, chews and tug toys.

Owners should be instructed to introduce feeding toys instead of regular food bowls. New toys and scheduled interactions with the owners should be part of the daily routine. Owners can hide food around the house or garden and encourage their pets to find those. The daily routine should not only meet the cat's or dog's needs, but it should also be predictable and consistent. Owners should strive to repeat the routine daily regardless of work schedule or day of the week. Therefore, when designing the routine, owners should consider all their pet's needs and the owner's work-and-life schedule. Then they should develop the routine in such a way that allows the owner to repeat it daily.

An essential part of the management should be training for both cats and dogs. While senior pets might be more challenging to train, especially those which suffer from early to moderate stages of CDS, it is possible. Cats should be trained as well. Training provides mental stimulation and positive and predictable interaction with the owners. Furthermore, training stimulates different brain centres simultaneously (e.g. auditory and visual cortices to perceive the information, prefrontal cortex to decipher the information, and motoric cortex to initiate a response) providing a robust activity.

A key point to discuss with owners is that changes should be done slowly and gradually. Ageing cats and dogs lose their ability to adapt to rapid changes. With sudden or rapid changes, they may become confused, agitated and anxious.

Owners should create a calm and predictable environment for their ageing pet. In particular, a specific location for rest and sleep should be set up for the pet. Owners should encourage the cat or dog to spend time there as part of the daily routine. This place should include a bed, toys and, possibly, a pheromone (e.g. Adaptil or Feliway) diffuser. The area should be calm and quiet. At night, owners should consider leaving a low light on, especially for ageing pets suffering from vision loss.

16.3.5.5 Future therapies

Current research into the management and prevention of CDS is ongoing. While these options are not currently available, they offer interesting possibilities.

Vaccinations against beta-amyloid protein deposition are one of those options. Currently, trials in senior dogs found an increase in clearance of beta-amyloid (primarily insoluble form) and a reduction in the clinical signs of CDS (Head *et al.*, 2008; Bosch *et al.*, 2013).

A more recent study investigated the effects of combined immunotherapy and behavioural enrichment for the management of CDS in dogs (Davis *et al.*, 2017). In this 20-month-long study, three study groups were compared to a control group: vaccines only, enrichment only, and vaccines and enrichment. The latter group showed the most improvement in reduction of beta-amyloid deposition and increase of brain-derived neurotrophic factor mRNA and improvement of clinical signs.

Recent studies investigated the use of stem cells from the skin (Valenzuela *et al.*, 2008) and olfactory mucosa (Veron *et al.*, 2014) as a treatment option for dogs with CDS. This area of science is still in its infancy and will require more research. However, it may provide promising results.

16.3.5.6 Adjunctive therapy

Many ageing cats and dogs that suffer from cognitive dysfunction may also suffer from concurrent mental diseases such as anxiety, phobias and panic attacks. It is essential to screen for these disorders as well as cognitive decline and other physical diseases.

In many cases, the veterinary surgeon must address secondary mental disorders. When doing so, caution should be exercised not to combine treatments that contradict each other. For example, when treating a senior cat with CDS using selegiline, a serotonergic medication such as fluoxetine should be avoided. Similarly, senior pets with CDS should not be treated with clomipramine for anxiety, given its anticholinergic effect.

Therefore, when treating an ageing cat or dog with concurrent diseases, the surgeon should focus on the main problem and then try managing the secondary problem using behavioural and environmental approaches and supplements and pheromones.

Finally, the doses of different medications may have to be adjusted (lower) to avoid side effects and address potential underlying physical disorders such as renal or hepatic diseases.

References

Araujo, J.A., Studzinski, C.M., Head, E., Cotman, C.W. and Milgram, N.W. (2005) Assessment of nutritional interventions for modification of age-associated cognitive decline using a canine model of human aging. *AGE* 27(1), 27–37. DOI: 10.1007/s11357-005-4001-z.

Araujo, J.A., Landsberg, G.M., Milgram, N.W. and Miolo, A. (2008) Improvement of short-term memory performance in aged beagles by a nutraceutical supplement containing phosphatidylserine, Ginkgo biloba, vitamin E, and pyridoxine. *The Canadian Veterinary Journal = La Revue Veterinaire Canadienne* 49(4), 379–385.

Araujo, J.A., Greig, N.H., Ingram, D.K., Sandin, J., de Rivera, C. *et al.* (2011) Cholinesterase inhibitors improve both memory and complex learning in aged beagle dogs. *Journal of Alzheimer's Disease* 26(1), 143–155. DOI: 10.3233/JAD-2011-110005.

Araujo, J.A., Faubert, M.L., Brooks, M.L., Landsberg, G.M. and Lobprise, H. (2012) NOVIFIT® (NoviSAMe®) tablets improve executive function in aged dogs and cats: implications for treatment of cognitive dysfunction syndrome. *The International Journal of Applied Research in Veterinary Medicine* 10(1), 90–98.

Bosch, M.N., Gimeno-Bayón, J., Rodríguez, M.J., Pugliese, M. and Mahy, N. (2013) Rapid improvement of canine cognitive dysfunction with immunotherapy designed for Alzheimer's disease. *Current Alzheimer Research* 10(5), 482–493. DOI: 10.2174/15672050113109990129.

Bottiglieri, T. (2013) Folate, vitamin B_{12}, and S-adenosylmethionine. *Psychiatric Clinics of North America* 36(1), 1–13. DOI: 10.1016/j.psc.2012.12.001.

Carrillo, M.C., Ivy, G.O., Milgram, N.W., Head, E., Wu, P. *et al.* (1994) (-)Deprenyl increases activities of superoxide dismutase (SOD) in striatum of dog brain. *Life Sciences* 54(20), 1483–1489. DOI: 10.1016/0024-3205(94)90015-9.

Christie, L.A., Studzinski, C.M., Araujo, J.A., Leung, C.S.K., Ikeda-Douglas, C.J. *et al.* (2005) Age-dependent spatial learning deficits: characterization of egocentric and allocentric spatial learning in the beagle dog. *Progress in Neuropharmacology and Biological Psychiatry* 29(3), 361–369.

Colle,M.-A., Hauw, J.-J., Crespeau, F., Uchihara, T., Akiyama, H. *et al.* (2000) Vascular and parenchymal Abeta deposition in the aging dog: correlation with behavior. *Neurobiology of Aging* 21(5), 695–704. DOI: 10.1016/S0197-4580(00)00113-5.

Cotman, C.W. and Head, E. (2008) The canine (dog) model of human aging and disease: dietary, environmental and immunotherapy approaches. *Journal of Alzheimer's Disease* 15(4), 685–707. DOI: 10.3233/JAD-2008-15413.

Cross, A.J., George, J., Woodward, M.C., Ames, D., Brodaty, H. *et al.* (2016) Potentially inappropriate medications and anticholinergic burden in older people attending memory clinics in Australia. *Drugs & Aging* 33(1), 37–44. DOI: 10.1007/s40266-015-0332-3.

Cummings, B.J., Satou, T., Head, E., Milgram, N.W., Cole, G.M. *et al.* (1996) Diffuse plaques contain C-terminal A beta 42 and not A beta 40: evidence from cats and dogs. *Neurobiology of Aging* 17(4), 653–659. DOI: 10.1016/0197-4580(96)00062-0.

Davis, P.R., Giannini, G., Rudolph, K., Calloway, N., Royer, C.M. *et al.* (2017) Aβ vaccination in combination with behavioral enrichment in aged beagles: effects on cognition, Aβ, and microhemorrhages. *Neurobiology of Aging* 49, 86–99. DOI: 10.1016/j.neurobiolaging.2016.09.007.

DeKosky, S.T., Williamson, J.D., Fitzpatrick, A.L., Kronmal, R.A., Ives, D.G. *et al.* (2008) Ginkgo biloba for prevention of dementia: a randomized controlled trial. *JAMA* 300(19), 2253–2262. DOI: 10.1001/jama.2008.683.

Denenberg, S. and Dubé, M.B. (2018) Tools for managing feline problem behaviours psychoactive medications. *Journal of feline medicine and surgery* 20(11), 1034–1045. DOI: 10.1177/1098612X18806760.

Denenberg, S., Liebel, F.X. and Rose, J. (2017) Behavioural and medical differentials of cognitive decline and dementia in dogs and cats. In: Landsberg, G.M., Madari, A. and Zilka, N. (eds) *Canine and Feline Dementia: Molecular Basis, Diagnostics, and*

Therapy. Springer International Publishing, Cham, Switzerland, pp. 13–58.
Fitzgerald, B.M. and Turner, D.C. (2000) Hunting behaviour of domestic cats and their impact on prey population. In: Turner, D.C. and Bateson, P. (eds) *The Domestic Cat: The Biology of Its Behaviour*, 2nd editon. Cambridge University Press, Cambridge, UK, pp. 151–175.
Gunn-Moore, D.A., McVee, J., Bradshaw, J.M., Pearson, G.R., Head, E. *et al.* (2006) Ageing changes in cat brains demonstrated by beta-amyloid and AT8-immunoreactive phosphorylated tau deposits. *Journal of Feline Medicine & Surgery* 8(4), 234–242. DOI: 10.1016/j.jfms.2006.01.003.
Gunn-Moore, D., Moffat, K., Christie, L.-A. and Head, E. (2007) Cognitive dysfunction and the neurobiology of ageing in cats. *Journal of Small Animal Practice* 48(10), 546–553. DOI: 10.1111/j.1748-5827.2007.00386.x.
Head, E. (2007) Combining an antioxidant-fortified diet with behavioral enrichment leads to cognitive improvement and reduced brain pathology in aging canines: strategies for healthy aging. *Annals of the New York Academy of Sciences* 1114, 398–406. DOI: 10.1196/annals.1396.004.
Head, E., Mehta, R., Hartley, J., Kameka, M., Cummings, B.J. *et al.* (1995) Spatial learning and memory as a function of age in the dog. *Behavioral Neuroscience* 109(5), 851–858. DOI: 10.1037/0735-7044.109.5.851.
Head, E., Hartley, J., Kameka, A.M., Mehta, R., Ivy, G.O. *et al.* (1996) The effects of l-deprenyl on spatial short term memory in young and aged dogs. *Progress in Neuro-Psychopharmacology and Biological Psychiatry* 20(3), 515–530. DOI: 10.1016/0278-5846(96)00014-0.
Head, E., Liu, J., Hagen, T.M., Muggenburg, B.A., Milgram, N.W. *et al.* (2002) Oxidative damage increases with age in a canine model of human brain aging. *Journal of Neurochemistry* 82(2), 375–381. DOI: 10.1046/j.1471-4159.2002.00969.x.
Head, E., Moffat, K., Das, P., Sarsoza, F., Poon, W.W. *et al.* (2005) Beta-Amyloid deposition and tau phosphorylation in clinically characterized aged cats. *Neurobiology of Aging* 26(5), 749–763. DOI: 10.1016/j.neurobiolaging.2004.06.015.
Head, E., Pop, V., Vasilevko, V., Hill, M., Saing, T. *et al.* (2008) A two-year study with fibrillar beta-amyloid (Abeta) immunization in aged canines: effects on cognitive function and brain Abeta. *Journal of Neuroscience* 28(14), 3555–3566. DOI: 10.1523/JNEUROSCI.0208-08.2008.
Heath, S.E., Barabas, S. and Craze, P.G. (2007) Nutritional supplementation in cases of canine cognitive dysfunction—A clinical trial. *Applied Animal Behaviour Science* 105(4), 284–296. DOI: 10.1016/j.applanim.2006.11.008.
Landsberg, G.M. and Malamed, R. (2017) Clinical picture of canine and feline cognitive impairment. In: Landsberg, G.M., Madari, A. and Zilka, N. (eds) *Canine and Feline Dementia: Molecular Basis, Diagnostics, and Therapy*. Springer International Publishing, Cham, Switzerland, pp. 1–12.
Landsberg, G.M., Denenberg, S. and Araujo, J.A. (2010) Cognitive dysfunction in cats: a syndrome we used to dismiss as 'old age'. *Journal of Feline Medicine and Surgery* 12(11), 837–848. DOI: 10.1016/j.jfms.2010.09.004.
Landsberg, G.M., Deporter, T. and Araujo, J.A. (2011) Clinical signs and management of anxiety, sleeplessness, and cognitive dysfunction in the senior PET. *Veterinary Clinics of North America: Small Animal Practice* 41(3), 565–590. DOI: 10.1016/j.cvsm.2011.03.017.
Levine, M.S., Lloyd, R.L., Hull, C.D., Fisher, R.S. and Buchwald, N.A. (1987) Neurophysiological alterations in caudate neurons in aged cats. *Brain Research* 401(2), 213–230. DOI: 10.1016/0006-8993(87)91407-7.
London, E.D., Ohata, M., Takei, H., French, A.W. and Rapoport, S.I. (1983) Regional cerebral metabolic rate for glucose in beagle dogs of different ages. *Neurobiology of Aging* 4(2), 121–126. DOI: 10.1016/0197-4580(83)90035-0.
Meleo, K.A. and Peterson, M.E. (2014) Treatment of insulinoma in the dog, cat, and ferret. In: Bonagura, J.B. and Twedt, D.C. (eds) *Current Veterinary Therapy XV. 2014*. Saunders Elsevier, pp. 130–134. Available at: www.currentveterinarytherapy.com
Messonier, S. (2001) *Cognitive Disorder (Senility). The Natural Health Bible for Dogs and Cats*. Prima Publishing, U.S., Rocklin, California, pp. 56–57.
Milgram, N.W. (2010) Neuropsychological function and aging in the cat.In: *Proceedings of the 15th Annual Conference on Canine Cognition and Aging*, Laguna Beach, California.
Milgram, N.W., Head, E., Zicker, S.C., Ikeda-Douglas, C., Murphey, H. *et al.* (2004) Long-Term treatment with antioxidants and a program of behavioral enrichment reduces age-dependent impairment in discrimination and reversal learning in beagle dogs. *Experimental Gerontology* 39(5), 753–765. DOI: 10.1016/j.exger.2004.01.007.
Milgram, N.W., Landsberg, G., Merrick, D. and Underwood, M.Y. (2015) A novel mechanism for cognitive enhancement in aged dogs with the use of a calcium-buffering protein. *Journal of Veterinary Behavior* 10(3), 217–222. DOI: 10.1016/j.jveb.2015.02.003.
Nakamura, S., Nakayama, H., Kiatipattanasakul, W., Uetsuka, K., Uchida, K. *et al.* (1996) Senile plaques in very aged cats. *Acta Neuropathologica* 91(4), 437–439. DOI: 10.1007/s004010050448.
Osella, M.C., Re, G., Odore, R., Girardi, C., Badino, P. *et al.* (2007) Canine cognitive dysfunction syndrome: prevalence, clinical signs and treatment with a neuroprotective nutraceutical. *Applied Animal*

Behaviour Science 105(4), 297–310. DOI: 10.1016/j.applanim.2006.11.007.

Pan, Y., Landsberg, G., Mougeot, I., Kelly, S., Xu, H. *et al.* (2018) Efficacy of a therapeutic diet on dogs with signs of cognitive dysfunction syndrome (CdS): a prospective double blinded placebo controlled clinical study. *Frontiers in Nutrition* 5(5), 127. DOI: 10.3389/fnut.2018.00127.

Parkinson, F.E., Rudolphi, K.A. and Fredholm, B.B. (1994) Propentofylline: a nucleoside transport inhibitor with neuroprotective effects in cerebral ischemia. *General Pharmacology: The Vascular System* 25(6), 1053–1058. DOI: 10.1016/0306-3623(94)90119-8.

Pugliese, M., Gangitano, C., Ceccariglia, S., Carrasco, J.L., Del Fà, A. *et al.* (2007) Canine cognitive dysfunction and the cerebellum: acetylcholinesterase reduction, neuronal and glial changes. *Brain Research* 1139, 85–94. DOI: 10.1016/j.brainres.2006.12.090.

Rème, C.A., Dramard, V., Kern, L., Hofmans, J., Halsberghe, C. *et al.* (2008) Effect of *S*-adenosylmethionine tablets on the reduction of age-related mental decline in dogs: a double-blinded, placebo-controlled trial. *Veterinary Therapeutics: Research in Applied Veterinary Medicine* 9(2), 69–82.

Ruehl, W.W., Neilson, J., Hart, B., Head, E., Bruyette, D.S. *et al.* (1997) Therapeutic actions of l-deprenyl in dogs: a model of human brain aging. *Advances in Pharmacology* 42, 316–319.

Siwak, C.T., Gruet, P., Woehrlé, F., Schneider, M., Muggenburg, B.A. *et al.* (2000a) Behavioral activating effects of adrafinil in aged canines. *Pharmacology Biochemistry and Behavior* 66(2), 293–300. DOI: 10.1016/S0091-3057(00)00188-X.

Siwak, C.T., Gruet, P., Woehrlé, F., Muggenburg, B.A., Murphey, H.L. *et al.* (2000b) Comparison of the effects of adrafinil, propentofylline, and nicergoline on behavior in aged dogs. *American Journal of Veterinary Research* 61(11), 1410–1414. DOI: 10.2460/ajvr.2000.61.1410.

Siwak, C.T., Tapp, P.D. and Milgram, N.W. (2003) Adrafinil disrupts performance on a delayed nonmatching-to-position task in aged beagle dogs. *Pharmacology Biochemistry and Behavior* 76(1), 161–168. DOI: 10.1016/S0091-3057(03)00211-9.

Sullivan, P.G. and Brown, M.R. (2005) Mitochondrial aging and dysfunction in Alzheimer's disease. *Progress in Neuro-Psychopharmacology and Biological Psychiatry* 29(3), 407–410. DOI: 10.1016/j.pnpbp.2004.12.007.

Taha, A.Y., Henderson, S.T. and Burnham, W.M. (2009) Dietary enrichment with medium chain triglycerides (AC-1203) elevates polyunsaturated fatty acids in the parietal cortex of aged dogs: implications for treating age-related cognitive decline. *Neurochemical Research* 34(9), 1619–1625. DOI: 10.1007/s11064-009-9952-5.

Takeuchi, Y., Uetsuka, K., Murayama, M., Kikuta, F., Takashima, A. *et al.* (2008) Complementary distributions of amyloid-beta and neprilysin in the brains of dogs and cats. *Veterinary Pathology* 45(4), 455–466. DOI: 10.1354/vp.45-4-455.

Tapp, P.D., Siwak, C.T., Gao, F.Q., Chiou, J.-Y., Black, S.E. *et al.* (2004) Frontal lobe volume, function, and beta-amyloid pathology in a canine model of aging. *Journal of Neuroscience* 24(38), 8205–8213. DOI: 10.1523/JNEUROSCI.1339-04.2004.

Tsakiris, S. and Deliconstantinos, G. (1985) Phosphatidylserine and calmodulin effects on Ca2+-stimulated ATPase activity of dog brain synaptosomal plasma membranes. *International Journal of Biochemistry* 17(10), 1117–1119. DOI: 10.1016/0020-711X(85)90045-X.

Valenzuela, M.J., Dean, S.K., Sachdev, P., Tuch, B.E. and Sidhu, K.S. (2008) Neural precursors from canine skin: a new direction for testing autologous cell replacement in the brain. *Stem Cells and Development* 17(6), 1087–1094. DOI: 10.1089/scd.2008.0008.

Vellas, B., Coley, N., Ousset, P.-J., Berrut, G., Dartigues, J.-F. *et al.* (2012) Long-Term use of standardised Ginkgo biloba extract for the prevention of Alzheimer's disease (GuidAge): a randomised placebo-controlled trial. *The Lancet Neurology* 11(10), 851–859. DOI: 10.1016/S1474-4422(12)70206-5.

Veron, A., Mengoli, M. and Bienboire-Frasini, D. (2014) Are nasal stem cells a promising approach in geriatric veterinary medicine. *Proceedings of International Congress on Semiochemistry and Management of Animal Populations*, Apt, France, p. 63.

Winblad, B., Fioravanti, M., Dolezal, T., Logina, I., Milanov, I.G. *et al.* (2008) Therapeutic use of nicergoline. *Clinical Drug Investigation* 28(9), 533–552. DOI: 10.2165/00044011-200828090-00001.

Appendices

Sarah Liversage and Sagi Denenberg*

*s.denenberg@bristol.ac.uk

A1 – GP Questionnaire – Cats

This questionnaire aims to identify any areas of concern you may have with your cat so that your veterinary surgeon can address them during your consultation.

Please answer Yes or No for every question below.

Have you noticed your cat showing any of the following?

	Yes	No
Disorientation such as aimless walking or staring into the distance		
Changes in vocalization		
Less active than before		
Not jumping onto/off surfaces as much		
Jumping onto a lower surface before jumping to a higher surface – i.e. jumping onto a chair before jumping onto the windowsill		
Taking longer to go up/down the stairs		
Has stopped going up/down the stairs		
No longer using raised resting areas or beds		
Limping		
Changes in sleep patterns – sleeping less or restless sleep		
Changes in sleep patterns – sleeping more		
Difficulty getting into the litter tray		
Urinating outside of the litter tray		
Passing faeces outside of the litter tray		
Changes in the frequency of urination		
Changes in the frequency of defecation		
Changes in appetite – increased		
Changes in appetite – decreased		
Difficulty chewing hard food		
Bad breath		
Changes in the amount they are drinking		
Changes in weight – loss of weight		
Changes in weight – gain in weight		

	Yes	No
Avoidance or aggression towards family members		
Avoidance or aggression towards other animals in the house		
Changes in its reaction to normal household noises		
Changes in its behaviour towards sudden loud noises		
Excessive licking of any areas of the body		
Any new lumps		
Any lumps which have changed in appearance		
Any changes in its coat		

Please list any other concerns you may have which are not covered in these questions:

A2 – GP Questionnaire – Dogs

This questionnaire aims to identify any areas of concern you may have with your dog so that your veterinary surgeon can address them during your consultation.

Please answer Yes or No for every question below.

Have you noticed your dog showing any of the following?

	Yes	No
Disorientation such as aimless walking or staring into the distance		
Changes in vocalization		
Less active than before		
Taking longer to navigate an obstacle, e.g. takes longer to get out of the door		
Misjudging jumps they used to do easily – not making it onto the sofa		
Taking longer to go up/down the stairs		
Has stopped going up/down the stairs		
Taking longer to get up after resting		
Limping		
Changes in sleep patterns – sleeping more		
Changes in sleep patterns – sleeping less or restless sleep		
Passing urine in the house		
Passing faeces in the house		
Changes in the frequency of urination		
Changes in the frequency of defecation		
Changes in appetite – increased		
Changes in appetite – decreased		
Struggles to use a bowl on the floor		
Difficulty chewing hard food or chews		
Bad breath		
Changes in the amount they are drinking		
Changes in weight – loss of weight		
Changes in weight – gain in weight		
Avoidance or aggression towards family members		
Avoidance or aggression towards people outside of the house		
Avoidance or aggression towards other animals in the house		
Avoidance or aggression towards other animals outside of the house		

	Yes	No
Avoidance or aggression when touched/groomed		
Changes in reaction to normal household noises		
Changes in behaviour towards sudden loud noises		
Excessive licking of any areas of the body		
Any new lumps		
Any lumps which have changed in appearance		
Any changes in their coat		

Please list any other concerns you may have which are not covered in these questions:

A3 – Behavioural Questionnaire – Cats

General information

Date:
Name:
Address:

Home phone:
Mobile:
Email:

Veterinarian's name:
Veterinary clinic:
Clinic's phone:
Clinic's email:

Pet information

Pet's name:
Date of birth or estimated age:
Breed:
Colour:
Sex: Neutered? At what age neutered?
Age at adoption:
Adopted from:

Home environment

(This section provides general information on your cat's environment and routine.)

Please list all family members, including age, their level of interaction with your cat, and how your cat responds to each one:

Please list all pets at home, their species and breeds, and how your cat interacts with them.
(If your cat has a problem with one of your other pets, please describe it below in **main problem** section.)

When your cat stays home alone, for how long, and where?

Briefly describe where your cat sleeps (both during the day and at night):

Briefly describe your cat's feeding routine including location, times, appetite, and type of bowl:

Do you use treats or feeding toys (e.g. Kitty Kong toys, Cat Activity Fun Board, or balls)?

If yes, briefly describe when, and your cat's favourite treats:

Is your cat fully house-trained?

If no, please describe where your cat is soiling, and specify if it is urine, stools or both. Please provide a diagram of your home and mark the locations of the litter box/es and of soiling. Use L for litter box, U for urine outside the box, and S for stools outside the box. Provide more details in the **Behaviour problem** section below:

Where is/are your cat litter box/es?

Do you use scratching posts?

If yes, please describe where and type of post(s):

Do you bar your cat from certain areas in the house?

If yes, please describe where and why:

Interactions

Please describe your cat's daily activities including play, grooming and sleep:

Please describe your cat's favourite play, game or toy:
Can you handle your cat safely (e.g. brush, pet and administer medication)?

If no, please give more details in the **Behaviour problem** section below.

Do you train your cat?

If yes, please briefly describe:

Please list the commands your cat knows, and the degree of responsiveness (e.g. responds sometimes, only with treats, or always):

Your cat's health

Does your cat have any current medical problems to your knowledge?

Do you know of any previous medical problems?

Is he/she on any current medication, herbal or homeopathic remedies?

Your cat's main behaviour problem(s)

(If your cat has more than one problem, please list them all separately from the most to least concerning to you.)

Please describe the problem(s):

When did this behaviour first start? If possible, describe the first incident.

Can you describe the last incident, and when did it occur?

When does the behaviour usually occur? Is it in any particular circumstances?

Describe where the behaviour occurs. Is it always in the same place?

Do you think it is becoming more frequent, less frequent, or staying about the same?

On average, how frequently does the problem occur?

Who is usually present at the time?

If your pet is an intact female, is the behaviour related to her heat cycle?

Do any related cats (e.g. parents or siblings) have similar problems?

Have there been previous attempts to manage this problem?

If yes, please describe; including training, tools, medication, or other options:

Has any treatment method improved or aggravated the situation?

Have you considered removing your cat from the home if the problem cannot be improved?

Reactivity

(Please describe briefly how your cat reacts to each of the following situations. Please leave blank if you have answered it above.)

Familiar people (including children) arriving at the home:

Unfamiliar people (including children) arriving at the home:

Car rides:

Loud noises (e.g., thunder, fireworks, vacuum cleaner, or other sudden loud sounds):

New environments/locations:

Changes in routine:

Being left alone at home:

During veterinary visits:

How long does it take your cat to settle down once he/she has reacted to any of the above situations?

Abnormal and repetitive behaviours
(These are behaviours that your cat may display in a repetitive manner and out of context. Specific behaviours may appear normal; however, it is important to consider the duration, frequency and intensity of the behaviour.)

Does your cat spin, circle or chase its tail?

Does your cat lick excessively? (e.g. itself, you, surfaces or objects)

Do you see frequent lip-licking, yawning, head and body shakes, stretching, or tail-flicking?

Does your cat follow you around the house constantly?

Does your cat spend long periods of time observing the street from the windows?

Do you notice any hallucinatory behaviours? (e.g. fly-snapping, or shadow-chasing)

Does your cat show skin rolling or rippling along the back?

What are your long-term expectations with regard to your cat's behaviour?

A4 – Behavioural Questionnaire – Dogs

General information

Date:
Name:
Address:

Home phone:
Mobile:
Email:

Veterinarian's name:
Veterinary clinic:
Clinic's phone:
Clinic's email:

Pet information

Pet's name:
Date of birth or estimated age:
Breed:
Colour:
Sex: Neutered? At what age neutered?
Age at adoption:
Adopted from:

Home environment

(This section provides general information on your dog's environment and routine.)

Please list other people that your dog may interact with (e.g. dog walker or a trainer):

Please list all pets at home, their species and breeds, and how your dog interacts with them.
(If your dog has a problem with one of your other pets, please describe it below in **main problem** section.)

When your dog stays home alone, for how long, and where?

Briefly describe where your dog sleeps (both during the day and at night):

Briefly describe your dog's feeding routine including location, times, appetite, and type of bowl:

Do you use treats or chews (e.g. Kong toys, rawhide, bones, or antlers)?

If yes, briefly describe when, and your dog's favourite treats or chews:

Is your dog fully house-trained?

If no, please describe where your dog is soiling, and specify if it is urine, stools or both. Please provide a diagram of your home and mark the locations of the soiling. Use U for urine, and S for stools. Provide more details in the **Behaviour problem** section below:

What is your dog's favourite elimination place?

Is your dog allowed on furniture (e.g. bed, sofa or chairs)?

If not, what do you do if you find your dog on furniture?

Do you bar your dog from certain areas in the house?

If yes, please describe where and why:

Interactions

Please describe your dog's exercise including walks (time, duration and location):

Please describe your dog's favourite play, game or toy:

Can you safely handle your dog (e.g. brushing, wiping feet, placing harness or collar, and administering medication)?

Do you train your dog (alone or with a trainer)?

If yes, please briefly describe:

Please list the commands your dog knows, and the degree of responsiveness (e.g. responds sometimes, only with treats, or always):

Your dog's health

Does your dog have any current medical problems to your knowledge?

Do you know of any previous medical problems?

Is he/she on any current medication, herbal or homeopathic remedies?

Your dog's main behaviour problem(s)

(If your dog has more than one problem, please list them all separately from the most to least concerning to you.)

Please describe the problem(s):

When did this behaviour first start? If possible, describe the first incident.

Can you describe the last incident, and when did it occur?

When does the behaviour usually occur? Is it in any particular circumstances?

On average, how frequently does the problem occur?

Do you think it is becoming more frequent, less frequent, or staying about the same?

Describe where the behaviour occurs. Is it always in the same place?

Who is usually present at the time?

If your pet is an intact bitch, is the behaviour related to her heat cycle?

Do any related dogs (e.g. parents or siblings) have similar problems?

Have there been previous attempts to manage this problem?

If yes, please describe; including training, tools, medication, or other options:

Has any treatment method improved or aggravated the situation?

Have you considered removing your dog from the home if the problem cannot be improved?

Reactivity

(Please describe briefly how your dog reacts to each of the following situations. Please leave blank if you have answered it above.)

Familiar people (including children) arriving at the home:

Unfamiliar people (including children) arriving at the home:

Going for a walk:

Meeting familiar people (including children) on walks:

Meeting unfamiliar people (including children) on walks:

Meeting familiar dogs on walks:

Meeting unfamiliar dogs and other animals on walks:

Fast-moving objects such as skateboards, cyclists or joggers:

Traffic (sounds and movements):

Car rides:

Loud noises (e.g., thunder, fireworks, vacuum cleaner, or other sudden loud sounds):

New environments/locations:

Changes in routine:

Being left alone at home:

During veterinary visits:

How long does it take your dog to settle down once he/she reacted to any of the above situations?

Abnormal and repetitive behaviours

(These are behaviours that your dog may display in a repetitive manner and out of context. Specific behaviours may appear normal; however, it is important to consider the duration, frequency and intensity of the behaviour.)

Does your dog spin, circle or chase its tail?

Does your dog lick excessively? (e.g., itself, you, surfaces or objects)

Do you see frequent lip-licking, yawning, head and body shakes, stretching, grinning or sneezing?

Does your dog follow you around the house constantly?

Does your dog spend long periods of time observing the street from the windows?

Do you notice any hallucinatory behaviours? (e.g. fly-snapping, or shadow-chasing)

Does your dog show skin rolling or rippling along the back?

What are your long-term expectations with regard to your dog's behaviour?

A5 – Cat Cognitive Dysfunction Questionnaire

Although it has not yet been formally identified, cats show signs of cognitive dysfunction in a similar way to dogs. Cognitive dysfunction is the medical term used for behavioural signs associated with the physical ageing of the brain in cats; think of it like cat dementia. The prevalence of cognitive dysfunction in cats is currently being investigated; however, it is thought that more than 55% of cats aged 11–15, and more than 80% of cats aged 16–20 show signs of cognitive dysfunction.

Behaviours that may be affected include:

- sleeping and activity patterns;
- eating and drinking habits;
- spatial awareness and orientation; and
- learning and memory.

This questionnaire aims to identify some of the behavioural changes associated with cognitive dysfunction and assist you and your veterinary surgeon through the diagnosis and management of this condition in your cat. For each question state Yes or No; if your answer is Yes, please state how often the behaviour is happening and if it has changed over the last six months.

Behaviour	No	Yes					Has this changed in the last six months?		
		Once a day	Once a week	Every two weeks	Once a month	Less frequently	Increased	Decreased	Same
Disorientation									
Have you noticed your cat pacing, walking around in circles or wandering with no apparent purpose?									
Have you noticed your cat walking into walls or doors?									
Does your cat go to the wrong side of a door when it is opened for them?									
Have you noticed your cat staring at the walls or floor?									
Have you noticed your cat meowing more than before or for no apparent reason?									
Interactions									
Have you noticed your cat struggling to recognize familiar people or pets?									
Have you noticed your cat avoiding being petted/stroked?									
Is your cat walking away while being petted/stroked more than they used to?									
Have you noticed that your cat does not want to play anymore?									
Have you noticed that your cat is not interacting with you as much?									
Sleep patterns									
Have you noticed that your cat is sleeping more during the day?									
Have you noticed that your cat is awake more at night?									
Has its normal sleep pattern changed?									
House-soiling									
Have you noticed your cat is passing urine outside of the litter tray when they have previously been litter-trained?									
Have you noticed your cat has started to pass faeces outside of the litter tray when they have been previously litter-trained?									
Has your cat stopped covering urine and faeces in the litter tray?									

Behaviour	No	Yes					Has this changed in the last six months?		
		Once a day	Once a week	Every two weeks	Once a month	Less frequently	Increased	Decreased	Same
Activity levels									
Is your cat more active than before?									
Is your cat less active than before?									
Does your cat appear less interested in the things they used to enjoy?									
Have you noticed your cat struggling to find something on the floor, like a piece of food?									
Medical									
Have you noticed an increase in the amount your cat is drinking?									
Have you noticed a change in your cat's appetite?									
Is your cat eating slower, especially when eating dry food?									
Have you noticed any repetitive behaviours such as excessive grooming in certain areas?									
Has your cat slowed down when they are going up or downstairs?									
Have you noticed your cat is struggling to get onto/off elevated surfaces?									
Have you noticed your cat is not using elevated resting spaces as much as it used to?									
Have you noticed your cat toileting next to the litter tray?									
Have you noticed your cat struggling to squat when in the litter tray?									
Have you noticed any changes in the frequency with which your cat is using the litter tray?									
Have you noticed any limping when your cat is walking around?									
Have you noticed any lumps which have got bigger recently?									
Have you noticed your cat licking their joints frequently?									
Have you noticed any abnormal behaviour? Please describe.									

A6 – Dog Cognitive Dysfunction Questionnaire

Dog cognitive dysfunction is the medical term for the behavioural signs associated with the physical ageing of the brain in dogs; think of it like doggie dementia. The prevalence of dog cognitive dysfunction has been estimated from studies to be between 14% and 60% in dogs over eight years old, with 68% of dogs between 15 and 16 years old showing signs.

Behaviours that may be affected include:

- sleeping and activity patterns;
- eating and drinking habits;
- spatial awareness and orientation; and
- learning and memory.

This questionnaire aims to identify some of the behavioural changes associated with dog cognitive dysfunction in order to assist you and your veterinary surgeon through the diagnosis and management of this condition in your dog. For each question state Yes or No; if your answer is Yes, please state how often the behaviour is happening and if it has changed over the last six months.

Questions	No	Yes					Has this changed in the last six months?		
		Once a day	Once a week	Every two weeks	Once a month	Less frequently	Increased	Decreased	Same
Disorientation									
Have you noticed your dog pacing, walking around in circles or wandering with no apparent purpose?									
Have you noticed your dog walking into walls or doors?									
Have you noticed your dog going to the wrong side of a door when it is opened?									
Have you noticed your dog staring at the walls or floor?									
Does your dog appear confused in a new environment, e.g. struggling to learn the layout of a holiday home?									
Have you noticed your dog barking or howling more than before or for no apparent reason?									
Interactions									
Have you noticed your dog struggling to recognize familiar people or pets?									
Have you noticed your dog avoiding being petted/stroked?									
Have you noticed your dog walking away while being petted/stroked more than they used to?									
Have you noticed your dog struggling to respond to cues they used to know such as Sit, Down or Come?									
Is your dog less playful?									
Is your dog showing less desire to interact with other dogs?									
Have you noticed your dog sniffing and exploring less on walks?									
Sleep patterns									
Have you noticed your dog sleeping more during the day?									
Have you noticed your dog pacing at night?									
Has its normal sleep pattern changed?									
House-soiling									
Have you noticed your dog urinating at home when it has previously been house-trained?									

Questions	No	Yes					Has this changed in the last six months?		
		Once a day	Once a week	Every two weeks	Once a month	Less frequently	Increased	Decreased	Same
Have you noticed your dog defecating at home when it has been previously house-trained?									
Is your dog asking to go outside during the night more frequently?									
Have you noticed your dog asking to go outside then coming back in and urinating or defecating in the house?									
Activity levels									
Is your dog more active than before?									
Is your dog less active than before?									
Have you noticed your dog showing less interest in things it used to enjoy?									
Have you noticed your dog struggling to find something on the floor, like a piece of food?									
Medical									
Have you noticed an increase in the amount your dog is drinking?									
Have you noticed a change in your dog's appetite?									
Have you noticed your dog eating more slowly, especially when eating dry food?									
Have you noticed any repetitive movements such as limb-shaking, head-bobbing or twitching?									
Have you noticed your dog struggling to get onto/off the sofa?									
Has your dog slowed down when going up or down the stairs?									
Have you noticed your dog limping when it walks or runs?									
Have you noticed any lumps that have got bigger recently?									
Have you noticed your dog struggling to squat to go to the toilet?									
Have you noticed any abnormal behaviour? Please describe.									

A7 – Behaviour Diary Template

In order to gain as much information as possible about your pet's behaviour problem, to monitor the progress of the problem, and help to increase the predictability of the problem, it is essential to maintain a diary.

The diary should include both normal and abnormal behaviours; for the abnormal behaviours, you should include a rough estimate of the duration and intensity of the behaviour. The intensity of the behaviour is subjective, and your assessment may not be the same as someone else's; this does not matter. The intensity scale is to track the overall trends in the behaviour, so do not worry if your intensity scale levels are different from those of someone else in your household. The important thing is that you can see improvements in the behaviour within your intensity scale.

Behaviours to track should include:

- Normal behaviours:
    - eating: appetite, speed of eating, what toys were used
    - sleeping: quality and quantity
    - playing: interest in play, how long they play for, if they play on their own or with other pets (where appropriate)
    - going for walks: interested in going, how they are on the walk, how quickly they settle after the walk
    - grooming: the amount of self-grooming, amount of mutual grooming between pets, amount of grooming you do
- Abnormal behaviours:
    - reaction to people
    - reaction to noises
    - reaction to interactions – familiar and unfamiliar people
    - reaction to other dogs/cats
    - house-soiling

A behaviour diary will help to identify all situations where the pet shows fidgeting, displacement behaviours and conflict-related behaviours. These behaviours indicate an increase in arousal levels and the potential for the pet's behaviour to escalate (for more information, see Section 7.4.3 and Handout B3 – Identifying Displacement and Conflict-related Behaviours). Once you start to track these behaviours, you will be able to identify situations where you will need to step in and help the pet.

Fidgeting: fidgeting is where the pet seems unable to settle down, rest and sleep. It can be seen as pacing, restlessness when trying to settle down, scratching themselves, and sometimes vocalizing, such as groaning.

Displacement behaviours: displacement behaviours are normal behaviours, and they are often seen within the normal behavioural repertoire of the pet. What makes them a displacement behaviour, rather than an appropriate behaviour, is that they are performed out of context.

Displacement behaviours are seen when there is an increase in arousal levels, and the pet crosses its emotional threshold.

Displacement behaviours include:

- yawning when not tired;
- licking lips when it does not have any food or water on the lips;
- shaking off as if coat is wet, when it is dry;
- looking at something out of the corner of the eye instead of looking straight at it;

- stretching when it has not been resting for an extended period; and
- sneezing when it does not have any allergies or anything irritating the nose.

Conflict-related behaviours: these are behaviours which are shown in situations where there are two or more competing emotional motivations. This causes the pet to be both interested in and hesitant about something at the same time.

Conflict-related behaviours can lead to an increase in arousal levels and can lead to the pet crossing its emotional or behavioural threshold.

Examples of conflict behaviours include:

1. The pet stretches towards a stranger offering a treat, but moves away as soon as it has taken the treat:
   - The pet might want the treat but not want to be that close to the stranger. To get the treat, it must be close to the stranger.

     This context causes conflict because the pet is torn between taking the treat while keeping its distance from the stranger.
2. Another dog approaches the pet to play:
   - The pet may approach the other dog to play but may have its hackles up or be growling.
   - This context causes conflict because the pet wants to play but does not know the other dog or how it will react.

You can keep your behaviour diary in any format you like – handwritten, Word document or Excel spreadsheet. Use the format which is going to be the easiest for you to complete regularly.

When completing your behaviour diary, consider using different-coloured fonts for different levels of arousal:

- green font for normal behaviour (e.g. no signs of anxiety, fear or arousal);
- yellow font when you notice a few displacement behaviours or increasing arousal, but you can still interact with the pet; and
- red font when you notice many displacement behaviours, high arousal, or when the pet will not listen to you.

This traffic-light system will allow you to quickly review the diary and track your progress from mostly red through to more yellow and finally more green behaviours throughout the behaviour modification programme.

An example of a diary would be:

					Sleeping	Situation 1	Situation 2
Date	Eating	Play	Walk	Grooming	15 – 16 hours	Reactions to dogs on walks	Reactivity to people moving past the house
19 Dec	Dry food in balls and interactive feeders; twice a day, ate everything	Played with toys in the house and garden	1 x 50 min road walk Pulling and sniffing the entire walk	Self-grooming in evening	8 hours over-night 9–11, 2–6, 14 hours total	Reaction to dog on walk – lip licking, stared pulled towards – easily distracted with food	Postman walking past fence – barking, jumping at the fence, running the fence line, not listening Took 5 mins to settle enough to take food
20 Dec	Slow feeder bowl Kong with peanut butter Ate everything	Tug with rope Played on his own Played with the other dog in the garden	1 x 60 min beach walk On long line, sniffing, digging and trotting	Self-grooming throughout the day	9 hours over - night, 8.30–10.30, 2–6, 8–9.30, 16.5 hours total	On lead dog on walk - looked at it but look at me immediately; rewarded with treat Off lead dog on walk – displacement behaviours seen (lip licking and yawn) Was able to respond to a touch cue and take a treat	Postman walking past – able to sit in front of me and take treats as he walked past – need to continually feed to keep his attention on me rather than the postman Displacement behaviours seen (lip licking, look out of the corner of his eye and full body shake once postman has gone)
21 Dec	Slow feeder bowl Kong and rawhide		No walk – has hydrotherapy at 10am	Shower before and after hydro, brushed when dry	9 hours over - night, 8–9, 12–6, 7–10, 18 hours total – always tired after hydro	Lip licking and yawning while getting into the pool – stopped once he was in and swimming Conflict as was offered high value treat to get into pool	No barking at people walking past he was sleeping after hydro

A8 – Pain Assessment

Capturing videos of your pet's movement (gait) and posture in different situations at home is invaluable for the assessment and diagnosis of pain-related changes. These changes could be very subtle, and your pet may hide these changes when in a veterinary setting as their emotions and behaviour will be different there. Even the most subtle changes in gait and posture could indicate the presence of pain. This pain will affect your pet's emotions and physical well-being.

Some common movement abnormalities that can indicate pain include, but are not limited to:

- Pacing – this is a type of gait where the dog or cat moves the right forelimb and right hindlimb at the same time, then moves the left forelimb and left hindlimb at the same time, which gives the gait a rocking motion. The pacing gait can indicate pain in the lower back or hips.
- Crabbing – this is a type of gait where the hind legs do not track behind the front legs correctly. This movement causes a gait where a dog or cat is moving forward, but their body is turned at a diagonal angle, and their hind legs can be seen off to one side as they move. The crabbing gait can indicate a problem with the pet's body structure or can indicate an orthopaedic or neurological problem.
- Bunny-hopping – this is a type of gait where both hind legs move together instead of independently. It is often seen when climbing stairs or running, where the pet moves its front legs independently in two movements but moves its hind legs together in one movement. The bunny-hopping type of gait often indicates pain in the hips or lower back.
- Low head carriage – this is where the pet tends to hold the head below the level of its back and will try to look up at you with its eyes rather than lifting the head. A low head carriage is often an indication of pain in the neck.
- Head-bobbing – this abnormality is seen when the pet drops its head as it places a forelimb on the ground. This is done to reduce the amount of weight being placed on that limb. It is an indication of forelimb pain.
- Weight distribution when standing – with your pet in a standing position, look at its feet. Does one foot look bigger than the others? Can you see more of the pad on one foot than on the others? Are the toes splayed? Is one foot placed underneath or to the side of the body? All of these could indicate there is pain on the limb.
- Different diameters of circling toward one side compared to the other – this is where the pet will turn in a smaller circle in one direction when compared to the other. This could indicate a muscular or joint issue.

Tips for getting the best videos of your pet moving:

1. Take all videos in landscape.
2. Keep the videos short – 30 seconds – 1 minute.
3. Keep the camera steady while filming – use a tripod or put the camera onto a steady, level surface.
4. Try not to angle the camera when taking videos – keep it perpendicular to your pet at all times (the camera may have to be low to the ground to avoid angling).
5. Two people are typically needed, one to walk with the pet and one to ensure you get the videos recording.
6. Use a flat, even terrain to move the pet on.
7. Ensure the area you use is well lit and that the pet stands out from the surroundings – avoid walking a black dog past a dark wall.
8. Try not to hold the dog lead too tight or use treats to encourage the pet to move – these will influence your pet's movement.

9. Get footage of your pet moving from the side – this may mean you have to kneel or get low to the ground to get the best video.
10. Try to capture all these videos three to four times, at similar times, on different days. For example, the first minute of the morning walk in the same area over four or five different days. This method would allow us to have an average over a few days, in case one day was different.

Below is a list of videos you should try capturing, so the possibility of pain can be assessed.

Walk and run: Capture a video of your pet walking and lightly running (trot) from around 5 metres away. Capture its movement from four different angles, moving towards you, moving away from you, moving from left to right and moving from right to left.

Jumping: Capture a video of your pet jumping onto and off surfaces. Ideally, capture when your pet leaves the surface, and then lands onto the next surface. This may be easier in two videos, where one video focuses on the front half of the body (head, neck, shoulders and front legs), while a second video should focus on the back, hind legs and abdomen. Capture this movement.

Stairs: Capture a video of your pet walking up and then down the stairs. Please only do this if it is safe for the pet to do so.

Rest: Capture a video of your pet lying down and then getting up. One video should focus on your pet's head and neck, and the second one on his feet.

Elimination: Capture a video of your pet eliminating (passing urine and stools). For dogs, try capturing leg-raising and crouching to defecate; for cats, try to capture it getting into and out of the litter tray, digging in the litter and eliminating.

Circling: Capture videos of your pet walking in circles; ensure you film it turning to the left and the right, in wide and tight circles.

A9 – Feeding Toys and Stimulation for Cats

In order to optimize and enrich your cat's environment, it needs to have access to various outlets which allow it to exhibit its normal behavioural repertoire and appropriately interact with you. Outlets which allow this include:

- feeding;
- play;
- environmental; and
- training.

Feeding

As cats are natural hunters, they may not get the chance to exhibit these behaviours if they are house cats or kept indoors for extended periods. Feeding your cat is an opportunity to mimic predatory behaviours with the use of food-dispensing toys, interactive bowls or lick mats. These can be bought, or you can make them yourself.

When looking at food-dispensing toys or interactive bowls, a lot of the toys and bowls available for small dogs will work well for cats too.

Food-dispensing toys are mainly used for dry food and treats.They can be bought or made. These are examples of feeding toys you can buy:

- Kitty KONG™;
- KONG Cat Wobbler™;
- KONG Cat Treat Dispensing Ball™;
- The Funkitty™ Twist 'n Treat™; and
- Nina Ottossonn DOG TREAT MAZE™.

Examples of feeding toys you can make include:

- egg box;
- empty bottle with holes in for dry food;
- paper rolls glued together with dry food in;
- empty cardboard box to climb into and find food; and
- small containers hidden with food inside.

Interactive bowls are available which can be used for a mixture of wet, dry or raw food. Examples include:

- TRIXIE Cat Activity Fun Board™;
- GREEN Slow Dog Feeder™ small; and
- Outward Hound Slo-Bowl Fun Feeder™.

Lick mats can be used for wet or raw diets. Examples include:

- LickiMat™;
- LickiMat™ Slomo; and
- SloDog - Slow Feeder Plate.

Play

Cats have a strong instinct to display predatory behaviours such as stalking, chasing, pouncing and biting prey. If your cat spends all or most of its day in the house, it may not get the opportunity to meet this need.

Toy-directed play can be used as a substitute for chasing and catching prey. Play can be solitary (the cat on its own with a toy) or social (with your or another cat, and a toy).

There are many different toys available, and some which you can make at home; which toy is best for your cat will depend on its individual preferences.

Examples of toys that cats can play on their own with include:

- balls such as KONG™ Moppy Ball;
- catnip stuffed toys such as KONG Kickeroo™ Mouse;
- PetStages® Tower of tracks; and
- all of the food-dispensing toys, interactive bowls and lick mats mentioned above.

Examples of toys you can interact and play with together include:

- KONG™ Fishing Pole Teaser; and
- Jackson Galaxy Air Prey Telescoping Wand.

Examples of toy you can make for your cat to play with on their own or with you include:

- boxes with holes in to explore;
- old socks with catnip in;
- pieces of string/wool glued into a ball; and
- a string with a toy or feathers tied to the end.

Tips for successful play:

- have a variety of different toys;
- rotate the toys to keep your cat interested in them;
- if you have multiple cats, ensure each cat has its toys in its resting area;
- set aside time to play with your cat – not all toys are for self-directed play, and so you will need to play with them; and
- if you are using a wand-type toy, allow your cat to catch the toy on the end of the wand so that it can complete the entire predatory behaviour sequence.

Environmental

Environmental outlets for your cat include resting places, scratching areas and possible access to cat grass.

Resting places: cats tend to prefer a resting area which is private and secure where it can go to when it wants to relax, rest and sleep. If you have an older cat or a kitten, it should have easy access to high resting areas via shelves or climbing trees – see below for more on these. If you have multiple cats, each cat should have access to its resting area, preferably in separate areas of the house, so it can be alone to rest and sleep if it wishes. In addition, each resting area should have more than one entry point so that access to or exit from this area cannot be blocked by the presence of another pet or people.

Within the resting area, there should be individual hiding places or resting places. Examples of these include:

- a cardboard box on its side with a pillow or fleece bed inside;
- a cat carrier with a pillow or fleece bed inside – if you use a wire carrier, ensure you cover it with a blanket to aid the need to hide;
- cat or small dog beds – these come in a variety of sizes and shapes;
- igloo-type beds – these can be bought or made;
- cat trees – cat trees have moved on from brown carpet-covered pieces of wood. There are many different materials in various styles available which will suit your home and your cat. Alternatively, you can make your own; and
- Shelves – these allow your cat to have access to high resting areas such as the top of bookshelves or a cupboard. You can buy specific cat shelves or use regular shelves with a non-slip surface attached.

Scratching

Cats scratch for multiple reasons and so having access to appropriate areas to scratch will ensure your cat can exhibit this part of the normal behavioural repertoire.

Every cat will have a preference as to what substrate they scratch on (e.g. rope, carpet, cardboard or wood) and whether they use a vertical or horizontal scratch post. You may have to provide a variety of scratching posts to find your cat's preference and be able to cater for it.

Cat grass

Some cats like to eat or chew fresh grass. Cat grass is available to buy, which is a mixture of grasses grown from seeds and includes wheat, barley, oats or rye. Cat grass is grown indoors, specifically for household pets.

Training

Reward-based training is a calm, positive way to interact with your cat and can be very rewarding for you and your cat.

Cats can be trained to perform several cues and tricks in the same way you would teach a dog; however, it may take longer to achieve the behaviours. Cues you can teach your cat include 'Sit', 'Come', 'Watch me', and 'Touch'.

A10 – Feeding Toys and Stimulation for Dogs

In order to optimize and enrich your dog's environment, it needs to have access to various outlets which allow it to exhibit its normal behavioural repertoire and appropriately interact with you. Outlets which allow this include:

- feeding;
- play;
- environmental; and
- training.

Feeding

Dogs are scavengers; however, they may not get the chance to exhibit these behaviours if they are fed once or twice a day from a bowl.

Food can be used to mimic scavenging behaviours with the use of food-dispensing toys, interactive bowls or lick mats. These can be bought, or you can make them yourself.

Food-dispensing toys are mainly used for dry food and treats. Examples of feeding toys you can buy include:

- KONG® Classic;
- *KONG Wobbler*™;
- Busy Buddy® Twist 'n Treat™;
- BUSTER food cube;
- Nina Ottosson DOG TORNADO; and
- Snuffle mat.

Examples of feeding toys you can make include:

- egg box;
- empty bottle with holes in for dry food;
- empty plastic bottle suspended on a rope;
- snuffle mat; and
- muffin tray with food in each section and a ball over.

Interactive bowls are available which can be used for a mixture of wet, dry, or raw food. Examples include:

- BUSTER DogMaze;
- GREEN Slow Dog Feeder™; and
- Outward Hound Slo-Bowl Fun Feeder™.

Lick mat can be used for wet or raw diets. Examples include:

- LickiMat™;
- LickiMat™ Slomo; and
- SloDog - Slow Feeder Plate.

Some of these toys, bowls and mats can be filled and frozen before given or hidden in the house or garden.

Play

Play is an enjoyable and stimulating way to interact with your dog. However, some dogs will be happy to play on their own with toys.

There are many different toys available to buy, and some which you can make at home; which toy is best for you and your dog will depend on your dog's preferences.

Examples of toys your dog can play with on their own include:

- balls such as KONG SqueakAir® Ball;
- KONG Phatz;
- KONG Wubba Weave with Rope; and
- all of the food-dispensing toys, interactive bowls and lick mats mentioned above.

Examples of toys you can interact and play with together include:

- ropes for tug and fetch; and
- all the toys which can be used for your dog to play on their own, with you, or another dog.

Examples of toys you can make for your dog to play with on their own or with you include:

- boxes with scrunched paper and toys in;
- old fabric made into tug toys or soft toys; and
- sandpits with a toy buried in.

Tips for successful play:

- have a variety of different toys;
- rotate the toys to keep your dog interested in them; and
- Set aside time to play with your dog – not all dogs will carry out self-directed play.

SAFETY: Always ensure the toys you give your dog are appropriate for the play; they should not be too small or easily broken. Ensure that they cannot be chewed, swallowed or cause injury. In addition, if they are too hard, they may cause damage to your dog's teeth while they are playing.

Environmental

Environmental outlets for your dog include secure outside access, outlets to perform normal behaviours (digging and chewing) and the opportunity to explore new environments.

Secure outside access: this provides your dog with the opportunity to explore and investigate while off-lead. Also, you do not need to supervise.

Outlets for normal behaviours: digging and chewing are normal behaviours. Therefore, your dog needs an outlet for these behaviours. A sandpit or designated area of the garden can provide the opportunity to dig. There are numerous products available for your dog to chew. Chews can be made of durable rubber or nylon, such as Nylabones, or a natural chew such as hooves, rawhides, antlers and bones. Every dog will have a personal preference as to which type of chew they like, and so you may have to provide a variety for them to choose from.

New environments: your dog should be provided with the opportunity to explore new environments. The frequency of visits to a new environment will be dependent on your dog's physical and mental health, and your ability to take it.

Training

There are many types of training and sports available to participate in with your dog. These include, but are not limited to: obedience, agility, flyball, tracking, gundog trials, herding, dancing to music, tricks and frisbee. What type of training or sport you do with your dog will depend on its physical and mental health.

A11 – Resources Available

Below you will find links to resources on the following:

1. Behavioural information – behaviour modification and pet training information.
2. Behavioural information – veterinary behaviour specialists and qualification information.
3. Veterinary behaviour drugs and supplements.
4. Product information.
5. Other useful websites.

1. Behavioural information – behaviour modification and pet training information

American Animal Hospital Association www.aaha.org/aaha-guidelines/behavior-management/behavior-management-home

Animal Behaviour and Training Council http://www.abtcouncil.org.uk

Association of Pet Behaviour Counsellors www.apbc.org.uk

Association of Pet Dog Trainers www.apdt.com

Canadian Association of Pet Dog Trainers www.cappdt.ca

CattleDog Publishing; Dr Sophia Yin www.drsophiayin.com

International Positive Dog Training Association www.ipdta.org

Karen Pryor Academy www.karenpryoracademy.com

Victoria Stilwell www.positively.com

2. Behavioural information – veterinary behaviour specialists and qualification information

Academy of Veterinary Behavioral Technicians www.avbt.net

American College of Veterinary Behaviorists www.dacvb.org

American Veterinary Society of Animal Behavior www.avsab.org

Animal Behaviour and Training Council Register of Veterinary Behaviourists www.abtcouncil.org.uk/veterinary-behaviourists

Certificated Clinical Animal Behaviourists (CCABs) www.asab.org/ccab

Australian and New Zealand College of Veterinary Scientists www.anzcvs.org.au/chapters/veterinary+behaviour+chapter

Clinical Animal Behaviour Group www.bristol.ac.uk/vet-school/services/behaviour-clinic

European College of Animal Welfare and Behavioural Medicine www.ecawbm.org

European Society of Veterinary Clinical Ethology www.esvce.org

Fellowship of Animal Behaviour Clinicians www.fabclinicians.org

International Association of Animal Behaviour Consultants www.iaabc.org

Royal College of Veterinary Surgeons and specialists in behavioural medicine www.findavet.rcvs.org.uk/find-a-vet-surgeon/by-specialist

Society of Veterinary Behavior Technicians www.svbt.org

3. Veterinary behaviour drugs and supplements

Medications:

Clomicalm® (clomipramine hydrochloride) www.elanco.us/products-services/dogs/clomicalm

Reconcile® (fluoxetine hydrochloride) www.reconcile.com

Selgian® (Selegiline Hydrochloride) www.noahcompendium.co.uk/?id=-474351

Vivitonin / Propentofylline www.noahcompendium.co.uk/?id=-456272

Pheromones:

Apadtil www.adaptil.com

Feliway www.feliway.com

Zenifel www.vetclick.com/news/introducing-zenifel-the-new-feline-facial-pheromone-plug-in-diffuser-p5386.php

Supplements:

Aktivait www.vetplusglobal.com/products/aktivait

Anxitane www.uk.virbac.com/products/calming/anxitane-tablets-helps-to-calm

Denamarin www.protexin.com/products/denamarin/6

Denosyl www.denosyl.com/

Nuracalm www.nutravet.co.uk/nutracalm

Senilife www.senilife.com

Zylkene www.zylkenepet.co.uk

4. Product information

Feeding toys/bowls:

Cat Activity Fun Board www.trixie.de

BUSTER products www.kruuse.com/frontpage/knowledge/intelligent-feeding

Busy Buddy products www.petsafe.net/busybuddy

GREEN slow feeder bowl www.companyofanimals.co.uk/product/green-slow-dog-feeder

KONG® www.kongcompany.com

LickiMat™, LickiMat™ Slomo, SloDog - Slow Feeder Plate www.innovativepetproducts.com

Nina Ottosson www.nina-ottosson.com

Outward Hound www.outwardhound.com

PetSafe FunKitty www.store.intl.petsafe.net/en-gb/play-challenge/cat-toys/l/funkittya

PetStages www.petstages.outwardhound.com

Snuffle Mats www.snufflemats.co.uk/

Head Halters:

Canny Collar www.cannyco.com

Dogmatic www.dogmatic.org.uk

Gentle leader www.petsafe.net/gentleleader
Halti headcollar www.companyofanimals.co.uk/product/halti-headcollar
Halti Opti ft www.companyofanimals.co.uk/product/halti-optifit
SnootLoop www.snootloop.com

Harnesses:

Freedom no-pull harness www.chemeyes.co.uk/product/freedom-no-pull-harness
Halti Front Control Harness www.companyofanimals.co.uk/product/halti-front-control-harness
Perfect Fit harness www.dog-games-shop.co.uk/perfect-fit-fleece-dog-harness
Petsafe Easy Walk® www.petsafe.net/easywalk
Positively No-Pull Harness www.positively.shop.musictoday.com/store
Rogz Control Harness www.rogz.com/product/control-harness
Ruffwear Front Range® Dog Harness www.ruffwear.co.uk/products/front-range-everyday-dog-harness

Muzzles:

Baskerville Classic www.companyofanimals.co.uk/product/baskerville-classic-muzzle
Baskerville Ultra www.companyofanimals.co.uk/product/baskerville-ultra-muzzle
BUMAS custom made muzzle www.bumas.uk/dog-muzzle?TABINDEX=0
Greyhound muzzles www.muzzlesforgreyhounds.com/muzzles
Heavy Duty Wire Muzzles www.campbellpet.com/collections/muzzles-dog-cat

Other products:

Microchip cat flap www.surepetcare.com/en-gb/pet-doors/microchip-cat-flap
Microchip pet feeder www.surepetcare.com/en-gb/pet-feeder
Pet fencing www.protectapet.com
Petporte smart flap® Microchip Cat Flap www.store.intl.petsafe.net/en-gb/doors/cat
Nylabone www.nylabone.com

5. Other useful websites

Canine arthritis management www.caninearthritis.co.uk
Dog dementia www.dogdementia.com
Doggone Safe! www.doggonesafe.com
Family Paws Parent Education www.familypaws.com/
Feline Advisory Bureau www.fabcats.org
International Cat Care www.icatcare.org
Ohio State University Indoor Pet Initiative www.indoorpet.osu.edu/cats
Veterinary Information Network www.vin.com

B1 – Body Language – Cat

Body language/behaviour seen		Underlying emotion/motivation				
		Calm	Attentive/high arousal	Anxious	Fearful – defensive	Fearful – offensive
Head	Ears	Relaxed Held in a neutral position	Forward-facing towards the point of interest	Swivelling independently Flattened back to their head when not moving	Pulled back Flat against the head	Tense Pulled back against the head
	Eyes	Blinking softly Half-closed Pupils appropriate for ambient light	Looking towards the point of interest Pupils appropriate for ambient light	Open Not blinking Pupils dilated	Wide open Not blinking Pupils fully dilated	Wide open Hard stare Pupils fully dilated
	Mouth	Closed	Closed	Closed with tension	Closed with tension Open with lips pulled back and teeth exposed while vocalizing	Closed with significant tension Open with lips pulled back and teeth exposed while vocalizing
	Face	No tension Whiskers in a neutral position	Some muscle tension Whiskers neutral or forward towards the point of interest	Muscle tension present Whiskers drawn back	Marked muscle tension Whiskers fully pulled back	Significant muscle tension Whiskers stiff and held out to the side

Body language/behaviour seen		Underlying emotion/motivation				
		Calm	Attentive/high arousal	Anxious	Fearful – defensive	Fearful – offensive
Body	Legs and back	Fully extended while lying	Bent while lying	Tucked under the body	Front legs fully extended and tense Back legs bent ready to move Possibly arched back	Significant muscle tension Possibly arch the back
	Position/stance	Standing Sitting Lying on the side	Standing Sitting Lying in an upright position angled towards the point of interest	Crouched/lowered to the floor Head held in line with the body	Standing or crouched Weight shifted backwards	Rigid body Standing with weight shifted forwards or crouched ready to pounce
	Fur	Laid flat against the body	Laid flat against the body	Laid flat against the body	Raised along the length of the body	Raised along the length of the body
Tail	Position and movement	Extended or wrapped around the body when resting Upright with the tip curled when standing/walking	Can be either extended or close to the body Tip may be twitching	Extended with a slow twitch	Curled under the body Side-to-side movements	Straight and stiff or curled under the body
	Fur	Laid flat against the tail	Laid flat against the tail	Laid flat against the tail	All fur standing upright	All fur standing upright
Movement		Resting Sleeping Slowly exploring	Resting Actively exploring	Alert Trying to move away	Motionless May try to move away	Motionless May suddenly move forward May strike out with front legs
Vocalization		Slow and calm meow Soft purr	Meow or quiet	May growl	Hissing, growling, yowling Spitting	Hissing, growling, yowling or silent

B2 – Body Language – Dog

Body language/behaviour seen		Underlying emotion/motivation: Calm	Attentive/high arousal	Anxious	Fearful – defensive	Fearful – offensive
Head	Ears	Relaxed; neutral position for the breed	Forward-facing towards the point of interest	Pulled back Pulled down close to the head	Pulled back flat against the head	Tense Upright Pointing forwards
	Eyes	Blinking softly Half-closed Pupils appropriate for ambient light	Looking towards the point of interest Pupils appropriate for ambient light	Wide and looking towards the point of interest Wide and looking out of the corner of the eye at the point of interest Pupils dilated	Wide and staring at point of interest Squinting, looking towards and away from the point of interest Pupils fully dilated	Widely open Pupils fully dilated Hard stare towards the point of interest
	Mouth	Closed or slightly open No tension Tongue may be out (depending on the temperature and panting)	Closed	Closed with tension Lip-licking Yawning May pant Corner of lips pulled back	Closed with marked tension Lips pulled back Teeth exposed	Open Tense lips, drawn back Teeth exposed Muzzle and nose wrinkled
	Face	No tension Whiskers in a neutral position	Whiskers neutral or forwards towards the point of interest May be some muscle tension	Muscle tension present Brows furrowed May turn head away	Marked muscle tension	Significant muscle tension Focused on the point of interest

Body language/behaviour seen		Underlying emotion/motivation Calm	Attentive/high arousal	Anxious	Fearful – defensive	Fearful – offensive
Body	Legs	Dependent on body position No tension or stiffness is seen	In an appropriate position ready to move dependent on body position	Tucked under the body Bent ready for movement	Back legs bent and tucked under the body	Significant muscle tension Straight front legs
	Position/stance	Standing Sitting Lying Walking	Standing Sitting Lying in an upright position Head and body angled towards the point of interest	Cowering May turn the head away from the point of interest	Cowering Turning away with the head facing the point of interest Lying on their side or back with hind leg raised May urinate	Standing upright Rigid body Weight shifted forwards ready to lunge
	Fur	Laid flat against the body	Laid flat against the body	Laid flat against the body (might shed more)	Raised along the length of the body (dorsal midline)	Raised along the length of the body Raised on the neck Potentially raised on the tail
Tail	Position and movement	Neutral position for the breed Broad side-to-side tail wag	Held upright Mostly still but possibly moving	Lowered Slow short wag of the tail	Curled under the body Small, slow and tight wags	High over the body Slow, tight wag
Movement		Resting Sleeping Actively exploring	Resting Actively exploring	Slow approach Move away Circling Hypervigilant	Motionless May try to move away	Motionless May suddenly lunge or bite
Vocalization		May bark if interacting	May bark	May bark	May make high-pitched bark	Silent Low growl

B3 – Identifying Displacement and Conflict-related Behaviours

Understanding arousal levels

The term arousal describes a physiological response to an emotional state. These physiological responses include increased pulse, respiration rate, blood pressure, and an increase in circulatory hormones such as cortisol and adrenaline (for more information see Section 7.4.3).

The change in emotional state can be a positive one such as excitement and may prepare the body to jump for joy; or it can be a negative one, such as anxiety or fear and prepare the body to run away. Following a trigger, it can take as little as three quarters of a second to mount an arousal response. However, it can take minutes, hours or even days for these levels to reduce again.

As the pet's arousal levels increase, it passes through two different thresholds: an emotional threshold and a behavioural threshold (see Figs 7.9A and B).

1. Emotional threshold: Above this level, the pet loses its ability to control its emotions. It will start displaying displacement behaviours or conflict behaviours (see below for more details). When it is at this level of arousal, you should still be able to interact with it and get it to respond to known cues (touch, watch, sit, etc.) and take treats.
2. Behavioural threshold: If the pet is continually exposed to various stimuli or does not have enough time for its arousal levels to reduce between each stimulus, it will cross the behavioural threshold. The pet will start to show behavioural signs of high arousal such as vocalizing, growling, snapping, biting, scratching and lunging. When it is at this level of arousal, it generally does not respond to known cues or take treats.

Which threshold the pet will pass through will depend on several factors such as:

- where its arousal level was before being exposed to the stimuli;
- any accumulative effect – every time the pet is exposed to a stimulus its arousal will increase. Over time, there is a cumulative effect which will increase arousal levels; and
- the intensity of the stimulus – it is possible for an individual stimulus to increase the pet's arousal levels past the behavioural threshold without any indication of it crossing its emotional threshold.

The pet can have chronic high arousal as it does not have sufficient time between exposures to simile to allow arousal levels to reduce. This could mean it remains above the emotional or behavioural threshold at all times.

Displacement behaviours

Displacement behaviours are normal behaviours, and they are often seen within the normal behavioural repertoire of the pet. What makes them displacement behaviours, rather than appropriate behaviour, is that they are performed out of context (see Section 7.3.3.2).

Displacement behaviours are seen when there is an increase in arousal levels, and the pet crosses its emotional threshold.

Displacement behaviours include:

- yawning when not tired;
- licking the lips when it does not have any food or water on the lips;

- shaking off as if the coat is wet when it is dry;
- looking at something out of the corner of the eye instead of straight at it;
- stretching when it has not been resting for an extended period; and
- sneezing when it is not allergic or does not have anything irritating its nose.

There are some things to look for, which will help you tell the difference between normal behaviour and displacement behaviour:

- Does the behaviour appear out-of-context (full-body shaking when dry)?
- Is the behaviour repetitive (e.g. the pet licks its lips several times in close succession)?
- Does the behaviour occur at the same time as other displacement behaviours (e.g. yawning and lip-licking)?
- Can you reproduce the behaviour by placing it in a similar situation (e.g. lip-licking and looking out of the corner of its eye when a dog approaches)?

If the answer is yes, then it is a displacement behaviour.

Conflict behaviours

Conflict-related behaviours are behaviours which are shown in situations where there are two or more competing emotional motivations; the pet is both drawn towards and repelled from something at the same time. Conflict-related behaviours lead to an increase in arousal levels (see Section 7.3.2).
Examples of conflict behaviours include:

1. The pet stretches towards a stranger offering a treat and moves away as soon as it has taken the treat.
    - The pet might want the treat but not be that close to the stranger. To get the treat, it must be close to the stranger.
      This context causes conflict because the pet is torn between taking the treat while keeping its distance from the stranger.
2. Another dog approaches the pet to play:
    - The pet may approach the other dog to play but may have its hackles up, or it may growl.
      This context causes conflict because the pet wants to play but does not know how the other dog will react.
3. Trimming the pet's nails:
    - The pet may want to be with you and have an interaction with you; however, it does not like its nails being trimmed.

C1 – Set Up to Succeed

To ensure both you and your pet get the most from a training session, there are several factors which should be considered before starting the session:

1. Meeting your pet's needs;
2. Ensuring your pet knows any cues you will use;
3. Preparation of rewards;
4. Allowing enough time; and
5. Training environment.

1. Meeting your pet's needs

Before you begin a training session, ensure that your pet has eliminated; they will not focus on the training if they need to pass urine.

Ensure that your pet has had some form of physical exercise. For cats, this may be a play session with you. For dogs, this may be a walk, run or play in the garden.

Ensure that your pet has not been fed for several hours before the training session; this will help with their motivation to work for the treats you are offering them. The duration of withholding food depends on your pet's age and physical health.

2. Ensuring your pet knows any cues you will use

If you are going to do a desensitization session with your pet, there are several behaviours they will need to know and be able to perform on cue before you start this form of training. In order to set your pet up to succeed, you need to ensure that your pet knows these cues and responds to them in a variety of environments with distractions before progressing with their desensitization training (see Handout C2 – How to Teach a 'Watch Me' and 'Touch' Cue).

3. Preparation of rewards

Which treats you use will be dependent on your pet's individual preferences. Some cats will work for a commercially available cat treat while other cats will only work for a prawn or some fish. Some dogs will work for pieces of cheese, liver or carrot while other dogs will only work for toys. You may need to try a variety of treats to find which your pet prefers and will work for the best.

For some training sessions (e.g. muzzle training, head-halter training or staying in one place), soft food such as peanut butter, cream cheese, paté or wet dog food on a wooden spoon or lick mat are useful to have to hand.

NB If using peanut butter, ensure it does not contain any artificial sweeteners, especially Xylitol, as these are toxic for dogs.

Whatever treat you use, ensure that you prepare enough small tasty treats to last the duration of the training session and have them to hand in a tub, a treat pouch or your pocket.

4. Allowing enough time

You should aim for each training session to last 10–15 minutes; after this length of time, your pet will need to have a break.

It is possible to do two sessions; however, there should be a 10–15-minute break between sessions where the pet is removed from the training environment and allowed to rest.

Ensure that you allocate enough time to get to the training environment, set up for the training session, carry out the training session and leave the training environment. If you travel to a field for the training, you may need to set aside up to two hours for the session.

Ideally, the training session should be carried out two to three times a week with at least one day between to allow arousal levels to reduce.

5. Training environment

The environment in which you carry out your training session will have a significant impact on how well your pet responds during the session.

The ideal training environment for initial training should be:

- quiet – no television or radio; minimal noises within the house; minimal outside noises; and
- minimal distractions including, but not limited to: other pets; other people; telephone/mobile phone which may ring; visitors; deliveries; post arriving.

Some training sessions need to be done outside the house. In these cases, an open field where you can see all around you, or a privately hired, secure paddock may be the best option.

If you can consider all of these points before starting a training session, you can be sure you have done everything possible to set your pet up to succeed in whatever training you are doing with them.

C2 – How to Teach a 'Watch Me' and 'Touch' Cue

Before each session, ensure that you have met your pet's needs and set them up to succeed; for example, they have had some physical exercise and have not been fed prior to the training session (see Handout C1 – Set Up to Succeed).

To teach the pet a 'Watch me' cue:

1. Choose a cue to use, such as 'Watch me', and a hand signal such as putting your finger on your nose or pointing at your face.
2. Have small tasty treats ready.
3. Take a treat and show it to the pet, keeping it far enough out of reach so that it does not take it.
4. Move the treat towards your face and show the pet the hand signal for 'Watch me'.
5. As it looks towards you, say 'Watch me' and give it the treat.
6. Repeat this several times until the pet can make eye contact with you as soon as it knows there is a treat in your hand, and you start to make the hand signal.
7. Test the pet; give the 'Watch me' cue and hand signal when you don't have a treat in your hand. If it looks at you, it has learnt the cue. If it does not look at you, go back to steps 3–7 until it can look at you when you test it again.
8. Slowly increase the level of distractions when training so that the pet learns to listen to the cue in many different situations. For example, if you are training in the kitchen, try moving into the lounge, by the door, in the garden, and then by the fence, building it up until you can practise the 'Watch Me' cue when out on a walk.

This cue can be added to your regular daily routine with your pet, such as before you open the door for it, before you give it food or a treat and before you give it affection. With dogs, you can use it before you attach the lead for a walk.

To teach the pet a 'Touch' cue:

1. Choose a cue to use, such as 'Touch', and a hand signal such as a flat hand held out to your side with your palm facing the pet.
2. Have small tasty treats ready.
3. With the pet in front of you, show it the hand signal.
4. When the pet moves to sniff your hand, say the cue word 'Touch' and give it a treat.
5. If the pet is not interested in approaching or sniffing your hand, you may need to hold a treat between your fingers, or rub soft food on your palm, to encourage it to move towards your hand.
6. If it is still not interested, you can move your hand closer to its nose, or even gently touch the nose.
7. Repeat this several times until the pet touches your hand as soon as you give the cue and show it the hand signal.
8. Test the pet; give the 'Touch' cue and hand signal when it has moved away from you – if the pet comes to you and touches its nose to your hand, it has learnt the cue. If it does not move towards you and touch your hand, go back to steps 5–8 until it can touch your hand when you test it again.

9. Slowly increase the level of distractions when training so that the pet learns to listen to the cue in many different situations. For example, if you are training in the kitchen, try moving into the lounge, by the door, in the garden, and then by the fence, building it up until you can practise the 'Touch' cue when out on a walk.

Again, this cue can be added to your regular daily routine with your pet as detailed above. A 'Touch' cue can be very useful for recalling your dog or changing direction on a walk.

C3 – Safe-haven

Safe-haven training will provide your pet with two separate places to go where they can spend time alone to rest, enjoy food dispensing toys, and sleep.

The two types of safe-haven you will provide your pet with are:

1. Safety/crisis management safe-haven
2. Everyday safe-haven

1. Safety/crisis management safe-haven training

The pet will be trained to use a safety/crisis management safe-haven as part of their everyday routine so that they become comfortable going there when you need to use it for safety or crisis management reasons. Situations where you may need to use a safety/crisis management safe-haven include when you can not supervise the pet in a high-risk situation; the pet may be exposed to a trigger, and its arousal level may cross the behavioural threshold; and, when your pet needs to rest or sleep, but the house is too busy to allow for rest or sleep.

You will need to consider safety (for all involved, including the pet) and practicality when choosing an area to use as a safety/crisis management safe-haven. You need to be able to leave the pet there knowing no one will accidentally enter the area or allow the pet out.

A bedroom, study or utility room work well if you can close the door. Alternatively, you can use a stair gate across the door to prevent any physical contact but allow the pet to see what is happening. The use of a door or stair gate will depend on the associated risks of having an open gate versus a closed, possibly locked, door. If using a room is not an option, a covered crate in the quietest area of the house will work well too. In some situations you may need to use a double stair gate situation to make sure people do not put their fingers through or similar.

Preparing safety/crisis management safe-haven

A safe-haven should have the following to create an ideal environment for resting and sleeping:

- Appropriate bedding;
- Fresh water;
- Food in feeding toys, slow feeders, and chews to keep the pet busy. These can be tethered in the room or crate to prevent the pet from taking them out;
- The windows closed to reduce noise;
- Curtains/blinds closed to darken the room – consider a blackout blind to block more light;
- A white noise machine to muffle any outside noises;
- Feliway™ (cats) or Adaptil™ (dogs) diffuser to help the pet feel comfortable in the room; and
- If the pet is likely to become distressed if the door is closed, a stair gate across the door to keep them there.

Training your pet to use the safety/crisis management safe-haven

Before each session, ensure you have met your pet's needs and set them up to succeed. For example, they have had physical exercise (play or walk) and have not been fed before the training session (see Handout C1–Set Up to Succeed).

Prepare some of their daily food in slow feeder bowls, feeding toys and chews. Soft food such as peanut butter, cream cheese, or paté can also be used in these.

NB If using peanut butter or other human foods ensure it does not contain any artificial sweeteners, especially Xylitol, as these are toxic for dogs.

The first time you use the safety/crisis management safe-haven, you will need to gauge how long the pet can stay in the area before they try to get out or vocalize. This is done in the following way:

1. Take the pet into the safe-haven and give them the prepared feeding toys, slow feeders or chews.
2. If you are using a stair gate, close the gate; if you are using the door, close the door as you leave the room.
3. Time how long it takes for the pet to come to the door and try to get out. This is how long they can cope with being in the room alone.
4. Repeat steps 1-3 several times over the next few days. Once you have done four to six timed sessions, work out the average of these times. You now have the average length of time your pet can stay in the safe-haven.
5. Before you start safety/crisis management safe-haven training, take a few minutes off of the average time calculated in step 4. This will be the length of time the pet can be left in the safe-haven for the initial training sessions. For example, if the pet shows restlessness or stands by the door, sniffing under the door, or panting after an average of 10 minutes, start the safe-haven training for 5 minutes per session.

The next steps of the safety/crisis management safe-haven training are:

1. Ensure you have met the pet's needs and set them up to succeed.
2. Take the pet into the safe-haven and give it the prepared feeding toys, slow feeders or chews.
3. Leave the pet alone in the area and close the door or gate behind you.
4. Leave the pet for the amount of time you have worked out in the steps above. Ideally, you can return to the room, open the door or gate and walk away. Do not encourage the pet to leave the safe-haven area; if it is settled, leave the pet there until it chooses to come out. Initially, the pet may leave as soon as you open the door; however, over time, the pet will build a positive association with the safe-haven and be comfortable enough to spend time there alone. The pet should eventually be comfortable enough to take itself off to the room to rest or sleep.
5. Repeat steps 1 – 4, while gradually increasing the amount of time before you re-enter the room by one to two minutes at a time.

Some pets may cope well with the training, and you can increase the time they are left quickly by a small amount every few days, while some may need a week or more at a particular time before you can extend the time. Do not be tempted to leave them for extended periods too quickly as this will undermine the training you have done and may prevent you from being able to use this safety/crisis management safe-haven again in the future.

2. Everyday safe-haven

The pet should also be trained to use an everyday safe-haven as part of their normal routine. It will become a place where it can go to rest or sleep, and the pet will not be approached or touched by anyone. Your pet is in control when they are here.

An everyday safe-haven does not have to be used in specific situations; it should be available at all times to allow your pet to choose whether it wants to interact with anyone or rest. This means that if you call the pet for a walk and it chooses to stay in its safe-haven, you respect its decision not to get up and you leave the pet to rest. However, if you call the pet for a walk and it comes to you, you can take them for a walk.

Preparing for everyday safe-haven training

The following needs to be considered when setting up an everyday safe-haven for your pet to rest and sleep:

1. Interacting with your pet – when your pet is in its everyday safe-haven, it should not be approached or touched. It is estimated that pets see a space of approximately 1.5-2 metres around them as their personal space.
2. Location – choose a place where your pet feels comfortable and will be able to rest. This may be next to your chair when you first start the training, which you can gradually move to a chosen place in the room.
3. Appropriate bedding – your pet should have access to comfortable bedding to encourage it to rest. Also, consider getting a new bed to use for this training, to avoid negative past association.
4. Feliway™ (cats) or Adaptil™ (dogs) diffuser to help the pet feel comfortable in the area.

If using a bed is not an option, a covered crate *with the door open* will work well too.

Training your pet to use an everyday safe-haven

The following steps will help you to train your pet to use its everyday safe-haven:

1. Ensure you have met the pet's needs and set it up to succeed.
2. Prepare some food dispensing toys which can be given while the pet is stationary on its bedding in the everyday safe-haven – stuffed Kong's work well for this exercise.
   NB: only do this if appropriate for your pet, and it will not put you or anyone else at risk.
3. Take the pet into the area where its everyday safe-haven will be and encourage it onto the bedding. You may need to lure the pet onto the bedding initially, but you must not force it to go or stay there.
4. Once on the bed, drop several small treats onto the bedding to encourage the pet to stay on the bed. Do not try to touch or interact with the pet while it is in the safe-haven.
5. If appropriate, offer a food-dispensing toy to encourage the pet to stay in the safe-haven.
6. Repeat this over several sessions, gradually reducing the number of treats given until the pet willingly goes to the everyday safe-haven to rest and have a food-dispensing toy.
7. It is essential that everyone follows a simple rule: that when your pet is in its safe haven, they do not impose anything on it. They stay away, and if they want something, they may ask in a friendly way, but must respect the response. For an animal to give something up that is in the safe-haven the animal must voluntarily move away in a relaxed way.
8. No one must be left in the same room as your pet and their safe-haven if they do not understand or cannot follow these rules.

If your pet gets off the bed at any point, allow it to move away; remember the everyday safe-haven should be a place where the pet feels comfortable to come and go at any time, knowing no harm will come to it.

Once the pet chooses to go to the safe-haven on its own, you can look at gradually moving the bedding towards your chosen location. You can move the bed a short distance towards the chosen location and repeating the steps above until the bedding is in the chosen location.

Once the pet can go to its everyday safe-haven and rest, you should notice it will be used by your pet when you have family members or visitors at the house, or anything that mildly disturbs it, although your pet will remain relaxed throughout. Any family or visitors to the house must respect your pet's needs to have a safe space where no one will approach or interact with it. If this is not possible and your visitors, or other family members, cannot respect your pet's needs to have a safe space, you may need to consider using a safety/crisis management safe-haven while these people are at the house.

C4 – Teaching a Pet how to Settle on Cue

Teaching the pet to settle down and relax on cue can be useful when you have a pet that is highly aroused and needs some help to calm down. It can be used in several different situations, including after being exposed to a trigger it has reacted to, during a training session to help reduce arousal levels, after a fun game and at bedtime.

The 'Settle' cue is a difficult exercise that may take several weeks, sometimes more, to achieve. What makes it difficult is that you are attempting to change emotions and reduce arousal levels rather than teaching a specific behaviour, such as 'Sit' or 'Down'.

Follow these steps to help you achieve success:

1. For the best results, this exercise should be done daily.
2. Before each training session, ensure you have met your pet's needs (see Handout C1 – Set Up to Succeed).
3. Each training session will take approximately 15–20 minutes, so ensure you have sufficient time.
4. Identify the time of the day when the pet is likely to sleep, regardless of your activities. Also, try identifying the pet's favourite sleeping area to use during the training exercise.
5. Use a distinctly coloured mat or towel, such as yellow or blue, which the pet can easily recognize on any surface.
6. Ask the pet to sit or lie on the mat.
7. When the pet sits on the mat, start petting it around the neck and shoulder area. Massaging this area helps to calm and relax it; however, some pets find this arousing. If your pet becomes aroused, try placing a hand on this area without moving it. If this is still too much stimulation, do not use any form of touch during the exercise.
8. Choose a verbal cue to use for this exercise, such as 'Settle'. Repeat the verbal cue in a calm and soft voice while gently massaging the neck.
9. The pet will start relaxing and may start falling asleep because it was going to rest at this time of the day anyway. You should continue with steps 7 and 8 very slowly and gently while the pet relaxes.
10. After several repetitions, you should notice that the pet relaxes and falls asleep quicker in every session.
11. After a few weeks, you can test the pet by altering one part of the exercise; change either the time or the location in which you practise the exercise. Do not change two things at once as this may confuse the pet, and you will not know if it has learnt the cue.
12. Ask the pet to sit on the mat and give the cue; see if the pet appears to settle down. For example, the body relaxes, it moves from sitting to lying down, or it takes a deep breath and slows its breathing rate; this will indicate that it has learnt the cue. The pet may not fall asleep, but it should appear to be more relaxed.

Over time, the goal is to transfer the association between the mat, massage, verbal cue and relaxation to other times and places where the pet needs to reduce its arousal levels. After the initial phase, practising this exercise at various times and locations helps to achieve better results when the pet is aroused. Once the pet can respond to the cue in the house, progress to the garden and other locations (e.g. walks, or in a field with dogs).

C5 – Muzzle, Head Halter and Body Harness Training

Muzzle

A muzzle is a very useful safety tool for many reasons, including:

- stopping physical harm if a dog tries to bite;
- decreasing the owner's anxiety around their dog;
- keeping unfamiliar people and dogs away from your dog while out walking; and
- stopping the dog from picking up and eating food and non-food items which could cause harm.

A muzzle should never be used to force a dog into situations where its anxiety and arousal levels increase or where it will be exposed to known triggers. Before exposing the dog to a situation with a muzzle on, stop and think: Would you expose the dog to that situation if they did not have a muzzle on? If the answer is no, then the dog should not be in that situation.

Once muzzle-trained, your dog should wear the muzzle randomly at home, when out walking or when doing something it likes. Frequent and routine muzzle use at home will help to reduce the chances of it associating the muzzle with any potential triggers. For example, a dog which only wears a muzzle at the veterinary practice may learn to associate the muzzle going on with going to the veterinary practice. If it randomly wears the muzzle as part of its daily routine, it will reduce the chances of creating this association.

Always use a basket-type muzzle. A basket muzzle allows the dog to open its mouth while wearing it. The dog can also take treats, drink and pant while wearing it. It also allows you to put treats through to reward the dog.

Each session should be five to ten minutes long; the session should stop after ten minutes regardless of the amount of progress made. It is possible to do two sessions; however, there should be a 10–15-minute break between sessions. The training sessions should be carried out every day.

Before each session ensure you have met your dog's needs and set it up to succeed. For example, the dog has had some play or physical exercise and has not been fed before the training session (see Handout C1 – Set Up to Succeed).

Prepare enough small tasty treats to last for the whole five- to ten-minute session and have them to hand in a treat pouch or pocket. Soft food such as peanut butter, cream cheese, paté or wet dog food should be to hand for use inside the muzzle.

NB If using peanut butter, ensure that it does not contain any artificial sweeteners, especially Xylitol, as these are toxic for dogs.

Stage 1 – introducing the muzzle

1. Choose a cue to use such as 'Muzzle', which will indicate that the muzzle is going to be used.
2. Have tasty treats ready.
3. Find a quiet place to train away from any distractions.
4. Sit with the dog and say 'Muzzle'. Show it the muzzle and give it a treat. Do not attempt to put it on; just show it to your dog.

5. Repeat this 15–20 times within a few minutes. During this time, do not expect any specific behaviour, such as 'Sit' or 'Down'; just show your dog the muzzle, say 'Muzzle' and give it a treat.
6. After 15–20 repetitions, the dog should start forming an association between seeing the muzzle and getting a treat.
7. Next, say 'Muzzle', then place the muzzle on the floor with some treats near it. Over time, move the treats closer to the muzzle and eventually inside the muzzle so that the dog gets used to touching the muzzle with its nose. Once the dog is comfortable approaching and touching the muzzle, progress to the next step.
8. Smear something the dog can lick, such as peanut butter, wet food, or paté, onto the inside of the muzzle and hold the muzzle in a position where the dog can get its nose into the muzzle (see Fig. C5.1). As the dog approaches, say the 'Muzzle' cue and allow the dog to lick the soft food from inside the muzzle. Do not push the muzzle onto its nose or try to do it up at this point; allow the dog to approach, put its nose in and move away in its own time.

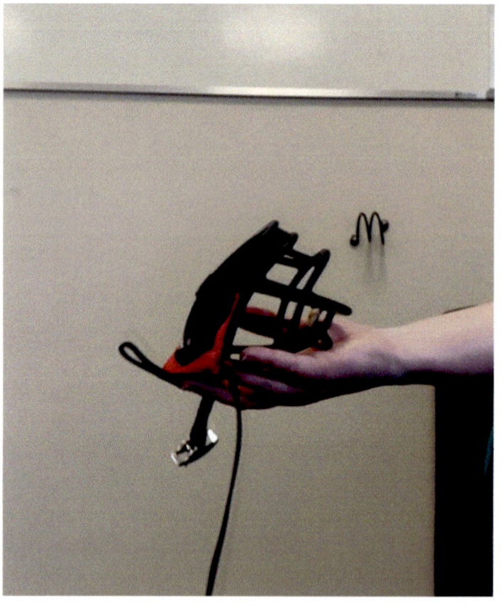

Fig. C5.1. Holding the muzzle for training.

9. Repeat this step several times, slowly moving the food further down into the muzzle so that the dog has to put its nose further into the muzzle each time.
10. Test the dog; hold the muzzle and say the 'Muzzle' cue; the dog should approach the muzzle and put its nose inside the muzzle. If the dog does not do this, go back and work through steps 8 and 9 until it responds to the muzzle cue.

Once the dog can put its nose in the muzzle on cue, you can move on to the next stage.

Stage 2 – getting used to the strap and buckle

This stage allows the dog to habituate to the noise of the clip or buckle, and the strap, being placed around its head.

1. Have tasty treats and soft food ready.
2. Find a quiet place to train away from any distractions.
3. Hold the muzzle where the dog can see it but does not try to put its nose into it. Do up the clip or move the buckle so it makes a noise, and give the dog a treat.

4. Next, hold the muzzle in a way that the dog can get its nose into it and you can move the straps. Rub soft food deep inside the end of the muzzle for the dog to lick. Say the 'Muzzle' cue, and while the dog is licking the inside of the muzzle, slowly move the straps. Do **not** try to do it up yet, just get the dog used to the straps moving around its neck while its nose is inside the muzzle.
5. Over several repetitions of step 4, slowly move the straps more until you can hold them behind the dog's head for a few seconds while it is licking the inside of the muzzle (see Fig. C5.2).

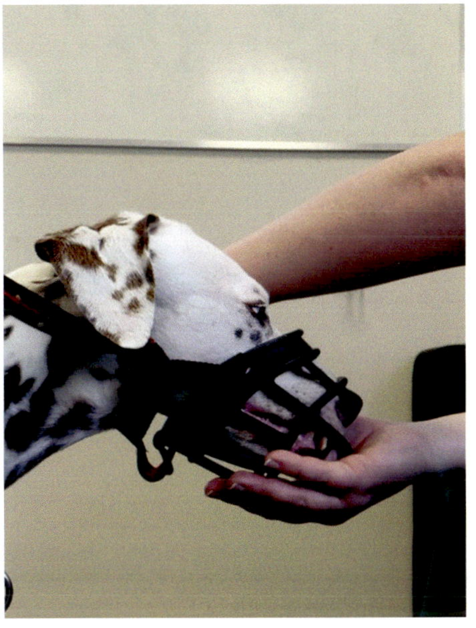

Fig. C5.2. Holding the straps behind the head.

Always release the straps before the dog finishes the food, so that it does not try to pull away from the muzzle.

Once you can hold the straps behind the dog's ears for a few seconds, you can move on to stage 3.

Stage 3 – fastening the muzzle and increasing the time wearing the muzzle

The most important aspect of stage 3 is to take your time – do not rush this stage as it could undo all of the muzzle training done thus far.

1. Have tasty treats and soft food ready.
2. Find a quiet place to train away from any distractions.
3. Place treats or soft food deep inside the muzzle for the dog to lick. Say the 'Muzzle' cue and while the dog is licking the inside of the muzzle, slowly move the straps and do the clip/buckle up. After three to five seconds, undo the muzzle and take it off. Repeat this several times until the dog is comfortable with closing the muzzle.
4. Slowly increase the time the dog spends wearing the muzzle. Increase it a few seconds at a time until the dog is comfortable wearing it for a few minutes.
5. At this early stage, keep feeding treats through the muzzle (see Fig. C5.3). Over time, you can decrease the number of treats given.

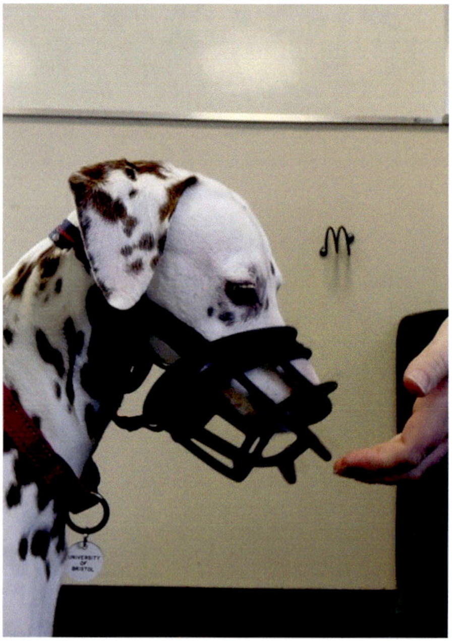

Fig. C5.3. Wearing the muzzle while taking treats.

6. When the dog is comfortable wearing the muzzle, you can introduce it at other times during the daily routine, such as when out walking or when you give affection. Put the muzzle on for short periods, allow the dog to sniff and receive treats with it on, then remove it.

Head halter

A head halter is a very useful safety and guidance tool which will help you control your dog. In addition to controlling the direction your dog moves in, a head halter can be used to redirect its gaze to you and so assist it when you need it to disengage with a potential trigger.

There are numerous types of head halter available, with the Halti® and Gentle Leader® being two of the most commonly used ones. Regardless of which brand you use, ensure you get the correct size; the neck strap should be up behind the ears, and snug enough for you to get two fingers under it, and the nose loop should be loose and away from the eyes but not reach the end of the nose. Most companies that produce head halters offer a sizing guide.

Each session should be five to ten minutes long; the session should stop after ten minutes regardless of the amount of progress made. It is possible to do two sessions; however, there should be a 10–15-minute break between sessions. The sessions should be carried out every day.

Before each session, ensure that your dog has had some play or physical exercise and the opportunity to eliminate. Ensure that the dog has not been fed prior to the session to increase its motivation to work for food.

Prepare enough small tasty treats to last for the whole five- to ten-minute session and have them to hand in a treat pouch or pocket. Soft foods such as peanut butter, cream cheese, paté or wet dog food on a wooden spoon or lick mat are useful to have to hand.

NB If using peanut butter, ensure that it does not contain any artificial sweeteners, especially Xylitol, as these are toxic for dogs.

Stage 1 – introducing the head halter

1. Choose a cue to use, such as 'Halter', which will indicate that the head halter is going to be used.
2. Have tasty treats ready.
3. Find a quiet place to train away from any distractions.
4. Sit with the dog and say the cue word; show it the head halter and give it a treat. Do not attempt to put it on; just show it to your dog.
5. Repeat this 15–20 times within a few minutes. During this time, do not expect any specific behaviour, such as 'sit' or 'down'; just show it the head halter, say the cue word and give it a treat.
6. After 15–20 repetitions, the dog should start forming an association between seeing the head halter and getting a treat.
7. Next, say the cue word, then place the head halter on the floor with some treats near it. Over time, move the treats closer to the head halter and eventually inside the nose loop of the head halter so that the dog gets used to touching the head halter with its nose. Once the dog is comfortable approaching and touching the head halter, progress to the next step.
8. Hold the head halter in a position where the dog can get its nose into the nose loop (see Fig. C5.4). Hold a treat near to the nose loop so that your dog has to put its nose through the nose loop to get the treat (see Fig. C5.5). As the dog approaches, say the cue word and allow it to take the treat. Do **not** push the head halter onto its nose or try to do it up at this point; allow the dog to approach, put its nose in the nose loop and move away in its own time.

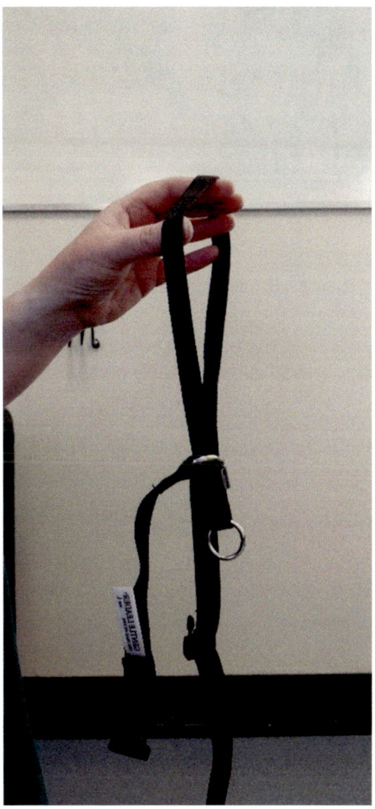

Fig. C5.4. Holding nose loop open.

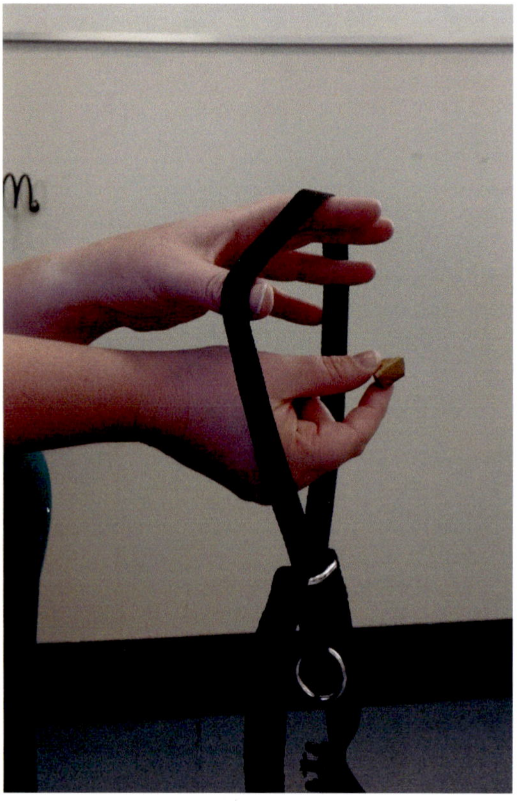

Fig. C5.5. Holding a treat through the nose loop.

9. Repeat this several times, slowly moving the food closer to you and further through the nose loop so that the dog has to put its nose further into the nose loop each time.
10. Test the pet; hold the head halter and say the cue word; the dog should approach the head halter and put its nose through the nose loop. If it does not do this, go back and work through steps 8 and 9 until it responds to the cue word.

Once the dog puts its nose in the nose loop on cue, you can move on to the next stage.

Stage 2 – getting used to the neck loop

This stage allows the dog to habituate to the noise of the clip and the strap being placed around its head.

It may be helpful to have a second person to give the dog treats for this stage or to have soft food on a wooden spoon that the dog can lick while you are training.

1. Have tasty treats and soft food ready.
2. Find a quiet place to train away from any distractions.
3. Hold the head halter where the dog can see it. Do up the clip and reward the dog.
4. Repeat this until the dog is looking for a treat when it hears the sound of the clip or buckle.
5. Hold the head halter in a way that the dog can get its nose through the nose loop and you can move the neck strap. Say the cue word; once the dog has its nose through the nose loop, give it a treat. Keep giving the dog treats or allow it to lick some soft food while you slowly move the straps. Do **not** try to clip it yet, just get the dog used to the neck strap around its neck while it has its head inside the nose loop.

6. Over several repetitions of step 5, slowly move the straps more until you can hold them behind its head for a few seconds while it receives treats or licks soft food.

Always release the neck strap before the dog finishes the food so that it does not try to pull away from the head halter.

Once you can hold the straps behind its ears for a few seconds, you can move on to stage 3.

Stage 3 – fastening the neck strap and increasing the time wearing the head halter

The most important aspect of stage 3 is to take your time; do not rush this stage as it could undo all of the head halter training done thus far.

1. Have tasty treats and soft food ready.
2. Find a quiet place to train away from any distractions.
3. Have some soft food ready for the dog to lick. While the dog is licking, say the cue word and slowly move the straps and do up the clip. After three to five seconds, undo it and take it off. Repeat this several times until the dog is comfortable with the head halter.
4. Slowly increase the time the dog spends wearing the head halter. Increase it by increments of a few seconds until it is comfortable wearing the head halter for a few minutes at a time.
5. At this early stage, keep feeding treats while the head halter is on. Over time, you can decrease the number of treats given.
6. When the dog is comfortable wearing the head halter, try scattering some treats on the floor to encourage it to move around with the head halter on.

Stage 4 – attaching the lead

Once the dog can wear the head halter and move around comfortably, the lead can be attached to the head halter.

1. Have tasty treats and soft food ready.
2. Find a quiet place to train away from any distractions.
3. Put the head halter on your dog.
4. Clip the lead on for a few seconds, give the dog some treats while it is attached, and then remove it. Do **not** move or pull on the lead; this step allows the dog to get used to the feeling of the lead attached to the head halter.
5. Gradually increase the length of time the lead is attached to the head halter. Always reward the dog for being comfortable wearing the head halter.
6. Once the dog is comfortable with the lead attached to the head halter, you can progress to holding the lead while it is attached to the head halter.

Once the dog is comfortable wearing the head halter with the lead attached, you can move on to train the dog how to walk on a loose lead (see Handout C10 – Training Loose-leash Walks).

Harness

A harness is a very useful safety tool which will help you control your dog by guiding its chest; it can be used in conjunction with a muzzle to have full control over the direction in which your dog moves.

There are numerous types of harness available; it can be trial and error to find which one fits your dog without restricting its movement. Regardless of which brand you use, ensure you get the correct size and fit; most companies which produce harnesses offer a sizing guide.

Each session should be five to ten minutes long; the session should stop after ten minutes regardless of the amount of progress made. It is possible to do two sessions; however, there should be a 10–15-minute break between sessions. The sessions should be carried out every day.

Before each session, ensure that your dog has had some play or physical exercise and the opportunity to eliminate. Ensure the dog has not been fed prior to the session to increase its motivation to work for food.

Prepare enough small tasty treats to last for the whole five- to ten-minute session and have them to hand in a treat pouch or pocket. Soft foods such as peanut butter, cream cheese, paté or wet dog food on a wooden spoon or lick mat are useful to have to hand.

NB If using peanut butter, ensure that it does not contain any artificial sweeteners, especially Xylitol, as these are toxic for dogs.

Before you start training your dog to wear a harness, you will need to ensure that you know how the harness is correctly put on and removed. Most manufacturers will have a written guide or video detailing the correct fit and placement. This handout is based on using an 'H-style' harness. It would be best to use a front-attached harness, which gives you better control and ability to guide your dog.

Stage 1 – introducing the harness

1. Choose a cue to use such as 'Harness', which will indicate that the harness is going to be used.
2. Have tasty treats ready.
3. Sit with the dog and say the cue word; show it the harness and give it a treat. Do not attempt to put it on; just show it to the dog.
4. Repeat this 15–20 times within a few minutes. During this time do not expect any specific behaviour, such as 'sit' or 'down', just show it the harness, say the cue word and give it a treat.
5. After 15–20 repetitions, the dog should start forming an association between seeing the harness and getting a treat.
6. Say the cue word, then place the harness on the floor with some treats near it. Over time, move the treats closer to the harness and eventually in the loops of the harness so that the dog gets used to touching the harness with its nose. Once the dog is comfortable approaching and touching the harness, progress to the next step.
7. Hold the harness by the strip that will sit along the dog's back, with the chest strap undone and in a position so the dog can get its nose into the neck loop.
8. Slowly move the treat closer to the neck loop so that the dog has to put its nose through the neck loop to get the treat. As the dog approaches say the cue word and allow the dog to take the treat. Do **not** push it over its head or try to do it up at this point. Allow the dog to approach, put its nose through the loop and move away in its own time.
9. Repeat this several times, slowly moving the food closer to you and further through the nose loop so that the dog has to put its nose further into the nose loop each time.
10. Test the pet; hold the harness and say the cue word; the dog should approach the harness and put its nose through the nose loop. If it does not do this, go back and work through steps 8 and 9 until the dog responds to the cue word.

Once the dog puts its nose in the nose loop on cue, you can move on to the next stage.

Stage 2 – getting used to the neck loop

This stage allows your dog to habituate to the noise of the clip and the strap being placed around its neck.

It may be helpful to have a second person giving the dog treats or to have soft food on a wooden spoon while you are training.

1. Have tasty treats and soft food ready.
2. Hold the harness where the dog can see it; do up the clip and reward it.
3. Repeat this until the dog is looking for a treat when it hears the clip.
4. Hold the harness in a way that the dog can get its nose through the nose loop. Say the cue word, and once the dog has its nose through the nose loop, give it a treat. Keep giving it treats or allow it to lick some soft

food while you slowly move the chest straps. Do not try to do it up yet, just get the dog used to the straps being moved around its chest while it has the neck loop on.
5. Over several repetitions of step 4, slowly move the straps more until you can hold it in the correct position for a few seconds while the dog receives treats or licks at soft food.

Always release the chest straps before the dog finishes the food so that it does not try to pull away from the harness.

Once you can hold the chest straps in position for a few seconds, you can move on to stage 3.

Stage 3 – fastening the chest strap and increasing the time wearing the harness

The most important aspect of stage 3 is to take your time – do not rush this stage as it could undo all of the harness training done so far.

1. Have tasty treats and soft food ready.
2. Have some soft food ready for the dog to lick. Say the cue word and while the dog is licking the treat with the neck loop on, slowly move the chest straps and do the clip up. After three to five seconds, undo it and take it off. Repeat this several times until the dog is comfortable wearing the harness.
3. Slowly increase the time the dog is wearing the harness. Increase in increments of a few seconds until the dog is comfortable wearing it for a few minutes at a time.
4. At this early stage, keep feeding treats while the dog is wearing the harness. Over time, you can decrease the number of treats given.
5. When the dog is comfortable wearing the harness, try scattering some treats on the floor to encourage it to move around while wearing the harness.

Stage 4 – attaching the lead

Once the dog can wear the harness and move around comfortably, the lead can be attached to the harness.

1. Have tasty treats and soft food ready.
2. Put the harness on the pet.
3. Clip the lead on for a few seconds; give the dog some treats while it is attached, then remove it. Do **not** move or pull on the lead; this step allows the dog to get used to the feeling of the lead attached to the harness.
4. Gradually increase the length of time the lead is attached to the harness; always reward the dog for being comfortable in the harness.
5. Once the dog is comfortable with the lead attached to the harness, you can progress to holding the lead while it is attached to the harness.

Once the dog is comfortable wearing the harness with the lead attached, you can move on to training it to loose-leash walk while wearing it (see Handout C10 – Training Loose-leash Walks).

C6 – Marker Training

Marker training is a training tool which is used to mark the exact point when the pet shows the desired behaviour. The marker is associated with a reward, and so it also predicts that a reward is coming. The combination of the marker being heard when the desired behaviour is performed and the learnt association that the marker precedes a reward reinforces the behaviour. This reinforcement will increase the chances of the pet showing the desired behaviour again in the future.

There are two stages to marker training:

1. conditioning the marker cue; and
2. using the marker.

Stage 1 – conditioning the marker cue

Conditioning the marker cue is the process of building an association between the marker cue and a reward through classical conditioning. Classical conditioning is where a neutral stimulus (the marker cue) is repeatedly associated with an unconditional stimulus (a treat). After enough repetitions of 'hearing the marker cue – get a reward', the marker cue predicts the reward and becomes a conditional stimulus.

One thing to bear in mind when choosing your maker cue is that it has to be with you every time you are training the pet and also in any other situations where you might want to reward appropriate behaviour. As such a standard clicker may not be the best option, you may forget when at home, when you go for a walk, or you may not have it when your pet shows the desired behaviour unexpectedly. Finger-snap or tongue-click will always be with you in all situations.

1. Before each session ensure you have met your pet's needs and set it up to succeed. For example, play with or exercise your pet and withhold food before the training session (see Handout C1 – Set Up to Succeed).
2. Select a marker cue: it can be a clicker, finger-snapping, tongue-clicking, or any other novel sound.
3. Prepare tasty treats that the pet will be willing to work hard to receive and have plenty ready before starting the training exercise.
4. Sit with the pet and give the marker cue followed by a treat (e.g. click and treat).
5. Repeat this 15–20 times within a few minutes. During this time, do not expect any specific behaviour, such as 'Sit', 'Down' or 'Come'. Give the marker cue followed by a treat, wait for the pet to finish the treat, and repeat.
6. After 15–20 repetitions, the pet should start forming an association between the marker cue and receiving a treat.
7. Test the pet: allow it to walk away and then give the marker cue. If the pet comes immediately back for a treat, it understands that the marker cue predicts a treat. If it does not respond to the marker cue, go back to step 5 and repeat steps 5–7.

Now the marker cue is conditioned, it can be used when training the pet.

A point to remember is that the pet must always get a treat when it hears the marker cue, even if it was given by mistake. Otherwise the marker cue will start to lose its meaning.

Stage 2 – using the marker

1. One of the best uses of the marker is to reinforce desired behaviours when the pet shows them voluntarily or at unexpected times. For example, the dog is sitting when observing other dogs instead of lunging. The marker allows you to reward the pet even when you were not prepared or did not ask the pet to show this behaviour. You can also use the marker when the pet shows desired behaviours voluntarily in their normal routine, as well as when you are working on a training session.
2. Ideally, you can choose two or three behaviours that you wish to encourage and focus on those. You can either ask your pet to perform the behaviour or wait for it to offer the behaviour; for example, when a cat walks into the room and calmly looks towards a second cat it used to attack. You can then use the marker to signal a calm look instead of an attack.
3. After you give the marker cue you need to find a treat to give the pet as the marker cue has been conditioned to predict a treat. You do not have to have one immediately to hand; you will have time to go to the cupboard and get one.
4. Over time, you can start using the marker cue to shape the pet's behaviour towards the final desired behaviour.

C7 – Response Substitution

Response substitution is a form of counter-conditioning which changes the pet's behavioural response to a trigger. This is done by teaching the pet to perform a behaviour on cue, which is incompatible with the behaviour they currently show when they see a trigger.

There are several keys to successful response substitution:

1. training the new behaviours;
2. understanding arousal levels and how to identify displacement and conflict behaviours;
3. how to use response substitution; and
4. ensuring the pet performs the behaviour.

1. Training the new behaviours

The first part of successful response substitution is to train the pet to perform a behaviour on cue, which can be used for response substitution. There are two basic cues which are instinctual for a pet to perform and so are easier for them to do when their arousal levels increase. These behaviours are 'Watch me' and 'Touch' (see Handout C2 – How to Teach a 'Watch Me' and 'Touch' Cue).

2. Understanding arousal levels and how to identify displacement and conflict behaviours

Understanding arousal levels

Arousal is a term used to describe a physiological response to a change in the emotional state of the pet, to prepare the body for action. These physiological responses include increased heart rate, increased respiration rate, increased blood pressure and an increase in circulatory hormones such as cortisol and adrenaline (see Section 7.4.3).

The change in emotional state can be a positive one such as excitement or expectation and prepare the body to jump for joy; or it can be a negative one, such as anxiety or fear and prepare the body to run away.

It can take as little as three quarters of a second to mount a full arousal response once the pet is exposed to a stimulus. However, it can take minutes, hours or even days for these levels to reduce again.

As the pet's arousal levels increase, they pass through two different thresholds: an emotional threshold and a behavioural threshold.

1. Emotional threshold: When the pet passes through the emotional threshold, it will show displacement behaviours or conflict behaviours (see below for more details). When it is at this level of arousal, you should still be able to interact with it and get it to respond to known cues (e.g. touch, watch or sit) and take treats.
2. Behavioural threshold: If the pet is continually exposed to various stimuli or does not have enough time for its arousal levels to reduce between each stimulus, it will cross its behavioural threshold. The pet will start to show behavioural signs of high arousal such as vocalizing, growling, snapping, biting, scratching and lunging. When it is at this level of arousal, it generally does not respond to known cues or take treats.

Which threshold the pet will pass through will depend on several factors, such as:

- where its arousal level was before being exposed to the stimuli;
- any cumulative effect – every time the pet is exposed to a stimulus its arousal will increase; over time, there is a cumulative effect which will increase arousal levels; and
- the intensity of the stimuli – it is possible for an individual stimulus to increase the pet's arousal levels past the behavioural threshold without any indication of it crossing its emotional threshold.

The pet can have chronic high arousal as it does not have sufficient time between exposures to allow its arousal levels to reduce; this could mean it remains above the emotional or behavioural threshold at all times.

Displacement behaviours

Displacement behaviours are normal behaviours, and they are often seen within the normal behavioural repertoire of the pet. What makes them a displacement behaviour, rather than an appropriate behaviour, is that it is performed out of context (see Handout B3 – Identifying Displacement and Conflict-related Behaviours).

Displacement behaviours are seen when there is an increase in arousal levels, and the pet crosses its emotional threshold.

Displacement behaviours include:

- yawning when not tired;
- licking lips when it does not have any food or water on its lips;
- shaking off as if it had a wet coat when it is dry;
- looking at something out of the corner of its eye instead of looking straight at it;
- stretching when it has not been resting for an extended period; and
- sneezing when it is not allergic or does not have anything irritating its nose.

There are some things to look for, which will help you tell the difference between normal behaviour and displacement behaviour:

- Does the behaviour appear out-of-context (full-body shaking when dry)?
- Is the behaviour repetitive (e.g. the pet licks its lips several times in close succession)?
- Does the behaviour occur at the same time as other displacement behaviours (e.g. yawning and lip-licking)?
- Can you reproduce the behaviour by placing it in a similar situation (e.g. lip-licking and looking out of the corner of its eye when a dog approaches).

If the answer is yes, then it is a displacement behaviour.

Conflict behaviours

Conflict-related behaviours are behaviours which are shown in situations where there are two or more competing emotional motivations; the pet is both drawn towards and repelled from something at the same time. Conflict-related behaviours lead to an increase in arousal levels.

Examples of conflict behaviours include:

- The pet stretches towards a stranger offering a treat, but moves away as soon as they have taken the treat:
    - The pet might want the treat but not be that close to the stranger; however, to get the treat, they must be close to the stranger.
      This context causes conflict because the pet is torn between taking the treat while keeping their distance from the stranger.
- Another dog approaches the pet to play:
    - The pet may approach the other dog to play but may have its hackles up or be growling while its tail is wagging.
      This context causes conflict because the pet wants to play but does not know how the other dog will react.

- Trimming the pet's nails:
  - The pet may want to be with you and have an interaction with you; however, they do not like their nails being trimmed.

3. How to use response substitution

Choose a behaviour to use in each situation your pet shows the behaviour you want to change. For example:

- Use 'Watch me' when the pet sees another dog.
- Use 'Sit' when the pet tries jumping on you.
- Use 'Touch' when you need to move the pet away from an area/situation.
- Use 'Turn around' when walking and you want to change direction.

The same cue must be used in the same situation; this will ensure there is consistency in the pet's training and will help them learn. If there are multiple people involved in the pet's training, they should also be consistent in their use of cues in each situation.

As soon as you notice an increase in your pet's arousal levels and see them displaying displacement behaviours, use response substitution. The longer you leave it to ask for response substitution behaviour, the more difficult it becomes for the pet to perform this behaviour.

Even if you ask for a response substitution behaviour but the pet's arousal levels were not going to increase any further, and they were not going to show the undesirable behaviour, you have just had an opportunity to train your pet in a different situation.

4. Ensure the pet performs the behaviour

There are going to be situations where the pet struggles to perform response substitution behaviour, especially if their arousal levels are increasing.

There are some things you can do to help the pet perform the behaviour you have asked for:

- Use a treat to lure it.
- Repeat the cue word – several times if needed.
- Use your hand to get it to look at you – for safety reasons the pet may need to be wearing a muzzle before you attempt this.
- Use a head collar to get it to look at you.
- Use a long line to ensure the pet returns to perform a touch cue.

Even if you have had to help the pet to perform the behaviour, reward it. The more it performs response substitution and is rewarded for it, the more likely it is to perform this behaviour in the future. The ideal outcome is that your pet sees a trigger and offers the desired behaviour without being asked to do it.

C8 – Litter Tray Training

Kittens tend to be attracted to an area where they can dig, scratch and bury things when they need to eliminate; this could be the litter tray you have provided or a plant pot.

To ensure your kitten learns to eliminate in the appropriate location and becomes litter-trained, the following need to be considered:

- choosing the desired location;
- litter-tray considerations;
- setting a routine;
- reinforcement of appropriate behaviours;
- cleaning soiled areas; and
- consistency.

1. Choosing the desired location

For your kitten to choose the litter tray over other areas to eliminate, it must have free access to the litter tray at all times. This may mean you have to have a litter tray in every room your kitten has access to, or you keep your kitten confined to one room with access to multiple trays while it is learning. You may need to consider removing plants or thick rugs from the room so that the only place your kitten can dig is in the litter tray.

Cats and kittens like privacy when they use the litter tray. When offering litter trays, ensure they are located in a quiet, private area of the room, where there is minimal traffic, human or animals.

Most cats/kittens will not eliminate near their food or water bowls. When providing a litter tray, ensure it is far enough away from the food and water – ideally on the opposite side of the room.

2. Litter-tray considerations

Normal elimination behaviour includes digging, squatting, eliminating and covering; litter trays need to be suitable to ensure your kitten can perform all of these normal behaviours.

Some things to remember when litter training are:

- Type of Litter tray – some litter trays have a high side which your kitten may not be able to climb. Consider a low-sided tray or cut the sides down to allow easier access. Some types of litter trays, such as self-cleaning trays, will move and make noise once your kitten has used it – not all kittens will like this, and some may develop an aversion to the tray because of this.
- Open or covered litter tray – you may need to provide your kitten with various types of litter trays while it develops its litter tray preferences.
- Number of litter trays – if you have more than one kitten, you should consider providing at least one litter tray per kitten. This can help to ensure that there is always a clean litter tray available when your kitten needs to eliminate.
- Size of the litter tray – the litter tray should be long enough for your kitten to stand and scratch in, so ideally it should be one and a half times the length of your kitten. As your kitten grows, it will need a bigger litter tray. Alternatively, you can provide an adult-sized litter tray from a young age.
- Depth of litter – the litter should be deep enough that your kitten can scratch and dig a hole to eliminate. As your kitten grows, it will need more litter in the tray to allow it to dig.

- Litter type – most cats prefer unscented, clumping litter; however, some cats prefer soil. Provide your kitten with a couple of options to allow it to choose.
- Plastic liners – some kittens find these aversive as their claws will catch in them when they dig.
- Litter tray hygiene – the litter tray will need to be scooped every time it is used to ensure your kitten always has access to a clean tray. Each litter tray should have its full content changed and be washed with mild, unscented soap once a week.

3. Setting a routine

Kittens usually need to eliminate after sleeping, eating or playing. You need to set up a routine in which you take your kitten to the desired location after each of these events.

If you notice your kitten starts to sniff and scratch at an area, take it to the litter tray.

The use of a safe-haven when you cannot supervise your kitten can be beneficial when house training (see Handout C3 – Safe-haven). Your kitten can be placed into their safe-haven with food and treats and litter tray access; it must be a comfortable place to rest for short periods when you cannot supervise. A safe-haven is not a place to leave your kitten for an extended period instead of training.

An example of a routine would be: wake up; take to litter tray; food and rest; take to litter tray; play in safe-haven with access to the litter tray; eat and rest with access to the litter tray.

4. Reinforcement of appropriate behaviours

As you will have a routine in place, you can be ready with tasty treats and go with your kitten when they need to eliminate. Every time your kitten eliminates in the litter tray, calmly praise and reward it once it has moved away from the tray._

5. Cleaning soiled areas

Your kitten may soil outside of the litter tray during training; do not punish your kitten for this. Punishment for eliminating outside of the litter tray will teach your kitten to stop eliminating in the presence of people and will cause anxiety associated with you.

The best way to address a mistake is to clean the area, be more aware of your kitten's routine and be prepared for the next time it will need to eliminate. Cleaning soiled areas should be done with a biological soap and water:

- The washing powder solution is made up of one part powder mixed with ten parts water – this solution can be made up and stored in a trigger-spray bottle.
- Remove as much urine/faeces from the area as possible with a disposable towel.
- Spray the area with the washing powder solution and scrub/clean well – if it is on a carpet or rug, make sure you get all the way down through the pile to the floor.
- You can repeat steps 1 and 2 if it is a particularly bad area.
- Dry the area with a disposable paper towel.
- Spray the area with disinfectant solution designed for use on pet-soiled areas, and allow it to air dry.
- Check all solutions on a hidden part of the surface before using to check they won't damage the finish.

6. Consistency

For your kitten to learn and become litter-trained, consistency is vital. Everyone who interacts with the kitten should be doing the same thing when litter training. This means they take the kitten to the litter tray when needed, stick to the same routine, and clean any mistakes without punishment. If there is inconsistency, your kitten will take longer to become litter-trained.

C9 – House Training Your Puppy

A puppy will learn which surface to eliminate on in two ways; by receiving positive reinforcement from you when it eliminates in the appropriate location and because the act of elimination is self-rewarding regardless of where it eliminates.

To ensure your puppy learns to eliminate in the appropriate location and becomes house-trained, the following need to be considered:

- choosing the desired location and surface;
- setting a routine;
- reinforcement of appropriate behaviours;
- cleaning soiled areas; and
- consistency.

1. Choosing a desired location and surface

Ease of access: most puppies will be trained to eliminate outside; ease of access to the outside needs to be considered. An eight-week-old toy breed will not be able to safely navigate steps to get outside when it needs to eliminate, while an eight-week-old large breed should be able to navigate one or two steps to get outside safely. Some alterations may need to be made to the access point to ensure your puppy can safely get outside when it needs to eliminate.

If it is cold or wet, some puppies may not want to go outside to eliminate; an area close to the door which has some shelter may be the best choice when you begin to house-train your puppy.

2. Setting a routine

If the door leading to the desired location is closed, you will need to be aware of your puppy's needs; this is where a routine helps.

Puppies usually need to eliminate after sleeping, eating or playing. You need to set up a routine in which you take your puppy to the desired location after each of these events.

The use of a safe-haven when you cannot supervise your puppy can be beneficial when house-training (see Handout C3 – Safe-haven). Your puppy can be put into its safe-haven with food, treats and chew toys. It must be a comfortable place to rest for short periods when you cannot supervise. A safe-haven is not a place to leave your puppy for an extended period instead of training.

An example of a routine would be: wake up; outside to eliminate; food and rest; outside to eliminate; chew toy in safe-haven; outside to eliminate; eat and rest; outside to eliminate.

3. Reinforcement of appropriate behaviours

As you will have a routine in place, you can be ready with tasty treats and can go outside with your puppy when it needs to eliminate. Every time your puppy eliminates in the desired location, calmly reward it.

You can add a cue word to the act of elimination so that you can get your puppy to eliminate on cue when it is older. This is done by saying the same cue word, such as 'Be quick' every time the puppy squats to eliminate.

4. Cleaning soiled areas

Your puppy is likely to soil at home during training; do not punish your puppy for this. Punishment for eliminating will teach your puppy to stop eliminating in the presence of people and will cause anxiety associated with you.

The best way to address a mistake is to clean the area, be more aware of your puppy's routine, and be prepared for the next time it will need to eliminate. Cleaning soiled areas should be done with biological soap and water:

- The washing powder solution is made up of one part powder mixed with ten parts water – this solution can be made up and stored in a trigger-spray bottle.
- Remove as much urine/faeces from the area as possible with a disposable towel.
- Spray the area with the washing powder solution and scrub/clean well – if it is on a carpet or rug, make sure you get all the way down through the pile to the floor.
- You can repeat steps 1 and 2 if it is a particularly bad area.
- Dry the area with a disposable paper towel.
- Spray the area with disinfectant solution that is designed for pet-soiled areas, and allow it to air dry.
- Check all solutions on a hidden part of the surface before using to check they won't damage the finish.

5. Consistency

For your puppy to learn and become house-trained, consistency is vital. Everyone who interacts with the puppy should be doing the same thing when house-training. This means they take the puppy to the same desired location, use the same cue word when it eliminates, stick to the same routine, and clean any mistakes without punishment. If there is inconsistency, your puppy will take longer to become house-trained.

C10 – Training Loose-leash Walks

Loose-leash walking is a skill your dog needs to learn to enable it to walk with you without pulling or tripping you over. Most dogs want to explore the environment at their own pace. As owners, we generally do not walk fast enough to keep up with it. This can lead dogs to pull in all directions to explore the environment.

This skill takes time, patience and consistency to teach as this is a difficult task for dogs to learn. It can take months for the dog to learn how to loose-leash walk.

To teach your dog loose-leash walking:

1. Before each session ensure you have met your pet's needs and set it up to succeed. For example, play with or exercise your dog and withhold food before the training session (see Handout C1 – Set Up to Succeed).
2. Choose a cue word to use such as 'Heel', 'Close' or 'Here'.
3. Have tasty treats ready.
4. Find a quiet place to train away from any distractions.
5. Make sure your dog has its collar, harness or head halter on and you have the leash to hand.
6. Attach the leash to your dog's collar, harness or head halter and stand still. As soon as your dog gives you attention, give it a treat; you can use its name to get its attention or use a 'Watch me' (see Handout C2 – How to Teach a 'Watch Me' and 'Touch' Cue).
7. Use a treat to lure your dog into the position next to you, where you want it to walk.
8. Make sure the leash is loose and that there is no pressure on your dog's collar/harness/head halter. While in this position, say the cue word and give your dog a treat.
9. Feed your dog a couple more treats for standing next to you with the leash loose.
10. Take one step forward, and as your dog takes a step with you, say the cue word and feed it another treat while they are still next to you. Try not to allow it to get ahead of you; feed it for staying next to you.
11. If your dog does not want to walk next to you, use a treat to lure it along.
12. Take another step forward; as your dog keeps moving with you, repeat the cue word and give it a few more treats for walking next to you.
13. Repeat steps 5–11 several times until it can stay next to you as you take a few steps after it hears the cue word.

Repeat step 4–12 until your dog can walk alongside you without pulling for up to about 20 paces before getting a treat, and if it pulls, it can move back into position to be able to move forward.

If at any time your dog walks ahead of you or pulls in another direction:

- stop walking or start walking in a different direction;
- use its name to get it to look at you;
- use a treat to lure it into position next to you again; and
- take one or two steps, say the cue word and reward your dog for walking with you.

If you reward your dog for returning to you before you start walking with it next to you, there is a chance that it will learn to pull to the end of the leash, then return to your side to get a treat. You will teach your dog to yo-yo to the end of the leash and back to you while walking.

Over time, your dog will learn that moving forward next to you is rewarding as it gets to continue its walk. At this point, you can slowly fade out the food rewards by increasing the number of steps you take between each treat.

Once you get to this stage in a quiet, controlled environment, slowly increase the level of distractions when training so that your dog learns to walk on a loose leash in many different situations. For example, if you are working in the house, move to the garden, then close to the fence, then a quiet road, then a slightly busier road and so on.

If your dog starts to pull, you may need to increase the frequency of the rewards again when they are loose-leash walking. If your dog is distracted by things in the environment, you may need to go back a step to a less distracting environment again and practise there again.

D1 – What are Desensitization and Counter-conditioning?

What is desensitization?

Desensitization is a structured behaviour modification programme used to reduce behavioural and emotional reactions through gradual exposure to the trigger in a controlled environment. Desensitization is often used in the treatment of fears and phobias and high arousal in many different situations.

What is counter-conditioning?

Counter-conditioning is a behaviour modification programme used for changing the pet's behavioural and emotional response to a trigger through teaching alternative behaviours and changing the current emotional association with the trigger.

There are two types of conditioning used when counter-conditioning:

- operant counter-conditioning – used to change the behavioural response; and
- respondent counter-conditioning – used to change the emotional response.

Operant counter-conditioning, also known as Response Substitution, is the process of teaching the pet to perform a behaviour on cue which is incompatible with the behaviour it currently shows when it sees a trigger (see Handout C7 – Response Substitution).

There are two cues which are commonly used as they are instinctual behaviours for dogs; these are 'Watch me' and 'Touch'. The 'Watch me' cue is used to get the pet to look at you, and the 'Touch' cue is used to get the pet to touch your hand with its nose. When used, both of these cues ensure the pet is no longer engaging with the trigger (see Handout C2 – How to Teach a 'Watch Me' and 'Touch' Cue). These signals can be used with cats as well.

Respondent counter-conditioning, also known as classical counter-conditioning, is the process of changing the pet's emotional response to seeing a trigger by pairing the sight or sound of a trigger with a reward. Food rewards are generally used, but some dogs will prefer a toy.

Marker training can be beneficial for this type of counter-conditioning. Marker training teaches the pet that a marker cue always precedes a positive reward; for example, hearing a click, get a food treat. Over time this pairing causes a positive emotional state when the pet hears the marker cue (see Handout C6 – Marker Training).

When used in counter-conditioning a marker cue can be given at the moment the pet becomes aware of the presence of a trigger but does not become over-aroused or show displacement and conflict behaviours (see 'Understanding arousal levels and how to identify displacement and conflict behaviours' below for more details). As the marker cue causes a positive emotional state, it will help to change the pet's emotional state when it is exposed to the trigger.

Before starting a desensitization and counter-conditioning programme

There are several steps which need to be completed before starting a desensitization and counter-conditioning programme:

1. training of necessary cues;
2. management and safety tools;
3. looking at the components of the trigger;
4. setting expectations;
5. understanding arousal levels and how to identify displacement and conflict behaviours; and
6. eliminating exposure to known triggers.

1. Training of necessary cues

Before starting a desensitization and counter-conditioning programme, the pet should learn to respond reliably to cues such as 'Watch me', 'Touch', 'Settle' and the marker. The pet should be taught these signals in a variety of situations and environments.

2. Management and safety equipment

When working on desensitization and counter-conditioning with a dog which shows high arousal, and possibly aggression, there are several tools which should be used to ensure the safety of yourself, your dog and other people or animals.

A muzzle

A muzzle is an essential safety tool when working with a dog which shows high arousal and aggression. The advantages of using a muzzle include preventing a bite, decreasing the owner's anxiety knowing the dog cannot bite, and keeping unfamiliar people and dogs away from the dog while out walking (see Handout C5 – Muzzle, head halter and body harness training).

Front-attached body harness

This harness has an additional clip on a strap which lies across the dog's chest, as well as the regular clip attached to the back of the harness between the dog's shoulders. The additional clip at the front of the dog's chest allows for extra control when walking and aids you in turning the dog towards you when needed (see Handout C5 – Muzzle, Head Halter and Body Harness Training).

Head collar

This is a very useful safety tool which will help you control your dog by guiding its head. A head halter allows you to control the dog's movement and direct its gaze towards you when you need to disengage it from the trigger (see Handout C5 – Muzzle, Head Halter and Body Harness Training).

When working on desensitization and counter-conditioning with a cat which shows high arousal, and possibly aggression, there are several tools which should be used to ensure the safety of yourself, your cat and other people or animals.

A solid door

This allows for exposure to scent and sound while reducing the risk of injury to all involved.

Glass or screen door

This allows controlled visual exposure to a trigger.

Heavy blanket or towel

If the cat shows aggression, the owner can cover the cat and remove it safely from the room, without risking a bite or a scratch.

Body harness

Similar to dogs, a cat can be taught to walk wearing a body harness. While this is more difficult than it is for dogs, with careful and patient teaching many cats will adapt.

3. Looking at the components of the trigger

For desensitization and counter-conditioning to be successful, each trigger should be broken down into its basic components. For pets showing aggression in the presence of unfamiliar people, possible components for this trigger include the proximity of the person, number of people, age of people, movement type and speed of movement (e.g. walking or jogging), any noise from them (e.g. talking, laughing or shouting), and any accessories with them (e.g. bicycle, umbrella or prams).

Next, a schedule of exposure can be drawn up to work through each component in a controlled and systematic way. This means working on the components separately, to begin with, starting with the least intense component to the most intense component. Once the pet is accustomed to the individual components separately, two components can be combined, then three and so on until the trigger has all of its various components combined.

4. Setting expectations

Before even beginning a desensitization and counter-conditioning programme, it is essential to have realistic expectations of what the pet may be able to achieve.

Even when the best desensitization and counter-conditioning programme has been followed to the letter, the pet may only get to a point where it can be near a trigger without crossing its behavioural threshold. The pet may never be able to interact with a trigger without crossing its behavioural threshold.

5. Understanding arousal levels and how to identify displacement and conflict behaviours

Arousal is a term used to describe a physiological response to a change in the emotional state of the pet, to prepare the body for action. This physiological response includes an increased heart rate, respiration rate, blood pressure and an increase in circulatory hormones such as cortisol and adrenaline. The change in emotional state can be a positive one, such as excitement or expectation, and prepare the body to jump for joy; or it can be a negative one, such as anxiety or fear and prepare the body to run away (for more information see Section 7.4.3).

It can take as little as three quarters of a second for the pet's arousal level to increase. However, it can take minutes, hours or even days for these levels to reduce again. As the pet's arousal level increases, it passes through two different thresholds; an emotional threshold and a behavioural threshold:

1. Emotional threshold: When the pet passes through the emotional threshold, it will start showing displacement behaviours or conflict behaviours. At this level of arousal, you should still be able to interact with the pet and get it to respond to known cues (e.g. 'Touch', 'Watch' and 'Sit') and take treats.
2. Behavioural threshold: If the pet is continually exposed to various or highly intense stimuli, or does not have enough time for its arousal levels to reduce between each stimulus, it will cross its behavioural threshold. The pet will start to show behavioural signs of high arousal such as vocalizing, growling, snapping, biting, scratching and lunging. At this level of arousal, the pet generally does not respond to known cues or take treats.

Which threshold the pet will pass through will depend on several things such as:

- where its arousal level was before being exposed to the stimuli;
- cumulative effect – every time the pet is exposed to a stimulus, its arousal will increase and, over time, there is a cumulative effect which will increase arousal levels; and
- the intensity of the stimuli – it is possible for an individual stimulus to increase the pet's arousal levels past the behavioural threshold without any indication of it crossing its emotional threshold.

The pet can have chronic high arousal as it does not have sufficient time between exposures to allow its arousal levels to reduce; this could mean it remains above the emotional or behavioural threshold at all times.

Displacement behaviours

Displacement behaviours are normal behaviours, and they are often seen within the normal behavioural repertoire of the pet. What makes them displacement behaviours rather than appropriate behaviours, is that the behaviour is performed out of context.

Displacement behaviours are seen when there is an increase in arousal levels, and the pet crosses its emotional threshold.

Displacement behaviours include:

- yawning when not tired;
- lip-licking without relation to food or water;
- shaking off as if the pet had a wet coat when it is dry;
- looking at something out of the corner of its eye instead of looking straight at it;
- stretching when it has not been resting for an extended period;
- sneezing when it is not allergic or does not have anything irritating its nose; and
- grinning when there is no nasal irritation.

Several observations may help you tell the difference between a normal behaviour and a displacement behaviour:

- Does the behaviour appear out-of-context (full-body shaking when the pet is dry)?
- Is the behaviour repetitive (e.g. the pet licks its lips several times in close succession)?
- Does the behaviour occur at the same time as other displacement behaviours (e.g. yawning and lip-licking)?
- Can you reproduce the behaviour by placing the pet in a similar situation (e.g. lip-licking and looking out of the corner of its eye when another dog approaches)?

If the answer is yes, then it is a displacement behaviour.

Conflict behaviours

Conflict-related behaviours are behaviours which are shown in situations where there are two or more competing emotional motivations. The pet is both drawn towards and repelled from something at the same time. Conflict-related behaviours lead to further increase in arousal levels. Examples of conflict behaviours include:

- The pet stretches towards a stranger offering a treat, but moves away immediately it has taken the treat:

    - The pet might want the treat but not be that close to the stranger; however, to get the treat, it must be close to the stranger. This context causes conflict because the pet is torn between taking the treat while keeping its distance from the stranger.
- Another dog approaches the pet to play:
    - The pet may approach the other dog to play but may have its hackles up or be growling. This context causes conflict because the pet wants to play but does not know how the other dog will react.
- Trimming the pet's nails:
    - The pet may want to interact with the owner; however, it does not like its nails being trimmed. The pet may mouth or lick the owner or vocalize.

6. Eliminating exposure to known triggers

Every time the pet is exposed to a trigger, its arousal levels will increase, and the pet will have the opportunity to perform the behaviour you are trying to change.

For the desensitization and counter-conditioning programme to be effective, it is essential to have low arousal levels. Therefore, preventing exposure to as many known triggers as possible is important while carrying out a desensitization and counter-conditioning programme.

D2 – Desensitization – People on Walks

Before starting a desensitization and counter-conditioning programme

There are several steps which need to be completed before starting a desensitization and counter-conditioning programme:

1. training of necessary cues;
2. management and safety tools;
3. looking at the components of the trigger;
4. setting expectations;
5. understanding what displacement and conflict behaviours are; and
6. eliminating exposure to unfamiliar people as much as possible.

Please see Handout D1 – What are Desensitization and Counter-conditioning? for full details on how to complete these steps.

Components of the trigger, in this presentation, can be:

1. a stationary person who ignores your dog;
2. a walking person who ignores your dog;
3. a stationary person who is talking;
4. a walking person who is talking;
5. a person who is making movements such as waving, jogging, etc.

NB Your pet may never be comfortable with a person touching/petting it; walking past within two metres may be the best outcome for this session.

Preparing for desensitization and counter-conditioning

When preparing, there are a few things which need to be done to set the session up. Desensitization is not a 'real-life' but a 'made-up' situation. These sessions need to be carried out in a calm, controlled environment without the risk of unexpected close interactions with other people on walks.

- Each session should be 10–15 minutes long. The session should stop after 15 minutes, regardless of the amount of progress made. It is possible to do two sessions; however, there should be a 10–15-minute break between sessions where your dog is removed from the training environment and allowed to rest away from any unfamiliar people. The sessions should be carried out two to three times a week with at least one day between to allow arousal levels to reduce.
- Find a suitable environment where a controlled session of gradual exposure can take place. An open field where you can see all around you or a privately hired paddock will work well for this.
- You will need the help of another person while you desensitize your dog. This person must be calm and ignore your dog throughout the session.
- Before each session, ensure your dog has had some physical exercise and the opportunity to eliminate.
- Ensure your dog has not been fed prior to the session to increase its motivation to work for food. Prepare enough small tasty treats to last for the whole 10–15-minute session and have them on hand in a treat pouch or pocket.

- Keep your dog on a lead, possibly with a head halter, to assist you with training and moving it if needed (see Handout C5 – Muzzle, Head Halter and Body Harness Training for more information).
- While working with your dog close to the other person, your dog must be on a lead and wearing a muzzle or head halter at all times.

See Handout C1 – Set Up to Succeed for more details.

Desensitization to a stationary person who ignores your dog

1. Gauge a distance to start the session where your dog shows minimal displacement behaviours when it sees the other person. This is done by slowly walking towards the person and watching for displacement or conflict behaviours.
   If you see displacement behaviours, ask for a 'Watch' or 'Touch' cue (see Handout C2 – How to Teach a 'Watch Me' and 'Touch' Cue):
   - If your dog responds to the cues, reward it and stay at this distance and use the 'Settle' cue to reduce your dog's arousal levels (see Handout C4 – Teaching a Pet How to Settle on Cue).
   - If your dog cannot perform these behaviours, you will need to walk away from the person and repeat the cues; you will either maintain the new distance or move further away depending on your dog's response.
2. At this distance, observe your dog's behaviour; see if it looks towards the person:
   - If your dog looks towards the person without showing displacement or conflict behaviours, use the marker cue to reinforce this calmer behaviour (see Handout C6 – Marker Training).
   - If you notice displacement behaviours, ask for a 'Touch' or 'Watch' to redirect your dog to you. Once you have its attention, give the 'Settle' cue to reduce your dog's arousal level before continuing with the exercise.
3. Once your dog is able to look at the person without showing displacement behaviours, move one step closer to the person.
4. Repeat steps 2 and 3 until you can be within eight metres (roughly the width of a standard road) of the person and not see any displacement behaviours.
5. Once your dog is able to do this, you can work towards walking closer to the person.

The distance moved in each session will depend on your dog's behaviour. Do not move closer until your dog is not showing any displacement or conflict behaviours when they see the stationary person.

If at any point during the sessions, your dog shows signs that it has crossed its behavioural threshold (e.g. growling, barking or lunging), ask for a 'Watch' or 'Touch' cue. If your dog responds to the cue, reward it, and then move away from the person. Once you have moved away, use the 'Settle' cue to reduce its arousal levels.

If your dog is completely ignoring you, turn around and move away from the person, even if you have to gently pull on the lead to get it to move away. Once you have moved away from the person, use the 'Settle' cue to reduce your dog's arousal levels.

If your dog is able to respond to the 'Settle' cue and you notice a reduction in its arousal levels, you can try the exercise again, but start at your current distance from the person. If your dog is unable to respond to the 'Settle' cue and is unable to respond to basic obedience cues, then end the session.

The next steps include similar desensitization to people who walk towards your pet, people that you stop to talk to, and then people who jog by your dog. As before, the first goal is to teach your pet to accept these people, and only if successful, the next goal is to interact with these people. You will need the help of other people to simulate these situations through the sessions.

Abbreviated exercise

Desensitization and counter-conditioning is the gold standard in behaviour modification. However, it can be challenging to organize the sessions as they are structured sessions in a controlled environment. An abbreviated version of the desensitization exercise is possible where you are not trying to teach your dog how to interact with the other person but help it to feel more positive when it sees other people (known as counter-conditioning). It is useful when used in addition to the desensitization programme.

1. Before each session, make sure your dog has had some exercise, had some playtime, eliminated and is hungry.
2. Plan on having 15–20 minutes for each session, ideally two to three times a week.
3. Prepare plenty of small tasty treats for a 20-minute session.
4. Go to an environment where your dog can view unfamiliar people in a controlled way; for example, quiet streets, behind a fence, or a footpath. Stand at a quiet location where you can avoid these people.
5. Start at a distance where your dog pays attention to the unfamiliar people. If your dog is not paying attention, you are too far; if your dog is showing displacement and conflict behaviours or crosses their behavioural threshold, you are too close.
6. Each time an unfamiliar person walks past and your pet is calmly looking; you can use the marker cue and give your dog a treat, praise or a pat. If you notice any signs of increased arousal (e.g. displacement or conflict), give your pet a signal such as 'Watch' or 'Touch', and then reward it.
7. After a few sessions, when your dog appears calm when it sees the unfamiliar people at that distance and is looking at you with anticipation for a treat, you can move slightly closer.
8. Repeat steps 6 and 7 until you can be within 8 metres (roughly the width of a standard road) of the unfamiliar people and not see any displacement or conflict behaviours.

Try this in several different locations so that your dog learns that dogs in all environments are positive.

D3 – Desensitization – Visitors at Home

Before starting a desensitization and counter-conditioning programme

There are several steps which need to be completed before starting a desensitization and counter-conditioning programme:

1. training of necessary cues;
2. management and safety tools;
3. looking at the components of the trigger;
4. setting expectations;
5. understanding what displacement and conflict behaviours are; and
6. eliminating exposure to any visitors to the house.

Please see Handout D1 – What are Desensitization and Counter-conditioning? for full details on how to complete these steps.

The components of this trigger, a visitor at home, can be broken down into:

1. car pulling up to the house;
2. car door closing;
3. a visitor walking to the front door;
4. doorbell or knocker;
5. family moving towards the front door;
6. front door opening;
7. a visitor walking in the home;
8. a visitor sitting in the home;
9. a brief interaction with your pet.

NB Your pet may never be comfortable with visitors coming into the house and trying to touch/pet it. The best outcome for this desensitization exercise may be that your pet does not become over-aroused when visitors arrive and rests in a different area/room.

Preparing for desensitization and counter-conditioning

When preparing, there are a few things which need to be done to set the session up. Desensitization is not a 'real-life' but a 'made-up' situation. These sessions need to be carried out in a calm, controlled environment without the risk of unexpected exposure to visitors.

- For all components, your pet should be away from the front door during the sessions. They should be at a safe distance from the front door, ideally with a safety gate between them and the door at all times – even when not working on a session.
- While working with dogs on components 1, 2, 3, 4 and 5, you should have your pet on a lead, possibly with a head halter, to assist you with training and moving it if needed (see Handout C5 – Muzzle, Head Halter and Body Harness Training for more information).
- When working with dogs on components 6, 7, 8 and 9, your pet must be on a lead with a muzzle or head halter on at all times during the sessions.

- Each session should be 10–15 minutes long; the session should stop after 15 minutes, regardless of the amount of progress made. It is possible to do two sessions; however, there should be a 10–15-minute break between sessions where the pet is removed from the training environment and allowed to rest away from any visitors. The sessions should be carried out two to three times a week with at least one day between to allow arousal levels to reduce.
- Before each session, ensure the pet has had some physical exercise and the opportunity to eliminate.
- Ensure the pet has not been fed prior to the session to increase its motivation to work for food. Prepare enough small tasty treats to last for the whole 10–15-minute session and have them on hand in a treat pouch or pocket.
- You will need the help of another person while you desensitize your dog. This person must be calm and ignore your dog throughout the session.
- Designate a space for your pet to go to when you have visitors – this can be a bed, crate or tether point. The place should be safe and secure for your pet, where visitors are not going to try to interact with it. The place should also be safe from any visitors you may have in the future, where they are not going to surprise your pet and put themselves at risk. At the beginning of each session, take your pet to this location so that they learn this is where they must be when you have visitors to the home.
- You will need to disconnect your current doorbell and muffle the knocker while you are doing this training exercise.

See Handout C1 – Set Up to Succeed for more details.

NB The distance the visitor moves in each session will depend on the behaviour of the pet; do not move on to the next component until the pet is not showing any displacement or conflict behaviours with the current component.

Stage 1 – car pulling up

This stage can be done with a family member or a visitor.

1. Start the session when your pet is in its safe space and you are in contact with the visitor. Have your visitor drive towards the house while you 'Watch' your pet for displacement or conflict behaviours.
   If you see displacement behaviours, ask your visitor to stop and give your pet a signal such as 'Watch' or 'Touch' (see Handout C2 – 'How to Teach a 'Watch Me' and 'Touch' Cue):
   - If the pet responds to the cues, reward it, and use the 'Settle' cue to reduce the pet's arousal levels (see Handout C4 – Teaching a Pet how to Settle on Cue).
   - If the pet cannot perform these behaviours, you ask the visitor to move away from the house. Once they have moved, repeat the cues; you will either maintain this new distance or ask the visitor to move further away depending on the pet's response.
2. At this distance, observe the pet to see if it looks towards the road:
   - If the pet looks in the direction of the car without showing displacement or conflict behaviours, use the marker cue to reinforce this calmer behaviour.
   - If you notice displacement behaviours, ask for a 'Touch' or 'Watch' to redirect the pet to you. Once you have the pet's attention, give the 'Settle' cue to reduce its arousal level before continuing with the exercise.
3. Once the pet is able to hear the visitors driving without showing displacement behaviours, ask the visitor to drive closer to the house.
4. Repeat steps 2 and 3 until the visitor can drive up to the house, and you do not see any displacement behaviours.

Once the pet is able to do this, you can move to the next component of the trigger.

Stage 2 – car door closing

This stage can be done with a family member or a visitor.

The steps followed will be the same as detailed above (e.g. teach your dog to stay in its place):

1. Gauge volume of the door closing; start by gently closing the door and see which volume leads to increased arousal.
2. Start at this volume level.
3. Gradually increase the force used to close the car door to increase the volume of the sound.

Stage 3 – doorbell or knocker

This stage can be done with a family member or a visitor.

The steps followed will be the same as detailed above:

1. Ask your visitor to ring the doorbell or knock once.
2. Teach your pet to go to its place and take treats.
3. Gradually increase the duration you expect your pet to stay in its place and settle once it hears the doorbell.

Alternatively, you can use a new doorbell sound and teach your pet to go to its safe place when it hears the doorbell. This is done by making the noise, leading your pet to its safe place and rewarding it. After multiple repetitions, your pet will learn to go to its safe place when it hears the doorbell.

Stage 4 – family moving towards the door

This stage should be done by everyone who lives with your pet and may open the front door.

The steps to follow will be the same as detailed above:

1. Gauge what movement/noise gets your pet's attention to the door.
2. Train at this level.
3. Gradually increase the intensity of the movement and noises made approaching the door.

Stage 5 – door opening; and Stage 6 – visitor walking in

Have the visitor approach the house, ring the doorbell and wait.

The steps you will follow once the person has approached the door will be the same as detailed above:

1. Gauge how far the door needs to open, or the visitor needs to step into the home before your pet's arousal levels increase.
2. Train at this distance.
3. Gradually increase the amount the door is opened or how far into the house the visitor walks.

If at any point the dog's arousal level increases and you have to ask for a 'Watch' or 'Touch', the visitor must stop moving, and, if asked, move further away while you reduce your pet's arousal levels. At no point should the visitor continue approaching if your pet's arousal levels are increasing.

Stage 7 – visitor sitting in the house

Once you have completed the previous stages and your pet does not show any displacement or intense arousal when the visitor enters the home, you can progress to having the visitor move into the lounge area and sit. Again, this will be done slowly and gradually and will follow the steps detailed above. Dogs should be on a lead and harness and wearing a muzzle, or a head halter. Cats should be restrained in a carrier or on a lead and harness.

Safety is paramount at this stage, if you feel that your pet is becoming too aroused, use the 'Watch' or 'Touch' cues to redirect its attention towards you and take it to its safe-haven away from the visitor. Any sudden movement from the visitor may increase your pet's arousal, so removing your pet would be the safe option.

If at any point during the sessions the pet shows signs that it has crossed its behavioural threshold (e.g. growling, barking or lunging), ask for a 'Watch' or 'Touch' cue. If the pet responds, reward it, and then increase the distance between your pet and the visitor. Once you have moved away (e.g. to a different room), use the 'Settle' cue to reduce their arousal levels.

If the pet completely ignores you, it should be moved further away. Once you have moved further away, use the 'Settle' cue to reduce its arousal levels. If the pet is able to respond to the 'Settle' cue and you notice a reduction in its arousal levels, you can try the exercise again but start at your current distance. If the pet is unable to respond to the 'Settle' cue and is unable to respond to basic obedience cues, then end the session.

Stage 8 – the visitor interacts with the pet

When your pet is calm (i.e. no displacement conflict behaviours) near the visitors, you can attempt to develop interactions between them. Your visitor should remain calm and slow, avoiding any sudden movements. You must use safety tools such as a body harness and a muzzle or a head halter. Similar to the above stages, continue slowly in moderate steps:

1. The visitor can start tossing treats on the floor close to your pet, without trying to interact with the pet directly.
2. If the pet takes the treats and shows no conflict when looking towards or approaching the visitors for more treats, you can continue.
3. Next, the visitor can ask the pet for a simple behaviour such as 'Watch' or 'Sit' (avoid direct contact such as 'Touch') and then toss treats for the pet.
4. If your pet responds calmly, the visitor can start offering treats such as soft food on a long wooden spoon, and later directly. If the pet does not show any displacement or conflict, you can proceed to the next step.
5. The visitor can start petting your pet. Start with a brief touch on the chin or the side of the neck. The visitor should move their hand slowly and in a way that your pet can see it and not be surprised. If the pet tries avoiding, your visitor should stop. If the pet accepts the touch, your visitor should only touch briefly and then give more treats.
6. Slowly increase the level of interaction, including offering toys and play.

D4 – Desensitization – New Baby

Before starting a desensitization and counter-conditioning programme

There are several steps which need to be completed before starting a desensitization and counter-conditioning programme:

1. training of necessary cues;
2. management and safety tools;
3. looking at the components of the trigger;
4. setting expectations;
5. understanding what displacement and conflict behaviours are; and
6. minimizing exposure to baby sounds and sights as much as possible.

Please see Handout D1 – What are Desensitization and Counter-conditioning? for full details of how to complete these steps.

Components of this trigger, a new baby, can include to following:

- the sight of the baby;
- the smell of the baby;
- sounds associated with the baby;
- more visitors to the house;
- novel items in the house; and,
- potentially, fewer interactions with you and less exercise.

Planning is essential when preparing your pet for the arrival of a baby; most of these components can be addressed before the baby is born. However, if you have already had your baby, then this training can still be used to desensitize your pet.

Preparing for a desensitization and counter-conditioning session

When preparing, there are a few things which need to be done to set the session up. Desensitization is not a 'real-life' but a 'made-up' situation. These sessions need to be carried out in a calm, controlled environment without the risk of unexpected exposure to the baby.

- Each session should be 10–15 minutes long; the session should stop after 15 minutes, regardless of the amount of progress made. It is possible to do two sessions; however, there should be a 10–15-minute break between sessions where the pet is removed from the training environment and allowed to rest. The sessions should be carried out two to three times a week with at least one day between to allow arousal levels to reduce.
- Before each session, ensure that your pet has had some physical exercise and the opportunity to eliminate.
- Ensure that your pet has not fed prior to the session to increase their motivation to work for food. Prepare enough small tasty treats to last for the whole 10–15-minute session and have them on hand in a treat pouch or pocket.
- If working with a dog, it would be useful to have your dog head-halter trained before starting this training; the head halter is a very useful tool to assist your dog with some cues you will be using (see Handout C5 – Muzzle, Head Halter and Body Harness Training for more details).

- If working with a dog which has shown avoidance or aggression towards babies or children in the past, then you will need to have it muzzle-trained before you begin the desensitization training (see Handout C5 – Muzzle, Head Halter and Body Harness Training for more details).
- If working with a cat, consider using a body harness or a carrier. The cat must be trained to wear the harness or spend time in a carrier before working on desensitization to babies.
- A life-sized doll is recommended to reduce exposing your baby to your pet during a session and to allow you to start training before your baby is born.
- This exercise would be easier with two people – one person to hold the baby (or doll) and a second person to work the pet. You can progress to one person holding the baby and working the pet once you have done the initial training.

See Handout C1 – Set Up to Succeed, for more details.

How to carry out desensitization and counter-conditioning to a new baby

Stage 1 – the sight of the baby

For safety reasons a life-sized doll is recommended for this stage. Dress the doll in baby clothes and wrap it in a blanket as you would your real baby.

The help of a second person to handle and train your pet is suggested. Your pet should be on a head halter or harness and lead in the same room as you and the doll.

1. Gauge a distance to start the session where the pet shows minimal displacement behaviours when it sees you holding the doll. If you see displacement behaviours (see Handout B3 – Identifying Displacement and Conflict-related Behaviours), ask your pet for a 'Watch' or 'Touch' cue (see Handout C2 – How to Teach a 'Watch Me' and 'Touch' Cue).
    - If the pet responds to the cues, reward it and stay at this distance and use the 'Settle' cue to reduce the pet's arousal levels (see Handout C4 – Teaching a Pet how to Settle on Cue).
    - If the pet cannot perform these behaviours, you or your helper will need to increase the distance between you and your pet and repeat the cues. Then, either maintain the new distance or move further away depending on the pet's response.
2. At this distance, watch the pet to see if it looks towards you and the doll.
    - If the pet looks at you without showing displacement or conflict behaviours, use the marker cue to reinforce this calmer behaviour.
    - If you notice displacement behaviours, you or your helper should ask for a 'Touch' or 'Watch' to redirect the pet. Once you have the pet's attention, give the 'Settle' cue to reduce its arousal level before continuing with the session.
3. Once the pet is able to look at you and the doll without showing displacement behaviours, slightly reduce the distance between the baby (or doll) and the pet.
4. Repeat steps 2 and 3 until your pet can be within one metre of you and the doll and not show any displacement behaviours.
5. Once the pet is able to do this, you can move on to getting your pet used to being next to you while you are holding the doll and petting the pet. A second person might be necessary to help you if your pet starts to show displacement or conflict behaviours as detailed above.

The distance moved in each session will depend on the behaviour of the pet. Do not move closer until the pet is not showing any displacement or conflict behaviours when it sees you and the doll.

If at any point during the sessions the pet shows signs of high arousal (e.g. displacement, growling, barking or lunging) ask for a 'Watch' or 'Touch' cue. If the pet responds to the cue, reward it for responding to the cue and then move slightly away. Once you have moved away, use the 'Settle' cue to reduce the pet's arousal levels.

If the pet is able to respond to the 'Settle' cue and you notice a reduction in its arousal levels, you can try the exercise again but start at your current distance from the baby. If the pet completely ignores you, you need to remove the pet to a different area or room and use the 'Settle' cue to reduce its arousal levels. If the pet is unable to respond to basic obedience or the 'Settle' cue, you should end the session.

Stage 2 – the smell of the baby

The same process can be repeated for your baby's smell, by allowing slow and controlled access to baby products, such as soaps, powder, shampoo, creams or clothing. Once the baby is born, pieces of clothing worn by your baby should be brought home before you leave the hospital and the controlled access detailed above followed to allow your pet time to explore the new scent without any risk to your baby.

Stage 3 – sounds associated with the baby

You can use recordings of your baby on your phone, or other baby sounds using a computer or CD. Ensure you have enough tasty treats, a feeding toy, chews and toys available to give your dog during the session.

1. Gauge the volume to start playing the noises, by watching your pet and noticing when it starts to show displacement behaviours as you slowly increase the volume of the noises.
   - If you see displacement behaviours, ask for a 'Watch' or 'Touch' cue.
   - If the pet responds to the cues, reward it and stay at this volume and use the 'Settle' cue to reduce the pet's arousal levels and give it a feeding toy to chew.
   - If the pet cannot perform these behaviours, you will need to reduce the volume and repeat the cues; you will either maintain the new volume or reduce it again depending on the pet's response.
2. At this volume, watch the pet to see if it looks towards the noises.
   - If it looks towards the noise without showing displacement or conflict behaviours, use the marker cue to reinforce this calmer behaviour and ensure it has a feeding toy or chew.
   - If you notice displacement behaviours, ask for a 'Touch' or 'Watch me' to redirect the pet to you. Once you have its attention, give the 'Settle' cue to reduce the pet's arousal level before giving it a feeding toy or chew.
3. Once the pet is able to hear the noises at this volume without showing displacement behaviours, you can increase the volume a little bit.

Try this in several different locations around the house so that your pet learns that it will hear these noises all over the house and receive reinforcement.

Stage 4 – more visitors to the house

When your baby comes home, there will be an increase in the number of visitors to the house. This might cause an increase in your pet's arousal levels and potential changes in behaviour.

Prior to the baby being born, ensure your pet has a safe-haven they are comfortable using and you have optimized their feeding routine with feeding toys and chews (see Handout C3 – Safe-haven, and A9 (Cat) and A10 (Dog) Feeding Toys and Stimulation, for more details).

Ask people to come for a visit more frequently in the weeks running up to the birth of your child and, if appropriate, allow your pet to interact with them for 10–15 minutes. Following the visit, place the pet in its safe-haven with feeding toys and chews. Over time, your pet will learn this routine.

Stage 5 – novel items in the house

Babies have many accessories associated with them which your pet may not have seen before. If you feel it is appropriate for your pet, you may want to have them on a harness or head halter and lead.

Try to get your pet used to these new items as soon as possible.

1. Allow your pet to approach an item in its own time – do not force your pet to approach something, especially if it shows displacement, conflict or even signs of fear.

2. If your pet approached the novel item and did not show any displacement or conflict, use the marker to reward that behaviour.
3. If you see displacement behaviours, ask for a 'Watch' or 'Touch' cue, reward your pet and allow it to continue approaching the item.
4. Allow your pet to approach, sniff and touch the novel items.
5. If your pet crosses the behavioural threshold, remove it from the room and consider the following before training again:
   - Was the room used big enough to allow the pet to move away?
   - Could the pet see the item as they entered the room, or did it startle them when they entered the room?
   - Would the pet be better off-lead when approaching the novel item?

Do not throw food near the novel item – this causes conflict as the pet will want the food but may not want to be near the novel object.

If any of the novel items move, such as a pram, you will need to repeat these steps while the items are moving.

Stage 6 – potentially fewer interactions with you and less exercise

A new baby will change your routine, and so you may not have time to play with or walk your pet as much as you did before.

Consider gradually reducing the amount of playtime and walks your pet has in the weeks running up to the birth. Alternatively, you could arrange for a dog walker, family member or friend to collect your pet and walk them for you.

A safe-haven and optimized feeding routine will be of great use as you can put your pet in their safe-haven with food toys while you are busy with your baby. Do not leave your pet shut in their safe-haven for extended periods as your pet will not want to go there in future.

D5 – Desensitization – Introducing a New Cat or Reintroducing Cats at Home

Before starting a desensitization and counter-conditioning programme

There are several steps which need to be completed before starting a desensitization and counter-conditioning programme:

1. training of necessary cues;
2. management and safety tools;
3. looking at the components of the trigger;
4. setting expectations;
5. understanding what displacement and conflict behaviours are; and
6. eliminating exposure between the cats in the house.

Please see Handout D1 – What are Desensitization and Counter-conditioning? for full details of how to complete these steps.

Components of this trigger, introduction or reintroduction of a cat, would include:

- scent and sounds – cats separated by a solid barrier;
- scent, sounds and sight – cats separated by a transparent barrier; and
- cats in the same room.

Preparing for a desensitization and counter-conditioning session

When preparing, there are a few things which need to be done to set the session up. Desensitization is not a 'real-life' but a 'made-up' situation. These sessions need to be carried out in a calm, controlled environment where accidental interactions between the cats are not possible.

- Each session should be 10–15 minutes long; the session should stop after 15 minutes, regardless of the amount of progress made. It is possible to do two sessions; however, there should be a 10–15-minute break between sessions where the pet is removed from the training environment and allowed to rest away from any other cats. The sessions should be carried out two to three times a week with at least one day between to allow arousal levels to reduce.
- Find a suitable environment where a controlled session of gradual exposure can take place. Initially, this will need to be with a solid barrier between the cats such as a closed door.
- Before each session, ensure both cats have had some physical exercise, such as a play session with you, and the opportunity to eliminate.
- Ensure neither pet has been fed prior to the session to increase their motivation to work for food. Prepare enough small tasty treats to last for the whole 10–15-minute session and have them to hand in a treat pouch or pocket. There are products available such as Webbox Lick-e-Lix, which work well for this exercise. Alternatively, feeding toys such as lick mats with wet food, paté or fish paste on are very useful for this exercise.

- NB Each cat is an individual so may prefer a play session with a toy over a food reward or feeding toy. You will have to take time to get to know your cat's preferences before starting this exercise.
- Having two people for this exercise is beneficial, one person to work with each cat. Each person will need treats or feeding toys prepared.
- It is recommended that both cats are trained to wear and walk in a harness before you get to Stage 3 – cats in the same room; see Handout C5 – Muzzle, Head Halter and Body Harness Training, for more details.

See Handout C1 – Set Up to Succeed, for more details.

How to carry out desensitization and counter-conditioning to the presence of other cats.

Stage 1 – scent and sound through a solid barrier

1. Prepare your training area before introducing the cats. Ensure you have treats, marker tools and feeding toys to hand. Ensure that the solid barrier between the cats is sturdy.
2. Bring the cats into separate areas. Maintain maximum distance from the solid barrier at this point.
3. Gauge a distance to start the sessions where the pets show minimal displacement behaviours when approaching the solid barrier. This is done by slowly walking towards the solid barrier and watching for displacement or conflict behaviours.
   If you see displacement behaviours (see Handout B3 – Identifying Displacement and Conflict-related Behaviours), ask for a 'Watch' or 'Touch' cue (see Handout C2 – How to Teach a 'Watch Me' and 'Touch' Cue).
   - If the pet responds to the cues, reward it and stay at this distance and use the 'Settle' cue to reduce the pet's arousal levels (see Handout C4 – Teaching a Pet how to Settle on Cue).
   - If the pet cannot perform these behaviours, you will need to walk away from the solid barrier and repeat the cues. Then, either maintain the new distance or move further away depending on the pet's response.
4. At this distance, offer a food toy or a small number of treats. Watch the pet to see if it looks towards or listens to sounds from behind the solid barrier.
   - If it orientates towards the solid barrier without showing displacement or conflict behaviours, use the marker cue to reinforce this calmer behaviour (see Handout C6 –Marker Training, for more details).
   - If you notice displacement behaviours, ask for a 'Touch' or 'Watch' to redirect the pet to you. Once you have its attention, give the 'Settle' cue to reduce the pet's arousal level before continuing with the exercise.
5. Once the pet is able to look at the solid barrier without showing displacement behaviours, move a step closer to the solid barrier.
6. Repeat steps 4 and 5 until you can have each cat next to the solid barrier on their respective sides and not see any displacement behaviours.
7. Once the pet is able to do this, you can work through the other components of the trigger.

Stage 2 – scent, sounds and sight – cats separated by a transparent barrier

Repeat the exercise detailed in stage 1; however, this time you will need a barrier that can prevent the cats from jumping over it (e.g. closed screen door or window). You can also place the cats in carriers so they can see but not reach each other. The cats must be used to their respective carriers before you start these sessions.

Stage 3 – cats in the same room

For this stage, the cats should be wearing a harness and lead. This will allow you to maintain safety or remove one, or both, cats if necessary. Start this exercise with the cats on opposite sides of the same room – ensure the room is large enough that each cat has room to move away.

The exercise will follow the same steps as detailed in stage 1. The distance moved in each session will depend on the behaviour of the pet; do not move closer until the cats do not show any displacement or conflict behaviours when watching each other. Each cat will progress at its own pace. You may have one cat moving closer within four sessions while the second cat may require six to eight sessions to move closer.

If at any point during the sessions the cats show signs of high arousal (e.g. displacement, growling, hissing or swiping), ask for a 'Watch' or 'Touch' cue. If the cats respond to the cue, reward them for responding to the cue and then increase the distance between the cats. You should then try to work on a 'Settle' exercise with each cat separately.

If the cats are completely ignoring you, move them to different areas, even if you have to gently pull on the lead or pick them up (separately, and only if safe to do so). Once you have moved away, use the 'Settle' cue to reduce their arousal levels.

If the cats are able to respond to the 'Settle' cue and you notice a reduction in their arousal levels, you can try the exercise again but start at your current distance between the cats. If the cats are unable to respond to basic obedience cues and the 'Settle', you should end the session.

NB If your cat chooses to move away at any point during the training, allow it to do so. Do not pull on the lead or force it to continue with the session. Use a 'Touch' cue to encourage it back to you and restart the training. If it moves away again, end the session.

Abbreviated exercise

Desensitization and counter-conditioning is the gold standard in behaviour modification. However, it can be challenging to organize the sessions as these are structured sessions in a controlled environment. An abbreviated version of the desensitization exercise is possible where you are not trying to teach the cats how to interact with each other but helping them to feel more positive when they see each other (known as counter-conditioning).

1. Before each session, make sure the cats have had some exercise, playtime, have eliminated and are hungry.
2. Plan on having 15–20 minutes for each session, ideally two to three times a week.
3. Prepare plenty of small tasty treats for a 20-minute session.
4. Set up an environment where one cat is moving freely in a closed room while the other cat is with you. The cat you work with should be the one that is more likely to chase or show aggression. Ensure neither cat can gain access to the other; this may mean you ensure anyone else in the house does not open the door where the other cat is.
5. Start at a distance where one cat pays attention to the other cat. If the cats ignore each other, you are too far from the barrier; if they show displacement and conflict behaviours or cross their behavioural threshold, you are too close to the barrier.
6. Each time the cat with you looks at or listens to the sounds of the other cat, use the marker cue and give your cat a treat, praise or a pat.
7. After a few sessions, when the cat appears calm when it hears the other cat at that distance and is looking at you with anticipation for a treat, you can move slightly closer.
8. Repeat steps 5, 6 and 7 until you can be next to the barrier and not see any displacement or conflict behaviours.

D6 – Desensitization – Dogs on a Walk

Before starting a desensitization and counter-conditioning programme

There are several steps which need to be completed before starting a desensitization and counter-conditioning programme:

1. training of necessary cues;
2. management and safety tools;
3. looking at the components of the trigger;
4. setting expectations;
5. understanding what displacement and conflict behaviours are; and
6. eliminating exposure to other dogs as much as possible.

Please see Handout D1 – What are Desensitization and Counter-conditioning? for full details on how to complete these steps.

Components of this trigger, dogs on walks, would include:

- stationary dog up to 8 metres away;
- stationary dog less than 8 metres away;
- walking dog up to 8 metres away;
- walking dog less than 8 metres away;
- dog making noises up to 8 metres away;
- dog making noises less than 8 metres away;
- dog making movements such as running/playing up to 8 metres away;
- dog making movements such as running/playing less than 8 metres away;
- brief sniffing and interaction.

The average road is approximately 8 metres wide. Getting to the point where you can walk your dog down the road, and it can pass another dog on the other side of the road, is a good starting point. You can then progress with further sessions to reduce this distance.

NB Your pet may never be comfortable with other dogs interacting with it; therefore, walking past within two metres may be the best outcome for this session.

Preparing for a desensitization and counter-conditioning session

When preparing, there are a few things which need to be done to set the session up. Desensitization is not a 'real-life' but a 'made-up' situation. These sessions need to be carried out in a calm, controlled environment without the risk of unexpected exposure to other dogs.

- Each session should be 10–15 minutes long; the session should stop after 15 minutes, regardless of the amount of progress made. It is possible to do two sessions; however, there should be a 10–15-minute break between sessions where your dog is removed from the training environment and allowed to rest away from any other dogs. The sessions should be carried out two to three times a week with at least one day between to allow arousal levels to reduce.

- Find a suitable environment where a controlled session of gradual exposure can take place; an open field where you can see all around you or privately hired paddock will work well for this.
- A calm, well-trained dog with a handler will be needed for this exercise. The handler of the second dog should keep the dog calm and focused and ignore your dog.
- Before each session, ensure both dogs have had some physical exercise and the opportunity to eliminate.
- Ensure neither pet has been fed prior to the session to increase their motivation to work for food. Prepare enough small tasty treats to last for the whole 10–15-minute session and have them to hand in a treat pouch or pocket.
- When working at a distance from the other dog, you should have your dog on a lead, possibly with a head halter, to assist you with training and moving it if needed (see Handout C5 – Muzzle, Head Halter and Body Harness Training, for more information).
- While working with your dog close to the other dog, your dog must be on a lead and wearing a muzzle or head halter at all times.

See Handout C1 – Set Up to Succeed, for more details.

How to carry out desensitization and counter-conditioning to the presence of other dogs

Stage 1 – stationary dog

1. Bring the dogs into the training area one at a time, ideally with the dog going in first and settling at the end of the training area. Maintain maximum distance between the dogs while doing this.
2. Gauge a distance to start the sessions where your dog shows minimal displacement behaviours when it sees the other dog. This is done by slowly walking towards the dog and watching for displacement or conflict behaviours.
   If you see displacement behaviours (see Handout B3 – Identifying Displacement and Conflict-related Behaviours), ask for a 'Watch' or 'Touch' cue (see Handout C2 – How to Teach a 'Watch Me' and 'Touch' Cue).
   - If your dog responds to the cues, reward it and stay at this distance and use the 'Settle' cue to reduce your dog's arousal levels (see Handout C4 – Teaching a Pet how to Settle on Cue).
   - If your dog cannot perform these behaviours, you will need to walk away from the dog and repeat the cues; you will either maintain the new distance or move further away depending on your dog's response.
3. At this distance, watch your dog; see if it looks towards the other dog.
   - If it looks at the dog without showing displacement or conflict behaviours, use the marker cue to reinforce this calmer behaviour.
   - If you notice displacement behaviours, ask for a 'Touch' or 'Watch' to redirect your dog to you. Once you have its attention, give the 'Settle' cue to reduce its arousal level before continuing with the exercise.
4. Once your dog is able to look at the other dog without showing displacement behaviours, move slightly closer to the dog (until you notice subtle signs of displacement behaviour).
5. Repeat steps 3 and 4 until you can be within 8 metres (approximately the width of a standard road) of the other dog and not see any displacement behaviours.
6. Once your dog is able to do this, you can work through the other components of the trigger. When working on direct interactions with the other dog, ensure you start with brief interactions coupled with a positive outcome. The other dog should be calm and friendly. Use a muzzle for safety.

The distance moved in each session will depend on your dog's behaviour; do not move closer until your dog is not showing any displacement or conflict behaviours when it sees the stationary dog.

If at any point during the sessions, your dog shows signs that it has crossed its behavioural threshold (e.g. displacement, growling, barking or lunging) ask for a 'Watch' or 'Touch' cue.

If your dog responds to the cue, reward it and then move away from the other dog. Once you have moved away, use the 'Settle' cue to reduce its arousal levels. If your dog is able to respond to the 'Settle' cue and you notice a reduction in its arousal levels, you can try the exercise again but start at your current distance from the other dog.

If your dog completely ignores you, turn around and move away from the other dog, even if you have to gently pull on the lead to get it to move away. Once you have moved away from the dog, use the 'Settle' cue to reduce its arousal levels. If your dog is unable to respond to basic obedience or the 'Settle' cue, you should end the session.

Abbreviated exercise

Desensitization and counter-conditioning is the gold standard in behaviour modification. However, it can be challenging to organize these sessions as they are structured sessions in a controlled environment. An abbreviated version of the desensitization exercise is possible where you are not trying to teach your dog how to interact with the other dog, but helping it to feel more positive when it sees other dogs (known as counter-conditioning).

1. Before each session make sure your dog has had some exercise, some playtime, has eliminated and is hungry.
2. Plan on having 15–20 minutes for each session, ideally two to three times a week.
3. Prepare plenty of small tasty treats for a 20-minute session.
4. Find an environment where your dog will see other dogs in a controlled way. Examples would be a footpath, pet shop, grooming salon or a veterinary surgery at times that you can see dogs walking by – the dogs which your dog sees during this exercise must be on a lead and under control to reduce the risk of an unplanned interaction.
5. Start at a distance where your dog pays attention to the other dogs. If your dog is not paying attention to the other dogs you are too far; if it is showing displacement and conflict behaviours or crosses its behavioural threshold, you are too close.
6. Each time an unfamiliar person walks past and your pet is calmly looking, you can use the marker cue and give the pet a treat, praise or a pat. If you notice any signs of increased arousal (e.g. displacement or conflict), give your pet a signal such as 'Watch' or 'Touch', and then reward it.
7. After a few sessions, when your dog appears calm when it sees the other dog at that distance and is looking at you with anticipation for a treat, you can move slightly closer.
8. Repeat steps 6 and 7 until you can be within 8 metres (roughly the width of a standard road) of the dog and not see any displacement or conflict behaviours.

Try this in several different locations so that your dog learns that dogs in all environments are positive.

D7 – Desensitization – Dogs on Property

Before starting a desensitization and counter-conditioning programme

There are several steps which need to be completed before starting a desensitization and counter-conditioning programme:

1. training of necessary cues;
2. management and safety tools;
3. looking at the components of the trigger;
4. setting expectations;
5. understanding what displacement and conflict behaviours are; and
6. eliminating exposure between the dogs in the house.

Please see Handout D1 – What are Desensitization and Counter-conditioning? for full details on how to complete these steps.

Components of this trigger, introduction or reintroduction of a dog, would include:

- scent and sounds – dogs separated by a solid barrier;
- scent, sounds and sight – dogs separated by a transparent barrier; and
- dogs in the same room.

Preparing for a desensitization and counter-conditioning session

When preparing, there are a few things which need to be done to set the session up. Desensitization is not a 'real-life' but a 'made-up' situation. These sessions need to be carried out in a calm, controlled environment without the risk of unexpected exposure to other dogs.

- Each session should be 10–15 minutes long; the session should stop after 15 minutes, regardless of the amount of progress made. It is possible to do two sessions; however, there should be a 10–15-minute break between sessions where your dog is removed from the training environment and allowed to rest away from any other dogs. The sessions should be carried out two to three times a week with at least one day between to allow arousal levels to reduce.
- Find a suitable environment (e.g. garden or lounge) where a controlled session of gradual exposure can take place. Initially, this will need to be with a solid barrier between the dog, such as a closed door.
- Before each session, ensure both dogs have had some physical exercise and the opportunity to eliminate.
- Ensure neither dog has been fed prior to the session to increase its motivation to work for food. Prepare enough small tasty treats to last for the whole 10–15-minute session and have them on hand in a treat pouch or pocket. Feeding toys such as lick mats with wet food, paté or fish paste on are very useful for this exercise. Each dog is an individual so may prefer a play session with a toy over a food reward or feeding toy. You will have to take time to get to know your dog's preferences before starting this exercise.
- You will need two people for this exercise, one person to work with each dog. Each person will need treats or feeding toys prepared.
- It is recommended that both dogs are trained to wear a harness and head halter for stages 1 and 2 (see Handout C5 – Muzzle, Head Halter and Body Harness Training, for more details).
- Both dogs should be muzzle-trained before you get to stage 3 (see Handout C5 – Muzzle, Head Halter, and Body Harness Training, for more details).

See Handout C1 – Set Up to Succeed, for more details.

How to carry out desensitization and counter-conditioning to the presence of other dogs

Stage 1 – scent and sound through a solid barrier

1. Prepare your training area before introducing the dogs; ensure you have treats, marker tools and feeding toys to hand. Ensure the solid barrier between the dogs is sturdy.
2. Bring the dogs into their separate areas; maintain maximum distance from the solid barrier at this point. It is advised to use a head halter for this exercise as it will give you more control over where your dog is looking.
3. Gauge a distance to start the sessions where your dog shows minimal displacement behaviours when it approaches the solid barrier. This is done by slowly walking towards the solid barrier and watching for displacement or conflict behaviours.
   If you see displacement behaviours (see Handout B3 – Identifying Displacement and Conflict-related Behaviours), ask for a 'Watch' or 'Touch' cue (see Handout C2 – How to Teach a 'Watch Me' and 'Touch' Cue).
   - If your dog responds to the cues, reward it and stay at this distance. Use the 'Settle' cue to reduce your dog's arousal levels (see Handout C4 – Teaching a Pet how to Settle on Cue).
   - If your dog cannot perform these behaviours, you will need to walk away from the solid barrier and repeat the cues; you will either maintain the new distance or move further away depending on your dog's response.
4. At this distance, offer a food toy or a small number of treats. Observe your dog's behaviour; see if it looks towards or listens to sounds from behind the solid barrier.
   - If your dog focuses on the solid barrier without showing displacement or conflict behaviours, use the marker cue to reinforce this calmer behaviour (see Handout C6 – Marker Training, for more details).
   - If you notice displacement behaviours, ask for a 'Touch' or 'Watch' to redirect your dog to you. Once you have its attention, give the 'Settle' cue to reduce its arousal level before continuing with the exercise.
5. Once your dog is able to look at the stolid barrier without showing displacement behaviours, move closer to the solid barrier.
6. Repeat steps 4 and 5 until you can have each dog next to the solid barrier on their respective sides and not see any displacement behaviours.
7. Once your dog is able to do this, you can work through the other components of the trigger.

Stage 2 – Scent, sounds and sight – dogs separated by a transparent barrier

Repeat the exercise detailed in Stage 1; however, this time use a transparent barrier, such as a stairgate or screen door, between the dogs.

Stage 3 – dogs in the same room

Repeat the exercise detailed in Stage 1; however, this time there is no physical barrier. Therefore, each dog should be on-lead, wearing a harness and muzzle, or a head halter so you can safely and effectively control them. You may need to remove one, or both, of the dogs if necessary and reduce any risk of injury.

Start this exercise with the dogs on opposite sides of the same room – ensure that the room is large enough so the dogs can keep their distance if they choose.

The distance moved in each session will depend on the behaviour of either dog, do not move closer until either dog is not showing any displacement or conflict behaviours when it looks at the barrier or other dog. Each dog will progress at its own pace; you may have one dog next to the barrier within four sessions, while the other dog may take six to eight sessions to get next to the barrier.

If at any point during the sessions, your dog shows signs that it has crossed its behavioural threshold (e.g. displacement, growling, barking or lunging) ask for a 'Watch' or 'Touch' cue. If your dog responds to the cue, reward it and then move away from the barrier or the other dog. Once you have moved away, use the 'Settle' cue to reduce its arousal levels.

If your dog is able to respond to the 'Settle' cue and you notice a reduction in its arousal levels, you can try the exercise again but start at your current distance from the barrier or other dog.

If your dog completely ignores you, turn around and move away from the barrier or other dog, even if you have to gently pull on the lead to get it to move away. Once you have moved away, use the 'Settle' cue to reduce its arousal levels. If your dog is unable to respond to basic obedience cues or the 'Settle' cue, you should end the session.

Abbreviated exercise

Desensitization and counter-conditioning is the gold standard in behaviour modification. However, it can be challenging to organize the sessions as it is structured sessions in a controlled environment. An abbreviated version of the desensitization exercise is possible where you are not trying to teach your dog how to interact with the other dog but helping it to feel more positive when it sees the other dog (known as counter-conditioning).

1. Before each session, make sure your dog has had some exercise, some playtime, has eliminated and is hungry.
2. Plan on having 15–20 minutes for each session, ideally two to three times a week.
3. Prepare plenty of small tasty treats for a 20-minute session.
4. Set up an environment where one dog is moving freely in a closed room, while the reactive dog is with you. Ensure neither dog can gain access to each other; this may mean you ensure anyone else in the house does not open the door where the other dog is.
5. Start at a distance where the reactive dog pays attention to the other dog. If the reactive dog is not paying attention to the other dog, you are too far from the barrier; if it is showing displacement and conflict behaviours or crosses its behavioural threshold, you are too close to the barrier.
6. Each time the reactive dog looks at or listens to the sounds of the other dog, you can use the marker cue and give the pet a treat, praise or a pat. If you notice any signs of increased arousal (e.g. displacement or conflict), give the dog a signal such as 'Watch' or 'Touch', and then reward it.
7. After a few sessions, when the reactive dog appears calm when it hears the other dog at that distance and is looking at you with anticipation for a treat, you can move slightly closer.
8. Repeat steps 5 and 6 until you can be next to the barrier and not see any displacement or conflict behaviours.

This abbreviated exercise should be repeated in various environments (the lounge, kitchen, garden and on a walk) so that the dogs learn to be around each other in multiple environments.

D8 – Desensitization – Handling

Before starting a desensitization and counter-conditioning programme

There are several steps which need to be completed before starting a desensitization and counter-conditioning programme:

1. training of necessary cues;
2. management and safety tools;
3. looking at the components of the trigger;
4. setting expectations;
5. understanding what displacement and conflict behaviours are; and
6. Minimizing or altogether avoiding handling in-between sessions.

Please see Handout D1 – What are Desensitization and Counter-conditioning? for full details on how to complete these steps.

Handling involves any interaction with your pet where you have to move or touch a part of its body, including brushing, putting on a harness, attaching a lead to a collar or harness, wiping its feet, and cleaning ears.

This handout will address brushing; however, the same steps should be followed for any other form of handling.

Components of this trigger, handling – brushing, would include:

- seeing the brush;
- brush moving toward your pet;
- brush touching your pet; and
- brush moving though its coat.

Preparing for a desensitization and counter-conditioning session

When preparing, there are a few things which need to be done to set the session up. Desensitization is not a 'real-life' but a 'made-up' situation. These sessions need to be carried out in a calm, controlled environment without the need for unnecessary or unexpected handling.

- Each session should be 10–15 minutes long; the session should stop after 15 minutes, regardless of the amount of progress made. It is possible to do two sessions; however, there should be a 10–15-minute break between sessions where your pet is removed from the training environment and allowed to rest alone or without interactions. The sessions should be carried out two to three times a week with at least one day between to allow arousal levels to reduce.
- Find a suitable environment where your pet can move away if it wants.
- Before each session, ensure your pet has had some physical exercise and the opportunity to eliminate.
- Ensure your pet has been fed before the session to increase its motivation to work for food. Prepare enough small tasty treats to last for the whole 10–15-minute session and have it on hand in a treat pouch or pocket. Feeding toys such as lick-mats with wet food, paté or fish paste on are very useful for this exercise.
- If working with a dog, it should be muzzle-trained before you start this exercise (see Handout C5 – Muzzle, Head Halter and Body Harness Training, for more details). A muzzle is for safety reasons, not to encourage you to push your dog further with the training.

See Handout C1 – Set Up to Succeed, for more details.

How to carry out desensitization to brushing

Stage 1 – seeing the brush

1. Choose a cue word to use, such as 'Brush', which will indicate the use of a brush.
2. Have tasty treats ready.
3. Sit with your pet and say 'Brush', show it the brush and give it a treat. Do not attempt to move the brush towards it; simply show the brush to your pet.
4. Repeat this 15–20 times within a few minutes. During this time, do not expect any specific behaviour, such as 'Sit' or 'Down', just show it the brush, say 'Brush' and give it a treat. Your pet should start forming an association between seeing the brush and getting a treat; you should see positive anticipation (excitement) when your pet hears the word 'Brush.
5. Next, say 'Brush', then place the brush on the floor with some treats near it. Once your pet seems more comfortable approaching the brush to take the treats, you should move the treats closer to the brush, and finally on the brush. Once your pet is comfortable approaching and touching the brush, progress to the next step.
6. Test your pet; hold the brush, and say the brush cue; your pet should approach and look at you for a treat. If it does not do this, go back and work through steps 4 and 5 until it can respond to the brush cue.

Stage 2 – brush moving towards your pet

If you are working with a dog, it should be wearing a muzzle for this stage.

1. Gauge a distance to start the training exercises where your pet shows minimal displacement behaviours when it sees the brush move towards it. This step is done by saying 'Brush', and moving the brush slowly towards your pet. Observe for the first signs of displacement or conflict behaviours and then stop.
   When you see displacement behaviours (see Handout B3 – Identifying Displacement and Conflict-related Behaviours), ask for a 'Watch' or 'Touch' cue (see Handout C2 – How to Teach a 'Watch Me' and 'Touch' Cue).
   a. If your pet responds to the cues, reward it and stay at this distance; use the 'Settle' cue to reduce your pet's arousal levels (see Handout C4 – Teaching a Pet how to Settle on Cue).
   b. If your pet cannot perform these behaviours, you will need to move the brush away and repeat the cues; you will either maintain the new distance or move further away depending on your pet's response.
2. Once you know the distance the brush can be from your pet before it shows increased arousal levels, observe your pet to see if it looks towards the brush.
   - If your pet looks at the brush without showing displacement or conflict behaviours, use the marker cue to reinforce this calmer behaviour (see Handout C6 – Marker Training, for more information).
   - If you notice displacement behaviours, ask for a 'Touch' or 'Watch' to redirect your pet to you. Once you have its attention, give the 'Settle' cue to reduce your pet's arousal level before continuing with the exercise.
3. Once your pet is able to look at the brush without showing any displacement behaviours, move the brush closer towards your pet. NB You may only be able to move the brush a few centimetres closer to your pet each time. Do not rush this process.
4. Repeat steps 2 and 3 until you can lightly touch your pet with the brush and not see any displacement behaviours.
5. Once your pet is able to do this, you can work on the next component.

The distance moved in each session will depend on the behaviour of your pet; do not move closer until your pet is not showing any displacement or conflict behaviours when it sees the brush.

If at any point during the sessions your pet shows signs that it has crossed its behavioural threshold (e.g. displacement, growling, barking or lunging) ask for a 'Watch' or 'Touch' cue.

If your pet responds to the cue, reward it for responding to the cue and then move the brush away. Once you have moved the brush, use the 'Settle' cue to reduce your pet's arousal levels. If your pet can respond to the 'Settle' cue and you notice a reduction in its arousal levels, you can try the exercise again but start with the brush further away and proceed at a slower pace than before.

If your pet completely ignores you, move the brush out of sight of your pet, and then use the 'Settle' cue to reduce its arousal levels. If your pet is unable to respond to basic obedience or the 'Settle' cue, you should end the session.

NB If your pet chooses to move away at any point during the training, allow it to do so. Do not follow your pet with the brush or force it to stay near you. Use a 'Touch' cue to encourage your pet back to you and restart the training. If it moves away again, stop the training session and try again on a different day.

D9 – Desensitization – Walks

Before starting a desensitization and counter-conditioning programme

There are several steps which need to be completed before starting a desensitization and counter-conditioning programme:

1. training of necessary cues;
2. management and safety tools;
3. looking at the components of the trigger;
4. setting expectations;
5. understanding what displacement and conflict behaviours are; and
6. Minimizing or altogether avoiding walks in between sessions.

Please see Handout D1 – What are Desensitization and Counter-conditioning? for full details on how to complete these steps.

Components of the trigger can be as follows:

- putting on the harness;
- putting on the lead;
- moving to the door;
- going through the door;
- leaving the property; and
- walking on the road.

Preparing for desensitization and counter-conditioning session

When preparing, there are a few things which need to be done to set the session up. Desensitization is not a 'real-life' but a 'made-up' situation. These sessions need to be carried out in a calm, controlled environment without the risk of unexpected setbacks when preparing for or going on a walk.

- Each session should be 10–15 minutes long; the session should stop after 15 minutes, regardless of the amount of progress made. It is possible to do two sessions; however, there should be a 10–15-minute break between sessions where your dog is removed from the training environment and allowed to rest in a calm and quiet area. The sessions should be carried out two to three times a week with at least one day between to allow arousal levels to reduce.
- Find a suitable environment where a controlled training session can take place – a quiet room in the house to start the sessions – and then choose a time of day when there will not be too much happening in the road outside your house.
- Before each session, ensure your dog has had some physical exercise (e.g. play in the home or garden) and the opportunity to eliminate.
- Ensure your dog has not been fed prior to the session to increase its motivation to work for food. Prepare enough small tasty treats to last for the whole 10–15-minute session and have them on hand in a treat pouch or pocket.

See Handout C1 – Set Up to Succeed, for more details.

NB Some dogs suffer from phobia when in busy environments (e.g. crowded streets with heavy traffic). These dogs may never feel comfortable on walks and will benefit from very short walks in quiet areas or exercise in the garden only.

Stage 1 – putting on the harness

Your dog may not enjoy a walk because it is not comfortable in the harness currently being used. Ensure the harness you use is the correct size, is properly fitted, and does not restrict the movement of the front legs while moving. You may need to consider getting a new harness for this exercise.

Please see Handout C5 – Muzzle, Head Halter and Body Harness Training, for details of how to get your pet used to wearing a harness.

Stage 2 – putting on the lead

Once your pet is used to wearing the harness, you can introduce the lead:

1. Choose a cue word to use, such as 'lead', which will indicate that the lead is going to be used.
2. Have tasty treats ready.
3. With your dog wearing the harness, say 'lead', show it the lead and give it a treat. Do not attempt to put it on; just show it to the dog.
4. Repeat this 15–20 times within a few minutes. During this time, do not expect any specific behaviour, such as 'Sit' or 'Down'; just show it the lead, say 'lead' and give it a treat. After 15–20 repetitions, your dog should start forming an association between seeing the lead and getting a treat.
5. Test your dog; hold the lead and say the 'lead' cue. Your dog should look at the lead, then immediately look at you expecting a reward. If it does not do this, go back and work through steps 3 and 4 until it can respond to the lead cue.

The next steps get your pet used to the lead being attached to the harness.

If you are working with a dog that shows aggression during handling and attaching a lead, it should be wearing a muzzle for this stage.

1. Gauge a distance to start the training exercises where your dog shows minimal displacement behaviours when it sees the lead. This is done giving the 'lead' cue and rewarding your dog while slowly moving the lead closer. You are looking for the first signs of displacement or conflict behaviours.
   If you see displacement behaviours (see Handout B3 – Identifying Displacement and Conflict-related Behaviours), ask for a 'Watch' or 'Touch' cue (see Handout C2 – How to Teach a 'Watch Me' and 'Touch' Cue).
   - If your dog responds to the cues, reward it and stay at this distance. Use the 'Settle' cue to reduce your dog's arousal levels (see Handout C4 – Teaching a Pet how to Settle on Cue).
   - If your dog cannot perform these behaviours, you will need to move the lead away and repeat the cues; you will either maintain the new distance or move further away depending on your dog's response.
2. Once you know the distance the lead can be from your dog before it shows increased arousal levels, carefully observe your dog to see if it looks towards the lead.
   - If it looks at the lead without showing displacement or conflict behaviours, use the marker cue to reinforce this calmer behaviour (see Handout C6 – Marker Training, for more information).
   - If you notice displacement behaviours, ask for a 'Touch' or 'Watch' to redirect your dog to you. Once you have its attention, give the 'Settle' cue to reduce its arousal level before continuing with the exercise.
3. Once your dog is able to look at the lead without showing displacement behaviours, move it closer towards your dog. Do not rush this process.
4. Repeat steps 2 and 3 until you can attach the lead to the harness and not see any displacement behaviours.
5. Once your dog is able to do this, you can work on the next component.

Stages 3 – moving to the door; 4 – going through the door; 5 – leaving the property; and 6 – walking on the road

These stages will follow the same steps as detailed in Stage 2.

The distance moved in each session will depend on the behaviour for your dog. Do not move closer until your dog is not showing any displacement or conflict behaviours when you move closer to the door and later leave home and walk on the street.

If at any point during the sessions your dog shows signs that it has crossed its behavioural threshold (e.g. displacement, avoidance, pulling, growling or barking), ask for a 'Watch' or 'Touch' cue.

If your dog responds to the cue, reward it and then move away from the door or closer to the home (if outside). Then give your dog the 'Settle' cue to reduce its arousal levels. If your dog is able to respond to the 'Settle' cue and you notice a reduction in its arousal levels, you can try the exercise again but start at your current distance from the door or the street.

If your dog completely ignores you, turn around and move away from the door, or walk into the home (if outside), even if you have to pull on the lead to direct it gently. Once you have moved away from the door or street, use the 'Settle' cue to reduce its arousal levels.

If your dog is unable to respond to basic obedience and the 'Settle' cue, you should end the session.

NB If your dog chooses to move away at any point during the training, allow it to do so. Do not follow, pull on the lead or force it to continue walking. Use a 'Touch' cue to encourage your pet back to you and restart the training. If it moves away again, stop the training session and, if appropriate, return home. You can try on a different day or time of day.

D10 – Desensitization – Cyclists, Joggers, Traffic

Before starting a desensitization and counter-conditioning programme

There are several steps which need to be completed before starting a desensitization and counter-conditioning programme:

1. training of necessary cues;
2. management and safety tools;
3. looking at the components of the trigger;
4. setting expectations;
5. understanding what displacement and conflict behaviours are; and
6. eliminating exposure to triggers as much as possible.

Please see Handout D1 – What are Desensitization and Counter-conditioning? for full details on how to complete these steps.

This handout will be based on cyclists; however, the same steps will be taken for joggers and traffic.

Components of the trigger, in this case, cyclists, can be as follows:

- cyclists in high-visibility cycling clothes;
- stationary bike, no cyclist;
- stationary cyclist with bike;
- cyclist walking slowly with bike;
- cyclist walking briskly with bike;
- cyclist riding bike slowly; and
- cyclist riding bike with increasing speed.

NB Your dog may never be comfortable with a cyclist coming past it within two metres; this may be the best outcome for this session.

Preparing for a desensitization and counter-conditioning session

When preparing, there are a few things which need to be done to set the session up. Desensitization is not a 'real-life' but a 'made-up' situation. These sessions need to be carried out in a calm, controlled environment without the risk of unexpected exposure to cyclists.

- Each session should be 10–15 minutes long; the session should stop after 15 minutes, regardless of the amount of progress made. It is possible to do two sessions; however, there should be a 10–15-minute break between sessions where your dog is removed from the training environment and allowed to rest in a calm and quiet area. The sessions should be carried out two to three times a week with at least one day between to allow arousal levels to reduce.
- Find a suitable environment where a controlled session of gradual exposure can take place; an open field where you can see all around you or a privately hired paddock will work well for this.

- You will need the help of a second person who acts as a cyclist. Throughout the whole exercise, the cyclist should ignore your dog, avoid sudden movements, and follow your instructions.
- Before each session, ensure that your dog has had some physical exercise and the opportunity to eliminate.
- Ensure your dog has not been fed prior to the session to increase its motivation to work for food. Prepare enough small tasty treats to last for the whole 10–15-minute session and have them on hand in a treat pouch or pocket.
- Ensure your dog is head halter- and muzzle-trained before starting this exercise (see Handout C5 – Muzzle, Head Halter and Body Harness Training, for more details).

See Handout C1 – Set Up to Succeed, for more details.

Stage 1 – cyclist in high-visibility cycling gear

1. With your dog wearing a head halter or harness and muzzle, gauge a distance to start the sessions where your dog shows minimal displacement behaviours when it sees the cyclist. This is done by slowly walking towards the cyclist and looking for displacement or conflict behaviours. If you see displacement behaviours, ask for a 'Watch' or 'Touch' cue (see Handout C2 – How to Teach a 'Watch Me' and 'Touch' Cue).
    - If your dog responds to the cues, reward it and stay at this distance. Use the 'Settle' cue to reduce your dog's arousal levels (see Handout C4 – Teaching a Pet how to Settle on Cue).
    - If your dog cannot perform these behaviours, you will need to move the lead away and repeat the cues; you will either maintain the new distance or move further away depending on your dog's response.
2. At this distance, observe your dog to see if it looks towards the cyclist.
    - If it looks at the cyclist without showing displacement or conflict behaviours, use the marker cue to reinforce this calmer behaviour (see Handout C6 – Marker Training).
    - If you notice displacement behaviours, ask for a 'Touch' or 'Watch' to redirect your dog to you. Once you have its attention, give the 'Settle' cue to reduce its arousal level before continuing with the exercise.
3. Once your dog is able to look at the cyclist without showing displacement behaviours, move closer to the cyclist.
4. Repeat steps 2 and 3 until you can be within two metres of the cyclist and your dog does not show any displacement behaviours. Two metres is used as it is approximately the width of the average cycling/walking path.
5. Once your dog is able to respond appropriately to a cyclist at a close distance, you can work through the next component.

The remaining components of the trigger are worked through by following the steps detailed above. The distance moved in each session will depend on the behaviour of your dog. Do not move closer until your dog is not showing any displacement or conflict behaviours when it sees a stationary cyclist.

If at any point during the sessions, your dog shows signs that it has crossed its behavioural threshold (e.g., displacement, pulling, growling, barking and lunging) ask for a "Watch" or "Touch" cue.

If your dog responds to the cue, reward it and then move away from the cyclist. Then give your dog the 'Settle' cue to reduce its arousal levels. If your dog is able to respond to the 'Settle' cue and you notice a reduction in its arousal levels, you can try the exercise again but start at your current distance from the cyclist.

If your dog completely ignores you, turn around and move away from the cyclist, even if you have to gently pull on the lead to get it to move away. Once you have moved away from the cyclist, use the 'Settle' cue to reduce its arousal levels. If your dog is unable to respond to basic obedience and the 'Settle' cue, you should end the session.

Abbreviated exercise

Desensitization and counter-conditioning is the gold standard in behaviour modification. However, it can be challenging to organize the sessions as they are structured sessions in a controlled environment and require the help of a second person. An abbreviated version of the desensitization exercise is possible where you are not trying to teach your dog how to interact, but to feel calm when it sees the cyclist (known as counter-conditioning).

1. Before each session, make sure your dog has had some exercise, some play time, has eliminated and is hungry.
2. Plan on having 15–20 minutes for each session, ideally two to three times a week.
3. Prepare plenty of small tasty treats for a 20-minute session.
4. Find an environment where your dog can see cyclists in a controlled way. For example, stand away from a cycling path or street corners. You should not be on the path or directly where cyclists pass so that you can reduce the risk of an unplanned interaction.
5. Start at a distance where your dog pays attention to cyclists. If your dog is not paying attention to the cyclists, you are too far; if your dog is showing displacement and conflict behaviours or crosses its behavioural threshold, you are too close.
6. Each time a cyclists goes past and your pet is calmly looking; you can use the marker cue and give the pet a treat, praise or a pat. If you notice any signs of increased arousal (e.g. displacement or conflict), give your pet a signal such as 'Watch' or 'Touch', and then reward it.
7. After a few sessions, when your dog appears calm when it sees cyclists at that distance and is looking at you with anticipation for a treat, you can move slightly closer.
8. Repeat steps 5, 6 and 7 until you can be within two metres of the cyclist and not see any displacement or conflict behaviours.

Try this in several different locations so that your dog learns that cyclists in all environments are positive.

D11 – Desensitization – Car Rides

Before starting a desensitization and counter-conditioning programme

There are several steps which need to be completed before starting a desensitization and counter-conditioning programme:

1. training of necessary cues;
2. management and safety tools;
3. looking at the components of the trigger;
4. setting expectations;
5. understanding what displacement and conflict behaviours are; and
6. minimizing unnecessary car rides as much as possible.

Please see Handout D1 – What are Desensitization and Counter-conditioning? for full details on how to complete these steps.

Components of the trigger can be as follows:

- putting on a car travel harness and lead on dogs, and cats should be in a secure carrier;
- moving towards the car;
- getting into the car;
- sitting in a stationary car, engine off, door open;
- sitting in a stationary car, engine off, door closed;
- sitting in a stationary car, engine idling, door open;
- sitting in a stationary car, engine idling, door closed;
- sitting in a car, moving in and out of the driveway; and
- car travel.

Preparing for a desensitization and counter-conditioning session

When preparing, there are a few things which need to be done to set the session up. Desensitization is not a 'real-life' but a 'made-up' situation. These sessions need to be carried out in a calm, controlled environment minimizing unnecessary car rides between sessions.

- Each session should be 10–15 minutes long; the session should stop after 15 minutes, regardless of the amount of progress made. It is possible to do two sessions; however, there should be a 10–15-minute break between sessions where your pet is removed from the training environment and allowed to rest in a calm and quiet area. The sessions should be carried out two to three times a week with at least one day between to allow arousal levels to reduce.
- Find a suitable environment where a controlled session can take place; a quiet room in the house to start the session, and then choose a time of day when there will not be too much happening in the road outside your house.
- Before each session, ensure that your pet has had some physical exercise and the opportunity to eliminate.
- Ensure that your pet has not been fed prior to the session to increase its motivation to work for food. Prepare enough small tasty treats to last for the whole 10–15-minute session and have them on hand in a treat pouch or pocket.

- If your dog shows aggression when getting into the car, it needs to be muzzle-trained before you start this exercise.

See Handout C1 – Set Up to Succeed, for more details.

NB Some pets suffer from motion sickness and will have difficulties to adjust to car rides. These pets are better placed high where they can see the road, instead of the footwell. Also, these pets may require medications to help with nausea.

Stage 1 – putting on the harness and lead

Some dogs do not enjoy a walk because it is not comfortable in the harness currently being used. Ensure the harness you use is the correct size, properly fitted and does not restrict the movement of the front legs while moving. You may need to consider getting a new harness for this exercise. Please see Handout C5 – Muzzle, Head Halter and Body Harness Training for details of how to get your pet used to wearing a harness. Cats will need to be comfortable spending time in a carrier (see Handout C3 – Safe-haven for more information on teaching cats to spend time in carriers).

Once your pet is used to wearing the harness, you can introduce the lead:

1. Choose a cue word to use, such as 'lead' which will indicate that the lead is going to be used.
2. Have tasty treats ready.
3. As your dog wears the harness, say 'lead', show it the lead and give it a treat. Do not attempt to put the lead on; just show it to your dog.
4. Repeat this 15–20 times within a few minutes. During this time, do not expect any specific behaviour, such as 'Sit' or 'Down'; just show it the lead, say 'lead' and give it a treat.
5. After 15–20 repetitions, your dog should start forming an association between seeing the lead and getting a treat.
6. Test your dog; hold the lead and say the 'lead' cue. Your dog should look at the lead, then immediately look at you expecting a reward. If it does not do this, go back and work through steps 3 and 4 until your dog can respond to the lead cue.

The next steps get your dog used to the lead being attached to the harness:

If you are working with a dog, it should be wearing a muzzle for this stage.

1. Gauge a distance to start the sessions where your dog shows minimal displacement behaviours when it sees the lead. This is done giving the 'lead' cue, slowly moving the lead towards your dog, and looking for the first signs of displacement or conflict behaviours.
   If you see displacement behaviours (see Handout B3 – Identifying Displacement and Conflict-related Behaviours), ask for a 'Watch' or 'Touch' cue (see Handout C2 – How to Teach a 'Watch Me' and 'Touch' Cue).
   - If your dog responds to the cues, reward it and stay at this distance; use the 'Settle' cue to reduce your dog's arousal levels (see Handout C4 – Teaching a Pet how to Settle on Cue).
   - If your dog cannot perform these behaviours, you will need to move the lead away and repeat the cues; you will either maintain the new distance or move further away depending on your dog's response.
2. Once you know the distance the lead can be from your dog before it shows increased arousal levels, watch your dog to see if it looks towards the lead.
   - If your dog looks at the lead without showing displacement or conflict behaviours, use the marker cue to reinforce this calmer behaviour (see Handout C6 – Marker Training for more information).
   - If you notice displacement behaviours, ask for a 'Touch' or 'Watch' to redirect your dog to you. Once you have its attention, give the 'Settle' cue to reduce its arousal level before continuing with the exercise.
3. Once your dog is able to look at the lead without showing displacement behaviours, move the lead closer towards your pet. Do not rush this process.
4. Repeat steps 2 and 3 until you can attach the lead to the harness and not see any displacement behaviours.
5. Once your dog is able to do this you can work on the next component.

Stages 2–9

The remaining components of a car ride will be addressed following the same steps detailed above in stage 1:

- Gauge the distance from the car before your pet starts showing increased arousal levels.
- Start the session at this known distance.
- Slowly move closer to the car using treats, affection and praise, and later build longer duration in the car throughout the various stages.

The distance moved in each session will depend on the behaviour of your pet. Do not move closer until your pet is not showing any displacement or conflict behaviours when it sees the car. Once your dog goes voluntarily into the car and rests on the seat, or your cat rests in its carrier inside the car, you can move to engine idling and, later, car travel.

If at any point during the sessions your pet shows signs that it has crossed its behavioural threshold (e.g. displacement, trying to escape, vocalizing or aggression) ask for a 'Watch' or 'Touch' cue.

If your pet responds to the cue, reward it for responding to the cue and then get out of the car if standing, or stop driving if moving. Once you have stopped the exercise, use the 'Settle' cue to reduce its arousal levels. If your pet is able to respond to the 'Settle' cue and you notice a reduction in its arousal levels, you can try the exercise again but start at your current position (e.g. continue the ride or walk towards the car if outside).

If your pet completely ignores you, stop the exercise and move away from the car (when possible). Once you have stopped, use the 'Settle' cue to reduce its arousal levels. If your pet is unable to respond to basic obedience and the 'Settle' cue, you should end the session.

NB If your pet chooses to move away at any point during the training or shows intense signs of fear, you should end the session. Do not pull on the lead or force it to continue with the session. Use a 'Touch' cue to encourage your pet back to you and restart the training. If it moves away again, stop the session and, if appropriate, return home.

D12 – Desensitization – Veterinary Visits

There are several steps which need to be completed before starting a desensitization and counter-conditioning programme:

1. training of necessary cues;
2. management and safety tools;
3. looking at the components of the trigger;
4. setting expectations;
5. understanding what displacement and conflict behaviours are; and
6. avoiding unnecessary visits to the vet when possible.

Please see Handout D1 – What are Desensitization and Counter-conditioning? for full details on how to complete these steps.

Components of the trigger, in this case veterinary visits, can be as follows:

- people in veterinary uniforms;
- getting out in the car park;
- walking into reception;
- waiting in reception;
- walking into the consulting room; and
- physical examination and handling.

NB Some pets struggle during veterinary visits due to earlier situations, such as car travel or the presence of other animals and people. You may need to work with your pet on desensitization and counter-conditioning to those triggers prior to desensitizing your pet to veterinary visits.

Preparing for desensitization and counter-conditioning session

When preparing, there are a few things which need to be done to set the session up. Desensitization is not a 'real-life' but a 'made-up' situation. These sessions need to be carried out in a calm, controlled environment, not in a busy office with many other pets and people present.

- Each session should be 10–15 minutes long; the session should stop after 15 minutes, regardless of the amount of progress made. It is possible to do two sessions; however, there should be a 10–15-minute break between sessions where your pet is removed from the training environment and allowed to rest in a calm and quiet area. The sessions should be carried out two to three times a week with at least one day between to allow arousal levels to reduce.
- This session is particular to the veterinary surgery environment; most veterinary surgeries will allow you access to the reception and a consultation room at quiet times of the day to carry out this training.
- Before each session, ensure your pet has had some physical exercise and the opportunity to eliminate.
- Ensure that your pet has not been fed prior to the session to increase its motivation to work for food. Prepare enough small tasty treats to last for the whole 10–15-minute session and have them on hand in a treat pouch or pocket.
- If your dog shows aggression on a veterinary visit it should be muzzle-trained before you start this exercise (see Handout C5 – Muzzle, Head Halter and Body Harness Training for more details).

- For additional control during this session, dogs should be trained to wear a head halter before you start this exercise (see Handout C5 – Muzzle, Head Halter and Body Harness Training for more details). Cats should be in a carrier until you are in the consulting room.
- For stage 1, access to a scrub top or lab coat will allow you to start this part of the training at home with the aid of a someone willing to dress as a member of the veterinary team. If this is not possible, you will have to discuss with your veterinary surgery if a member of staff can help you with this session. The person helping with this exercise should ignore you and your pet at all times during the sessions.

See Handout C1 – Set Up to Succeed, for more details.

Stage 1 – people in veterinary uniforms

With your dog wearing a head halter or harness and muzzle (if aggressive), or your cat in a carrier or wearing a harness, gauge a distance to start the sessions where your pet shows minimal displacement behaviours when it sees the veterinary staff member. This is done by slowly walking towards the veterinary staff member and watching for displacement or conflict behaviours (see Handout B3 – Identifying Displacement and Conflict-related Behaviours).

If you see displacement behaviours, ask for a 'Watch' or 'Touch' cue (see Handout C2 – How to Teach a 'Watch Me' and 'Touch' Cue).

- If your pet responds to the cues, reward it and stay at this distance and use the 'Settle' cue to reduce your pet's arousal levels (see Handout C4 – Teaching a Pet how to Settle on Cue).
- If your pet cannot perform these behaviours, you will need to walk away from the veterinary staff and repeat the cues. You will either maintain the new distance or move further away depending on your pet's response.

1. At this distance, watch your pet to see if it looks towards the veterinary staff.

- If your pet looks at the veterinary staff without showing displacement or conflict behaviours, use the marker cue to reinforce this calmer behaviour (see Handout C6 – Marker Training for more information).
- If you notice displacement behaviours, ask for a 'Touch' or 'Watch' to redirect your pet to you. Once you have its attention, give the 'Settle' cue to reduce its arousal level before continuing with the exercise.

2. Once your pet is able to look at the veterinary staff without showing displacement behaviours, move slightly closer.
3. Repeat steps 1 and 2 until you your pet is close to the veterinary staff but not in reach of them or making physical contact.
4. Once your pet is able to do this, you can work through the next component.

Stages 2–5 (getting out in the car park; walking into reception; waiting in reception; walking into the consulting room)

The remaining components of a veterinary visit will be addressed by following the same steps detailed above in stage 1:

- Gauge the distance, first to the practice entrance, and later from other people and the consulting room.
- Start the session at this known distance.
- Slowly move closer to the practice entrance and later into the consulting room using treats, affection and praise; and later build longer duration in the consulting room, before moving to the final trigger: physical examination and handling.

Stage 6 – physical examination and handling

This stage should start at home as soon as possible.

If your dog shows aggression during an examination, it needs to be muzzle-trained before starting this session. Your dog should be wearing a muzzle for all examination sessions.

Each area which is to be examined can be given a cue word to provide your pet with predictability. For example, examining the ears:

1. Choose a cue word to use such as 'ear', which will indicate that the ear is going to be touched.
2. Have tasty treats ready.
3. Sit with your pet and say 'ear' and give it a treat. Do not attempt to touch the ear at this point.
4. Repeat this 15–20 times within a few minutes. During this time, do not expect any specific behaviour, such as 'Sit' or 'Down'; just say 'ear' and give it a treat.
5. After 15–20 repetitions, your pet should start forming an association between the word 'ear' and getting a treat.
6. Test your pet; say the 'ear' cue; your pet should approach and look at you for a treat. If it does not do this, go back and work through steps 3 and 4 until it can respond to the 'ear' cue.
7. Once your pet responds to the cue, you can start introducing physical handling; give the cue word 'ear', gently touch the ear, and immedicably reward your pet.
8. Over multiple sessions, increase the amount of contact you have with the ear, start moving the ear and eventually lifting the ear as your vet would do during an examination.

These steps should then be repeated for other parts of the body, mimicking a full examination.

The progress made in each session will depend on the behaviour of your pet. Do not move closer or increase handling until your pet is not showing any displacement or conflict behaviours.

If at any point during the sessions your pet shows signs that it has crossed its behavioural threshold (e.g. displacement, trying to escape, vocalizing or aggression) ask for a 'Watch' or 'Touch' cue.

If your pet responds to the cue, reward it for responding to the cue and then move away from the trigger or stop handling it. Once you have done this, use the 'Settle' cue to reduce its arousal levels.

If your pet completely ignores you, move it further away, or you move further away from the pet (if at home). If you are at the veterinary surgery, you may have to gently pull on the lead to get it to move away. Once you have moved away from the trigger, use the 'Settle' cue to reduce its arousal levels.

If your pet is able to respond to the 'Settle' cue and you notice a reduction in its arousal levels, you can try the exercise again but starting at your current distance from the trigger or just saying the cue word for the body part you are working on, and provide treats.

If your pet is unable to respond to basic obedience or the 'Settle' cue, you should end the session.

NB If your pet chooses to move away at any point during the training or shows intense signs of fear, you should end the session. Do not pull on the lead or force it to continue with the session. Use a 'Touch' cue to encourage your pet back to you and restart the training. If it moves away again, stop the session and, if appropriate, return home.

D13 – Desensitization – Noises

Before starting a desensitization and counter-conditioning programme

There are several steps which need to be completed before starting a desensitization and counter-conditioning programme:

1. training of necessary cues;
2. management and safety tools;
3. looking at the components of the trigger;
4. setting expectations;
5. understanding what displacement and conflict behaviours are; and
6. eliminating exposure to any visitors to the house.

Please see Handout D1 – What are Desensitization and Counter-conditioning? for full details on how to complete these steps.

The components of this trigger, noises, can be broken down into:

- volume of the noise;
- duration of the noise; and
- combination of noises.

NB Some pets show noise aversion as a result of pain. Loud sounds such as gunshots, fireworks or thunder are very loud and may surpass 100 dB. Some pets may also react to other components during sound events. For example, thunderstorms also include rain, lightning, changes in barometric pressure, and strong winds, all of which can scare the pet.

Preparing for desensitization and counter-conditioning session

When preparing, there are a few things which need to be done to set the session up. Desensitization is not a 'real-life' but a 'made-up' situation. These sessions need to be carried out in a calm, controlled environment minimizing other sounds between sessions.

- Source a sounds CD, download a recording, or use online sources of the known noises to which your pet becomes over-aroused when it hears them.
- Each session should be 10–15 minutes long; the session should stop after 15 minutes, regardless of the amount of progress made. It is possible to do two sessions; however, there should be a 10–15-minute break between sessions where your pet is removed from the training environment and allowed to rest in a calm and quiet area. The sessions should be carried out two to three times a week with at least one day between to allow arousal levels to reduce.
- Before each session, ensure that your pet has had some physical exercise and the opportunity to eliminate.
- Ensure that your pet has not been fed prior to the session to increase its motivation to work for food. Prepare enough small tasty treats to last for the whole 10–15-minute session and have them on hand in a treat pouch or pocket.
- Prepare a variety of feeding toys and stimulation for your pet prior to each session (see Handouts A9 (Cats) and A10 (Dogs) – Feeding Toys and Stimulation for more details).

See Handout C1 – Set Up to Succeed, for more details.

Stage 1 – volume of noises

Before you expose your pet to any noises, ensure it is calm and has access to feeding toys.

1. Gauge the volume of the noise to start the session. This is done by playing the noises at the lowest volume level possible and slowly increasing the volume, while you observe your pet for displacement or conflict behaviours.

   If you see displacement behaviours, ask for a 'Watch' or 'Touch' cue (see Handout C2 – How to Teach a 'Watch Me' and 'Touch' Cue).
   - If your pet responds to the cues, reward it, and use the 'Settle' cue to reduce your pet's arousal levels (see Handout C4 – Teaching a Pet how to Settle on Cue).
   - If your pet cannot perform these behaviours, you will need to decrease the volume then repeat the cues; you will either maintain the new volume or decrease the noise further depending on your pet's response.
2. At this volume, watch your pet to see if it responds to the noises.
   - If your pet looks in the direction of the noises without showing displacement or conflict behaviours, use the marker cue to reinforce this calmer behaviour (see Handout C6 – Marker Training).
   - If you notice displacement behaviours, ask for a 'Touch' or 'Watch' to redirect your dog to you. Once you have its attention, give the 'Settle' cue to reduce its arousal level before continuing with the exercise.
3. After several repetitions of training at this volume, your pet should be able to hear the noises at this volume without showing displacement behaviours and continue to interact with the feeding toy. This is the point where you can progress.
4. Increase the volume until your pet shows interest in the noises again; repeat steps 1 and 2 until you can play the noises at a reasonable volume without your pet showing displacement behaviours.

Stage 2 – duration of the noise

Follow the same approach above when desensitizing the pet to the duration of the noise:

- gauge duration;
- train at this duration; and
- gradually increase duration.

Stage 3 – combination of noises

Once you have worked on individual noises, you can move to stage 3 – combining different noises. Follow the same approach as stage 1, but play multiple sounds at the same time. For example, you can desensitize your pet to rain and thunder individually, and later to both at the same time.

NB This stage could take multiple sessions over several weeks or months – it is crucial you do not rush this training as you could increase your pet's sensitivity to the noises instead of reducing it.

If at any point during the sessions your pet shows signs that it has crossed its behavioural threshold (e.g. displacement, trying to escape, vocalizing or aggression) ask for a 'Watch' or 'Touch' cue.

If your pet responds to the cue, reward it for responding to the cue and then decrease the volume of the noises. Once you have decreased the volume, use the 'Settle' cue to reduce its arousal levels. If your pet is able to respond to the 'Settle' cue and you notice a reduction in its arousal levels, you can try the exercise again but start at your current volume.

If your pet completely ignores these cues, reduce the volume of the noises even more – consider turning them off. Once you have done this, use the 'Settle' cue to reduce its arousal levels. If your pet is unable to respond to basic obedience and the 'Settle' cue, you should end the session.

D14 – Desensitization – Separation-related Problems

Before starting a desensitization and counter-conditioning programme

There are several steps which need to be completed before starting a desensitization and counter-conditioning programme:

1. training of necessary cues;
2. management and safety tools;
3. looking at the components of the trigger;
4. setting expectations;
5. understanding what displacement and conflict behaviours are; and
6. eliminating exposure to any visitors to the house.

Please see Handout D1 – What are Desensitization and Counter-conditioning? for full details on how to complete these steps.

The components of this trigger, separation-related problems, can be broken down into:

- owner in the room but not interacting with your pet;
- separation through a transparent barrier; the owner is at home;
- separation through a solid barrier; the owner is at home;
- separation; the owner is not at home;
- duration of separation; the owner is not at home._

Preparing for desensitization and counter-conditioning session

When preparing, there are a few things which need to be done to set the session up. Desensitization is not a 'real-life' but a 'made-up' situation. These sessions need to be carried out in a calm, controlled environment minimizing unnecessary departures or separation between sessions.

- Your pet should be trained to use a safe-haven for this session – see Handout C3 Safe-haven for more details.
- If appropriate for your pet, it should be receiving medication from your veterinary surgeon to aid with this training.
- Initially, each session should be 10–15 minutes long; the session should stop after 15 minutes, regardless of the amount of progress made. It is possible to do two sessions; however, there should be a 10–15-minute break between sessions where your pet is removed from the training environment and allowed to rest in a calm and quiet area. The sessions should be carried out two to three times a week with at least one day between to allow arousal levels to reduce.
- Before each session, ensure your pet has had some physical exercise and the opportunity to eliminate.
- Ensure that your pet has not been fed prior to the session to increase its motivation to work for food. Prepare enough small tasty treats to last for the whole 10–15-minute session and have them on hand in a treat pouch or pocket.

- Prepare a variety of feeding toys and stimulation for your pet prior to each session (see Handouts A9 (Cats) and A10 (Dogs) – Feeding Toys and Stimulation for more details).

See Handout C1 – Set Up to Succeed, for more details.

Stage 1 – separation from the owner

Before you expose your pet to any form of separation, ensure it is settled in its safe-haven and has access to feeding toys.

1. Gauge where you need to start this session; some pets will need to be in constant visual contact with you and cannot be left alone in a room while others can be left alone in a room for a couple of minutes. Observe for any displacement or conflict behaviours as you walk towards the exit from the room where your pet stays (see Handout B3 – Identifying Displacement and Conflict-related Behaviours). When you see displacement behaviours, stop the movement and ask for a 'Watch' or 'Touch' cue (see Handout C2 – How to Teach a 'Watch Me' and 'Touch' Cue).
   - If your pet responds to the cues reward it, and use the 'Settle' cue to reduce your pet's arousal levels (see Handout C4 – Teaching a Pet how to Settle on Cue).
   - If your pet cannot perform these behaviours, you will need to move closer to your pet, and repeat the cues. You will either maintain the new distance or move closer depending on your pet's response.
2. At this distance, observe your pet to see if it responds to you ignoring it.
   - If your pet looks towards you without showing displacement or conflict behaviours, use the marker cue to reinforce this calmer behaviour (see Handout C6 – Marker Training).
   - If you notice displacement behaviours, ask for a 'Touch' or 'Watch' to redirect your dog to you. Once you have its attention, give the 'Settle' cue to reduce its arousal level before continuing with the exercise.
3. After several repetitions of training at this distance, your pet should be able to interact with the feeding toys without showing displacement behaviours. This is the point where you can progress.
4. Increase the distance from your pet until it shows interest in you again; this may only be one step at this early stage of the desensitization programme. Repeat steps 1 and 2 until you stand at this distance without your pet showing displacement behaviours.
5. Once you can leave the room your pet is in, and it continues to interact with its feeding toys without showing displacement behaviours, you can build the duration you are away from it. This is done by following steps 1 – 4 but increasing the duration you are away from your pet instead of increasing the distance you are from your pet.

Stage 2 – separation through a transparent barrier; the owner at home

Follow the same steps as in stage 1:

- gauge distance you can move from the barrier;
- train at this distance;
- gradually increase the distance; and
- gradually increase the duration you are away from your pet.

Stage 3 – separation through a solid barrier; the owner is at home

You can start this stage once your pet is calm when it's away from you for several minutes but can see the opening (transparent barrier). Follow the same approach as stage 2.

Stage 4 – separation, the owner is not at home

You can only work on this stage once your pet is able to stay in a different area of the home (e.g. its safe-haven) without you for an extended duration. Follow the same steps as the previous stages. Start desensitizing your pet to noises and behaviours related to departure. For example, wearing a coat or shoes, taking keys and opening the door.

1. Start by leaving your pet in its safe-haven with feeding toys. Ideally, you can leave a camera facing your pet, and watch it on your phone or computer.
2. As the pet settles into chewing its toy, pretend to leave the house. For example, make noises with your keys or open the door.
3. If you see that your dog stops chewing its toy, or starts vocalizing, stop and wait to see your pet's response.
4. If your pet settles and goes back to rest or to chew its toy, continue the exercise. If your pet does not settle and appears over-aroused, go to it and give it the 'Settle' cue. Once your pet settles, you can continue the exercise.
5. Once your pet is settled when it hears one sound, you can desensitize it to other sounds, and later a combination of the sounds.

NB It may take multiple sessions, over weeks or months, before you will be able to leave your pet alone at home. It is crucial you do not rush this training as you could increase your pet's sensitivity to you leaving instead of reducing it.

Stage 5 – duration of separation; the owner is not at home

Once your pet is calm when you leave the house, you can continue and desensitize your pet for more extended periods of being alone at home. Follow the same approach as above, starting with a short duration and slowly increasing.

Ideally, you can set a camera facing your pet and watch it on your phone or computer. Aim to return before your pet becomes agitated. The first few sessions may be a trial and error as you gauge how long your pet can be left alone. Start with short periods based on the previous stages (i.e. leaving the pet alone when you are at home). It is better to start with short periods and take longer to desensitize your pet than starting with long periods and increasing the pet's sensitivity to being left alone at home.

If at any point during the sessions your pet shows signs that it has crossed its behavioural threshold (e.g. displacement, trying to escape, vocalizing or aggression) ask for a 'Watch' or 'Touch' cue.

Index

Note: Page numbers in **bold** type refer to **figures**
Page numbers in *italic* type refer to *tables*

LARGEMOUTH BASS AQUACULTURE

LARGEMOUTH BASS AQUACULTURE

Edited by

James Tidwell, Shawn Coyle and Leigh Anne Bright

5m Publishing

First published 2019

Published by
5M Publishing Ltd,
Benchmark House,
8 Smithy Wood Drive,
Sheffield, S35 1QN, UK
Tel: +44 (0) 1234 81 81 80
www.5mpublishing.com

A Catalogue record for this book is available from the British Library

ISBN 9781789180480

Book layout by Servis Filmsetting Ltd, Stockport, Cheshire
Printed and bound in Wales by Gomer Press Ltd
Photos by the authors unless otherwise indicated
Bass drawing on the front cover by Rick Hill, Kentucky Division of Fish and Wildlife Resources
Front cover design by Patrick Tidwell

Contents

Contributors

Phillip W. Bettoli, Department of Biology, Tennessee Technological University, Cookeville, Tennessee, USA

Leigh Anne Bright, Kentucky State University, Division of Aquaculture, Frankfort, Kentucky, USA

Angela Caporelli, Kentucky Department of Agriculture, Frankfort, Kentucky, USA

Shawn D. Coyle, Kentucky State University, Division of Aquaculture, Frankfort, Kentucky, USA

Robert M. Durborow, Kentucky State University, Aquaculture Research Center, Frankfort, Kentucky, USA

Carole R. Engle, Engle-Stone Aquatic$, LLC, Adjunct Faculty, Virginia Seafood AREC, Virginia Polytechnic Institute and State University, Blacksburg, Virginia, USA

Boris Gomelsky, Kentucky State University, Division of Aquaculture, Frankfort, Kentucky, USA

Todd S. Harmon, Walt Disney World, Animal Programs, Lake Buena Vista, Florida, USA

Habte-Michael Habte-Tsion, Aquaculture Research Center, Kentucky State University, Frankfort, Kentucky, USA

Chengyue Liu, Fisheries College, Ocean University of China, Qingdao, China

Michael D. Matthews, A.E. Wood Fish Hatchery, San Marcos, Texas, USA

Leandro E. Miranda, US Geological Survey, Mississippi Cooperative Fish and Wildlife Research Unit, Mississippi State University, Mississippi, USA

Kathryn M. Mitchell, Kentucky State University, Aquaculture Research Center, Frankfort, Kentucky, USA

John G. Nickum, Retired, National Aquaculture Coordinator, Department of the Interior, U.S Fish and Wildlife Service, Washington D.C., USA

Eric Peatman, Auburn University, School of Fisheries, Aquaculture and Aquatic Sciences, Auburn, Alabama, USA

Waldemar Rossi Jr., Aquaculture Research Center, Kentucky State University, Frankfort, Kentucky, USA

Kenneth J. Semmens, Kentucky State University, Division of Aquaculture, Frankfort, Kentucky, USA

James H. Tidwell, Kentucky State University, Aquaculture Research Center, Frankfort, Kentucky, USA

Joseph R. Tomasso, School of Fisheries, Aquaculture and Aquatic Sciences, Auburn University, Auburn, Alabama, USA

Yangen Zhou, Key Laboratory of Mariculture (Ocean University of China), Ministry of Education, China

CHAPTER 1

Largemouth bass natural history

Leandro E. Miranda[1] *and Phillip W. Bettoli*[2]

[1]US Geological Survey, Mississippi Cooperative Fish and Wildlife Research Unit, Mississippi State, Mississippi, USA

[2]Department of Biology, Tennessee Technological University, Cookeville, Tennessee, USA

1.1 Introduction

The largemouth bass (*Micropterus salmoides*) stands out as one of North America's most popular sport-fish. Its common name, and other vernacular names (Table 1.1, Cloutman and Olmsted, 1983), reflect the striking size of its jaws, with the lower jaw projecting very strongly, and the maxilla in the adult extending beyond the hind margin of the eye. It is a member of the family Centrarchidae, a diverse and prominent family endemic to North America. The family consists of seven genera, among them the black basses, genus *Micropterus*, which includes multiple species. Evidence suggests that the ancestral *Micropterus* began allopatric speciation about 10 million years ago, driven by vicariance caused by sea-level fluctuations (Near et al., 2003; Smith et al., 2015). It is estimated that the largemouth bass separated from the Florida bass *M. floridanus* less than 5 million years ago (Smith et al., 2015).

The largemouth bass was first described by French naturalist Bernard Germain de Lacépède in his 1800 book *Histoire Naturelle des Poissons, Volume III*. The description was made in France based on a drawing and accompanying manuscript notes sent from the vicinity of Charleston, South Carolina (Henshall, 1881). The local name of the fish was "trout," as it still is in some southern states. Lacépède named it *Labrus salmoides*, trout-like wrasse, in accordance with its general appearance and vernacular name. The genus name *Micropterus* is also attributed to Lacépède and his 1801 book *Histoire Naturelle des Poissons, Volume IV*, but he associated the name with the smallmouth bass *Micropterus dolomieu*. *Micropterus* means "small fin," named after a specimen that happened to have a deformed (trimmed) dorsal fin (Henshall, 1881). The largemouth bass was not associated with the genus *Micropterus* until the 1870s, having some bewildering classifications in the interval that included genus names such as *Bodianus*, *Calliurus*, *Lepomis*, *Etheostoma*, *Cichla*, *Huro*, *Grystes*, *Centrarchus*, and *Dioplites*.

Whereas the genus classification was settled, ichthyologists have not always agreed on the number of *Micropterus* species. Ramsey (1975) commented that when compared with the speciose North American genus *Notropis* (more than 100 valid named species) and genus *Etheostoma*

Table 1.1 Selected attributes of largemouth bass natural history.

Attribute	Description
Scientific name	*Micropterus salmoides*
Common name (English)	Largemouth bass
Common name (French)	Achigan à grande bouche
Common name (Spanish)	Lobina negra
Other vernacular names	Bigmouth, widemouth, bucketmouth, green bass, green trout, pond trout, Oswego bass, Welshman
Age of the species	<5 million years
Native range	Eastern North America
Native range area	3,297,900 km^2
Naturalized range	>50 countries in all continents but Antarctica and Australia
Environment	Warm, eutrophic, mostly lentic, and shallow
Habitat	Submerged plants and underwater structures
Sexuality	Monomorphic, mostly monogamous
Nesting	Excavated substrate in shallow water
Age at sexual maturity	1–4 years old depending on growth rate
Size at maturity	Minimum length near 200–250 mm TL
Contribution of gonads to body weight during spawning season	As high as 10–13% female; <2% males
Fecundity	$F = 0.00003*TL^{3.407}$
Diameter of mature eggs	0.75–1.5 mm
Diameter of water-hardened eggs	1.5–2 mm
Spawning temperature	Start 14–16°C; peaks 18–20°C
Length of spawning season	30–120 days, depending on latitude
Nest spacing	3–6 m apart
Nest guarding	Males, possibly females
Egg hatching	3–4 days
Total length of larvae at hatch	4 mm TL
Total length of larvae at swim-up	6 mm TL
Average length at age 1, 2, and 3	102, 202, 273 mm TL
Maximum size and age	787 mm TL, 10.1 kg, 24 years
Weight-length relationships for fish >150 mm TL	$W = 0.000002965*L^{3.273}$
Weight-length relationships for fish 25–150 mm TL	$W = 0.000020216*L^{2.858}$
Age 0 mortality	10–20% per week
Age 1+ mortality	35–37% per year
Diet	Invertebrates to about 35 mm TL; switch to fish diet at 35–160 mm TL; mostly fish afterwards
Daily ration	2–6% of body weight
Gape width	Gape width = -5.59 + 0.14*TL (all units in mm)
Optimum temperature for growth	25–30°C
Temperature tolerance	Juveniles stop feeding below 6°C; can tolerate spells up to 40°C
Dissolved oxygen tolerance	Growth reduced below 4 mg/l; prolonged exposure below 1 mg/l is lethal
Salinity tolerance	up to 8–12 ppt

(over 80 species), the half-dozen or so species of *Micropterus* would seem to have presented a relatively straightforward problem in taxonomic definition. Nevertheless, over 40 years later the number of extant species has increased to nine (Near and Koppelman, 2009), and as many as eight additional species are being considered (Baker et al., 2013; Long et al., 2015). Until recently the Florida bass had been considered a subspecies of largemouth bass, but has now been given species status (Kassler et al., 2002); therefore, facts about largemouth bass assembled during the 20th century and reported herein reflect these two species as one.

1.2 Geography

1.2.1 Native range

Encompassing an area of 3,297,900 km^2 over the eastern half of North America, the largemouth bass has the widest native distribution of the black basses (MacCrimmon and Robbins, 1975; Lee et al., 1980; Pyron, 1999). The eastern limit of its native range is the Atlantic seaboard extending northward from the St. Mary's River in Georgia to the James River in Virginia in coastal watersheds (Figure 1.1). The southern limits of the native range are the Gulf of Mexico

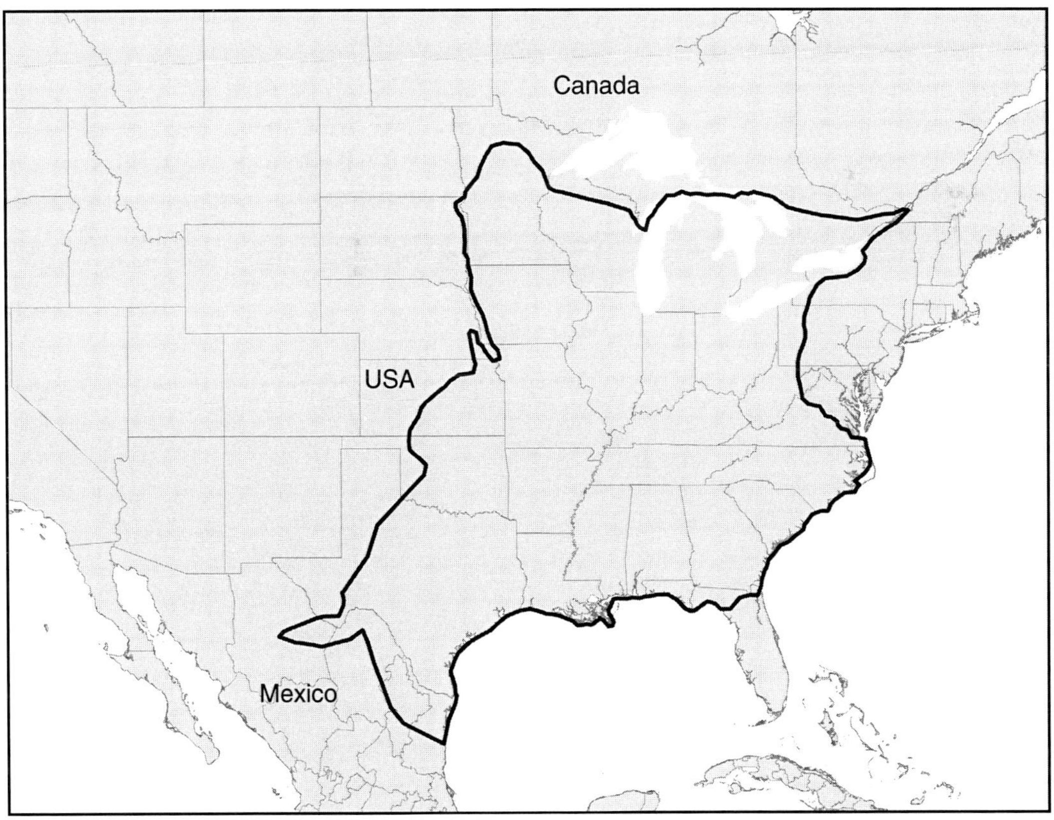

Figure 1.1 Native range of largemouth bass in North America (modified from Lee et al., 1980).

drainages from the Suwanee River in Florida to northern Mexico. The exact southwestern limit is obscured by early transplants, but would appear to have been the Rio Conchos, a tributary of the Rio Grande in north central Mexico, to the Rio Soto La Marina, a tributary of the Gulf of Mexico in northern Mexico. The western limit includes much of the western Mississippi River Basin extending into the Great Plains region where the precise boundary is variable depending on annual precipitation. It likely extends from the confluence of the Rio Conchos and Rio Grande in a northeasterly direction through central Texas, western Oklahoma, central Kansas, extreme eastern Nebraska, western Iowa, and most of Minnesota and Wisconsin south of the Rainy River and Lake Superior drainages. The northern boundary includes much of the Great Lakes basin, exclusive of Lake Superior but including the upper St. Lawrence River. The northeastern limit is the Ottawa River system southward into the St. Lawrence River and the Chaudiere River south of Quebec City. This northeastern limit extends south into the upper Ohio River drainage in western New York, western Pennsylvania, Ohio, West Virginia, and possibly western Maryland. The species is not native to the New England states or the Atlantic seaboard north of the James River in Virginia, and was absent, except peripherally, from much of the Appalachian and Ozark Mountains.

1.2.2 Naturalized range

The native range has been extended through intentional and unintentional transfers in North America, and to every continent but Antarctica and Australia. Extensions of self-sustaining populations of largemouth bass beyond its native range have been mostly the result of intentional transfers but, occasionally, have resulted from natural movements through manmade waterways or other connections. The widespread construction of reservoirs throughout most of the 20th century created favorable habitats in regions otherwise unsuited for the species (Moyle, 1986; Gido and Brown, 1999). Largemouth bass stockings were sanctioned by US government actions beginning in 1871, and by 1900 largemouth bass were found in all conterminous states of the USA (MacCrimmon and Robbins, 1975; Moyle, 1976). The species has also become established across southern regions of Canada warm enough to support it, and most of Mexico and Central America (Lee et al., 1980). Beginning in the late 1800s, the species was introduced into Europe, southern Africa, South America, parts of Asia and many oceanic islands, and by the end of the 20th century it was established in over 50 countries (MacCrimmon and Robbins, 1975; Welcomme, 1992; Rahel, 2007). The goals of introductions have included improving recreational fishing, improving local fish assemblages, and aquaculture. However, in some countries the largemouth bass is listed as a nuisance species because of its effects on native fish communities (Jackson, 2002), and is currently targeted for eradication in Japan (Tsunoda et al., 2010).

1.3 Habitat

The largemouth bass is a warmwater generalist that inhabits a wide variety of habitats, partially accounting for its broad spatial distribution (Pyron, 1999). Generally, it seems to be better adapted to warm and eutrophic waters than most other *Micropterus* species, excluding Florida bass, although throughout its range it co-occurs with many of its congeners. The species is often common in natural lakes, wetlands, backwaters, slow moving streams, and coastal marshes, and has thrived in artificial impoundments small and large (Warren, 2009). In streams, they occupy various lotic habitats but are most common in low-gradient streams and slow-moving pools; avoiding low-order streams. The species is often found along shallow littoral areas associated with submerged aquatic vegetation; with underwater structures including woody debris, rocks, and flooded terrestrial vegetation; and with steep bank slopes or undercut banks (Annett et al., 1996; Raibley et al., 1997).

Largemouth bass can tolerate a fairly broad range of conditions (Chapter 4). Although they can tolerate the high temperatures (near 40°C; Beitinger et al., 2000) associated with shallow waters in their southern range, the duration and severity of winters has been associated with the northern limits of their geographical distribution (Miranda, 2014). Prolonged stints with temperatures <6°C reportedly limit food intake and cause increased mortality of juveniles (Garvey et al., 1998). Although largemouth bass can tolerate a wide range of dissolved oxygen concentrations, their growth is reduced substantially at levels below 4 mg/l (Stewart et al., 1967) and prolonged exposures to levels below 1.0 mg/l are considered lethal (Moss and Scott, 1961). Although activity levels and foraging success may vary with water clarity (Reid et al., 1999; Shoup and Wahl, 2009), largemouth bass can thrive in both clear and turbid waters. The pH level affects juveniles more than adults; juvenile mortality has been reported at pH levels lower than 5 due to increased energy demand and reduced feeding (Orsatti and Colgan, 1987; McCormick and Jensen, 1992). Largemouth bass inhabiting coastal marshes can tolerate, at least temporarily, salinities up to 8–12 ppt, with juveniles being more tolerant than adults (Meador and Kelso, 1990).

1.4 Feeding

1.4.1 Adult diets

It could be argued that few freshwater fishes have a broader diet than adult largemouth bass, which is partly related to their wide geographic distribution. In addition to fish prey, the literature has documented adult largemouth bass consuming terrestrial insects, aquatic insects, mollusks, crayfish, reptiles, amphibians, birds, and even small mammals (Hodgson and Hansen, 2005; Purdom et al., 2015). That said, the diet of adult largemouth bass in all but the least productive aquatic systems consists primarily of fish. In southern US waters, important fish prey includes gizzard shad (*Dorosoma cepedianum*) and threadfin shad (*D. petenense*); other centrarchids, especially bluegills (*Lepomis macrochirus*); and various minnow (Cyprinidae) species.

In less productive aquatic systems at higher latitudes, largemouth bass will rely heavily on zooplankton, and aquatic and terrestrial insects (Hodgson and Kitchell, 1987), in addition to whatever fishes are present (for example, yellow perch [*Perca flavescens*]), including juvenile largemouth bass (Clady, 1974). In coastal lakes in New England with access to the Atlantic Ocean, introduced largemouth bass readily prey upon anadromous river herring (alewife [*Alosa pseudoharengus*] and blueback herring [*A. aestivalis*]; Yako et al., 2000). On the Pacific coast, introduced largemouth bass prey upon Pacific salmon (Tabor et al., 2007), as well as other native and introduced fish species.

When transplanted abroad, adult largemouth bass prey upon whatever suitably size fish prey are available. For instance, introduced largemouth bass in Cuba preyed heavily upon several species of topminnows (Cyprinodontidae; Rivero, 1937). In Puerto Rico, introduced adult largemouth bass preyed on other introduced species, such as threadfin shad, sunfish, tilapia (*Oreochromis mossambicus* and *Coptodon rendalli*), and peacock bass (*Cichla ocellaris*), as well as native species, such as the bigmouth sleeper (*Gobiomorus dormitor*) (Bacheler et al., 2004). In a South African river, introduced largemouth bass adults relied primarily on dragonflies (Odonata) and river crabs (*Potamonautes sidneyi*) during low-flow seasons but availed themselves of juvenile estuarine fishes entering the river during periods of high flows (Wasserman et al., 2011). As these and numerous other articles will attest, the largemouth bass in its native and introduced range is an extremely opportunistic feeder that will prey on fish when present, but readily switch to other food resources when necessary.

Perhaps the only factor curbing what a largemouth bass will consume, be it fish or some other prey item, is its gape limitation. First described in detail by Lawrence (1958), the size of prey fishes of various species that can be consumed by largemouth bass is gape limited, although the mouth morphology of largemouth bass allows them to consume larger prey than other predatory species of similar length, such as smallmouth bass (*M. dolomieu*), muskellunge (*Esox masquinongy*), and walleye (*Sander vitreus*). The gape width of largemouth bass increased rapidly from about 3% to 10% in largemouth bass 50 to 140 mm total length (TL), and reached 13% by about 550 mm TL (Hill et al., 2004). Although largemouth bass are physically capable of ingesting very large prey, they typically prey upon fish with body depths well below the maximum size that could be ingested (Hambright, 1991).

1.4.2 Ontogenetic dietary shifts

Like most other fish species, at hatching a larval largemouth bass must rely on its yolk sac for nutrition for several days. Once yolk-sac absorption is complete, largemouth bass fry that are about 6 mm TL leave the nest and become swim-up fry. At this critical period, the fry must switch to exogenous feeding. They may feed initially on small zooplankton such as rotifers (Wickstrom and Applegate, 1989), but fry quickly switch as they grow in length to larger microcrustacean zooplankton (copepod nauplii, adult copepods, and cladocerans) and immature aquatic insects (Parmley et al., 1986). If zooplankton are abundant and a largemouth bass hatches earlier in the growing season than other competitors for zooplankton prey (for example, juvenile clupeids and other centrarchids), growth can be rapid (1.0–1.4 mm per day; Goodgame and Miranda, 1993; Dorsey, 1997).

At a length of about 25 mm TL, largemouth bass will start to prey on fish if suitably sized prey are abundant and readily available and they will stop preying on zooplankton at about 35 mm TL (Huskey and Turnigan, 2001). In southern US waters, age 0 bluegills and shads are typical fish prey of fingerling largemouth bass. The onset of piscivory, which has been the subject of intense study for decades (Keast and Eadie, 1985; Bettoli et al., 1992; Mittelbach and Persson, 1998; Yasuno et al., 2012), has profound ramifications for individuals as well as the entire cohort of largemouth bass hatched in a given year. Specifically, a fingerling that switches to piscivory early (that is, at a small size) will grow much faster than a bass feeding on insects or zooplankton and it will likely maintain and increase that growth advantage over the course of the first growing season and beyond (Olson, 1996; Ludsin and DeVries, 1997).

As noted in the previous section, piscivores, such as largemouth bass, face gape limitations when consuming fish prey (Mittelbach and Persson, 1998; Nowlin et al., 2006) and faster growth by piscivorous fingerlings allows them to consume a broader suite of potential prey fishes throughout the growing season than smaller nonpiscivorous fingerlings. Conversely, if largemouth bass hatch late in the spring their potential fish prey (for example, age 0 shads and sunfishes) may be too large and grow too fast to be vulnerable to predation (Olson, 1996). Faster growth and larger size often equate to better survival of juvenile largemouth bass through their first growing season (Shelton et al., 1979; Maceina et al., 1988). Switching early to piscivory and achieving larger sizes also promotes the deposition of lipids and higher lipid reserves can increase overwinter survival in many species, including age 0 largemouth bass (Miranda and Hubbard, 1994; Ludsin and DeVries, 1997; Biro et al., 2004).

Hatching early in systems with abundant fish prey does not guarantee early onset of piscivory by largemouth bass, with all of its attendant advantages. Savino and Stein (1982) demonstrated in a laboratory study that the predatory success of largemouth bass feeding on bluegills declined with increases in structural complexity. Bettoli et al. (1992) and others subsequently demonstrated in field studies that structural complexity in the form of aquatic vegetation delays the onset of piscivory in largemouth bass. For instance, largemouth bass collected from densely vegetated habitats in Lake Conroe, Texas, did not become piscivorous (that is, at least 60% of fish with some stomach contents had fish remains in the gut) until reaching lengths of 160 mm; whereas, largemouth bass collected from vegetation-free habitats were piscivorous at 80 mm. Concomitant with the earlier onset of piscivory were significantly greater mean lengths at age 1 (~200 mm versus ~130 mm). As a final note, early onset of piscivory does not necessarily guarantee that a largemouth bass does not revert back to relying on invertebrate food resources. For instance, Huskey and Turnigan (2001) observed that following the onset of piscivory 122–317 mm TL largemouth bass relied more on crayfish prey than fish in their diet in a lake in Florida.

In the context of aquaculture, piscivory by largemouth bass has long received attention because largemouth bass (like most piscivorous species) will readily resort to cannibalism (Stranahan, 1906). If given the opportunity, largemouth bass 10–14 mm long in laboratory aquaria will cannibalize 6 mm TL individuals (Johnson and Post, 1996). In hatcheries, cannibalism will arise to problematic levels unless the fingerlings are routinely graded to achieve homogenous size groups (Nelson et al., 1974; Bondari, 1983) and sufficient quantities of natural forage (or pelleted feed) are provided.

1.4.3 Feeding behavior

Unlike a classic ambush predator, such as northern pike (*E. lucius*; Harper and Blake, 1991), largemouth bass are opportunistic, mobile predators that rely mostly on visual cues when stalking their prey. Suction feeding (that is, rapid expansion of the buccal cavity) is employed by many piscivorous fishes and other species rely primarily on ram feeding (that is, forward motion of the body or jaws to engulf prey); most species, including largemouth bass, can employ a combination of these two modalities (Gardiner and Motta, 2012). Largemouth bass can successfully forage in a variety of habitats with diverse levels of structural complexity, at diverse depths and water clarities, and at diverse light levels. Their ubiquitous distribution and the wide array of prey they consume reflect their plasticity in feeding behavior (Almeida et al., 2012). Although they rely mostly on visual cues, largemouth bass are capable of feeding at very low light levels (McMahon and Holanov, 1995) and when deprived of sight, they can locate and successfully ingest fish prey using their lateral line system (Gardiner and Motta, 2012). When largemouth bass grow large enough to reduce their risk of being preyed upon by other piscivores (including their own kind), they are able to utilize a broader range of habitats and prey to support their diets (Ward and Neumann, 1998; Huskey and Turnigan, 2001).

In their native habitats, largemouth bass have coevolved with their principal prey species and prey fish have developed behavioral strategies to reduce their predation risk. Perhaps the best studied largemouth bass predator–prey system involves bluegill as the prey. For instance, bluegill will inhabit beds of vegetation and exhibit distinct swimming behaviors to reduce their predation risk when in the presence of largemouth bass (Savino and Stein, 1989). Potential prey species that did not coevolve with largemouth bass lack the behavioral traits necessary to reduce their predation risk. For instance, early efforts to control nuisance aquatic vegetation by stocking grass carp *Ctenopharyngodon idella* consistently failed when small (< 200 mm TL) fish were stocked because of heavy predation by largemouth bass (Shireman et al., 1978). Many other accounts exist of naive fish species lacking an appropriate repertoire of behaviors to reduce largemouth bass predation, to the detriment of local populations (Rivero, 1937; Azuma and Motomura, 1998; Jang et al., 2006).

1.5 Bioenergetics

The bioenergetics of largemouth bass have not been as well-studied as their food habits and foraging behavior; nevertheless, a sizeable literature on the thermal ecology and bioenergetics of largemouth bass extends back at least four decades (reviewed by Bevelhimer and Breck, 2009). One of the earliest largemouth bass bioenergetics models was produced by Rice et al. (1983) and subsequently validated by Rice and Cochran (1984). Other bioenergetics models for largemouth bass have been produced and evaluated by Carline (1987) and Whitledge and Hayward (1997). In those and other studies of bioenergetics, the goal often is to model growth and consumption as a function of fish size, temperature, and perhaps the genetic traits of the fish stock (Venables et al., 1977). Of particular interest to aquaculturists is the temperature at which daily ration, food conversion, and growth are maximized for fish at different life history stages. The temperature at which growth is optimized can be measured directly, in a hatchery setting, or indirectly by estimating the final temperature preference. The temperature that a fish will ultimately gravitate towards when given a choice is termed the final preferendum; that thermal endpoint can also be defined as the temperature at which the acclimation temperature of a fish equals the temperature selected acutely in a laboratory gradient. The final preferendum is usually a good predictor of the temperature that maximizes growth and fitness of individuals (Jobling, 1981; Kelsch, 1996).

Temperatures that optimized growth were reported to be 27°C for largemouth bass fry (Strawn, 1961) and ~25°C for juveniles and subadults (Niimi and Beamish, 1974). Tidwell et al. (2003) reported that feed conversion and growth by fingerling largemouth bass were similar at

26 and 32°C and both were higher than at 20°C. Díaz et al. (2007) stated the final preferendum of fingerling largemouth bass was similar to the range of temperatures that optimized growth (28–29°C). The final preferendum for largemouth bass has also been reported to be ~30°C (juvenile and subadults in field; Neill and Magnuson, 1974), 27–32°C (adults in laboratory; Venables et al., 1978), 32.2°C (juveniles in laboratory; Cincotta and Stauffer, 1984), and 27.1–30.5°C (juveniles in laboratory; Koppelman et al., 1988).

Neal and Noble (2006) applied a bioenergetics model to ascertain why non-native largemouth bass in Puerto Rico had short lifespans (few fish lived beyond age 3) and slow growth. They concluded that multiple spawning events each year directed more energy to reproduction than somatic growth; water temperatures that never cooled below 23°C were also implicated. They reported that largemouth bass across the globe achieved their maximum size at a latitude of about 28°N (peninsular Florida; northern Mexico); shorter growing seasons at higher latitudes decreased the maximum size that largemouth bass achieved.

Bioenergetics models require information on (or predict) daily rations. Although daily rations of largemouth bass fed *ad libitum* can reach 5 or 6% of body weight·d^{-1} (Cochran and Adelman, 1982; Carline, 1987), daily rations in field and hatchery settings are usually closer to 2% (Whitledge and Hayward, 1997).

1.6 Reproduction

1.6.1 Sexual dimorphism and monogamy

Dimorphism evident in many fish taxa is commonly manifested as size, color, or shape variations (Hedrick and Temeles, 1989; Parker, 1992). In *Micropterus*, sexual dimorphism is not evident as it is in other centrarchid genera, particularly *Lepomis* (Ehlinger et al., 1997). In fact, outside of the breeding season when gametes may be extruding, the only positive way to determine the sex of largemouth bass is through meticulous examination of the vent (Benz and Jacobs, 1986).

The monomorphism exhibited by largemouth bass has usually been associated with monogamous species (Clutton-Brock, 1989). Evidence suggests that *Micropterus* males are only rarely bigamous (Ridgway et al., 1989; Wiegmann et al., 1992). However, males may have more than one female mate as a result of extended or disrupted breeding seasons. In a largemouth bass population in South Carolina studied through genetic analyses, eggs in nearly 90% of nests were almost exclusively the product of one male and one female. The other 10% of the nests included eggs from 1 male and 2–3 females (DeWoody et al., 2000).

1.6.2 Nesting habitat

Largemouth bass nest on the substrate of shallow areas of lakes, rivers, and backwaters (Breder, 1936; Annett et al., 1996). Nests are excavated over a variety of substrates but coarse gravel and sand and the roots and stems of aquatic vegetation tend to be used most often (Allan and Romero, 1975; Annett et al., 1996). Although nests have been reported in water deeper than 5 m, most nests are constructed in shallower water and average 0.5–2 m deep (Kramer and Smith, 1962; Heidinger, 1975). Most males select nest sites near cover where they are less exposed to nest incursion by egg predators (Vogele and Rainwater, 1975; Annett et al., 1996). Average nest spacing ranged from 6 to 9 m in an Arkansas reservoir or about 15 nests/100 m transect (Hunt and Annett, 2002). Other studies have reported lower densities of 1–3 nests/100 m of shoreline (Vogele and Rainwater, 1975).

1.6.3 Age and size at maturity

Largemouth bass typically reach sexual maturity at ages 1–5 and at minimum sizes near 200–250 mm TL. In fast-growing populations in the lower latitudes of their native range, largemouth bass can reach 250 mm and become sexually mature by age 1 (Clugston, 1964; Nieman et al., 1979). In higher latitudes fish grow slower and maturity is often delayed to ages 3–5 for males and ages 4–5 for females (Kelley, 1962; Scott and Crossman, 1973).

1.6.4 Gametogenesis

The ovaries of largemouth bass are bilobed, elongated nearly circular in cross section, and can make up as much as 10–15% of the body weight during the spawning season (Timmons et al., 1980; Miranda and Muncy, 1987). Male testes make up a smaller fraction of the body weight, peaking at 1.5–2% (Bennett and Gibbons, 1975; Brown and Murphy, 2004). Fecundity increases with female size exponentially, but is highly variable, even for fish of the same age or size (Kelley, 1962; Heidinger, 1975; Timmons et al., 1980). Fecundity estimates compiled by Bishop (1968) and Carlander (1977) from various water bodies in the USA indicated ovaries of female bass contained 2,000–145,000 eggs. Warren (2009) used published data to derive an equation that estimated fecundity (f) from total length as:

$$f = 0.00003 * TL^{3.407}$$

This equation predicts that females can produce an average of about 2,000 eggs at 200 mm TL, 8,000 at 300 mm, and 47,000 at 500 mm.

Mature eggs in the ovaries range 0.75–1.5 mm in diameter; after they are fertilized and water-hardened they increase to 1.5–2 mm (Kelley, 1962; Meyer, 1970; Heidinger, 1975). After they are fertilized, the eggs settle to the bottom of the nest and adhere to the substrate. The eggs lie with the oil globule up, and water-harden within 15 min. Sperms have an ovoid head approximately 0.002 mm long, with a tail 0.02 mm long (Carr, 1942). Sperms are viable for only a minute or so after they are released.

1.6.5 Spawning season

Once they reach maturity, largemouth bass spawn annually. Spawning typically occurs from early spring to mid-summer, extending for less than 1 month to several months depending on latitude (Conover, 1992; Waters and Noble, 2004; Rogers et al., 2006). Spawning begins when water temperature rises to 14–16°C, peaks at 18–20°C, and dwindles as water warms up to and exceeds 25°C. Large adults reportedly spawn before smaller adults (Miranda and Muncy, 1987). The male guards the eggs and continues to guard the young fish for several weeks after they hatch

(Heidinger, 1976). During this stage, male largemouth bass show heightened aggression and demonstrate a high susceptibility to angling (Suski and Philipp, 2004).

Duration and timing of spawning by largemouth bass at the population and individual levels depend on many interacting factors. Duration, as estimated from the range of number of daily growth rings in otoliths of fish from the same cohort, exhibits a latitudinal gradient: 26 days in New York (Schmidt and Fabrizio, 1980), 36–51 days in Illinois (Miller and Storck, 1982; Kohler et al., 1993), 60–71 days in Mississippi (Goodgame and Miranda, 1993), 68–75 days in Texas (Isely and Noble, 1987; Maceina et al., 1988), and over 120 days in Puerto Rico (Ozen and Noble, 2002). This gradient may represent an adaptation to length of the growing season (Conover and Present, 1990).

In theory, a cohort may follow one of two primary sequences of events during the first year of life, depending on how early in the reproductive season they hatch (Ludsin and DeVries, 1997). An early hatched cohort should begin feeding on invertebrates and make the transition to piscivory during summer, allowing for rapid growth the remainder of the year. Alternatively, a late-hatched cohort is less prone to make the transition to piscivory because fish prey may be too large, leading to slower growth, higher exposure to predation, and comparatively lower contribution to the new year class (Ludsin and DeVries, 1997).

1.6.6 Nesting, spawning behavior, and parental care

Largemouth bass are solitary nesters. Males use caudal sweeping to excavate circular, depression nests 0.5–1.0 m diameter (Kramer and Smith, 1962; Cooke et al., 2001). Nests are usually spaced out 3–6 m apart. The males normally guard an area about 2 m diameter around the nest (Annett et al., 1996). If there is a visual obstruction or barrier, nests tend to be excavated closer together (Vogele and Rainwater, 1975).

When a female joins the male, they slowly circle the nest, side by side. Male courtship behaviors include opercle flaring, hovering, flashing, and herding potential female partners with gentle nudges and nipping (Allan and Romero, 1975; Cooke et al., 2001). Spawning occurs with both fish tilted laterally so their vents are close together. Both parents shudder as eggs and sperm are released simultaneously (Heidinger, 1975).

The male then takes a position over the eggs and continuously fans them with his fins until they hatch (Cooke et al., 2001). The current created by the fanning keeps the eggs free of silt and ensures that they are always in contact with freshwater. Depending on water temperature, in the southern US eggs generally hatch in 3–4 days (Heidinger, 1975). The male will continue to guard the fry until they disperse from the nest. Nesting success may be reduced if the temperature drops below 14–15°C. This temperature usually causes the male to leave the nest (Kelley, 1968; Allan and Romero, 1975). Without a guard the eggs will not be fanned or protected and the likelihood of suffocation and predation increases. During the spawning season the males reportedly do not eat and many males may die during this period likely due to poor body condition (Heidinger, 1975).

Whereas most accounts indicate that parental care in largemouth bass is provided exclusively by males (Breder, 1936; Heidinger, 1975; Cooke et al., 2006), DeWoody et al., (2000) documented biparental care. Most of the nests examined by DeWoody et al. (2000) in a South Carolina reservoir were attended by a female and a guardian male. The attendant female generally faced the nest while 1–2 m away and the attendant male positioned over the nest, but these positions were occasionally reversed. The guardian male showed no aggression towards the female, and the attendant female actively chased away conspecific nest intruders and predators. Nests with attendant females occurred across several stages of brood development, indicating that nest guarding by the female extended well past spawning, and into incubation of eggs to the free-swimming fry stage of the brood. A few nests that lacked parental males were guarded exclusively by females. Biparental care may not be of general occurrence across largemouth bass populations, but the existence of biparental care in largemouth bass is consistent with several reproductive life history traits including large body size, large eggs, sexual monomorphism, monogamy, and extended parental care (DeWoody et al., 2000).

1.6.7 Early larvae

Newly hatched larvae measure about 4 mm TL (Heidinger, 1975). Depending on temperature, the larvae remain in the nest for about 5–10 more days until they become free-swimming fry, schooling above the nest. After another day or two, parents move the fry to allow them to forage while still providing parental care (Cooke et al., 2002). Initially the fry form tight schools or "fry balls" that begin to forage on zooplankton, but as they grow, schools become broader and looser. Schools break up 20–30 days after hatching when fish are about 20–25 mm TL. Largemouth bass may be one of the most attentive parents in the centrarchid family, often remaining with schooling fry for several days or weeks after hatching (Breder, 1936). On average, largemouth bass may invest 3–6 weeks in parental care from spawning to fry dispersal (Kramer and Smith, 1962; Cooke et al., 2006).

1.7 Growth and Mortality

1.7.1 Maximum size and age

The largest largemouth bass on record was caught by angling in a pond in the state of Georgia, USA, in 1932. It weighted 10.1 kg with an estimated length of 787 mm TL (IGFA, 2015). This record was recently tied by a largemouth bass caught in Lake Biwa, Japan (IGFA, 2015). Even bigger largemouth bass may have once lived. For instance, Smith (1907) reported that "examples weighing as much as 20–25 lbs [9.1–11.3 kg] have been taken in lakes" in Florida. In 1907 only two species of *Micropterus* were recognized – largemouth bass and smallmouth bass. The oldest largemouth bass aged was a 23- or 24-year-old individual measuring 584 mm TL that was collected in the state of New York (Green and Heidinger, 1994). The largest largemouth bass in Canada was caught in Ontario in 1948 and weighed 4.7 kg (Scott and Crossman, 1973).

The maximum age of largemouth bass also follows a latitudinal distribution. In northern latitudes including Minnesota, Wisconsin, and Ontario longevity can be 13–16 years (Carlander, 1977), but in Puerto Rico few largemouth bass live beyond age 3 (Neal and Noble, 2006). There is evidence that at least in some populations older individuals are mostly females (Heidinger, 1975; Webb and Reeves, 1975; Carlander, 1977).

1.7.2 Growth rate

Growth rates of largemouth bass vary greatly across their range, with populations in southern latitudes having some of the highest growth rates (Beamesderfer and North, 1995). The variability in growth rates is due mostly to the longer growing season and higher temperatures in southern latitudes (Clugston, 1964; Coutant and DeAngelis, 1983), although local forage availability can account for much of the variability (Keast and Eadie, 1985; Hoyle and Keast, 1987; Garvey and Stein, 1996). Largemouth bass generally do not grow in temperatures less than 5–10°C and reach maximum growth rates near 25–30°C depending on fish size (see Bioenergetics section). Growth rates generally decrease in temperatures above 30°C, and growth ceases at temperatures > 36°C (Stuber et al., 1982).

Beamesderfer and North (1995) surveyed the literature on largemouth bass in North America searching for estimates of mean length at age. Median length at age of 698 populations ranged from 102 mm at age 1 to 514 mm at age 15 (Figure 1.2). Lengths were inversely correlated with latitude and elevation and directly correlated with air temperature and degree-days. However, these variables accounted for only part of the observed variability in growth rates. Other research suggests that the unexplained variability may also be related to trophic state of the water body, water quality, habitat availability, prey abundance, and fish community composition (Miranda and Durocher, 1986; McCauley and Kilgour, 1990; Meador and Kelso, 1990; Bettoli et al., 1992; Putman et al., 1995). Considering these sources of variability, Helser and Lai (2004) reported that growth across North America varied by more than 120% in terms of average maximum attainable size (L_∞; 360–800 mm) and by more than 88% in terms of the Brody growth coefficient (K; 0.091 to 0.670 per year).

1.7.3 Weight–length relationship

In many cases, size is more relevant than age because physiological and ecological factors are more size-dependent than age-dependent. Weight–length relationships have several applications including estimation of weight from length, estimation of body condition, and morphological comparisons between populations (Froese, 2006). The weight (W) of largemouth bass is

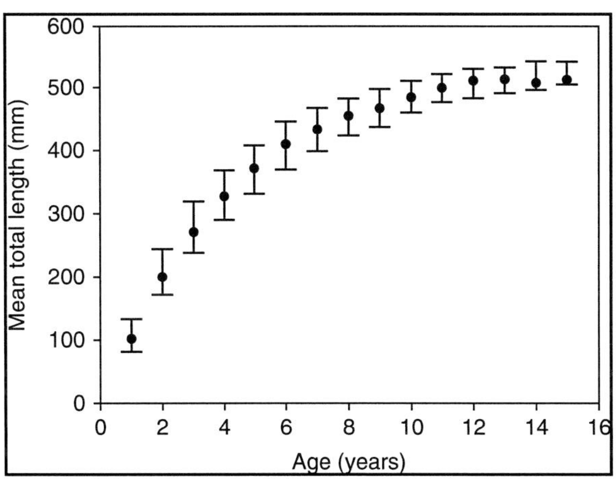

Figure 1.2 Relationship between total length and age of largemouth bass in North America. Values represent median length at age and whiskers indicate 25–75 percentiles. Estimates represent 698 populations compiled by Beamesderfer and North (1995).

exponentially related to their length (L) according to the equation $W = aL^b$, where a is the intercept and b is the slope. The slope is an indicator of condition and growth pattern. When $b = 3$, the growth is considered isometric (that is, all fish dimensions increase at the same rate as fish get longer), hypoallometric if $b < 3$ (that is, the fish increases less in weight than predicted by its increase in length, becoming relatively more elongated as it grows), and hyperallometric if $b > 3$ (that is, the fish increases more in weight than predicted by its increase in length, becoming more roundish as it grows). Based on the assumption that heavier fish of a given length are in better condition, when comparing two populations, the one with the larger b may be considered to be in better condition. A standard weight–length equation commonly used for largemouth bass is $W = 0.000002965{*}L^{3.273}$ where weight is in grams and total length in millimeters (Neumann et al., 2012). This equation is suitable for fish > 150 mm TL, and because it was developed to score body condition, it yields the 75th percentile weight. For fish 25–150 mm TL, we derived the 75th percentile equation $W = 0.000020216{*}L^{2.858}$ with fish collected in Alabama, Georgia, Iowa, and Mississippi (unpublished data).

1.7.4 Age 0 mortality

Juveniles of highly fecund organisms such as fish can experience high mortality rates. Small size and high abundance often render these organisms more susceptible to high rates of mortality during early life stages than during later stages (Houde, 1989). Miller and Kramer (1971) estimated a 9–23% per week embryo mortality, and Miranda et al. (1984) estimated a 13–21% weekly mortality of juveniles in the months after hatching. Length differences within a cohort often result from interactions between time of hatching and subsequent growth. Largemouth bass hatched earlier in the season obtain an initial length advantage over those hatched later, an advantage that may be maintained and increased through the first year of life (Shelton et al., 1979; Miller and Storck, 1984; Isely and Noble, 1987). Time of hatching can affect the ability of young largemouth bass to switch to a fish diet early in the growing season and eventually affect their survival to age 1. Bass that achieve a large length during their first growing season may be less vulnerable to overwinter predation and starvation than smaller members of their cohort (Gutreuter and Anderson, 1985; Goodgame and Miranda, 1993). Post et al. (1998) reported that overwinter mortality was size dependent, strongly affecting bass entering the winter at < 50–60 mm TL.

1.7.5 Age 1+ mortality

Most mortality estimates for largemouth bass available in the literature have been derived through catch-curve analysis, which estimates overall natural and fishing mortality for fish age 1 or older (Miranda and Bettoli, 2007). This analysis assumes constant recruitment and mortality over all age groups. Fewer studies have estimated fishing mortality, which along with overall mortality can be used to derive conditional natural mortality. Conditional natural mortality reflects potential deaths during an interval, say 1 year, had natural mortality been the only acting force of mortality (Miranda and Bettoli, 2007). Beamesderfer and North (1995) reported that conditional annual natural mortality in 40 largemouth bass populations in North America averaged 37% (25–75 percentiles: 21–47). In a separate review, Allen et al. (2008) reported total and fishing mortalities for over 30 largemouth bass populations and based on those estimates conditional annual natural mortality averaged 35% (25–75 percentiles: 27–42).

1.8 Role of stocking

Hatchery-reared largemouth bass have been stocked to mitigate for projects that drastically alter natural habitats and their native fish communities and sport-fisheries. Perhaps one of the best-known examples of mitigation stocking has been the decades-long stocking of largemouth bass into Lake Mead in Nevada–Arizona, which commenced in the 1930s and continued through the 1980s (McCall, 1980). However, at the present time most largemouth bass and Florida bass in North America are stocked to either increase fishable stocks, influence the genetic characteristics of the receiving stock, or to meet both objectives.

A rich literature exists on the efficacy of stocking largemouth bass and Florida bass (hereafter referred to simply as "largemouth bass") at different life-history stages to increase the number and standing crop of largemouth bass in receiving systems. In some instances, stocking adult (~300 mm TL) largemouth bass provided an immediate, albeit short-term, boost to fishing success (Buynak et al., 1999). In other studies, stocking adult largemouth bass had no effect on the resident population (Alford et al., 2009). Most hatchery-reared largemouth bass are stocked as fingerlings or advanced fingerlings and the verdict on those efforts is checkered, at best. For every report of a reasonable contribution of stocked largemouth bass to year-class strength or the fishery (for example, Buynak and Mitchell, 1999; Colvin et al., 2008; Mesing et al., 2008), the literature is replete with observations that persistence of stocked fingerlings after a year or two was negligible (for example, Buckmeier and Betsill, 2002; Hoffman and Bettoli, 2005; Hartman and Janney, 2006; Diana and Wahl, 2008; Ashe et al., 2016).

Several factors can contribute to low contributions of stocked fish. Fingerling largemouth bass harvested from culture ponds or raceways and transported to stocking sites are invariably stressed and will suffer high immediate mortality if remedial measures are not undertaken such as anesthetizing fish before and during hauling, transporting at cool temperatures, and adding salt to the water (Carmichael, 1984; Carmichael et al., 1984). Diana and Wahl (2009) estimated that stress associated with hauling and stocking accounted for up to 50% of the mortality of the fingerling largemouth bass they stocked, especially at water temperatures above 24°C. Porak et al. (2002) also noted highly variable, and occasionally very high (83%), stocking mortality of stocked fingerling largemouth bass.

Once stocked, inexperienced largemouth bass inevitably face a suite of potential predators that will readily prey upon them and high predation is usually cited as the reason for failed stocking programs (Schlechte et al., 2005). For instance, Buckmeier et al. (2005) estimated that nearly 28% of stocked fingerling (30–46 mm TL) largemouth bass were lost to predation within 12 h of stocking. Resident juvenile and adult largemouth bass, in particular, will readily prey upon stocked fingerlings, as will other piscivores (for example, white bass [*Morone chrysops*]) and zooplanktivores/insectivores such as bluegill (Buckmeier et al., 2005; Diana and Wahl, 2009).

To reduce predation losses, researchers and managers have investigated stocking larger, advanced (> 75 mm TL) fingerlings (Buynak and Mitchell, 1999; Mesing et al., 2008; Diana and Wahl, 2009), as well as stocking fish into structurally complex habitats (Buckmeier et al., 2005; Ashe et al., 2016) or at times coinciding with adequate prey resources (Hoxmeier and Wahl, 2002; Mesing et al., 2008). In a novel approach to produce advanced (~100 mm TL) fingerlings for stocking early in the growing season when suitable prey may be more abundant, Matthews and Stout (2013) manipulated water temperatures and photoperiods to induce captive broodstock to spawn in the fall. Stocking fish that are reared on or trained to consume live forage (instead of just pelleted-food) has also been investigated because pellet-reared largemouth bass may delay their transition to feeding on natural prey (Porak et al., 2002) and suffer higher mortality (Heidinger and Brooks, 2002; Pouder et al., 2010; Rachels et al., 2012). Allowing stocked fish to briefly recover and habituate to their new environment in predator-exclusion pens has also been examined, especially in systems with low habitat complexity and high predator densities (Schlechte et al., 2005; Schlechte and Buckmeier, 2006).

Despite the plethora of largemouth bass stocking programs that experienced poor survival and low contributions to year-class strength, the ability of hatchery fish to alter the genetic composition of receiving populations is indisputable. Specifically, the production and stocking of vast numbers of Florida bass, which began in the early 1970s and continues to this day, are an important component of the fisheries management programs in several states, such as Texas, Oklahoma, and Tennessee. The introgression of Florida bass genes into northern and intergrade largemouth bass populations has increased the maximum size that largemouth bass achieve in states outside the native range of Florida bass. For instance, the Tennessee state record largemouth bass caught in 1954 (6.6 kg) was eclipsed in 2015 by a 6.9 kg F1 hybrid largemouth bass caught in a reservoir that had been stocked with more than 2 million Florida bass and F1 hybrid fry and fingerlings since 2000. The Texas state record fish caught in 1943 (6.1 kg) was bested by a 6.4 kg fish in 1980 and the current state record (8.3 kg) was caught in 1992. The 50 heaviest largemouth bass caught in Texas have all been caught after Texas initiated its Florida bass stocking program in the 1970s and the catches of trophy (> 5.9 kg) largemouth bass were greater in reservoirs stocked with fingerling Florida bass (Myers and Allen, 2005). Oklahoma experienced a similar phenomenon after its Florida bass stocking program commenced; a forty-year old record was broken in 1983 and by the 1990s most of the largest fish caught possessed some Florida bass genes.

Given the preponderance of evidence that survival of stocked fingerling largemouth bass is often poor, how have agencies managed to produce significant introgression of the Florida bass genome into resident stocks of northern or intergrade largemouth bass? As Dunham et al. (1992) and others have reported, introgression is promoted by long-term stocking programs (6–15 years) consisting of many stocking events and high stocking numbers (up to 100,000 per stocking site [10–41 per hectare]; Buckmeier et al., 2003). The exception to that rule is when newly impounded waters are stocked for a few years with Florida bass as the reservoir basin fills (Maceina et al., 1988). It is indisputable that the maximum size and catches of trophy largemouth bass have increased in the tier of states in the southern USA with large Florida bass stocking programs; however, introduced non-native genes outside of their native range will persist through many generations (Johnson and Fulton, 2004; Naninni et al., 2014). As such, many authors have cautioned against the introduction of possible maladaptive genes (Philipp et al., 2002). To address those concerns in part, many US fisheries agencies have policies that either prohibit the introduction of Florida bass into their waters, or restrict their introductions into waters deemed suitable from a thermal standpoint. For instance, the Oklahoma Department of Wildlife Conservation determines which waters are stocked based on heating degree days; Florida bass will not thrive in cooler waters that support native largemouth bass populations; therefore, they are stocked where the thermal environment is more conducive to their growth and survival. The Tennessee Wildlife Resources Agency follows a similar strategy (that is, relying on heating degree days to determine which waters are and are not stocked).

1.9 Conclusion

A few years ago, the first author was pulling a seine in Represa Mourão, a small hydropower reservoir in Parana State in southern Brazil. Filled with the anticipation of catching a rich and diverse assemblage of unfamiliar taxa, he was extremely disappointed, but surprised, and yet even comforted by the catch of only two species, both familiar friends and invitees from other continents: largemouth bass and Nile tilapia (*Oreochromis niloticus*). This collection in a remote reservoir in Brazil illustrates the adaptive capacities of largemouth bass and tilapia, two of the most introduced fish taxa on the planet (Welcomme, 1992). Both species have demonstrated their resilience in diverse abiotic and biotic environments. The versatility of largemouth bass can be attributed to a merely average fecundity that is reinforced by parental care, to a diverse diet, to rapid early growth, and to flexible habitat utilization. Success in spreading largemouth bass outside their native range can also be linked to the relative ease with which juveniles are cultured in earthen ponds and transported to release sites (Chapter 7 and 11). The impetuses for spreading the species include its aesthetic qualities, taste, and gameness. The largemouth bass is an aesthetically pleasing fish considering its desirable shades of bronze, black, and greenish colors over an attractive trout-like shape. Relative to taste, the meat is white, flaky, and low in oil content making largemouth bass a good culinary fare if properly cleaned soon after being caught. And as to gameness, we leave you with a quote from Henshall (1881, emphasis added) "I consider him, *inch for inch* and *pound for pound*, the gamest fish that swims. The royal Salmon and the lordly Trout must yield the palm to a [largemouth bass] of *equal weight*."

References

Alford, J.B., O'Keefe, D.M. and Jackson, D.C. (2009) Effects of stocking adult largemouth bass to enhance fisheries recovery in Pascagoula River floodplain lakes impacted by Hurricane Katrina. *Proceedings of the Annual Conference of Southeastern Fish and Wildlife Agencies* 63, 104–110.

Allen, M.S., Walters, C.J. and Myers, R. (2008) Temporal trends in largemouth bass mortality, with fishery implications. *North American Journal of Fisheries Management* 28, 418–427.

Allan, R.C. and Romero, J. (1975) Underwater observations of largemouth bass spawning and survival in Lake Mead. In: Stroud, R.H. and Clepper, H. (eds) *Black Bass Biology and Management.* Sport Fishing Institute, Washington, DC, pp. 104–112.

Almeida, D., Almodóvar, A., Nicola, G.G., Elvira, B. and Grossman, G.D. (2012) Trophic plasticity of invasive juvenile largemouth bass *Micropterus salmoides* in Iberian streams. *Fisheries Research* 113, 153–158.

Annett, C., Hunt, J. and Dibble, E.D. (1996) The complete bass: habitat use patterns of all stages of the life cycle of largemouth bass. In: Miranda L.E. and DeVries, D.R. (eds) *Multidimensional Approaches to Reservoir Fisheries Management.* American Fisheries Society, Symposium 16, Bethesda, MD, pp. 306–314.

Ashe, D.E., Driscoll, M.T. and Schlechte, J.W. (2016) Stocking contributions of fingerling largemouth bass in three aquatic vegetation types in Toledo Bend Reservoir, Texas-Louisiana. *Journal of the Southeastern Association of Fish and Wildlife Agencies* 3, 46–49.

Azuma, M. and Motomura, Y. (1998) Feeding habits of largemouth bass in a non-native environment: the case of a small lake with bluegill in Japan. *Environmental Biology of Fishes* 52, 379–389.

Bacheler, N.M., Neal, J.W. and Noble, R.L. (2004) Diet overlap between native bigmouth sleepers (*Gobiomorus dormitor*) and introduced predatory fishes in a Puerto Rico reservoir. *Ecology of Freshwater Fish* 13, 111–118.

Baker, W.H., Blanton, R.E. and Johnston, C.E. (2013) Diversity within the redeye bass, *Micropterus coosae* (Perciformes: Centrarchidae) species group, with descriptions of four new species. *Zootaxa* 3635, 379–401.

Beamesderfer, R.C. and North, J.A. (1995) Growth, natural mortality, and predicted response to fishing for largemouth bass and smallmouth bass populations in North America. *North American Journal of Fisheries Management* 15, 688–704.

Beitinger, T.L., Bennett, W.A. and McCauley, R.W. (2000) Temperature tolerances of North American freshwater fishes exposed to dynamic changes in temperature. *Environmental Biology of Fishes* 58, 237–275.

Bennett, D.H. and Gibbons, J.W. (1975) Reproductive cycles of largemouth bass (*Micropterus salmoides*) in a cooling reservoir. *Transactions of the American Fisheries Society* 104, 77–82.

Benz, G.W. and Jacobs, R.P. (1986) Practical field methods of sexing largemouth bass. *The Progressive-Fish Culturist* 48, 221–225.

Bettoli, P.W., Maceina, M.J., Noble, R.L. and Betsill, R.K. (1992) Piscivory in largemouth bass as a function of aquatic vegetation abundance. *North American Journal of Fisheries Management* 12, 509–516.

Bevelhimer, M.S. and Breck, J.E. (2009) Centrarchid energetics. In: Cooke, S.J. and Phillip, D.P. (eds) *Centrarchid Fishes: Diversity, Biology and Conservation.* Wiley-Blackwell, Chichester, pp. 165–206.

Biro, P.A., Morton, A.E., Post, J.R. and Parkinson, E.A. (2004) Over-winter lipid depletion and mortality of age-0 rainbow trout (*Oncorhynchus mykiss*). *Canadian Journal of Fisheries and Aquatic Sciences* 61, 1513–1519.

Bishop, H. (1968) Largemouth bass culture in the southwest. *Proceedings of the North Central Warmwater Fish Culture Workshop*, Ames, IA, pp. 24–27.

Bondari, K. (1983) Training and growth of artificially fed largemouth bass in culture tanks. *Aquaculture Research* 14, 145–149.

Breder, C.M., Jr. (1936) The reproductive habits of the North American sunfishes (family Centrarchidae). *Zoologica* 21, 1–48.

Brown, M.L. and Murphy, B.R. (2004) Seasonal dynamics of direct and indirect condition indices in relation to energy allocation in largemouth bass *Micropterus salmoides* (Lacépède). *Ecology of Freshwater Fish* 13, 23–36.

Buckmeier, D.L. and Betsill, R.K. (2002) Mortality and dispersal of stocked fingerling largemouth bass and effects on cohort abundance. In: Philipp, D.P. and Ridgway, M.S. (eds) *Black Bass: Ecology, Conservation, and Management.* American Fisheries Society, Symposium 31, Bethesda, MD, pp. 667–676.

Buckmeier, D.L., Schlechte, J.W. and Betsill, R.K. (2003) Stocking fingerling largemouth bass to alter genetic composition: efficacy and efficiency of three stock rates. *North American Journal of Fisheries Management* 23, 523–529.

Buckmeier, D.L., Betsill, R.K. and Schlechte, J.W. (2005) Initial predation of stocked fingerling largemouth bass in a Texas reservoir and implications for improving stocking efficiency. *North American Journal of Fisheries Management* 25, 652–659.

Buynak, G.L. and Mitchell, B. (1999) Contribution of stocked advanced-fingerling largemouth bass to the population and fishery at Taylorsville Lake, Kentucky. *North American Journal of Fisheries Management* 19, 494–503.

Buynak, G.L., Mitchell, B., Michaelson, D. and Frey, K. (1999) Stocking subadult largemouth bass to meet angler expectations at Carr Creek Lake, Kentucky. *North American Journal of Fisheries Management* 19, 1017–1027.

Carlander, K.D. (1977) *Handbook of Freshwater Fishery Biology, Volume 2.* The Iowa State University Press, Ames, IA.

Carline, R.F. (1987) Simplified method based on bioenergetics modeling to estimate food consumption by largemouth bass and northern pike. *Transactions of the American Fisheries Society* 116, 224–231.

Carmichael, G.J. (1984) Long distance truck transport of intensively reared largemouth bass. *The Progressive Fish-Culturist* 46, 111–115.

Carmichael, G.J., Tomasso, J.R., Simco, B.A. and Davis, K.B. (1984) Characterization and alleviation of stress associated with hauling largemouth bass. *Transactions of the American Fisheries Society* 113, 778–785.

Carr, M.H. (1942) The breeding habits, embryology, and larval development of the large-mouthed black bass in Florida. *Proceedings of the New England Zoölogical Club* 20, 43–77.

Cincotta, D.A. and Stauffer, J.R. (1984) Temperature preference and avoidance studies of six North American freshwater fish species. *Hydrobiologia* 109, 173–177.

Clady, M.D. (1974) Food habits of yellow perch, smallmouth bass, and largemouth bass in two unproductive lakes in northern Michigan. *The American Midland Naturalist* 91, 453–459.

Cloutman, D.G. and Olmsted, L.L. (1983) Vernacular names of freshwater fishes of the southeastern United States. *Fisheries* 8 (2), 7–11.

Clugston, J.P. (1964) Growth of the Florida largemouth bass *Micropterus salmoides floridanus* (LeSueur), and northern largemouth bass, *M. salmoides* (Lacépède), in subtropical Florida. *Transactions of the American Fisheries Society* 93, 146–154.

Clutton-Brock, T.H. (1989) Mammalian mating systems. *Proceedings of the Royal Society of London B* 236, 339–372.

Cochran, P.A. and Adelman, I.R. (1982) Seasonal aspects of daily ration and diet of largemouth bass (*Micropterus salmoides*), with an evaluation of gastric evacuation rates. *Environmental Biology of Fishes* 7, 265–275.

Colvin, N.E., Racey, C.L. and Lochmann, S.E. (2008) Stocking contribution and growth of largemouth bass stocked at 50 and 100 mm into backwaters of the Arkansas River. *North American Journal of Fisheries Management* 28, 434–441.

Conover, D.O. (1992) Seasonality and the scheduling of life history at different latitudes. *Journal of Fish Biology* 41(sB), 161–178.

Conover, D.O. and Present, T.M.C. (1990) Countergradient variation in growth rate: compensation for length of growing season among Atlantic silversides from different latitudes. *Oecologia* 83, 316–324.

Cooke, S.J., McKinley, R. and Phillip, D.P. (2001) Physical activity and behavior of a centrarchid fish, *Micropterus salmoides*, during spawning. *Ecology of Freshwater Fish* 10, 227–237.

Cooke S.J., Philipp, D.P. and Weatherhead, P.J. (2002) Parental care patterns and energetics of smallmouth bass (*Micropterus dolomieu*) and largemouth bass (*Micropterus salmoides*) monitored with activity transmitters. *Canadian Journal of Zoology* 80, 756–770.

Cooke S.J., Philipp, D.P., Wahl, D.H. and Weatherhead, P.J. (2006) Parental care energetics of six syntopic centrarchid fishes. *Oecologia* 148, 235–249.

Coutant, C.C. and DeAngelis, D.L. (1983) Comparative temperature-dependent growth rates of largemouth and smallmouth bass fry. *Transactions of the American Fisheries Society* 112, 416–423.

DeWoody, J., Fletcher, D., Wilkins, D., Nelson, W. and Anise, J. (2000) Genetic monogamy and biparental care in an externally fertilizing fish, the largemouth bass. *Proceedings of the Royal Society of London B* 267, 2431–2437.

Diana, M.J. and Wahl, D.H. (2008) Long-term stocking success of largemouth bass and the relationship to natural populations. In: Allen, M.S., Sammons, S.M. and Maceina, M.J. (eds) *Balancing Fisheries Management and Water Uses for Impounded River Systems*. American Fisheries Society, Symposium 62, Bethesda, Maryland, pp. 413–426.

Diana, M.J. and Wahl, D.H. (2009) Growth and survival of four sizes of stocked largemouth bass. *North American Journal of Fisheries Management* 29, 1653–1663.

Díaz, F., Denisse Re, A., González, R.A., Sánchez, L.N., Leyva, G. and Valenzuela, F. (2007) Temperature preference and oxygen consumption of the largemouth bass *Micropterus salmoides* (Lacépède) acclimated to different temperatures. *Aquaculture Research* 38, 1387–1394.

Dorsey, L.G. (1997) Population dynamics and habitat use of age-0 largemouth bass and spotted bass in Normandy Reservoir, Tennessee. MSc thesis. Tennessee Technological University, Cookeville, TN.

Dunham, R.A., Turner, C.J. and Reeves, W.C. (1992) Introgression of the Florida largemouth bass genome into native populations in Alabama public lakes. *North American Journal of Fisheries Management* 12, 494–498.

Ehlinger, T.J., Gross, M.R. and Philipp, D.P. (1997) Morphological and growth rate differences between bluegill males of alternative reproductive life histories. *North American Journal of Fisheries Management* 17, 533–542.

Froese, R. (2006) Cube law, condition factor and weight–length relationships: history, meta-analysis and recommendations. *Journal of Applied Ichthyology* 22, 241–253.

Gardiner, J.M. and Motta, P.J. (2012) Largemouth bass (*Micropterus salmoides*) switch feeding modalities in response to sensory deprivation. *Zoology* 115, 78–83.

Garvey, J.E. and Stein, R.A. (1996) Linking bluegill and gizzard shad prey assemblages to growth of age-0 largemouth bass in reservoirs. *Transactions of the American Fisheries Society* 127, 70–83.

Garvey J.E., Wright, R.A. and Stein, R.A. (1998) Overwinter growth and survival of age-0 largemouth bass (*Micropterus salmoides*): revisiting the role of body size. *Canadian Journal of Fisheries and Aquatic Sciences* 55, 2414–2424.

Gido, K.B. and Brown J.H. (1999) Invasion of alien fish species in North American drainages. *Freshwater Biology* 42, 387–398.

Goodgame, L.S. and Miranda, L.E. (1993) Early growth and survival of age-0 largemouth bass in relation to parental size and swim-up time. *Transactions of the American Fisheries Society* 122, 131–138.

Green, D.M. and Heidinger, R.C. (1994) Longevity record for largemouth bass. *North American Journal of Fisheries Management* 14, 464–465.

Gutreuter, S.J. and Anderson, R.O. (1985) Importance of body size to the recruitment process in largemouth bass populations. *Transactions of the American Fisheries Society* 114, 317–327.

Hambright, K.D. (1991) Experimental analysis of prey selection by largemouth bass: role of predator mouth width and prey body depth. *Transactions of the American Fisheries Society* 120, 500–508.

Harper, D.G. and Blake, R.W. (1991) Prey capture and the fast-start performance of northern pike *Esox lucius*. *Journal of Experimental Biology* 155, 175–192.

Hartman, K. and Janney, E.C. (2006) Relative persistence and dispersal of age-0 and age-1 largemouth bass stocked into two Ohio River embayments. *Journal of Freshwater Ecology* 21, 627–637.

Hedrick, A.V. and Temeles, E.J. (1989) The evolution of sexual dimorphism in animals: hypotheses and tests. *Trends in Ecology and Evolution* 4, 136–138.

Heidinger, R.C. (1975) Life history and biology of largemouth bass. In: Stroud, R.H. and Clepper, H. (eds) *Black Bass Biology and Management*. Sport Fishing Institute, Washington, DC, pp. 11–20.

Heidinger, R.C. (1976) Synopsis of biological data on the largemouth bass, *Micropterus salmoides* (Lacépède) 1802. *Fisheries Synopsis 115*. Food and Agriculture Organization of the United Nations, Rome.

Heidinger, R.C. and Brooks, R.C. (2002) Relative contribution of stocked minnow-fed and pellet-fed advanced fingerling largemouth bass to year-classes in Crab Orchard Lake, Illinois. In: Philipp, D.P. and Ridgway, M.S. (eds) *Black Bass Ecology, Conservation, and Management*. American Fisheries Society, Symposium 31, Bethesda, MD, pp. 703–714.

Helser, T.E. and Lai, H.-L. (2004) A Bayesian hierarchical meta-analysis of fish growth: with an example for North American largemouth bass, *Micropterus salmoides*. *Ecological Modelling* 178, 399–416.

Henshall, J.A. (1881) *Book of the Black Bass, Comprising its Complete Scientific and Life History Together with a Practical Treatise on Angling and Fly Fishing and a Full Description of Tools, Tackle and Implements*. Robert Clarke & Company, Cincinnati, OH.

Hill, J.E., Nico, L.G., Cichra, C.E. and Gilbert, C.R. (2004) Prey vulnerability to peacock cichlids and largemouth bass based on predator gape and prey body depth. *Proceedings of the Annual Conference Southeastern Association of Fish and Wildlife Agencies* 58, 47–56.

Hodgson, J.R. and Hansen, E.M. (2005) Terrestrial prey items in the diet of largemouth bass, *Micropterus salmoides*, in a small north temperate lake. *Journal of Freshwater Ecology* 20, 793–794.

Hodgson, J.R. and Kitchell, J.F. (1987) Opportunistic foraging by largemouth bass (*Micropterus salmoides*). *The American Midland Naturalist* 118, 323–336.

Hoffman, K. and Bettoli, P.W. (2005) Growth, dispersal, mortality, and contribution of largemouth bass stocked into Chickamauga Lake, Tennessee. *North American Journal of Fisheries Management* 25, 1518–1527.

Houde, E.D. (1989) Subtleties and episodes in the early life of fishes. *Fish Biology* 35 (Supplement A), 29–38.

Hoyle, J.A. and Keast, A. (1987) The effect of prey morphology and size on handling time in a piscivore, the largemouth bass (*Micropterus salmoides*). *Canadian Journal of Zoology* 65, 1972–1977.

Hoxmeier, R.J.H. and Wahl, D.H. (2002) Evaluation of supplemental stocking of largemouth bass across reservoirs: effects of predation, prey availability, and natural recruitment. In: Philipp, D.P. and Ridgway, M.S. (eds) *Black Bass Ecology, Conservation, and Management. American Fisheries Society*, Symposium 31, Bethesda, MD, pp. 639–647.

Hunt, J. and Annett, C.A. (2002) Effects of habitat manipulation on reproductive success of individual largemouth bass in an Ozark reservoir. *North American Journal of Fisheries Management* 22, 1201–1208.

Huskey, S.H. and Turnigan R.G. (2001) Variation in prey-resource utilization and oral jaw gape between two populations of largemouth bass, *Micropterus salmoides*. *Environmental Biology of Fishes* 61, 185–194.

IGFA (2015) Top ten record largemouth bass. International Game Fish Association. Available at: https://www.igfa.org/Fish/lmbass2015 (accessed 11 June 2017).

Isely, J.J. and Noble, R.L. (1987) Use of daily otolith rings to interpret development of length distributions of young largemouth bass. In: Summerfelt, R.C. and Hall, G.E. (eds) *The Age and Growth of Fish*. The Iowa State University Press, Ames, IA, pp. 475–481.

Jackson, D.A. (2002) Ecological effects of *Micropterus* introductions: the dark side of black bass. In: Phillip, D.P. and Ridgway, M.S. (eds) *Black Bass: Ecology, Conservationk and Management*. American Fisheries Society Symposium 31, Bethesda, Maryland, MD, pp. 221–232.

Jang, M.-H., Joo, G.-J. and Lucas, M.C. (2006) Diets of introduced largemouth bass in Korean rivers and potential interactions with native fishes. *Ecology of Freshwater Fish* 15, 315–320.

Jobling, M. (1981) Temperature tolerance and the final preferendum – rapid methods for the assessment of optimum growth temperatures. *Journal of the Fisheries Research Board of Canada* 19, 439–455.

Johnson, J.M. and Post, D.M. (1996) Morphological constraints on intracohort cannibalism in age-0 largemouth bass. *Transactions of the American Fisheries Society* 125, 809–812.

Johnson, R.L. and Fulton, T. (2004) Incidence of Florida largemouth bass alleles in two northern Arkansas populations of largemouth bass, *Micropterus salmoides* Lacépède. *The American Midland Naturalist* 152, 425–429.

Kassler, T.W., Koppelman, J.B., Near, T.J., Dillman, C.B., Levengood, J.M., Swofford, D.L., Van Orman, J.L., Claussen, J.C. and Philipp, D.P. (2002) Molecular and morphological analyses of the black basses: implications for taxonomy and conservation. In: Philipp, D.P. and Ridgway, M.S. (eds) *Black Bass Ecology, Conservation, and Management*. American Fisheries Society, Symposium 31, Bethesda, MD, pp. 291–322.

Keast, A. and Eadie, J.M. (1985) Growth dispensation in year-0 largemouth bass: the influence of diet. *Transactions of the American Fisheries Society* 114, 204–213.

Kelley, J.W. (1962) Sexual maturity and fecundity of the largemouth bass, *Micropterus salmoides* (Lacépède), in Maine. *Transactions of the American Fisheries Society* 91, 23–28.

Kelley, J.W. (1968) Effects of incubation temperatures on survival of largemouth bass eggs. *The Progressive Fish-Culturist* 30, 159–163.

Kelsch, S.W. (1996) Temperature selection and performance by bluegills: evidence for selection in response to available power. *Transactions of the American Fisheries Society* 125, 948–955.

Kohler, C.C., Sheehan, R.J. and Sweatman, J.J. (1993) Largemouth bass hatching success and first-winter survival in two Illinois reservoirs. *North American Journal of Fisheries Management* 13, 125–133.

Koppelman, J.B., Whitt, G.S. and Philipp, D.P. (1988) Thermal preferenda of northern, Florida, and reciprocal F_1 hybrid largemouth bass. *Transactions of the American Fisheries Society* 117, 238–244.

Kramer, R.H. and Smith, J.L. (1962) Formation of year classes in largemouth bass. *Transactions of the American Fisheries Society* 9, 29–41.

Lawrence, J.M. (1958) Estimated sizes of various forage fishes largemouth bass can swallow. *Proceedings of the Annual Conference of Southeastern Association of Game and Fish Commissioners* 11, 220–225.

Lee, D.S., Gilbert, C.R., Hocutt, C.H., Jenkins, R.E., McAllister, D.E., and Stauffer, J.R. (1980) *Atlas of North American Freshwater Fishes*. North Carolina State Museum of Natural History, Raleigh, NC.

Long, J.M., Allen, M.S., Porak, W.F. and Suski, C.D. (2015) A historical perspective of black bass management in the United States. In: Tringali, M.D., Long, J.M., Allen, M.S. and Birdsong, T. (eds) *Black Bass Diversity: Multidisciplinary Science for Conservation*. American Fisheries Society, Bethesda, MD, pp. 99–122.

Ludsin, S.A. and DeVries, D.R. (1997) First-year recruitment of largemouth bass: the interdependency of early life stages. *Ecological Applications* 7, 1024–1038.

MacCrimmon, H.R. and Robbins, W.N. (1975) Distribution of black basses in North America. In: Stroud, R.H. and Clepper, H. (eds) *Black Bass Biology and Management.* Sport Fishing Institute, Washington, DC, pp. 56–66.

Maceina, M.J., Murphy, B.R. and Isely, J.J. (1988) Factors regulating Florida largemouth bass stocking success and hybridization with northern largemouth bass in Aquilla Lake, Texas. *Transactions of the American Fisheries Society* 117, 221–231.

Matthews, M.D. and Stout, R.B. (2013) Out-of-season spawning method for Florida largemouth bass to produce advanced-sized fingerlings by early spring. *North American Journal of Aquaculture* 75, 524–531.

McCall, T.C. (1980) Fishery investigation of Lake Mead, Arisona-Nevada, from Separation Rapids to Boulder Canyon, 1978–1979. Agency report submitted to the U.S. Department of the Interior, Water and Power Resources Service, Boulder City, NV.

McCauley, R.W. and Kilgour, D.M. (1990) Effect of air temperature on growth of largemouth bass in North America. *Transactions of the American Fisheries Society* 119, 276–281.

McCormick, J.H. and Jensen, K.M. (1992) Osmoregulatory failure and death of first-year largemouth bass (*Micropterus salmoides*) exposed to low pH and elevated aluminum, at low temperature in soft water. *Canadian Journal of Fisheries and Aquatic Sciences* 49, 1189–1197.

McMahon, T.E. and Holanov, S.H. (1995) Foraging success of largemouth bass at different light intensities: implications for time and depth of feeding. *Journal of Fish Biology* 46, 759–767.

Meador, M.R. and Kelso W.E. (1990) Growth of largemouth bass in low-salinity environments. *Transactions of the American Fisheries Society* 119, 545–552.

Mesing, C.L., Cailteux, R.L., Strickland, P.A., Long, E.A. and Rogers, M.W. (2008) Stocking of advanced-fingerling largemouth bass to supplement year-classes in Lake Talquin, Florida. *North American Journal of Fisheries Management* 28, 1762–1774.

Meyer, F.A. (1970) Development of some larval centrarchids. *The Progressive Fish-Culturist* 32, 130–136.

Miller, K.D. and Kramer, R.H. (1971) Spawning and early life history of largemouth bass (*Micropterus salmoides*) in Lake Powell. In: Hall, G.E. (ed.) *Reservoir Fisheries and Limnology.* American Fisheries Society, Special Publication 8, Bethesda, MD, pp. 73–83.

Miller, S.J. and Storck, T. (1982) Daily growth rings in otoliths of young-of-the year largemouth bass. *Transactions of the American Fisheries Society* 111, 527–530.

Miller, S.J. and Storck, T. (1984) Temporal spawning distribution of largemouth bass and young-of-year growth, determined from daily otolith rings. *Transactions of the American Fisheries Society* 113, 571–578.

Miranda, L.E. (2014) Changes in latitudes, changes in attitudes. *Lakeline* 34, 28–31.

Miranda, L.E. and Bettoli, P.W. (2007) Mortality. In: Guy, C. and Brown, M. (eds) *Analysis and Interpretation of Freshwater Fisheries Data.* American Fisheries Society, Bethesda, MD, pp. 229–278.

Miranda, L.E. and Durocher, P.P. (1986) Effects of environmental factors on growth of largemouth bass in Texas reservoirs. In: Hall, G.E. and Van Den Avyle, M.J. (eds) *Reservoir Fisheries Management: Strategies for the 80's.* American Fisheries Society, Bethesda, MD, pp. 115–121.

Miranda, L.E. and Hubbard, W.D. (1994) Length-dependent winter survival and lipid composition of age-0 largemouth bass in Bay Springs Reservoir, Mississippi. *Transactions of the American Fisheries Society* 123, 80–87.

Miranda, L.E. and Muncy, R.J. (1987) Recruitment of young-of-year largemouth bass in relation to size structure of parental stock. *North American Journal of Fisheries Management* 7, 131-137.

Miranda, L.E., Shelton, W.L. and Bryce, T.D. (1984) Effects of water level manipulation on abundance, mortality, and growth of young-of-year largemouth bass in West Point Reservoir, Alabama-Georgia. *North American Journal of Fisheries Management* 4, 314–320.

Mittelbach, G.G. and Persson, L. (1998) The ontogeny of piscivory and its ecological implications. *Canadian Journal of Fisheries and Aquatic Sciences* 55, 1454–1465.

Moss, D.D. and Scott, DC (1961) Dissolved oxygen requirements of three species of fish. *Transactions of the American Fisheries Society* 90, 377–393.

Moyle, P.B. (1976) Fish introductions in California: history and impact on native fishes. *Biological Conservation* 9, 101–118.

Moyle, P.B. (1986) Fish introductions into North America: patterns and ecological impact. In: Mooney, H.A. and Drake J.A. (eds) *Ecology of Biological Invasions of North America and Hawaii*. Springer-Verlag, Berlin, pp. 27–43.

Myers, R.A. and Allen, M.S. (2005) Factors related to angler catch of trophy largemouth bass in Texas reservoirs. *Lake and Reservoir Management* 21, 309–315.

Naninni, M.A., Diana, M.J., Claussen, J.E., Philipp, D.P. and Wahl, D.H. (2014) Assessing the long-term reproductive contribution of stocked fish to largemouth bass populations. *Transactions of the American Fisheries Society* 143, 606–612.

Neal, J.W. and Noble, R.L. (2006) A bioenergetics-based approach to explain largemouth bass size in tropical reservoirs. *Transactions of the American Fisheries Society* 135, 1535–1545.

Near, T.J., Kassler, T.W., Koppelman, J.B., Dillman, C.B. and Philipp, D.P. (2003) Speciation in North American black basses, *Micropterus* (Actinopterygii: Centrarchidae). *Evolution* 57, 1610–1621.

Near, T.J. and Koppelman, J.B. (2009) Species diversity, phylogeny, and phylogeography of Centrarchidae. In: Cooke, S.J. and Phillip, D.P. (eds) *Centrarchid Fishes: Diversity, Biology and Conservation*. Wiley-Blackwell, Chichester, pp. 1–38.

Neill, W.H. and Magnuson, J.J. (1974) Distributional ecology and behavioral thermoregulation of fishes in relation to heated effluent from a power plant at Lake Monona, Wisconsin. *Transactions of the American Fisheries Society* 103, 663–710.

Nelson, J.T., Bowker, R.G. and Robinson, J.D. (1974) Rearing pelleted-fed largemouth bass in a raceway. *The Progressive Fish-Culturist* 36, 108–110.

Neumann, R.M., Guy, C.S. and Willis, D.W. (2012) Length, weight, and associated indices. In: Zale, A.V., Parrish, D.L. and Sutton, T.M. (eds) *Fisheries Techniques, 3rd edition*. American Fisheries Society, Bethesda, MD, pp. 637–676.

Nieman, D.A., Clady, M.D. and Gebhart, G.E. (1979) Sexual maturity of small yearling largemouth bass in Oklahoma. *Proceedings of the Oklahoma Academy of Sciences* 59:51–52.

Niimi, A.J. and Beamish, F.W.H. (1974) Bioenergetics and growth of largemouth bass (*Micropterus salmoides*) in relation to body weight and temperature. *Canadian Journal of Zoology* 52, 447–456.

Nowlin, W.H., Drenner, R.W., Guckenberger, K.R., Lauden, M.A., Alonso, G.T., Fennell, J.E. and Smith, J.L. (2006) Gape limitations, prey size refuges, and top-down impacts of piscivorous largemouth bass in shallow pond ecosystems. *Hydrobiologia* 563, 357–369.

Olson, M.H. (1996) Ontogenetic niche shifts in largemouth bass: variability and consequences for first-year growth. *Ecology* 77, 179–190.

Orsatti, S.D. and Colgan, P.W. (1987) Effects of sulphuric acid exposure on the behaviour of largemouth bass, *Micropterus salmoides*. *Environmental Biology of Fishes* 19, 119–129.

Ozen, O. and Noble, R.L. (2002) Relationship between water level fluctuations and largemouth bass spawning in a Puerto Rico reservoir. In: Philipp, D.P. and Ridgway, M.S. (eds) *Black Bass Ecology, Conservation, and Management*. American Fisheries Society, Symposium 31, Bethesda, MD, pp. 213–220.

Parker, G.A. (1992) The evolution of sexual size dimorphism in fish. *Journal of Fish Biology* 41, 1–20.

Parmley, D., Alvarado, G. and Cortez, M. (1986) Food habits of hatchery-reared Florida largemouth bass. *The Progressive Fish-Culturist* 48, 264–267.

Philipp, D.P., Claussen, J.E., Kassler, T.W. and Epifanio, J.M. (2002) Mixing stocks of largemouth bass reduces fitness through outbreeding depression. In: Philipp, D.P. and Ridgway, M.S. (eds) *Black Bass Ecology, Conservation, and Management.* American Fisheries Society, Symposium 31, Bethesda, MD, pp. 349–364.

Porak, W.F., Johnson, W.E., Crawford, S., Renfro, D.J., Shoeb, T.R., Stout, R.B., Krause, R.A. and DeMauro, R.A. (2002) Factors affecting survival of largemouth bass raised on artificial diets and stocked into Florida lakes. In: Philipp, D.P. and Ridgway, M.S. (eds) *Black Bass Ecology, Conservation, and Management.* American Fisheries Society, Symposium 31, Bethesda, MD, pp. 649–665.

Post, D.M., Kitchell, J.F. and Hodgson, J.R. (1998) Interactions among adult demography, spawning date, growth rate, predation, overwinter mortality, and the recruitment of largemouth bass in a northern lake. *Canadian Journal of Fisheries and Aquatic Sciences* 55, 2588–2600.

Pouder, W.F., Trippel, N.A. and Dotson, J.R. (2010) Comparison of mortality and diet composition of pellet-reared advanced-fingerling and early cohort age-0 wild largemouth bass through 90 days poststocking at Lake Seminole, Florida. *North American Journal of Fisheries Management* 30, 1270–1279.

Purdom, T., Schoofs, A., Hodgson, J.R., Maki, T. and Hodgson, J.Y. (2015) A thirty year diet record of largemouth bass (*Micropterus salmoides*) from a small north temperate lake. *Bios* 86, 20–30.

Putman, J.H., Pierce, C.L. and Day, D.M. (1995) Relationships between environmental variables and size-specific growth rates of Illinois stream fishes. *Transactions of the American Fisheries Society* 124, 252–261.

Pyron, M. (1999) Relationships between geographical range size, body size, local abundance, and habitat breadth in North American suckers and sunfishes. *Journal of Biogeography* 26, 549–558.

Rachels, K.T., Taylor, G.R., Baumhoer, B.M., Shresta, S. and Lochmann, S.E. (2012) Pellet-reared largemouth bass competitive ability at various levels of exposure to live forage. *Proceedings of Annual Conference of the Southeastern Association of Fish and Wildlife Agencies* 66, 16–19.

Rahel, F.J. (2007) Biogeographic barriers, connectivity and homogenization of freshwater faunas: it's a small world after all. *Freshwater Biology* 52, 696–710.

Raibley, P.T., Irons, K.S., O'Hara, T.M., Blodgett, K.D. and Spark, R.E. (1997) Winter habitats used by largemouth bass in the Illinois River, a large river-floodplain ecosystem. *North American Journal of Fisheries Management* 17, 401–412.

Ramsey, J.S. (1975) Taxonomic history and systematic relationships among species of *Micropterus.* In: Stroud, R.H. and Clepper, H. (eds) *Black Bass Biology and Management.* Sport Fishing Institute, Washington, DC, pp. 67–75.

Reid, S.M., Fox, M.G. and Whillans, T.H. (1999) Influence of turbidity on piscivory in largemouth bass (*Micropterus salmoides*). *Canadian Journal of Fisheries and Aquatic Sciences* 56, 1362–1369.

Rice, J.A. and Cochran, P.A. (1984) Independent evaluation of a bioenergetics model for largemouth bass. *Ecology* 65, 732–739.

Rice, J.A., Breck, J.E., Bartell, S.M. and Kitchell, J.F. (1983) Evaluating the constraints of temperature, activity, and consumption on growth of largemouth bass. *Environmental Biology of Fishes* 9, 263–275.

Ridgway, M.S., Goff, G.P. and Keenleyside, M.H.A. (1989) Courtship and spawning behavior in smallmouth bass (*Micropterus dolomieui*). *The American Midland Naturalist* 122, 209–213.

Rivero, L.H. (1937) The introduced largemouth bass, a predator upon native Cuban fishes. *Transactions of the American Fisheries Society* 66, 367–368.

Rogers, M.W., Allen, M.S. and Porak, W.F. (2006) Separating genetic and environmental effects on temporal spawning distributions of largemouth bass. *Canadian Journal of Fisheries and Aquatic Sciences* 63, 2391–2399.

Savino, J.F. and Stein, R.A. (1982) Predator-prey interactions between largemouth bass and bluegills as influenced by simulated submersed vegetation. *Transactions of the American Fisheries Society* 111, 255–266.

Savino, J.F. and Stein, R.A. (1989) Behavior of fish predators and their prey: habitat choice between open water and dense vegetation. *Environmental Biology of Fishes* 24, 287–293.

Schlechte, J.W. and Buckmeier, D.L. (2006) A pond evaluation of habituation as a means to reduce initial mortality associated with poststocking predation of hatchery-reared largemouth bass. *North American Journal of Fisheries Management* 26, 119–123.

Schlechte, J.W., Betsill, R.K. and Buckmeier, D.L. (2005) A laboratory evaluation of poststocking predatory losses for cultured largemouth bass. *Transactions of the American Fisheries Society* 134, 141–148.

Schmidt, R.E. and Fabrizio, M.C. (1980) Daily growth rings on otoliths for aging young-of-the-year largemouth bass from a wild population. *The Progressive Fish-Culturist* 42, 78–80.

Scott, W.B. and Crossman, E.J. (1973) *Freshwater Fishes of Canada.* Fisheries Research Board of Canada Bulletin 184, Ottawa.

Shelton, W.L., Davies, W.D., King, T.A. and Timmons, T.J. (1979) Variation in the growth of an initial year class of largemouth bass in West Point Reservoir, Alabama and Georgia. *Transactions of the American Fisheries Society* 108, 142–149.

Shireman, J.V., Colle, D.E. and Rottmann, R.W. (1978) Size limits to predation on grass carp by largemouth bass. *Transactions of the American Fisheries Society* 107, 213–215.

Shoup, D.E. and Wahl, D.H. (2009) The effects of turbidity on prey selection by piscivorous largemouth bass. *Transactions of the American Fisheries Society* 138, 1018–1027.

Smith, H.M. (1907) *The Fishes of North Carolina.* North Carolina Geological and Economical Survey, Raleigh, NC.

Smith, J.A., Nelson-Maney, N., Parsons, K.J. and Albertson, R.C. (2015) Body shape evolution in sunfishes: divergent paths to accelerated rates of speciation in the Centrarchidae. *Evolutionary Biology* 42, 283–295.

Stewart, N.E., Shumway, D.L. and Doudoroff, P. (1967) Influence of oxygen concentration on the growth of juvenile largemouth bass. *Journal of the Fisheries Research Board of Canada* 24, 475–494.

Strawn, K. (1961) Growth of largemouth bass fry at various temperatures. *Transactions of the American Fisheries Society* 90, 334–335.

Stuber, R.J., Gebhart, G. and Maughan, O.E. (1982) Habitat suitability index models: largemouth bass. FWS/OBS-82/10.16, U.S. Fish and Wildlife Service, Washington, DC.

Suski, C.D. and Philipp, D.P. (2004) Factors affecting the vulnerability to angling of nesting male largemouth and smallmouth bass. *Transactions of the American Fisheries Society* 133, 1100–1106.

Tabor, R.A., Footen, B.A., Fresh, K.L., Celedonia, M.T., Mejia, F., Low, D.L. and Park, L. (2007) Smallmouth bass and largemouth bass predation on juvenile chinook salmon and other salmonids in the Lake Washington Basin. *North American Journal of Fisheries Management* 27, 1174–1188.

Tidwell, J.H., Coyle, S.D., Bright, L.A., Van Arnum, A. and Yasharian, D. (2003) Effect of water temperature on growth, survival, and biochemical composition of largemouth bass *Micropterus salmoides. Journal of the World Aquaculture Society* 34, 175–183.

Timmons, T.J., Shelton, W.L. and Davies, W.D. (1980) Gonad development, fecundity, and spawning season of largemouth bass in newly impounded West Point Reservoir, Alabama-Georgia. Technical Paper 100, U.S. Fish and Wildlife Service, Washington, DC.

Tsunoda, H., Mitsuo, Y., Ohira, M., Doi, M. and Senga, Y. (2010) Change of fish fauna in ponds after eradication of invasive piscivorous largemouth bass, *Micropterus salmoides*, in north-eastern Japan. *Aquatic Conservation: Marine and Freshwater Ecosystems* 20, 710–716.

Venables, B.J., Pearson, W.D. and Fitzpatrick, L.C. (1977) Thermal and metabolic relations of largemouth bass, *Micropterus salmoides*, from a heated reservoir and a hatchery in north central Texas. *Comparative Biochemistry and Physiology Part A: Physiology* 57, 93–98.

Venables, B.J., Fitzpatrick, L.C. and Pearson, W.D. (1978) Laboratory measurement of preferred body temperature of adult largemouth bass (*Micropterus salmoides*). *Hydrobiologia* 58, 33–36.

Vogele, L.E. and Rainwater, W.C. (1975) Use of brush shelters as cover by spawning black basses (*Micropterus*) in Bull Shoals Reservoir. *Transactions of the American Fisheries Society* 104, 264–269.

Ward, S.M., and Neumann, R.M. (1998) Seasonal and size-related food habits of largemouth bass in two Connecticut lakes. *Journal of Freshwater Ecology* 13, 213–220.

Warren, M.L., Jr. (2009) Centrarchid identification and natural history. In: Cooke, S.J. and Phillip, D.P. (eds) *Centrarchid Fishes: Diversity, Biology and Conservation*. Wiley-Blackwell, Chichester, pp. 375–535.

Wasserman, R.J., Strydom, N.A. and Weyl, O.L.F. (2011) Diet of largemouth bass, *Micropterus salmoides* (Centrarchidae), an invasive alien in the lower reaches of an Eastern Cape River, South Africa. *African Zoology* 46, 378–386.

Waters, D.S. and Noble, R.L. (2004) Spawning season and nest fidelity of largemouth bass in a tropical reservoir. *North American Journal of Fisheries Management* 24, 1240–1251.

Webb, J.F. and Reeves, W.C. (1975) Age and growth of Alabama spotted bass and northern largemouth bass. In: Stroud, R.H. and Clepper, H. (eds) *Black Bass Biology and Management*. Sport Fishing Institute, Washington, DC, pp. 204–215.

Welcomme, R.L. (1992) A history of international introductions of inland aquatic species. *ICES Marine Science Symposium* 194, 3–14.

Whitledge, G.W. and Hayward, R.S. (1997) Laboratory evaluation of a bioenergetics model for largemouth bass at two temperatures and feeding levels. *Transactions of the American Fisheries Society* 126, 1030–1035.

Wickstrom, G.A. and Applegate, R.L. (1989) Growth and food selection of intensively cultured largemouth bass. *The Progressive Fish-Culturist* 51, 79–82.

Wiegmann, D.D., Baylis, J.R. and Hoff, M.H. (1992) Sexual selection and fitness variation in a population of smallmouth bass, *Micropterus dolomieui* (Pisces: Centrarchidae). *Evolution* 46:1740–1753.

Yako, L.A., Mather, M.E. and Juanes, F. (2000) Assessing the contribution of anadromous herring to largemouth bass growth. *Transactions of the American Fisheries Society* 129, 77–88.

Yasuno, N., Chiba, Y., Shindo, K., Fujimoto, Y., Shimada, T., Shikano, S. and Kikuchi, E. (2012) Size-dependent ontogenetic diet shift to piscivory documented from stable isotope analyses in an introduced population of largemouth bass. *Environmental Biology of Fishes* 93, 255–266.

CHAPTER 2

History of largemouth bass production

James H. Tidwell[1] *and John G. Nickum*[2]

[1]Kentucky State University, Aquaculture Research Center, Frankfort, Kentucky, USA
[2]Retired, National Aquaculture Coordinator, Department of the Interior, U.S. Fish and Wildlife Service, Washington, DC, USA

2.1 Introduction

The art of aquaculture, in general, likely began in China and dates back 4,000–5,000 years (Stickney, 1979). These early efforts focused primarily on common carp (*Cyprinus carpio*). There is evidence of pond aquaculture in Egypt dating back over 2,000 years and their culture included tilapia. For a comprehensive review of the history of aquaculture see Stickney and Treece (2012). The general focus of this historical account is the development of the aquaculture of the largemouth bass including its production as a food-fish. However, this industry largely evolved from procedures developed for producing juvenile largemouth bass for pond and reservoir stocking as sport-fish. In fact, sport-fish stocking has been the main driver for the development of culture methods for many species of fishes.

While we know that efforts to reproduce largemouth bass extend back to at least the mid-1800s, written reports are difficult to find. What was documented was often in hatchery records or organizational reports, not in publications available to the general public. There are many gaps in the records of fish culture in general, including the history of largemouth bass culture. Techniques that individual culturists developed for their own use were hopefully passed along orally, or went with them to their graves.

Especially in the era of immediate access to information, it is easy to miss or minimize the contributions of those who have come before us, especially if their work is not available in electronic form. This would be a serious mistake. Let this chapter pay tribute to the culturist, hatchery managers, fishery managers, and researchers who have contributed to the knowledge base for the largemouth bass, now extending back over 150 years.

2.2 Background

The largemouth bass is a member of the sunfish family, Centrarchidae, which also includes the "bream" species like bluegill as well as rock bass and crappies. All are native to North America. The largemouth bass is a member of the genus Micropterus whose members are collectively known as the black bass. The largemouth bass is *Micropterus salmoides*, meaning small fin and a salmon-like body. The largemouth bass was described in 1802 by Lacépède. While native to the drainages of North America east of the Rocky Mountains, the largemouth bass has been widely transplanted. Heidinger (1976) listed 37 countries where the largemouth bass could now be found. Within the USA, intentional stocking programs were initiated in 1871 or 1872, and by 1900 largemouth bass were found in all 48 of the contiguous states.

In the 19th century largemouth bass were harvested recreationally as a sport-fish but were also commercially harvested as a food-fish. In the 1800s all fisheries were widely considered to be inexhaustible resources (Clepper, 1966). However, by the mid to late 1800s it began to be realized that this was a fallacy and efforts were initiated to control harvests and increase stocking programs. Declines in fish populations supporting sport-fisheries led managers to focus on fish propagation and stocking as a primary management approach for maintaining "fishable" populations. This pattern was applied first to brook trout, American shad, and Atlantic salmon. Depletion of largemouth bass and smallmouth bass populations later led managers and culturists to attempt similar practices for bass.

2.3 Early culture

Exactly when American fish culturists first tried to propagate largemouth bass is unknown. Efforts of these early hatchery workers were not recorded. We can safely conclude that largemouth bass culture began sometime in the latter half of the 19th century. American fish culture for any species was essentially non-existent prior to 1850, although a presentation about propagating brook trout has been reported to have been made in South Carolina in 1804. A publication titled *A Treatise on the Artificial Propagation of Certain Kinds of Fish, with the Description and Habits of Such Kinds as are Most Suitable for Pisciculture* was produced by Dr. Theodatus Garlick in 1857, but focused primarily on his experiments with brook trout (Davis, 1961). Information on salmonid propagation efforts in Europe dated back to the 14th century and came to North America with European immigrants. Although salmonids were the focus of early fish culture efforts, the popularity of black basses as warmwater sport-fishes stimulated the curiosity of anglers and encouraged scientists to conduct practical experiments on the culture of bass and other species of value.

2.4 Hatchery scale-up

In 1870, the American Fish Culturist Association was formed (later to become the American Fisheries Society). Its primary function was to serve as a way to share information on artificial fish propagation and one of the first topics addressed was black bass culture (Moffitt, 2001). The journal *The Progressive Fish-Culturist* was their primary conduit for information dissemination and many of the fundamental papers on LMB propagation and culture were published there.

In 1871, the federal government became directly involved. The Office of the Commissioner of Fish and Fisheries (commonly known as the U.S. Fish Commission) was established with a mandate of enquiring into the causes in the decrease of food-fishes and to recommend remedies. In 1872, the Commission undertook the propagation of food-fish. Millions of eggs were hatched and fingerlings stocked. Much of the focus was still on salmonids, such as Atlantic salmon, Pacific coho, and Chinook salmon. However, largemouth bass were also produced (along with many others). For the fiscal year 1897, the U.S. Fish Commission reported that 95,358 largemouth bass eggs, fry, and juveniles were distributed. That same year, the U.S. Commission of Fish and Fisheries published *A Manual of Fish-Culture.* Methods for propagating "black basses, crappies, and rock bass" were of sufficient interest to warrant a 25-page chapter in that manual. Many of the pond-based culture methods described in that chapter are still used in present day hatcheries.

In 1898, the state of New York reduced the number of black bass a fisherman could catch per day and also recognized a need to devise a means "for the hatching of bass artificially" (Long et al., 2015). State fish agencies in New York, New Jersey, and the New England states developed state fish culture and management programs and also fostered early private fish farms. The emphasis, however, was on brook trout, the native freshwater salmonid in northeastern America, and to a lesser extent, the American shad. Old government reports also indicate an interest in the common carp.

2.5 Legacy of overfishing

While overfishing was recognized as having a negative impact on fish populations, during the late 1800s it also began to be recognized that man's impact on the environment could also negatively impact fish populations. Logging and mining increased sediment run-off, manufacturing produced chemical effluents, and dam construction changed flowing water environments (lotic ecosystem) to more of a still water environment (lentic ecosystem). Black bass were proposed as suitable species for stocking into these new stillwater conditions. Unlike trout and shad, bass could establish self-reproducing populations (Long et al., 2015). Supplying juvenile fish to stock into these systems, and other impoundments developed during the country's expansion west, created a need for black bass hatchery programs. By the 1900s, black bass had been stocked into 26 states outside of their native range (Robbins and MacCrimmon, 1974).

Although the average citizen and fisherman primarily still saw recreational fishing as a source of food, certain individuals and groups began to call for a halt to the commercial harvest of black bass and to push for their status as a recreational only (game fish) species. The Izaak Walton League was formed in 1922 and worked with the states to pass laws protecting black bass from commercial harvest for food-fish markets.

As these state laws were promulgated, a new set of issues developed. Black bass harvested illegally in one state began to be "bootlegged" across state lines and sold in another state where sales were still legal. This led to a federal statute known as the Black Bass Act 1926, which made it a federal offense for fish caught illegally in one state to be sold into a different state. For many years this basically ended the status of black bass as a commercial food-fish species.

2.6 Government intervention and expansion

As the country moved from the 1920s into the depression era of the 1930s, President Franklin Roosevelt launched his New Deal programs. Several of the programs included water development projects, including the Tennessee Valley Authority (TVA) Act 1933 and the Flood Control Act 1936. Both of these supported the construction of large dams, which impounded large reservoirs. However, it was feared that the rapid filling off these large water bodies would result in biological deserts (Miranda, 1996). To prevent this, fish hatcheries were often constructed on site as part of the overall project.

These New Deal programs not only supported the construction of huge reservoirs but also the building of a large number of small farm ponds. Farm pond construction was promoted to control soil erosion, as well as a self-sustaining source of food, by the Soil Conservation Service in 1954. The number of farm ponds estimated to exist in 1934 was 20,000. By 1965, this number had increase to 2,000,000 (Swingle, 1970). The largemouth bass was the species most often stocked into these ponds (Swingle, 1970). The number of state and federal hatcheries producing largemouth bass grew from fewer than 100 in 1900 to 99 federal hatcheries and over 500 state hatcheries by 1950. The number of private bass hatcheries has not been documented, but they could be found in most states across the South and the Midwest.

Research on fisheries management, and the biology of fish that supported recreational fisheries, was stimulated by the establishment of the US Fish and Wildlife Service Cooperative Fishery Research Units beginning in the early 1960s. Co-op Units were located at land-grant universities across the USA and provided research, graduate level training, and extension on matters of interest to state and federal agencies. Research on largemouth bass issues was a major part of the programs in Missouri, New York, Texas, Oklahoma, and several other states. Much of the research focused on strategies to use the enormous reproductive potential of natural reproduction, rather than hatchery propagation, to increase recruitment.

2.7 Modern culture of the largemouth bass

However, the demand for fingerling largemouth bass to stock ponds and reservoirs continued to increase. Robbins and MacCrimmon (1974) reported that > 35 million largemouth bass were stocked annually between 1966 and 1970. Despite increased demand, culture methods remained essentially those in use during the late 1800s. If a production system works predictably and produces fish relatively efficiently, "Why change?" Hatchery managers and fish farmers saw no compelling reason to change when the old system worked.

While managers agreed that stocking new water was beneficial, the positive effects of continued supplemental stocking came to be considered as questionable (Long et al., 2015). Most of the fingerlings stocked in these early stocking programs were small (< 25–50 mm). However, researchers indicated that the best success came when stocking large size largemouth bass fingerlings (178–229 mm). This created an increased demand for the production of these advanced fingerlings.

As discussed previously, first attempts at largemouth bass culture mimicked the techniques that had been developed for trout culture. However, there are fundamental differences between these fishes in large-scale reproduction and fry rearing techniques. Stripping eggs and milt from bass that appeared ready to spawn revealed a major problem immediately: bass anatomy does not lend itself to egg or milt stripping procedures. It did not matter how "ripe" the bass were, they could not be stripped. Although "ripe" female bass release eggs and attentive males would rush in to fertilize them in a pond or lake environment, attempts to strip milt from mature bass, or other centrarchid fishes, simply did not work.

A second difference between trout and bass involved larval and fry feeding. Trout have large eggs and larval yolk sacs. With these stored reserves, trout fry can survive for weeks without exogenous feeding. In contrast, bass eggs are small, and fry have very little stored energy and nutrient reserves in their yoke sacs; therefore, they must begin feeding soon after hatching, typically in no more than 3–4 days. Largemouth bass are primarily reared in nursery ponds, relying on natural or enhanced zooplankton populations. Brine shrimp, rotifers, copepods, and other forms of zooplankton have been used in tank or trough systems and shown to be technically feasible for first-feeding bass, but have not yet proven practical at production scale. Bass have to undergo a feed-training regime at 3.5–5 cm, while trout can be trained to take artificial feeds at swim-up (first-feeding).

In review, there was a steady increase in the demand for hatchery production of largemouth bass dating back to the 1800s. By the 1900s, black bass had been artificially propagated and stocked into scores of states, including > 25 outside of their natural range. In the 1930s the federal government supported the construction of both small impoundments on farms as well as large reservoirs, requiring millions of largemouth bass fingerlings for stocking. Most of these were small fingerlings (5–8 cm), but fisheries managers found that larger fingerlings (18–22 cm) were much more successful after stocking. In the 1960s and 1970s, the work of Jack Snow

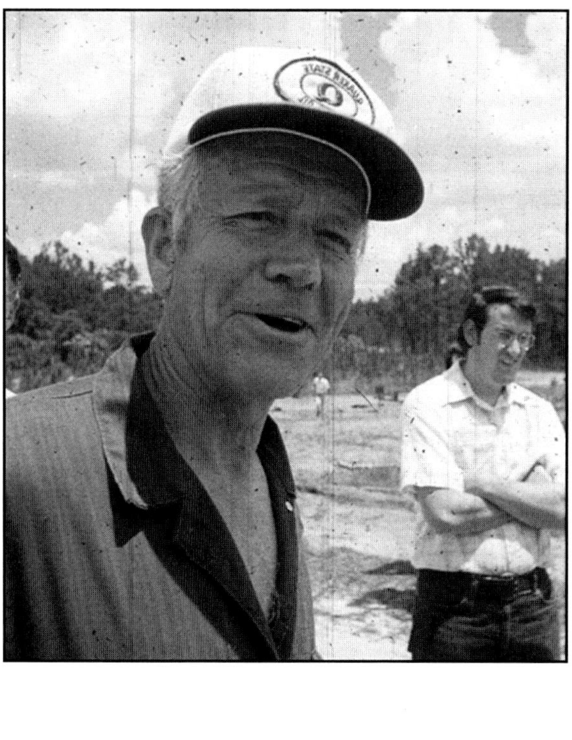

Figure 2.1 Jack Snow of the Marion National Fish Hatchery in Marion, Alabama. Photo courtesy of the Auburn University Fisheries and Allied Aquacultures Image Gallery.

(Figure 2.1) and colleagues at the Marion National Fish Hatchery in Alabama resulted in the development of the "Marion Method" (Snow 1960, 1963, 1968, 1975) with which large numbers of advanced and large largemouth bass fingerlings could be produced per unit of pond space.

2.8 Largemouth bass as a food-fish

So, when did largemouth bass begin to be grown for food-fish markets? While federal and state hatcheries sometimes document their production through reports and technical advancements through publications, private hatcheries largely do not. We know that private hatcheries have also been producing largemouth bass likely back to the 1800s. They have utilized the technologies developed and shared by the public hatcheries while also making and refining their own technologies and innovations. As discussed previously, there has been resistance to the sale of largemouth bass in the USA back to at least the 1920s. However, what is actually legal and what is actually illegal is not always well defined and differs between states. Producers might choose to not ask and raise the issue. This is the fisheries version of "don't ask, don't tell." If the questions were asked, the assumption is they would be ruled illegal due the legislation from the 1920s banning the harvest and sales of black bass as commercial fisheries. It is likely that large markets for largemouth bass developed early in Toronto, Canada not only because it is a large population center of ethnic Asians, but also because they were in close proximity to, but still outside of, the US border. Very little of the history of the production of largemouth bass as a food-fish in the USA has been captured in written form. So, the question is, when did largemouth bass begin being raised as a food-fish?

Bardach et al. (1972) in their early classical work on aquaculture, reported that in the 1950s, several centrachids were evaluated for commercial production by Auburn University. The bluegill (*Lepomis macrochirus*) and the flier (*Centrarchus macropterus*) were rejected as unsuited for culture, but they found that the crappies and largemouth bass showed potential. The authors reported that the LMB in the 1970s was much more common in commercial fish culture in Europe than in its native land. They indicated that the LMB had been stocked in Latin America and Africa and in 1965 experimental culture was initiated in Tunisia. In Europe, they were used as a predator in polyculture to control unwanted trash fish and the excessive reproduction of the other polyculture species. The commercial international seafood supplier Sea Port (2018) indicates that the largemouth bass was introduced in to Taiwan in the 1970s. They have been raised there since that time and currently are the source of fish for their commercial export of whole frozen largemouth bass. In the USA, Bardach et al. (1972) reported that in the early 1970s, a few commercial fish hatcheries, particularly in Arkansas, were already raising edible size centrarchids, including the largemouth bass. However, they were being marketed to and through fee fishing ponds. Major limitations noted were that the production rate of food size largemouth bass was only 44 kg/ha (Bardach et al., 1972) and their sale in some areas was forbidden.

Because of a lack of written information, the authors of this chapter conducted a number of interviews with both private producers and government officials to try to establish some aquaculture dates and timelines. A longtime fish producer in northern Ohio indicates that he sold his first load of largemouth bass food-fish in the mid-1980s. The fish were sold into an Asian market that was already in existence, but was still relatively small. To "break into" this market required traveling to New York or Toronto for face-to-face meetings with the buyer. Only then could any fish be sold. His first loads of live largemouth bass went to Toronto, Canada.

An Ohio grower also indicated that he had started feed-training largemouth bass fingerlings back in 1979, using moist cat food. Around 1985, he sold some third-generation feed-trained fish to producers in Arkansas. As documented in Chapter 5, the use of domesticated feed-trained brooders makes for rapid progress in the feed-training success of offspring and adaptation to production conditions. The producer reported that initially, there were a lot of problems with "liver-disease" (this was probably glycogen deposition from using high carbohydrate feeds, see Chapter 7). By 1995, there was a lot of interest in the state (Ohio) from producers requesting help getting into largemouth bass production. He indicated though that these efforts were all "grass roots" with little or no support from state agencies or universities.

In another interview, a large fish hatchery in Arkansas reported that they began selling largemouth bass into the Asian food-fish market before 1998. Prior to that they had already been raising feed-trained largemouth bass fingerlings. The first fish they sold into the food-fish market were retired broodfish. Their business had concentrated on sport-fish as their selling price was more than double what food-fish sold for. As the largemouth bass became more domesticated, and their techniques improved, the fish performed better on feed and survivals increased. With that, the farm moved into producing large quantities of largemouth bass for the food-fish market in 1998. Initial fish for these markets were sold at 225–340 g. However, markets later expressed a desire for larger sizes. The producer indicated that at the time of interview (2018), there is still unfulfilled demand for food-fish largemouth bass. Limitations on expansion include high production costs, primarily due to high feed costs, poor labor availability, and government regulations. He indicated that he was not sure if consumers would continue to pay the high selling prices imposed by these high production costs. This farm not only sells fish into Toronto markets, but also reports significant markets on the west coast, including San Francisco, Oakland, San Diego, and San Jose (California).

To understand the history of the development of the largemouth bass as a food-fish, we need to understand some aspects of the ethnic Asian market which is by far the primary outlet. The market is covered more thoroughly in Chapter 12. While these markets may be relatively new to us, they are actually part of a culture whose desire for live seafood goes back millennia. In an interview with food writer Wendy Goodfriend, Lisa Li, who grew up in Guanghou China explained "in Chinese culture, we like to get our protein as close to live as possible" (Goodfriend, 2018). What could be fresher than a fish that was swimming less than an hour before you eat it? The cultural context is captured even more when they discuss a Chinese New Year's Eve feast where a whole fish is the traditional last course. The word fish (*yu*) is also the Chinese word for abundance, making a simply dressed, steamed whole fish a symbolic way to end the meal. Serving the fish whole represents "completeness." It is essential that the fish be served with head and tail still attached to make sure the coming year has both a good beginning and a good end. At the New Year's Eve dinner, the head of the fish is always pointed toward the oldest or most honored guest. It is also a tradition to not finish the fish course on New Year's Eve, but to leave some uneaten for the next day so that the abundance of *yu* will continue into the New Year (Goodfriend, 2018).

A significant change in the live largemouth bass market occurred when, at the beginning of 2013, the New York State Department of Environmental Conservation opened the market in New York City for hatchery-raised largemouth bass. They required that bass be in labeled containers, purchase and sales records must be maintained by distributors, and fish can be sold live but must be killed before being transferred to the retail customers. This change was opposed by sport-fishing advocates who argued that the rule change would create a black market that could damage the states recreational fisheries (ActivistAngler, 2013). The counter argument was made by aquaculturists in New York that the ready availability of legal farm-raised LMB would actually lessen the demand for black market fish and relieve pressures on the natural fisheries (Figura, 2012).

2.9 Conclusion

The history of largemouth bass aquaculture dates back to the mid-1850s. Techniques were adapted from those developed in Europe for salmonids. Expansion of hatchery production occurred as the country expanded westward, the farm pond program of the 1930s led to the construction of thousands of small ponds, and New Deal programs constructed large reservoirs. Most of these activities were based on small fingerlings. However, larger fingerlings were shown to be more effective in stocking programs. Snow and associates at the Marion Lab in Alabama established feed-training procedures that allowed larger sizes to be produced at higher densities. Larger fish began to be marketed into ethnic Asian markets in the 1970s. In 2013, the New York market was allowed to sell farm-raised largemouth bass. The market for live largemouth bass is likely approaching 1,000,000 kg/year.

References

ActivistAngler (2013) New York permits sale of bass, encourages black market. Available at: http://activistangler.squarespace.com/journal/2013/3/4/new-york-permits-retail-sale-of-bass-encourages-black-market.html (accessed 23 August 2018).

Bardach, J.E., Ryther, J.H. and McLarney, W.O. (1972) *Aquaculture: the Farming and Husbandry of Freshwater and Marine Organisms*. John Wiley and Sons, Inc., London.

Clepper, H.E. (1966) *Origins of American Conservation*. The Ronald Press Company, New York.

Davis, R.E. (1961) Daily rhythms in the behavior of two freshwater fishes, *Lepomis macrochirus* and *Micropterus salmoides*. PhD thesis, University of Wisconsin-Madison.

Figura, D. (2012) Commercial bass hatchery owner says column about selling bass fillets was one-sided. Available at: http:// http://blog.syracuse.com/outdoors/2012/06/commercial_bass_hatchery_owner.html (accessed 23 August 2018).

Goodfriend, W. (2018) Buy a live fish in Oakland Chinatown for a traditional Chinese New Year's Feast. Bay Area Bites. KQED Food. Available at: https://www.kqed.org/bayareabites/56072/ (accessed 23 August 2018).

Heidinger, R.C. (1976) Synopsis of biological data on the largemouth bass *Micropterus salmoides* (Lacépède) 1802. *FAO Fisheries Synopsis no. 115*. FAO, Rome.

Long, J.M., Allen, M.S., Porak, W.F. and Suski, C.D. (2015) A historical perspective of black bass management in the United States. *American Fisheries Society Symposium* 82, 99–122.

Miranda, L.E. (1996) Development of reservoir fisheries management paradigms in the twentieth century. In: Miranda, L.E. and DeVries, D.R. (eds) *Multidimensional Approaches to Reservoir Fisheries Management*. American Fisheries Society Symposium 16, Bethesda, MD.

Moffitt, C.M. (2001) *Reflections: A Photographic History of Fisheries and the American Fisheries Society in North America.* American Fisheries Society, Bethesda, MD.
Robbins, W.H. and MacCrimmon, H.R. (1974) *The Blackbass in America and Overseas.* Biomanagement and Research Enterprises, Sault Ste. Marie, Ontario.
Sea Port (2018) Products – largemouth bass. Available at: http://www.cport.net/product/view/largemouth-bass (accessed 24 August 2018).
Snow, J.R. (1960) An exploratory attempt to rear largemouth black bass fingerlings in a controlled environment. *Proceedings of the Southeastern Association of Game and Fish Commissioners* 14, 253–257.
Snow, J.R. (1963) Results of further experiments on rearing largemouth bass fingerlings under controlled conditions. *Proceedings of the Southeastern Association of Game and Fish Commissioners* 17, 191–203.
Snow, J.R. (1968) Production of six- to eight-inch largemouth bass for special purposes. *The Progressive Fish-Culturist* 30(3), 144–152.
Snow, J.R. (1975) Hatchery propagation of the black basses. In: Stroud, R.H. and Clepper, H.E (eds) *Black Bass Biology and Management.* Sport Fishing Institute, Washington, DC, pp. 344–356.
Stickney, R.R. (1979) *Principles of Warmwater Aquaculture.* John Wiley and Sons, Chichester.
Stickney, R.R. and Treece, G.D. (2012) History of aquaculture. In: Tidwell, J.H. (ed.) *Aquaculture Production Systems.* Wiley–Blackwell, Oxford, pp. 15–50.
Swingle, H.S. (1970) History of warmwater pond culture in the United States. *A Century of Fisheries in North America. American Fisheries Society, Special Publication* 7, 95–105.

CHAPTER 3

Largemouth bass production in China

Yangen Zhou[1] *and Chengyue Liu*[2]

[1]Key Laboratory of Mariculture (Ocean University of China), Ministry of Education
[2]Fisheries College, Ocean University of China, Qingdao, China

3.1 History of largemouth bass production in China

The largemouth bass (*Micropterus salmoides*) is a freshwater fish native to North America. It has been widely stocked into a number of other countries, primarily as a sport-fish. Around 1970, it was introduced into Taiwan from North America. The first successful artificial spawning in Taiwan occurred in 1983 (Liao, 2000). It was then introduced into Guangdong Province, China, in 1983, and has since become a popular culture species across the whole country (Bai et al., 2008; Bai and Li, 2013b; Ma et al., 2003; Lou, 2000; Zhang and He, 1994).

While largemouth bass has become an economically important freshwater species in many parts of China when compared to some other cultured species, it has a slower growth rate, advanced age at sexual maturity, a high feed conversion ratio, and low resistance to stress. For a time, these issues restricted the further development of the species in China. However, in 2010, a new breeding variety "Youlu No. 1" was produced by the Pearl River Fisheries Research Institute, Chinese Academy of Fishery Sciences, Guangzhou, China. The culture of this new genetic variety has become popular across large areas of Guangdong, Jiangsu, and Hunan provinces (Liang et al., 2007). The Youlu No. 1 variety has demonstrated three advantages over other varieties: (1) a desirable body shape, with a low rate of deformities; (2) faster growth and high production rates (kg/ha); and (3) minimal growth differences among individuals, producing high yields while maintaining size uniformity (Bai and Li, 2013a).

3.2 Largemouth bass production areas in China

With the continuous development of improved farming technologies, this species can now be cultured in most provinces of China, including those in the north, such as Liaoning Province, Heilongjiang Province, and Xinjiang Uygur Autonomous Region (Zhan, 2001; Zhang et al., 2017). However, the main largemouth bass culturing areas are Foshan city in Guangdong

Table 3.1 Area of production and yields of largemouth bass across China in 2007 and 2013.

Province	City	Culture method	2007[1]		2013[2]		Diet
			Area (km^2)	Annual yield (10^3t)	Area (km^2)	Annual yield (10^3t)	
Guangdong	Foshan	Pond culture	40	90	47	100	Frozen fish
Zhejiang	Huzhou	Pond culture	14	15	14	18	Frozen fish
Jiangsu	Wujiang	Cage and pond culture	7	11	17	14	Frozen fish
Jiangsu	Nanjing	Pond culture	5	6	13	8	Frozen fish
Jiangsu	Suzhou	Cage and pond culture	–	–	10	8	Frozen fish
Sichuan	Mianyang	Cage and pond culture	3	3	4	4	Frozen fish with feed
Sichuan	Jianyang	Cage culture	0.1	0.1	0.1	0.1	Frozen fish with feed
Sichuan	Guangyuan	Cage culture	0.1	0.1	0.1	0.1	Frozen fish with feed
Total				125.5		152.2	

Sources: [1]Bai *et al.* (2009), [2]Bai and Li (2013).

Province, Huzhou city in Zhejiang Province, Wujiang district and Nanjing in Jiangsu Province, and Mianyang city in Sichuan Province (Figure 3.1) (Bai et al., 2009; Li et al., 2012). Table 3.1 shows that the production of largemouth bass in China increased 23.7% between 2007 to 2013, going from 125,500 metric tons (MT) to 152,200 MT. If we compare the data in Tables 3.1 and 3.2, they indicate that in 2007 and 2013 largemouth bass production accounted for 80% and 45% of total freshwater bass production, respectively. In these data other fish included in the freshwater bass category included the roughskin sculpin (*Trachidemus fasciatus*), the Asian seabass (*Lates calcarifer*), and the European perch (*Perca fluviatilis*).

3.3 Largemouth fry and fingerling rearing

Reproduction of largemouth bass in China begins with broodfish stocked into spawning ponds. Resulting fry can then be cultured to sizes suitable for feed training (~2 cm) either in nursery ponds or in concrete tanks.

3.3.1 *Spawning ponds*

For fry production, the selected broodfish are placed in the spawning pond. The density of broodfish is 0.45–0.60 fish/m^2 at about 300 kg/ha. The ratio of males to females is 4 : 6. The reason for fewer male fish in the pond, is to prevent unnecessary energy loss caused by male to male territoriality and aggressive interactions. Largemouth bass spawning ponds should have an area of 2,000–3,300 m^2 (0.2–0.3 ha), water depths ranging 1.3–1.5 m, and an adequate supply of high-quality water. A pond of this size and depth has three advantages: (1) it is easy to seine; (2) the temperature at the bottom remains suitable; and (3) the dissolved oxygen (DO) is sufficient, which is beneficial to the spawning of the fish.

Generally, the spawning ponds have 2–3 aerators, and aerators are turned on in the evening. With rainy and cloudy weather, aerators may be turned on during the day to maintain

Table 3.2 Annual outputs of bass (freshwater) in different provinces of China (10^3 t).

Province	Year											
	2003	2004	2006	2007	2008	2009	2010	2011	2013	2014	2015	2016
Beijing	0.28	0.15	0.13	0.03	0.06	0.02	0.05	0.05	0.19	0.19	0.00	0.01
Tianjing	0.15	0.00	0.17	0.09	0.00	0.00	0.00	0.00	0.76	0.00	0.80	0.92
Hebei	0.02	0.03	0.02	0.01	0.02	0.03	0.01	0.04	0.03	0.04	0.19	0.25
Shanxi	0.01	0.00	0.00	0.01	0.02	0.02	0.04	0.03	0.04	0.04	0.02	0.02
Liaoning	0.09	0.07	0.19	0.05	0.07	0.18	0.22	0.11	0.14	0.17	0.10	0.09
Jilin	0.01	0.00	0.01	0.03	0.04	0.26	0.16	0.15	0.05	0.04	0.03	0.04
Heilongjiang	0.00	0.00	0.03	0.01	0.01	0.01	0.04	0.01	0.01	0.01	0.01	0.01
Shanhai	0.00	0.69	0.70	0.49	0.28	0.37	0.36	0.20	0.25	0.34	0.37	0.01
Jiangsu	10.77	12.83	14.23	14.23	20.15	19.65	22.68	27.18	34.86	34.97	36.21	36.88
Zhejiang	8.86	9.36	11.49	10.29	11.43	14.24	15.01	18.07	18.16	18.58	21.34	29.06
Anhui	1.24	0.82	1.31	1.27	0.99	2.55	2.49	4.11	0.82	4.97	5.85	5.93
Fujian	6.38	4.03	6.44	5.40	4.39	6.44	7.63	7.98	10.18	10.41	11.08	11.27
Jiangxi	2.18	6.55	11.37	12.70	13.92	15.14	16.00	17.22	20.19	21.01	21.78	22.70
Shandong	0.80	0.77	0.86	0.79	0.29	0.39	0.74	0.54	0.71	0.73	0.60	0.59
Henan	0.02	0.06	0.25	0.28	0.25	0.28	0.13	0.27	0.38	0.41	0.57	0.83
Hubei	0.96	0.47	0.90	1.18	1.61	2.04	2.94	2.42	3.34	3.56	3.84	4.39
Hunan	1.03	1.30	1.14	0.94	1.01	0.99	1.29	1.68	1.54	1.43	1.51	3.09
Guangdong	89.22	94.81	104.54	101.36	102.72	101.47	104.71	115.57	231.84	237.70	227.94	234.69
Guangxi	3.20	3.22	0.64	0.51	0.55	0.57	0.61	0.80	0.74	0.75	0.77	0.72
Chongqing	0.03	0.05	0.11	0.14	0.17	0.33	0.33	0.74	0.94	1.08	1.61	1.96
Sichuan	1.03	1.37	5.42	7.06	8.38	8.31	8.78	9.40	10.95	11.43	12.23	12.39
Guizhou	0.03	0.11	0.79	0.45	0.00	0.88	1.10	1.34	2.48	2.75	4.79	6.44
Yunan	0.00	0.01	0.02	0.01	0.03	0.04	0.01	0.01	0.51	0.12	0.19	0.18
Shaanxi	0.01	0.13	0.10	0.06	0.08	0.08	0.08	0.05	0.10	0.00	0.11	0.11
Gansu	0.00	0.00	0.01	0.01	0.00	0.01	0.01	0.01	0.00	0.00	0.00	0.00
Ningxia	0.00	0.00	0.00	0.00	0.00	0.00	0.00	0.00	0.00	0.16	0.25	0.31
Xijiang	0.06	0.04	0.07	0.12	0.15	0.20	0.58	0.36	0.66	0.87	0.89	1.10
Total	**126.37**	**136.87**	**160.96**	**157.49**	**166.60**	**174.47**	**185.94**	**208.33**	**339.84**	**351.77**	**353.08**	**374.06**

Source: China Fisheries Statistics Yearbook.

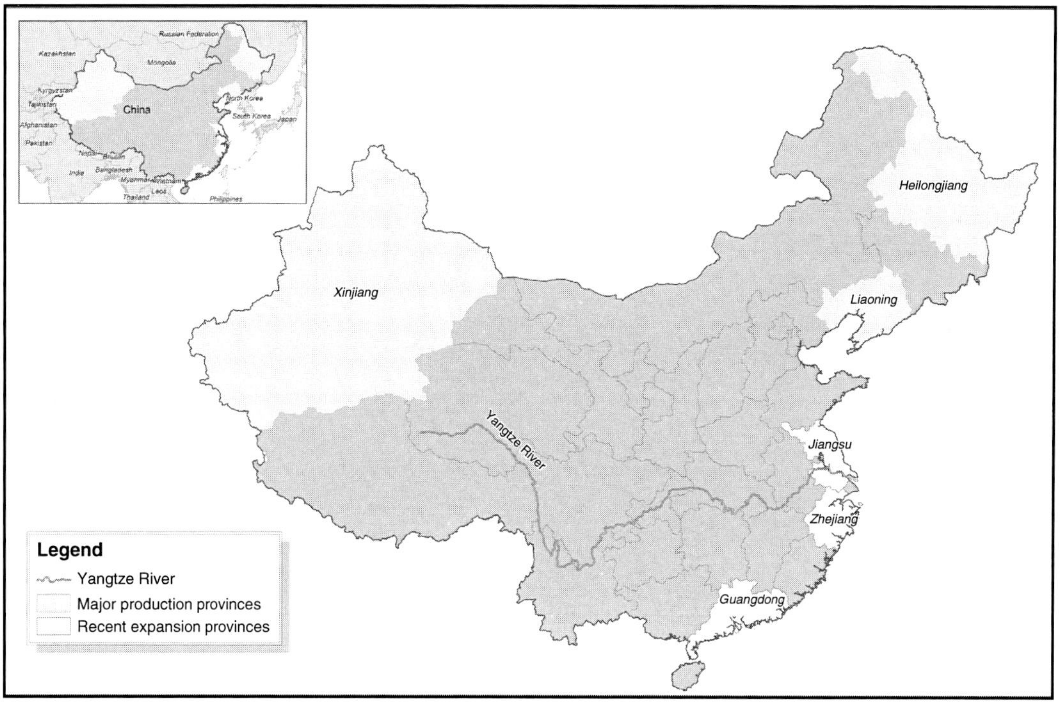

Figure 3.1 Main Chinese largemouth bass production regions and northern regions of recent expansion.

DO concentrations. The water in the pond is kept clear, with a transparency of ≥ 30 cm. The water quality of the pond should be maintained in the range of: pH 7.0–7.8, ammonia-nitrogen < 0.4 mg/l, and nitrite concentration < 0.3 mg/l.

After spawning and with fry-swim up, the fry deplete their yolk-sac storage of endogenous nutrition and switch to exogenous feeding. However, in this species the fry cannot be immediately trained to accept artificial feeds and must be cultured on natural foods until they reach a size when they can be acclimated to artificial diets. This period of natural foods is considered the nursery phase. In China, there are two main nursey methods used to rear largemouth bass fry. These methods are concrete tanks and nursery ponds. In general, the fry survival rate is greater when reared in concrete tanks (> 80%) compared with ponds (~50%), but the production costs are higher (Li, 2008; Wu, 1993).

3.3.2 Fry rearing in concrete tanks

The size of the concrete tanks used to rear largemouth bass fry in China ranges from 20 to 30 m^2. Walls should be smooth to prevent skin abrasions. Initially, the water depth is 20–25 cm, and then increases with new water input to 50–70 cm. Fry density at stocking is approximately 600 fish/m^2. Fry initially are fed small zooplankton, such as rotifers and caudate (salamander) larvae that have been harvested from ponds, and can be fed 2–3 times daily. Later, when fish fry reach 1.5–2.0 cm in length, larger zooplankton such as cladocerans, copepods, or rotifer should be provided. Wickstrom and Applegate (1989) reported that six genera of invertebrates served as feed sources for largemouth bass fry during a 25 d period. In that trial, the fry preferred to eat the cladoceran *Moina brachiate*. When fish length exceeds 2 cm, they can be fed with water earthworm (Oligochaeta), and then begin acclimation to frozen fish or commercial food. However, in 2017 the Chinese government started to prohibit the feeding of frozen fish for aquaculture, so fingerlings are now all acclimated to artificial feeds (Li, 2008; Wu, 1993). If the fingerlings are reared over the winter in tanks, they should be in a greenhouse to maintain warm temperature and reduce the impact of seasonal weather changes.

3.3.3 Fry rearing in nursery ponds

The stocking density of nursery ponds ranges from 40,000 to 70,000 fish/1,000 m^2 (400,000–700,000 fish/ha). Fry stocked together should be derived from the same batch to ensure a consistent size and prevent cannibalism. Since largemouth bass fry mainly feed on plankton, a certain degree of water fertilization must be maintained. Fish reaching a mean body length of 1.5 cm are ready to be trained to accept commercial feeds (Li, 2008; Wu, 1993).

As noted previously, the largemouth bass requires a training period for acclimation to commercial feed. In China, the feed-training procedure usually takes place in the concrete tanks previously described for use in the nursery phase of fry rearing or in large plastic tanks. On some small farms with limited resources a corner of the fry pond is cordoned off with netting or a simple net-pen is constructed. These enclosures are shaded by a roof. The feed-training procedure is as follows: The water should be rich by using fertilizer to promote natural productivity in pond. The fish fry (about 1.32 cm) are fed red insect powder (dried chironomids) along with commercial fry feed powder or fish paste. If the fish fry eats the fish paste well, you can add the fry feed powder to the fish paste, and increase the amount of feed powder in the mix day by day.

After about 1 week, the mix comprises approximately 60–70% feed powder. The fish are usually then ready to transition to commercial feed. After 7–10 d, the amount of commercial feed is slowly increased until the fish are completely acclimated to it. In general, fry at sizes ranging from 1.98 cm to 2.64 cm should be completely acclimated to commercial feed. It should be noted that in China the fish are then size graded and the small fish fry are put through feed-training again. After a second feed acclimation period of 7–10 d, these fish should also be trained and can be transferred to be cultured in ponds or cages. There the fish are fed three times per day (morning, noon, and night), using the feeding rule of "slow, quick, and slow" until most fish are not coming to surface for more feed. Since this species has the characteristic of avoiding strong light, it is better to offer most of the feed in the morning or at night (Bai and Li, 2013a).

3.4 Pond and cage culture

Pond and cage culture (Figures 3.2 and 3.3) are the main production systems for the rearing of largemouth bass in most culturing provinces in China. Pond culture mostly occurs in southern China, such as Guangdong Province (Li et al., 2012). Cage culture is distributed across the Yangtze River regions (Figure 3.1) which contain lakes and reservoirs, such as Sichuan Province (Bai et al., 2009; Li and Li, 2000; Zhan, 2001).

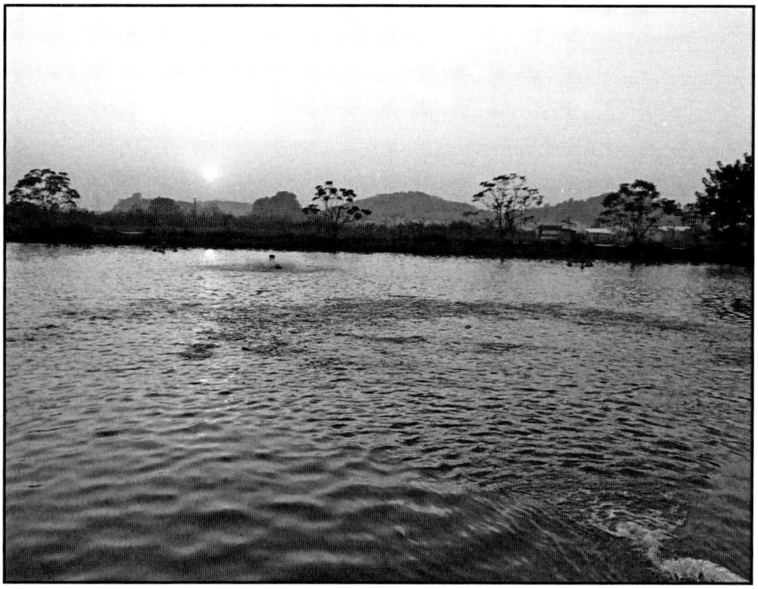

Figure 3.2 Largemouth bass pond aquaculture in Jiangmen, Guangdong province.

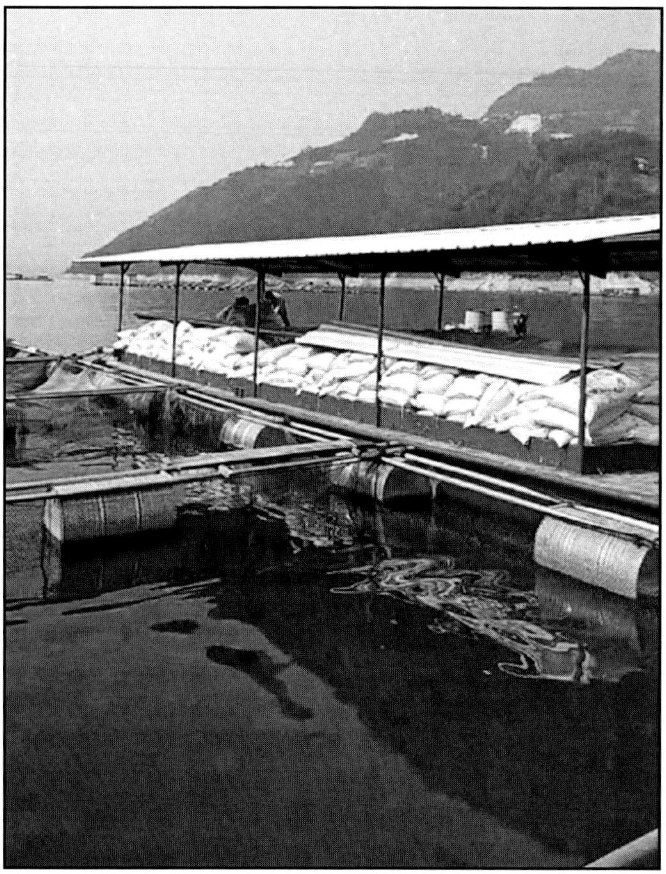

Figure 3.3 Largemouth bass cage aquaculture in Nanning, Guangxi province.

3.4.1 Pond aquaculture

Aquaculture ponds used in largemouth bass production must maintain good water quality. The pond bottom is usually comprised of fine sand and gravel, with low levels of silt. The pond size is usually 2,000–3,500 m^2 (0.2–0.35 ha) and water depth is 1.5–2.0 m. Ponds are routinely disinfected before use.

The stocking densities of largemouth bass in ponds are: if stocking 8–10 cm juveniles 1,500–2,300 per 1,000 m^2 (15,000–23,000/ha); or if stocking 15 cm juveniles 1,000–1,500 per 1,000 m^2 (10,000–15,000/ha). To help maintain water quality, approximately 200–250 large-size silver carp (*Hypophthalmichthys molitrix*), crucian carp (*Carassius auratus*), and bighead carp (*Aristichthys nobilis*) can be placed in the pond (a total of 600–1,000 carp/ha).

3.5 Pond polyculture

Ponds for extensive polyculture production should exceed 2,500 m^2 (0.25 ha) in surface area to ensure adequate space for polyculture. The ponds should not contain snakehead (*Ophiocephalus argus*), catfish (*Parasilurus asotus*), or other aggressive and carnivorous fish. Approximately 100–150 juvenile largemouth bass 5–6 cm in size are stocked per 1,000 m^2 (1,000–1,500/ha) on an annual basis in April or May. The size (average individual weight) of other fish in the polyculture pond, such as grass carp (*Ctenopharyngodon idella*), silver carp, bighead carp, carp (*Cyprinus carpio*), and bighead carp should not exceed 150 g each (Li et al., 2012; Zhan, 2001).

3.6 Cage culture

Cages are constructed of polyethylene no-knot mesh and are generally 2 m × 2 m × 2 m or 3 m × 3 m × 2.5 m in size. The mesh size used is dependent on the size of fingerlings being stocked. A cage with 1 cm mesh is suitable for 8 cm fish, while 2.5–3.0 cm mesh should be used when fish exceed 15 cm. The cage mesh is suspended within a floating closed frame that provides some shaded area with good air flow. Cages should be located in open water, in an area with good air movement, a water depth > 3.5 m, and limited water flow (< 0.1 m/s) (Bai et al., 2009).

Largemouth bass density in culture cages is determined by the size of fish being stocked, with densities decreasing as fish size increases. The cages are initially stocked with 8–10 cm juveniles at approximately 300 fish/m^2. When the juveniles reach 30–50 g average weight, the density is decreased to 150–200 fish/m^2. When fish weight reaches 150 g the density is reduced to 100 fish/m^2 (Bai et al., 2009; Li and Li, 2000; Zhan, 2001).

3.7 Feed types and sources

Until 2016, largemouth bass culturing in China was still dominated by frozen trash fish feed, or a mix of frozen trash fish and formulated diets (Zhu et al., 2006). However, with the development of intensive high-density largemouth bass culture, formulated diets have become more popular (Li et al., 2012; Zhou et al., 2015).

Currently there are more than a hundred commercial aquaculture feed companies in China. Commercial largemouth bass feeds are produced by both domestic and international feed companies. Currently largemouth bass are primarily fed floating feed. The domestic feed producer TECH-BANK Food Co. Ltd. has produced the extruded floating pellets for largemouth bass since 2015. The protein content of commercial feed for largemouth bass feeds ranges from 44% to 48%. The main protein source in the feeds is still fish meal.

3.7.1 Frozen fish feed

As stated, in the past largemouth bass in China were largely fed frozen trash fish during grow out. When feeding frozen fish, the feed conversion ratio (FCR) exceeded 4.0 but was still reasonably profitable. However, since 2017 the Chinese government has prohibited the feeding of frozen fish in aquaculture for several reasons. First, it is difficult to guarantee the quality and quantity of frozen fish. Second, feeding frozen fish can transfer diseases. Finally, when feeding frozen fish, water quality can easily be negatively impacted.

3.7.2 Formulated diets

In recent years, commercial feeds for largemouth bass have been more fully developed. Using commercial pelleted feeds, feed conversion ratios (FCR) of 1.1–1.3 have been achieved. The three primary advantages associated with the use of commercial feeds are: (1) reduced labor requirements for feeding; (2) maintenance of better water quality; and (3) reductions in disease (Yang et al., 1995).

3.8 Markets and product forms

Largemouth bass as a food-fish is rich in protein, lipids, and essential amino acids. The market demand for largemouth bass in China has increased considerably in recent years. Live largemouth bass are primarily transported in refrigerated containers. Long-distance transport using refrigerated containers involves three phases: live fish holding, packaging, and transportation.

Of the largemouth bass cultured in the Pearl River Delta, 5–8% are sold into the local aquatic product markets in the cities of Beijing, Xi'an, Zhengzhou, and Shanghai. In the provinces of Jiangsu and Zhejiang, production has increased in recent years. Most of these fish are sold into the growing nearby markets of Nanjing, Hangzhou, and Shanghai, with a small amount being sold in Beijing and Xi'an (Bai and Li, 2013b).

The size of fish desired by the different regions and markets varies. In northern markets, such as Beijing and Zhengzhou, the primary demand is for large fish (> 500 g), and they are often used in restaurants. However, in Shanghai, Jiangsu, Zhejiang, and Xi'an, smaller fish (< 400 g) are more popular (Zhou et al., 2015). The fish are transported live by specialized transport companies and marketed live for preparation at home.

Different regions also have different cooking preferences for largemouth bass. In Guangdong province, people prefer to steam them or eat them raw (sashimi). In other provinces, varied preparations, such as steaming or dry frying are utilized.

3.9 Conclusion

With improvements in culture technologies, genetics, and changes in the modes of transportation and marketing, the economics of largemouth bass aquaculture in China has continuously improved. This has supported a steady and stable development of the largemouth bass aquaculture industry. However, some challenges remain for the largemouth bass aquaculture industry in China (Bai and Li, 2013b).

3.9.1 Genetic challenges

The foundation population originally introduced from North American was very small. Since that time there has been little attention paid to broodstock management or breeding and genetics. The rate of survival has decreased, the age at sexual maturity has increased, and disease resistance has decreased.

The development and dissemination of improved genetic varieties is required. Even if a new breeding variety, such as Youlu No. 1, is developed, currently the hatchery production of largemouth bass is on small farms. National and provincial level hatcheries are needed for this species.

3.9.2 Feed challenges

Currently, largemouth bass feeds in China still contain about 30% fish meal. Commercial feeds for largemouth have improved. However, the diet formulations for largemouth still need to be optimized for satisfying their nutrient requirements (Chen et al., 2012; Li et al., 2017).

The development and optimization of commercial feeds is required. Research and development of feeds for this species have progressed rapidly among some Chinese companies in recent years. However, there is still a need to improve and optimize feed formulations specific for this species (Li and Chen, 2011). Also, from a genetic breeding standpoint, the adaptability of largemouth bass individuals to accept commercial feed varies greatly. Therefore, there is a need to combine improved diet formulation, improved feed processing technology, and improved genetics to build a new largemouth bass aquaculture model (Bai and Li, 2013b).

3.9.3 Disease challenges

To increase yields and profits, the culture density of largemouth bass has been continuously increasing. With the genetic degradation of the species, disease issues are a frequent problem. Currently there are several common diseases, including parasites, viral and bacterial diseases, as well as a "multi-pathogen comprehensive disease phenomenon" (Bai and Li, 2013b). Disease susceptibility and its interaction with nutrition and genetics need to be better understood.

Better disease control is required. Appropriate stocking densities need to be established for this species. Overstocking at unsustainable densities is a problem for Chinese aquaculture farmers. More sustainable stocking densities would reduce the use of chemicals and drugs. Increased use of ecological control techniques such as probiotics and prebiotics should be evaluated. Moreover, the Chinese government should strengthen its support of research on disease control of this species, establish rapid detection technologies, and speed up the research and development of vaccines, especially those targeting viral disease (Bai and Li, 2013b).

3.9.4 Industrial management challenges

There are no large companies or enterprises rearing this species. Cultivation of largemouth bass is almost entirely by small farmers. Therefore, there is little supply chain management and the industrial chain is short and the level of technology development is low. This also contributes to the market price fluctuations which lead to fluctuations in production (Bai and Li, 2013b).

Industrial management and brand establishment should be improved. There is a need to establish the model of "company + farmer." Larger companies could provide high-quality fingerlings and high-quality feeds. Larger companies could also support advanced breeding technologies and provide market consultation to farmers. This model has been put into operation in Pearl River Delta of China. Branding and marketing of the largemouth bass could help to avoid large fluctuations in market price. In addition, there is a need to study the food science aspects of the species, including processing and cooking techniques. Also, there is a need to promote the use of the largemouth bass in traditional dishes, to develop unique dishes and preparations featuring the culinary attributes of the largemouth bass (Bai and Li, 2013b).

References

Bai, J. and Li, S.J. (2013a) *Research on Genetic Breeding in Largemouth Bass.* Ocean Press, Beijing.

Bai, J.J. and Li, S. (2013b) Current status and development trend on China largemouth bass industry. *Chinese Fisheries Economics* 5, 104–108.

Bai, J., Lutz-Carrillo, D.J., Quan, Y. and Liang, S. (2008) Taxonomic status and genetic diversity of cultured largemouth bass *Micropterus salmoides* in China. *Aquaculture* 278, 27–30.

Bai, J.J., Li, S.J., Zheng, G. and Xie, J. (2009) The culturing status and technology of Largemouth bass in China. *Chinese Fisheries Economics* 7, 15–17.

Chen, N.S., Xiao, W.W., Liang, Q.L., Zhou, H.Y., Ma, X.L. and Zhao, M. (2012) Effects of dietary lipid to protein ratios on growth performance, body composition and non-specific immunity of largemouth bass (*Micropterus salmoides*). *Journal of Fisheries of China* 36, 1270–1280.

Li, E.C. and Chen, L.Q. (2011) Research advances on nutrient requirements of *Micropterus salmoides. Modern Agricultural Science and Technology* 21, 312–318.

Li, J., Lei, G., Li, X., Bi, X. and Lin, M. (2012) Current situation and development suggestion of largemouth bass in Guangdong. *Chinese Fisheries Economics* 33, 2–5.

Li, S. (2008) Breeding techniques of largemouth bass. *Contemporary Aquaculture* 33, 26–28.

Li, X. and Li, D. (2000) Three culturing patterns of largemouth bass. *Agriculture of Hunan* 6, 19–25.

Li, Z.F., Gong, W.B., Wang, J.L., Wang, G.J., Yu, D.G. and Xie, J. (2017) Evaluation of effects of frozen fresh fish and artificial compound feed on muscle quality and health status of *Micropterus salmoides. Chinese Journal of Animal Nutrition* 29, 4180–4188.

Liang, S.X., Bai, J.J., Xing, Y.E., Lao, H.H. and Jian, Q. (2007) RAPD analysis of genetic diversity for cultured largemouth bass *Micropterus salmoides. Journal of Dalian Fisheries University* 22, 260–263.

Liao, L.C. (2000) The state of finfish diversification in Asian aquaculture. *Cahiers Options Méditerranéennes* 7, 109–125

Lou, Y. (2000) Present situation and countermeasure of the study on fish introduction in China. *Journal of Fisheries of China* 24, 185–192.

Ma, X.F., Xiong, B.X. and Wang, M.X. (2003) Intentionally introduced and transferred fishes in China's inland waters. *Asian Fisheries Science* 16, 279–290.

Wickstrom, G.A. and Applegate, R.L. (1989) Growth and food selection of intensively cultured largemouth bass fry. *North American Journal of Aquaculture* 51, 79–82.

Wu, Q. (1993) Reproduction habits, early embryonic development of *Micropterus salmoides* and relation between its incubation and water temperature. *Transaction of Oceanology and Limnology* 1, 64–70.

Yang, H., Lou, R., Tang, X. and Xu, Y. (1995) Studies on the feeding of largemouth bass. *Journal of Shanghai Fisheries University* 4, 194–198.

Zhan, X. (2001) Several breeding techniques for largemouth bass. *Rural Things* 2, 35–36.

Zhang, K., Yu, D., Xie, J., Wang, G., Yu, E., Gong, W., Li, Z., Nan, W., Yun, X. and Wang, C. (2017) Energy evaluation of largemouth bass (*Micropterus salmoides*) aquaculture system in the Pearl River Delta, China. *Journal of Fisheries of China* 41, 1424–1433.

Zhang, Y. and He, Y. (1994) Study on culture techniques of largemouth bass (*Micropterus salmoides*). *Journal of Zhanjiang Ocean University* 14, 23–28.

Zhou, Z., Hu, D., Zhu, Q. and Wang, S. (2015) The prospects of diet and current status for largemouth bass in Huzhou. *Chinese Fisheries Economics* 31, 4–6.

Zhu, X.P., He-Jun, D.U., Zheng, G.M., Jiao, Z.Y., Chen, S. and Chen, Z.A. (2006) Genetic diversity analysis of largemouth bass (*Micropterus salmoides*) cultured in ponds. *Journal of Dalian Fisheries University* 21, 341–345.

CHAPTER 4

Environmental requirements for the culture of largemouth bass

Joseph R. Tomasso

School of Fisheries, Aquaculture and Aquatic Sciences, Auburn University, Auburn, Alabama, USA

4.1 Introduction

Largemouth bass are adapted to temperate, freshwater environments. Since temperate aquatic environments characteristically exhibit extensive variability in physiochemical characteristics, it is not surprising that largemouth bass are tolerant to wide ranges of specific characteristics. In this chapter, the preferences and limits of largemouth bass to water quality characteristics important to aquaculture will be summarized.

4.2 Temperature

Temperature is the predominant physiochemical characteristic in aquaculture operations. It affects the amount of oxygen a given amount of water will hold, the rate of photosynthesis and decomposition, the ionization of ammonia, and the metabolic rate of the fish. Changing temperatures are also major cues for reproduction. Fry (1947, 1971) characterized the role of temperature as an environmental controller, and as such, should be given primary consideration when siting an aquaculture operation.

Largemouth bass eggs spawned at 17–21°C exhibited good hatching (≥ 90%) when incubated between 13 and 24°C. By slowly (0.2°C/h) changing from spawning to incubation temperature, the range of good hatching was extended to 10–27°C (Kelley, 1968). When tested under constant-temperature conditions ranging from 15 to 36°C, fry grew best in 25–27°C water (Coutant and DeAngelis, 1983).

Largemouth bass fingerlings (mean 9.1 g) were cultured in tanks for 97 days on a commercial salmonid diet at either 20, 26, or 32°C (Tidwell et al., 2003). Survival averaged 94% and was not affected by water temperature. Weight gain in the 26 and 32°C treatments was similar and averaged 647% while weight gain in the 20°C treatment averaged 325%. Across the three treatments, feed conversion ratio ranged from 1.0 to 1.2 and was lowest in the 26°C treatment. Condition

Table 4.1 Temperatures of importance to the culture of largemouth bass *Micropterus salmoides.*

Temperature (°C)	Action	References
2.0	Temperature at which 48% of Florida subspecies died after 5 days exposure	Carmichael et al., 1988
10.0–27.0	Good (≥ 90%) hatching success when acclimated to hatching temperature at 0.2°C/h	Kelley, 1968
25.0–27.0	Best temperature range for fry growth	Coutant and DeAngelis, 1983
26.0	Best temperature for fingerling growth based on a 97-day growth trial	Tidwell et al., 2003
28.1–28.6	Best temperature for growth based on temperature preference	Díaz et al., 2007
37.3	Chronic thermal maximum for northern subspecies	Fields et al., 1987
39.2	Chronic thermal maximum for Florida subspecies	Fields et al., 1987

factor (K) ranged from 1.3 to 1.4 and was lowest in the 20°C treatment. In aggregate, these results indicate that 26°C is the best temperature of the three tested in which to grow largemouth bass fingerlings. A study by Díaz et al. (2007) using a temperature preference approach estimated the optimum temperature for growth to be between 28.1 and 28.6°C.

Two subspecies of largemouth bass, the northern largemouth bass (*Micropterus salmoides salmoides*) and the Florida largemouth bass (*Micropterus salmoides floridanus*), are recognized and cultured in the USA (Philipp et al., 1985). As the names imply, one subspecies is native to more northern areas while the other is native to more southern areas. The two subspecies do differ from each other in characteristics that may be important to aquaculture. For instance, when water temperature is reduced to 2°C (at a rate of 1°C/day) and then held for 5 days, about one-half of the exposed Florida largemouth bass fingerlings died while only 4–5% of northern fish died (Carmichael et al., 1988). Interestingly, hybrids of the subspecies (both originals and reciprocals) exhibited low-temperature tolerance similar to the northern subspecies. When water temperature was increased at a rate of 1°C/day, the northern subspecies was the most susceptible to high temperature while the Florida subspecies was most resistant and the hybrids were intermediate (Fields et al., 1987). Table 4.1 summarizes temperatures of importance to the culture of largemouth bass.

4.3 Dissolved oxygen

Fish, like all animals, require oxygen to transfer energy efficiently from molecules making up food to molecules that can transfer the energy to the host of physiological processes within the organism. Most oxygen in culture water comes from two sources. First, oxygen diffuses from the atmosphere down a pressure gradient into the water (mechanical aerators simply enhance this process). Second, oxygen is produced within the water by photosynthetic activity of algae. Some intensive aquaculture systems may also add pure oxygen. Oxygen dissolved in the water will enter a fish by diffusing down a pressure gradient across the gills into the blood of the fish. Once in the fish, the oxygen is transported to the tissues where it is needed, at which point it further diffuses down a pressure gradient into the tissue that will consume it. It should be noted that the driving force for delivering oxygen to the tissues is passive (diffusion down a pressure gradient). The pressure gradient is maintained by a high concentration of oxygen in the water (because of constant inputs) and a low concentration of oxygen in the tissues (because of constant consumption). There is no active uptake system for oxygen. Hence, acceptable environmental oxygen levels must be maintained at all times or the fish will not have adequate oxygen to function to its potential (Colt and Tomasso, 2001).

When discussing oxygen concentrations required for fishes, temperature must be an integral part of the discussion for two reasons. First, increasing temperature increases the metabolic rate of fishes, which is reflected in increased oxygen needs (Fry, 1947, 1971). Second, warmer water holds less oxygen than cooler water (Table 4.2 this volume, discussed in Colt and Tomasso, 2001). Taken together, fish in warmwater have a higher oxygen requirement in an environment with a decreased pressure gradient with which to deliver the oxygen to the tissues. For example, oxygen consumption of largemouth bass fingerlings acclimated for 30 days to 20, 23, 26, 29, and 32°C demonstrated a linear increase in oxygen consumption (from 46 to 86 mg O_2/kg/h) over the range of acclimation temperatures, an 87% increase (Díaz et al., 2007).

Largemouth bass embryo development and egg hatching as a function of temperature and dissolved oxygen concentrations were investigated in a comprehensive study by Dudley and Eipper (1975). Their results indicated that dissolved oxygen concentrations should be above 2.0, 2.1, and 2.8 mg/l for incubation temperatures of 15, 20 and 25°C, respectively, for successful hatching. However, the investigators observed many abnormally developed larvae. A further analysis of the results suggested that dissolved oxygen concentrations of 2.0, 2.5, and 3.5 mg/l for incubation temperatures of 15, 20, and 25°C, respectively, are adequate to reduce the incidence of abnormally developed larvae to the level found in incubation water containing 90% oxygen saturation. The Dudley and Eipper study also indicated that vertical movement of the hatching chamber in the water column was detrimental to hatching.

Critical oxygen levels (the lowest dissolved oxygen level at which fish consistently survived for 24 h) for largemouth bass fingerlings were determined by Moss and Scott (1961). Fish acclimated to 25, 30, and 35°C demonstrated critical oxygen levels of 0.92, 1.19, and 1.40 mg/l, respectively. These values fit well with residual oxygen concentrations (dissolved oxygen concentrations at time of death from hypoxia) of ~0.7 mg/l for largemouth bass fingerlings acclimated to 22°C (Carmichael et al., 1988).

Table 4.2 Dissolved oxygen saturation in pure water at selected temperatures under an air atmosphere at 760 mm Hg pressure (modified from Boyd, 1979).

Temperature (°C)	Dissolved oxygen (mg/l)	Temperature (°C)	Dissolved oxygen (mg/l)
8	11.5	22	8.5
10	10.9	24	8.3
12	10.4	26	8.0
14	10.0	28	7.8
16	9.6	30	7.5
18	9.2	32	7.3
20	8.8	34	7.1

Table 4.3 Dissolved oxygen concentrations of importance to the culture of largemouth bass *Micropterus salmoides*.

Dissolved oxygen (mg/l)	Action	Reference
2.0, 2.5, 3.5	Minimum oxygen levels in 15, 20, and 25°C water, respectively, for good hatching success and normally developed larvae	Dudley and Eipper, 1975
0.92, 1.19, 1.40	Critical levels of dissolved oxygen (the lowest level at which fish consistently survived for 24 h) at 25, 30, and 35°C	Moss and Scott, 1961
0.7	Residual oxygen concentration (oxygen concentration at time of death) at 22°C	Carmichael et al., 1988
1.5	Residual oxygen concentration at 22°C in the presence of 0.7 mg/l un-ionized ammonia	Carmichael et al., 1988
1.6	Reduced growth and feed conversion at 26°C	Stewart et al., 1967
4.0	Concentration at which fingerling growth and feed conversion did not differ from fish in higher oxygen concentrations at 26°C	Stewart et al., 1967

In a short-term (11–15 day) laboratory study at 26°C (Stewart et al., 1967), largemouth bass fingerling growth was shown to increase with increasing dissolved oxygen levels in a near-linear fashion up to air saturation levels (~8.2 mg/l dissolved oxygen). Feed conversion also improved as dissolved oxygen levels increased. Dissolved oxygen levels as low as 1.6 mg/l did not affect survival but did affect growth and feed conversion. The authors indicated 4 mg/l as an oxygen level above which growth and feed conversions did not differ markedly. Interestingly, dissolved oxygen levels above air saturation levels (achieved using pure oxygen) had a detrimental effect on growth and feed conversion. The high pressure gradient in the supersaturated water may have suppressed ventilation (breathing) activity of the fish because oxygen was flowing quickly into the blood. However, a consequence of reduced ventilation is reduced release of carbon dioxide which can lead to metabolic pH disturbances in the fish (Wood, 1991) and perhaps have an impact on growth and feed conversion.

Table 4.3 summarizes dissolved oxygen levels of importance to largemouth bass. It appears that largemouth bass are fairly tolerant of low dissolved oxygen concentrations. However, oxygen levels affect fish health and immune systems as well as survival, growth and feed conversion. It is advised that culturists design production systems to maintain dissolved oxygen levels well above minimums discussed here.

4.4 Dissolved solids

Surface and ground waters contain dissolved substances that are derived from the environment as the water passes through, on and below the surface of the Earth. When speaking of freshwater, the term "total dissolved solids" is used to denote all dissolved solids, regardless of the specific nature, found in a sample. When speaking of sea water, the term "salinity" is used to describe the total concentration of a very specific set of ions and complex ions that exist in specific ratios to each other (Spotte, 1979). The terms salinity and total dissolved solids are often used interchangeably, but doing so can be misleading.

Table 4.4 Major ions, their chemical forms, and concentrations found in full-strength sea water (adapted from Bowen, 1966, and Spotte, 1979).

Ion	Major form	mg/l	Ion	Major form	mg/l
Chloride	Cl^-	19,000	Potassium	K^+	380
Sodium	Na^+	10,500	Bromide	Br^-	65
Magnesium	Mg^{++}	1,350	Carbon	CO_3H^-	28
Sulfur	$SO4^{--}$	885	Strontium	Sr^{++}	8
Calcium	Ca^{++}	400	Silicon	$Si(OH)_4$	3

Within freshwater, two important ions are calcium and magnesium. Collectively, they make up the hardness of the water. Hardness is expressed as milligram per liter of equivalent calcium carbonate (Boyd, 1979). The environmental calcium is especially important in fish culture because it helps reduce water and ion flux across the gills, reducing the energy requirements to maintain homeostasis in the fish (Weirich et al., 1992; Grizzle et al., 1993). Water hardness requirements for the culture of freshwater fishes are not well defined. The recommended hardness for the culture of striped bass *Morone saxatilis* juveniles is 150 mg/l as calcium carbonate (Hall, 1991). Largemouth bass appear to do well in a range of hardnesses.

Seawater contains 35 g/l sea salt (Spotte, 1979). Sea salt contains over 60 elements. Table 4.4 lists some of the elements and their major forms found in seawater. In the tidal areas of rivers entering estuaries, it is common to find an extended continuum of sea water to freshwater. Largemouth bass are often found in the continuum (Meador and Kelso, 1989, 1990; DeVries et al., 2015). Freshwater fishes do have a limit to the salinity they can tolerate for extended periods of time. This limit corresponds to 10–12 g/l salinity, the point where water begins leaving the fish osmotically across the gills. Long-term survival above 10–12 g/l requires physiological mechanisms characteristic of estuarine and seawater-adapted fishes (Colt and Tomasso, 2001). Salinity is expressed as parts per thousand, grams per liter, or per mille (‰). For practical purposes, all mean the same thing (gram of sea salt per liter of solution).

In a laboratory study by Meador and Kelso (1990), largemouth bass (185–289 mm total length) were collected from a freshwater lake and a 2 g/l salinity marsh. The fish were then cultured for 120 days at 0, 4, 8, or 12 g/l salinity (22°C). Fish from the freshwater lake grew equally well in 0 and 8 g/l salinity. Growth was lower in 8 g/l, and no fish survived the study in 12 g/l. Fish from the marsh grew equally well in 0, 4, and 8 g/l salinity, while no fish survived the study in 12 g/l. These results indicate the potential to grow largemouth bass in low-salinity water.

4.5 pH, carbon dioxide, and alkalinity

The negative logarithm of the hydrogen ion concentration of a solution is defined as pH. It presents on a scale of 1 to 14. Solutions with a pH below 7 are acidic, solutions with a pH above 7 are basic (alkaline), and solutions with a pH of 7 are neutral. The further the number is from seven, the stronger the acid or base. The sensitivity of largemouth bass to pH is not well defined. However, anecdotal evidence indicates that they do well in the range of 6.5 to 9.0 recommended for hatchery operations (Piper et al., 1982).

When discussing pH and culture conditions, it is important to distinguish between chronic and transient exposure. During pond culture, fish are typically exposed to a daily cycle of pH with lowest pH just after sunrise and highest pH just before sunset (see below in the discussion of alkalinity). In raceway culture, using well or stream water, or recirculating culture, the fish may be exposed to constant pH values. Largemouth bass appear to do well in pond culture and can tolerate a wide range of pH values, including short term exposures of up to 10 (characteristic of low alkalinity ponds). However, continuous exposure to high or low pH water may have detrimental effects.

Two major detrimental effects can be attributed to extreme culture pH values. At the low end, bicarbonate (H_2CO_3) in solution will dehydrate to form free carbon dioxide (CO_2). This process increases in rate as pH falls below 7.0 (Boyd, 1979). As the partial pressure of carbon dioxide increases in the culture water, it inhibits the excretion of carbon dioxide from the fish by way of the gills. As carbon dioxide builds up in the blood, it interferes with oxygen transport. At the high end, pH will increase the fraction of ammonia in its toxic form (see below discussion on ammonia). Consequently, extreme pH situations, especially during continuous exposure, need to be monitored and managed. Little work has been conducted to understand the sensitivity of largemouth bass to carbon dioxide. However, one study using corticosteroid hormones as indicators of stress reported that largemouth bass appeared unstressed (pH ~7.3) when exposed to 35 mg/l carbon dioxide but slightly stressed when exposed to 135 mg/l (Carmichael et al., 1984).

An example of a management strategy is one used in the author's lab for recirculating systems. In this case, we set pH limits of 7.5 and 8.0. The range is applied to both freshwater and seawater systems and considers three aspects of pH and culture – low pH increases free carbon dioxide concentrations, high pH increases the fraction of ammonia in its toxic form, and the pH range that supports efficient biofilter function (Spotte, 1979). We monitor pH daily, or every few days. Functioning biofilters will suppress pH as hydrogen ions are released in the nitrification process. Buffering capacity is less in freshwater than saltwater, so pH will fall faster in freshwater systems. When pH reaches 7.5, we add adequate sodium bicarbonate to raise the pH to near 8.0.

The total titratable base in an aqueous solution is referred to as total alkalinity (Boyd, 1979). It is expressed as equivalent calcium carbonate. In ponds, alkalinity interacts with algal photosynthesis in that periods of high net carbon dioxide production by algae (evening) tend to reduce pond pH while periods of high net algal carbon dioxide consumption (daytime with sunshine) tend to allow pH to rise. The degree of the daily pH shift is partly a function of the alkalinity – high alkalinity ponds have a higher buffering capacity and lower pH shift, lower alkalinity ponds have a lower buffering capacity and broader pH shift (Boyd and Tucker, 2014). The alkalinity of culture water has no direct impact on the culture animals. It is the pH that is important, so managing alkalinity is an indirect way of managing pH. Managing alkalinity by adding lime to ponds is discussed in Boyd (1979) and Boyd and Tucker (2014).

4.6 Nitrogenous wastes

Fish feed contains protein to support fish development, growth and health. When feed is introduced into a pond or other culture unit, most (hopefully) of the feed is consumed by the fish. The remainder is consumed by the decomposer community in the pond. By either route, part of the protein is retained in additional biomass (fish or decomposer growth) and part is used as an energy source. Largemouth bass, being carnivores, will use more protein for energy than omnivores, such as catfish. Hence, catfish feeds have a lower level of protein than feed for carnivorous fishes. When protein is metabolized for energy, it is first reduced to its component amino acids which, in turn, are deaminated. The deamination step produces ammonia, which is very toxic to animals and must be excreted. Once in the culture water, ammonia is normally removed by the processes of the nitrogen cycle in ponds, which includes the process of nitrification, or removed simply by nitrification in recirculating systems (Spotte, 1979; Boyd and Tucker, 2014). If the nitrogen cycle and nitrification are working correctly, the concentration of ammonia in the culture water remains low. However, if feed inputs exceed the capacity of the ammonia removal systems or if some other factors affect the systems (for example, rapid temperature change), a buildup of ammonia may occur in the culture system.

In aqueous solution, ammonia exists in two forms – ammonia (NH_3) and ammonium (NH_4^+). Together, these two chemical species are referred to as total ammonia. NH_3 is the toxic form of ammonia because it is capable of diffusing across the gill membrane (Tomasso, 1994; Wright and Wood, 2009). The toxicity of ammonia to fishes depends largely on the pH of the culture water because the pH controls the proportion of the total ammonia that is in the toxic form (Table 4.5). Temperature has a lesser effect on ionization. As can be seen in Table 4.5, the percent of ammonia in the toxic form rises sharply as pH rises above 8, so ammonia levels should be carefully monitored when culturing fish at constant pH values above 8. Transient pH values above 8 such as during daily pH cycling in ponds may not be detrimental because the animals have an opportunity to excrete ammonia during the periods of lower pH.

Limited studies (unpublished, Carmichael and Tomasso) indicate that largemouth bass have a 72 h median-lethal concentration (the concentration of a poison that will kill one-half of exposed animals in 72 h) of 15.3 mg/l total ammonia-nitrogen at pH 8.0 and temperature 25°C. Of this total, 0.82 mg/l is in the un-ionized, or toxic, form (see Table 4.5). Recommendations for "safe" levels vary, but a rule of thumb is to keep ambient levels no higher than one-tenth and preferably below one-twentieth of lethal levels (0.082 and 0.041 mg/l, respectively).

The process of nitrification is mediated by nitrifying bacteria (Spotte, 1979; Boyd and Tucker, 2014). During this process, ammonia is oxidized to nitrite (NO_2^-) and then to nitrate (NO_3^-). In a balanced pond or recirculating system, ammonia and nitrite concentrations are low and nitrate either accumulates or is removed by assimilation into aquatic plants. As noted above, perturbations of the nitrification process may lead to increases in ammonia concentrations. It

Table 4.5 The percent of total ammonia in aqueous solution that is in the un-ionized (NH_3) form at five pH values and three temperatures (modified from Emerson et al., 1975)

pH	Percent in un-ionized form				
	10°C	15°C	20°C	25°C	30°C
6	00.019	00.027	00.040	00.057	00.081
7	00.186	00.273	00.396	00.566	00.799
8	01.830	02.670	03.820	05.380	07.460
9	15.700	21.500	28.400	36.300	44.600
10	65.100	73.300	79.900	85.100	89.000

may also lead to increases in nitrite concentrations. Nitrite, like ammonia, may be toxic to fish. Conversely, nitrate is not very toxic.

Nitrite is highly toxic to many species of fishes (Tomasso, 1994). However, largemouth bass is not one of them. Palachek and Tomasso (1984) reported a 96 h median-lethal concentration to largemouth bass fingerlings of 140 mg/l nitrite-N, compared to 7.1 mg/l for channel catfish (*Ictalurus punctatus*). The basis for the large interspecies difference in toxicity was later shown to be related to differences in chloride-uptake mechanisms (Tomasso and Grosell, 2005). It is doubtful that nitrite will reach detrimental levels in largemouth bass culture systems. The most obvious clinical sign of nitrite toxicity is the presence of brown blood brought about by nitrite-induced oxidation of the iron in hemoglobin (Tomasso, 1994). If a culturist suspects nitrite toxicity, a brownish coloration to the blood or gills would serve as a presumptive diagnosis.

No work has focused on nitrate toxicity to largemouth bass. However, work on the closely related Guadalupe bass (*Micropterus treculi*) showed a 96 h median-lethal concentration of 1,261 mg/l nitrate-nitrogen (Tomasso and Carmichael, 1986). This value fits well with other toxicity values for freshwater fishes reviewed in Camargo et al. (2005). Nitrate does not appear to be a consideration from a toxicity perspective; however, nitrate is a fundamental plant nutrient, so high environmental nitrate levels can be expected to affect phytoplankton growth in any culture system receiving sunlight.

4.7 Gas supersaturation

Atmospheric gases over water tend toward an equilibrium with gases dissolved in the water. Biological and chemical activity in the water consume dissolved gases (particularly oxygen), usually keeping the total gas pressure in the water below that of the air above it and providing a pressure gradient for further diffusion from the atmosphere. Occasionally, culture water may become gas supersaturated – the total gas pressure in the water is higher than in the atmosphere above it. Gas supersaturation is an unstable condition in which the excess gas in the water is prone to form bubbles (much like the bubbles that form when a carbonated drink is opened). If these dissolved gases diffuse across the gills into the fish, and then bubbles form, capillary and small vessel circulation will be inhibited (termed gas bubble disease) resulting in death of the culture animals.

Gas bubble disease is not usually a problem in ponds given the large surface area that is the interface between the water and atmosphere. Also, mechanical and wind aeration promote degassing from water to atmosphere down the pressure gradient. Problems with supersaturation tend to occur in hatcheries, holding facilities and recirculating systems where water is pumped or heated. Heating reduces the ability of water to hold dissolved gases, so increasing the temperature of saturated water puts it in a supersaturated condition (this is why bubbles form on the sides of a saucepan when heating water on a stove). Pumps with air leaks on the low-pressure side will draw in air and then force it into the water on the high-pressure side resulting in supersaturation. Another common way water is supersaturated in fish production facilities is filling empty pipes with water with the end valves closed, pressurizing the air in the pipes. Colt and Tomasso (2001) and Hargreaves and Tomasso (2004) discuss supersaturation in more detail.

No controlled studies of the effects of gas supersaturation on largemouth bass were found. However, anecdotal reports from hatcheries clearly indicate that largemouth bass are susceptible to gas supersaturation and exposure should be avoided.

Largemouth bass are also susceptible to swim bladder stress syndrome (Carmichael and Tomasso, 1984), a malady that may be mistaken for gas bubble disease. This syndrome is characterized by overinflated swim bladders that may cause the fish to broach. It is distinct from gas bubble disease in that no emboli form in the blood. The etiology of swim bladder stress syndrome is not clear; however, it appears to be more related to handling stress than gas supersaturation.

A final consideration when discussing gas supersaturation is oxygen supersaturation, which can occur when pure oxygen is being used to maintain proper oxygen levels in water. This often occurs in transport tanks when oxygen is being metered into the tanks at too high a rate. Measured oxygen levels can reach two or more times the saturation level for aeration systems; however, the total gas pressure does not exceed atmospheric pressure though because oxygen is displacing nitrogen in the water. Oxygen supersaturation can cause developmental problems if transporting eggs, embryos or fry; however, it is generally not a problem when transporting fingerlings.

4.8 Hydrogen sulfide

Hydrogen sulfide (H_2S) is a toxic gas produced by way of anaerobic activity of bacteria. It is sometimes found in well water and in anaerobic pond bottoms where organic material has collected. A common problem in warmwater pond culture is the release of hydrogen sulfide from the sediments when fingerling ponds are drained to collect fish. Raking pond bottoms and allowing the ponds to remain empty between production cycles reduces the accumulation of organic material and incidence of hydrogen sulfide release.

Maintaining aerobic conditions will promote the oxidation of sulfides to sulfates, which are not toxic. Hydrogen sulfide exists in a pH- and temperature-dependent equilibrium with the HS^- ion. The non-ionic species is the toxic form because it is gill permeable (similar to ammonia). At pH 7 and temperature 25°C, about one-half of the sulfide is in the toxic form (Table 4.6). At a pH of 9, only about 1% is (Wedemeyer, 1996). The USEPA (1986) recommends a maximum

Table 4.6 Effect of pH on the percentage of total hydrogen sulfide and total chlorine in the toxic forms (H_2S and HOCl, respectively).

pH	Percent in toxic forms	
	H_2S	HOCl
5	99	100
6	91	97
7	51	76
8	9	23
9	1	3

Source: Hydrogen sulfide information adapted from Wedemeyer (1996) at 25°C. Chlorine information adapted from Boyd and Tucker (2014) at an unreported temperature.

safe exposure level for aquatic animals of 0.002 mg/l H_2S-S. Tucker (1993) suggests half the USEPA maximum.

4.9 Chlorine

Chlorine is a very effective disinfectant. However, it is also very toxic to aquatic animals. Chlorine can be applied as a liquid, gas, or solid. Regardless of the form of application, an equilibrium forms in the water between the highly toxic hypochlorous acid (HOCl) and less toxic OCl^-. The pH of the water determines the nature of the equilibrium with more HOCl present at high pH values (Table 4.6). The equilibrium is at molar equality at a pH of about 7.5 (Boyd and Tucker, 2014).

Recommended maximum exposure levels for aquatic animals range from 0.001 to 0.10 mg/l total chlorine (summarized in Colt and Tomasso, 2001). Chlorine can be removed by activated carbon, aeration, or sunlight. Simple-to-use test kits are commercially available and should be used after any process in which chlorine is used.

4.10 Copper sulfate

Copper sulfate is commonly added to aquaculture ponds for the control of algae and external parasites. Caution must be exercised when using copper sulfate because copper is very toxic to fish and water chemistry has a large impact on both toxicity and effective concentrations. For example, the 96 h median-lethal concentration of copper (from copper sulfate) to channel catfish increases 20-fold (0.05 to 0.98 mg/l) as the alkalinity is increased from 16 to 240 mg/l as $CaCO_3$ (Straus and Tucker, 1993). The Biotic Ligand Model (DiToro et al., 2000) was developed to integrate the effects of multiple water quality characteristics on both toxicity and effectiveness. Calculating effective and safe levels of copper sulfate for pond application is complex. Inexperienced culturists are encouraged to contact their local extension office for guidance.

4.11 Formalin

Formalin is a water solution containing formaldehyde at saturation level (about 37%). Since malachite green was banned from use, formalin has become the standard antifungal treatment and preventative for fish eggs. It is also used for the treatment of ectoparasites on fish. The 24 h median-lethal concentration for formalin to largemouth bass fingerlings is about 140 µl/l. For ectoparasite control, fish are usually exposed to high concentrations (150–250 µl/l) for about 1 h.

An interesting aspect of formalin use with largemouth bass is that fingerlings are about twice as resistant to formalin as are tadpoles (*Rana berlandieri*). A common problem during largemouth bass fingerling production is that large numbers of tadpoles are harvested from ponds along with the fish – at times the biomass of tadpoles exceeds the biomass of fingerlings. Separating the fish and tadpoles is time-consuming and stressful to the fish. Carmichael and Tomasso (1983) demonstrated that separation could be accomplished by exposing mixed groups of largemouth bass

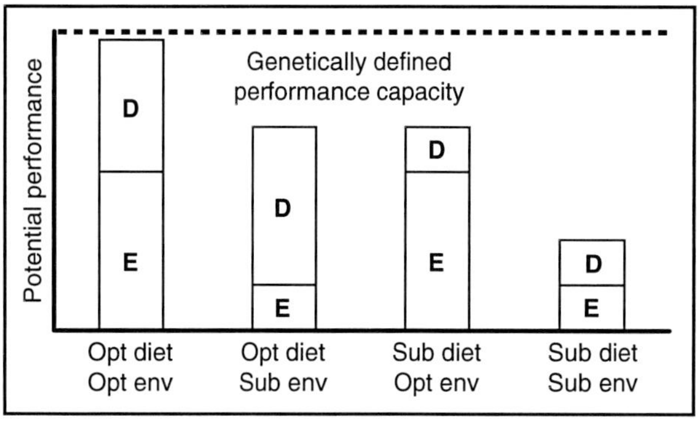

Figure 4.1 Conceptualization of the relationship among genetically defined performance capacity (dashed line), diet, and environment. Suboptimal diets (sub diet) and suboptimal environments (sub env) can reduce performance compared to optimal diets (opt diet) and optimal environments (opt env). The relative contributions of diet and environment shown here are for illustration and not based on experimentation.

fingerlings and tadpoles to 200 µl/l formalin for one hour followed by flushing with 6.9 turnovers per hour. By the end of 24 h, all of the tadpoles were dead and washed toward the drain end of the tank. As with copper sulfate, inexperienced culturists are advised to contact their local extension office for guidance and the latest regulations regarding the use of formalin on food-fish.

4.12 Conclusion

The largemouth bass is a hardy temperate species that is tolerant of a range of water quality. This chapter has highlighted several aspects of the environmental requirements of the species. Several other resources (Williamson et al., 1993; Colt and Tomasso, 2001; Hargreaves and Tomasso, 2004; Boyd and Tucker, 2014) provide additional details and insight.

This chapter has focused on the environment for producing largemouth bass. However, it is important to put environment into perspective. Schreck (1981) used the concept of performance capacity to describe the relationship of a fish to its environment. Essentially, an animal has a genetically defined maximum capacity to perform (survive, grow, reproduce, and so on). Maximum performance capacity is reduced by suboptimal environments or stress. This concept was later put into an aquaculture context (Tomasso, 1995). Figure 4.1 shows the performance capacity concept and how two broad categories (environment and nutrition) can have an impact on performance. In summary, maintaining environments (and diets) as close to optimum as possible will result in better performance (survival, growth, reproduction, feed conversion).

References

Boyd, C.E. (1979) *Water Quality in Warmwater Fish Ponds.* Alabama Agricultural Experiment Station, Auburn, AL.

Boyd, C.E. and Tucker, C.C. (2014) *Handbook for Aquaculture Water Quality.* Available through http://was.org.

Bowen, H.J.M. (1966) *Trace Elements in Biochemistry.* Academic Press, New York.

Camargo, J.A., Alonso, A. and Salamanca, A. (2005) Nitrate toxicity to aquatic animals: a review with new data for freshwater invertebrates. *Chemosphere* 58, 1255–1267.

Carmichael, G.J. and Tomasso, J.R. (1983) Use of formalin to separate tadpoles from largemouth bass fingerlings after harvesting. *Progressive Fish-Culturist* 45, 105–106.

Carmichael, G.J. and Tomasso, J.R. (1984) Swim bladder stress syndrome in largemouth bass. *Texas Journal of Science* 35, 315–321.

Carmichael, G.J., Tomasso, J.R., Simco, B.A. and Davis, K.B. (1984) Confinement and water quality-induced stress in largemouth bass. *Transactions of the American Fisheries Society* 113, 767–777.

Carmichael, G.J., Williamson, J.H., Woodward, C.A.C. and Tomasso, J.R. (1988) Responses of northern, Florida, and hybrid largemouth bass to low temperature and low dissolved oxygen. *Progressive Fish-Culturist* 50, 225–231.

Colt, J.E. and Tomasso, J.R. (2001) Hatchery water supply and treatment. In: Wedemeyer, G.A. (ed.) *Fish Hatchery Management.* American Fisheries Society, Bethesda, MD, pp. 91–186.

Coutant, C.C. and DeAngelis, D.L. (1983) Comparative temperature-dependent growth rates of largemouth and smallmouth bass fry. *Transactions of the American Fisheries Society* 112, 416–423.

DeVries, D.R., Wright, R.A., Glover, D.C., Farmer, T.M., Lowe, M.R., Norris, A.J. and Peer, A.C. (2015) Largemouth bass in coastal estuaries: a comprehensive study from the Mobile-Tensaw River delta, Alabama. *American Fisheries Society Symposium* 82, 297–309.

Díaz, F., Re, A.D., Gonzáles, R.A., Sánchez, L.N., Leyva, G. and Valenzuela, F. (2007) Temperature preference and oxygen consumption of largemouth bass *Micropterus salmoides* (Lacépède) acclimated to different temperatures. *Aquaculture Research* 38, 1387–1394.

DiToro, D.M., Allen, H.E., Bergman, H.L., Meyer, J.S., Santore, R.C. and Paquin, P. (2000) *The Biotic Ligand Model: A Computational Approach for Assessing the Ecological Effects of Copper and Other Metals in Aquatic Systems.* International Copper Association Limited, New York.

Dudley, R.G. and Eipper, A.W. (1975) Survival of largemouth bass embryos at low dissolved oxygen concentrations. *Transactions of the American Fisheries Society* 104, 122–128.

Emerson, K., Russo, R.C., Lund, R.E. and Thurston, R.V. (1975) Aqueous ammonia equilibrium calculations: effect of pH and temperature. *Journal of the Fisheries Research Board of Canada* 32, 2379–2383.

Fields, R., Lowe, S.S., Kaminski, C., Whitt, G.S. and Philipp, D.P. (1987) Critical and chronic thermal maxima of northern and Florida largemouth bass and their reciprocal F_1 and F_2 hybrids. *Transactions of the American Fisheries Society* 116, 856–863.

Fry, F.E.J. (1947) Effects of environment on animal activity. *University of Toronto Studies Biological Series* 55, 1–62.

Fry, F.E.J. (1971) The effects of environmental factors on the physiology of fish. In: Hoar, W.S. and Randall, D.J. (eds) *Fish Physiology*, Volume VI. Academic Press, New York, pp. 1–98.

Grizzle, J.M., Cummins, K.A. and Ashfield, C.J. (1993) Effects of environmental concentrations of calcium and sodium on the calcium flux in stressed 34-day-old striped bass. *Canadian Journal of Zoology* 71, 1379–1384.

Hall, L.W., Jr. (1991) A synthesis of water quality and contaminants data on early life stages of striped bass, *Morone saxatilis. Reviews in Aquatic Sciences* 4, 261–268.

Hargreaves, J.A. and Tomasso, J.R. (2004) Environmental biology. In: Tucker, C.S. and Hargreaves, J.A. (eds) *Biology and Culture of Channel Catfish.* Elsevier, New York, pp. 36–68.

Kelley, J.W. (1968) Effects of incubation temperature on survival of largemouth bass eggs. *Progressive Fish-Culturist* 30, 159–163.

Meador, M.R. and Kelso, W.E. (1989) Behavior and movements of largemouth bass in response to salinity. *Transactions of the American Fisheries Society* 118, 409–415.

Meador, M.R. and Kelso, W.E. (1990) Growth of largemouth bass in low-salinity environments. *Transactions of the American Fisheries Society* 119, 545–552.

Moss, D.D. and Scott, D.C. (1961) Dissolved-oxygen requirements of three species of fish. *Transactions of the American Fisheries Society* 90, 377–393.

Palachek, R.A. and Tomasso, J.R. (1984) Toxicity of nitrite to channel catfish, largemouth bass, and tilapia: evidence for a nitrite-exclusion mechanism. *Canadian Journal of Fisheries and Aquatic Sciences* 41, 1739–1744.

Philipp, D.P., Childers, W.F. and Whitt, G.S. (1985) Correlations of allele frequencies with physical and environmental variables for populations of largemouth bass *Micropterus salmoides* (Lacépède). *Journal of Fish Biology* 27, 347–365.

Piper, R.G., McElwain, I.B, Orme, L.E., McCraren, J.P., Fowler, L.G. and Leonard, J.R. (1982) *Fish Hatchery Management.* U.S. Department of the Interior, U.S. Fish and Wildlife Service, Washington, DC.

Schreck, C.B. (1981) Stress and compensation in teleostean fishes: response to social and physical factors. In: Pickering, A.D. (ed.) *Stress and Fish.* Academic Press, New York, pp. 295–322.

Spotte, S. (1979) *Fish and Invertebrate Culture: Water Management in Closed Systems*, 2nd edn. John Wiley and Sons, New York.

Stewart, N.C., Shumway, D.L. and Doudoroff, P. (1967) Influence of oxygen concentrations on the growth of juvenile largemouth bass. *Journal of the Fisheries Research Board of Canada* 24, 475–494.

Straus, D.L. and Tucker, C.S. (1993) Acute toxicity of copper sulfate and chelated copper to channel catfish *Ictalurus punctatus*. *Journal of the World Aquaculture Society* 24, 390–395.

Tidwell, H.H., Coyle, S.D., Bright, L.A., VanArnum, A. and Yasharian, D. (2003) Effect of water temperature on growth, survival, and biochemical composition of largemouth bass *Micropterus salmoides*. *Journal of the World Aquaculture Society* 34, 175–183.

Tomasso, J.R. (1994) Toxicity of nitrogenous wastes to aquaculture animals. *Reviews in Fisheries Science* 2, 291–314.

Tomasso, J.R. (1995) Environmental requirements of aquaculture animals: a conceptual summary. *World Aquaculture* 27, 27–31.

Tomasso, J.R. and Carmichael, G.J. (1986). Acute toxicity of ammonia, nitrite, and nitrate to Guadalupe bass. *Bulletin of Environmental Contamination and Toxicology* 36, 866–870.

Tomasso, J.R. and Grosell, M. (2005) Physiological basis for large differences in resistance to nitrite among freshwater and freshwater-acclimated euryhaline fishes. *Environmental Science and Technology* 39, 98–102.

Tucker, C.S. (1993) Water analysis. In: Stoskompf, M. (ed.) *Fish Medicine.* W.B. Saunders, Philadelphia, PA, pp. 166–197.

USEPA (1986) *Quality Criteria for Water.* EPA 440/5–86–001, U.S. Environmental Protection Agency, Washington, DC.

Wedemeyer, G.A. (1996) *Physiology of Fish in Intensive Culture Systems.* Chapman and Hall, New York.

Weirich, C.R, Tomasso, J.R. and Smith, T.I.J. (1992) Confinement and transport-induced stress in white bass *Morone chrysops* X striped bass *Morone saxatilis*: effect of calcium and salinity. *Journal of the World Aquaculture Society* 23, 49–57.

Williamson, J.H., Carmichael, G.J., Graves, K.G., Simco, B.A. and Tomasso, J.R. (1993) Centrarchids. In: Stickney, R.R. (ed.) *Culture of Nonsalmonid Freshwater Fishes*, 2nd edn. CRC Press, Ann Arbor, MI, pp. 145–197.

Wood, C.M. (1991) Branchial ion and acid-base transfer in freshwater teleost fish – environmental hypoxia as a probe. *Physiological Zoology* 64, 68–102.

Wright, P.A. and Wood, C.M. (2009) A new paradigm for ammonia excretion in aquatic animals: role of Rhesus (Rh) glycoproteins. *Journal of Experimental Biology* 212, 2303–2312.

CHAPTER 5

Reproduction and genetics

Boris Gomelsky,[1] Kenneth J. Semmens,[1] Eric Peatman,[2] Shawn D. Coyle,[1] and Michael D. Matthews[3]

[1]Kentucky State University, Division of Aquaculture, Frankfort, KY, USA
[2]Auburn University, School of Fisheries, Aquaculture and Aquatic Sciences, Auburn, AL, USA
[3]A.E. Wood Fish Hatchery, San Marcos, TX, USA

5.1 Reproduction

5.1.1 Natural spawning

5.1.1.1 Introduction

Natural spawning (allowing broodfish to select a mate) is recommended for largemouth bass. This section focuses on natural spawning techniques in ponds and raceways. Largemouth bass fingerlings are rarely reared to a size > 5 cm in the same ponds in which they are spawned because competition for food and cannibalism limit production numbers. Instead, fry are produced in several ways and then stocked into nursery ponds. Using a separate spawning phase allows fry production intensification so that adequate fry can be produced for the nursery phase. Advanced fry (10–20 mm) may be produced through the spawning/rearing method by allowing broodfish to spawn naturally in ponds and harvesting large fry and broodfish after 40–50 d (Hutson, 1990). Alternatively, pond or raceway spawning methods are used to produce eggs or swim-up fry that are transferred to incubation tanks or stocked directly to nursery ponds. Commonly, fry are collected from the spawning ponds and stocked into fingerling production ponds (Piper et al., 1982; Simco et al., 1986). More controlled raceway spawning paired with indoor incubation to swim-up allows for more consistency in fry size and accuracy in numbers stocked.

5.1.1.2 Broodstock selection, care and maintenance

If pond space allows, broodfish should be separated into ponds by year class and gender. This allows the allocation of forage based on broodfish needs, prevents unexpected spawning and minimizes handling during harvest and pairing of broodfish. Older fish generally ripen and spawn earlier than younger fish which, when different age groups are mixed in spawning ponds, can increase size disparity in fry populations promoting cannibalism (Piper et al., 1982). It has been recommended that largemouth bass broodfish be stocked at 200–350 kg/ha with equal numbers of males and females (Hutson, 1990). Glenewinkel et al. (2011) recommended stocking 140 kg females/ha and equal numbers of males to females regardless of the weight of males.

Secondary sex characteristics are poorly defined in largemouth bass. Several methods have been suggested for distinguishing between male and female fish (Snow, 1963). Mature fish can be sexed with reasonable accuracy just prior to spawning. At other times, morphological differences are not distinct enough for this to be done. Broodfish are selected for spawning in the early spring when water temperatures are consistently above 15°C. In spawning condition, females are easily distinguishable from males or unripe females by examining them side-by-side belly up. Ripe females exhibit distended, soft, pendulous ovarian region, and a swollen, red, protruding vent. Ripe males usually release a small amount of milt when palpated. To palpate fish, turn the fish belly up and slowly but firmly apply pressure along the sides or middle of the abdominal region. For spawning, only use males that freely express milt when palpated.

In the southern half of the USA, largemouth bass can attain sexual maturity at 1 year of age if a minimum size of 180 g is reached (Swingle, 1950). Since growth is slower in the northern part of its range, 2 years may be required. Snow (1965) reported that good results can be obtained from 1-year-old fish which have reached a minimum size of 320 g. A key factor in producing bass which will spawn at 1 year of age is supplying an ample quantity of forage fish of a suitable size when water temperatures are > 15°C. As much as 20% of the body weight of the fish may be consumed per day under optimal conditions. It is suggested that 1 kg of gain in bass weight requires about 5.1 kg of forage consumption (Piper et al. 1982). When producing broodstock on forage, stocking densities of 250–370 handpicked fingerlings per hectare have been used successfully (Snow, 1961).

Eggs are formed in the late summer and fall prior to spawning the following spring. Adequate nutrition during the period of egg formation is necessary for normal development. While artificial food can be used, growth is slower and egg quality generally not as good as from fish fed a natural diet (Snow, 1970). However, there are several advantages of using broodstock habituated to artificial diets. Artificial diets can be fed in the spawning ponds without contaminating the environment with unwanted fish. Feeding artificial diets also greatly reduces the possibility of bass tapeworm infestation and bacterial disease can be treated by feeding medicated feed (Snow, 1970). Some management initiatives may necessitate the use of forage fish for maintaining genetically "wild type" broodstock; although bass produced for food-fish purposes are generally the progeny of several generations of feed trained or "domesticated" broodstock.

Species of forage fish that appear to be best for propagation as bass food include the goldfish (*Carassius auratus* [Linnaeus]), common carp (*Cyprinus carpio*), fathead minnow (*Pimphales promelas*), and golden shiner (*Notemigomis crysoleueas*). Goldfish are preferred by some managers because of ease of spawning, high production rates, and rapid growth. Carp have similar characteristics although they tend to outgrow bass to a greater degree and do not spawn over as long a period as goldfish. Fathead minnows and golden shiners seldom get too large for bass to swallow but do not yield as much weight per unit area. Bluegill (*Lepomis macrochirus*) spawn at higher water temperatures where offspring are not large enough for forage until late in the summer. Where legally allowed, tilapia (*Oreochromis* spp.) are an excellent forage species, being prolific, fast growing, and disease resistant. The primary disadvantage being low tolerance to water temperatures below 12°C. Goldfish, carp, and tilapia also inhibit the development of aquatic vegetation when present at densities of > 224 kg/ha (Snow, 1961).

The use of anesthetics is recommended when handling largemouth bass broodfish. Handling large broodfish by hand can increase the chance of stress, injury, and disease, which will delay and likely reduce spawning success and fry production. Skaggs et al. (2017) showed that handling and holding largemouth bass broodfish out of water for 60 s increased the stress response significantly to impact spawning. MS-222 is an approved sedative for warmwater fish. Dosing concentrations of 15–330 mg/l are permitted and has a 21 d withdraw period. Dosage required to sedate bass broodfish for handling is 25 mg/l and complete sedation requires 50 mg/l. Aqui-S®E (AquaTactics Fish Health, Kirkland, WA) is a relatively new anesthetic for fish which currently can only be used under the Investigational New Animal Drug (INAD) program. Dosing concentrations of 10–100 mg/l are permitted and requires a zero withdraw period if the fish are sedated less than 15 min or requires a 3 d withdraw period in all other applications. Aqui-S concentrations diminish over time in water so is not recommended for longer sedation periods. A dose of 30 mg/l on largemouth bass will effectively sedate fish for capture, measurement, and distribution for spawning.

5.1.1.3 Spawning behavior

Spawning activity of largemouth bass is closely related to rising water temperatures following winter. Largemouth bass are relatively synchronous regionally in their reproductive cycle. Bass typically spawn from early spring into the summer, displaying latitude variation between northern and southern climates with spawning times ranging from February to July within the USA (Heidinger, 1975). A water temperature of 18°C is generally recognized as the spawning temperature of this species. Often, spawning will not take place until the second or third time the temperature warms to this level. Spawning activity tends to peak when a majority of the fish are stimulated to spawn as temperature rises but spawning may continue for weeks after the "main spawn" has occurred. The length of the spawning season is generally 3–4 weeks (Waters and Noble, 2004).

Largemouth bass are classified as fractional, batch or "multiple" spawners. Only a portion of the eggs are released during a spawning event and the females spawn more than once during the spawning season. The eggs are released at intervals, usually over several days or weeks. This allows more, smaller, and immature eggs to be carried in a limited abdominal cavity space as the intervals allow the smaller eggs time to mature. Eggs mature at different times, thus avoiding complete loss of a season's spawning to predators or weather perturbations. Females normally release about one-half of their total eggs during the first spawn and one-half of the remaining eggs during the second spawn. A third spawn up to a month later to release the remaining eggs is common (Davis and Lock, 1997). This behavior reduces the efficacy of using hormone injection for artificial spawning, as only a portion of the oocytes respond and as a result is generally not practiced in commercial production (Mayes et al., 1993).

The eggs of largemouth bass require a relatively long period for development beginning in the fall and continuing through the winter and spring. Largemouth are seasonal spawners, where after spawning no more eggs will develop until water temperatures begin to decrease during the following fall. Largemouth bass eggs are demersal and adhesive. Fertilized eggs range in diameter from 1.2 to 1.8 mm. Smaller and younger fish produce smaller eggs. The number of fertilized eggs per milliliter averaged 571 for 1-year-old fish as compared to 374/ml for fish 3 years old (Snow, 1970). Egg counts of samples from ovaries of unspawned fish indicate a potential to yield

30,000 to 45,000 per 454 grams of body weight. Even higher numbers have been reported in some instances (Davis and Lock, 1997).

Largemouth bass are nest builders and guarders. The male selects and prepares the nest site guarding it against intruders. Preferred sites are protected locations in shallow water over firm bottom or a fibrous substrate such as tree roots. Largemouth bass will preferentially use artificial spawning substrates such as Blocksom or Spawntex™ mats (Isaac and Staats, 1992). These substrates are generally placed 1.8 m apart in raceways to reduce male territory aggressive behavior and 3–6 m apart in ponds at water depths of 0.5–1.0 m and close to the pond bank to allow easy observation. Mats can then be transferred indoors or directly to other ponds for hatching.

When broodstock are first stocked into ponds or raceways for spawning typically they school together initially. After a couple of days, males begin to select and guard spawning sites. Once the nest is established the male becomes territorial and stays in close proximity to the nest attempting to entice a female to spawn. Following a short courtship, a female lays eggs on the nest and the guarding male fertilizes them. After spawning is completed, the male continues to guard the nest. Spawning can occur at any time of day. Maintaining clear water and using a flashlight helps to locate spawns. If water is stained or murky it may be necessary to use spawning mats and gently lift up each mat to examine for eggs. If a guarding male does not readily abandon a nest being examined a spawn is likely present.

Spawns should be collected as early in the morning as possible so that subsequent spawning activities can resume quickly. Spawning mats can be collected by one person by lifting each mat out of the water and quickly submerging it in a tub of the same water. If two people are available, it may be preferable not to lift the mats out of the water. This can be accomplished by one person lifting the mat and another sinking a tub underneath the mat to retrieve it. Both people then raise the tub to the water surface and slowly pour off the excess water before transport.

Incubation time varies with temperature. Heidinger (1975) summarized several studies which give incubation times ranging from 317 h (13 d) at 10°C to 49 h (4 d) at 28°C. Bass eggs incubated at 17.7°C required 3–4 d to hatch and only 2 d to hatch at 22.2°C (Matthews et al., 2012). Newly hatched fry swim-up in 7–9 d at 18–20°C and in 5–7 d at 22–24°C (Matthews and Stout, 2013). Maintaining consistent water temperatures during egg incubation is recommended and incubating bass eggs at 22–23°C increases hatch rates over lower incubation temperatures in intensive culture programs and reduces dependence on chemical treatments (Matthews et al., 2012).

Ponds should be stocked with spawns (eggs or fry) from three consecutive days or fewer to reduce size variability and subsequent cannibalism before fingerlings are harvested. This 3 day "rule" can be increased to ~ seven days if the eggs and fry are manipulated by reducing temperatures of one group to elongate time to swim-up and increasing temperature on another group to shorten time to swim-up. At hatching, the fry are quite small ranging from 3 to 5.5 mm. Growth and development continue during the yolk sac absorption period which may require 120 h or longer. When ready for first feeding a size of 5.5 to 6.5 mm has been attained and color has changed from amber or cream color to some shade of brown.

5.1.1.4 Spawning methods

Spawning methods used for largemouth bass fry production are based on the available facilities infrastructure and production goals of the hatchery. The scale of hatchery operations varies from small private producers with only a small pond or two and production goals of a few thousand fingerlings to large state and federal hatcheries with highly sophisticated indoor and outdoor facilities and production goals of several million. In recent years, new technologies have led to refinement of culture methods and improvements in bass fingerling production. The appropriate technology is a site based decision largely determined by resource availability. Hatchery production of largemouth bass involves three main culture methods: spawn and rear, egg or fry transfer and intensive culture.

For best results, spawning ponds should be prepared each year. Earthen ponds should be drained and allowed to dry and the bottoms disked and packed. Bottoms and sides of ponds should be sprayed with an approved herbicide to control unwanted vegetation. If lined ponds are used, they should be cleaned of bottom sediments including removal of sediments from drain boxes or kettles. Pond filling should ideally begin 1–7 d before broodfish are stocked. Incoming water should be filtered through a 1,000 μm sock filter to prevent unwanted organisms from entering the pond. In plastic-lined ponds spawning substrate should be provided. The number of pans or mats placed in each pond should equal the number of males.

The spawn-and-rear method is the oldest and simplest approach to largemouth bass culture. Broodfish are stocked into spawning ponds when water temperatures approach 18°C and are allowed to pair-up and spawn freely. Stocking densities are typically 25–100 broodfish/ha (White, 1981). Broodfish are left in the pond until the fingerlings reach a size large enough for harvest and either distribution or subsequent feed training which is generally 30–45 d after broodfish have been stocked (Hutson, 1990). The spawning/rearing method offers some advantages over spawning-only ponds as the larger fry (> 15 mm) produced are easier to count accurately providing more control over stocking densities and fry survival in rearing ponds increases with stocking size (Kurten, 2001). The spawning/rearing method typically yields mixed-age fry that should be graded before the next rearing stage. Owing to cannibalism of fingerlings by the broodstock, this method is only effective for fingerlings up to 25 mm. Ponds are typically fertilized to stimulate primary productivity and subsequent production of zooplankton and larval insects to provide food for the developing fry and fingerlings.

For the egg transfer method, ponds are stocked with broodstock as described for the spawn-and-rear method although the stocking densities of broodstock are generally 100–200 broodfish/ha. Ponds are managed for water clarity and are not fertilized. Fibrous spawning mats such as Blocksom or Spawntex™ are used as a removable substrate for bass to spawn for egg collection (Isaac and Staats, 1992). Spawning mats are checked daily for eggs. Nests with spawns are transferred from spawning ponds into fertilized nursery ponds where the eggs hatch and the fry remain and grow to the target size (Hutson, 1983). The disadvantage of this method is that the number of fry to hatch successfully is unknown and may be too high or too low relative to the carrying capacity of the pond. This makes management difficult, production unpredictable and could require significantly more pond hectares than other methods.

For the fry transfer method, ponds are managed and stocked as described above for the egg transfer method, but the swim-up fry are transferred from spawning ponds to fertilized nursery ponds. Where eggs or fry are harvested directly from spawning ponds, these ponds are usually managed for water clarity as it is important to be able to observe fry and spawning activity. These ponds are unlikely to require fertilization, since fry will be removed before they begin feeding. To visually identify schooling swim-up fry, managers often use a tool to silhouette the fry.

Examples include: white boat paddles or bucket lids attached to a long handle. These are pulled under the water surface near the shoreline. Free-swimming schools of fry remain near the nest for several days following swim-up where they can be collected by dip netting, seining, trapping or pond draining (Snow, 1975; White, 1981; Hutson, 1990). Largemouth bass swim-up fry can be enumerated using a standard weight index of 275 fry/g (Glenewinkel et al., 2011).

The fry transfer method allows for stocking densities to be tailored for specific production goals, such as fingerling size (White, 1981). Also, ponds can be more easily stocked with fry of similar size and age to minimize cannibalism, which can significantly reduce fish yield. Unfortunately, spawns can be missed in the fry transfer method resulting in fry size differences and cohort cannibalism. Mixed fry sizes become more pronounced as the spawning season progresses due to the mixing of fry from subsequent spawns, as a result most hatcheries using this method only transfer fry to nursery ponds from the earliest fish to spawn within a few days of each other. Another disadvantage is reduced spawning by males protecting broods where the removal of spawning substrates containing eggs and replacement stimulates continued spawning of males.

Methods for indoor incubation of largemouth bass eggs were developed to improve efficiency and ameliorate inconsistent production results associated with other methods (Snow, 1972). Broodfish stocking densities in ponds are similar to those of the egg transfer method while densities in raceways varies by facility. Broodfish are spawned in ponds or tanks and the eggs are collected and incubated under controlled conditions in either vertical-tray incubators (Snow, 1972), hatching jars (Sarti, 1986), or on spawning mats suspended in raceways (Matthews and Stout, 2013). Hatching in tanks is preferred as fry of similar age and known number can be stocked into a nursery pond. If eggs are to be incubated in trays or hatching jars the mats are typically dipped in a solution of 45 g/l sodium sulfite to remove the adhesiveness of the eggs followed by a light water spray to remove the eggs from spawning mats. However, Matthews and Stout (2013) attributed a poor hatch rate of eggs (50%) to egg damage caused by the removal process and discouraged this process. Swim-up fry are either stocked into prepared nursery ponds or cultured in tanks on a combination of natural and artificial foods (Snow, 1965; Skudlarek, et al. 2013).

5.1.1.5 Preliminary experiments on tank spawning largemouth bass

Developing technologies for intensive fry production, such as controlled indoor spawning, egg incubation, and fry rearing, could improve the reliability of bass fingerling production. Currently the majority of commercial largemouth bass production in the USA occurs in the southeastern states. Bass producers in more northerly locations possess marketing advantages in proximity to large urban markets; although, spawning dates are later compared to more southern states. Early spawning allows for the production of larger first-year fingerlings by the end of the first summer growing season (Pine et al., 2000). The delayed temperature-dependent spawning of largemouth bass in northern areas can "domino" through the production cycle, causing fish to not achieve market size (0.50–0.75 kg) by the end of the second year (Tidwell et al., 1998).

Preliminary trials were conducted to examine the feasibility of a simple method to manipulate water temperature to induce early spawning of largemouth bass and subsequent egg incubation in temperature controlled tanks (unpublished data, Coyle and Tidwell). Nine 19,000 l fiberglass tanks located outdoors were filled to a depth of 0.7 m. Each of the tanks contained four spawning mats (Spawntex™) and four pairs of largemouth bass broodfish were stocked into each tank. Three treatments were evaluated in triplicate tanks. The control treatment was uncovered tanks to simulate natural temperature conditions. For the second treatment, tanks were covered with clear plastic stretched over PVC pipe to create a passive "greenhouse." In the third treatment, the water surface was covered with a blue solar swimming pool cover. Spawning mats were examined each morning for eggs then transferred indoors for incubation.

The use of passive solar heating warmed water to suitable spawning temperatures for largemouth bass approximately 2–3 weeks earlier than natural conditions. The greenhouse treatment was more effective at reducing spawning time than the solar cover treatment, but due to algae growth in the greenhouse tanks it may be more practical to use solar covers, which did not allow algae growth. Collecting eggs on mats allowed for easy transfer indoors and subsequently provided increased control over water temperature and disease.

5.1.1.6 Controlled indoor spawning

Where suitable facilities exist, spawning largemouth bass in raceways offers several advantages to spawning ponds for fry production. Broodfish can be used more intensively in a smaller culture space freeing up pond space for additional fingerling growout. In ponds, females may only spawn one time due to the large variability of conditions possible in a natural environment. Spawning in controlled environments increase the likelihood of females spawning multiple times, and as a result, more fry can be produced per kilogram of broodfish (Isaac and Staats, 1992). Controlled spawning reduces the spawning season duration and number of broodfish required (Mayes et al., 1993; Matthews and Stout, 2013), so nursery ponds can be stocked within a shorter time frame, yielding more uniform size and number of fry.

Presently, the maximum number of spawns per female is unknown and likely varies widely among females. In one trial (personal communication, Matthews), 14 female Florida largemouth bass were allowed to spawn over a 115 d period. During this time, an average of seven spawns per female were collected from in a single 24 m raceway. These females, averaging 2 kg each, collectively produced 1.13 million eggs, 40,464 eggs/kg female, 11,000 eggs/spawn, and 80,929 eggs/female. These results are averages, meaning an individual female could have spawned more than seven times. However, in production typical spawning periods are much shorter (21–28 d) and the number of spawns per female are less than two (Matthews and Stout, 2013).

Broodstock can be stocked at a 1 : 1 female to male sex ratio in indoor raceways with the number of spawning mats, with their proper separation, dictating the number of males. Stocking with a 3 : 2 female to male sex ratio increases the number of spawns collected (personal communication, Matthews). In a 26 × 4 m raceway, 20 mats, 10 per side, can be evenly spaced (~2 m apart) along the length of each long wall. Broodstock need time to acclimate to the artificial environment. This could take 3 to 8 weeks for fish the first time they are spawned indoors. Broodfish used again in subsequent years become habituated to spawning in raceways and, if kept indoors all year, can begin spawning within 1 to 3 d. If kept in gender segregated ponds outside, broodstock may still require 1 to 2 weeks of acclimation and courtship behavior before spawning. Co-mingling bass broodstock, prior to the addition of spawning structures, reduced spawning latency by approximately 2 weeks (Jackson, 1979; Matthews and Stout, 2013). Bass can be paired and placed in a clean-bottomed spawning raceway without mats with minimal risk of spawning on the bare raceway floor.

Broodstock should not be fed during spawning as it is difficult to clean spawning raceways and can increase the numbers of bacteria and parasites present, which could reduce hatch rates and fry survival. During a prolonged spawning period, spawning mats can be removed and the broodfish fed. After feeding broodfish in spawning tanks the raceway should be cleaned (preferably with a vacuum or siphon as not to drastically alter the water level or crowd and stress the bass) before spawning resumes. Bass should be given 4 d to feed and 3 to 4 d to clear their digestive tracts before replacing mats.

The raceways should be checked each morning and mats containing spawns removed and hung vertically in an "incubation" tank or raceway. Spawns are transferred in water and remain in the transfer tubs less than 15 min. Each incubation tank should be filled with enough water to completely immerse the spawning mat. Incoming water is screened through 500 µm mesh to exclude unwanted organisms. The drain pipe should include a saran-screen guard to prevent fry escapement and an air ring at the base to help prevent clogging of the screen. A divider screen at the end of the tank is also recommended. Low pressure air is gently bubbled in front of the divider screen to help prevent clogging. Air is also bubbled along one side, down the length of the trough, to keep the water moving around the mats and to mix therapeutic chemicals if required. A supported wire is stretched along the length of the trough allowing the spawning mats to be vertically suspended in the water. A 4.5 m trough supplied with 15 to 40 l/min can hold 20–30 spawning mats without overcrowding hatched fry. An example of spawns in concrete raceways is shown in Figure 5.1.

Spawns from up to 3 d old apart can be incubated together in the same trough depending on temperature and required chemical treatments. Spawns can be treated with approved chemicals to control "fungus" water mold from growing. Typically, the eggs hatch in 2–4 d after spawning depending on water temperature and swim-up fry are typically ready for harvest 7–10 d

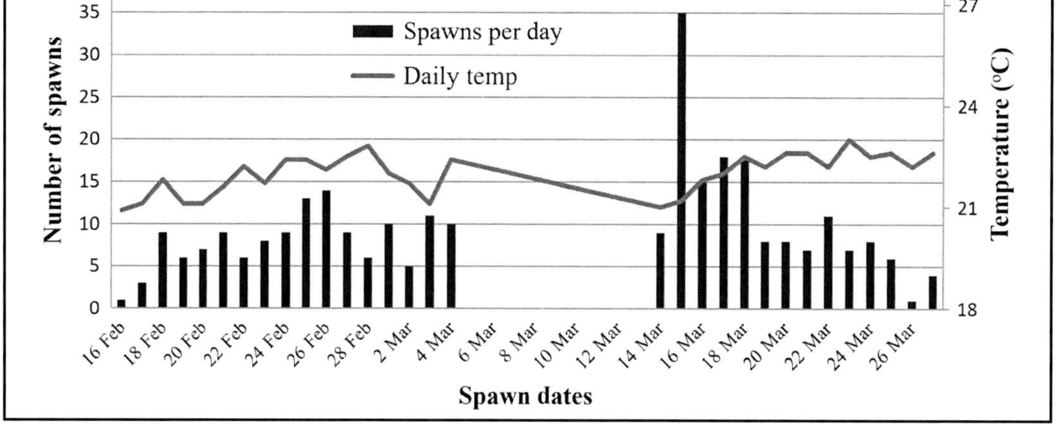

Figure 5.1 Results from spawning 101 females using a 3 : 2 female to male ratio in four indoor 24 m concrete raceways for 17 days producing 136 spawns. Mats were removed, bass were fed koi, and mats replaced after seven days. Spawning resumed two days after mats were replaced for 14 d producing 155 more spawns from the same broodfish. Water temperature was recorded each morning from 16 February to 4 March and 14 to 28 March.

post-stock. Take caution incubating bass eggs at water temperatures above 26°C. The increased temperature promotes accelerated hatch and fry growth, quickly reducing yolk sac volume and reducing the time frame for "first feeding." The yolk-sac may be depleted before body structures required to capture and utilize live prey items are developed. The occurrence of physical deformities also increases. The hatched fry initially appear as small golden globules along the sides of the troughs and edges of the mats. The color of the fry darkens over time and they become dark-gray. Mats are removed from troughs when the fry begin to swim freely in the water column. Mats should be examined for trapped fry during removal; this is especially important when different aged spawns are incubated together. Avoid vigorous rinsing of mats to prevent injury to fry and releasing unhatched eggs which may foul the tanks.

5.1.1.7 Out of season spawning

Out of season spawning of largemouth bass using photoperiod and temperature manipulation was first described by Carlson (1973). It is relatively common to delay spawning of bass by holding at water temperatures below 17°C in order to avoid unpredictable spring temperature fluctuations and/or maximize sequential hatchery production of other species (Brauhn et al., 1972). A limiting factor in delayed spawning is suitable pond water temperatures for adequate zooplankton quantities and sizes during the subsequent nursery phase. Since zooplankton population dynamics are dependent on water temperature, out-of-season spawning of bass is limited by seasonal zooplankton abundance. Zooplankton abundance is highest during the spring "bloom" which corresponds with natural spawning. In regions having sufficient periods of suitable water temperature zooplankton blooms also occur in the fall proving an opportunity for out-of-season spawning and subsequent fingerling production of largemouth bass.

The development of a technique that successfully produces bass spawns in September and October is described in detail by Matthews and Stout (2013). Spawning and rearing bass in the fall allowed for production of 100 mm bass by the following March and better utilized pond space in the fall. Protocols, stocking ratios, and stocking rates are the same as described earlier in this chapter in the controlled indoor spawning section, but requires the addition of temperature and daylight manipulation to naturally induce spawning. Water temperatures were systematically lowered to 12°C over a 4 week period, held there for 3 weeks, then increased over a 4 week period back to ambient.

The amount of daylight was manipulated using black plastic to completely block light and simulate the dark period of winter. Raceways had 10 h of light for the first four weeks, 8 h for 3 weeks (held at 10 to 12°C), increased to 10 h for 2 weeks and then increased to 14 h for the last 2 weeks of conditioning. The 14 h of light were maintained throughout spawning. An example of spawns collected over a single out of season spawning period is shown in Figure 5.2.

Observations between multiple seasons of spring spawning and out of season spawning showed no obvious differences in fry size (300 fry/g), health, or behavior. The only obvious difference was the average number of fry/spawn. Spring production averaged 6,000 to 12,000 fry/spawn while out of season produced 4,000 to 7,000 fry/spawn. Florida largemouth bass production at the A.E. Wood State Fish Hatchery in San Marcos, Texas, and Texas Freshwater Fisheries Center, Athens, Texas, similarly average 8,000 to 12,000 fry/spawn during spring production. The reduced fry/spawn numbers from the out of season spawning remains unknown but could

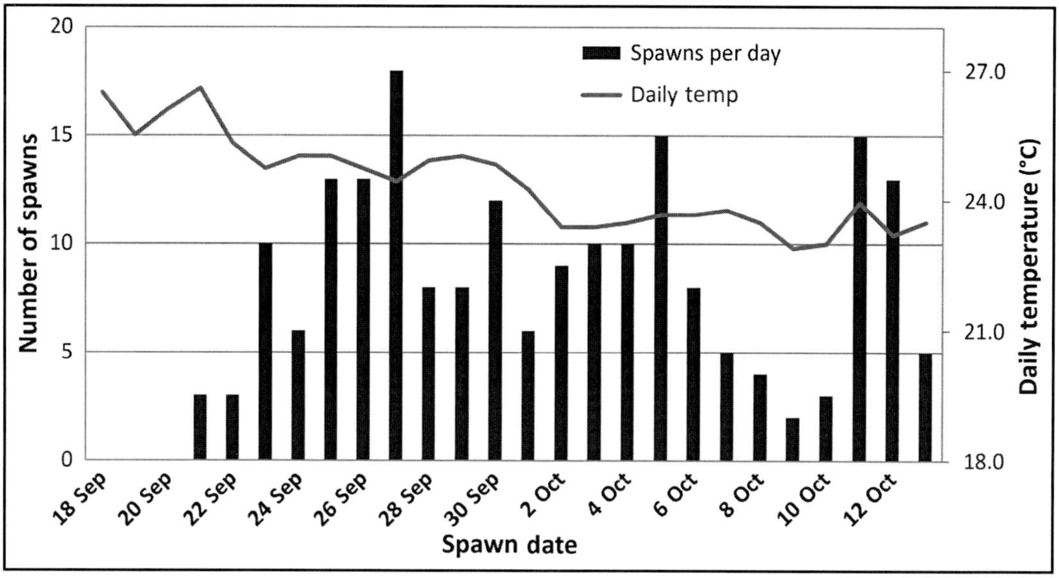

Figure 5.2 Results of spawning female LMB "out of season" in indoor raceways with morning water temperatures shown on the right-hand y axis.

possibly be a result of regressed gonad development typically observed during July–October (Brauhn et al., 1972; Rosenblum et al., 1994; Gross et al., 2002). Comparisons are further complicated by differing production requests (numbers required) and removing mats after production numbers were achieved. The data in Table 5.1 represent production totals achieved in a specific short time frame and should not be considered maximum values.

5.1.1.8 Disease control methods for eggs and fry

Although possible, newly hatched fry kept in clean tanks with adequate water quality are not typically infested with parasites or have bacterial infections. However, eggs are very susceptible to fungus which, if left untreated, can cause up to 100% mortality. Water mold, commonly referred to as fungus due to visual characteristics, is caused by eight species of mold from the family Saprolegniaceae, but only *Saprolegnia* sp., *Achlya* sp., and *Aphanomyces* sp. are of concern in freshwater aquaculture (Tucker and Robinson, 1990; Woo and Bruno, 1999). There are several options for treatment depending on location and water quality, which can be found at https://www.fws.gov/fisheries/aadap/home.htm. Temperature, hydrogen peroxide, and formalin are effective at controlling Saprolegnia infestations (Marking et al., 1994). Water mold can grow at water temperatures of 5–30°C (Koeypudsa et al., 2005). However, by incubating bass eggs at water temperatures above 20°C the eggs hatch in ~48 h, greatly reducing water mold-induced mortality and the need for chemical treatment.

One experiment evaluated the effects of water temperature and hydrogen peroxide on hatch rates. Florida largemouth bass eggs were incubated under four treatments; ambient temperature (17.9–19.2°C), ambient temperature plus hydrogen peroxide (100 mg/l), heated water (22.1–23.6°C), and heated water plus hydrogen peroxide. The four treatments yielded hatch rates of 49, 79, 79, and 91% hatch, respectively (Matthews et al., 2012). Hydrogen Peroxide (35% active)

Table 5.1 Example of actual spring and fall production totals and corresponding averages for Florida largemouth bass spawned in indoor 24 m raceways. Requests for larger amounts of fry in the fall account for the greater total fry and fry/female averages. The spawning data listed represents multiple years, but all fall within a 21 to 36 d spawning duration.

Raceway unit		Total spawns	Spawns/ female	Fry/g	Fry/ spawn	Total fry	Fry/ female	Spawning females
Spring spawn								
	R	34	1.1	300	12,010	372,324	11,635	32
	R	34	1	300	12,426	410,042	11,715	35
	R	41	1.4	300	11,047	408,726	13,624	30
	R	15	0.4	300	10,819	162,284	4,271	38
	R	37	1.0	300	11,205	414,586	11,205	37
	R	32	0.9	300	10,821	346,268	10,184	34
Average					11,388	352,372	10,439	
Fall spawn								
	R	36	1.2	300	4,807	173,049	5,768	30
	R	68	2.7	300	6,545	314,153	12,566	25
	R	81	3.7	300	5,189	254,274	11,558	22
	R	86	2.3	300	7,065	586,380	15,431	38
	R	106	2.9	300	7,367	744,063	20,110	37
	R	94	2.8	300	8,112	697,621	20,518	34
Average					6,514	461,590	14,325	

is approved for use on bass eggs at 750 to 1,000 mg/l, but may be toxic to newly hatched fry (personal communication, Matthews).

Another trial evaluated the use of salt to control water mold (*Saprolegnia*) during the incubation of largemouth bass eggs. Northern largemouth bass eggs were collected from a newly transferred spawn mat for the experiment. Twenty eggs were placed into each of eighteen 2 l containers to be hatched at different salinities. Salinity concentrations of 0–10 ppt, in increments of 2 ppt, were evaluated with three replicates per treatment. Eggs were initially stocked into 1 l of water and then the salinity was gradually increased, to prevent osmotic shock, until the desired concentration was reached. The eggs were monitored daily for hatching and presence of swim-up of fry. The salt treatments found to be most effective for control of water mold (*Saprolegnia*) were 4 and 6 ppt, resulting in 9.2 and 5.0% greater swim-up rates, respectively (personal communication, Coyle and Tidwell).

5.1.2 Artificial spawning

Largemouth bass is a difficult fish species to reproduce artificially for a number of reasons. While spawning hormones have been utilized, it is difficult to predict reaction of fish to hormonal stimulation. This reaction cannot be standardized and depends on many factors; such as preparedness of fish to spawning and conditions of fish rearing (temperature and photoperiod, presence of brooders of opposite sex, density, and others). This difficulty is rooted in a complex spawning behavior of largemouth bass, which includes building of nests by males and a period of courtship. Hormonal injection results in final maturation and ovulation of only a small portion of oocytes in the ovaries. This reaction to hormone injection is consistent with the fact that largemouth bass females are intermittent (partial) spawners. During the spawning season, a female may spawn with several males in several locations over a period of time. Even if the fish culturist is able to induce ovulation in female bass, and collect adequate numbers of viable eggs, obtaining suitable volume of viable milt is a problem. Hormonal injection results in release of very small amount of sperm. In many cases there is no apparent release of milt at all after hormonal injection. As a result, sperm is not stripped from males, and must be obtained with other methods.

Artificial spawning of largemouth bass has been used almost exclusively in cases when it was essential for the purposes of research. These cases included distant hybridization or application of some chromosome set manipulation methods (induced triploidy and gynogenesis) when there was a need for influence on gametes or early embryos. Below, the experience of artificial reproduction of largemouth bass is summarized. (In this section only the methods of artificial breeding are only described. Results of experiments on distant hybridization, triploidy and gynogenesis are presented in section 5.2.)

Stevens (1970) and Wilbur and Langford (1975) (cited in Heidinger, 1976) were the first to show that injection of human chorionic gonadotropin (HCG) with dose of 4,000 IU per one kg of fish weight can result in final oocyte maturation and ovulation in females and spermiation in males of the largemouth bass.

Beaty and Childers (1980) injected largemouth bass females with 4,000 IU/kg for induction of eggs ovulation in order to produce interspecies hybrids (female largemouth bass × male smallmouth bass). Gomelsky et al. (2004) also reported production of the same type of hybrids (largemouth bass × smallmouth bass) by artificial spawning. Largemouth bass females were injected with HCG with dose 4,000 IU/kg; largemouth bass and smallmouth bass males were injected with HCG at dose 2,000 IU/kg. Eggs were stripped 30–36 h after injection (Figure 5.3). Largemouth bass and smallmouth bass males did not release sperm after injection. Therefore, males were dissected and removed testes were macerated and washed with 0.85% saline solution. In further studies on largemouth bass × smallmouth bass hybridization (Stilwell, 2008) largemouth bass females were also injected with HCG with a dose of 4,000 IU/kg; eggs were stripped 30–36 h after injection. In order to investigate influence different types of hormones on spermiation in males, injections with HCG (2,000 IU/kg), LHRHa (100 μg/kg) and carp pituitary extract (CPE, 3 mg/kg) were tested. Largemouth bass and smallmouth bass males did not produce sperm by stripping after injection of any of these hormones. Therefore, males were sacrificed and their testes were dissected out and macerated through a 500 μm screen using 0.85% saline solution. In total, approximately 7,000 actively feeding largemouth fry and 2,000 largemouth bass × smallmouth bass fry were produced in this study (Stilwell, 2008).

In a study on triploidy induction in largemouth bass, Garrett et al. (1992) injected females and males with HCG at dose of 4,000 IU/kg. Sperm was stripped from males, collected by pipette and used for fertilization of eggs stripped from females. Injection of HCG at the same dose was also used by Fries et al. (2002) in another study on induced triploidy in largemouth bass. It was estimated that 200–2,000 eggs were obtained from one female; about 40–60% of stripped eggs were not viable. The average number of viable fry per female obtained by hand-stripping after HCG injections was less than 12. Fry production increased up to about 1,000

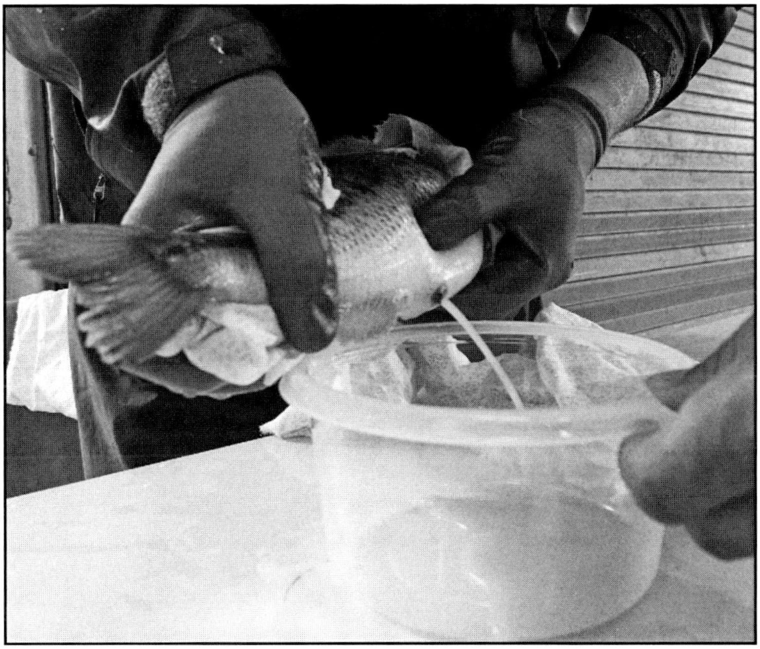

Figure 5.3 Stripping eggs from a largemouth bass female after hormonal injection.

in further trials when instead of hormone injections fish were allowed to enter into spawning behavior in a natural manner prior to hand-stripping.

Neal et al. (2004) also used artificial spawning in studies on induced triploidy in largemouth bass. Both largemouth bass males and females were injected intramuscularly with 5 mg/kg of CPE and with 50 μg/kg of LHRH in the dorsal lymphatic node. Injection of these hormones induced production of free-flowing gametes in more than half of fish. Peak gamete production occurred within 21–24 h following injection at water temperatures ranging 23–28°C. Males produced very low volume of sperm which was collected by pipette. Before fertilization of eggs, sperm was mixed with about 10 ml of 0.3% NaCl to increase the volume. In a further study on induced triploidy Neal (2014) induced ovulation and spermiation in largemouth bass females and males by injection of Ovaprim with initial dose of 0.1 ml/kg and resolving dose of 0.5 ml/kg with 8 h between two injections. The testes were removed and macerated with approximately 10 ml of 0.3 NaCl solution. For fertilization, macerated testes were mixed with water poured through a fine mesh over the eggs.

In a study on induced gynogenesis in largemouth bass, Glennon et al. (2012) injected females with HCG at a dose of 4,000 IU/kg to induce ovulation. The time between hormonal injection and ovulation was 36–40 h. For induction of gynogenetic development, largemouth eggs were inseminated with UV-irradiated white bass or striped bass sperm.

A recent study (personal communication, Semmens and Gomelsky) at Kentucky State University compared HCG and Ovaprim® (Western Chemical, Inc.) as inducing agents for artificial spawning of largemouth bass. Ovaprim® is a commercial product containing salmon gonadotropin releasing hormone analog (20 μg/ml) and dopamine antagonist (10 mg/ml). In late April of 2017, largemouth bass (36 females and 36 males) were injected with the two inducing agents in two trials spaced a week apart. Mean weight of females was 1,139 g while mean weight of males was 979 g. All fish were given a single intramuscular injection early in the morning (approximately 7 am) and examined for a response the following day. HCG was applied at a rate of 4000 IU/kg for females and 2000 IU/kg for males while Ovaprim® was applied at a rate of 0.5 ml/kg to both males and females. The response rate for HCG and Ovaprim® was 89% and 78% with a mean weight of eggs 31.2 and 26.8 g per female, respectively (Table 5.2). The number of eggs per female was similar for both treatments and ranged from 5,600 to 40,500 and from 5,000 to 44,000 for HCG and Ovaprim®, respectively. The mean latent period for egg ovulation was also similar for both treatments being 33.4 and 34.4 h for HCG and Ovaprim®, respectively.

In this study, regardless of inducing agent, it was not possible to strip sperm from the males. Therefore, males were euthanized, dissected and the testes were extracted as a source of sperm (Gomelsky et al., 2004; Neal, 2014). Testicular tissue was screened through a fine mesh (high density polyethylene filter cloth 540 μm mesh) to create a suspension containing sperm. The mesh retaining tissue was rinsed with 6 ml saline (0.85%) per testes of one male. Average weight of testes was 4.9 g with a range of 2.8 to 6.5 g among both treatments. Testes from one male was used to fertilize ≤ 75 g of eggs; testes from two males were used for larger spawns. For artificial fertilization of eggs, ~200 ml of water was added to suspension of sperm in saline solution and then this mixture was added to the eggs and gently stirred with a feather for 1 min (Figure 5.4).

Subsequently, 700 ml of a fuller's earth slurry (25 g/l) was added to prevent egg adhesiveness and clump forming. The mixture was stirred for approximately 20 min and loaded into

Table 5.2 Egg ovulation response of largemouth bass females to two hormonal treatments and results of eggs artificial fertilization and incubation.

Parameter	Hormonal treatment	
	HCG	Ovaprim®
Mean weight of females (g)	1132±55*	1146±62
Number of injected females	18	18
Number of females releasing eggs	16	14
Response rate (%)	88.9	77.8
Mean latent period (h)	33.4±0.55	34.4±0.74
Range of latent period (h)	30.2–36.4	27.1–37.8
Total weight of eggs released (g)	499	375
Mean weight of eggs per female (g)	31.2±4.6	26.8±5.2
Number of eggs in 1 g (before fertilization)	572±28	658±21
Total number of eggs collected	295,506	240,532
Number of eggs collected per female (mean)	18,469±3,191	17,181±3,316
Number of eggs collected per female (range)	5,600–40,500	5,000–44,000
Number of eggs taken for fertilization	292,887	222,761
Number of incubation jars	5	3
Mean number of eggs incubated per jar	58,577±18,080	74,254±50,123
Total number of collected swim-up larvae	13,047	14,286
Number of swim-up larvae per female (mean)	815	1,020
Yield of swim-up larvae (%)**	4.5	6.4

Notes: *Mean values ± SE are presented in table. **From the number of eggs taken for fertilization.

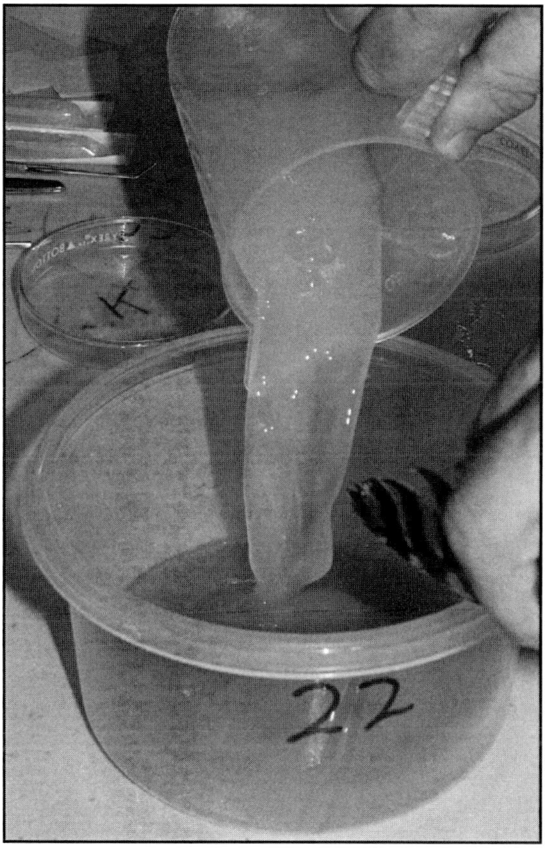

Figure 5.4 Fertilization of eggs with suspension of sperm.

a McDonald hatching jar for incubation. The yield of swim-up larvae was 4.5 and 6.4% for HCG and Ovaprim® treatments, respectively, with corresponding numbers of swim-up larvae per female of 815 and 1,020. There was no possibility to determine fertilization rate at cleavage stage since eggs at that time were heavily coated with fuller's earth particles. However, it can be suggested that low yield of larvae was caused by low fertilization rate. Inability to strip sperm from males can be considered as one of the main obstacles for practical application of induced spawning for production of mass quantities of fry in largemouth bass.

5.2 Genetics

5.2.1 Genetics and domestication

It is estimated that only about 15% of all aquaculture production is based on genetically improved stocks. However, when fish are cultivated in captivity even for a relatively short period, they are under strong and permanent "domestication" pressure, even if unintentional. Domestication can be defined as "a process by which a population of animals becomes adapted to man and the captive environment by some combination of genetic changes occurring over generations and environmentally induced developmental events recurring during each generation" (Price, 1984). Selection of fish for fitness under new conditions (ability to survive under high density, ability to consume artificial diet and so on) occurs permanently.

In 1960s–1970s, the intensive method of largemouth bass production had been developed. This method includes training of largemouth fingerlings to take artificial feed (for details see Chapter 6). Apparently, the changes in outcomes in training largemouth bass to artificial feed can be a good example of selection of fish for fitness under new conditions. Heidinger (2000) noted that one can expect in excess of 60% of the fingerlings to learn to accept the prepared diet while those fingerlings that have been produced from first- or second-generation hatchery-reared broodfish tend to have training rates in excess of 90%. Currently, broodstocks of largemouth bass have been raised on artificial diets for more than 7–8 generations at about ten different fish hatcheries in the US southern region. During this time, not only the percentage of fish accepting prepared diet has increased but the training process of fingerlings to accept artificial diet became much easier. Possibly, to some extent these changes can be attributed to some progress in training techniques (for example, by development of high-quality floating pellets). However, undoubtedly the underlying genetic composition of the fish themselves has changed as a result of domestication.

There are several examples in the literature, when the effects of animal domestication have been extremely rapid, and within even just a few generations of selection large changes occurred (Jensen and Wright, 2014). For example, selection of silver foxes for tameness for only several (4–6) generations resulted in profound changes in animal behavior and physiology (Trut, 1999; Trut et al., 2009). Along with progress in selection, animals rapidly acquired morphological traits, which are typical for some breeds of domesticated dog (for example, floppy ears and rolled tails). The level of corticosteroids (stress indicators) in the blood was significantly lower than in unselected animals. This research demonstrated that domesticated animals were less stressed by being kept in captivity. It would be incorrect to make direct analogies from domestication of mammals to domestication of largemouth bass. However, it can be suggested that adaptation of largemouth bass to new conditions has also caused many relatively rapid changes in fish behavior and physiology.

5.2.2 Florida and northern largemouth bass

In bass, the most common and best studied hybridization event occurs between the subspecies/species of largemouth bass, *Micropterus salmoides salmoides* (northern largemouth [NLMB]) and *Micropterus salmoides floridanus* (Florida largemouth bass [FLMB]). These two fish are now commonly recognized to represent separate species (Near et al., 2003; Barthel et al., 2015), although variable classifications are still seen in the literature. First described by Bailey and Hubbs (1949), the ranges of NLMB and FLMB bass were originally delineated based on morphometric and meristic techniques. They restricted FLMB to peninsular Florida, and NLMB to the majority of the midwestern, eastern, and southeastern US regions, outside of Alabama, Georgia, and South Carolina where a natural intergrade between the two was identified. Interestingly, Bailey and Hubbs (1949) refer to the already well-established larger maximum size of the FLMB (Hubbs, 1932), referring to it as a "giant" and commenting on differences in physiology between northern and Florida forms. They also comment on the difficulty of establishing the original boundaries between the subspecies given "extensive stocking." These themes, touched on in brief almost 70 years ago, have dominated the genetics of largemouth bass in intervening years and have continuing importance for genetic improvement and selection of largemouth bass as an aquaculture species.

5.2.2.1 Stocking of Florida and northern largemouth bass: controversy and consequences

Transport and stocking of largemouth bass (whether FLMB or NLMB) in non-native waters has been something of a long-standing tradition in the USA, sometimes directed by angling enthusiasts themselves and often as part of widespread state agency-directed efforts to improve recreational fishing. By the time Philipp et al. (1983) revisited the distribution of Florida/Northern alleles in 1983 using allozyme markers, stocking had led to hybridization between *M. salmoides* and *M. floridanus* far beyond the natural integrade zone. FLMB have been stocked most extensively throughout the southeastern USA, particularly in manmade reservoirs. Stocking has also occurred in the US Midwest, California, Japan, China, the Caribbean islands, South America, and elsewhere. One consequence of such widespread stocking is that geographical region can no longer be safely used as an indicator for determining the type of resident largemouth bass, status of introgression, degree of inbreeding, domestication and so on. Genetic testing is a pre-requisite before sourcing largemouth bass for a hatchery or aquaculture facility (see marker discussion below).

Much of the evidence for differential performance of FLMB and NLMB comes not from carefully controlled pond or tank studies, but rather from reservoir assessment reports following stocking. The ideological divide over stocking FLMB is best encapsulated in Maceina and Murphy (1992) where the authors spar with Philipp and Whitt over potential positive and negative effects of stocking outside the native range. While not advocating indiscriminate stocking, Maceina and Murphy argue that the reservoirs created by impoundment are unnatural habitats for native NLMB and, in some cases, more ideally suited for FLMB, using the success of FLMB and FLMB × NLMB hybrids in Texas reservoirs as evidence (Maceina et al., 1988). Philipp working with several coauthors has proposed vigorously that introducing FLMB in waters outside peninsular Florida has deleterious fitness consequences for recipient populations (Philipp, 1991) due to swamping of native populations through hybridization, outbreeding depression, lowered reproductive success, heightened susceptibility to disease, and so on (Fields et al., 1987; Cooke et al., 2001; Grant et al., 2003; Goldberg et al., 2005). However, Maceina and Murphy (1992) point out that many of these experiments involve stocking FLMB outside their thermal optima (for example, Central Illinois, Wisconsin), potentially biasing against the success of FL alleles. While this ongoing debate may seem to reside primarily in the realm of conservation and fisheries management, there are definite spill-over effects as state fisheries biologists weigh potential consequences of escapement from largemouth bass hatcheries and farms during permitting processes and regulate the movement of NLMB and FLMB. For example, the state of Florida, as part of a genetics conservation program, has declared it illegal to possess NLMB or their hybrids within the native range of FLMB and is restricting transport of bass among different genetic regions within the state (Porak et al., 2015). Other states, when faced with permitting largemouth bass aquaculture facilities, are likely to be heavily influenced by the "outbreeding depression" literature regarding non-native bass hybridization.

5.2.3 Differential performance of largemouth bass genotypes

Studies in both reservoir and aquaculture settings have highlighted differences in behavioral and production-important traits in FLMB, NLMB, and their hybrids. Results in these studies have been conflicting, and, oftentimes, a sufficient body of literature is not available to resolve differing findings. Differences in thermal optima for NLMB and FLMB are expected to impact performance and must be accounted for in comparing genetics stocks. Fields et al. (1987) reported that NLMB had chronic and critical thermal maxima significantly lower than NLMB × FLMB hybrids, FLMB × NLMB hybrids (note female in cross is listed first), and FLMB. Even outside these maxima, suboptimal temperatures undoubtedly affect performance. Studies also often fail to provide the domestication history of genetic strains/species they compared. A comparison between a NLMB under domestication for 10 generations with wild spawned FLMB and their hybrids is not an accurate reflection of genetic potential, but rather a testament to the importance of domestication.

With these caveats, the literature does provide importance insights into the comparative growth and performance of bass genetic stocks. The higher catchability and trainability of NLMB have long been noted. Zolczynski and Davies (1976) found faster growth in NLMB than FLMB or their hybrid in the first summer of growth. Many studies, both reservoir and aquaculture, point out the faster initial growth of NLMB, a favorable aspect for food production where the larger eventual size of FLMB over 10+ years is of little consequence. Similarly, Williamson and Carmichael (1990) found that NLMB had faster growth, 40% lower feed conversion ratio, lower mortality during net confinement, better feed training success, and other benefits in concluding that they were superior to FLMB and F_1 hybrids as potential aquaculture candidates. Here, more detail about source of stocks would have been helpful. They state that fish used in their trials came from wild populations. Given the large natural range of NLMB, for example, one wonders the aquaculture suitability of broodstock from Louisiana for a Texas growout facility versus broodstock sourced from northern Minnesota. Both are technically NLMB. Recent genetic analyses (Li et al., 2015) have revealed (not unexpectedly) that southern NLMB share a greater proportion of alleles with FLMB than do NLMB. Further studies comparing performance of various NLMB sourced across their natural range would be helpful in evaluating aquaculture broodstock candidates.

A 1990 study in Texas ponds (Kleinsasser et al., 1990) found that the FLMB × NLMB cross was superior for growth in its second year (641.1 g), having a significantly higher ending weight than NLMB (462.4 g), the reciprocal hybrid NLMB × FLMB (506.8 g), or FLMB (403.3 g). The wary, skittish nature of FLMB was noted as a cause for its poor showing (403 g average ending weight). Kubitza and Lovshin (1997) examined the impact of strain on feed training success. They utilized Fx hybrid crosses (roughly 70/30 FL/N or 70/30 N/FL contributions). They found comparable acceptance of a pelleted diet by both crosses. While the literature remains fairly sparse and confusing on this subject, the general consensus is that the faster initial growth, superior feed trainability, and more aggressive nature of the NLMB make it the preferred largemouth bass candidate for aquaculture. However, as described above, further intra-NLMB studies are needed and the geographic location and configuration of a grow-out facility may ultimately dictate the optimal genotype. Within the right thermal window, FLMB × NLMB hybrids deserve additional research and scrutiny as well (Bonvechio and Rydell, 2016).

5.2.4 Genetic markers: ancestry, parentage and beyond

The potential for success in selective breeding is governed in large part by the presence of sufficient genetic variation in founding populations. Loss of genetic variation is often attributable to a lack of knowledge of base populations or hatchery practices that introduce artificial genetic bottlenecks (Bai et al., 2008). The long history of movement and stocking of largemouth bass (as documented above) makes uninformed assumptions about broodstock or fingerling origin or levels of diversity fraught with peril. The propensity of NLMB and FLMB to hybridize, the presence of natural intergrades, and lack of clear morphological features distinguishing largemouth bass forms, has long necessitated chemical and molecular testing to clearly delineate ancestry. Beginning with the work of Philipp et al. (1983), where 28 enzyme loci were examined, largemouth bass genetic testing has followed the progression of the advance of molecular genetic techniques from allozymes, to microsatellites and then to single-nucleotide polymorphism (SNP) markers.

In their 1983 work, Philipp et al. screened 28 enzymes, but identified only two, isocitrate dehydrogenase-B and aspartate aminotransferase-B, with fixed allelic differences useful for determining the contribution of the subspecies to the gene pool of various populations throughout the USA. Other enzymes were useful in demonstrating genetic distinctness among populations, although not necessarily correlated with NLMB/FLMB composition. Allozyme analyses became the gold standard for population genetics research and for testing commercial populations for the next two decades. However, with only two diagnostic loci, clear detection of hybridity across the largemouth bass genome was inconsistent at best. As sequencing technologies allowed the identification of simple sequence repeats, or microsatellites, these markers were developed for largemouth bass. Lutz-Carrillo (2008) developed 52 microsatellite markers for FLMB and demonstrated their utility in other largemouth bass. Seyoum et al. (2013) developed an additional 18 microsatellites, focusing on development of multiplex panels with similar annealing temperatures and cycling parameters. These microsatellites included no fixed loci, but several loci possessed clear allelic frequency distribution differences between FLMB and NLMB (and other black basses). Microsatellites have well-established pros and cons as a marker technology. Their allelic richness makes each locus highly informative. However, they suffer from null alleles, expense of reagents, difficulty in multiplexing, and the high labor cost associated with careful scoring of loci. Furthermore, changes in technology for sequencing have made it more difficult to maintain microsatellite running capabilities in many labs.

The dramatic decline in sequencing costs associated with next generation sequencing has increased the accessibility of SNP markers for population genetics (Hohenlohe et al., 2011). SNPs are valued for their even genome-wide distribution, abundance, ease of multiplexing, and low genotyping error rate. Li et al. (2015) described the work conducted to develop diagnostic SNP marker panels for largemouth bass at Auburn University. Two panels of 25 and 38 fixed SNP loci can clearly distinguish purity and hybridity (including multi-generation backcrosses) across the genome. In daily running, the single 38-plex panel is sufficient for these purposes. Over 5,000 largemouth bass from rivers, reservoirs, hatcheries, and ponds across the USA, China, and Japan have been genotyped to date with these markers. The short, discrete nature of SNP loci also allow use of highly degraded samples, allowing DNA to be collected by swab sampling, use of cruder (and cheaper) DNA extraction techniques, and even for genotypes to be obtained from long term formalin-fixed museum samples.

Once questions of FLMB/NLMB purity and hybridity have been answered, genetic markers are often needed to determine parentage. As hatchery configuration and space restraints often preclude 1 : 1 mating schemes, so raceways, tanks, or ponds are used for communal spawning. Identification of superior broodstock (for example, walk-back selection) based on progeny performance in a common-garden growout necessitates the use of markers to establish parentage. Parentage analyses are also critical in determining effective numbers of breeders contributing to offspring to avoid inbreeding and ensuring broodstock maintain essential genetic diversity. Austin et al. (2012) screened broodstock and fingerlings at the Richloam Fish Hatchery in Florida with microsatellite loci to assess hatchery effects on genetic diversity and to determine sibling relationships. While they concluded that their current raceway breeding practices were sufficient to maintain diversity, they found that the use of nine microsatellite loci was insufficient to allow parentage assignment for individual fingerlings. A subsequent study, Hargrove and Austin (2017) used a different set of microsatellites to examine parentage, demonstrating that most broodfish contributed to reproduction, and that most spawns could be attributed to one pair of parents. Similarly, SNP markers recently have been developed and demonstrated for parentage analyses in FLMB (Zhao et al., 2018), with downstream applications in hatchery management, selection, and parentage-based tagging in reservoirs.

Further aquaculture applications for molecular tools in largemouth bass lie in the realm of marker-assisted selection for trait performance. In this, Chinese aquaculturists appear to be leading the way. NLMB were introduced into China in 1983 and now account for 100,000 tons of annual aquaculture production. Genetic analyses show a distinct signature of genetic bottlenecking due to the founder effect (Bai et al., 2008). Recent research has identified SNPs and other polymorphisms linked to growth traits and early efforts are underway to use these as a basis for selective breeding (Li et al., 2009, 2017). Other more cryptic literature from China references long-term selection of largemouth bass for growth.

5.2.5 Potential for selective breeding and continued genetic improvement

Selective breeding for largemouth bass has been sporadic and poorly reported, often residing in "grey" literature of state hatchery reports or conference communications. While selection for pelleted feed acceptance has a long history (Snow, 1960; Kubitza and Lovshin, 1997), foundational stocks were often not rigorously evaluated, record keeping was sporadic, and the current genetic integrity of these lines is often difficult to ascertain. Private hatcheries have also carried out selection, but often their goals have been aimed primarily at trophy bass production for recreational angling rather than shorter-term aquaculture growout potential, and their success is difficult to rigorously evaluate. Clearly, the need and potential remains for a well-controlled, multi-generation selective breeding program for largemouth bass and/or the FLMB × NLMB hybrid aimed at food-fish production.

As noted, a comparison of the growth potential of NLMB sourced from different regions and river systems is needed. Studies examining the heritability of traits important for aquaculture production are also needed (growth, disease resistance, fillet yield, and so forth). The ongoing ShareLunker program in the state of Texas, has recently reported that angler return of trophy fish caught in Texas reservoirs for use as hatchery broodstock has yielded offspring significantly heavier than resident cohorts (1.19 kg versus 0.99 kg at age 4) within several reservoirs (Baird et al., 2016), indicating that, even in large, highly variable environments, genetic contributions to growth can be realized. As with much of aquaculture, the development of a long-term, well-structured selection program for largemouth bass, is hindered by economic constraints. Investment in additional hatchery and grow-out facilities, record keeping, and molecular marker analysis must be offset by a return from a higher priced fingerling, lowered costs of production, or higher yields. The small size of the largemouth bass market, at least in the USA at this writing, likely makes it difficult to realize an economic gain on large-scale investments in genetic selection. Development and release of improved lines may be better achieved through developing partnerships with existing university programs or U.S. Department of Agriculture research labs focused on aquaculture. Once a stable breeding program is developed with well-established lines or strains, additional gains may be realized through all female bass production (Bonvechio and Rydell, 2016), potentially augmented by use of molecular markers to develop monosex all-female breeding populations as described below (gynogenesis). Towards that end, efforts are ongoing to develop high density genetic maps for largemouth bass with markers linked to sex determination (Peatman lab at Auburn University).

5.2.6 Production and evaluation of triploids

Studies on induced triploidy in largemouth bass were initiated based on the suggestion that sterile triploids could have better growth parameters than normal fertile diploids. Also, stocking of sterile triploids into water bodies outside native range could minimize impacts on genetic pools of local populations. Garrett et al. (1992) produced triploid progenies of largemouth bass using hydrostatic pressure for retention of second polar body in freshly fertilized eggs. Pressure levels from 4,000 pounds per square inch (psi) to 8,000 psi (281–563 kg/cm^2) were tested; pressure shock durations were 3 min for pressure levels from 4,000 to 6,500 psi (457 kg/cm^2) and 1 min for 8,000 psi, respectively. In all experimental variants pressure shock was applied 5 min after fertilization; pre-shock water temperature was 21–25°C. Ploidy of 1- or 2-month-old fish was determined by measurement of DNA content by flow cytometric analysis. All applied treatments produced triploids in experimental groups. A treatment of 8,000 psi (or 563 kg/cm^2) was considered as the best; it yielded 100% triploids and a relatively low mortality. Parameters of pressure determined by Garrett et al. (1992) were usually used in later studies on inducement of triploidy in largemouth bass. Fries et al. (2002) used pressure shock with these parameters (initiation: 5 min after fertilization, duration: 1 min, intensity – 563 kg/cm^2) for production triploids. Results of flow cytometric analysis showed that triploidy induction technique was effective; overall success rate was 95.5%.

Neal et al. (2004) used the same parameters of pressure shock (5 min after insemination, duration 1 min, 563 kg/cm^2) for production triploids in largemouth bass in Puerto Rico. Flow cytometry analysis revealed 100% triploid fingerlings in pressure-treated group. Also, a method of fish ploidy determination based on erythrocyte lengths on blood smears was developed. Neal and Noble (2008) have presented comparative data on growth and maturation of 1-year-old diploid and triploid largemouth bass raised in a reservoir in Puerto Rico. No difference in growth rate between 1-year-old diploid and triploid fish was detected. Diploid females had much better developed ovaries than triploid females and had mean gonadosomatic indices of 1.98 and 0.29%, respectively. In a further study, Neal (2014) had not detected differences in growth rate between diploid and triploid largemouth bass at fish age 2 years and older. Maximum sizes, which were attained by diploid and triploid fish, were similar. Most of females with total length 250 mm and larger were mature while no triploid females displayed maturing ovaries. Diploid males had significantly larger mean gonadosomatic index than triploid males. These data showed that retardation in gonad development in triploid largemouth bass did not result in increased growth rate compared to normal diploids.

5.2.7 Sex control

Largemouth bass are sexually dimorphic. Females of largemouth bass demonstrate faster growth rate and attain larger size than males. Therefore, it would be attractive to produce and raise all-female progenies. Also, raising monosex (either all-female or all-male progenies) would restrict unwanted reproduction.

Artificial sex regulation in fish is connected mainly with elaboration and application of the hormonal sex reversal method. Hormonal sex reversal is a change from the normal process of sex differentiation under the influence of steroid sex hormones (or some other substances) so that genotypic females develop testes or genotypic males develop ovaries. Sex reversal changes only fish phenotype while the genotypic formula of sex chromosomes remains the same. Hormonal sex reversal may be used in two different ways for sex regulation. The direct method for producing monosex (all-female or all-male) populations involves hormonal treatment of all reared fish during the period of sex differentiation. The indirect method, or genetic sex regulation, involves crossing normal fish with previously obtained sex-reversed fish. Most studies performed in largemouth bass until now were aimed at direct feminization or masculinization of fish by treatment of estrogens or androgens, respectively. These studies performed are briefly reviewed below.

Garrett (1989) performed a series of experiments on hormonal sex control of largemouth bass. In one experiment, largemouth bass fry were fed with hormone-enriched live brine shrimp (Artemia) from beginning of active feeding for 10 weeks. Two estrogens (17α-estradiol and estrone) and two androgens (17α-methyltestosterone and androsterone) were used for sex reversal. For enrichment, each hormone was dissolved in 95% ethanol and added to brine shrimp culture media to concentration of 5 mg/l; in the control variant only ethanol was added without any hormone. Feeding largemouth bass fry with hormone administration through brine shrimp was highly effective for sex reversal. Experimental groups, which consumed androgen-treated (with both methyltestosterone and androsterone) brine shrimp, consisted of males only while groups fed with estrogen-treated (with both estradiol and estrone) brine shrimp consisted only of females. The sex ratio in control group was significantly skewed towards males (89% males). It was suggested that skewed sex ratio in control group has resulted from androgen influence via water vapor since the control jar was adjacent to the jars with hormone-treated brine shrimp. In a later similar experiment, which used hormone concentration of 10 mg/l for Artemia enrichment, the control container was placed approximately 2 m away from hormone-treated containers and resulting sex ratio in control group was close to expected 1 : 1; hormonal influence in that experiment was again 100% effective in all experimental groups. In another experiment performed by Garrett (1989) 20–30 mm 5-week-old largemouth bass fry nursed in a pond were fed with hormone-containing food for 6 weeks. The same two estrogens (17α-estradiol and estrone) and two androgens (17α-methyltestosterone and androsterone) were used for sex reversal. Two doses of 17α-methyltestosterone (50 and 100 mg/kg of food) were evaluated while for the other three hormones only one dose of 100 mg/kg was used. Treatments of androgens resulted in sex reversal of most of the genotypic females (90–98% of males in androgen-treated groups). In the control group the sex ratio did not differ significantly from 1 : 1. Estrogens appeared to be ineffective for sex reversal in genotypic males; fish sex ratios in groups receiving estradiol or estrone with diet did not differ significantly from 1 : 1.

Porter (1996) studied effectiveness of feeding largemouth bass fry with 17α-methyltestosterone (MT) with doses of 30 and 50 mg/kg for periods of 4, 6, or 10 weeks. Hormonal treatment started when fish had mean total length about 25 mm. Sex of fish in hormonally treated and control groups was determined based on two criteria: gonad morphology (structure) and histology. Morphologically, "V-shaped" testes were distinguished from "Y-shaped" ovaries. Histologically, testes were identified by the absence of oogonia. In control variants about 50% of fish were identified as males based both on gonad morphology and histology. In experimental groups receiving MT in their food, 96–100% of fish were identified as males based on gonad histology; however, about 50% of these fish had gonads with the morphological structure of ovaries.

Al-Ablani and Phelps (2001) indicated that 17α-estradiol and diethylstilbestrol were both effective in producing 100% feminization in 40 d-old largemouth bass fry when fed at concentrations of 100, 200, or 400 mg/kg of diet for 40 d. Arslan et al. (2009) reported that feeding of 40 d-old largemouth fry with 17α-estradiol at a concentration of 200 mg/kg for 30, 45, or 60 d resulted only in slight increases in the frequency of females (up to 59.8–70.5%) in experimental groups. Feeding of fry of the same age with diets containing MT at a concentration 60 mg/kg for 30, 45, or 60 d did not result in a shift in sex ratios. The three- or six-time immersions of largemouth fry in a MT solution of 1 mg/l for 5 h between 40 and 46 or 54 d post-hatching were also not effective in inducing sex reversal.

As mentioned above, the indirect method of sex control, or genetic sex regulation, involves crossing normal fish with previously obtained sex-reversed fish. Genetic sex regulation is regarded as the preferred method since there is no need to treat all reared fish with a hormone and hormonally treated fish are not used for human consumption. The scheme of crosses used to produce all-female progenies depends on the type of heterogamety in given fish species. In fishes, both male (XY males, XX females) and female (WZ females, ZZ males) heterogamety are described; sometimes different types of heterogamety are revealed in closely related species. In the case of female homogamety, all-female progenies may be produced by crossing normal females XX with sex-reversed XX males (neomales) obtained by hormonal sex reversal of genotypic females. In the case of female heterogamety the scheme for production of all-female progenies is more complex. In this case it needs to identify WW females either in progenies obtained by crossing sex-reversed WZ males with normal WZ females or in meiotic gynogenetic progenies. Cross of WW females with normal ZZ males should produce females (WZ) only.

One of the basic methods for determining the type of heterogamety in fish is based on sex composition of gynogenetic progenies. In the case of male heterogamety (XY/XX), gynogenetic progenies usually consist of females only; the presence of both females and males indicates female heterogamety in a given species (WZ/ZZ). Gynogenetic development in fish is usually induced by insemination of eggs with genetically inactivated (by UV-irradiation) sperm while restoration of diploidy is caused by suppression either second meiotic division in eggs (meiotic gynogenesis) or first mitotic (cleavage) division in haploid embryos (mitotic gynogenesis).

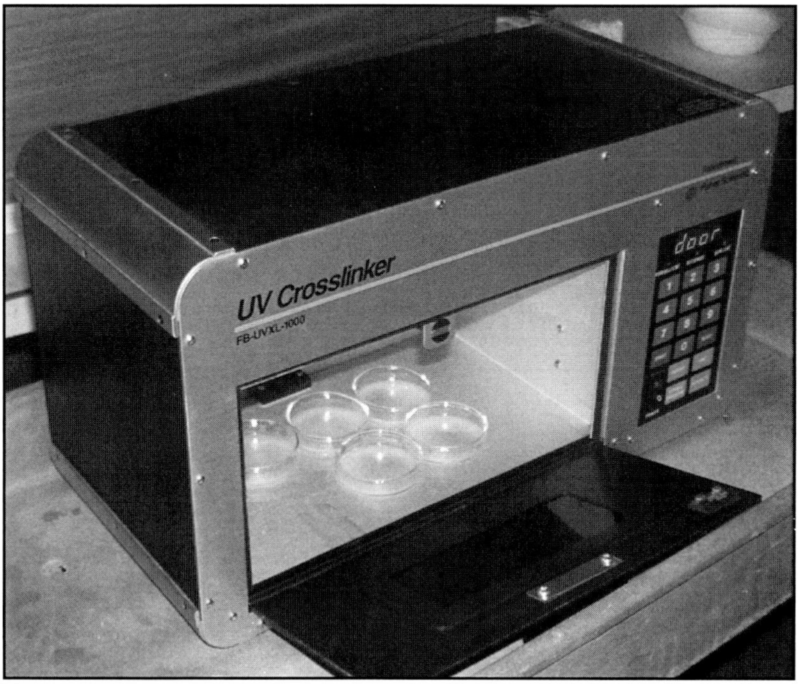

Figure 5.5 Petri dishes with diluted white bass sperm are placed into Crosslinker for UV-irradiation.

Only one study on induced meiotic gynogenesis in largemouth bass has been performed so far (Glennon et al., 2012). In this study, gynogenetic development was induced by insemination of largemouth bass eggs with genetically inactivated (by UV-irradiation) sperm from white bass or striped bass. Sperm was irradiated at a dose of 1,000 J/m^2 with a FisherBiotech UV microprocessor-controlled Crosslinker (FB-UVXL-1000). For irradiation, 2 ml of sperm diluted 10-fold with 0.85% NaCl solution was placed in 6 cm-diameter glass Petri dishes (Figure 5.5).

Suppression of the second meiotic division in largemouth bass eggs was achieved by hydrostatic pressure; pressure shock of 8,000 psi for 1 min was initiated 5 min after the eggs were inseminated with irradiated sperm (Figure 5.6).

Fifteen 1 year old fish of gynogenetic origin were dissected for sex determination; seven fish were male and eight fish were female. Another six gynogenetic fish were sexed live using ultrasound investigation and were identified as females. In total, of the 21 gynogenetic fish analyzed, 7 fish (33.3%) were male and 14 fish (66.7%) were female. Based on presence of males in meiotic gynogenetic progeny the existence of female heterogamety (WZ/ZZ) in largemouth bass was suggested (Glennon et al., 2012). In meiotic gynogenetic progeny obtained later all seven analyzed fish were female (Robert Glennon, personal communication). Based on this information, it may be stated that existence of female heterogamety in largemouth bass suggested earlier (Glennon et al., 2012) needs further confirmation.

5.2.8 Interspecies hybridization

Childers (1975) noted that hybridization of largemouth bass with fish of other species is a rare phenomenon under natural conditions. However, many different interspecies hybrids of largemouth

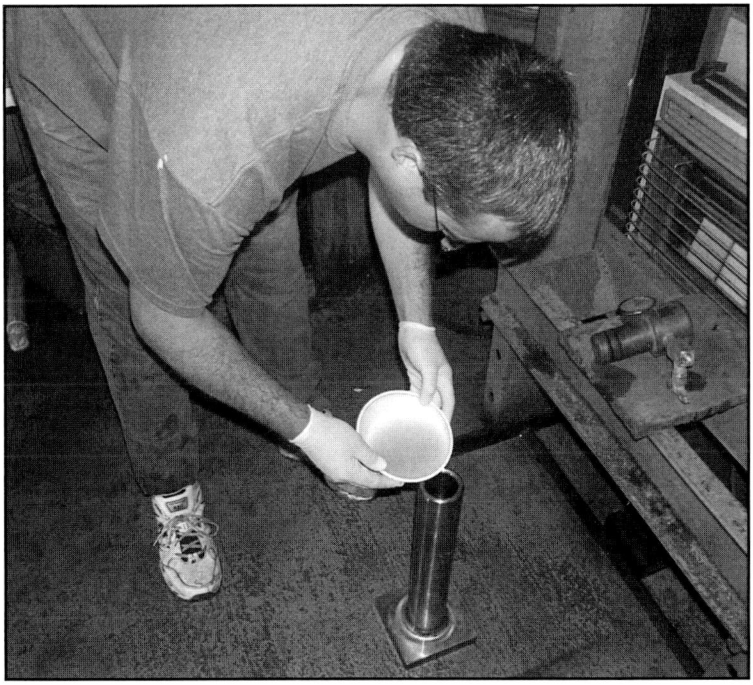

Figure 5.6 Largemouth bass eggs inseminated with irradiated white bass sperm are placed into pressure chamber for applying of hydrostatic shock.

bass with fishes of genus *Lepomis* and other fish of genus *Micropterus* have been obtained artificially. In many cross combinations, the obtained hybrids had low viability and poor growth rate. The only hybrids, which appeared to have some superior characteristics, were those obtained by cross of largemouth bass females with smallmouth bass (*Micropterus dolomieui*) males. Hybrids obtained by reciprocal cross (females smallmouth bass × males largemouth bass) were inviable. Childers (1975) and Beaty and Childers (1980) described that largemouth bass × smallmouth bass hybrids demonstrated better growth rate than pure largemouth bass. However, further studies (Buck and Hooe, 1986; Stilwell, 2008) have not confirmed these observations. In these studies, growth rate of hybrids was similar to or slower than that of largemouth bass. There are other factors which make production and raising of these hybrids impractical. Largemouth bass × smallmouth bass hybrids can be produced only by artificial spawning. Also, Gomelsky et al. (2004) showed these hybrids are fertile and can backcross with parental species. Thus, possible escapement of artificially obtained hybrids could result in genetic contamination of natural populations.

References

Al-Ablani, S.A. and Phelps, R.P. (2001) Induction of feminization in largemouth bass (*Micropterus salmoides*) by oral administration of estradiol-17 beta or diethylstilbestrol and associated pathological effects. *Journal of Aquaculture in the Tropics* 16, 185–195.

Arslan, T., Phelps, R.P. and Osborne, J.A. (2009) Effects of oestradiol-17β or 17α-methyltestosterone administration on gonadal differentiation of largemouth bass *Micropterus salmoides* (Lacépède). *Aquaculture Research* 40, 1813–1822.

Austin, J.D., Johnson, A., Matthews, M., Tringali, M.D., Porak, W.F. and Allen, M.S. (2012) An assessment of hatchery effects on Florida Bass (*Micropterus salmoides floridanus*) microsatellite genetic diversity and sib-ship reconstruction. *Aquaculture Research* 43, 628–638.

Bai, J., Lutz-Carrillo, D.J., Quan, Y. and Liang, S. (2008) Taxonomic status and genetic diversity of cultured largemouth bass *Micropterus salmoides* in China. *Aquaculture* 278, 27–30.

Bailey, R.M. and Hubbs, C.L. (1949) The black basses (*Micropterus*) of Florida, with description of a new species. *University of Michigan Occasional Papers of the Museum of Zoology* 516, 1–40.

Baird, M.S., Bister, T.J., Farooqi, M.A., Hungerford, T.J., Schlechte, J.W., Lutz-Carrillo, D.J. and Martinez, J.G. (2016) Comparison of Growth of Selectively Bred and Resident Largemouth Bass in Texas Small Impoundments. *Journal of the Southeastern Association of Fish and Wildlife Agencies* 3, 57–63.

Barthel, B.L., Allen, M.S., Porak, W.F. and Kerns, J. (2015) Florida Bass *Micropterus floridanus* (LeSueur, 1822). In: Tringali, M.D., Long, J.M., Birdsong, T.W. and Allen, M. S. (ed.) *Black bass diversity: multidisciplinary science for conservation.* American Fisheries Society, Symposium 82, Bethesda, MD, pp. 43–53.

Beaty, P.R. and Childers, W.F. (1980) Hybridization of Northern largemouth bass (*Micropterus salmoides salmoides*) and Northern smallmouth bass (*Micropterus dolomieui dolomieui*). Illinois Natural History Survey, Final Report to the Bass Research Foundation, Starkville, MS.

Bonvechio, T.F. and Rydell, J.J. (2016) Use of a female-only stocking strategy to establish a trophy largemouth bass in a small Georgia impoundment. *Journal of the Southeastern Association of Fish and Wildlife Agencies* 3, 136–143.

Brauhn, J.L., Holz, D. and Anderson, R.O. (1972) August spawning of largemouth bass. *Progressive Fish Culturist* 34, 207–209.

Buck, D.H. and Hooe, M.L. (1986) Comparative growth of Northern largemouth bass and F_1 hybrid largemouth bass through three growing seasons. *Transactions of the American Fisheries Society* 115, 296–304.

Carlson, A.R. (1973) Induced spawning of largemouth bass [*Micropterus salmoides* (Lacépède)]. *Transactions of the American Fisheries Society* 102, 442–444.

Childers, W.F. (1975) Bass genetics as applied to culture and management. In: Clepper, H. (ed.) *Black Bass Biology and Management.* Sport Fishing Institute, Washington, DC, pp. 362–372.

Cooke, S.J., Kassler, T.W. and Philipp, D.P. (2001) Physiological performance of largemouth bass related to local adaptation and interstock hybridization: implications for conservation and management. *Journal of Fish Biology* 59, 248–268.

Davis, J.T. and Lock, J.T. (1997) Culture of largemouth bass fingerlings. Southern Regional Aquaculture Center (SRAC), SRAC Publication No. 201, Stoneville, MS.

Fields, R., Lowe, S.S., Kaminski, C., Whitt, G.S. and Philipp, D.P. (1987) Critical and chronic thermal maxima of northern and Florida largemouth bass and their reciprocal F_1 and F_2 hybrids. *Transactions of the American Fisheries Society* 116, 856–863.

Fries, L.T, Kurten, G.L, Isaak, J. Jr., Engelhardt, T., Lyon, D. and Smith, D.G. (2002) Mass production of polyploid Florida largemouth bass for stocking public waters in Texas. In: Philipp, D.P. and Ridgway, M.S. (eds) Black Bass: *Ecology Conservation and Management,* American Fisheries Society, Symposium 31, Bethesda, MD, pp. 393–399.

Garrett, G.P. (1989) Hormonal sex control of largemouth bass. *The Progressive Fish-Culturist* 51, 146–148.

Garrett, G.P., Birkner, M.C.F. and Gold, J.R. (1992) Triploidy induction in largemouth bass, *Micropterus salmoides. Journal of Applied Aquaculture* 1, 27–34.

Glenewinkel, H., Barkoh, A., Engeling, T., Hall, L., Paret, J. and Owens, T. (2011) Guidelines for the culture of black bass. Management data series No. 267, Texas Parks and Wildlife, Inland Fisheries Division, Austin, TX, USA.

Glennon, R.P., Gomelsky, B., Schneider, K.J., Kelly, A.M. and Haukenes, A. (2012) Evidence of female heterogamety in largemouth bass, based on sex ratio of gynogenetic progeny. *North American Journal of Aquaculture* 74, 537–540.

Goldberg, T.L., Grant, E.C., Inendino, K.R., Kassler, T.W., Claussen, J.E. and Philipp, D.P. (2005) Increased infectious disease susceptibility resulting from outbreeding depression. *Conservation Biology* 19, 455–462.

Gomelsky, B., Dabrowski, K., Garcia-Abiado, M.A., Stilwell, W., Tidwell, J.H. and Coyle, S.D. (2004) Ploidy of backcross hybrids of largemouth bass and smallmouth bass. *North American Journal of Aquaculture* 66, 133–136.

Grant, E.C., Philipp, D.P., Inendino, K.R. and Goldberg, T.L. (2003) Effects of temperature on the susceptibility of largemouth bass to largemouth bass virus. *Journal of Aquatic Animal Health* 15, 215–220.

Gross, T.S., Wieser, C.M., Sep´ulveda, M.S., Wiebe, J.J., Schoeb, T.R. and Denslow, N.D. (2002) Characterization of annual reproductive cycles for pond reared Florida Largemouth Bass *Micropterus salmoides floridanus*. In: Philipp, D.P. and Ridgway, M.S. (eds) *Black Bass: Ecology, Conservation, and Management*. American Fisheries Society, Bethesda, MD, USA, pp. 205–212.

Hargrove, J.D. and Austin, J.D. (2017) Parentage and mating patterns in a Florida Largemouth Bass (*Micropterus salmoides floridanus*) hatchery. *Aquaculture Research* 48, 3272–3277.

Heidinger, R.C. (1975) Life history and biology of the largemouth bass. In: Clepper, H. and Stroud, R.H. (eds) *Black Bass Biology and Management*, Sport Fishing Institute, Washington, DC, pp. 11–20.

Heidinger, R.C. (1976) *Synopsis of Biological Data on the Largemouth bass, Micropterus salmoides (Lacépède) 1802*, FAO Fisheries Synopsis No. 115, Rome.

Heidinger, R.C. (2000) Black bass/largemouth bass culture. In: Stickney, R.R. (ed.) Encyclopedia of Aquaculture, John Wiley & Sons, New York, pp. 108–117.

Hohenlohe, P.A., Amish, S.J., Catchen, J.M., Allendorf, F.W. and Luikart, G. (2011) Next-generation RAD sequencing identifies thousands of SNPs for assessing hybridization between rainbow and westslope cutthroat trout. *Molecular Ecology Resources* 11, 117–122.

Hubbs, C.L. (1932) The Species of Black Bass. *Transactions of the American Fisheries Society* 61, 86–88.

Hutson, P.L. (1983) Smallmouth bass culture in Texas. Management Data Series 35, Texas Parks and Wildlife Department, Austin, TX, USA.

Hutson, P.L. (1990) Florida Largemouth Bass culture in Texas. Management Data Series No. 35. Texas Parks and Wildlife Department, Austin, TX, USA.

Isaac, Jr., J. and Staats, V.H. (1992) Florida Largemouth Bass raceway spawning substrate evaluation. *Proceeding of the Annual Conference of the Southeastern Association of Fish and Wildlife Agencies* 46, 453–457.

Jackson, U.T. (1979) Controlled spawning of largemouth bass. *Progressive Fish-Culturist* 41, 90–95.

Jensen, P. and Wright, D. (2014) Behavioral genetics and animal domestication. In: Grandin, T. and Deesing, M.J. (eds) *Genetics and the Behavior of Domestic Animals*, 2nd edn. Academic Press, London, pp. 41–79.

Kleinsasser, L.J., Williamson, J.H. and Whiteside, B.G. (1990) Growth and catchability of northern, Florida, and F1 hybrid largemouth bass in Texas ponds. *North American Journal of Fisheries Management* 10, 462–468.

Koeypudsa, W., Phadee, P., Tangtrongpiros, J. and Hatai, K. (2005) Influence of pH, temperature, and sodium chloride concentration on growth rate of *Saprolegnia* sp. *Journal of Scientific Research at Chulalongkorn University* 30, 123–130.

Kubitza, F. and Lovshin, L.L. (1997) Effects of initial weight and genetic strain on feed training largemouth bass *Micropterus salmoides* using ground fish flesh and freeze dried krill as starter diets. *Aquaculture* 148, 179–190.

Kurten, G. (2001) Evaluation of stocking, harvest and zooplankton variables in ponds for rearing Florida largemouth bass fingerlings. Management Data Series No. 195. Texas Parks and Wildlife Department, Austin, TX, USA.

Li, C., Gowan, S., Anil, A., Beck, B.H., Thongda, W., Kucuktas, H., Kaltenboeck, L. and Peatman, E. (2015) Discovery and validation of gene-linked diagnostic SNP markers for assessing hybridization between Largemouth bass (*Micropterus salmoides*) and Florida bass (*M. floridanus*). *Molecular Ecology Resources* 15, 395–404.

Li, S., Liu, H., Bai, J. and Zhu, X. (2017) Transcriptome assembly and identification of genes and SNPs associated with growth traits in largemouth bass (*Micropterus salmoides*). *Genetica* 145, 175–187.

Li, X.H., Bai, J.J., Ye, X., Hu, Y.C., Li, S.J. and Yu, L.Y. (2009) Polymorphisms in the 5′ flanking region of the insulin-like growth factor I gene are associated with growth traits in largemouth bass *Micropterus salmoides. Fisheries Science* 75, 351–358.

Lutz-Carrillo, D.J., Hagen, C., Dueck, L.A. and Glenn, T.C. (2008) Isolation and characterization of microsatellite loci for Florida largemouth bass, *Micropterus salmoides floridanus*, and other micropterids. *Molecular Ecology Resources* 8, 178–184.

Maceina, M.J. and Murphy, B.R. (1992) Stocking Florida largemouth bass outside its native range. *Transactions of the American Fisheries Society* 121, 686–691.

Maceina, M.J., Murphy, B.R. and Isely, J.J. (1988) Factors regulating Florida largemouth bass stocking success and hybridization with northern largemouth bass in Aquilla Lake, Texas. *Transactions of the American Fisheries Society* 117, 221–231.

Marking, L.L., Rach, J.J. and Schreier, T.M. (1994) Evaluation of antifungal agents for fish culture. *The Progressive Fish-Culturist* 56, 225–231.

Matthews, M.D. and Stout, R.B. (2013) Out-of-season spawning method for Florida largemouth bass to produce advanced-sized fingerling by early spring. *North American Journal of Aquaculture* 75, 524–531.

Matthews, M.D., Sakmar, J.C. and Trippel, N. (2012) Evaluation of hydrogen peroxide and temperature to control mortality caused by saprolegniasis and to increase hatching success of largemouth bass eggs. *North American Journal of Aquaculture* 74, 463–467.

Mayes, K.B, Rosenblum, P.M. and Brandt, T.M. (1993) Raceway spawning of Florida Largemouth Bass: effects of acclimation time and hormone treatment on spawning success. *The Progressive Fish-Culturist* 55, 1–8.

Neal, J. W. (2014) Comparison of diploid and triploid largemouth bass growth and maturation in Puerto Rico. *Journal of the Southeastern Association of Fish and Wildlife Agencies* 1, 1–6.

Neal, J.W. and Noble, R.L. (2008) Comparison of diploid and triploid largemouth bass growth and maturation through age 1 in Puerto Rico. *North American Journal of Fisheries Management* 28, 688–693.

Neal, J.W., Neal, D.M., Noble, R.L. and McGee, M.V. (2004) Artificial propagation and induction of triploidy in largemouth bass *Micropterus salmoides* and ploidy discrimination using erythrocyte length. *Journal of the World Aquaculture Society* 35, 46–54.

Near, T. J., Kassler, T.W., Koppelman, J. B., Dillman, C.B. and Philipp, D.P. (2003) Speciation in North American black basses, *Micropterus* (Actinopterygii: Centrarchidae). *Evolution* 57, 1610–1621.

Philipp, D.P. (1991) Genetic implications of introducing Florida largemouth bass, *Micropterus salmoides floridanus. Canadian Journal of Fisheries and Aquatic Sciences* 48, 58–65.

Philipp, D.P., Childers, W.F. and Whitt, G.S. (1983) A biochemical genetic evaluation of the northern and Florida subspecies of largemouth bass. *Transactions of the American Fisheries Society* 112, 1–20.

Pine, W.E., Ludsin, S.A. and DeVries, D.R. (2000) First-summer survival of largemouth bass cohorts: is early spawning really best? *Transactions of the American Fisheries Society* 129, 504–513.

Piper, R.G., McElwain, I.B., Orme, L.E., McCraren, J.P., Fowler, L.G. and Leonard, J.R. (1982) *Fish Hatchery Management.* United States Department of the Interior, Fish and Wildlife Service, Washington, DC, USA.

Porak, W.F., Barthel, B.L., Stout, R.B., Tringali, M.D., Matthews, M., Pouder, W.F. and Philipp, D.P. (2015) The development of a genetic conservation program for the FLMB in its native range. In: Tringali, M.D., Long, J.M., Birdsong, T.W. and Allen, M.S. (eds) *Black bass diversity: multidisciplinary science for conservation.* American Fisheries Society, Symposium 82, Bethesda, MD, pp. 585–600.

Porter, M.D. (1996) Effect of methyltestosterone on largemouth bass, *Micropterus salmoides. Journal of Applied Aquaculture* 6, 39–45.

Price, E.O. (1984) Behavioral aspects of animal domestication. *The Quarterly Review of Biology* 59, 1–32.

Rosenblum, P.M., Brandt, T.M. Mayes, K.B. and Hutson, P. (1994) Annual cycles of growth and reproduction in hatchery-reared Florida Largemouth Bass, *Micropterus salmoides floridanus,* raised on forage or pelleted diets. *Journal of Fish Biology* 44, 1045–1059.

Sarti, M.J. (1986) Largemouth bass raceway spawning at Jake Wolf Memorial Fish Hatchery. In: Sweet, R. (ed.) *Midwest Black Bass Culture.* Missouri Department of Conservation, Kansas City, MO, USA, pp. 35–36.

Seyoum, S., Tringali, M.D., Barthel, B.L., Davis, M.C, Schmitt, S.L., Bellotti, P. S. and Porak, W.F. (2013) Isolation and characterization of eighteen microsatellite loci for the Largemouth Bass, *Micropterus salmoides,* and cross amplification in congeneric species. *Conservation Genetics Resources* 5, 697–701.

Simco, B.A., Williamson, J.H., Carmichael, G.J. and Tomasso, J.R. (1986) Centrarchids. In: Stickney, R.R. (ed.) *Culture of Non-Salmonid Freshwater Fishes.* CRC Press, Boca Raton, FL, USA. pp. 73–89.

Skaggs, J.Y., Quintana, S., Shaw, M., Allen, N., Trippel, A. and Matthews, M. (2017) Effects of common angler handling techniques on Florida largemouth bass behavior, feeding, and survival. *North American Journal of Fisheries Management* 37, 263–270.

Skudlarek, N., Coyle, S. and Tidwell, J.H. (2013) Development of first-feeding protocols for indoor larviculture of largemouth bass (*Micropterus salmoides*). *Journal of Applied Aquaculture* 25, 9–23.

Snow, J.R. (1960) An exploratory attempt to rear largemouth black bass fingerlings in a controlled environment. *Proceedings of the Southeastern Association of Game and Fish Commissioners* 14, 253–257.

Snow, J.R. (1961) Forage fish preference and growth rate of largemouth bass fingerlings under experimental conditions. *Proceedings Southeastern Association Game and Fish Commissioners* 15, 303–313.

Snow, J.R. (1963) A method of distinguishing male bass at spawning time. *The Progressive Fish-Culturist* 25, 49.

Snow, J.R. (1965) Results of further experiments on rearing Largemouth Bass fingerlings under controlled conditions. *Proceedings Southeastern Association Game and Fish Commissioners* 17, 191–203.

Snow, J.R. (1970) Fecundity of largemouth bass, *Micropterus salmoides* (Lacépède), receiving artificial food. *Proceedings Southeastern Association Game and Fish Commission* 24, 550–559.

Snow, J.R. (1972) Controlled culture of largemouth bass fry. *Proceedings Southeastern Association Game and Fish Commissioners* 26, 392–398.

Snow, J.R. (1975) Hatchery propagation of the black basses. In: Clepper, H. (ed.) *Black Bass: Biology and Management.* Sport Fishing Institute, Washington, DC, pp. 344–356.

Stevens, R.E. (1970) Hormonal relationships affecting maturation and ovulation in largemouth bass (*Micropterus salmoides* Lacépède). PhD Thesis, North Carolina State University, Raleigh, NC, USA.

Stilwell, W.E. IV (2008) Evaluation of largemouth bass × smallmouth bass (*Micropterus salmoides* × *M.*

dolomieui) hybrid based on results of artificial spawning and early growth characteristics. MSc thesis. Kentucky State University, Frankfort, KT, USA.

Swingle, H.S. (1950) Relationships and dynamics of balanced and unbalanced fish populations. Bulletin No. 274, Alabama Agricultural Experiment Station, Auburn, AL, USA.

Tidwell, J.H., Coyle, S.D. and Webster, C.D. (1998) Effects of stocking density on third-year growth of largemouth bass, *Micropterus salmoides*, fed prepared diets in ponds. *Journal of Applied Aquaculture* 8(4), 39–45.

Trut, L.N. (1999) Early canid domestication: the farm-fox experiment. *American Scientist* 87, 160–169.

Trut, L., Oskina, I. and Kharlamova, A. (2009) Animal evolution during domestication: the domesticated fox as a model. *BioEssays* 31, 349–360.

Tucker, C.S., and Robinson, E.H. (1990) *Channel Catfish Farming Handbook*. Van Nostrand Reinhold, New York,.

Waters, D.S. and Noble, R.L. (2004) Spawning season and nest fidelity of largemouth bass in a tropical reservoir. *North American Journal of Fisheries Management* 24(4), 1240–1251.

White, B.L. (1981) Culture of Florida largemouth bass. In: Hutson, P.L. and Lillie, J. (eds) Midwest Black Bass Culture. Texas Parks and Wildlife Department, Austin, TX, USA, pp. 146–159.

Wilbur, R.L. and Langford, P. (1975) Use of human chorionic gonadotropin (HCG) to promote gametic production in male and female largemouth bass. *Proceedings of the Annual Conference Southeastern Association of Game and Fish Commissioners* 28, 242–250.

Williamson, H. and Carmichael, G.J. (1990) An aquacultural evaluation of Florida, Northern and hybrid largemouth bass, *Micropterus salmoides. Aquaculture* 85, 247–257.

Woo, P.T.K. and Bruno, D.W. (1999) *Fish Diseases and Disorders*: *Viral, bacterial, and fungal infections*. CAB International, New York.

Zhao, H., Li, C., Hargrove, J.S., Bowen, B., Thongda, W., Zhang, D., Mohammed, H., Beck, B.H., Austin, J.D. and Peatman, E. (2018) SNP marker panels for parentage assignment and traceability in the Florida Bass (*Micropterus floridanus*). *Aquaculture* 485, 30–38.

Zolczynski Jr., S.J. and Davies, W.D. (1976) Growth characteristics of the northern and Florida subspecies of largemouth bass and their hybrid, and a comparison of catchability between the subspecies. *Transactions of the American Fisheries Society* 105, 240–243.

CHAPTER 6

Production of feed trained largemouth bass fingerlings: nursery phase through feed training

Shawn D. Coyle[1] and Michael D. Matthews[2]

[1]Kentucky State University, Aquaculture Research Program, Frankfort, Kentucky, USA
[2]A.E. Wood Fish Hatchery, San Marcos, Texas, USA

6.1 Introduction

Largemouth bass fingerlings have been produced by state and federal hatcheries since the 1890s for stocking programs (Lydell, 1903; Turner and Kraatz, 1921). Before the 1960s, hatcheries relied solely on live feeds, beginning with zooplankton and then switching to forage fish until the desired stocking size was reached. Unlike channel catfish (*Ictalurus punctatus*) and rainbow trout (*Oncorhynchus mykiss*), newly hatched largemouth bass fry (swim-up stage) cannot be easily trained to accept prepared diets (Brandt et al., 1987; Williamson et al., 1993). Therefore, bass fry are usually raised in fertilized nursery ponds until they reach 25–50 mm TL (1–2 g) (Tidwell et al., 2000). Fry stocking densities in ponds are commonly 125,000–500,000 fry/ha to produce 25–50 mm fingerlings. In well managed ponds, growth rates of 1.0–1.5 mm/d and target lengths of 38 mm can be achieved in 30–45 d after fry stocking (Hutson, 1990). Previously, fingerlings were then transferred to growout ponds where they were raised to larger sizes on forage fish. However, this extensive production method requires many ponds for both the bass and the forage fish, as it requires approximately 5–10 kg forage fish to produce a 1 kg bass (Nelson et al., 1974).

Studies have examined largemouth bass production on artificial feeds since the 1960s (Snow, 1968a, 1970a; Snow and Maxwell, 1970; McCraren, 1975; Snow and Wright, 1975; Sloane, 1993). Today many federal, state, and private hatcheries produce 10–15 cm fingerlings on feed for stock enhancement programs and for further growout. To economically produce large numbers of fish of this size requires that fingerlings be feed-trained to accept artificial feeds. This allows much higher stocking densities, which produces more advanced fingerlings from finite pond resources especially if forage fish production is considered. Feed training is the production phase where pond-reared juveniles are crowded into tanks at high densities and presented highly palatable food items at frequent intervals. Juveniles are gradually transitioned to a 100% artificial feed over 10–14 d. Several studies have tested different initial food items, such as ground fish, fish eggs, moist pellets, and freeze-dried krill (FDK) for feed-training largemouth bass fingerlings (Snow, 1965; Anderson, 1974; Kubitza and Lovshin, 1997a).

Advances in hatchery design have also contributed to the intensification of largemouth bass production. For example, spawning bass in raceways has reduced dependence on spawning ponds for fry production (Isaac and Staats, 1994; Mayes et al., 1993; Lyon et al., 2002) and allowed production intensification of 25–50 mm fingerlings. Techniques to intensively spawn bass "out-of-season," enabling managers to stock 100 mm fingerling in early spring, have been developed (Matthews and Stout, 2013). Lined ponds have reduced water and maintenance requirements compared to typical earthen hatchery ponds and advances in pond aeration systems, better harvest structures, and research into pond fertilization and management have improved outcome predictability for rearing fry and fingerlings. Approved chemical treatments, antibiotics, and vaccines increase egg, fry, and fingerling survival. In this chapter, we summarize some of these advances in knowledge about largemouth bass nursery and feed training and simultaneously point out those areas where improvements are still needed.

6.2 Nursery phase

The nursery phase is the most vulnerable time in production as largemouth bass have relatively small larvae that do not accept artificial diets at first feeding. Developing and sustaining desirable phytoplankton and zooplankton populations is essential for high survival and fast growth of largemouth bass fry in nursery ponds, because these fish rely completely on naturally occurring foods (Kurten, 1995). Largemouth bass fry are small to medium size (6–7 mm TL at swim-up) for a warmwater, freshwater fish, compared to 10–12 mm TL for channel catfish and 2–6 mm TL for sunshine bass (*Morone chrysops* × *M. saxatilis*) fry (Ludwig, 1999). Fry size at first feeding determines what size zooplankton are required, which is the basis for species-specific nursery pond management. Larval stages are critical times for fish survival because of higher predation and starvation risks (Hubbs and Blaxter, 1986; Dabrowski, 1989; Timmerman et al., 2000). Ready access to a suitable food source is especially critical to larval fish survival, since they have a relatively short time to feed before succumbing to an energy deficit incurred from unsuccessful attempts to capture food (Laurence, 1969).

Production methods during the nursery phase are now designed to produce 25–50 mm TL fingerlings, which can be successfully habituated to commercial diets. Purely pond-based nursery culture generally has been limited to smaller fingerlings, because when fish near 50 mm TL zooplankton abundance becomes insufficient (grazing pressure plus seasonal changes) and cannibalism increases. Production procedures described by Piper et al. (1982) are still used today and are summarized in the following paragraphs.

Fry are stocked in fertilized nursery ponds at rates varying from 100,000–200,000/ha. Production rates for small largemouth bass in fertilized nursery ponds ranges from 34–168 kg/ha depending on fish size, nursery pond productivity, and natural food availability. Some producers have successfully feed-trained largemouth bass fingerlings ≤25 mm, which increases acceptable stocking densities and potentially decreases required time in nursery ponds, but also increases time required to feed train (Matthews, 2009). If a fingerling size > 50 mm is desired, the fry stocking density should be reduced proportionally.

Bass fry numbers are estimated in various ways. One method used at the Peter W. Pfeifer Fish Hatchery in Frankfort, Kentucky, consists of counting a known number (usually 1,000) into a “dish pan” containing water and then placing fry in other dish pans until the densities appear to be equal. This method allows fry to be transferred in water using small pitchers or cups. Largemouth bass fry can also be enumerated volumetrically (Swanson, 1982) or gravimetrically. Lyon et al. (2002) reported an average weight of 0.0036 g (275 fry/g) and an average length of 7 mm at swim-up for Florida largemouth bass (FLMB). A prepared pond should be completely stocked in one day to ensure early growth uniformity and to reduce cannibalism.

The amount of time required for bass fry to grow to a target size depends mainly on stocking density, water temperature, food supply, and initial stocking size. Normally, 30–45 d are required at 18–24°C. Survival rates are usually 75–90%. Largemouth bass must be harvested once zooplankton are depleted as bass become very cannibalistic and many fish can be lost in just a couple of days (Heidinger, 2000a). Typical yields from stocking 80,000 fry/0.4 ha earthen pond are 48,000, 25–40 mm fingerlings after a 25–35 d growout period in central Florida (Matthews and Stout, 2013) and stocking ~200,000 fry/0.4 ha lined pond are 132,000, 25–42 mm fingerlings after a 27–38 d growth period (Matthews, 2015).

Variable growth among bass fingerlings is common, but if size difference become too great cannibalism can cause heavy losses. If this occurs, the pond must be harvested, and fingerlings size graded and separated into size groups (Figure 6.1). It is therefore important to stock equal-sized

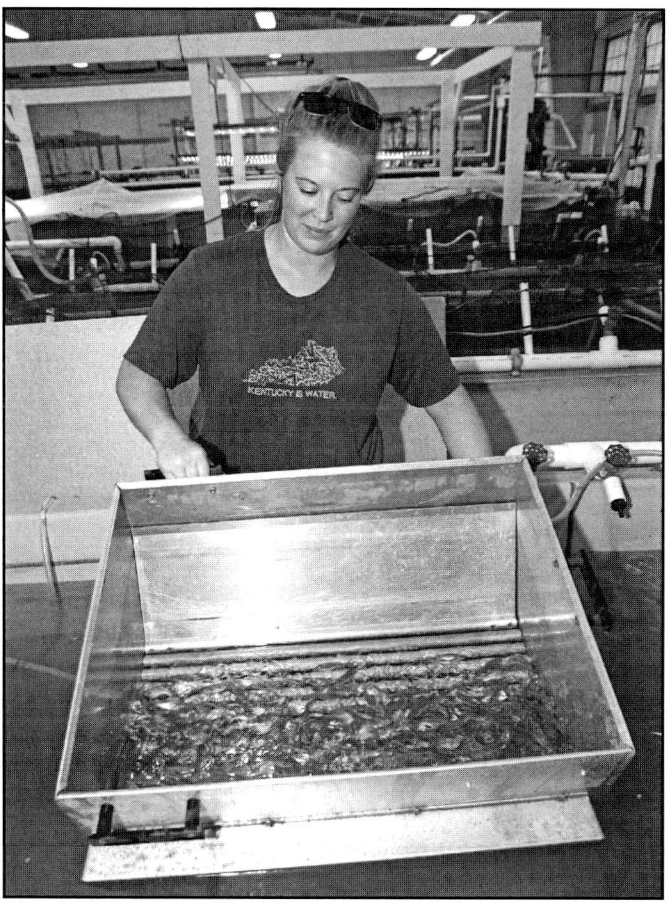

Figure 6.1 Grading feed-trained largemouth bass with a floating adjustable box grader.

largemouth bass, ideally cohorts within 2–3 d of swim-up. Size variation among cohabitating predator species often results in smaller fish becoming prey (Cooper, 1937; Wright, 1970; Snow, 1971). Cooper (1937) found cannibalism among age 0 largemouth bass in ponds occurred when fish lengths differed by a factor of 1.6. Factors encouraging size differences, such as stocking densities disproportional to prey availability, and size variation at stocking, accentuate differences in survival probabilities for faster and slower growing individuals.

Herbicide application to nursery ponds is sometimes used to prevent fingerling entrapment within filamentous algae mats during pond draining and harvest. However, avoid herbicide use if possible, as applications typically increase production costs and reduce dissolved oxygen and zooplankton densities (Summerfelt et al., 1994). If herbicides are applied, use them near the end of production when fingerlings have more likely converted to consuming insect larvae (for example, chironomid) and negative effects may not be as significant (Fairchild, 1982; Piper et al., 1982; Parmley et al., 1986).

Largemouth bass fingerlings are cultured throughout the USA and across the world using vastly different water sources and culture facilities. As a result, many culture practices are site-specific, and universal management techniques have not been developed. Consequently, most culture practices for largemouth bass have developed from trial and error rather than experimental design. Heidinger (2000b) suggested each largemouth bass fingerling producer needs to develop a fertilization regime that works well for his or her own unit.

6.3 Pre-season pond management and selection

If using earthen ponds, proper management begins before water is added. With older impermeable ponds, it has been suggested to dry and disk pond bottoms during winter to promote aerobic breakdown of nutrient-rich sediments (Piper et al., 1982). Drying ponds in the fall has also been suggested to eliminate predaceous insects, fish, and diseases (Davis and Lock, 1997). Relatively new ponds with little organic material buildup are less likely to require drying and disking. Some nutrients are desirable for fingerling culture because they promote phytoplankton growth on which zooplankton graze, but an overabundance tends to produce growth of undesirable blue-green and filamentous algae. Additionally, by excess nutrient removal through oxidation, the pond manager has more control over fertilization timing and zooplankton succession.

Piper et al. (1982) suggested seeding the edges of ponds with ryegrass (9–11 kg/ha) if it is to remain dry for several months. Snow (1975) also recommended ryegrass or wheat be sowed in largemouth bass nursery ponds to produce a green cover crop before filling and stocking. This cover prevents pond dike erosion and provides an organic fertilizer source when the pond is flooded in spring (Davis and Lock, 1997). Grass should be cut and partially dried before pond filling, or rapid decay may deplete dissolved oxygen (Piper et al., 1982). Bowling et al. (1984) evaluated largemouth bass fingerling production in similarly fertilized ponds with and without a green ryegrass cover crop. Ponds with cover crop were dried, disked, and then seeded with 9.0 kg seed/ha in fall. At harvest, there were no differences in fingerling production or zooplankton numbers between ponds seeded with ryegrass and control ponds. The authors concluded the added expense of a cover crop was not justified. However, erosion control benefits may outweigh costs for hatcheries with erodible levees.

Agricultural lime application (1,120–3,363 kg/ha) during the fallow time may be necessary to improve buffering capacity of ponds with soft-water. Boyd (1990) recommended freshwater ponds be limed to enhance fertility where water supplies have a total alkalinity < 20 mg/l. Wyatt et al. (2000) compared using hydrated lime and agricultural lime in earthen largemouth bass rearing ponds. Three treatments were evaluated: agricultural lime broadcast at 30.5 kg/ha, hydrated lime broadcast at 30.5 kg/ha, and agricultural lime applied at 2,245 kg/ha to the corners of ponds. Mean water quality and fish production variables were statistically similar among treatments. Zooplankton densities were lower in the hydrated lime treatment compared to agricultural lime treatments, and the hydrated lime elevated pH for several days after application. The effects of hydrated lime use on fish production were unclear due to high within-treatment variations in fish survival. However, all three methods of liming successfully elevated pond water alkalinity from 12 mg/l (incoming) to > 20 mg/l.

Fish hatchery ponds are increasingly being lined with a variety of impervious materials, usually plastics. Lining ponds offers several advantages over earthen ponds. Seepage is reduced or eliminated, erosion is substantially reduced, and herbicide needs are largely eliminated. The need to dry and disk pond bottoms is eliminated, disinfection is easier and harvest is simplified. However, accumulated sediments in lined ponds require periodic removal to prevent difficulties at fingerling harvest. Although there are no side-by-side comparisons of lined vs. un-lined ponds, generally, lined ponds reduce fertilization requirements and produce more uniform results. Well-managed lined ponds can have exceptional yields of 32 mm bass fingerlings, as high as 450,000 fish/ha and 190 kg/ha (Smith et al., 2000).

Ponds to be fertilized should be carefully selected. Fertilization may be economically impractical if a pond is too large or too small. Do not fertilize muddy or turbid ponds with poor light penetration, those containing filamentous algae, or rooted macrophytes, or those with a history of low dissolved oxygen. Ponds which have a high water-exchange-rate or low water temperature from shading or spring source water may yield poorly relative to amount of fertilizer applied. Some largemouth bass fingerling producers do not use fertilizer in nursery ponds as off-cycle or rotational growout ponds provide enough fertility to support objectives. Most managers select ponds for fertilization based on past performance, overall condition, water color, and the absence of filamentous algae.

6.4 Nursery pond fertilization

Appropriate pond fertilization programs depend mainly on local conditions. The level of intensification depends on the level of hatchery modernization. Earthen ponds are inherently less predictable in response to fertilization than lined ponds and seem more vulnerable to predacious insects and nuisance organisms. Conversely, earthen ponds may be better buffered against water quality changes and nutrient pulses. Pond size and shape uniformity within a hatchery may dictate whether routine fertilization regimens can be applied to all ponds. Local costs and fertilizer availability may drive the choice of which to use.

Fertilization promotes fish production by increasing the quantity and quality of naturally occurring food organisms. Numerous factors affect fertilizer use, and responses are not predicable under all conditions. Physical and biological factors influencing appropriate fertilizer use are: pond depth, shoreline amount, water exchange rate, turbidity, water temperature, plant and animal types already present, and food habits of the cultured fish (Piper et al., 1982). Chemical factors to consider are water and bottom mud composition such as: nitrogen, phosphorus, pH, alkalinity, calcium, and magnesium (Boyd, 1979). Another factor to consider is pond age: older ponds are generally more fertile than new ponds (Mischke and Zimba, 2004). Application rates and frequencies vary depending on region and natural pond productivity, therefore, universal rates applicable to all hatcheries are difficult to recommend.

Where facilities, budget, and trained staff exists, fertilization program dependability can be enhanced by basing application rates on target nutrient levels and periodically monitoring and validating those levels (Anderson and Tave, 1993). In some cases, cost savings may be made by reducing or eliminating unnecessary fertilization or critical supplements may be added that dramatically improve production. Owing to the vast differences in natural pond fertility, research results should be considered with respect to local conditions, and results may only be applicable where they were observed.

6.4.1 Organic fertilizers

Organic fertilizers are widely used for fertilizing largemouth bass nursery ponds (Piper et al., 1982; Parmley et al., 1986; Young and Flickinger, 1989; Hutson, 1990). The rationale for organic fertilization is to stimulate autotrophic production by supplying nutrients for phytoplankton uptake and to stimulate heterotrophic production of bacteria, fungi, and invertebrates, which serve as food for zooplankton and fish (Geiger, 1983a; Boyd, 1990; Harding and Summerfelt, 1994).

Organic fertilizers may accelerate zooplankton production by supplying a direct food source for the zooplankton even before phytoplankton bloom development, and provide a carbon source for potentially carbon-limited phytoplankton and heterotrophic pathways (Snow, 1975; Piper et al., 1982; Boyd, 1990). Organic fertilizers have been recommended particularly to enhance zooplankton production in new or sterile ponds (Piper et al., 1982).

Simco et al. (1986) indicated an initial application of 1,500 kg/ha alfalfa hay produces a more immediate zooplankton response than inorganic fertilizer. The rationale being that zooplankton feed primarily on detritus while inorganic fertilizer must be incorporated into phytoplankton pathways before becoming available to zooplankton. Boyd (1990) recommended using organic fertilizers to reduce occurrences of high pH in ponds by providing a reserve of carbon dioxide for phytoplankton. Chironomid larvae are known to use organic matter in the pond substrate (Oliver, 1971); therefore, organic fertilizers may be especially important late in culture when largemouth bass shift to a diet dominated by insect larvae (Fairchild, 1982; Parmley et al., 1986).

Organic fertilizers used in largemouth bass fingerling ponds are typically locally available agricultural grains or by-products such as soybean meal, rice bran, cottonseed meal (CSM), alfalfa meal (AFM), chopped hay, or animal manures. Generally, choice of organic fertilizer is based on local availability, cost, and what has worked best previously. Organic fertilizer carbon, nitrogen, and phosphorus content and decay rates can vary considerably (Boyd, 1990; Anderson and Tave, 1993; Wedemeyer, 2001).

Barkoh (1996) conducted a side-by-side comparison of AFM and CSM in plastic-lined largemouth bass fingerling rearing ponds which were also fertilized with inorganic nitrogen and phosphorus. CSM provided better water quality and fish production in these ponds compared to

AFM. These results agreed with similar findings for two fertilizers in palmetto bass *Morone saxatilis* × *M. chrysops* fingerling growout in plastic-lined ponds (Buurma et al., 1996). Additionally, CSM is generally cheaper than AFM.

Kurten et al. (1999) reported earthen largemouth bass nursery ponds fertilized with either CSM, rice bran, or AFM, produced similar fish yield, growth, survival, and zooplankton densities. In another trial, CSM and inorganic fertilizer, AFM and inorganic fertilizer, and inorganic fertilizer alone were compared, and no significant difference in fish production was found (Kurten et al., 1995). The authors hypothesized eliminating organic fertilizers may reduce production cost and improve oxygen levels without adversely affecting production.

A subsequent trial evaluated the effect of fertilizing earthen largemouth bass nursery ponds with either inorganic fertilizer alone or inorganic fertilizer plus CSM on plankton population dynamics, water quality dynamics, and fingerling production. Supplementing ponds with CSM enhanced largemouth bass fingerling production by increasing fish harvest weight, reducing pH, and increasing desirable zooplankton densities but also reduced overall oxygen (O_2) levels compared to ponds fertilized with only inorganic fertilizer (Kurten et al., 1999). This study also validated that CSM can provide a significant source of carbon dioxide and can ameliorate high pH. Fertilization cost was 260% higher with added CSM. The authors concluded higher production cost and potential low dissolved oxygen should be weighed against the gain in fish production when deciding whether to use organic fertilizer.

Organic fertilizers are seldom applied based on estimated nutrient composition, and application rates are commonly reported on weight per surface area (kg/ha) making comparisons of fertilizers and application rates difficult, especially between ponds of variable depth but similar surface area. However, some studies have calculated the nutrient composition of organic fertilizers and based applications on weight per volume. Barkoh et al. (2005) found best water quality, phytoplankton standing crop, and zooplankton densities are achieved when organic meal application rates were based on nitrogen content.

Barkoh et al. (1994) compared pond productivity and largemouth bass fingerling production in ponds fertilized with either chicken manure or plant meals (consisting of equal parts by weight of CSM, AFM, and wheat shorts). Liquid inorganic fertilizer (10–34–0; $N–P_2O_5–K_2O$) was also applied to all ponds at a rate and ratio of N : P = 470 : 750 µg/l/week. Moist chicken manure (75% moisture) was applied at N : P = 219 : 67 µg/l the first week, 158 : 49 µg/l the second week, and 105 : 32 µg/l/week in subsequent weeks. Plant meals were added at a weekly rate of N : P = 2,442 : 149 µg/l/week for the first two weeks and at 1,221 : 75 µg/l/week in subsequent weeks. Largemouth bass fingerling (mean size 51–55 mm) yield was significantly greater in plant meal fertilized ponds (133.8 kg/ha) compared to ponds fertilized with chicken manure (84 kg/ha). Ponds fertilized with plant meals had higher chlorophyll-*a* concentrations and lower dissolved oxygen concentrations than ponds fertilized with chicken manure. Phytoplankton standing crop was also consistently higher in plant meal fertilized ponds, likely from higher nitrogen content of the plant meal regime compared to chicken manure. Zooplankton densities were generally adequate (717–923 organisms/l) in all ponds and did not follow a consistent pattern over time. With no difference in zooplankton food base between treatments, the authors suggested that observed differences in yield may have been from differences in heterotrophic production. Food habit studies have established immature insects, such as chironomids and chaoborins, are important food items for post-larval largemouth bass (Hodson and Strawn, 1968;

Noriega-Curtis, 1979; Parmley et al., 1986). Benthic invertebrate numbers were not measured in this study, although they may have contributed to reported yield differences.

Combining organic and inorganic fertilizers is a common practice, particularly in hatchery ponds where draining is frequent and time for suitable food supply development is limited. It has been reported a combination of organic meal and superphosphate in a 3 : 1 ratio provides higher fish production than organic material alone (Piper et al., 1982). While costs associated with organic fertilizer application are higher, the high value of a largemouth bass crop justifies the expense. Simco et al. (1986) recommended a combination of organic and inorganic fertilizers in largemouth bass nursery ponds: begin fertilization 2–3 week before stocking by initially applying 168 kg/ha peanut hay; 10 d later, add 100 kg/ha 16–20–0 inorganic fertilizer followed by a second application 10 d later at 50 kg/ha. Kurten (2001a) reported high production rates of 32 mm TL largemouth bass fingerlings (400,000 fish/ha; 140 kg/ha) was achieved by an initial application of 57 kg/ha CSM, 0.08 mg P/l, and 0.3 mg N/l at pond filling (8 d before stocking fry) followed by a large fertilizer dose consisting of 227 kg/ha CSM, 0.16 mg P/l, and 0.6 mg N/l 2 d before stocking fry. Thereafter, ponds were fertilized twice weekly with 57 kg/ha CSM, 0.08 mg P/l and 0.3 mg/l N until 1 week before harvest.

Disadvantages of organic fertilizers are they are more expensive than inorganic fertilizers, may deplete oxygen during decomposition, may stimulate filamentous algae growth, and require more labor to apply (Piper et al., 1982; Culver et al., 1993; Middleton and Reeder, 2003). Owing to these concerns, there has been an increase in research emphasis and use of liquid inorganic fertilizers to supply nitrogen and phosphorus directly to phytoplankton (Boyd, 1979, 1990).

6.4.2 Inorganic fertilizers

Inorganic fertilizers are relatively inexpensive sources of nitrogen, phosphorus, and, sometimes, potassium that stimulate phytoplankton growth directly. Their contributions to ambient pond nutrient concentrations are easier to calculate and trace than organic fertilizers based on their known composition. Once in solution, inorganic nutrients stimulate phytoplankton growth and reproduction, which subsequently support populations of zooplankton (Piper et al., 1982). They may also accelerate organic material breakdown, including organic fertilizers (Boyd, 1990). Excessive use of inorganic fertilizers can lead to high pH and ammonia levels which may negatively impact fish survival (Boyd, 1990; Bergerhouse, 1994; Barkoh, 1996).

The most important limiting nutrients in freshwater are nitrogen and phosphorus, and typically aquatic algae contain a N : P mass ratio of 7 : 1 (Wetzel, 2001). Absolute concentrations and ratios of nitrogen and phosphorus can influence phytoplankton succession and dominance patterns (Welch, 1980; Wetzel, 2001). This consideration should drive the choice of inorganic fertilizer and application rates. However, inorganic fertilization programs should be site specific, as soil and water chemical composition differs widely across different geographical areas.

Phosphorus is generally considered to be the most essential limiting element in freshwater pond fertilization for phytoplankton growth (Boyd, 1990). Phytoplankton growth can be limited at phosphorus concentrations < 20–35 μg P/l (Sommer, 1985; Wetzel, 2001). Phosphorus is an active chemical which cannot exist alone except under very specialized conditions (Boyd, 1990).

Most applied phosphorus eventually collects in sediments in the form of insoluble compounds that become unavailable to the water column. Calcium may precipitate phosphorus in hard water, resulting in greater daily decline rates (Boyd, 1990). Phosphoric acid has been recommended as the best phosphorus source for pond fertilization (Anderson and Tave, 1993) because of its high solubility.

Phosphorus fertilizers are commonly used to stimulate phytoplankton production in largemouth bass nursery ponds (Parmley et al., 1986; Young and Flickinger, 1989; Kurten, 1995). Applying the appropriate phosphorus regime to your culture strategy can be challenging. Too little phosphorus will not sustain adequate phytoplankton production and limits zooplankton production (Kurten, 1995). Adding too much phosphorus can allow high levels to be discharged into receiving waters during pond drainage or can promote excessive blooms of unwanted blue-green and filamentous algae (Seymour, 1980; Culver et al., 1993).

Snow (1970a) suggested fertilization of largemouth bass nursery ponds, after filling, at 8 kg/ha superphosphate (35 μg P/l for an average pond depth of 1 m) and 9 kg/ha nitrogen at weekly intervals until abundant zooplankton is established, typically requiring three or four applications. After the zooplankton bloom becomes established, Snow (1970a) recommended biweekly fertilizer applications to sustain the bloom until about 10 d before anticipated harvest. Several workers have recommended applications of 1 mg/l phosphorous pentoxide (P_2O_5; 0.22 mg P/l) periodically during production (Piper et al., 1982; Geiger, 1983a, 1983b).

Parmley et al. (1986) used 1 mg P_2O_5/l (0.22 mg P/l) two to three times weekly for largemouth bass fingerling production. Young and Flickinger (1989) reported applying 1.0 mg H_3PO_4/l (0.32 mg P/l) three times weekly pre-stocking and twice weekly post-stocking to largemouth bass nursery ponds. Hutson (1990) recommended phosphorus application rates for largemouth bass nursery ponds of 1.00 mg P/l (from phosphoric acid) for initial fertilization and 0.33 mg P/l three times weekly for follow-up applications. Culver et al. (1993) and Anderson and Tave (1993) recommended lower phosphorus fertilization rates, suggesting 30 μg P/l as a target concentration for phosphorus, to avoid high pH and problems with excessive filamentous algae.

Culver et al. (1993) reported increased production and decreased production costs by eliminating organic fertilizers and relying solely on inorganic fertilizer in percid production ponds. This work was revolutionary in that the authors suggested applying fertilizer on an as needed basis according to chemical analysis of nutrient concentration. Although phosphorus is generally the most limiting nutrient in ponds, Mischke and Zimba (2004) reported ponds in the Yazoo-Mississippi River flood plain were more nitrogen limited than phosphorus limited. They recommended applying inorganic fertilizer at an initial rate of 20 kg/ha N and 2 kg/ha P (0.5 mg N/l and 0.05 mg P/l assuming a pond depth of 1 m) followed by subsequent weekly applications of one-half the initial rate for 3–4 weeks in nursery ponds for channel catfish.

Boyd (1990) recommended applying 0.5–1.0 mg N/l in ponds with low nitrogen concentrations to stimulate phytoplankton growth and to reapply at this rate at weekly intervals to sustain the bloom. If the hatchery pond is 1 m deep, apply nitrogen at 2.8–11.8 kg/ha (0.28–1.18 mg N/l) (Boyd, 1990). Using a typical N : P phytoplankton mass ratio of 7 : 1 (Wetzel, 2001) and a minimum algal requirement of 35 μg P/l (Sommer, 1985) supports a rate of 245 μg N/l as an appropriate target for nitrogen maintenance concentrations in fertilized ponds to stimulate algal productivity. These rates are lower in nitrogen than the weekly restoration targets 600 μg N/l and 30 μg/l phosphorus suggested by Culver et al. (1993) for percid fingerling growout ponds.

Urea has been recommended as the best nitrogen source (Anderson and Tave, 1993; Boyd and Daniels, 1994).

Kurten (1995) presented a case study where phosphoric acid (1.0 mg P/l) and ammonium nitrate (0.5 mg N/l) were applied weekly to largemouth bass spawning/rearing ponds over several years. An excess of filamentous algae (*Hydrodictyon* and *Anabaena* spp.) was a recurrent problem in these ponds and hindered fry harvest. While monitoring nutrient levels in spawning and rearing ponds, unexpectedly high phosphorus levels were found. Five weeks after initial fertilization, phosphorus concentrations up to 4.0 mg P/l were measured. Filamentous algae also appeared 4–5 week after initial fertilization following the clear-water phase associated with increased zooplankton densities and grazing (Parmley and Geiger, 1985; Lampert et al., 1986). Kurten (1995) reported phosphorus concentrations in those ponds rarely declined < 0.5 mg P/l between applications. The following year, weekly phosphorus application rates were reduced to 0.5 mg P/l and applied only when individual pond concentrations fell below 0.25 mg P/l. This change alleviated filamentous algae problems although fry production was low.

The following year, an experiment was conducted to determine if lower phosphorus concentration would prevent filamentous algae problems without reducing phytoplankton and zooplankton populations and subsequent largemouth bass fingerling production. Target phosphorus concentrations of 0.5 and 1.0 mg P/l were maintained based on weekly additions following water quality analysis. All ponds received the same nitrogen and organic fertilization regime. Both treatments provided adequate phosphorus for phytoplankton and zooplankton development and were low enough to avoid excessive filamentous algae growth. Total lengths, weight, and number of fingerling largemouth bass at harvest were similar between the two treatments. However, zooplankton succession differed. Phytoplankton biomass and zooplankton densities increased more rapidly and reached higher maxima in high phosphorus ponds, although they were sustained longer in low phosphorus ponds. In high phosphorus ponds, initial rotifer and cladoceran blooms rapidly overgrazed phytoplankton and limited food for latter copepod populations. These results suggest, in this particular situation, the lower phosphorus application rate was beneficial from the provision of a more stable zooplankton population over the longer culture periods typically used for largemouth bass fingerling production.

As most waters have an ample potassium supply, it is generally considered to be less important than nitrogen or phosphorus for plankton growth. However, in waters deficient, or where heavy fertilization with N and P is employed, it may be beneficial to add potassium. The ratio of 4–4–1, N_2–P_2O_5–K_2O, has been reported to produce favorable plankton growth for fingerling production ponds (Piper et al., 1982). The fertilizer grade most commonly used providing this ratio is 20–20–5.

6.4.3 Timing of filling ponds

The size and quantity of zooplankton available must be appropriate to the size and quantity of bass fry present, necessitating precise timing of pond filling and fertilization (Bishop, 1968; Simco et al., 1986). Filling time likely differentiates management strategies used for culturing different species of warmwater fish more than any other variable. Filling time directly affects zooplankton succession patterns in rearing-ponds. This is important because prey size largely determines consumption by fish (Geiger, 1983a).

Previous work has shown that phytoplankton and zooplankton abundance in ponds declines sharply 4–5 weeks after filling (Geiger et al., 1985; Culver, 1988). Zooplankton egg-to-egg generation times, and time to peak reproduction, are therefore important given the short time to maximize zooplankton populations in rearing ponds (Geiger, 1983b). Rotifers have a short egg-to-egg generation time of 2–3 d, while cladocerans and copepods have egg-to-egg generation times of 7 d and 14 d, respectively (Allan, 1976). At 20°C, time of peak reproduction is 3.5 d for rotifers, 14–15 d for cladocerans, and about 24 d for copepods (Allan, 1976). Accordingly, if copepod nauplii abundance is desired at stocking, it may be beneficial to fill and fertilize ponds 14–20 d in advance.

Recommended time intervals between filling and stocking for largemouth bass nursery ponds vary widely. Parmley et al. (1986), based on a detailed evaluation of largemouth bass food habits over 33 d, suggested stocking fry 8–14 d following filling to provide appropriate zooplankton succession in terms of prey type, size, and overall abundance. Heidinger (2000a) suggested largemouth bass nursery ponds should be filled with water 10–20 d before stocking. Davis and Lock (1997) suggested ponds should be filled no more than 14 d before stocking to reduce predaceous insect build up. As there are many variables affecting fertilization response and zooplankton population progression beyond filling time, this too should be a site-based management decision considering all available information.

Filling time also depends on the water source, as surface waters from reservoirs or streams usually contain nutrients and may contain zooplankton; thus, allowing ponds to be filled closer to stocking compared to ponds filled with well water (Brewer and Rees, 1990). Filling time also depends on management strategy for dealing with filamentous algae and predaceous insects. Fairy shrimp (Anostraca) and predaceous insects can become troublesome soon after ponds are filled. Fairy shrimp compete with desirable crustacean zooplankton for available food resources and predaceous insects may feed directly on larval fish (Geiger, 1983a). Filling ponds immediately before stocking allows less time for establishment of unwanted organisms but also does not allow time for desirable zooplankton populations to develop properly. If possible, filtering incoming water through a filter sock can be an effective method of excluding unwanted and predaceous insects.

Some producers fill ponds slowly, a process known as "puddle culture," to more quickly establish a bloom. The concept being water temperatures may increase faster and sunlight can penetrate more completely through the water column in shallow water. Barkoh et al. (1994) evaluated pond volume manipulation effects in producing largemouth bass fingerlings. Stage-filled ponds filled to one-third volume the first week, to two-third volume the second week, and then completely filled the fourth week were compared to ponds fully filled initially. Largemouth bass fry (0.0025 g; 7 mm TL) were stocked at 88,462–94,392 fry/ha at 9–13 d after initiation of pond filling. During the first 18 d, temperature and dissolved oxygen in stage-filled ponds were 22–24°C and 5.0–8.0 mg/l, respectively compared to 19–20°C and 2.3–5.0 mg/l in full ponds. Yield (mean size 53–55 mm) was significantly greater in stage filled ponds (133.8 kg/ha) compared to full ponds (99.0 kg/ha). Additionally, since fertilization rates were based on water volume, stage filled ponds reduced the fertilizer cost per kilogram largemouth bass by 50%. With puddle culture, it is important to watch upcoming weather patterns, as unseasonably cold weather could cause shallow ponds to become colder than full ponds.

6.4.4 Monitoring and managing zooplankton densities

Availability of zooplankton in sufficient abundance and appropriate size is necessary for successful nursery culture of largemouth bass fingerlings. This can be challenging considering the dynamic nature of the sequential changes in feeding habits of the fish and prey availability during nursery culture. Fortunately, much of this timing is predetermined based on water temperature, as fish spawning temperatures coincide with natural cyclic increases in prey availability. Also, as zooplankton population dynamics typically follow predictable succession patterns, species composition can be manipulated with management practices tailored to the nutritional needs and preferences of the cultured species.

Several authors have indicated rotifers are target prey for largemouth bass fry for only a short time (Applegate et al., 1967; Parmley et al., 1986; Wickstrom and Applegate, 1989). Wickstrom and Applegate (1989) reported largemouth bass swim-up fry initially consume rotifers, switching to copepods and cladocerans soon thereafter. Copepod nauplii are reported to be major prey items for first-feeding largemouth bass fry (Parmley et al., 1986). At 2 weeks post swim-up, moderate cladoceran concentrations of > 100/l are required to sustain good numbers of largemouth bass fry. Cladoceran densities typically increase quickly, attain their maximum density, and then decline rapidly over only a few days (Parmley and Geiger, 1985; Kurten, 1995).

When fish predation is sufficient to control zooplankton populations, rotifers usually displace cladocerans over time (Geiger, 1983a). Bass fry then switch to larger invertebrates (for example, insect larvae; Morris and Clayton, 2009). Insect larvae become increasingly important in smallmouth bass *Micropterus dolomieu* diets once they reach 20 mm TL (Farquhar and Guest, 1991). This is likely also the case for largemouth bass fry (Parmley et al., 1986; Kurten, 2001b).

Parmley et al. (1986) described feeding habits of largemouth bass fry as they grew from an initial size of 5 mm to 25 mm TL in nursery ponds and provide a detailed examination of the relationship between composition and abundance of available crustacean zooplankton prey and predation by young hatchery reared largemouth bass. Fish 4.5–5.5 mm TL collected from nest sites contained no food items in their guts. No rotifers were found in fish gut contents at any sampling even though they were present in high numbers in ponds. Fish began feeding at a mean TL of 6.7 mm and exhibited positive selection for copepod nauplii. Sequentially, selection shifted to copepod adults for 7.5–10.5 mm fish, to adult copepods and cladocerans for 10.9–20.4 mm fish, and lastly, to predominantly immature insects for fish > 22.8 mm. Although selection values were negative for 7.5–10.5 mm fish feeding on cladocerans, 30% more cladocerans than copepod adults were consumed. Copepods may provide more energy on a dry weight basis than cladocerans, but copepods are also known to be faster moving and better able to avoid attack (O'Brien, 1979; Parmley et al., 1986). Young bass fry are opportunistic sight-based strike-feeders and are likely better adapted to feeding on slower constantly moving cladocerans than swifter, intermittently moving copepods (O'Brien, 1979; Parmley et al., 1986).

Elliot (1976) examined stomach contents of a school of largemouth bass fry (25.3 mm; mean weight 0.18 g) over 24 h. Fry fed continuously on limnetic zooplankton throughout the day and did not feed at night. Although rotifers and copepod nauplii were more abundant than any of the other prey groups, they were not consumed. Daphnia and calanoid copepods were the most abundant and were eaten nearly proportional to their abundance. The fry fed selectively on the largest prey (*Leptodora* spp. and cyclopoids) and selected against the smallest (*Bosmina* spp.). Largemouth bass fry appear to be opportunistic predators feeding predominantly on the most available prey of a suitable size, yet actively select larger, more visible prey. Based on feeding habit studies, it appears first feeding largemouth bass fry prefer copepod nauplii for about 1 week, then transition to copepod adults and cladocerans for the next 2–3 weeks. By week 4, they should be 25 mm, and insect larvae such as chironomids become more important.

Kurten (2001a) examined the relationships between fingerling harvest variables and fingerling stocking variables and zooplankton densities for 197 largemouth bass rearing ponds over a 6 year period with a production goal of 38 mm fingerlings. Harvest biomass and harvest length appeared to be improved by lengthening the interval between pond filling and fish stocking. Interestingly, zooplankton densities at stocking and 7 d after stocking were weak indicators of harvest variables. Low correlation of fish production and zooplankton variables and the indication that lengthening the pond filling to stocking interval improves production and size indicate managing for larger pond invertebrates may improve fish production above managing for zooplankton alone (Kurten, 2001a).

Successful culture of planktivorous fry depends heavily on zooplankton composition and density established in rearing ponds during the 4–6 week culture period (Geiger, 1983a). Fish number and age affect the zooplankton number needed for successful culture. In general, 100–500 zooplankton/l of suitable size and species should be present throughout culture (Geiger and Turner, 1990). Generally, planktivorous fish preferentially consume the largest zooplankton they can capture and ingest. This creates a succession pattern where there is an increase in the proportion of smaller zooplankton over time as larger zooplankton are selectively removed. An increase in numbers of smaller zooplankton usually indicates predation pressure by fish is too great, and it is time to harvest (Morris and Mischke, 1999). Further fertilization is usually not warranted by this point.

The culturist should periodically check zooplankton population densities in fertilized nursery ponds. A practical method for visually assessing zooplankton densities is to examine ponds at night using a spot light where a trained eye can observe and estimate density, type and can distinguish the presence of undesirables, such as clam and fairy shrimp. Traditional plankton nets with detachable collecting containers are often used for collecting plankton from ponds to determine species composition (Hoff and Snell, 2004). Sampling zooplankton populations using towable nets provides good qualitative data, but it may be difficult to estimate density (number of zooplankton per liter).

Techniques showing promise for quantitative analyses are using pumps and tube-samplers (Morris and Mischke, 1999). Farquhar and Geiger (1984) described a pump system and Graves and Morrow (1988) evaluated a simple tube sampler and reported good quantitative estimates. Pump systems are more elaborate and therefore more expensive. Tube samplers can be made of 25–50 mm polyvinyl chloride pipe equipped with a check valve on the bottom end of the pipe. The tube is then lowered into the water column and either filtered through a plankton net or collected in a bucket for further sampling, enumeration, and identification of zooplankton taxa. Consistency in sampling is important to obtaining good quantitative samples. As zooplankton may not be uniformly distributed throughout the pond, it is important to obtain samples from several locations (Morris and Mischke, 1999). Zooplankton are known to migrate vertically within the water column throughout the day, so data should be collected and compared over time (Morris and Mischke, 1999).

Hatcheries frequently inoculate or supplement largemouth bass rearing ponds with zooplankton from dedicated, heavily fertilized zooplankton ponds. This strategy is based on the belief this practice will enhance zooplankton populations or provide significant amounts of additional food. Martinez et al. (2005) confirmed this practice enhanced the initial and later zooplankton density in largemouth bass ponds. However, the expense and time required to inoculate ponds was not warranted, because fish production was not significantly enhanced.

6.4.5 Clam shrimp and fairy shrimp

Clam shrimp (Conchostraca) and fairy shrimp can reduce fish production in largemouth bass nursery ponds. Fairy shrimp are known to compete with desirable crustacean zooplankton for available food resources thus limiting zooplankton production (Geiger, 1983b). Large numbers of clam shrimp can also greatly reduce zooplankton densities and impede fish harvest by clogging screens and suspending sediment (McCraren et al., 1977; Czarnezki et al., 1994). High clam shrimp densities cause excessive turbidity, which interferes with photosynthesis (McCraren and Phillips, 1977). Clam shrimp and fairy shrimp can be controlled with chemicals, such as Dylox; however, these chemicals are not approved as pesticides in ponds and also kill *Cladocera* (McCraren and Phillips, 1977) which are important food for largemouth bass fry.

Fairy shrimp and clam shrimp characteristically inhabit temporary ponds and pools and are most plentiful in spring and early summer (Pennak, 1978; Czarnezki et al., 1994). Drying and freezing are reported as a stimulus for hatching their eggs in spring (Weaver, 1943; Czarnezki et al., 1994). Czarnezki et al. (1994) successfully controlled clam shrimp in walleye nursery ponds by refilling ponds either immediately after harvest or during summer and keeping ponds full through winter, thus interrupting the clam shrimp reproductive cycle. However, the authors cautioned this practice may reduce zooplankton numbers, as winter drying also promotes hatching of zooplankton eggs (Pennak, 1978; Geiger, 1983a).

Kurten et al. (1996, 1997, 1998) examined several strategies for controlling clam shrimp and fairy shrimp in largemouth bass rearing ponds. In the first study, ponds were filled and fertilized either 7 or 14 d before stocking fish. Shortening the pre-stocking interval from 14 to 7 d allowed largemouth bass fingerlings to prey on and reduce densities of smaller clam and fairy shrimp, but did not eliminate them completely and did not improve fish production (Kurten et al., 1996). In a second study, ponds were flooded at 28 d and 14 d before stocking fish and fertilized at 14 d before stocking (Kurten et al., 1997). The 14 d pre-fertilization interval (incubated ponds) allowed shrimp to complete their life cycle, and shrimp were nearly absent by fish stocking. Zooplankton densities were higher, and shrimp were absent in incubated ponds at fish harvest which alleviated enumeration and screen clogging problems, but fish production was not improved. In a third study, the pre-fertilization interval was reduced to 7 d and was not superior to the 14 d pre-fertilization interval (Kurten et al., 1998). The authors concluded filling ponds and allowing the clam and fairy shrimp to complete their life cycle before pond fertilization improved ability to harvest and enumerate largemouth bass, and such a strategy was not detrimental to production.

6.5 Feed training

As in the propagation of other widely cultured species an evolution to more intensive culture methods for largemouth bass has slowly occurred. Demand for largemouth bass has stimulated the development of intensive production practices at both private and public hatcheries. Primary obstacles to intensive production of piscivorous fish are cannibalism and the failure of fry and fingerlings to voluntarily accept commercially available formulated feeds. To overcome this problem, feed training techniques have been developed over time that have become standard practice in largemouth bass production.

Prior to the 1960s, state and federal hatchery programs stocked fingerling largemouth bass (25–50 mm) directly from nursery ponds into managed lakes and reservoirs for stock enhancement (Snow, 1965). Small fish were used due to poor acceptance of formulated feeds and increased cannibalism of cohorts in pond reared populations larger than 50 mm. Subsequently, in the 1970s, fisheries managers determined that survival of stocked largemouth bass fingerlings was low when stocking small fish and requested hatchery managers produce larger fingerlings (100 mm) for stocking programs (Snow, 1975).

The transition to stocking larger bass fingerlings was to improve sportfish recruitment based on the supposition that larger fish would be less vulnerable to predation and would benefit from the ability to utilize larger prey items. However, the food preferences of largemouth bass > 50 mm shifts from primarily insects to small fish, requiring the use of forage fish which greatly increased production costs (Snow, 1971). The desire to produce larger largemouth bass fingerlings for stock enhancement programs prompted a considerable amount of research effort on production techniques to produce bigger (≥ 100 mm) largemouth bass cost effectively (Snow and Maxwell, 1970; Snow, 1973). One of the primary areas of research was developing technologies to improve success during the feed-training phase of largemouth bass production.

Early researchers wrote "how to" papers to achieve the crucial step in getting fish to recognize and accept non-living food items (Snow, 1968a; Snow, 1970a; Snow and Maxwell, 1970). Weaning fry from live feeds to dry diets is one of the most expensive processes with farming predatory fishes (Curnow et al., 2006). The costs associated with this process are mainly associated with labor, the high prices of live food, and mortality during habituation (Baskerville-Bridges and Kling, 2000; Callan et al., 2003). Seed stock costs are a relatively large percentage of operating cost and minimizing mortality is an important goal for increasing farming profitability (Fletcher et al., 2007). Engle and Southworth (2008) estimated that the cost of raising 100 mm largemouth bass fingerlings on forage results in a more than 100-fold increase in the cost per fingerling compared to feed-training and raising them on feed. Production efficiency is also greatly improved by feed-training largemouth bass fingerlings compared to raising them on forage fish. For example, it is possible to produce up to 123 kg/ha of largemouth bass when they are pond-reared together with forage fish (Snow, 1970b; Sloane and Lovshin, 1995). However, when trained to accept dry, pelleted commercial feeds, largemouth bass productivity ranges from 2,700 to 7,281 kg/ha in a 117 to 153 growing period (Kubitza, 1995; Sloane and Lovshin, 1995).

Owing to increased production efficiency, feed-training largemouth bass fingerlings has become a standard practice among hatchery managers with goals of producing fish > 50 mm.

However, the procurement cost of feed-trained largemouth bass fingerlings for commercial food-fish producers remains relatively high (approximately US$0.25 per each 50 mm fish; personal communication, Robert Mayer, Mayer's Fish Farm, Bardstown, Kentucky), suggesting productivity and success during feed-training likely have a major impact on production costs of fingerlings.

6.5.1 Feed training diets

Feed consumption is influenced by several factors including: flavor, taste, and smell. Many natural ingredients, such as meals, hydrolysates, and oils, derived from fish and crustaceans are highly palatable and can increase feeding response and feed intake (Barrows, 2000). Several studies have described and tested different initial food items, such as using ground fish, fish eggs, moist pellets, and freeze-dried krill (FDK) for feed training largemouth bass fingerlings (Snow, 1965; Anderson, 1974; Willis and Flickinger, 1981; Brandenburg et al., 1979; Kubitza and Lovshin, 1997a, 1997b).

Krill (*Euphausia* sp.) are a group of oceanic planktonic crustaceans having commercial fishery value primarily for use as food for aquaculture. There are two primary species of commercial importance: the Antarctic krill (*E. superba*) and the Northern Pacific krill (*E. pacifica*). The latter is smaller and better sized for use as a feed training diet for largemouth bass. Sloane (1993) was one of the first to utilize FDK as a training diet for largemouth bass; however, only 13% of the fish were successfully transitioned to the dry diet (feed trained). Kubitza and Lovshin (1997a) reported 27% feed training success when using only FDK to transition largemouth fingerlings to a dry diet. In another experiment, Kubitza and Lovshin (1997b) reported 77% success rate when they incorporated FDK into specially formulated training diets using "gradual feed ingredient transition."

Primarily because of the effectiveness and ease of use, FDK has become one of the most popular feed training diets for largemouth bass. However, the cost of FDK (≥ 40 $US/kg; Argent Chemical Laboratories, Redmond, Washington) can be a significant expense in the feed training phase. Engle and Southworth (2008) evaluated the costs of raising largemouth bass fingerlings and determined that the cost of krill was the greatest cost (77% of total costs) followed by labor for the feed training phase of production. Campbell and Phelps (2002) evaluated the use of dried shrimp (*Penaeus* sp.) to replace krill as a feed training diet for largemouth bass. The motivation for this work was that FDK was considerably more expensive than dried shrimp. The authors reported that the feed training success was 81% for fish fed FDK and 78% for those fed dried shrimp. The authors concluded that replacing FDK with dried shrimp reduced the cost of feed training diets by 82%.

Kubitza et al. (1997) compared the feed training success of largemouth bass fed with ground fish and reported percent feeders was 75% when ground fish was the starter diet compared to 41% for FDK. An unpublished study (Coyle and Tidwell), evaluated ground fathead minnows (*Pimephales promelas*) as an alternative to FDK for feed training largemouth bass. The minnows were ground in a blender and used to top coat and soften 1.5 mm floating pellets for one hour prior to feeding. The relative proportion of ground minnows to dry feed was reduced by 25% every three days from the initial 20% by wet weight ground minnows to 80% dry diet. This technique was compared to using FDK in decreasing proportions as described by Kubitza and

Lovshin (1997a). Feed training success was greater for the fish fed the pellets top coated with minnows (75%) than for those receiving the krill (41%).

Skudlarek et al. (2007) evaluated the modification of a commercial dry pellet to see if its acceptance as an initial training diet could be improved. In the control (CTL), fingerlings were initially fed FDK then gradually transitioned to a 1.5 mm commercial diet (Steelhead; Skretting USA, Murray, Utah, USA). For days 1–3, fish were fed only FDK (10% initial body weight/day [BW/d] divided equally between three feedings), for days 4–6 they were fed a mixed ration containing 75% FDK and 25% commercial diet (75 : 25 ration), for days 7–9 a 50 : 50 ration, for days 10–12 a 25 : 75 ration, and then for days 13–18 they were fed only the commercial diet. In the second treatment (DRY), only the dry commercial pellet was fed throughout the experiment. In Treatment 3 (MST), the commercial pellets were moistened with water prior to feeding. In Treatment 4 (OIL), pellets were top dressed with menhaden fish oil (Rangen Inc., Buhl, Idaho, USA), to soften the pellet and potentially increase palatability. The DRY treatment resulted in a decrease in feed training success (82%) compared to other treatments which averaged 95%. The MST and OIL treatments may be advantageous due to reduced feed cost. The OIL treatment may be preferable to the MST as it would reduce the likelihood of nutrients leaching out of the pellets during water softening. Previous studies showed that semi-moist or soft diets perform better than dry/hard diets during feed training largemouth bass (Snow, 1965; Lovshin and Rushing, 1989; Sloane, 1993).

FDK is one of the most popular training diets used for habituating largemouth bass to artificial diets. Several alternatives to FDK have proven successful as feed training stimulants for largemouth bass. Ground fish and dried shrimp were both found to be more effective than FDK. Use of a floating diet rather than a sinking pellet may be advantageous and softening or oil coating pellets appears to be beneficial. A summary of some studies evaluating feed training diets and protocols is presented in Table 6.1.

6.5.2 Other factors affecting success during feed training

Training success can be related to many variables such as initial fish size and condition, the acceptability of the training diet, the suitability of the training system, and the genetic potential of the particular strain (Williamson, 1983). The size of fingerlings at the onset of feed-training is known to be an important factor in successful-feed training (Snow, 1965). Largemouth bass fry are approximately 3–4 mm TL at hatch and 5–6 mm TL at swim-up. The size of the fry harvested from nursery ponds for feed-training is dependent on the food availability and duration of the nursery period. Most producers feed-train largemouth bass fingerlings at sizes ranging from 25 to 50 mm when feed-training is more successful.

However, sometimes it may be advantageous to wean fry onto artificial diets as early as possible and may be necessary to harvest nursery ponds before bass fry reach sizes > 25 mm due to natural food depletion or other management considerations. Early reports documented attempts to feed-train smaller bass fingerlings using common carp, (*Cyprinus carpio*) eggs. Brandenburg et al. (1979) cultured 20 mm largemouth bass on common carp eggs with a mean training success of 52%. In another report (Willis and Flickinger, 1981), largemouth bass fry > 10 mm were trained to accept carp eggs with a success rates of 49–97% which increased as the initial fry size increased from 10 to 30 mm. An initial size of 10 mm was determined to be the minimum

Table 6.1 Select studies showing different training diets and protocols for feed training largemouth bass fingerlings.

Citation	Initial size	Water temp. (°C)	Stocking density	Training diet	Times fed per day	Disease treatment	Feed trained (%)
Campbell & Phelps (2002)	40 mm (1.0 g)	22	3.5 g/l	Dried shrimp	5	Prophylactic; 2 mg/l potassium permanganate daily for the first 7 days	78.0
Willis & Flickinger (1981)	20 mm	22	13 fish/l	Carp eggs	12	None	79.0
Williamson (1983)	0.45 g	23	7.0 g/l	Biodiet	Cont. for 6 h/d (15% SB/d)	Flexibacter columnaris; 5 mg/l copper sulfate once daily for a week	43.1
Williamson & Carmichael (1990)	0.27 g	23	3.3 g/l	Biodiet	Cont. for 12 h/d (20% SB/d)	None reported	96.0
Brandenburg et al. (1979)	20 mm	27	4 fish/l	Carp eggs	4 (15% BW/d)	None reported	52.0
Kubitza & Lovshin (1997a, 1997b)	1.4 g			FDK			58.0

Notes: SB, stocked biomass of fish; BW/d, body weight per day; FDK, freeze-dried krill.

threshold for successful training to carp eggs, likely due to the inability of smaller fish to ingest the 1.0–1.3 mm diameter eggs. In an unpublished study (Coyle and Tidwell), a feed training trial evaluated two size groups of pond-reared largemouth bass fingerlings harvested from the same nursery pond and size-graded into two groups with initial weights of 0.9 g (21 mm) and 1.4 g (28 mm). The percent training success was greater for the larger size fish (88%) compared to the smaller group (59%).

Kubitza and Lovshin (1997b) compared the feed training success of two genetic strains and different initial sizes of largemouth bass. Both strains were northern × Florida hybrids. Fish of 0.2, 0.4, 0.6, 0.9, and 1.4 g initial weight were fed using gradual feed ingredient transition (GFIT) with diets containing 80, 60, 40, 20, and 0% ground fish or 70, 50, 30, 10, and 0% krill meal. Feed-training success of the two strains was similar. Average percent feeders were 58% and 53% starting bass on FDK and ground fish, respectively. Percent feeders increased from 7% to 52% as initial fish weight increased from 0.2 to 1.4 g for fish started on FDK. Percent feeders increased from 59% to 88% as initial fish weight increased from 0.9 to 1.4 g among fish started on ground fish. In this study the feed-training diet and the initial size of the fish had more to do with success than the strain; however, domestication is thought to be important to feed-training success and is discussed later in this chapter. As a rule of thumb, pond-reared fingerlings should be a minimum of 20 mm TL or around 1 g to optimize feed-training success.

Williamson and Carmichael (1990) evaluated two wild (undomesticated) strains of FLMB and northern largemouth bass (NLMB) subspecies and first-generation hybrids under intensive conditions to determine their respective suitability for commercial aquaculture. Feed-training trials used a semi-moist diet fed via electronically controlled automatic feeders set to deliver approximately 20% of the fish biomass daily over 12 h at 15 min intervals. The northern strain had the highest percent feed-trained (96%), with the hybrids intermediate (91%) and worst performance in the Florida strain (80%). In addition, the northern strain grew faster, converted food to biomass more efficiently, resisted net-stress better and tolerated high ammonia, low temperature and low oxygen better. The northern strain largemouth bass is generally considered to be the better subspecies for commercial food-fish production in the USA.

Willis and Flickinger (1981) conducted a series of trials to evaluate factors influencing feed-training success in largemouth bass and made several important observations. The authors reported improved feed-training success with red rearing containers over white containers and reported that partially covering the containers greatly improved feed-training success. Improved success in the covered tanks was thought to be due to the lower light intensities of 6–12 lux compared to uncovered tanks (62 lux). Deeper tanks were found to be preferable over shallow tanks and rectangular tanks were better than round tanks in these trials. It was suggested that because largemouth bass do not eat food from the tank bottom the deeper tanks increased the time that food remained in the water column as the training diets were sinking pellets. The initial size of pond reared fry ranged from 9–30 mm, with improvements in feed-training success as the size increased to 20 mm. Training success was generally > 90% (on carp eggs) for fry > 20 mm.

Most early published reports used sinking pellets (Biodiet™ or Oregon Moist Pellet) during feed-training of largemouth bass because that was all that was commercially available at the time.

Manufacturing methods used to produce fish feeds have improved greatly over the past 50 years. Most fish feed manufactures now offer extruded floating feeds in sizes as small as 0.8–1.2 mm where previously high protein floating feeds for carnivorous species were limited to sizes ≥ 2.5 mm. Young largemouth bass generally only strike at pellets on the surface or as they slowly sink, and do not readily eat pellets on the tank bottom (McCraren, 1975; Flickinger et al., 1975; Willis and Flickinger, 1981). Kubitza and Lovshin (1997a) indicated that the tendency to float was one of the positive attributes of FDK as a training diet. Skudlarek et al. (2007) reported feed training success of 97% using FDK as the initial training diet and transitioning to a commercial 1.5 mm floating diet. Fish were observed to ingest and reject pellets many times before they would consume them. Floating pellets remain accessible for an extended time and may increase the success of feed-training largemouth bass.

Temperature is the single most pervasive environmental factor for poikilothermic animals (Stickney, 1979). Temperature significantly affects the growth and body composition of fish by controlling feed consumption and food retention time (Coutant, 1975). In a study performed by Tidwell et al. (2003), it was shown that higher culture temperatures (26 and 30°C) significantly increased growth and production of juvenile largemouth bass compared to those reared at 20°C. However, feed training is typically practiced at ambient pond and/or well water temperatures of < 24°C. The ground water temperature for the Mississippi River valley alluvial aquifer in eastern Arkansas, one of the major commercial production areas in the USA for juvenile largemouth bass, averages 22.1°C. Water temperature is important during the feed training phase as it influences appetite and starvation time.

Coyle et al. (2009) evaluated the effect of water temperatures on feed training success and growth of largemouth bass juveniles. Bass fingerlings (2 g) were stocked at 700 fish/m^3. Three water temperatures were evaluated (20, 24, and 28°C). Fingerlings were initially fed FDK then gradually transitioned to a 1.5 mm commercial floating pellet containing 45% protein and 12% fat according to a schedule modified by Kubitza and Lovshin (1997a). For days 1–3, fish were fed only FDK, for days 4–6 they were fed 75% FDK and 25% commercial diet (75 : 25 ratio), for days 7–9 a 50 : 50 ratio, for days 10–12 a 25 : 75 ratio, and then for days 13–24 they were fed only the commercial diet. One week of receiving only the formulated diet was long enough to ensure that feeders and non-feeders could be easily differentiated. Initially bass were fed a daily ration of 10% initial BW/d, divided into two equal feedings at 0900 and 1600 hours. On day 8, owing to an increase in feed consumption, the daily ration was increased to 15% initial BW/d in all treatments.

Average weight and feed trained percentage increased with increasing water temperature. The percentage of fish successfully feed trained averaged 70, 82, and 90% for the 21, 24, and 28°C treatments, respectively. Individual weights averaged 5.4, 6.8, and 7.8 g for fish feed trained at 21, 24, and 28°C, respectively. The results of this experiment indicate that water temperature has a significant impact on feed training success and growth rate of largemouth bass fingerlings during the feed training phase. Given that increasing water temperature increases the energy demand for maintenance and activity of fish (Weatherley and Gill, 1987), at some point further increases would not be productive. It is unknown if higher temperatures than those evaluated in this study would be beneficial or detrimental during feed training largemouth bass. Training success in this study was 70–90%, which is higher than many published reports, but is comparable to previous feed training experiments at this laboratory using the same strain, similar size fish and a floating pellet as the training diet (Skudlarek et al., 2007). According to Heidinger (2000b), most established producers of largemouth bass are approximately 75% successful in training pond reared fingerlings to feed on a prepared diet. It is not known if the increased percentage of feed trained fingerlings that could be produced by increasing water temperatures would justify the increased cost associated with heating water.

6.5.3 Feed training improvements over time may be related to domestication

Reported feed-training success of largemouth bass in the published literature is highly variable, ranging from 13–90% (Lovshin and Rushing, 1989; Sloane, 1993; Kubitza and Lovshin, 1997b; Skudlarek et al., 2007). Many early publications (1970–1990) reported feed-training success of only 25–50% whereas today most private and public hatcheries achieve 70–90%. These improvements are partially due to the development of better technologies through applied research, but non-systematic selection and domestication have also likely contributed.

Little research has been conducted on the genetic aspects of largemouth bass culture traits. One possible explanation for the 90% feed-training success reported by Coyle et al. (2009) and Skudlarek et al. (2007) could be domestication. Snow (1965) reported that offspring from pellet-trained broodfish survived better under hatchery conditions. He recommended a "genetic approach" to developing a strain of largemouth bass more readily adapted to the controlled, intensive culture environment. Subsequently, Williamson (1981) reviewed several reports from researchers and federal fish hatcheries during the 1970s, indicating better survivals of largemouth bass fingerlings from feed-trained parents and suggested that adaptability to eat artificial food was a heritable trait. It was also suggested that first generation largemouth bass from the wild did not feed-train as readily as those reared under hatchery conditions for several generations.

Williamson (1983) compared the feed-training success of two genetic strains of largemouth bass from different National Fish Hatcheries in Texas. The San Marcos strain (San Marcos National Fish Hatchery, Texas) were descendants of the Marion strain (Marion National Fish Hatchery, Alabama) developed by J.R. Snow in 1966 from a single pair of broodfish in response to a request by the U.S. Bureau of Sport Fisheries and Wildlife for the development of a national reference strain. Offspring of the single mating were maintained as the only source of bass at the Marion hatchery and were the progeny used in Snow's pioneering work in intensive largemouth bass culture (Snow, 1968a, 1968b, 1968c, 1970a, 1970b, 1973, 1975; Snow and Maxwell, 1970). The ancestors of the pairing are thought to have originated from waters near the hatchery in 1950. From 1950 to 1966, Marion broodfish were selected based on appealing body conformation (short, deep bodies and small heads). The Marion strain was later determined to be from a naturally occurring intergrade or hybrid population of the NLMB and FLMB subspecies (Harvey et al., 1980). The second strain evaluated was the Inks Dam strain (Inks Dam National Fish Hatchery, Texas). Broodfish from the Inks Dam strain were of northern origin and had always been maintained on forage.

The fingerlings of both strains were pond reared to 0.48 and 0.45 g for the Inks Dam and San Marcos strains, respectively. Fingerlings were fed Biodiet (Bioproducts, Warrenton, Oregon, USA) continuously during daylight hours with automatic feeders at 15% of the initial fish biomass daily. The training success for the San Marcos strain was 43% and for the Inks Dam strain was 23%. This represents an 84% difference in feed training success between the two strains, supporting the hypothesis that genetics may play a major role in determining hatchery performance between different strains of largemouth bass.

An unpublished study (Coyle and Tidwell), compared feed-training success of two strains of largemouth bass, "wild" and "domestic," and found survival to be greater in the domestic strain (60%) than the wild strain (34%). Conversely, the average weights were greater for the wild strain (1.9 g) than the domestic strain (1.6 g) at the end of the training period (both groups averaged 1.1 g at stocking). The wild strain were sourced from Barren River reservoir in Kentucky and are known to be 100% northern subspecies *Micropterus salmoides salmoides*. The domestic strain were sourced from the Pfeiffer Fish Hatchery, Frankfort, Kentucky, and were the same strain as used in Coyle et al. (2009) and Skudlarek et al. (2007). The domestic strain was progeny from a line of largemouth bass broodfish that had been pellet-raised in Kentucky for over 15 generations and were hybrids of the original Marion strain (natural northern-Florida hybrid) and wild broodfish sourced from Kentucky waters (personal communication, Mike Larimore, Hatchery Manager, Pfeiffer Fish Hatchery, Frankfort, Kentucky). Although little is known about the selection process involved in creating the Pfeiffer line, it is apparent that approximately 40 years of non-systematic selection have occurred for attributes that allow for survival in a semi-intensive aquaculture environment. It seems likely that domestication may, at least in part, explain the high feed-training success in Coyle et al. (2009) and Skudlarek et al. (2007).

To further evaluate the effect of domestication on feed-training success in largemouth bass a second study was conducted to compare growth and survival of wild, domestic, and both hybrid crosses during the feed-training phases. The domestic strain was the same as described above having been raised on pelleted feeds for more than five generations. Wild largemouth bass broodfish were collected from Barren River reservoir in Kentucky, which has been impounded over 60 years and has not received supplemental stocking. Broodfish from both strains were paired and pond-spawned. Swim-up fry from each group were transferred to fertilized nursery ponds for 6 weeks, then harvested by seine, and stocked into tanks for feed-training.

Fingerlings of similar size (average individual weight 0.9 g) were stocked in 190 l tanks at a rate of 150 fish per tank. Dechlorinated municipal water, maintained at 27°C, was supplied at 1.5 l/min to each tank. Each of the four genetic groups (Domestic♀ × Domestic♂, Domestic♀ × Wild♂, Wild♀ × Wild♂, and Wild♀ × Domestic♂) were randomly stocked into four replicate tanks. Fingerlings were fed twice daily at a rate of 10% of initial biomass per day. They were fed FDK for the first 3 d, then gradually weaned to a floating commercial diet (45% protein, 16% fat), according to previously established procedures. After 21 d, all fish in each tank were removed, individually weighed, and measured for total length.

Final average individual weight (g) was significantly greater for the Wild♀ × Wild♂ strain (2.95 g) compared to other groups: Domestic♀ × Domestic♂ (2.70 g), Domestic♀ × Wild♂ (2.53 g), and Wild♀ × Domestic♂ (2.55 g). Percent survival was significantly lower for the Domestic♀ × Domestic♂ group (86.9%) compared to the other groups, which averaged 97–100%. Reduced survival in the Domestic♀ × Domestic♂ group was primarily due to *Aeromonas hydrophila* infection which was isolated.

The faster growth of the Wild × Wild fish supports results from a previous study that compared fish of Barren River origin with domestic fish from the same commercial strain. However, in that previous study survival of the wild strain fish was lower than in the Domestic strain fish, in contrast to the superior survival of wild strain fish in the present study. Previous studies have reported improvements in feed-training success in subsequent generations of feed-trained largemouth bass. However, in the present study, feed-training success for the wild group was very high (99%). Based on these studies, the effect of non-selective domestication on feed training success is not clear. These data indicate it may be beneficial to evaluate the culture potential of various wild strains of largemouth bass geographically for selective breeding aimed at commercial aquaculture.

Domestication of largemouth bass may be beneficial for food-fish production but could be detrimental to genetic diversity of natural populations for stock enhancement programs (Lorenzen et al., 2012). The goal of domesticating bass for better and more consistent feed-training relates to food-fish production and generally not for fisheries management strategies.

6.5.3.1 Effect of diet on health

Low survival of pellet-reared Florida bass stocked in lakes (Porak et al., 2002) lead to the discovery of "pale liver syndrome" caused by inadequate nutrition in artificial diets used for production. The bass were fed commercial diets designed for trout and striped bass that contained unsuitable carbohydrate and fatty acid profiles leading to bass-glycogen storage disease and bass-fatty liver disease (Cardeilhac, 2009).

Seven years of testing a largemouth bass diet found that dietary carbohydrate content reduced to 12%, high protein content ~60% and reduction of dietary linoleic acid concentrations in a palatable dry pellet corrected "pale liver syndrome" and produced healthy 100 mm FLMB (Cardeilhac et al., 2004; Cardeilhac, 2009). The two diets resulting from this work are known as Diet 11 and Diet 12 or "Richloam bass diets" and are commercially available from Skretting USA, Tooele, Utah, USA. Richloam bass diets are milled once a year, typically in the fall.

Feed selection (brand) for feed training and growout needs to consider production purpose, intensity, water quality conditions, and longevity of "on feed" duration. Price is also a factor to consider but should be carefully weighed against final product health. Nutritional requirements should dictate feed selection, but once bass are feed trained they will eat many brands of feed. Csargo et al. (2013a) compared Otohime, Bio-Oregon, and Purina's Aquamax as initial feeds for feed training 3 g bass fingerlings. All three diets achieved > 90% survival, but the Otohime and Bio-Oregon feed produced significant increases in weight and condition factor (K).

The duration the bass remain on artificial feed and the nutrient content of the feed require consideration for best results. More research of long-term effects on differing feeds is needed. Florida bass reared on the Richloam bass diet for up to six months remained healthy, but the 3 mm maximum pellet size limited further usage (personal communication, Matthews).

6.5.3.2 Feed training in large-scale intensive culture systems

Small to moderate numbers of largemouth bass are feed trained annually at hatcheries producing warmwater sport-fish and several of the previously proposed feed training protocols involve hand feeding in combination with small battery-operated belt feeders. Feed training several hundred thousand bass fingerlings in large modern hatcheries requires a modified approach to be successful using minimal labor. It is important to start with a known number of robust, healthy fingerlings that are of similar length. *Artemia* (brine shrimp, a freshwater invertebrate similar in size to the zooplankton found in nursery ponds) are used to assist in transitioning bass feeding on microscopic invertebrates to artificial diets.

During feed training, bass fingerlings should be fed 24 h a day, and uneaten feed must be removed regularly to ensure water quality remains adequate. Successful feed training starts with the correct stocking density, ranging from 11 to 16 fingerlings/l of water. By nature, bass are very aggressive and survival depends of how successful they are at capturing prey. By stocking training tanks at high densities, competition helps stimulate bass to take prepared diets. Besides density, temperature can impact feed training success with optimal temperatures ≥ 22°C. Bass not transitioning to the artificial feed will get weak and aggregate to the surface and sides of the tank eventually moving to the back of the tank and clogging the outlet screens. These fish should be manually removed as they are vectors for bacterial diseases such as *Flavobacterium columnare*.

Typical success of FLMB subjected to feed training using the following protocol is about 60% and ranged from 35 to 97% over 8 years and more than 70 trials (Matthews, unpublished data). The fingerlings in these trials were all F1 generation spawned from wild caught FLMB broodfish. Higher success rates are expected in hatchery produced broodfish specifically selected for feed trainability for the use in food-fish propagation. Although larger fish (35 mm) commonly have greater training success than smaller fish, fish as small as 25 mm can be successfully trained. The following protocol can be modified to fit site specific conditions and is given to serve as a guide that has worked successfully in an intensive culture hatchery. The time frames listed are flexible and the progression and acceptance of feed items is more important to monitor as no two groups of fish train alike.

Before pond harvest

1 Start one to two heated vats of *Artemia* (45 g/vat) 24 to 36 h prior to harvest. Need to be ready when the bass are stocked into the feed training tank.
2 Set up feed training schedule for the next 14 d. Bass need to be fed every 30 min for the first 2 to 4 d (longer if smaller than 0.45 g or if the water is consistently less than 20°C).
3 Make sure all equipment; vacuum hoses, feed cart, buckets, small plastic beakers, graduated cylinders, mixing spoons and screen/feeder brush are ready.

Feed training

1 The bass start out on *Artemia* and a diet of Otohime C-1 (Marubeni Nisshin Feed Co., Tokyo, Japan). Amount depends on the number of fish and volume in the tank. There are ~275,000 cysts per gram. At 85% hatch a 15 l vat yields 701,000 *Artemia*/l. Sample counts (*Artemia*/ml) of each batch of *Artemia* is recommended. An *Artemia* hatching vat stirred by aeration filled with 15 l of water and 45 g of *Artemia* cysts feeds 75,000 bass fry for 2 d depending on tank volume. The larger the tank, the more *Artemia* required. If bass are held at an 11 to 16 fish/l density, calculate and add enough *Artemia* to the tank to reach > 100 *Artemia*/l. *Artemia* incubated at 26.7°C hatch in 18 to 24 h.
2 Otohime C-1 is fed every half-hour and *Artemia* every hour. The *Artemia* are mixed in with the feed every hour for the first 48 h. Feed only Otohime every hour on day 3 and 4. Bass should be given 10% of their BW/d. This allows maximum exposure to the feed as it slowly falls to the bottom of the tank at which time the bass lose interest. After 4 d start mixing in 1 mm Richloam bass diet (Skretting USA, Tooele, Utah, USA). The ratio of these feeds and duration used is dependent on initial fish size and to a lesser degree water temp. Larger fish (> 2 g) need 6 to 8 d to feed train while smaller bass (< 2 g) need to stay on the C-1 feed longer requiring 8–10 d. Temperatures below 20°C may extend these intervals. Start mixing with 75% C-1 and 25% Diet 11. Slowly start decreasing the amount of C-1 and increasing the amount of Diet 11 until a 0% C-1 and 100% Diet 11 ratio is reached.
3 The bass need to be hand fed for the first 6 to 8 d (preferably for the first 14 d) or until all fish are actively feeding. The feed needs to be placed "in front of the fish's nose" by taking a small amount of feed in a plastic beaker mix it with 1 l of water and "slurry feed" the corners, sides, middle, and in front of the screen if fish have their nose in the screen.
4 After the first 24 h, the feed can be offered dry (not slurried in water) in the corners, sides, middle, and in front of the screen. It is best to slurry one time then dry feed the next.
5 The bass need to be fed every 60 min during the transition from Otohime to their final diet.
6 Once the bass are actively feeding the feed can be placed in an automatic feeder. Still hand feed several times a day to observe the fish.
7 The goal is to get the bass on the 1 mm bass diet as soon as possible without sacrificing feed training percentage. This protocol typically yields a 60% feed training percentage.

Gut contents should be examined under a dissecting scope 40 h from the start of feed training. Length and weight should be recorded as well. Gut contents should be examined every 24 h from this point. Size somewhat dictates this but usually at 112 h full guts can be found in 80% or more of the surviving bass. *Artemia* and small amounts of food are usually found as early as 40 h from the onset of feeding. It is best to measure gut contents 10 min after a good feeding. Feed trained bass get thick from head to tail and can easily be distinguished from non-feed trained bass. Once trained and actively feeding, spread the bass out (decrease density) and feed them often. Growth rates of 1 to 2 mm/d are possible if water quality remains acceptable. The Richloam Diet is over 60% digestible protein, so ammonia can spike to unacceptable levels quickly if left unchecked (Csargo et al., 2013b).

6.5.3.3 Intensive indoor production of largemouth bass swim-up fry on artificial feed

The intensification of larval rearing techniques for largemouth bass has been identified as a priority area of research for commercialization of the species (Dupree and Huner, 1984). Developing technologies for intensive fry production, such as controlled indoor spawning, egg incubation, and fry rearing, could improve the reliability of bass fingerling production. Out of season spawning in indoor raceways allows for large-scale fry production (Matthews and Stout, 2013) and recent research at Kentucky State University was successful in developing a protocol for raising bass fry entirely indoors, eliminating the need for nursery ponds, by habituating largemouth bass fry to dry diets at smaller sizes than previously considered to be possible (Skudlarek et al., 2013). When combined, these technologies could enable largemouth bass fingerling production to occur at any time of the year.

In pond-based fingerling production systems, largemouth bass swim-up fry normally begin to feed on naturally occurring zooplankton in ponds. In intensive indoor hatchery systems, there is no nursery pond phase and bass fry are fed newly hatched brine shrimp nauplii (*Artemia* sp.) at the time of swim-up. Preliminary trials indicated that first feeding largemouth bass fry are large enough to consume *Artemia* nauplii, thus eliminating the need to culture live rotifers, as is the case with striped bass *Morone saxatilis* (Webster and Lovell, 1990). Live brine shrimp nauplii (*Artemia* sp.) comprise approximately 85% or more of the prepared live foods fed to larval fish worldwide (Sorgeloos, 1980). Determination of the proper combination of live food and larval diets for the first 2–3 weeks after hatch allows the nursery pond stage to be eliminated, thereby increasing control and predictability. This combination has proven effective in the other freshwater predators such as striped bass (Webster and Lovell, 1990) and walleye *Stizostedion vitreum* (Nickum, 1986).

A series of experiments were conducted to investigate live foods, natural foods, prepared diets, and optimal feeding schedules required to raise largemouth bass fry from first feeding until fully habituated to a commercial dry diet (Skudlarek et al., 2013). In each experiment, largemouth bass eggs were hatched under controlled conditions and swim-up fry were transferred to a recirculating system and stocked at 50 fry/l into either 3 l (Trials 1 and 2) or 10 l (Trial 3) acrylic aquaria. Trial 1 was a preliminary trial to screen six candidate diets to evaluate whether largemouth bass fry could be transitioned directly to prepared diets or if they required live foods. In Trial 2 the necessary duration for feeding live *Artemia* (1, 2, or 3 weeks) and the appropriate size of commercial diets (> 200 or 200–360 µm) were determined. Based on the results of Trials 1 and 2, largemouth bass fry in Trial 3 were fed *Artemia* for two weeks then transitioned either to a commercial marine finfish starter (Otohime; 200–360 µm), decapsulated *Artemia* cysts (Decap), a commercial trout starter, or freeze-dried copepods for one week. Fish were then fed a commercial trout starter for 2 weeks.

In Trial 1, Otohime and decapsulated *Artemia* cysts performed better than other diets tested. However, survivals even in these treatments were relatively low (6–8%). In Trial 2, fry fed *Artemia* for 2 weeks then transitioned to diet sizes of 200–360 µm performed better than other combinations tested. In Trial 3, survival was significantly better for fry fed Decap and Otohime. Average individual weight was significantly higher for fry fed Decap and trout starter. Use of decapsulated *Artemia* or Otohime fry diet as transitional feeds produced the best combination of high survival and average weight. These data indicate that live food is likely necessary for the first two weeks followed by a gradual transition to either decapsulated *Artemia* cysts or Otohime (200–360 µm) for one week then transition to trout starter. This protocol yielded survival rates of approximately 70% and may have significant potential for improving the reliability of largemouth bass fingerling production.

In Skudlarek et al. (2013), *Artemia* were fed to excess and optimal bass stocking and prey densities were not determined. Subsequently two independent feeding trials were conducted to determine optimal fry and *Artemia* densities for the first 2 weeks of largemouth bass larviculture. In the first trial, largemouth bass swim-up fry (9 mg) were stocked in a factorial arrangement at densities of 20, 40, and 80 fry/l and *Artemia* nauplii feed rates of 5, 10, and 20 nauplii/ml were administered twice daily. The results for Trial 1 indicated that after 14 days the lowest fish densities and the highest *Artemia* densities (20 fry/l fed 20 *Artemia*/ml and 40 fry/l fed 20 *Artemia*/ml) resulted in higher average weights (39 and 40 mg, respectively). There were no statistical differences in survival between treatments, which averaged 51–83%.

Based on these results, Trial 2 evaluated lower fish densities and higher *Artemia* densities. The second trial evaluated fry stocking densities of 10, 20, and 40 fry/l and *Artemia* nauplii feed rates of 20, 30, and 40 nauplii/ml administered twice daily. Results for Trial 2 again indicated that the lowest fish densities and the highest *Artemia* densities (10 fry/l fed 30 *Artemia*/ml, 10 fry/l fed 40 *Artemia*/ml, and 20 fry/l fed 40 *Artemia*/ml) resulted in significantly higher average weights (40, 43, and 40 mg, respectively). There were no significant differences in survival, which averaged 81–94%. Based on these data, fry stocking densities of 10–20/l in combination with *Artemia* feed rates of 20–40 nauplii/ml twice daily appear suitable for rearing largemouth bass fry for the first two weeks of feeding. This protocol yielded survivals of 60–80% in experimental units.

The last trial in this series (Coyle and Tidwell, unpublished data) evaluated two strains of largemouth bass for their adaptability to these intensive protocols. The two strains were followed from hatch through to the transition to 1.5 mm floating pelleted feeds at which point they would be considered commercially marketable fingerlings to food-fish producers. The domestic strain was the one cultivated by fish farmers in the region. Wild largemouth bass broodfish were collected from Barren River reservoir, Kentucky, USA. Broodfish from both strains were pond-spawned in separate outdoor ponds provided with Spawntex™ spawning mats. Fertilized eggs from the two strains were collected on mats from outdoor tanks on the same day, transferred indoors and incubated in separate 380 l tanks maintained at 26°C and supplied with dechlorinated municipal water in a flow-through system. Swim-up fry were fed live *Artemia* nauplii twice daily for two weeks and then restocked into eight separate 150 l tanks with four replicate tanks per strain. Fry were then fed decapsulated *Artemia* cysts for one week, transitioned to a commercial trout starter (no. 0) for 2 weeks, then fed the same formulation in a no. 1 crumble (1 week), and finally transitioned to a 1.5 mm floating trout diet (1 week). At this point, all fish in each tank were removed, counted, and individually weighted to determine survival and average weight.

After 5 weeks of receiving only dry feed, survival of the domestic strain (60%) was higher than the wild strain (40%). However, the wild strain (1.9 g) had higher average individual weight than the domestic (1.6 g). In general, the results of this study show that the described technique for feeding largemouth bass swim-up fry may have potential for scale up. Once habituated to trout starter (400 μm) and fed for 2 weeks, fry appeared to retain this learned feeding behavior and are easily transitioned to first a no. 1 crumble or a 0.8 mm floating pellet (1 week), and finally transitioned to a 1.5 mm floating diet (1 week).

A commercial scale trial of this protocol was conducted which identified some constraints to scale-up. Current bottleneck issues appear to be synchronization of the spawn needed to maintain appropriate fry densities in larger tanks. Labor associated with waste removal (siphoning) is demanding because of the need to feed to excess, particularly when transitioning to fry starter. The lack of a commercially available fish grader of the appropriate size (< 8/64") is also a problem as size variability inevitably leads to reduced survival due to cannibalism. These constraints appear to be researchable questions. Further development may lead to the intensive commercial production of feed-trained largemouth bass juveniles entirely under controlled conditions.

6.5.3.4 Disease control

Stress or injury to largemouth bass fingerlings during pond harvest, transportation, size grading, and routine husbandry practices, such as tank cleaning, can result in mortality during feed-training. In addition to directly causing mortality, stressors caused by poor handling combined with the stress associated with the feed-training process can result in disease outbreaks. Also, the better the condition the fingerlings are in, the more successfully they will adapt to formulated feeds and intensive culture conditions. Poor condition at nursery pond harvest can result from declining food availability or overpopulated ponds. Fingerlings in poor condition seldom have the energy reserves needed to tolerate harvest stresses, and adapt to a new culture environment, and transition to a different food source.

The most prevalent diseases during the feed-training processes in largemouth bass are columnaris disease and hemorrhagic septicemia caused by the bacteria *Flavobacterium columnare* and *Aeromonas hydrophila*, respectively. These bacteria are ubiquitous and are considered opportunistic pathogens meaning that they occur at increased frequency when one or more stressors occur. These can include environmental changes, behavioral or physiological stressors or changes in water temperature. Additionally, because of high fish densities and high nutrient loads, fungal infections (*Saprolegnia* sp.) and parasitic protozoans such as *Trichodina* sp. and *Ichthyophthirius multiphiliis* can cause disease-related mortality in largemouth bass during feed-training.

In the past, a number of compounds were used to alleviate stress, prophylactically prevent, or therapeutically treat disease in largemouth bass fingerlings. However, the use of many of these compounds is no longer permitted. Accordingly, refer to Chapter 10 in this book that discusses disease and chemotherapeutic use in largemouth bass. Disease outbreaks can be minimized by implementing least-stress harvesting and husbandry procedures, combined with prophylactic static salt baths (0.7% for 4 h) administered after unavoidable stressful procedures such as weighing and measuring (Malison and Held, 1996).

Lange (2003) conducted a series of experiments evaluating preventative treatments to reduce the mortality associated with columnaris disease during feed-training largemouth bass. The three treatments evaluated were a one-time attenuated immersion vaccine for *F. columnare* (VAC; Intervet/Schering-Plough, Keniworth, New Jersey, USA), a 20 mg/l Oxytetracycline bath (OTC bath) for 10 min every 3 d or feeding Oxytetracycline top-coated on the training diets at a rate of 5.5 g active ingredient (AI) per 100 kg fish (OTC fed). A low level of columnaris disease occurred during feed-training, and survivals ranged from 87.1 to 96.6% with no differences between the treatments. Following feed-training, a *F. columnare* challenge was performed where fish were intentionally exposed to live cultures. Following the 20 d challenge, survivals were—OTC bath treated fish (92%) > OTC fed fish (72%) > VAC fish (55%) > control fish (38%).

Bass intensively reared in indoor raceways require grading to keep size ranges small to avoid predation-induced disease outbreaks. This additional handing can also increase the risk of disease. Bebak et al. (2009) followed Florida bass fry 7–9 d post-hatch immersion vaccinated with AQUAVAC-COL (Intervet/Schering-Plough, Kenilworth, New Jersey, USA), reared in nursery ponds for ~33 d, feed trained in 4,914 l raceways, and reared for an additional 44 d in cohabitation with sham-vaccinated bass had significantly less mortality from *F. columnare* than the sham-vaccinated fish. However, producers will need to weigh the cost of the vaccine against possible additional fish production and labor costs.

Chemical bath treatments for fingerlings may also be effective. Bowker et al. (2013) reported results from four separate chloramine-T (20 mg/l) trials and three separate hydrogen peroxide (150 mg/l and two at 50 mg/l) trials on bass and Bluegill (*Lepomis macrochirus*). Both chemicals were effective in controlling *F. columnare* disease when used as 60 min bath treatments on three consecutive or alternate days. Identifying and beginning treatment early greatly increases the chances of survival. No withdrawal period is required with either of these chemicals.

In large volume tanks, it may be necessary to use an antibiotic feed additive to treat *F. columnare.* Matthews et al. (2013) reported Aquaflor (florfenicol, 50%) top-coated feed at 10 mg/kg of fish body weight effectively controlled columnaris disease in both feed-trained bass and bluegill (10 d treatment). The use of Aquaflor requires a Veterinarian Feed Directive (VFD) which can be obtain through a licensed vet. There is a 15 d withdraw period after treatment meaning fish require 15 d post-treatment before they can be processed, sold live for food, or stocked in public waters.

6.5.3.5 Cannibalism and size grading

Cannibalism has been reported in many species of cultured fish (Nishimura and Hoshino, 1999). Cannibalism can cause significant losses especially during intensive culture of carnivorous fishes and can be affected by several factors including fish age and size uniformity, food availability and stocking density (Baras and Jobling, 2002). Not all fish start to exhibit cannibalism at the same size nor is cannibalism equally intense in different species or life stages. The impact of intracohort cannibalism is dictated by the time when it emerges. Intracohort cannibalism in largemouth bass has been reported to begin as early as 9 d after swim-up (Johnson and Post, 1996).

As discussed earlier, in largemouth bass there is a natural dietary conversion from consuming invertebrates to consuming fish that occurs sometime in their first year usually at around 40 mm TL (Olson, 1996). It is during this natural transition that feed training typically occurs. It is also during this transition that cannibalism can become pronounced. Increased size variability between cohorts is a normal occurrence, due to differential growth among individuals within the population (Jensen, 1990). Early cannibalism may promote growth heterogeneity and accentuate size variability because digestible nutrients are often higher in fish than in plankton prey (Kubitza and Lovshin, 1997b). Due in part to their increased tendency for cannibalism at sizes > 40 mm; largemouth bass nursery ponds are typically harvested at this size and the fish are brought into the hatchery for feed training.

Predator to prey size ratios vary substantially between fish species and life stages. Cannibalism is limited by mouth gape size and allometric growth of mouth parts. It is well known that piscivorous fish are size selective predators and seek out as large a prey item as they can efficiently consume (Werner and Hall, 1974; Mittlebach, 1981; Hambright, 1991). This size selectivity is based on the optimal allocation of time spent searching for and handling food items related to energy return. This allows them to take in the maximum nutrition with least expenditure of energy in feeding. As the name implies, largemouth bass are capable of consuming large food items relative to their size. Largemouth bass swallow prey whole, therefore mouth diameter (gape) limits prey size. Johnson and Post (1996) used morphological measurements to predict a threshold predator-prey size relationship. According to these calculations largemouth bass can swallow prey items with a length approximately 60% of their total length.

Timmerman et al. (2000) evaluated factors limiting prey size swallowed by juvenile largemouth bass (> 31 mm TL) and determined there was a large individual variation in gape size which may contribute to improved feeding success and growth potential for some cohorts within a population which may contribute to eventual cannibalism. Empirical evidence suggests that largemouth bass juvenile populations should have no more than a 20% variability in TL to reduce the occurrence of cannibalism (Timmerman et al., 2000).

Size variability is common among many species of same-age farmed fish and cannibalistic species need to be mechanically size graded more frequently to maintain survival rates (Kelly and Heikes, 2013). Fish graders consist of smooth steel bars equally spaced to allow a portion of the population to pass through while retaining the larger fraction. Several commercial graders are available, although many producers make their own graders to fit their specific needs. Mixed sizes of fish may require grading through more than one size of grader.

The two types of graders that are most commonly used for grading largemouth bass in tanks prior to and during the feed training phase are floating box graders and panel or drag graders. Box graders are designed to float in a tank. The frame typically holds interchangeable inserts made of 4.8 mm aluminum bars with 0.4 mm spacing between the bars. Fish are placed into the floating box grader where large fish are retained and smaller fish pass down through the grader. The process can be repeated with a smaller size grader. Panel graders are often used in vats or trough type raceway tanks and consist of evenly spaced bars welded or bolted to a rectangular frame with rubber flanges attached to the outside of the panels to allow them to fit tightly against the tank walls. Like box graders the larger fish are retained as the panel is pulled from one end of the tank to the other. Panel graders typically require less handling of the fish and cause less stress than box graders.

A series of sizes of graders are necessary as pond-reared nursery-phase largemouth bass populations may consist of several size groupings of fish possibly from several spawns. It is also important to size grade again after the feed training phase to ensure size uniformity before stocking back out into ponds for first year growth and again after harvest from first year ponds prior to stocking second year ponds for food-fish production. Table 6.2 provides bar grader sizes for different length largemouth bass modified from Kelly and Heikes (2013). These should be considered estimates as individual populations of fish may be different as passing through the grader depends on the individual condition or body width of the fish not the length. Prior to and after feed training most food-fish producers grade off the largest 1–2% and either discard

Table 6.2 Bar grader size to retain largemouth bass fingerlings of different total length.

Bar width in inches	Size retained in inches (cm)
10/64–11/64	1.00 (2.5)
12/64–13/64	1.50 (3.75)
14/64–15/64	2.00 (5.0)
18/64	2.75 (6.875)
21/64	3.00 (7.5)
44/64	6.00 (15.0)
60/64	8.00 (20.0)

them as cannibals or use them for recreational sales. Next, they typically attempt to separate the remaining population into two groups, the larger fraction and the smaller, by experimenting with different size grader bars.

Factors other than size variability are also likely to affect cannibalism in largemouth bass but have not been fully studied. In better studied species, it has been determined that cannibalism can be triggered or enhanced by a wide range of biotic and abiotic factors that influence food requirements and access. The influence of genetics on cannibalism is somewhat controversial. One idea is that some fish may have a greater genetic propensity toward cannibalism ('natural born killer' hypothesis), and the other that cannibals are the winners of an intense initial competition ('lottery winner' hypothesis) (Baras and Jobling, 2002).

It has been shown that some strains of fish are more prone to cannibalism than others of the same species and that domestication may reduce or exacerbate the condition depending upon the selection process criteria (Hecht and Pienaar, 1993). Selection for or against cannibalism in largemouth bass may be based on the ultimate goals of the producers. Food-fish producers may desire uniform growth with little competition and discard cannibals when found, whereas producers supplying managed trophy fisheries may wish to select for the most aggressive fish within a population.

Cannibalism can also be influenced by population density. Generally, under conditions where food is adequately provided, increased stocking densities result in a lower incidence of dominance hierarchies and reduced cannibalism in predatory fish (Petit et al., 2001). However, factors that induce changes in spatial distribution, such as water flow and light intensity, may affect cannibalism by increasing the chances of encounter between cannibals and prey. Also, environmental factors that increase feed intake in largemouth bass such as increased water temperature and 24 h light may have an effect (Petit et al., 2001). Any restriction of food availability may enhance cannibalism through both food shortage and the resulting increase in differential growth.

6.5.3.6 Post-feed training

After the 25–50 mm largemouth bass fingerlings are trained to accept a prepared diet, they are size graded. This allows the separation of cannibals (large) and non-feeders (small). The uniform trained fish are then typically stocked back into ponds at first year growout densities of 33,000–44,000 fingerlings/ha. However, sometimes only 50% of the fingerlings will continue to feed on the prepared diet when stocked at these pond densities after only a 2 week feed-training period (Heidinger, 2000a). This problem is thought to be related to when fingerling producers use primarily automatic feeders during feed training. It does not seem to be as big of a problem when bass are trained by hand feeding. To ameliorate this problem, some producers confine fish to one area of the pond with a net or concentrate the fingerlings at much higher densities of 110,000–220,000/ha in small ponds, for a few weeks or until the fingerlings reach > 75 mm. During this period, the fingerlings are fed several times per day as reinforcement training. If well water or ample surface water to supply flow-through tanks is available, concentrating the feed-trained fingerlings indoors in tanks for an additional two weeks transition at densities of 1–3 fish/l provides the producer with better disease control options, such as daily formalin (25 ppm) and/or salt (5 ppt) treatments, and reduces handling stress when ultimately moving the fish back out into ponds at the reduced density for further growout.

During this phase, it is advisable to feed by hand only two or three times per day. Many commercial producers of feed-trained bass use automatic feeders to deliver small amounts of feed at frequent intervals throughout the daylight hours. This approach conditions the fish to respond to the equipment as their food stimulus and not directly with hatchery personnel, and frequent feeding in a small area allows a small number of more aggressive fish or "bullies" to patrol the feeding area. Hand feeding helps the fish to identify with people as their food providers and feeding less frequently with greater amounts of food spread more uniformly over the water surface promotes equal distribution of feeding opportunity. At this stage they should already be feed-trained; the goal here is to strengthen the learned behavior without promoting size disparity.

6.6 Conclusion

Meeting the challenges of intensifying largemouth bass culture will require further research into all facets of existing culture techniques for the species. Much can be learned by reviewing the techniques developed, investigated, and highlighted in this chapter; however, incorporating and applying these methods will depend largely on the level of hatchery design and infrastructure development. Aquaculture facilities with good water supplies, large raceways, many troughs and tanks, and control over environmental conditions can intensify production at every step along the way to producing market-size largemouth bass. Currently, the highest level of intensification consists of spawning broodfish in raceways, harvesting eggs and hatching them in troughs, stocking lined ponds with fry for fingerling production, and then transitioning fingerlings to commercial diets for growout to market or stocking-size. Aquaculturists should realize that each of these steps poses challenges and opportunities for optimization. Timing and understanding the environmental conditions and variability unique to each hatchery are crucial to developing a successful program. Managing natural food production and pond fertility will always be a significant aspect and challenge of production because fry do not readily take to artificial diets.

We suggest the following research priorities for intensifying largemouth bass production. These are provided in order of production sequence and with the previous caveat on hatchery site specificity. These questions plague all hatcheries, but their degree of importance must be prioritized individually. What is the optimum density of broodfish for spawning ponds and raceways to produce adequate numbers of high quality fry in the least amount of space? Are there suitable feed substitutes to managing natural food for initial fry and fingerling production? What are the optimum timing and fertility levels in ponds to best product the most desirable food organisms? What is the optimum and acceptable water quality for managing each life stage? How can nuisance organisms be managed effectively? What is the optimum production size for stock enhancement or the commercial market?

References

Allan, J.D. (1976) Life history patterns in zooplankton. *The American Naturalist* 110 (971), 165–180.

Anderson, R.J. (1974) Feeding artificial diets to smallmouth bass. *The Progressive Fish-Culturist* 36 (3), 145–151.

Anderson, R.O. and Tave, D. (1993) *Strategies and Tactics for Management of Fertilized Hatchery Ponds.* Haworth Press Inc., New York.

Applegate, R.L., Mullan, J.W. and Morais, D.I. (1967) Food and growth of six centrarchids from shoreline areas of Bull Shoals Reservoir. *Proceedings of the Annual Conference Southeastern Association of Game and Fish Commissioners* 20, 469–482.

Baras, E. and Jobling, M. (2002) Dynamics of intracohort cannibalism in cultured fish. *Aquaculture Research* 33 (7), 461–479.

Barkoh, A. (1996) Effects of three fertilization treatments on water quality, zooplankton, and striped bass fingerling production in plastic-lined ponds. *The Progressive Fish-Culturist* 58 (4), 237–247.

Barkoh, A., Anderson, R.O. and Rabeni, C.F. (1994) Effects of pond volume manipulation on production of fingerling largemouth bass *Micropterus salmoides*. *Journal of Applied Aquaculture* 2 (3–4), 151–170.

Barkoh, A., Hamby, S., Kurten, G. and Schlechte, J.W. (2005) Effects of rice bran, cottonseed meal, and alfalfa meal on pH and zooplankton. *North American Journal of Aquaculture* 67 (3), 237–243.

Barrows, F.T. (2000) Feed additives. In: Stickney R.R. (ed.), *Encyclopedia of Aquaculture*. John Wiley and Sons Inc., New York, pp. 335–340.

Baskerville-Bridges, B. and Kling, L.J. (2000) Early weaning of Atlantic cod (*Gadus morhua*) larvae onto a microparticulate diet. *Aquaculture* 189, 109–117.

Bebak, J., Matthews, M. and Shoemaker, C. (2009) Survival of vaccinated, feed-trained largemouth bass fry (*Micropterus salmoides floridanus*) during natural exposure to *Flavobacterium columnare*. *Vaccine* 27 (32), 4297–4301.

Bergerhouse, D.L. (1994) Lethal effects of elevated pH and ammonia on early life stages of hybrid striped bass. *Journal of Applied Aquaculture* 2, 81–100.

Bishop, H. (1968) Largemouth bass culture in the southwest. *Proceedings of the North Central Warmwater Fish Culture Workshop*, Ames, IA.

Bowker, J.D, Carty, D., Trushenski, J.T., Bowman, M.P., Wandelear, N. and Matthews, M. (2013) Controlling mortality caused by external columnaris in largemouth bass and bluegill with chloramine-T or hydrogen peroxide. *North American Journal of Aquaculture* 75, 342–351.

Boyd, C.E. (1979) *Water Quality in Warmwater Fish Ponds*. Auburn University Agricultural Experiment Station, Auburn, AL.

Boyd, C.E. (1990) *Water Quality in Ponds for Aquaculture*. Alabama Agricultural Experiment Station. Auburn University. Auburn, AL.

Boyd, C.E. and Daniels, H.V. (1994) Liming and fertilization of brackishwater shrimp ponds. *Journal of Applied Aquaculture* 2, 221–234.

Bowling, C.W., Rutledge, W.P. and Geiger, J.G. (1984) Evaluation of ryegrass cover crops in rearing ponds for FLMB. *The Progressive Fish-Culturist* 46, 55–57.

Brandenburg, A.M., Ray, M.S. and Lewis, W.M. (1979) Use of carp eggs as a feed for fingerling largemouth bass. *The Progressive Fish Culturist* 41(2), 97–98.

Brandt, T.M., Jones Jr., R.M. and Anderson, R.J. (1987) Evaluation of prepared feeds and attractants for largemouth bass. *The Progressive Fish-Culturist* 49, 198–203.

Brewer, D.L. and Rees, R.A. (1990) Pond culture of phase I striped bass fingerlings. In: Harrell, R.M., Kerby, J.H. and Minton, R.V. (eds.) *Culture and Propagation of Striped Bass and its Hybrids*, American Fisheries Society, Bethesda, MD, pp. 99–120.

Buurma, B.J., Barkoh, A. and Alexander, G. (1996) Effects of cottonseed and alfalfa meals as fertilizers on production of palmetto bass *Morone saxatilis* X *M. chrysops* fingerlings in plastic-lined ponds. *Journal of Applied Aquaculture* 6 (3), 59–70.

Callan, C., Jordaan, A. and Kling, L.J. (2003) Reducing *Artemia* use in the culture of Atlantic cod (*Gadus morhua*). *Aquaculture* 219, 585–595.

Campbell, L.T. and Phelps, R.P. (2002) Use of shrimp *Penaeus* spp. to replace krill *Euphausia* spp. in a feed training diet for largemouth bass. *North American Journal of Aquaculture* 64, 294–296.

Cardeilhac, P.T. (2009) Development of a pelleted feed for the intensive culture of FLMB (*Micropterus salmoides floridanus*). Improved Hatchery Capabilities of Florida Largemouth Bass, Florida Fish and Wildlife Conservation Commission Final Report for Grant Number f-129-R, Contract 7063.

Cardeilhac, P., Dickson, H., Stout, R. and Hardin, S. (2004) A pelleted feed for the high-volume production of largemouth fingerlings free of pale liver syndrome. *International Association for Aquatic Animal Medicine* 35, 12–13.

Cooper, G.P. (1937) Food habits, rate of growth and cannibalism of young largemouth bass (*Aplites salmoides*) in state-operated rearing ponds in Michigan during 1935. *Transactions of the American Fisheries Society* 66, 242–266.

Coutant, C.C. (1975) Responses of bass to natural and artificial temperature regimes. In: Stroud, R.H. and Clepper, H. (eds.), *Black Bass Biology and Management*, Sport Fishing Institute, Washington, DC, pp. 272–285.

Coyle, S.D., Patton, S., Schneider, K. and Tidwell, J.H. (2009) The effect of water temperature on growth and survival of largemouth bass during feed training. *North American Journal of Aquaculture* 71, 256–259.

Csargo, I. J., Brown, M.L. and Ward, M.J. (2013a) Evaluation of four commercial grower diets for production of largemouth Bass. *Journal of Applied Aquaculture* 25 (1), 35–49.

Csargo, I.J., Brown, M.L. and Ward, M.J. (2013b) Practical comparison of commercial starter diets for feed training Largemouth Bass fingerlings. *Journal of Applied Aquaculture* 25 (1), 24–34.

Culver, D.A. (1988) Plankton ecology in fish hatchery ponds in Narrandera, NSW, Australia. *Internationale Vereinigung für Theoretische und Angewandte Limnologie: Verhandlungen* 23 (2), 1085–1089.

Culver, D.A., Madon, S.P. and Qin, J. (1993) Percid pond production techniques: timing, enrichment, and stocking density manipulation. *Journal of Applied Aquaculture* 2, 9–31.

Curnow, J., King, J., Partridge, G. and Kolkovski, S. (2006) Effects of two commercial microdiets on growth and survival of barramundi (*Lates calcarifer* Bloch) larvae within various early weaning protocols. *Aquaculture Nutrition* 12 (4), 247–255.

Czarnezki, J.M., Hamilton, E.J. and Wagner, B.A. (1994) Water management to control clam shrimp, *Cyzicus morsie*, in walleye, *Stizostedion vitreum*, production ponds. *Journal of Applied Aquaculture* 2, 234–242.

Dabrowski, K. (1989) 12th Annual Larval Fish Conference: Formulation of bioenergetic model for coregonine early life history. *Transactions of the American Fisheries Society* 118, 138–150.

Davis, J.T. and Lock, J.T. (1997) Culture of largemouth bass fingerlings. Southern Regional Aquaculture Center (SRAC), SRAC Publication No. 201, Stoneville, MS.

Dupree, H.K. and Huner, J.V. (1984) Propagation of black bass, sunfishes, tilapias, eels, and hobby fishes. In: Dupree, H.K. and Huner, J.V. (eds.) *Third Report to the Fish Farmers*, U.S. Department of the Interior, Fish and Wildlife Service, Washington, DC, pp. 119–135.

Elliot, G.V. (1976) Diel activity and feeding of schooled largemouth bass fry. *Transactions of the American Fisheries Society* 105, 624–627.

Engle, C. and Southworth, B. (2008) *Cost of Raising Largemouth Bass Fingerlings*. Publication ETB260, University of Arkansas at Pine Bluff, Cooperative Extension Service, Pine Bluff, AK.

Fairchild, G.W. (1982) Population responses of plant-associated invertebrates to foraging by largemouth bass fry (*Micropterus salmoides*). *Hydrobiologia* 96, 169–176.

Farquhar, B.W. and Geiger, J.G. (1984) Portable zooplankton sampling apparatus for hatchery ponds. *The Progressive Fish-Culturist* 46, 209–211.

Farquhar, B.W. and Guest, W.C. (1991) Food habits and feeding selectivity of smallmouth bass in culture ponds. In: Jackson, D.C. (ed.) *The First International Smallmouth Bass Symposium*. Mississippi State University, Starkville, MS, pp. 24–26.

Fletcher Jr., R.C., Roy, W., Davie, A., Taylor, J., Robertson, D. and Migaud, H. (2007) Evaluation of new microparticulate diets for early weaning of Atlantic cod (*Gadus morhua*): implications on larval performance and tank hygiene. *Aquaculture* 263 (1–4), 35–51.

Flickinger, S.A., Anderson, R.J. and Puttmann, S.J. (1975) Intensive culture of smallmouth bass. In: Clepper, H. (ed.) *Black Bass Biology and Management*. Proceedings of the National Symposium on the Biology and Management of the Centrarchid Basses, Sport Fishing Institute, Washington, DC, pp. 373–379.

Geiger, J.G. (1983a) Zooplankton production and manipulation in striped bass rearing ponds. *Aquaculture* 35, 331–351.

Geiger, J.G. (1983b) A review of pond zooplankton production and fertilization for the culture of larval and fingerling striped bass in ponds. *Aquaculture* 35, 353–369.

Geiger, J.G. and Turner, C.J. (1990) Pond fertilization and zooplankton management techniques for production of fingerling striped bass and hybrid striped bass. In: Harrell, R.M., Kerby, J.H. and Minton, R.V. (eds.) *Culture and Propagation of Striped Bass and its Hybrids,* American Fisheries Society, Bethesda, MD, pp. 79–98.

Geiger, J.G., Fitzmayer, K., Turner, C.J. and Nichols, W.C. (1985) Feeding habits of larval and fingerling striped bass and zooplankton dynamics in fertilized rearing ponds. *The Progressive Fish-Culturist* 47, 213–223.

Graves, K.G. and Morrow, J.C. (1988) Technical notes: Tube sampler for zooplankton. *The Progressive Fish-Culturist* 50, 182–183.

Hambright, K.D. (1991) Experimental analysis of prey selection by largemouth bass: role of predator mouth width and prey body depth. *Transactions of the American Fisheries Society* 120, 500–508.

Harding, L.M. and Summerfelt, R.C. (1994) Effects of fertilization and of fry stocking density on pond production of fingerling walleye, *Stizostedion vitreum. Journal of Applied Aquaculture* 2, 59–80.

Harvey, W.D., Greenbaum, I.F. and Noble, R.L. (1980) Electrophoretic evaluation of five hatchery stocks of largemouth bass in Texas. *Annual Proceedings of the Texas Chapter of the American Fisheries Society* 3, 49–63.

Hecht, T. and Pienaar, A.G. (1993) A review of cannibalism and its implications in fish larviculture. *Journal of the World Aquaculture Society* 24, 246–261.

Heidinger, R.C. (2000a) A white paper on the status and needs of largemouth bass culture in the north central region. North Central Regional Aquaculture Center, Carbondale, IL.

Heidinger, R.C. (2000b) Black bass/largemouth bass culture. In: Stickney, R.R. (ed.), *Encyclopedia of Aquaculture*, Wiley, New York, pp. 108–117.

Hodson, R.G. and Strawn, K. (1968) Food of young-of-the-year largemouth and spotted bass during the filling of Beaver Reservoir, Arkansas. *Proceedings of the Southeastern Association of Game and Fish Commissioners* 22, 510–516.

Hoff, F.H. and Snell, T.W. (2004) *Plankton Culture Manual*, sixth edition. Florida Aqua Farms Inc., Dade City, Florida.

Hubbs, C. and Blaxter, J.H.S. (1986) Ninth larval fish conference: Development of sense organs and behaviour of Teleost larvae with special reference to feeding and predator avoidance. *Transactions of the American Fisheries Society* 115, 98–114.

Hutson, P.L. (1990) FLMB culture in Texas. Management Data Series No. 35. Texas Parks and Wildlife Department, Austin, TX.

Isaac Jr., J. and Staats, V.H. (1994) FLMB raceway spawning substrate evaluation. *Proceeding of the Annual Conference of the Southeastern Association of Fish and Wildlife Agencies* 46, 453–457.

Jensen, G.L. (1990) *Sorting and Grading Warmwater Fish*. Southern Regional Aquaculture Center (SRAC), SRAC Publication No. 391, Stoneville, Mississippi.

Johnson, J.M. and Post, D.M. (1996) Morphological constraints on intracohort cannibalism in age-0 largemouth bass. *Transactions of the American Fisheries Society* 125 (5), 809–812.

Kelly, A.M. and Heikes, D. (2013) *Sorting and Grading Warmwater Fish*. Southern Regional Aquaculture Center (SRAC), SRAC Publication No. 391, Stoneville, Mississippi.

Kubitza, F. (1995) Intensive culture of largemouth bass *Micropterus salmoides*: production of advanced juveniles and food-size fish. PhD dissertation, Auburn University, Auburn, AL.

Kubitza, F. and Lovshin, L.L. (1997a) The use of freeze-dried krill to feed train largemouth bass (*Micropterus salmoides*): feeds and training strategies. *Aquaculture* 148, 299–312.

Kubitza, F. and Lovshin, L.L. (1997b) Effects of initial weight and genetic strain on feed training largemouth bass *Micropterus salmoides* using ground fish flesh and freeze dried krill as starter diets. *Aquaculture* 148, 179–190.

Kubitza, F., Lovshin, L.L. and Lovell, R.T. (1997) Identification of feed enhancers for juvenile largemouth bass *Micropterus salmoides*. *Aquaculture* 148, 191–200.

Kurten, G. (1995) Comparison of two target phosphorus concentrations for fertilizing Florida largemouth bass spawning ponds. *The Progressive Fish-Culturist* 57, 277–286.

Kurten, G. (2001a) Evaluation of stocking, harvest and zooplankton variables in ponds for rearing Florida largemouth bass fingerlings. Management Data Series No. 195. Texas Parks and Wildlife Department, Austin, TX.

Kurten, G. (2001b) Evaluation of fertilization of Florida largemouth bass fingerling rearing ponds at the A.E. Wood fish hatchery: a baseline study. Management Data Series No.190. Texas Parks and Wildlife Department, Austin, TX.

Kurten, G., Hall, L. and Thomson, N. (1995) Comparison of cottonseed meal and alfalfa meal for fertilizing earthen largemouth bass spawning and rearing ponds. Management Data Series No. 113. Texas Parks and Wildlife Department, Austin, TX.

Kurten, G., Hall, L. and Thompson, N. (1996) Evaluation of a shorter pond filling-stocking interval to control fairy shrimp and clam shrimp densities in Florida largemouth bass rearing ponds. Management Data Series No.123. Texas Parks and Wildlife Department, Austin, TX.

Kurten, G., Hall, L. and Thompson, N. (1997) Comparison of two pond filling strategies to control fairy shrimp and clam shrimp in Florida largemouth bass fingerling rearing ponds. Management Data Series No.138, Texas Parks and Wildlife Department. Austin, TX.

Kurten, G., Hall, L. and Thompson, N. (1998) Evaluation of a 14 day pre-fertilization period to control fairy shrimp and clam shrimp in Florida largemouth bass fingerling rearing ponds. Management Data Series No.156. Texas Parks and Wildlife Department, Austin, TX.

Kurten, G., Hall, L. and Thompson, N. (1999) Evaluation of cottonseed meal supplementation of inorganically fertilized Florida largemouth bass spawning ponds. *North American Journal of Aquaculture* 61, 115–125.

Lampert, W., Fleckner, W., Rai, H. and Taylor, B.E. (1986) Phytoplankton control by grazing zooplankton: a study on the spring clear-water phase. *Limnology and Oceanography* 31, 478–490.

Lange, M.D. (2003) Methodologies to reduce mortalities due to *Flavobacterium columnare* during the feed-training and cage-culture of largemouth bass (*Micropterus salmoides*). Master's Thesis, Kentucky State University, Frankfort, KT.

Laurence, G.C. (1969) The energy expenditure of largemouth bass larvae, *Micropterus salmoides*, during yolk absorption. *Transactions of the American Fisheries Society* 98, 398–405.

Lorenzen, K. Beveridge, M.C.M. and Mangel, M. (2012). Cultured fish: integrative biology and management of domestication and interactions with wild fish. *Biological Reviews* 87, 639–660.

Lovshin, L.L. and Rushing, J.H. (1989) Acceptance by largemouth bass fingerlings of pelleted feeds with a gustatory additive. *The Progressive Fish Culturist* 51, 73–78.

Ludwig, G.M. (1999) *Zooplankton Succession and Larval Fish Culture in Freshwater Ponds*. Southern Regional Aquaculture Center (SRAC). SRAC Publication No. 700, Stoneville, MS.

Lydell, D. (1903) *The Habits and Culture of the Black Bass*. U.S. Fish Commission Bulletin for 1902, Government Printing Office, Washington, DC.

Lyon, D.D., Wyatt, T.A. and Pence, N.E. (2002) Reproductive performance of Florida largemouth bass at two sex ratios in indoor raceways. Management Data Series No. 205. Texas Parks and Wildlife Department, Austin, Texas.

Malison, J.A. and Held, J.A. (1996) Habituating pond-reared fingerlings to formulated feed. In: Summerfelt, R.C. (ed.) *Walleye Culture Manual*. North Central Regional Aquaculture Center (NCRAC), NCRAC Culture Series 101, Iowa State University, Ames, IA, pp. 199–204.

Martinez, J.G., Wyatt, T. and Kurten, G. (2005) Effect of inoculation and supplemental feeding of zooplankton on Florida largemouth bass (*Micropterus salmoides floridanus*) fingerling production in plastic-lined ponds. Management Data Series No. 237. Texas Parks and Wildlife Department, Austin, TX.

Matthews, M. (2009) Feed training juvenile largemouth bass *Micropterus salmoides floridanus* in intensive culture. American Fisheries Society, Fish Culture Section, Aquaculture Application Note #2, Bethesda, MD.

Matthews, M.D. (2015) Evaluating hatchery produced Florida largemouth bass *Micropterus salmoides floridanus* for fisheries management. Dissertation, University of Florida, Gainesville, FL.

Matthews, M.D. and Stout, R.B. (2013) Out-of-season spawning method for Florida largemouth bass to produce advanced-sized fingerlings by early spring. *North American Journal of Aquaculture* 75, 524–531.

Matthews, M.D., Bowker, J.D., Carty, D.G., Wandelear, N., Bowman, M.P., Sakmar, J.C. and Childress, K. (2013) Efficacy of Aquaflor (50% Florfenicol) – medicated feed to control mortality associated with *Flavobacterium columnare* infection in Florida largemouth bass and bluegill. *North American Journal of Aquaculture* 75, 385–392.

Mayes, K.B, Rosenblum, P.M. and Brandt, T.M. (1993) Raceway spawning of FLMB: effects of acclimation time and hormone treatment on spawning success. *The Progressive Fish-Culturist* 55, 1–8.

McCraren, J.P. (1975) Feeding young bass. *Farm Pond Harvest* 9, 10–12.

McCraren, J.P. and Phillips, T.R. (1977) Effects of Masoten (Dylox) on plankton in earthen ponds. *Proceedings of the Southeastern Association of Fish and Wildlife Agencies* 31, 441–448.

McCraren, J.P., Millard, J.L. and Woolven, A.M. (1977) Masoten (Dylox) as a control for clam shrimp in hatchery production ponds. *Proceedings of the Southeastern Association of Fish and Wildlife Agencies* 31, 329–331.

Middleton, R.J. and Reeder, B.C. (2003) Dissolved oxygen fluctuations in organically and inorganically fertilized walleye (*Stizostedion vitreum*) hatchery ponds. *Aquaculture* 219, 337–345.

Mischke, C.C. and Zimba, P.V. (2004) Plankton community responses in earthen channel catfish nursery ponds under various fertilization regimes. *Aquaculture* 233, 219–235.

Mittlebach, G.G. (1981) Foraging efficiency and body size: a study of optimal diet and habitat use by bluegills. *Ecology* 62 (5), 1370–1386.

Morris, J.E. and Clayton, R.D. (2009) Centrarchid aquaculture. In: Cooke, S.J. and Philipp, D.P. (eds) *Centrarchid Fishes: Diversity, Biology, and Conservation.* John Wiley and Sons, Chichester, pp. 293–311.

Morris, J.E. and Mischke, C.C. (1999) *Plankton Management for Fish Culture Ponds.* Technical Bulletin Series #114. Iowa State University, Ames, IA.

Nelson, J.T., Bowker, R.G. and Robinson, J.D. (1974) Rearing pellet-fed largemouth bass in a raceway. *The Progressive Fish-Culturist* 36, 108–110.

Nickum, J. (1986) Walleye. In: Stickney, R.R. (ed.) *Culture of Non-Salmonid Freshwater Fishes.* CRC Press, Boca Raton, FL, pp. 115–126.

Nishimura, K. and Hoshino, N. (1999) Evolution of cannibalism in the larval stage of pelagic fish. *Evolutionary Ecology* 13, 191–209.

Noriega-Curtis, P. (1979) Primary productivity and related fish yield in intensely manured fishponds. *Aquaculture* 17, 335–344.

O'Brien, W.J. (1979) The predator-prey interactions of planktivorous fish and zooplankton. *American Scientist* 67, 572–581.

Oliver, D.R. (1971) Life history of Chironomidae. *Annual Review of Entomology* 16, 211–230.

Olson, M.H. (1996) Ontogenetic niche shifts in largemouth bass: variability and consequences for first-year growth. *Ecology* 77 (1), 179–190.

Parmley, D., Alvarado, G. and Cortez, M. (1986) Food habits of small hatchery-reared Florida largemouth bass. *The Progressive Fish-Culturist* 48, 264–267.

Parmley, D. and Geiger, J.G. (1985) Succession patterns of zooplankton in fertilized culture ponds without fish. *The Progressive Fish-Culturist* 47, 183–186.

Pennak, R.W. (1978) Fresh-water Invertebrates of the United States, 2nd edition. John Wiley and Sons, New York, New York.

Petit, G., Beauchaud, M. and Buisson, B. (2001) Density effects on food intake and growth of largemouth bass (*Micropterus salmoides*). *Aquaculture Research* 32, 495–497.

Piper, R.G., McElwain, I.B., Orme, L.E., McCraren, J.P., Fowler, L.G. and Leonard, J.R. (1982) *Fish Hatchery Management.* United States Department of the Interior, Fish and Wildlife Service, Washington, D.C.

Porak, W.F., Johnson, W.E., Crawford, S., Renfro, D.J., Schoeb, T.R., Stout, R.B., Krause, R.A. and DeMauro, R.A. (2002) Factors effecting survival of largemouth bass raised on artificial diets and stocked into Florida lakes. In: Philipp, D.P. and Ridgway, M.S. (eds) *Black Bass: Ecology, Conservation, and Management.* American Fisheries Society, Bethesda, MD, pp. 649–665.

Seymour, E.A. (1980) The effects and control of algal blooms in fish ponds. *Aquaculture* 19, 55–74.

Simco, B.A., Williamson, J.H., Carmichael, G.J. and Tomasso, J.R. (1986) Centrarchids. In: Stickney, R.R. (ed.) *Culture of Non-Salmonid Freshwater Fishes*. CRC Press, Boca Raton, FL, pp. 73–89.

Skudlarek, N.A., Cochran, N.J., Larimore, M., Marple, S., Coyle, S. and Tidwell, J.H. (2007) Alternatives to freeze–dried krill in the feed training phase of largemouth bass. *North American Journal of Aquaculture* 69, 395–399.

Skudlarek, N., Coyle, S.D. and Tidwell, J.H. (2013) Development of first-feeding protocols for indoor larviculture of largemouth bass (*Micropterus salmoides*). *Journal of Applied Aquaculture* 25, 9–23.

Sloane, M.B. (1993) Performance of training and growout diets for Largemouth Bass. MS thesis, Auburn University, Auburn, AL.

Sloane, M.B. and Lovshin, L.L. (1995) Feed training and intensive production of advanced largemouth bass fingerlings: a review. *Reviews in Fisheries Science* 3 (1), 65–89.

Smith, D., Barkoh, A. and Stacell, M. (2000) Effects of plastic-lined pond sediments on production of Florida Largemouth Bass fingerlings. Management Data Series No. 168. Texas Parks and Wildlife Department. Austin, TX.

Snow, J.R. (1965) Results of further experiments on rearing largemouth bass fingerlings under controlled conditions. *Proceedings Southeastern Association Game and Fish Commissioners* 17, 191–203.

Snow, J.R. (1968a) The Oregon moist pellet as a diet for largemouth bass. *The Progressive Fish-Culturist* 30, 235.

Snow, J.R. (1968b) Production of six to eight-inch largemouth bass for special purposes. *The Progressive Fish-Culturist* 30, 144–152.

Snow, J.R. (1968c) Some progress in the controlled culture of largemouth bass, *Micropterus salmoides* (Lac.). *Proceedings Southeastern Association Game and Fish Commissioners* 22, 380–387.

Snow, J.R. (1970a) Culture of largemouth bass. Proceedings of the 1970 Workshop on Fish Feed Technology and Nutrition. *Resource Publication, U.S. Bureau Sportfish Wildlife* 102, 86–102.

Snow, J.R. (1970b) Fecundity of largemouth bass, *Micropterus salmoides* (Lacépède), receiving artificial food. *Proceedings Southeastern Association Game and Fish Commissioners* 24, 550–559.

Snow, J.R. (1971) Harvest and feeding habits of largemouth bass in Murphy Flowage, Wisconsin. Technical Bulletin No. 50, Wisconsin Department of Natural Resources, Madison, WI.

Snow, J.R. (1973) Controlled culture of largemouth bass fry. *Proceedings Southeastern Association Game and Fish Commissioners* 26, 392–398.

Snow, J.R. (1975) Hatchery propagation of the black basses. In: Clepper, H. (ed.) *Black Bass: Biology and Management*. Sport Fishing Institute, Washington, DC, pp. 344–356.

Snow, J.R. and Maxwell, J.I. (1970) Oregon moist pellet as a production ration for largemouth bass. *The Progressive Fish-Culturist* 32, 101–102.

Snow, J.R. and Wright, C.F. (1975) Rearing of largemouth bass fingerlings in cages. *Proceedings Southeastern Association of Game and Fish Commissioners* 29, 74–81.

Sommer, U. (1985) Comparison between steady state and non-steady state competition: experiments with natural phytoplankton. *Limnology and Oceanography* 30, 335–346.

Sorgeloos, P. (1980) The use of brine shrimp *Artemia* in aquaculture. In: Persoone, G., Sorgeloos, P., Roels, O. and Jaspers, E. (eds) *The Brine Shrimp Artemia, Vol. 3, Ecology, Culturing, Use in Aquaculture*. Universa Press, Wetteren, pp. 25–46.

Stickney, R.R. (1979) *Principles of Warmwater Aquaculture*. Wiley, New York.

Summerfelt, R.C., Clouse, C.P. and Harding, L.M. (1994) Pond production of fingerling walleye, *Stizostedion vitreum*, in the northern Great Plains. *Journal of Applied Aquaculture* 2, 33–58.

Swanson, R. (1982) Bass propagation at the Las Animas Fish Hatchery. In: Hutson, P.L. and Lillie, J. (eds) *Midwest Black Bass Culture*. Texas Parks and Wildlife Department, Austin, Texas and Kansas Fish and Game Commission, Pratt, KS, pp. 25–63.

Tidwell, J.H., Coyle, S.D. and Woods, T.A. (2000) *Species Profile Largemouth Bass*. Southern Regional Aquaculture Center (SRAC). SRAC Publication No. 722, Stoneville, MS.

Tidwell, J.H., Coyle, S.D., Bright, L.A., VanArnum, A. and Yasharian, D. (2003) Effect of water temperature on growth, survival and biochemical composition of largemouth bass (*Micropterus salmoides*). *Journal of the World Aquaculture Society* 34, 175–183.

Timmerman, C.M., Annett, C.A. and Bailey, C.F. (2000) Determination of factors limiting prey size swallowed by larval and small juvenile largemouth bass. *Transactions of the American Fisheries Society* 129, 618–622.

Turner, C.L. and Kraatz, W.C. (1921) Food of young large-mouth black bass in some Ohio waters. *Transactions of the American Fisheries Society* 50, 372–380.

Weatherley, A.H. and Gill, H.S. (1987) *The Biology of Fish Growth*. Academic Press, London.

Weaver, C.R. (1943) Observations on the life cycle of the fairy shrimp *Eubranchipus vernalis*. *Ecology* 24, 500–502.

Webster, C.D. and Lovell, R.T. (1990) Comparison of live brine shrimp nauplii and nonliving diets as first food for striped bass larvae. *The Progressive Fish-Culturist* 52, 171–175.

Wedemeyer, G. (2001) *Fish Hatchery Management*, second edition. American Fisheries Society, Bethesda, MD.

Welch, E.B. (1980) *Ecological Effects of Waste Water*. Cambridge University Press, New York.

Werner, E.E. and Hall, D.J. (1974) Optimal foraging and size selection of prey by the bluegill sunfish (*Lepomis macrochirus*). *Ecology* 55, 1042–1052.

Wetzel, R.G. (2001) *Limnology: Lake and River Ecosystems*, 3rd edn. Academic Press, New York.

Wickstrom, G.A. and Applegate, R.L. (1989) Growth and food selection of intensively cultured largemouth bass fry. *The Progressive Fish-Culturist* 51 (2), 79–82.

Williamson, J.H. (1981) Training northern largemouth bass fingerlings on OMP. *Proceedings of the Catfish Farmers American Research Workshop* 3, 68–69.

Williamson, J.H. (1983) Comparing training success of two strains of largemouth bass. *The Progressive Fish-Culturist* 45 (1), 3–7.

Williamson, J.H. and Carmichael, G.J. (1990) An aquacultural evaluation of Florida, northern, and hybrid largemouth bass, *Micropterus salmoides*. *Aquaculture* 85 (1–4), 247–257.

Williamson, J.H., Carmichael, G.J., Graves, K.G., Simco, B.A. and Tomasso, J.R. (1993) Centrarchids. In: Stickney, R.R. (ed.) *Culture of Non-Salmonid Freshwater Fishes*, 2nd edition. CRC Press, Boca Raton, FL, pp. 145–197.

Willis, D.W. and Flickinger, S.A. (1981) Intensive culture of largemouth bass fry. *Transactions of the American Fisheries Society* 110, 650–655.

Wright, L.D. (1970) Forage size preference of the largemouth bass. *The Progressive Fish-Culturist* 32, 39–42.

Wyatt, T., Hall, L. and Thompson, N. (2000) Effects of hydrated lime and agricultural lime on water quality, zooplankton density, and Florida largemouth bass fingerling production in earthen ponds. Final Report, Texas Parks and Wildlife Department, Austin, TX.

Young, C.H. and Flickinger, S.A. (1989) Zooplankton production and pond fertilization for largemouth bass fingerling production. *Proceedings of the Annual Conference Southeastern Association of Fish and Wildlife Agencies* 42, 66–73.

CHAPTER 7

Culture methods

James H. Tidwell

Kentucky State University, Aquaculture Research Center, Frankfort, Kentucky, USA

7.1 First-year ponds

As noted previously, the primary focus of this book is a review of the culture of the largemouth bass as a food-fish. However, food-fish culture evolved out of production of sport-fish for stocking. Because of this, production methods so far remain largely the same during the early stages. Largemouth bass require two growing seasons to reach food-fish target sizes (≥ 0.5 kg). Production of largemouth bass as food-fish can be broken up into five phases including a hatching phase, a nursery phase (when fingerlings feed on zooplankton), a feed-training phase, then first-year growth and second-year growth. The first phase (fry) is covered in Chapter 5. Nursery and feed-training are the subject of Chapter 6. This chapter will review production procedures after the fish are trained to accept artificial diets.

After the initial feed-training period, fingerlings are usually graded to ensure non-feeders are separated out and that fingerlings stocked together are as uniform in size as possible. This helps to reduce the likelihood of cannibalism and possibly improves overall growth, as larger fish can dominate feeding areas. Research has suggested that feed-trained fingerlings of 4–5 cm can be stocked into prepared ponds at 50,000–75,000/ha (Tidwell et al., 2000). Some producers add an intermediate step to "reinforce" feed-training during the transition from feed-training to tanks to ponds (Heidinger, 2000). One option for this is a short period (2–4 weeks) in small ponds (0.01 ha) at very high densities (250,000 fish/ha) with frequent feedings. Another method is to cordon off a section of the first-year production pond using a seine as a block-net. All of the fish are confined within this area for several weeks until actively feeding. Water quality, especially dissolved oxygen, must be closely monitored during these high-density periods.

Once fish are released into the open pond for first-year growth, they are fed high-protein, low-carbohydrate, floating diets two to three times per day (see Chapters 8 and 9). Fish are fed to apparent satiation at each feeding. Feed response will vary based on environmental changes such as sunlight, water temperature, and/or changes in other water quality variables. If feeding response is reduced for several consecutive days without obvious external factors such as weather changes, the producer should suspect and monitor for water quality problems and/or disease onset.

Fish spawned in the spring, feed-trained in tanks, then cultured in ponds should reach 15–20 cm by the fall of this first year. Fish that do not reach a minimum size of 20 cm can be marketed for sport-fish stocking at this stage and this is a significant market outlet. If fish are to be grown on to food-fish sizes (> 0.5 kg), a second growing season will be required.

Kubitza and Lovshin (1997) evaluated various stocking densities for the production of advanced juvenile (100–200 g) largemouth bass during the first summer growing season. largemouth bass fingerlings were feed trained from May to June and stocked into ponds at various densities as they became available. The study evaluated a range of stocking densities from 17,000 fish/ha to 67,136 fish/ha. At harvest, average weights were generally higher (202–225 g) for largemouth bass fingerlings stocked at densities of 17,000 to 18,680 fish/ha. Medium densities of 20,533 to 34,124 fish/ha resulted in 184 to 189 g fish, while higher densities of 39,016 to 67,136 fish/ha resulted in smaller fish ranging from 85 to 130 g. Fish stocked at the lower densities also grew considerably faster (1.36–1.56 g/d) than the medium (0.87–1.18 g/d) and the high density (0.68–0.95 g/d). Gross yield was generally less for fish stocked at the lower densities (2,743–3,219 kg/ha) than for the medium (4,050–5,007 kg/ha) and high densities (3,832–7,281 kg/ha). The authors suggested stocking densities of 15,000 to 20,000 fish/ha to maximize average weight gain of first-year largemouth bass and achieve fingerling sizes needed for second-year growth to food-fish sizes. The authors reported that the feeding response of first-year largemouth bass during summer was noticeably higher in the early morning compared to evening feedings, especially when evening water temperatures exceeded 30°C.

Experience and collaboration with commercial producers suggests that lower stocking densities produce more predictable outcomes with fewer incidences of water-quality problems and disease outbreaks (personal communication, Robert Mayer, Kentucky). Following a 15–20 d period of high-density (110,000 fish/ha) feed-training-reinforcement, producers typically stock first year ponds at 26,000–34,000 fish/ha based on the availability of pond space and the number of surviving feed-trained fingerlings. These stocking densities are considerably lower than recommended in much of the research literature. This is largely based on the need to produce market-size fish of > 568 g by the end of the second summer growing season. This minimum market size is not based on the average weight of the group, but on the smallest fish in the group. Buyers do not want fish in the load that are smaller than what they consider marketable size. Owing to inevitable size variability, the average harvest size may be > 600 g to ensure that the smallest fish in a group are > 568 g at the end of the second growing season. This requires that largemouth bass fingerlings attain a minimum size of 20 cm (approximately 150 g) and preferably 25 cm (> 200 g) by the end of first-year growth.

Stocking densities can also be based on assumed maximum carrying capacities, which are dependent on farm infrastructure, acceptable risk, and producer experience. If management determines that 5,600 kg/ha is the targeted maximum carrying capacity for that farm, then stocking densities can be back calculated. For example, for a 5,600 kg/ha carrying capacity, a first-year fingerling target size of 250 g, and an assumed survival of 100%, then the appropriate stocking density would be 22,400 fish/ha. If a 90% survival is assumed, the density would be 24,800 fish/ha.

Another variable that needs to be considered is the length of the local growing season, or the number of days in which the water temperature is above 18°C. Largemouth bass are considered warmwater fish, with optimal water temperatures for growth of 26–28°C. However, largemouth bass will actively feed at water temperatures > 18°C. In Kentucky, these conditions (water temperatures > 18°C) exist May through October, or approximately 160 d. The spawning season for largemouth bass in the region is usually early May. This means that the locally produced feed-trained fingerlings are not available until the second week in July (based on one week of egg incubation, a 4–6 week nursery period, and 2 weeks of feed training). As a result, most largemouth bass producers in the central and north central USA purchase feed-trained fingerlings from more southerly states with earlier spawning seasons. This functionally extends the local growing season, producing a larger first-year fingerling.

7.2 Second-year ponds

As discussed, to reach a final target size of > 0.5 kg largemouth bass in temperate zone ponds requires at least a second year of growth. First year fish can be thinned to grow-out densities either in the fall or spring. For second-year growout densities, Heidinger (2000) recommended a density of 4,950 fish/ha. However, Tidwell et al. (1998a) reported no significant differences in the average harvest weight or survival during second-year growout of largemouth bass fingerlings stocked at either 6,175 or 12,350 fish/ha. In that trial, Tidwell et al. (1998a) followed fish stocked in their second summer at two densities for a full 13 month period (May–May). Fish were fed a 44% protein diet once daily to satiation. In terms of water quality, overall means for total ammonia-nitrogen, nitrite-nitrogen, and un-ionized ammonia did not differ between ponds stocked at the different densities. Survival also did not differ among fish stocked at the two densities and averaged 93%, overall. At harvest, there were no significant differences in weight gain or average weight (Table 7.1). In other better studied culture species, a higher stocking density usually results in smaller harvest weights (Tucker and Robinson, 1991).

Total yield was greater for largemouth bass stocked at 12,350/ha than at 6,175/ha (4,598 kg/ha and 2,354 kg/ha, respectively). Also, at the higher stocking density feed was more efficiently utilized, as indicated by a lower feed conversion ratio (FCR) (2.3) compared to the low stocking

Table 7.1 Initial individual weight (mean ± SE), final individual weight, final lengths, percentage, survival, average individual gain, total yield, and feed conversion ratio (FCR) for largemouth bass fed prepared diets for one year in ponds. Means within a row followed by the different letters are significantly different ($P \leq 0.05$).

	Stocking rate (fish/ha)	
	6,175/ha	12,350/ha
Stocking weight (g)	124 ± 4	122 ± 2
Final weight (g)	406 ± 32	406 ± 22
Weight gain (%)	282 ± 29	283 ± 23
Final length (cm)	29.3 ± 0.8	29.1 ± 0.5
Survival (%)	93.9 ± 8.5	91.7 ± 6.7
Total yield (kg/ha)	2,354 ± 242b	4,598 ± 418a
FCR	3.3 ± 0.3a	2.3 ± 0.2b

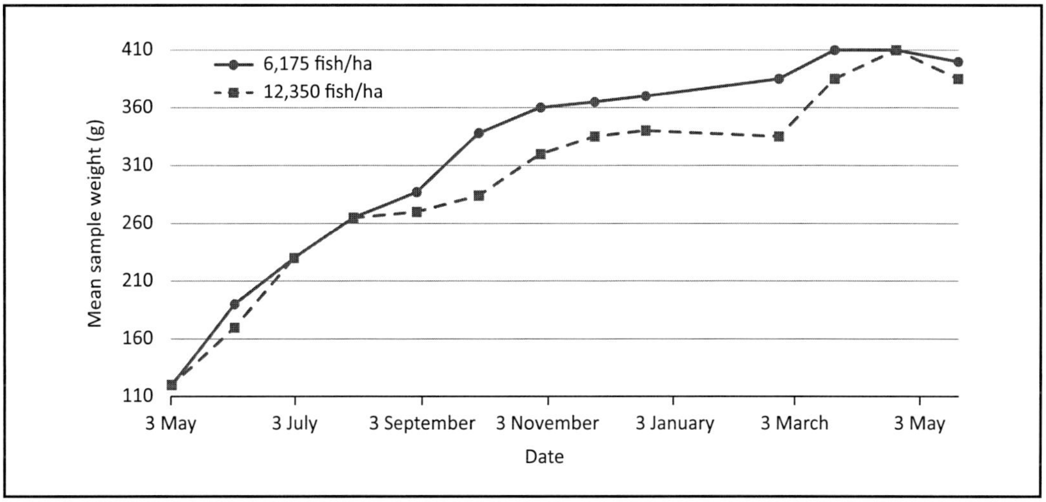

Figure 7.1 Mean sample weights of largemouth bass stocked at 6,175 or 12,350 fish/ha during second-year growth in ponds. There were no significant differences ($P > 0.05$) in average weights at any sampling date.

density (3.3) (Table 7.1) Again, these results differ from the better studied channel catfish, where higher stocking densities usually result in higher FCRs due to reduced feed intake, reduced availability of natural food items, and decreased efficiency of feed conversion (Tucker and Robinson, 1991).

Tidwell et al. (1996) had previously reported that the most active feeding period for largemouth bass during second-year growth was June–July (water temperatures > 25°C). However, in Tidwell et al. (1998b) the fish stocked at the lower density gained weight more rapidly in fall months during the period of declining water temperatures (September–November), while those stocked at the higher density gained weight more rapidly during the rising water temperatures of spring (March–May) (Figure 7.1). However, at final harvest, average weights of fish in the two treatments was similar.

Stocking largemouth bass juveniles at the higher density (12,350/ha) resulted in higher net and gross yields, and more efficient feed conversion than stocking at the low density. The average standing crop at harvest of largemouth bass stocked at 12,350/ha (4,600 kg/ha) in Tidwell et al. (1998b) was comparable to yields reported in channel catfish culture (Busch, 1985) (4,000–6,000 kg/ha). Optimal stocking density is normally a compromise between higher total unit production rates (kilograms per hectare), offset by reduced individual growth of higher densities, and deterioration of water quality at higher densities (Tucker and Robinson, 1991). In Tidwell et al. (1998a) measured water quality variables were not significantly impacted, and average fish size and survival at harvest were not reduced at the higher stocking density and the FCR was actually improved. These factors may indicate that the optimal stocking density for largemouth bass growout may be greater than 12,350/ha.

Engle et al. (2013) evaluated three largemouth bass stocking densities over a 2 year period. These included the same stocking densities of 6,175 and 12,350 fish/ha as Tidwell et al. (1998a) plus a higher density of 18,525 fish/ha. The study was stocked in late October with first-year largemouth bass fingerlings averaging 57 g. Mean weight after the second summer of production ranged from 426 to 515 g. Largemouth bass growth differed significantly among densities, with the low density having the highest growth rate and the high density the lowest growth. The medium density (12,350 fish/ha) was similar in production to the low-density treatment (6,175 fish/ha), supporting the findings of Tidwell et al. (1998a). FCR was significantly higher for the low density as compared to the medium and high densities. The optimum temperature for maximum feeding of largemouth bass ranged from 27 to 30°C in Engle et al. (2013), which was higher than the optimal temperatures of 25 to 28°C previously reported (Kubitza and Lovshin, 1997; Nelson et al., 1974).

In an earlier study, Kubitza and Lovshin (1997) evaluated largemouth bass (mean = 62.4 g) stocked at densities of 2,470 and 7,410 fish/ha during the second summer growing season. Growth rate and final weight for second-year largemouth bass were 1.47 g/d and 370 g, respectively, at the low stocking density, and 1.16 g/d and 307 g at the high stocking density. Gross yield was 738 kg/ha at the low stocking density and 1,742 kg/ha at the higher density. FCR and survival rates were similar and averaged 1.5 and 78% overall. The authors reported daily feed consumption increased rapidly during April and May as the water temperatures reached > 18°C, but dropped slightly and remained relatively constant during periods when afternoon water temperatures exceeded 29°C. The authors reported an increase in daily feed consumption in September in response to decreasing water temperatures followed by a decline as water temperatures dropped below 25°C. These results differ from Tidwell et al. (1998b) and Engle et al. (2013), suggesting a density effect on growth rates of largemouth bass even at relatively low stocking densities.

When discussing appropriate stocking densities, it is also important to consider the desired target weight at harvest. It is particularly problematic to compare and make suggestions related to stocking density if the fish do not reach market size. Even though there was no significant difference in average weight between largemouth bass stocked at the two densities of 6,175 of 12,350 fish/ha by Tidwell et al. (1998a) and Engle et al. (2013); the fish in neither study reached the current target market size for food-fish (568 g) after two summer growing seasons. Second-year largemouth bass in Kubitza and Lovshin (1997) study only reached 307–370 g. The reason the fish in these studies did not attain market size is likely because the 1 year-old largemouth bass stocked were too small (Kubitza and Lovshin, 1997, 62.4 g; Tidwell et al., 1998a, 122.1 g; Engle et al., 2013, 57 g). Cochran et al. (2009) achieved average weights of 516 to 546 g for second-year using fingerlings stocked at 210 g.

Under commercial culture conditions it is common for a small percentage of the fish (10–20%) to not reach the target size of 568 g following the second summer growout. Producers have to grade off those smaller fish and either stock them into a separate pond for continued growth during the third year or sell them into the recreational sport-fish market. This situation creates an inherent advantage for large farms which supply largemouth bass into both the food-fish and sport-fish markets.

Commercial producers commonly stock second-year largemouth bass at densities of 6,600 to 9,600 fish/ha to achieve a final weight of 600 g, reduce the numbers of undersized fish, and lower biomass densities (personal communication, Robert Mayer, Kentucky). For example, using an assumed 90% survival and a 600 g average weight this equates to biomass densities at harvest of 3,565 kg/ha and 5,185 kg/ha, respectively, for fish stocked at 6,600 and

9,600 fish/ha, respectively. These are reasonable biomass densities for largemouth bass produced in aerated ponds.

7.3 Third-year ponds

While largemouth bass can achieve target sizes of 0.7–1.1 kg in a second year of pond growout, there are markets that desire even larger fish. These include food-fish markets but also corrective pond stocking and trophy sport-fish ponds. Tidwell et al. (1998b) evaluated the effect of stocking density on third-year growth of largemouth bass in ponds.

The pattern of weight gain during third year growth (Figure 7.2) differed from that reported during second-year growth. The primary difference was during the period of August to November. In second-year fish, those stocked at the lower density gained more weight, while in third-year fish those stocked at the higher density gained more weight. Since increased density did not reduce average fish size, treatment densities resulted in large differences in total biomass densities with the high-density treatment producing significantly greater total yields.

The differences in feed conversions in ponds stocked at different densities were large (9.6 and 3.8 in low- and high-density ponds, respectively). The FCR for third-year bass at high density (3.8) was much higher than reported for second-year bass at high density (2.3; Tidwell et al., 1998a). This agrees with Lovell (1989) who stated that growth rate and feed conversion efficiencies generally decrease as fish sizes increase. In terms of fish growth, while density did not have a significant impact, overall growth was slow averaging 154 g of absolute growth and only 41% weight gain over the period of third-year growth.

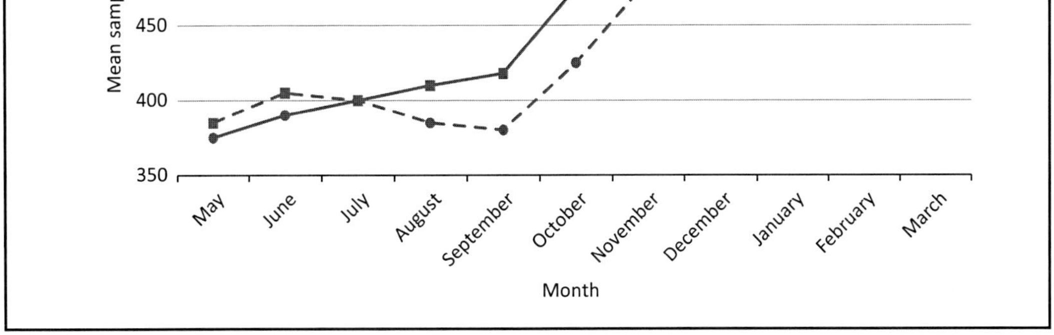

Figure 7.2 Mean sample weights of largemouth bass stocked at 3,750 and 7,500 fish/ha during third-year growth in ponds. There were no significant differences ($P > 0.05$) in average weights at any sampling date.

Engle et al. (2013) evaluated the production performance of largemouth bass stocked at three stocking densities during their third year of growth. Stocking densities of 6,175, 12,350 and 18,525 fish/ha were evaluated over a period of 2 years. Gross yields were significantly greater at higher densities, achieving 9,096 kg/ha at the highest density. Average harvest weight was lower at the high stocking density and ranged from 744 to 896 g. Third-year growth rates in Engle et al. (2013) ranged from 0.8 to 1.0 g/d, which were considerably better than growth rates reported for third-year largemouth bass by Tidwell et al. (1998a) of 0.40 and 0.52 g/d for largemouth bass stocked at densities of 3,750 and 7,500 fish/ha, respectively. There was no significant difference in survival rates among the three densities which averaged 70% overall. The FCR was significantly greater for the low density (3.6) as compared to the medium and high densities, which both averaged 2.5.

Engle et al. (2013) reported gross yields of 9,096 kg/ha and 65% survival for largemouth bass stocked at 18,525 fish/ha after three growing seasons. This reported yield and stocking densities are higher than other previous reports (Tidwell et al., 1998b) and are higher than those commonly used on commercial farms. The focus of the research of Engle et al. (2013) was to evaluate the potential for largemouth bass to be produced for a fillet market and the authors reported the lowest breakeven price was at the medium stocking density (US$7.26/kg) due to better feed conversion efficiency compared to the lowest density (US$9.34/kg) and larger average weights and slightly better survival compared to the highest density (US$7.61/kg).

It is important to evaluate the economic risks associated with intensive pond culture of largemouth bass, as the production costs and value are both high compared to many other commonly cultured food-fish. Ultimately management decisions such as intensification level are site based decisions related to acceptable risk as determined by the operator.

7.4 Recycle systems

Pond culture of finfish, although generally considered the most economical approach to fish production, requires significant land, labor, and water resources, has a greater range of potential environmental impacts and harvest is highly vulnerable to weather (Tucker and Hargreaves, 2012). Considering the relative high value of largemouth bass it might be possible and economically advantageous to intensify and better control largemouth bass production by culturing the fish indoors in temperature-controlled tanks; however, very little research has been conducted on rearing largemouth bass indoors. Indoor controlled environment production using recirculating aquaculture system (RAS) technologies could potentially reduce the growout period by maintaining ideal temperatures year-round and "eliminating" winter.

Widespread usage of RAS technology has not yet been adopted. In the 2013, USDA census of aquaculture, farmers reported that 35.8% of the total value of US aquaculture products was raised in ponds compared to only 8.7% for RAS systems (USDA, 2014). However, RAS systems allow for year-round production with consistent volumes of product throughout the year as compared to seasonal availability and slow winter growth, which are a characteristic of pond production. Recirculating technologies can also allow for greater economies of scale with higher production per unit area, production per unit water volume, and per unit worker than ponds (Ebeling and Timmons, 2012).

To achieve financial feasibility, RAS systems require high stocking densities per unit of volume. In pond culture of largemouth bass the maximum harvest density reported is equivalent to approximately 0.5–0.91 kg/m^3 (5,000–9,100 kg/ha, Tidwell et al., 1996; Engle et al., 2013) whereas reported maximum densities for species well suited to high-density culture in RAS, such as tilapia (*Oreochromis* sp.), are 50–100 kg/m^3 (Ebeling and Timmons, 2012). High population densities are known to affect fish health, food intake, and growth (Petit et al., 2001). Fish living in crowded conditions can become stressed from altered social interactions, restrictions of their ability to move freely or to otherwise behave normally (Wedemeyer, 1996). Baker and Ayles (1990) reported that the level of antagonistic interaction between cohorts of arctic charr (*Salvelinus alpines*) and rainbow trout (*Oncorhynchus mykiss*) changed with changes in stocking density.

No previous published studies were found evaluating growout of largemouth bass to food-fish sizes in RAS. The determination of appropriate stocking densities is the logical first step in determining the species suitability to RAS production. Watts et al. (2016) conducted a study to compare the growth, feed conversion, and survival of 1 year-old largemouth bass during second-year growth stocked at three different densities in an RAS. Largemouth bass fingerlings (112.0 ± 38.0 g) were randomly stocked into nine 900 l tanks to achieve densities of 30, 60, or 120 fish/m^3 with three replicate tanks per density. The RAS consisted of a 3,000 l sump, 0.25 hp pump, bead filter for solids removal, mixed-moving-bed biofilter for nitrification and a 400 W UV light for sterilization. Fish were fed a commercially available floating diet (45% protein and 16% lipid) once daily to apparent satiation. At harvest all fish were counted, individually weighed, and measured.

Harvest data indicated that biomass densities significantly increased with stocking rate achieving 6.2 kg/m^3 at 30 fish/m^3, 13.2 kg/m^3 at 60 fish/m^3, and 22.9 kg/m^3 at 120 fish/m^3 (Table 7.2). The stocking densities evaluated in this trial had no significant impact ($P > 0.05$) on survival, average harvest weight, uniformity index (UI_{10}, Bell, 2002) or FCR, which averaged 93%, 294 g, 26.2 and 1.8, respectively (Table 7.2).

Although survival and feed conversion were acceptable, after 6 months of culture the largemouth bass did not achieve target sizes of 500 g, which is considered a marketable-size in most

Table 7.2 Means (± SD) of average harvest weight (AHW) (g), minimum/maximum of individual harvest weight (g), total production (kg/m^3), survival (%), feed conversion ratio (FCR), percent weight gain (% wt gn), and uniformity index$_{10}$ (%) of largemouth bass raised in tanks at three densities and fed a commercially available extruded pellet diet.[a]

	30/m^3	60/m^3	120/m^3
AHW (g)	301.3 ± 31.9^a	298.7 ± 20.1^a	283.5 ± 17.5^a
Min/max (g)	151/492	124/556	108/598
Total production (kg/m^3)	7.6 ± 1.0^c	16.4 ± 1.1^b	28.2 ± 3.9^a
Surv (%)	90.7 ± 4.6^a	98.7 ± 2.3^a	89.3 ± 7.1^a
FCR[b]	2.0 ± 0.3^a	1.6 ± 0.1^a	1.7 ± 0.3^a
% wt gn[c]	269.0 ± 28.5^a	266.7 ± 17.9^a	253.1 ± 15.6^a
UI_{10} (%)[d]	25.1 ± 5.9	27.1 ± 2.7	26.5 ± 8.8

Notes: [a]Values within columns within trials followed by different superscripts are significantly different ($P \leq 0.05$). [b]FCR = g dry feed fed/g wet weight gain. [c]Percentage weight gain (% wt gn) = (average harvest weight (g)/ average stock weight (g)) × 100. [d]UI_{10} (%) = (n_{10}/N) × 100, where n_{10} is fish number (frequency) between "mean × 0.9" and "mean × 1.1" and N is total fish number measured.

food-fish marketplace. It appears that intraspecific competition within tanks resulted in increased size variation as densities increased. The UI_{10} for body weight was 25 at 30/m^3, 27 at 60/m^3, and 27 at 120/m^3. Observations indicate that each tank had one or two fish that did achieve market size, but the remainder of the population did not. The size ranges are illustrated by minimum and maximum sizes (min/max) (Table 7.2) and again increase as densities increased, although average weights did not differ significantly. Smaller fish were observed to often show signs of tail biting and bullying from cohorts.

Petit et al. (2001) compared juvenile largemouth bass growth and size variation in aquaria stocked at different densities. The authors evaluated initial biomass densities of 1, 2, and 3 kg/m^3 compared to the initial biomass densities of 2.6, 5.1, and 10.2 kg/m^3 evaluated in this trial. In agreement with the current study, they reported no differences in average weight although the coefficients of variation (CV) of weight increased with stocking densities. Increases in the CV for weight within a population are known to be indicative of the establishment of hierarchies which can suppress the growth of cohorts (Brett, 1979). Petit et al. (2001) also observed antagonism during feeding, reporting that one or a few fish ate first and that dominant fish ate more than the others. The authors fed a sinking feed once per day and reported that their feeding method may have influenced antagonism and weight variability.

Extruded floating pellets are typically used in commercial production of largemouth bass in ponds as it allows the farmer to see how much, and how actively, the fish eat. However, it may be beneficial to feed a slow sinking pellet to largemouth bass in RAS to reduce the ability of a few fish to prevent others from access to feed on the water surface. Perhaps multiple daily feedings would allow more aggressive individuals to become satiated reducing antagonism during subsequent feedings.

Development of genetic strains of largemouth bass better suited for high-density tank culture would likely also be beneficial. Production in RAS would allow the largemouth bass to be produced in closer proximity to their primary markets (Toronto, New York) reducing transport stress and the subsequent negative impacts on survival in these live markets.

Other production systems are successfully utilized in China, such as net-pens in lakes and reservoirs. These are reviewed in Chapter 3.

For fish cultured in high-density environments such as tanks and raceways, different species have different tolerances in terms of crowding. Fish densities can be based on water quality and water flow. In raceway culture, a "flow index" is determined based on species and size and flow rate (Fornshell et al., 2012). However, some species require a certain amount of "personal space", independent of water quality. In raceway systems an independent index determined for different species termed a density index looks at the effect of the physical proximity of individual fish. The largemouth bass, as a top-level carnivore, may be a species which does not tolerate physical crowding well.

As part of evaluating largemouth bass for culture in tank-based systems, Park et al. (2015) conducted two trials. In the first trial, experimental treatments were based on initial biomass densities of 15, 20, 25, 30, 35, and 40 kg/m^3. Tanks were 190 l (18 tanks), 9 g fish were stocked, and these densities equated to 300, 400, 500, 600, 700, and 800 fish per tank. Fish were fed a diet containing 45% protein and 15% lipid twice daily for 60 days. Results were based on survival, growth, and feed conversion. However, size variability was also important as cannibalism on small cohorts could be a problem.

At harvest, survival was good in all treatments (95–97%) as were feed conversions (0.96–1.13). CV for individual growth measures did not indicate greater size variability among the different density treatments.

A subsequent study was conducted by the same research group to approximate the maximum yield and final size distribution patterns in stocker size largemouth bass (Park et al., 2017). Fingerling largemouth bass (37 g) were stocked into 165 l tanks (18 tanks) at 4.5, 9.1, 18.8, 36.5, 54.6, and 73 kg/m^3 (three replicates of each). This equated to 22, 44, 88, 176, 264, and 352 fish per tank. Fish were fed the same diet (46/16) twice daily for 60 d.

At harvest, survivals ranged from 82–97%, specific growth rate from 1.16 to 1.45%/day, final weights of 64–75 g, and FCR from 1.00 to 1.45. Best results were achieved in tanks with initial stocking rates of 18–36 kg/m^3. It was determined that a maximum yield of approximately 70 kg/m^3 was achievable for largemouth bass of this size.

There is some commercial production of largemouth bass advanced fingerlings in RAS to supply growout ponds with one year old fish. A producer in Kentucky is using reconditioned hog barns for largemouth bass advanced fingerling production and growing largemouth bass food-fish in renovated manure or lagoon ponds. This system has the advantage of requiring fewer ponds and provides the advantage of year-round feeding of first-year fish ensuring that they reach > 200 g during the first year.

7.5 Conclusion

Although the largemouth bass has been cultured for over 100 years, most of the production methods used today in the USA are derived from pond methods used to raise small fingerlings for sport-fish stocking. These systems have not changed radically and neither have the fish. There is increasing interest and activity in producing the largemouth bass in other types of production systems. This will likely require that genetic lines of largemouth bass be developed which are selected and adapted for more intensive culture conditions. In China (Chapter 3) the fish is widely produced in cages and net-pen systems and there are genetically improved strains being developed and utilized.

References

Baker, R.F. and Ayles, G.B. (1990) The effects of varying density and loading level on the growth of Arctic charr (*Salvelinus alpinus* L.) and rainbow trout (*Oncorhynchus mykiss*). *World Aquaculture* 21 (1), 58–62.

Bell, D.D. (2002) Cage management for layers. In: Bell, D.D. and Weaver, W.D. (eds) *Commercial Chicken Meat and Egg Production*. Springer, Boston, MA, pp. 1007–1040.

Brett, J.R. (1979) Environmental factors in growth. In: Hoar, W.S., Randall, D.J. and Brett, J.R. (eds) *Fish Physiology* Vol. III. Academic Press, New York, pp. 599–675.

Busch, R.L. (1985) Channel catfish culture in ponds. In: Tucker, C.S. (ed.) *Channel Catfish Culture*. Elsevier Science, Amsterdam, pp. 13–84.

Cochran, N.J. Coyle, S.D. and Tidwell, J.H. (2009) Evaluation of reduced fish meal diets for second year growout of the largemouth bass, *Micropterus salmoides. Journal of the World Aquaculture Society* 40, 735–743.

Ebeling, J.M. and Timmons, M.B. (2012) Recirculating aquaculture systems. In: Tidwell, J.H. (ed.) *Aquaculture Production Systems*. Wiley-Blackwell, Ames, IA, pp. 245–277.

Engle, C.R., Stone, N. and Xie, L. (2013) Feasibility of pond production of largemouth bass, *Micropterus salmoides*, for the filet market. *Journal of the World Aquaculture Society* 44, 805–813.

Fornshell, G., Hinshaw, J. and Tidwell, J.H. (2012) Flow-through raceways. In: Tidwell, J.H. (ed.) *Aquaculture Production Systems*. Wiley-Blackwell, Ames, IA, pp. 173–190.

Heidinger, R. (2000) Black bass/largemouth bass culture. In: Stickney, R.R. (ed.) *Encyclopedia of Aquaculture*. Wiley-Interscience Publication, New York, pp. 108–117.

Kubitza, F. and Lovshin L.L. (1997) Pond production of pellet-fed advanced juvenile and food-size largemouth bass. *Aquaculture* 149, 253–262.

Lovell, R.T. (1989) *Nutrition and Feeding of Fish*. Van Nostrand Reinhold, New York.

Nelson, J.T., Bowker, R.G. and Robinson, J.D. (1974) Rearing pellet fed largemouth bass in a raceway. *Progressive Fish Culturist* 36, 108–110.

Park, J., Renukdas, N., Luna, T. and Roy, L.A. (2015) The effects of biomass density on size variability and growth performance of juvenile largemouth bass, *Micropterus salmoides*, in a semi-closed recirculating system. *Journal of the World Aquaculture Society* 46 (3), 283–291.

Park, J., Renukdas, N., Luna, T. and Roy, L.A. (2017) Maximum yield approximation and size distribution patterns of stocker size largemouth bass, *Micropterus salmoides* reared in a semi-closed indoor system. *Aquaculture Research* 48 (3), 780–791.

Petit, G., Beauchaud, M. and Buisson, B. (2001) Density effects on food intake and growth of largemouth bass (*Micropterus salmoides*). *Aquaculture Research* 32, 495–497.

Tidwell, J.H., Webster, C.D. and Coyle, S.D. (1996) Effects of dietary protein level on second year growth and water quality for largemouth bass (*Micropterus salmoides*), raised in ponds. *Aquaculture* 145, 213–223.

Tidwell, J.H., Coyle, S.D. and Webster, C.D. (1998a) Effects of stocking density on third-year growth of largemouth bass, *Micropterus salmoides*, fed prepared diets in ponds. *Journal of Applied Aquaculture* 8, 39–45.

Tidwell, J.H., Webster, C.D., Coyle, S.D. and Schulmeister, G. (1998b) Effect of stocking density on growth and water quality for largemouth bass *Micropterus salmoides* growout in ponds. *Journal of the World Aquaculture Society* 29, 79–83.

Tidwell, J.H., Coyle, S.D. and Woods, T.A. (2000) Species profile-largemouth bass. Publication Number 732, Southern Regional Aquaculture Center, Stoneville, Mississippi, USA.

Tucker, C. and Hargreaves, J. (2012) Ponds. In: Tidwell, J. H. (ed.) *Aquaculture Production Systems*. Wiley-Blackwell, Ames, IA, pp. 191–244.

Tucker, C.S. and Robinson, E.H. (1991) *Channel Catfish Farming Handbook*. Chapman and Hall, New York.

USDA (United States Department of Agriculture) (2014) National Agriculture Statistics Service, 2013 Census of Agriculture. USDA, Washington, DC.

Wedemeyer, G. (1996) *Physiology of Fish in Intensive Culture Systems*. Springer Science, New York.

Watts, C.T., Bright, L.A., Coyle, S.D. and Tidwell, J.H. (2016) Evaluation of stocking density during second year growth of largemouth bass, *Micropterus salmoides*, raised in a recirculating aquaculture system. *Journal of the World Aquaculture Society* 47 (4), 538–543.

CHAPTER 8

Largemouth bass nutrition

Waldemar Rossi Jr. and Habte-Michael Habte-Tsion

Aquaculture Research Center, Kentucky State University, Frankfort, Kentucky, USA

8.1 Introduction

Perhaps the first study on the nutritional requirements of largemouth bass (*Micropterus salmoides* L.), using formulated diets, was published by Anderson et al. (1981). These authors used semi-purified diets to evaluate the protein requirements of largemouth bass at ages 0 (~2 g) and one (~6 g). Although the importance of the knowledge on nutritional requirements for the expansion of largemouth bass production in the United States has been recognized since the 1980s (JSA, 1984), the first summary report on the subject was not published until almost 20 years later (Tidwell et al., 2002). Even then, only limited information was available regarding the nutritional requirements of the species. Today, because of increased interest on the production of food-size fish in North America and Asia, and the global need to optimize cost-effective feed formulations for maximum production performance and minimum nutrient output to the environment, more is known about the nutritional requirements of largemouth bass. However, much work lies ahead.

This chapter will summarize information on known nutritional requirements of largemouth bass, as well as raw material utilization and nutritional value, and feed additives. A brief discussion on recent findings from immunonutrition and nutrigenomics studies is also included.

8.2 Digestive tract

The digestive tract of largemouth bass can be divided into mouth, buccal cavity, esophagus, stomach, anterior and posterior intestine, and rectum. Auxiliary digestive organs include the liver, gallbladder, and distinct pancreas. Pyloric caeca are also present and can contain more than 20 digitiform tubules opening into the anterior intestine immediately posterior to the pyloric constriction of the stomach (Sarbahi, 1951) (Figure 8.1). As a general characteristic of predatory fish species, the digestive tract of largemouth bass is short, extending only slightly beyond

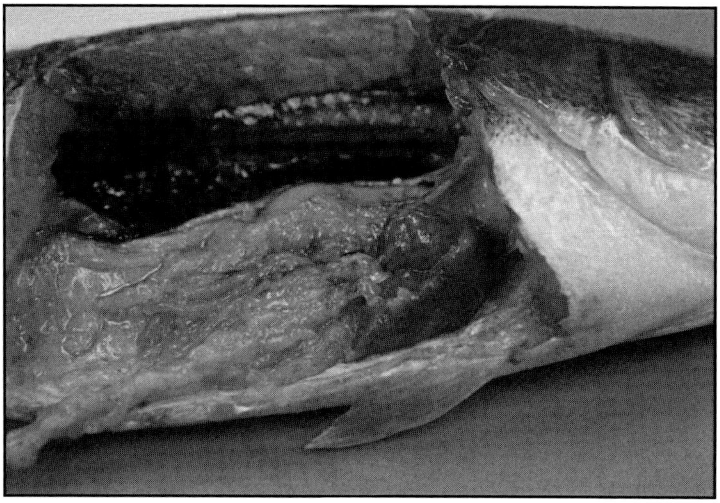

Figure 8.1 Dissection of largemouth bass intraperitoneal cavity showing the gallbladder, liver, and caeca.

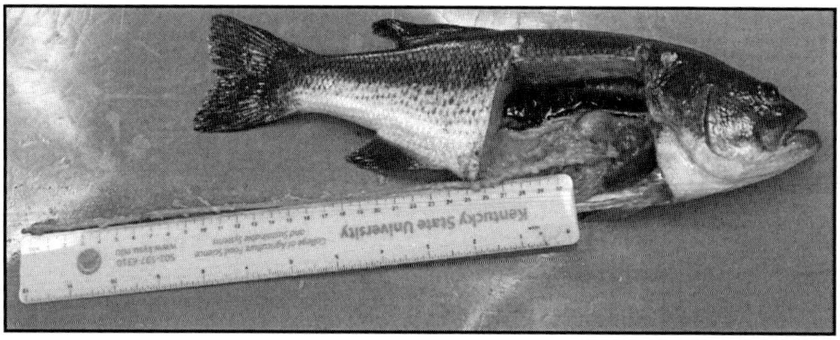

Figure 8.2 Dissection of largemouth bass intraperitoneal cavity showing the relative length of the intestine.

its total length (Figure 8.2). The activities of digestive enzymes including pepsin, trypsin (gastric and pancreatic), lipase and amylase have long been reported in largemouth bass (Sarbahi, 1951; McGeachin and Debnam, 1960).

8.3 Nutritional requirements

8.3.1 Protein and essential amino acids

As a carnivorous species, largemouth bass appears to be highly responsive to dietary protein, even at late growout phases near market sizes (400–700 g). In general, the available literature indicates that largemouth bass require between 40 to 50% dietary crude protein (CP) for maximum production performance. Most requirement studies were conducted using juvenile fish, and the observed differences in requirement values are likely due to factors including initial fish size, ingredient composition and digestibility of experimental diets, feeding rate, dietary non-protein energy, and possibly genetics.

Brecka et al. (1996) evaluated four semi-purified diets formulated to contain 31, 34, 37, or 40% CP and an estimated 3.27 kcal/g digestible energy (DE) in largemouth bass (12.2 g MIW).

Diets containing 37 or 40% CP and energy-to-protein ratios of 8.8 and 8.2 kcal DE/g, respectively, were found to support maximum growth of the fish. Portz et al. (2001) assessed the dietary protein and energy requirements of largemouth bass (14.5 g MIW) and concluded that a minimum of 43.6 and 44.8% dietary CP was required to maximize growth and minimize feed conversion ratio (FCR). The authors also indicated that DE : CP ratios ranging from 8.9 to 9.6 kcal/g would support FCR values between 0.96 and 1.10.

Slightly higher dietary CP levels have been recommended. In the study of Huang et al. (2017), largemouth bass (8.7 g MIW) were fed eight diets containing 42, 45, 48, and 51% CP and two lipid levels (8 or 12%). The authors recommended 48–51% CP and 12% lipid as most suitable levels. Likewise, in a study evaluating different dietary lipid-to-protein ratios in largemouth bass (10.1 g MIW), Chen et al. (2012a) concluded that the lipid-to-protein ratio supporting the best growth performance was 0.23, corresponding to a diet containing 46.3% digestible protein (DP), 10.1 of digestible lipid, 4.1 kcal/g DE, and 8.7 kcal DE/g DP.

Information on the dietary protein requirement of largemouth bass at larger sizes (> 100 g) might be limited to the study of Tidwell et al. (1996). In a 12 month pond feeding trial, largemouth bass (122.1 g MIW) were fed diets containing 42, 44, or 47% CP. The highest weight gain and lowest FCR were observed in fish fed the 47% CP diet, indicating that diets formulated to contain over 45% CP can support relatively faster growth rates and higher feed efficiency during growout.

Based on the essential amino acid (EAA) requirements of aquatic species reported to date, it can be assumed that largemouth bass require all ten classic EAAs (that is, arginine [Arg], histidine [His], isoleucine [Ile], leucine [Leu], lysine [Lys], methionine [Met], phenylalanine [Phe], threonine [Thr], tryptophan [Trp], and valine [Val]). However, to date, quantitative requirement values have only been determined for Arg, Lys, and Met. In general, amino acid requirement studies have been carried out for 8 to 10 weeks utilizing semi-purified diets containing both peptide-bound and crystalline sources of amino acids that, together, follow the relative ratios found in largemouth bass muscle.

Zhou et al. (2012) determined the Arg requirement of largemouth bass (~25 g mean initial weight [MIW]) using 46% CP and 12% lipid diets containing Arg from 1.7 to 3.0%. The available dietary Arg requirement for maximum weight gain was found to be 1.91% (4.16% of CP).

In Dairiki et al.'s (2007) study, largemouth bass (1.29 g MIW) were fed diets containing 43% CP, 9% lipid, and Lys ranging from 1.2 to 3.5%. The dietary Lys requirement for maximum growth was found to be 2.10% (4.9% of CP), while 1.69% dietary Lys (3.9% of CP) was required to minimize FCR. Using larger fish (14.1 g MIW) and diets formulated to contain 40% CP, 12% lipid, and Lys from 1.0 to 3.0%, Woodward et al. (personal communication) estimated the dietary Lys requirement for maximum growth and feed efficiency of largemouth bass to be 1.6 and 1.7% (4.0 and 4.3% of CP), respectively.

The Met requirement of largemouth bass was first reported by Chen et al. (2010) who fed largemouth bass (37.9 g MIW) 44% CP and 9.2% lipid diets containing Met from 0.6 to 1.6% and a constant level of 0.3% cysteine (Cys). The dietary Met maximizing the performance of the fish was found to be 1.2% (2.8% of CP), corresponding to a total sulfur amino acid (TSAA) requirement of 1.5% (3.4% of CP). A second assessment of the Met requirement of largemouth bass (6.0 g MIW) was conducted by Rossi et al. (2018) using 42% CP, 13% lipid diets containing Met from 0.5 to 1.3% and a constant level of 0.26% Cys. The dietary Met supporting maximum weight gain and feed efficiency was found to be 0.85% (2.0% of CP), corresponding to a dietary TSAA requirement of 1.1% (2.6% of CP). Results from the same study also suggested that dietary Cys could spare around 40% of the Met requirement of largemouth bass.

The study of Frederick et al. (2016) indicated that taurine (Tau) is not essential in the diet of largemouth bass and that the species is capable of synthesizing it. Although not strictly an amino acid due to the lack of a carboxyl group, Tau has been found to be dietary indispensable for an increasing number of fish species (reviewed by Salze and Davis, 2015), or to spare dietary Met in Nile tilapia (*Oreochromis Niloticus*) fed marginally deficient diets (Michelato et al., 2018). Hypothetically, any species capable of synthesizing Tau through the transsulfuration pathway might spare Met with dietary Tau to some extent, but has not yet been assessed in largemouth bass.

8.3.2 Lipids and essential fatty acids

Lipids comprise the most concentrated source of chemical energy and supply essential fatty acids, phospholipids, and sterols in feeds. In general, total lipid content found in isolipidic formulations for largemouth bass have ranged from 8.5 to 14% (Coyle et al., 2000; Subhadra et al., 2006; Tidwell et al., 2007; Yun et al., 2013; Yadav et al., 2018). However, findings from a limited number of studies evaluating diets containing ≥ 40% CP suggest dietary lipid in the higher end of that range for maximum production performance of largemouth bass (Chen et al., 2012a; Huang et al., 2017).

Bright et al. (2005) fed 43% CP diets containing lipid from 8.2 to 24% (dry matter basis) to largemouth bass (16.3 g MIW) and found no effects on production performance – although the reported FCR and protein efficiency ratio (PER) appeared to be correlated (negatively and positively, respectively) to dietary lipid. The authors also observed higher whole-body fat in fish fed diets containing ≥ 21% lipid.

Considering the upper-tolerance limit for total digestible carbohydrates in largemouth bass (see Section 8.3.4), total digestible lipid content in formulations for this species should be based on digestible carbohydrate and protein contents, and energy-to-protein ratio. For instance, based on the energy of combustion of 5.65, 4.20, and 9.50 kcal/g of protein, carbohydrate, and lipid, respectively (Merrill and Watt, 1955), diets formulated to contain 35 to 45% DP, 10% digestible carbohydrates, and a DE : DP ratio of 8.7 (Chen et al., 2012a), would require digestible lipid ranging from 7 to 10%.

Most studies evaluating essential fatty acid (EFA) requirements in largemouth bass have indicated that highly unsaturated fatty acids (HUFA) of both n-6 (arachidonic acid, ARA) and n-3 (eicosapentaenoic acid, EPA; docosahexaenoic acid, DHA) series are dietary dispensable. These findings support the notion that as a freshwater species, largemouth bass EFA requirements can be satisfied by the dietary supply of 18-carbon HUFA precursors, namely linoleic acid (LA, 18:2 n-6) and α-linolenic acid (ALA, 18:3 n-3).

Subhadra et al. (2006) fed largemouth bass (5.0 g MIW) with 47% CP and 14% lipid diets containing 30% solvent-extracted fish meal and supplemented with canola oil, chicken oil, or menhaden oil. The authors found no significant differences in production performance of the fish fed the experimental diets containing different levels of ARA (0–2.0%), EPA (0–13.8%), and DHA (0–5.3% of total fatty acids). Likewise, Tidwell et al. (2007) fed largemouth bass (15.7 g MIW) diets containing ARA, EPA, and DHA ranging from 0.2, 0.9, and 0.9% to 28.9,

11.0, and 3.9% of total fatty acids, respectively, and observed no dietary effects on production performance.

Notwithstanding the above, positive responses to supplemental EPA and DHA rich oils have been observed in largemouth bass. In the study of Yadav et al. (2018), largemouth bass (13.8 g MIW) fed 45% CP and 12% lipid diets containing 1 or 2% EPA+DHA displayed higher weight gain and feed efficiency compared to fish fed a control diet devoid of n-3 HUFA. These results indicate that the supplementation of ~1% EPA+DHA to nutrient-dense feeds may maximize production performance of largemouth bass.

Since the utilization of high-performance feeds is a common practice in the rearing of largemouth bass fingerlings and early grow-out of juveniles, more studies on the potential benefits of supplemental n-3 HUFA in feeds are recommended. Additionally, from a consumer perspective and in view of the health benefits associated with the consumption of n-3 HUFA, the evaluation of finishing feeds designed to modulate the concentrations of these fatty acids in largemouth bass muscle is also warranted.

8.3.3 Vitamins and minerals

Information on the dietary vitamin and mineral requirements of largemouth bass is limited although supplementation in commercial feeds is a common practice to ensure adequate supply. The available information on dietary vitamin requirements of largemouth bass is summarized in Table 8.1. Despite discrepancies among different studies, the vitamins A, E, and C might be the only vitamins with more than a single requirement estimate for largemouth bass.

Table 8.1 Summary of dietary vitamin requirements of largemouth bass.

Vitamin	Recommended level (unit/kg)	Reference
A	6,000 IU	Qi (2014)
	2,600–3,550 IU	Lian et al. (2017)
D	2,200 IU	Qi (2014)
E	150 IU	Qi (2014)
	73–108 mg	Li et al. (2018)
K	10 mg	Qi (2014)
Ascorbic acid	780 mg	Qi (2014)
	≥ 1,000 mg	Xie et al. (2006)
	148 mg	Chen et al. (2015)
	> 700 mg*	Yuan et al. (2015)
Biotin	2.0 mg	Qi (2014)
Choline	2,500 mg	Qi (2014)
Cyanocobalamin (B_{12})	0.01mg	Qi (2014)
Folic acid	5.0 mg	Qi (2014)
Niacin	200 mg	Qi (2014)
Pantothenic acid	60 mg	Qi (2014)
Pyridoxine (B_6)	20 mg	Qi (2014)
Riboflavin	20 mg	Qi (2014)
Thiamine	30 mg	Qi (2014)

Note:*Diets containing oxidized fish oil.

The production performance of largemouth bass was significantly enhanced in response to dietary vitamin A in the range of 415 to 2,755 IU/kg, tending to plateau at higher levels (3,000–4,000 IU/kg diet) and the optimum requirement was determined to range between 2,600 and 3,550 IU of vitamin A/kg (Lian et al., 2017). However, Qi (2014) reported higher dietary vitamin A requirement (6,000 IU/kg diet) for largemouth bass.

Reported signs of vitamin C deficiency in largemouth bass include anorexia, poor survival and growth, lordosis, and skin darkening along with sluggish behavior and exophthalmia (Chen et al., 2015). Chronic mortality in ponds has been observed in largemouth bass fed diets containing vitamin C at 100 mg/kg (Porak et al., 2002). Reported dietary requirement values for vitamin C in largemouth bass are quite variable and range from 148 mg/kg (Chen et al., 2015) to over 1,000 mg/kg (Xie et al., 2006). However, it appears that a level of 1,000 mg/kg of vitamin C in more stable forms (for example, Stay C, 35%) can be recommended to support adequate health and growth of largemouth bass even when semi-purified diets are used. The vitamin E requirement for largemouth bass was reported to range from 73 to 108 mg by Li et al. (2018). The review of Qi (2014) gathered most of the known vitamin requirements for largemouth bass. The dietary levels (dry matter basis) of supplemental vitamins used in practical or semi-purified diets in the Kentucky State University Aquatic Animal Nutrition Laboratory are presented in Table 8.2.

Largemouth bass dietary requirements (mg/kg, dry matter basis) for manganese (180.0), copper (8.0), cobalt (1.5), iodine (6.0), iron (66.0), zinc (150.0), and selenium (0.3) have been reported (Qi, 2014). Except for the relatively higher dietary requirement for manganese and zinc, values for the other microminerals are within requirement ranges reported for other fish species (Watanabe et al., 1997; NRC, 2011). To date, it appears that dietary requirements for macrominerals in largemouth bass are still lacking in the literature. Results from a recent study indicated that soybean meal-based diets containing ≥ 0.60% non-phytate phosphorus can support adequate production performance and health of largemouth bass, but ~0.8% non-phytate phosphorus was required to maximize whole-body phosphorus and ash contents (Miller et al., personal communication).

Table 8.2 Dietary levels (dry matter basis) of supplemental vitamins in practical diets for largemouth bass (Kentucky State University Aquatic Animal Nutrition Laboratory).

Vitamin	Unit	Unit/kg of diet
A	IU	9,920
D	IU	661
E	IU	529
K	IU	5.5
Ascorbic acid	mg	1,050
Biotin	mg	0.5
Choline	mg	1,800
Cyanocobalamin (B_{12})	mg	0.04
Folic acid	mg	13.2
Niacin	mg	331
Pantothenic acid	mg	159
Pyridoxine (B_6)	mg	38
Riboflavin	mg	79
Thiamine	mg	49

8.3.4 Carbohydrates

No dietary requirement for carbohydrates (CHO) has been reported for aquatic animals. However, digestible CHO are widely utilized in aquaculture feeds for two main reasons: (1) they comprise the least expensive sources of dietary energy; (2) starch gelatinization during processing increases water stability and adds buoyancy to finished feeds.

Carnivorous fish species generally utilize digestible CHO poorly as a source of energy. At dietary levels exceeding tolerance limits, digestible CHO can also be detrimental to the health and production performance of fish. Goodwin et al. (2002) reported a case of unexplained mortality of largemouth bass in the farm of a major producer in the USA. After thorough examination, the cause of the escalated mortality was attributed to the increased accumulation of glycogen in the liver and subsequent necrosis of hepatic tissue. In a follow-up feeding trial with diets containing 21, 27, and 35% nitrogen-free extract (NFE), the authors reported higher liver glycogen levels in fish fed diets containing > 21% NFE. After the producer switched to a commercial feed containing approximately 45% CP, 25% lipid, and 22% CHO no signs of liver pathology were found in 16 month-old fish.

Perhaps, the study of Goodwin et al. (2002) was the first indicating an upper tolerance limit for dietary CHO in largemouth bass and their findings were corroborated by later studies. Tan et al. (2005) fed largemouth bass (8.0 g MIW) with diets ranging from 15 to 23% CHO and found the best growth and feed efficiency at the dietary CHO level of 19%. Similar responses were found by Amoah et al. (2008) after feeding largemouth bass (128.5 g MIW) with diets containing 13 to 25% NFE. Lower growth rates and higher FCR were observed in fish fed the diet containing 25% NFE; and a positive correlation between liver vacuolization and dietary NFE was found. The authors recommended < 20% NFE in feeds for largemouth bass.

Although most studies evaluating dietary CHO in largemouth bass have recommended NFE ≤ 20%, good production performances of largemouth bass have been observed with diets containing as much as 35% NFE (Tidwell et al., 1996; Hulefeld et al., 2017, unpublished). Discrepancies in dietary CHO tolerance of largemouth bass may be attributed to the variable chemical composition and digestibility of the NFE fraction of feeds (Morales et al., 1994; Sanz et al., 1994; Rahman et al., 2016). Factors such as processing temperature have been found to influence NFE digestibility (Hernández et al., 2010). Therefore, caution should be exercised when limiting CHO in largemouth bass feeds solely based on NFE.

Formulations based on digestible CHO rather than NFE values may help in optimizing CHO inclusion in largemouth bass feeds. For instance, when largemouth bass (28.36 g MIW) were fed diets containing digestible starch from 5.9 to 21.7%, growth and PER of the fish was maximized at the digestible starch levels of 9.2 and 10.1%, respectively (Gou et al., 2015). Similarly, Lin et al. (2018) fed largemouth bass (16.9 g MIW) with semi-purified diets containing 5, 10, or 20% wheat starch and observed better production performance in fish fed the diets containing 5 and 10% starch. Overall, these findings suggest that best production performance of largemouth bass can be achieved when dietary digestible CHO is ≤10%.

Literature information on the effects of dietary fiber and other non-starch polysaccharides in largemouth bass is extremely scarce. Qian (2000) indicated that crude fiber should be kept below 3.5% in diets for largemouth bass.

8.3.5 Energy

Based on the levels of dietary protein, carbohydrate (measured as nitrogen free extract [NFE]), and lipid reported by different studies (Coyle et al., 2000; Subhadra et al., 2006; Tidwell et al., 2007; Csargo et al., 2013; Yun et al., 2013; Hulefeld et al., 2017, unpublished; Yadav et al., 2018) and the respective physiological fuel values (4, 4, and 9 kcal/g) of these components, DE in practical diets for largemouth bass has ranged from 3.5 to 4.6 kcal/g. Considering the DE : DP ratio of 8.7 kcal/g found to maximize the production performance of largemouth bass in the study of Chen et al. (2012a), diets formulated to contain DP in the range of 35 to 45% should contain DE ranging from 3.1 to 4.0 kcal/g. This range of DE appears to be in close agreement with that estimated from practical diets.

8.4 Raw materials utilization

Digestibility and availability coefficients of practical ingredients in largemouth bass have been reported (Portz and Cyrino, 2004; Masagounder et al., 2009) and are summarized in Table 8.3. Irrespective of all potential sources of variation including raw material origin and quality, fecal collection method and experimental protocol, the reported coefficients for the same raw material-type are fairly similar and within ranges found in the literature for other fish species (NRC, 2011).

Several plant-protein feedstuffs have been utilized in diet formulations for largemouth bass with soybean meal (SBM) being the most widely used and often constitutes the main source of dietary protein. Contrary to some carnivorous species such as Atlantic salmon (*Salmo salar*), largemouth bass appear to tolerate high dietary levels of SBM. For instance, fish meal (FM) levels in SBM-based diets for largemouth bass have been reduced to as low as 8% without detrimental effects on production performance (Cochran et al., 2009; Kolimadu et al., 2018; Hulefeld et al., 2017, unpublished).

The utilization of protein feedstuffs of animal origin has been proven effective in diets for largemouth bass. The inclusion of poultry by-product meal (PBM) in low FM, plant-based formulations appears to sustain adequate palatability and nutritional value for the species (Tidwell et al., 2005; Cochran et al., 2009). Tidwell et al. (2005) demonstrated that PBM could replace all dietary FM (included at 30%) in a SBM-based diet fed to largemouth bass without negatively affecting production performance. Insect meals are regarded as promising feed ingredients and are becoming increasingly more available for use in aquaculture feeds. A high nutritional value of defatted black soldier fly meal to largemouth bass was demonstrated in the study of Walling et al. (2017), as nearly 100% of dietary FM (included at 40%) was successfully replaced with the insect meal.

Literature information on lipid utilization shows that a wide range of practical lipid sources can be utilized in diets for largemouth bass as long as adequate amounts of n-6 and n-3 fatty acids are present. Lipids sources evaluated in studies have included marine oils derived from fish and algae, vegetable oils derived from canola, soybean, palm, linseed, and sunflower, and oils and fats derived from the rendering of terrestrial animals (Coyle et al., 2000; Bright et al., 2005; Subhadra et al., 2006; Tidwell et al., 2007; Laporte and Trushenski, 2011; Yun et al., 2013;

Table 8.3 Apparent digestibility and availability coefficients (%) of practical feedstuffs in largemouth bass.

Ingredient	FM	PBM	MBM	SBM	CGM	Corn	Wheat
Energy	78.3–87.4	85.2–87.0	72.3	75.4–79.8	76.5	53.0	55.3
Dry matter	70.0–77.6	82.6–83.4	58.2	70.4–79.0	75.3	50.0	55.5
Protein	87.7	81.5	–	94.3	93.6	–	–
Lipid	98.2	98.2	–	93.3	83.4	–	–
Calcium	62.8	86.7	–	81.1	74.5	–	–
Phosphorus	72.3	93.9	–	88.0	82.8	–	–
Arginine	92.5–93.9	91.2–94.7	83.6	97.0–97.8	98.4	91.8	92.7
Histidine	85.8–91.9	93.1–93.5	86.0	91.0–96.4	91.9	90.5	91.9
Isoleucine	88.9–92.6	85.8–90.6	83.4	94.2–96.5	94.9	81.9	85.4
Leucine	85.7–93.1	88.6–91.0	84.3	94.1–97.6	88.9	91.9	90.8
Lysine	94.8–95.8	90.8–95.4	85.8	95.7–96.1	95.9	80.1	82.7
Methionine	82.7–91.8	71.3–92.7	85.3	80.3–94.3	83.1	85.1	90.4
Phenylalanine	91.1–91.7	87.5–90.1	83.5	94.5–94.7	93.1	89.0	91.5
Threonine	88.0–93.5	86.1–92.6	82.6	93.6–96.3	95.5	78.4	85.2
Tryptophan	82.2–92.5	51.5–92.8	89.0	86.6–96.9	80.0	–	83.8
Valine	91.7–92.0	83.0–89.0	82.1	93.7–98.6	97.1	90.6	89.3
Alanine	87.5–91.7	87.6–90.7	83.3	92.6–99.4	97.0	87.9	83.6
Aspartate	85.0–91.0	82.0–91.9	82.3	96.0–99.6	93.8	86.0	87.8
Cysteine	41.5–82.9	50.4–82.3	53.6	51.2–94.7	56.2	80.1	90.4
Glutamate	91.1–93.2	87.5–92.9	83.3	96.8–99.8	93.1	94.2	97.6
Glycine	88.2–91.4	91.0–93.1	80.6	93.0–99.9	99.4	81.2	85.7
Proline	90.8–92.8	89.2–91.6	80.3	95.3–99.9	97.9	90.2	95.6
Serine	87.3–92.1	77.0–91.7	81.1	95.5–99.7	91.8	88.5	92.9
Tyrosine	91.7–95.9	92.5–96.2	79.5	95.7–98.2	94.7	80.6	86.3

Note: FM = fish meal; PBM = poultry by-product meal; MBM = meat and bone meal; SBM = soybean meal; CGM = corn gluten meal.

Source: Summarized from Portz and Cyrino (2004) and Masagounder et al. (2009).

Kolimadu et al., 2018; Yadav et al., 2018). More recently, hydrogenated soybean oil was found to be a suitable alternative lipid source in the diet of largemouth bass (Laporte and Trushenski, 2011).

8.5 Feed additives

A limited number of studies have evaluated different feed additives in the diet of largemouth bass. Kubitza et al. (1997) concluded that the dietary inclusion of inosine-5-monophosphate at 2,800 mg/kg enhanced feed intake in juvenile fish by 23%. Liu et al. (2015) included ethoxyquin from 0 to 1,500 mg/kg in the diet of largemouth bass and observed higher survival and antioxidant protection at the ethoxyquin level of 300 mg/kg. Likewise, Yu et al. (2018) found that the inclusion of butylated hydroxytoluene (BHT) at a level of 150 mg/kg in the diet improved lipid metabolism and antioxidant response of the fish. Li et al. (2017) found that diets supplemented with selenium-yeast enhanced lipid metabolism and antioxidant response of largemouth bass and recommended 1.29 mg Se/kg. When fed diets supplemented with hydrolyzed yeast at 30g/kg, largemouth bass displayed significant improvements in growth, feed intake and intestinal health (Zheng et al., 2015). Similarly, Zhou et al. (2018a) concluded that dietary brewer's yeast hydrolysate might beneficially modulate the gut microbiota of largemouth bass. Niu et al. (2010) found that the supplementation of phytase at 1,000 FU/kg improved growth, FCR and protease activity in both the stomach and pyloric caeca of largemouth bass.

8.6 Immunonutrition and nutrigenomics

Based on our comprehension of the linkage between nutrition, immunology and genetics (specific signaling molecules), appropriate feeds and feeding regimes give optimum fish health. Immunomodulatory nutrients supply the basic requirements for the fish immune system to realize its function as well as to protect tissues from collateral damage (Figure 8.3). In addition, to prevent diseases, nutrition research is investigating how nutrition can optimize and maintain cellular, tissue, organ and whole-body homeostasis. This requires understanding how nutrients act at the molecular level and, to this end, the use of nutrigenomics is becoming increasingly more common in fish nutrition research to characterize gene products, their physiological functions, and their interactions with nutrients.

The role of dietary EAA on fish immune response and signaling molecules related to immune and metabolic functions has received little attention (Habte-Tsion et al., 2015, 2016). The exception is research on the role of Arg (Liang et al., 2016, 2018; Figure 8.4). In a study on largemouth bass, dietary Arg improved serum protein content, serum lysozyme and respiratory burst activities of head kidney leucocytes (Zhou et al., 2012), indicating the immunomodulatory function of this amino acid in this species. Moreover, dietary Arg and carbohydrate/lipid ratios differentially regulated the mRNA expression of growth-related genes such as growth hormone (GH), insulin-like growth factor-I (IGF-I), and insulin in largemouth bass (Chen

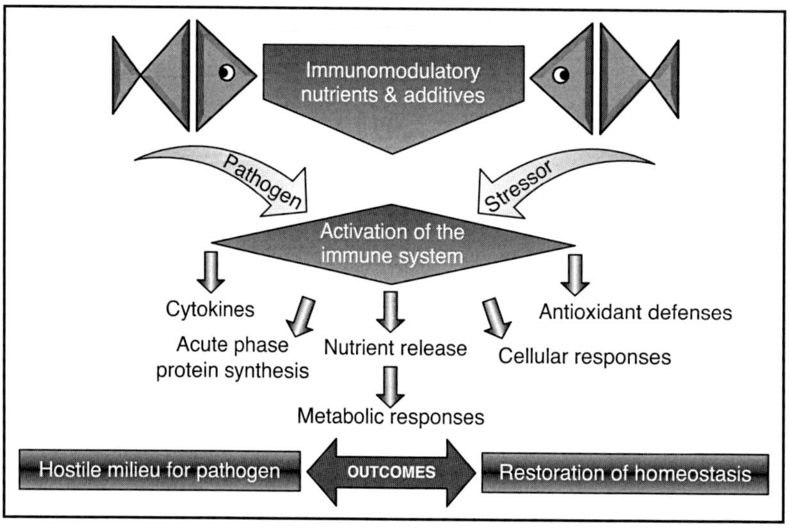

Figure 8.3 Concept of fish immunonutrition in preventive health
Source: Fish immune system and its nutritional modulation for preventive health care; Viswanath Kiron; Animal Feed Science and Technology; Volume 173 Issue 1–2 (2012)

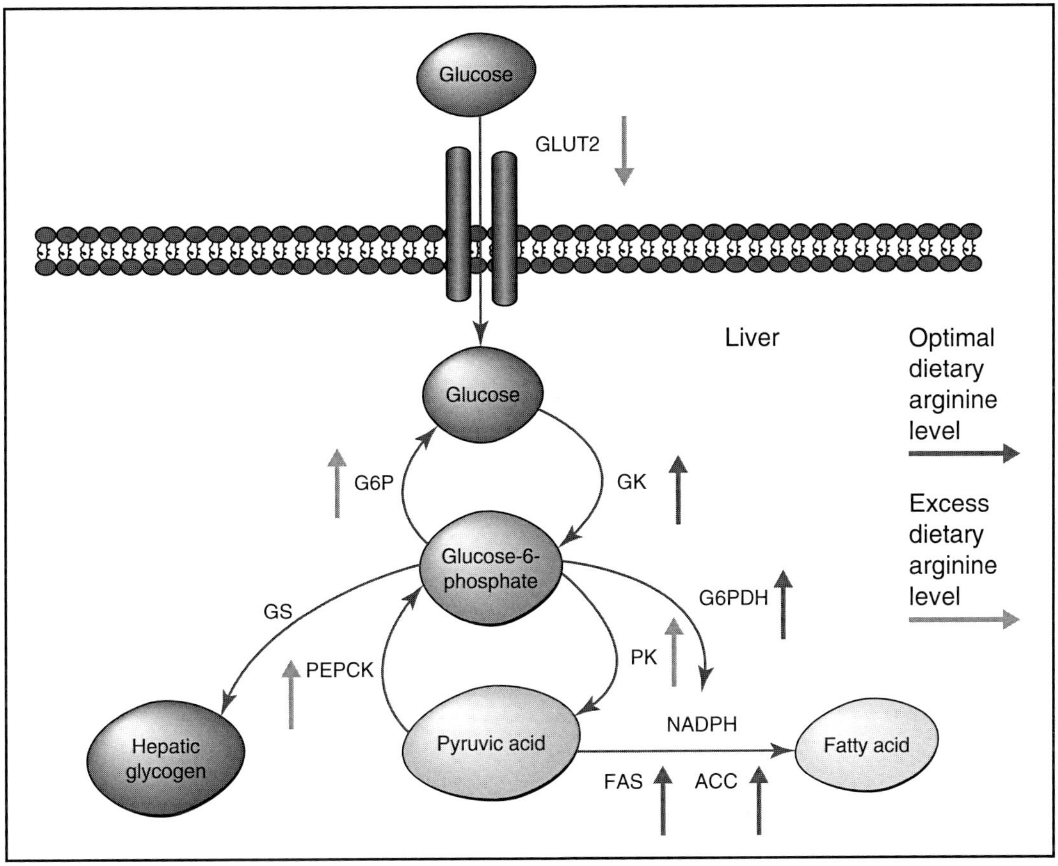

Figure 8.4 The concept of nutrigenomics: glucose and lipid metabolism signaling pathway, adopted from Liang et al. (2017). Optimal dietary arginine level (1.62%) elevated the relative expression of glucokinase (GK), glucose-6-phosphate dehydrogenase (G6PDH), fatty acid synthase (FAS), and acetyl CoA carboxylase (ACC) in fish. High dietary arginine level (2.70%) increased the relative gene expressions of phosphoenolpyruvate carboxykinase (PEPCK), glucose 6-phosphatase (G6P) and pyruvate kinase (PK), and lowered glucose transporter 2 (GLUT 2) in fish.

Source: Dietary arginine affects the insulin signaling pathway, glucose metabolism and lipogenesis in juvenile blunt snout bream Megalobrama amblycephala: Hualiang Liang, Habte-Michael Habte-Tsion, et al. Scientific Reports, volume 7, Article number: 7864 (2017) – Creative Commons.

et al., 2012b). Chen et al. (2012b) suggested that dietary Arg level might exert an independent and positive effect on the GH and IGF-I transcription, which confirms the fundamental role of the endocrine system in the regulation of the nutrient metabolism and somatic growth of largemouth bass.

Lipids are the energy dense macronutrients in feeds that fulfil both energy and EFA requirements of fish. A number of studies have been conducted with largemouth bass to evaluate alternative lipid sources (terrestrial plant and animal oils/fats) and EFA requirements (Coyle et al., 2000; Bright et al., 2005; Subhadra et al., 2006; Tidwell et al., 2007; Yun et al., 2013; González-Félix et al., 2016; Huang et al., 2017; Liu et al., 2017; Yadav et al., 2018), but only few reports are available regarding immunomodulatory effects (Subhadra et al., 2006; Chen et al., 2012a; Zhu et al., 2018). Subhadra et al. (2006) used diets supplemented with 10% lipid as canola (CAN), chicken (CHK), menhaden fish oil (MFO) or CHK + MFO (50/50%), and reported no significant differences in immune parameters (hematocrit, hemoglobin, mean corpuscular hemoglobin content and serum lysozyme activity) of largemouth bass fed the test diets, but lysozyme activity was lower in fish fed a commercial trout diet compared to fish fed the CHK + MFO (50/50%) diet. The report also added that largemouth bass fed diets with 10% MFO or CAN had higher alternative complement activity than fish fed diets with CHK. In addition, an increased oxidative stress was reported in largemouth bass fed oxidized lipid that stimulated hepatic antioxidant defenses (Chen et al., 2012c). Zhu et al. (2018) found no significant effects of dietary lipids on the peroxide (malondialdehyde, MDA) and antioxidant responses (superoxide dismutase and glutathione peroxidase) except catalase activity. However, there is no report regarding the molecular effects of dietary lipid and fatty acids on largemouth bass.

Microminerals are supplemented to aquaculture feeds due to their essential roles, and their low and/or variable levels in practical feedstuffs (Hunt, 2003). Elements including iron (Lim et al., 2001), zinc (Sanchez-Dardon et al., 1999) and selenium (Fontagné-Dicharry et al., 2015) have been shown to have immunomodulatory functions in other fish species. However, currently there is no report regarding the effects of microminerals on the immunity and target genes of largemouth bass.

Reports of vitamin deficiency in fish farms are often linked to vitamins C and E (Hardy, 2001), and these two vitamins are frequently studied in relation to their effects on immune responses. Chen et al. (2015) reported that optimum dietary vitamin C supplementation not only increased antioxidant capacities of the liver and muscle of largemouth bass, but also exerted a sparing effect on vitamin E utilization in plasma and liver, thereby decreasing lipid peroxidation (MDA concentration). Vitamins A (Lian et al., 2017) and C (Xie et al., 2006) improved the growth, antioxidant capacity and nonspecific immunity of largemouth bass; while dietary vitamin E and selenium were found to protect largemouth bass from oxidative damage in the study of Chen et al. (2013).

Plant-protein feedstuffs are promising sources of amino acids for aquaculture feeds mainly due to their quality, competitive price and availability (Collins et al., 2012; Slawski et al., 2013; Zhou et al., 2018b). However, a major concern is the presence of antinutritional factors (ANFs) in these ingredients, including protease inhibitors, non-starch polysaccharides and phytic acid, which can adversely affect the growth and health of fish. Hence, besides novel processing technologies designed to reduce ANF levels and improve the nutritional value of traditional ingredients, nutrigenomic tools are very important to predict long-term detrimental effects (for example, subtle physiological changes) of dietary modifications on farmed aquatic animals, including largemouth bass.

8.7 Conclusion

Culture of largemouth bass as food-fish continues to expand and knowledge on nutritional needs of the species is a premise for efficient and profitable production of nutritious fish to consumers.

As for any farmed fish, the optimization of feeds for largemouth bass relies upon accurate information on nutritional requirements, quality and nutritional value of feed ingredients, proper use of key feed additives that aid in supporting optimum production performance and health, and precise formulation of feeds for different life stages.

Research on EAA requirements of largemouth bass must be intensified as only three out of ten EAA have been studied to date. As aquaculture feeds continue to depart from the use of traditional marine-based proteins to the use of terrestrial plant and animal-based protein sources, proper supplementation of EAA based on quantitative requirements is critical for supporting growth and feed efficiency, and to minimize nutrient load to receiving waters.

Information on mycotoxin effects on health and production performance of largemouth bass, as well as upper limits thereof in feeds for this species is lacking. This is of particular importance considering that mycotoxin occurrences in feeds are increasingly more common, primarily due to the extensive use of plant-based ingredients prone to contamination.

Finally, yet importantly, information on the immunonutrition and nutrigenomics of largemouth bass also needs to be expanded. It is reasonable to assume that, as for other species, both approaches represent new tools allowing nutritionists to prevent or attenuate challenges related to health and production of largemouth bass.

References

Amoah, A., Coyle, S.D., Webster, C.D., Durborow, R.M., Bright, L.A. and Tidwell, J.H. (2008) Effects of graded levels of carbohydrate on growth and survival of largemouth bass, *Micropterus salmoides. Journal of the World Aquaculture Society* 39, 397–405.

Anderson, R.J., Kienholz, E.W. and Flickinger, S.A. (1981) Protein requirements of smallmouth bass and largemouth bass. *Journal of Nutrition* 111, 1085–1097.

Brecka, B.J., Wahl, D.H. and Hooe, M.L. (1996) Growth, survival, and body composition of largemouth bass fed various commercial diets and protein concentrations. *The Progressive Fish-Culturist* 58, 104–110.

Bright, L.A., Coyle, S.D. and Tidwell, J.H. (2005) Effect of dietary lipid level and protein energy ratio on growth and body composition of largemouth bass *Micropterus salmoides. Journal of the World Aquaculture Society* 36, 129–134.

Chen, N., Ma, J.-Z., Zhou, H.-Y., Zhou, J., Qiu, X.-J., Jin, L.-N. and Lin, L.-F. (2010) Assessment of dietary methionine requirement in largemouth bass, *Micropterus salmoides. Journal of Fisheries of China* 34, 1244–1253.

Chen, N.-S., Xiao, W.-W., Liang, Q.-L., Zhou, H.-Y., Ma, X.-L. and Zhao, M. (2012a) Effects of dietary lipid to protein ratios on growth performance, body composition and non-specific immunity of largemouth bass (*Micropterus salmoides*). *Journal of Fisheries of China* 36, 1270–1280.

Chen, N.-S, Jin, L.-N., Zhou, H.-Y. and Qiu, X.-J. (2012b). Effects of dietary arginine levels and carbohydrate-to-lipid ratios on mRNA expression of growth-related hormones in largemouth bass, *Micropterus salmoides.* General and Comparative Endocrinology 179, 121–127.

Chen, Y.-J., Liu, Y.-J., Yang, H.-J., Yuan, Y., Liu, F.-J., Tian, L.-X., Liang, G.-Y. and Yuan, R.-M. (2012c) Effect of dietary oxidized fish oil on growth performance, body composition, antioxidant defence mechanism and liver histology of juvenile largemouth bass *Micropterus salmoides. Aquaculture Nutrition* 18, 321–331.

Chen, Y.-J., Liu, Y.-J., Tian, L.-X., Niu, J., Liang, G.-Y., Yang, H.-J., Yuan, Y. and Zhang, Y.-Q. (2013) Effect of dietary vitamin E and selenium supplementation on growth, body composition, and antioxidant defense mechanism in juvenile largemouth bass (*Micropterus salmoide*) fed oxidized fish oil. *Fish Physiology and Biochemistry* 39 (3), 593–604.

Chen, Y.-J., Yuan, R.-M., Liu, Y.-J, Yang, H.-J., Liang, G.-Y. and Tian, L.-X. (2015) Dietary vitamin C requirement and its effects on tissue antioxidant capacity of juvenile largemouth bass, *Micropterus salmoides*. *Aquaculture* 435, 431–436.

Cochran, N.J., Coyle, S.D. and Tidwell, J.H. (2009) Evaluation of reduced fishmeal diets for second year growout of the largemouth bass, *Micropterus salmoides*. *Journal of the World Aquaculture Society* 40 (6), 735–743.

Collins, S.A., Desai, A.R., Mansfield, G.S., Hill, J.E., Van Kessel, A.G. and Drew, M.D. (2012) The effect of increasing inclusion rates of soybean, pea and canola meals and their protein concentrates on the growth of rainbow trout: concepts in diet formulation and experimental design for ingredient evaluation. *Aquaculture* 344, 90–99.

Coyle, S.D., Tidwell, J.H. and Webster, C.D. (2000) Response of largemouth bass *Micropterus salmoides* to dietary supplementation of lysine, methionine, and highly unsaturated fatty acids. *Journal of the World Aquaculture Society* 31, 89–95.

Csargo, I.J., Brown, M.L. and Ward, M.J. (2013) Evaluation of four commercial grower diets for production of largemouth bass. *Journal of Applied Aquaculture* 25, 35–49.

Dairiki, J.K., Dias, C.T.D.S. and Cyrino, J.E.P. (2007) Lysine requirements of largemouth bass, *Micropterus salmoides*: a comparison of methods of analysis of dose-response trials data. *Journal of Applied Aquaculture* 19 (4), 1–27.

Fontagné-Dicharry, S., Godin, S., Liu, H., Prabhu, P.A.J., Bouyssiére, B., Bueno, M., Tacon, P., Médale, F. and Kaushik, S.J. (2015) Influence of the forms and levels of dietary selenium on antioxidant status and oxidative stress-related parameters in rainbow trout (*Oncorhynchus mykiss*) fry. *British Journal of Nutrition* 113 (12), 1876–1887.

Frederick, C.A., Coyle, S.D., Durborow, R.M., Bright, L.A. and Tidwell, J.H. (2016) Effect of taurine supplementation on growth response and body composition of largemouth bass. *North American Journal of Aquaculture* 78 (2), 107–112.

González-Félix, M.L., Maldonado-Othón, C.A. and Perez-Velazquez, M. (2016) Effect of dietary lipid level and replacement of fish oil by soybean oil in compound feeds for the shortfin corvina (*Cynoscion parvipinnis*). *Aquaculture* 454, 217–228.

Goodwin, A.E., Lochmann, R.T., Tieman, D.M. and Mitchell, A.J. (2002) Massive hepatic necrosis and nodular regeneration in largemouth bass fed diets high in available carbohydrate. *Journal of the World Aquaculture Society* 33, 466–477.

Gou, S., Chen, N., Xu, X., Liu, Z. and Yin, J. (2015) Effects of dietary digestible starch levels on growth performance, body composition, and non-specific immunological index of largemouth bass (*Micropterus salmoides*). *Journal of Fisheries of China* 39, 1499–1510.

Habte-Tsion, H.-M., Ge, X.-P., Liu, B., Xie, J., Ren, M.-C., Zhou, Q.-L., Miao, L.-H., Pan, L.-K. and Chen, R. (2015) A deficiency or an excess of dietary threonine level affects weight gain, enzyme activity, immune response and immune-related gene expression in juvenile blunt snout bream (*Megalobrama amblycephala*). *Fish & Shellfish Immunology* 42, 439–446.

Habte-Tsion, H.-M., Ren, M.-C., Liu, B., Ge, X.-P., Xie, J. and Chen, R. (2016) Threonine modulates immune response, antioxidant status and gene expressions of antioxidant enzymes and antioxidant-immune-cytokine-related signaling molecules in juvenile blunt snout bream (*Megalobrama amblycephala*). *Fish & Shellfish Immunology* 51, 189–199.

Hardy, R.W. (2001) Nutritional deficiencies in commercial aquaculture: likelihood, onset and identification. In: Lim, C., Webster, C.D. (eds) *Nutrition and Fish Health*. The Haworth Press, Inc., Binghamton, New York, pp. 131–147.

Hernández, A., Bórquez, A., Alcaíno, L., Morales, J., Dantagnan, P. and Saez, P. (2010) Effects of autoclaving on the apparent digestibility coefficient of dehulled pea seed meal (*Pisum sativum* L.) in rainbow trout (*Oncorhynchus mykiss* W.). *Ciencia e Investigación Agraria* 37 (3), 39–46.

Huang, D., Wu, Y., Lin, Y., Chen, J., Karrow, N., Ren, X. and Wang, Y. (2017) Dietary protein and lipid requirements for juvenile largemouth bass, *Micropterus salmoides*. *Journal of the Aquaculture Society* 48, 782–790.

Hunt, J.R. (2003) Bioavailability of iron, zinc, and other trace minerals from vegetarian diets. *American Journal of Clinical Nutrition* 78, 633S–639S.

JSA (Joint Subcommittee on Aquaculture) (1984) Largemouth bass species plan. In: *National Aquaculture Development Plan*, Vol. II. US. Department of the Interior, Washington, DC, pp. 68–75.

Kiron, V. (2012) Fish immune system and its nutritional modulation for preventive health care. *Animal Feed Science and Technology* 173, 111–133.

Kolimadu, G., Rossi Jr., W., Kumar, V. and Habte-Tsion, H-M. (2018) Assessing the nutritional value of novel soybean meals in the diet of largemouth bass *Micropterus salmoides*. *Aquaculture America 2018 Abstract Book*, p. 252.

Kubitza, F., Lovshin, L.L., Lovell, R.T. (1997) Identification of feed enhancers for juvenile largemouth bass *Micropterus salmoides*. *Aquaculture* 148, 191–200.

Laporte, J. and Trushenski, J. (2011) Growth performance and tissue fatty acid composition of largemouth bass fed diets containing fish oil or blends of fish oil and soy-derived lipids. *North America Journal of Aquaculture* 73 (4), 435–444.

Li, N., Zheng, Y., Wu, X., Wang, X., Xue, M. and Wu, L. (2017) Tolerance of selenium-yeast in diets of largemouth bass (*Micropterus salmoides*). *Chinese Journal of Animal Nutrition* 29, 1949–1960.

Li, S., Lian, X., Chen, N., Wang, M. and Sang, S. (2018) Effects of dietary vitamin E level on growth performance, feed utilization, antioxidant capacity and nonspecific immunity of largemouth bass, *Micropterus salmoides*. *Aquaculture Nutrition* (https://doi.org/10.1111/anu.12802).

Lian, X., Chen, N., Wang, M., Yan, C., Ding, G. (2017) Dietary vitamin A requirement of largemouth bass (*Micropterus salmoides*). *Chinese Journal of Animal Nutrition* 29, 3819–3830.

Liang, H.-L., Habte-Tsion, H.-M., Ge, X.-P., Ren, M.-C., Xie, J., Miao, L.-H., Zhou, Q.-L., Lin, Y., Pan, W.-J. (2017) Dietary arginine affects the insulin signaling pathway, glucose metabolism and lipogenesis in juvenile blunt snout bream *Megalobrama amblycephala*. *Scientific Reports* 7, 7864, doi:10.1038/s41598–017–06104–3.

Liang, H.-L., Ji, K., Ge, X.-P., Ren, M.-C., Liu, B., Xi, B.-W. and Pan, L.-K. (2018) Effects of dietary arginine on antioxidant status and immunity involved in AMPK-NO signaling pathway in juvenile blunt snout bream. *Fish and Shellfish Immunology* 78, 69–78.

Liang, H.-L., Ren, M.-C., Habte-Tsion, H.-M., Ge, X.-P., Xie, J., Mi, H.-F., Xi, B.-W., Miao, L.-H., Liu, B., Zhou, Q.-L. and Fang, W. (2016) Dietary arginine affects growth performance, plasma amino acid contents and gene expressions of the TOR signaling pathway in juvenile blunt snout bream, *Megalobrama amblycephala*. *Aquaculture* 461, 1–8.

Lim, C., Klesius, P.H. and Shoemaker, C.A. (2001) Dietary iron and fish health. In: Lim, C. and Webster, C.D. (eds) *Nutrition and Fish Health*. The Haworth Press, Inc., Binghamton, New York, pp. 189–199.

Lin, S.-M., Shi, C.-M., Mu, M.-M., Chen, Y.-J. and Luo, L. (2018) Effect of high dietary starch levels on growth, hepatic glucose metabolism, oxidative status and immune response of juvenile largemouth bass, *Micropterus salmoides*. *Fish and Shellfish Immunology* 78, 121–126.

Liu, J., Ai, L., Wang, J., Han, F., Xue, M., Zheng, Y., Wu, X. and Zhang, Y. (2015) Evaluation of ethoxyquin in diets of largemouth bass (*Micropterus salmoides*). *Chinese Journal of Animal Nutrition* 27, 1152–1162.

Liu, Z., Chen, N., Wang, M., Lian, X., Yan, C. and Yin, J. (2017) Suitable dietary starch source and supplementation level for largemouth bass (*Micropterus salmoides*). *Journal of Fishery Sciences of China* 24, 317–331.

Liu, K., Liu, H., Chi, S., Dong, X., Yang, Q. and Tan, B. (2017) Effects of different dietary lipid sources on growth performance, body composition and lipid metabolism-related enzymes and genes of juvenile golden pompano, *Trachinotus ovatus*. *Aquaculture Research* 49, 717–725.

Masagounder, K., Firman, J.D., Hayward, R.S., Sun, S. and Brown, P.B. (2009) Apparent digestibilities of common feedstuffs for bluegill *Leponis macrochirus* and largemouth bass *Micropterus salmoides* using individual test ingredients. *Aquaculture Nutrition* 15, 29–37.

McGeachin, R.L. and Debnam Jr., J.W. (1960) Amylase in fresh water fish. *Experimental Biology and Medicine* 103, 814–815.

Merrill, A.L. and Watt, B.K. (1955) *Energy Values of Foods – Basis and Derivation*. USDA Agriculture Handbook No. 74. U.S. Government Printing Office, Washington, DC.

Michelato, M., Furuya, W.M. and Gatlin III, D.M. (2018) Metabolic responses of Nile tilapia *Oreochromis niloticus* to methionine and taurine supplementation. *Aquaculture* 485, 66–72.

Morales, A.E., Cardenete, G., Higuera, d.l. M. and Sanz, A. (1994) Effects of dietary protein source on growth, feed conversion and energy utilization in rainbow trout, *Oncorhynchus mykiss*. *Aquaculture* 124, 117–126.

Niu, J.-F, Wu, R.-Q, Xie, J., Wang, G.-J. and Guan, S.-J. (2010) Effects of phytase on growth and digestive enzyme activities in largemouth bass *Micropterus salmoides*. *Journal of Dalian Fisheries University* 25, 132–136.

NRC (2011) *Nutrient Requirements of Fish and Shrimp*. National Academies Press, Washington, DC.

Porak, W.F., Johnson, W.E., Crawford, S., Renfro, D.J., Schoeb, T.R., Stout, R.B., Krause, R.A., and DeMauro, R.A. (2002) Factors affecting survival of largemouth bass raised on artificial diets and stocked into Florida lakes. In: Philipp, D.P. and Ridgway, M.S. (eds) *Black Bass: Ecology, Conservation, and Management. American Fisheries Society Symposium 31*, American Fisheries Society, Bethesda, MD, pp. 649–665.

Portz, L., Cyrino, J. and Martino, R. (2001) Growth and body composition of juvenile largemouth bass *Micropterus salmoides* in response to dietary protein and energy levels. *Aquaculture Nutrition* 7, 247–254.

Portz, L. and Cyrino, J.E. (2004) Digestibility of nutrients and amino acids of different protein sources in practical diets by largemouth bass *Micropterus salmoides* L. *Aquaculture Research* 35, 312–320.

Qi, G. (2014) Advances in nutrient requirements of largemouth bass (*Micropterus salmoides*). *Guangdong Feed* 9, 40–42.

Qian, G.-Y. (2000) Effects of dietary protein, fibre and fat on the growth of largemouth bass (*Micropterus salmoides*). *Acta Zoonutrimenta Sinica* 02. Available at: http://en.cnki.com.cn/Article_en/CJFDTOTAL-DWYX200002011.htm.

Rahman, M.M., Lee, K.-J. and Lee, S.-M. (2016) Effect of dietary carbohydrate sources on apparent nutrient digestibility of olive flounder (*Paratichthys olivaceus*) feed. *Fisheries and Aquatic Sciences* 19, 1–5.

Rossi Jr., W., Kumar, V. and Woodward, B. (2018) Dietary methionine requirement of largemouth bass *Micropterus salmoides* L. *Aquaculture America 2018 Abstract Book*, p. 406.

Salze, G.P. and Davis, D.A. (2015) Taurine: a critical nutrient for future fish feeds. *Aquaculture* 437, 215–229.

Sanchez-Dardon, J., Voccia, I., Hontela, A., Chilmonczyk, S., Dunier, M., Boermans, H., Blakley, B. and Fournier, M. (1999) Immunomodulation by heavy metals tested individually or in mixtures in rainbow trout (*Oncorhynchus mykiss*) exposed in vivo. *Environmental Toxicology Chemistry* 18, 1492–1497.

Sanz, A., Morales, A.E., Higuera, d.l. M. and Cardenete, G. (1994) Sunflower meal compared with soybean meal as partial substitutes for fish meal in rainbow trout (*Oncorhynchus mykiss*) diets: protein and energy utilization. *Aquaculture* 128, 287–300.

Sarbahi, D.S. (1951) Studies of the digestive tracts and digestive enzymes of the goldfish, *Carassius auratus* (Linnaeus) and the largemouth black bass, *Micropterus salmoides* (Lacépède). *The Biological Bulletin* 100: 3.

Slawski, H., Nagel, F., Wysujack, K., Balke, D.T., Franz, P. and Schulz, C. (2013) Total fish meal replacement with canola protein isolate in diets fed to rainbow trout (*Oncorhynchus mykiss* W.). *Aquaculture Nutrition* 19, 535–542.

Subhadra, B., Lochmann, R., Rawles, S. and Chen, R. (2006) Effect of dietary lipid source on the growth, tissue composition and haematological parameters of largemouth bass (*Micropterus salmoides*). *Aquaculture* 255, 210–222.

Tan, X.-Y., Liu, Y.-J., Tian, L.-X., Yang, H.-J., Liang, G.-Y., Luo, Z., Huang, J.-W. and Guo, R. (2005) The effects of dietary carbohydrate levels on the growth, nutrient composition of juvenile largemouth bass *Micropterus salmoides. Acta Scientiarum Naturalium Universitatis Sunyatseni* 44, 258–263.

Tidwell, J.H., Coyle, S. and Bright, L.A. (2007) Effects of different types of dietary lipids on growth and fatty acid composition of largemouth bass. *North American Journal of Aquaculture* 69 (3), 257–264.

Tidwell, J.H., Coyle, S.D., Bright, L.A. and Yasharian, D. (2005) Evaluation of plant and animal source proteins for replacement of fish meal in practical diets for the largemouth bass *Micropterus salmoides. Journal of the World Aquaculture Society* 36, 454–463.

Tidwell, J.H., Coyle, S.D. and Webster, C.D. (2002) Centrarchids: largemouth bass, *Micropterus salmoides*. In: Webster, C.D. and Lim, C.E. (eds) *Nutrient Requirements and Feeding of Finfish for Aquaculture.* CABI Publishing, New York, pp. 374–380.

Tidwell, J.H., Webster, C.D. and Coyle, S.D. (1996) Effects of dietary protein level on second year growth and water quality for largemouth bass (*Micropterus salmoides*) raised in ponds. *Aquaculture* 145, 213–223.

Walling, C.T., Kumar, V., Rossi, W., Bright, L.A., Tidwell, J.H. (2017) Evaluation of black soldier fly *Hermetia illucens* larvae as a fish meal replacement in practical diets for largemouth bass *Micropterus salmoides. Aquaculture America 2018 Abstract Book*, p. 506.

Watanabe, T., Kiron, V. and Satoh, S. (1997) Trace minerals in fish nutrition. *Aquaculture* 151, 185–207.

Xie, Y.-R., Wu, R.-Q., Xie, J., Wang, G.-J., Ye, F.-L., Chen, G. and Guan, S.-J. (2006) Effect of dietary vitamin C on growth and non-specific immunity of largemouth bass, *Micropterus salmoides. South China Fisheries Science* 2, 40–45.

Yadav, A.K., Rossi Jr., W., Kumar, V., Habte-Tsion, H-M. (2018) Responses of juvenile largemouth bass *Micropterus salmoides* to dietary EPA and DHA-rich oils. *Aquaculture America 2018 Abstract Book*, p. 527.

Yu, L.L., Yu, H.H., Liang, X.F., Li, N., Wang, X., Li, F.H., Wu, X.F., Zheng, Y.H., Xue, M. and Liang, X.F. (2018) Dietary butylated hydroxytoluene improves lipid metabolism, antioxidant and anti-apoptotic response of largemouth bass (*Micropterus salmoides*). *Fish and Shellfish Immunology* 72, 220–229.

Yun, B., Xue, M., Wang, J., Fan, Z.-Y., Wu, X.-F., Zheng, Y.-H and Qin, Y.-C. (2013) Effects of lipid sources and lipid peroxidation on feed intake, growth, and tissue fatty acid composition of largemouth bass (*Micropterus salmoides*). *Aquaculture International* 21, 97–110.

Yuan, R.-M., Liu, Y.-J., Wang, G.-P., Jiang, R.-L., She, Z.-J., Liang, G.-Y., and Tian, L.-X. (2016) Effects of dietary oxidized fish oil and vitamin C on growth and antioxidant ability of largemouth bass (*Micropterus salmoides*). *Guangdong Agricultural Sciences* 1, 136–144.

Zheng, Y., Peng, C., Wu, X., Han, F., Xue, M., Wang, J. and Hu, L. (2015) Effects of hydrolysed yeast on growth performance, lipids metabolism and intestinal structure of largemouth bass (*Micropterus salmoides*). *Chinese Journal of Animal Nutrition* 27, 1605–1612.

Zhou, H., Chen, N., Qiu, X., Zhao, M. and Jin, L. (2012) Arginine requirement and effect of arginine intake on immunity in largemouth bass, *Micropterus salmoides*. *Aquaculture Nutrition* 18, 107–116.

Zhou, M., Liang, R., Mo, J., Yang, S., Gu, N., Wu, Z., Babu, S.-V, Li, J., Huang, Y. and Li, L. (2018a) Effects of brewer's yeast hydrolyzate on the growth performance and intestinal bacterial diversity of largemouth bass (*Micropterus salmoides*). *Aquaculture* 484, 139–144.

Zhou, Q.L., Habte-Tsion, H.-M., Ge, X.P., Xie, J., Ren, M.C., Liu, B., Miao, L. and Pan, L. (2018b) Graded replacing fishmeal with canola meal in diets affects growth and target of rapamycin pathway gene expression of juvenile blunt snout bream, *Megalobrama amblycephala*. *Aquaculture Nutrition* 24 (1), 300–309.

Zhu, T., Jin, M., Sun, P., Li, C., Ma, H., Luo, J., Yuan, Y. and Zhou, Q. (2018) Effects of dietary lipid level on morphology indexes, tissue fatty acid composition, serum biochemical indexes and liver antioxidant indexes of largemouth bass (*Micropterus salmoides*). *Chinese Journal of Animal Nutrition* 30 (1), doi: 10.3969/j.issn.1006–267x.2018.01.000.

CHAPTER 9

Practical feeds and feeding

James H. Tidwell

Kentucky State University, Aquaculture Research Center, Frankfort, Kentucky, USA

9.1 Evaluation of largemouth bass on feed

The largemouth bass is highly regarded as a sport-fish in the USA and around the world. The species has been cultured since the late 1800s (Heidinger, 2000). Federal hatcheries began producing the fish in the early 1900s, but all early work was in support of stocking programs. Because of the Farm Pond Program of the 1930s there was a greater impetus for increased production of stocker largemouth bass (Simco et al., 1986). Most of this production targeted large numbers of small juvenile fish (2.5–5.0 cm) to establish new sport fisheries. Later, to give management options for sport-fish stocking, larger fingerlings (> 10 cm) were needed (Simco et al., 1986).

This greater need for larger sizes presented a problem for hatchery managers. The largemouth bass is known for its aggressive, predacious nature. During early life, the fry are raised in fertilized ponds where they feed on zooplankton, microcrustaceans, and small insects. However, at about 3.8–5.0 cm the fingerlings switch to becoming more piscivorous. If fingerlings are left in the ponds, small sized natural foods become depleted and losses to cannibalism significantly reduce production (Simco et al., 1986).

Different approaches to largemouth bass fingerling production have been utilized. If the number of required fingerlings is small the Spawning-Rearing Pond System can be utilized. Broodfish are stocked at 25–100 broodfish/ha and the pond is fertilized to promote zooplankton blooms. Fingerlings are harvested at ≤ 5.0 cm and ≤12,000 fingerlings/ha are produced. However, predation on fry by the broodfish can be severe. Another method is the Fry Transfer Method. To maintain water clarity, ponds are not fertilized. Schools of fry are captured and transferred to separate fingerling rearing ponds which are fertilized to establish and maintain zooplankton blooms. If target sizes are 2.5–5.0 cm rearing ponds can be stocked at 120,000–240,000 fry/ha. However, if the target size is 10 cm fingerlings, stocking sizes as low as 24,000/ha may be required. Properly managed rearing ponds yield 30–150 kg/ha of fingerlings at 3.8–5.0 cm total length (TL). To produce 10 cm fingerlings 50% survival is considered acceptable, yielding < 5,000 10 cm fish from a 1 ha pond.

As long as the food provided is limited to natural foods, production will be low. In species feeding low on the food chain, organic and inorganic fertilizers can increase primary productivity. The target fish species still relies on natural foods but the carrying capacity of the pond can be increased. As a top predator, largemouth bass may not respond to pond fertilization as well as species feeding lower on the food chain. Because of this, production of largemouth bass fingerlings, especially of advanced sizes (≥ 10 cm), requires a very large amount of pond resources to produce even relatively low numbers of fish.

In other species, a shift to prepared (pelleted) feeds is the most effective way to intensify production (that is, produce more kilograms of fish per hectare of pond). In some species, such as rainbow trout and channel catfish, first feeding fry will readily accept artificial diets. For the largemouth bass, a shift to a pelleted feed requires that the fish first be "trained" to accepted non-living food. This can be done during a critical period of development when in nature the fish are going through a changeover from consuming zooplankton and small insects to being a piscivore and feeding on other fish. This natural "reprogramming" phase can be hijacked to now program the fish to accept artificial diets. This process is very important to the modern intensive production of largemouth bass and it has an entire chapter devoted to it (see Chapter 6). Once trained to accept artificial feeds, largemouth bass retain the learned behavior indefinitely (McCraren, 1974). The remainder of this chapter will focus on feeding fish after feed training and the development of practical diets.

As previously stated, to increase the number of advanced fingerlings (≥ 10 cm) that could be produced per unit of hatchery pond space, an Intensive Culture System for largemouth bass was needed. As early as the 1930s, Langlois (1932, 1933) conditioned largemouth bass fingerlings to consume ground fish. In a series of studies J.R. (Jack) Snow at the Marion National Fish Hatchery in Alabama developed the "Marion Program" which established the basic procedures used today to produce large numbers of advanced fingerlings (15–20 cm) using artificial diets (Simco et al., 1986).

Early feeding trials by Snow (1963, 1968) first utilized a manufactured artificial diet developed for salmon, the Oregon Moist Pellet (OMP). It was felt that the soft texture was more acceptable to the largemouth bass than the hard-dry pellets used for trout and catfish. Snow and Maxwell (1970) reported that they produced 3,000 kg/ha of 10–23 cm fish feeding this diet. This represents a 1,900% increase in production per unit of pond area over the 150 kg/ha reported for fertilized ponds (Simco et al., 1986). However, diets with > 10% moisture levels tend to be expensive and require refrigerated storage. As largemouth bass have become more adapted to intensive culture conditions, succeeding generations have become more amenable to hard-dry pellets.

Growout to sizes for advanced stockers (15–20 cm) for corrective stocking can be achieved in the first summer of growth. However, to achieve sizes desired for food-fish (600–900 g) requires a second summer of growth in temperate ponds (see Chapter 7). Current procedures are variations of the following steps. After feed training fish can be maintained in tanks actively feeding on pellets for up to 2 weeks. Fingerlings can then be stocked into ponds for first-year growth at 50,000–75,000/ha. They are fed two to three times per day using a 2.3 mm diameter pellet containing 40 to 48% protein diet with 8 to 10% fat. Most producers currently use commercial diets formulated for salmonids. However, diets formulated specifically for largemouth bass are becoming commercially available. Feed the fish all they will actively consume at each feeding. Largemouth bass will feed voraciously on some days and not so actively on others. Differences are likely associated with water temperature, sunlight, and or water quality changes (Tidwell et al., 2000).

9.2 Feeding rates

In terms of feeding rates, a number of different factors come into play. Small fish need high protein levels in small pellets, and a feed volume at a high percentage of their body weight (BW) per day. As they grow the protein requirement decreases, the pellets get larger, and their food consumption as a percentage of BW decreases. Davis and Lock (1997) indicated that after being stocked into ponds the fish should be consuming about 15% of total biomass daily and that rate will gradually drop to about 5% of biomass per day. However, the total amount of feed being fed (kg/ha pond/d) will increase as the fish get larger. According to Boyd (1990) when feeding rates exceed about 30 kg feed/ha/d episodes of low oxygen can become a problem. Simco et al. (1986) reported that standing crops of 1,684 to 2,245 kg/ha of largemouth bass might be raised before low oxygen levels become a limiting factor. That equates to a feeding rate of approximately 20 kg/ha/d in unaerated ponds.

Under conditions where aeration is available and oxygen levels are monitored and managed, total ammonia-nitrogen becomes the limiting factor to acceptable feed rates and biomass densities. Kubitza and Lovshin (1997) reported maximum daily feed rates of 87 kg/ha for first-year largemouth bass stocked at 67,136 fish/ha and having a gross yield of 7,281 kg/ha at harvest. The authors reported having total ammonia-nitrogen (TAN) values of 4.0 mg/l in the same pond in October; demonstrating the risks associated with high stocking densities and associated high feed rates. Tidwell et al. (1996) also reported elevated levels of TAN during cooler water temperatures and lower feeding rates of fall and winter in intensively fed largemouth bass ponds receiving high protein diets (47%) and having total gross yields at harvest of 5,330 kg/ha. The authors suggested that high ammonia readings in the fall was likely due to reduced assimilation of ammonia by phytoplankton and reduced bacterial nitrification at cool temperatures (Tucker and Robinson, 1990). Cochran et al. (2009) reported maximum TAN readings of < 0.5 mg/l in intensively fed second-year largemouth bass ponds achieving gross yields at harvest of < 3,020 kg/ha. More recently much higher feeding and production rates have been achieved (Chapter 7).

Efficient feeding practices can be as important as having a diet properly formulated for the species being fed. A perfect diet that is not fed efficiently decreases feed conversion efficiency and increases the cost of production. In largemouth bass feed costs were estimated at 51% of total operating costs. (Engle et al., 2013). Under commercial culture conditions largemouth bass are usually fed floating feeds to satiation and feeding rates are limited by stocking densities which are limited by targeted biomass densities of usually > 5,600 kg/ha. During the early fall when water temperatures drop to 20°C, largemouth bass will normally consume approximately 1% of their BW which can be used to estimate total standing crop.

9.3 Feeding frequency

Feeding frequency refers to the number of times a day that fish are fed in culture systems. Feeding frequency is an essential consideration in fish feed management as it affects growth, feed conversion, water quality as well as profit maximization. The optimal interval between meals is related to environmental factors, such as water temperature and water quality, as well as the diet fed, the size of the fish and the species. Other factors that can affect optimization of the feeding regime are the nutrient density of the feed, the maximum voluntary food intake in one meal, and the evacuation rate of the stomach. These parameters have not been studied in largemouth bass, but have for better studied finfish species from which inferences can be made.

Riche et al. (2004) determined that gastric evacuation rate and return of appetite following a satiation meal for Nile tilapia (*Oreochromis niloticus*) to be 4 h at 28°C suggesting that tilapia should be fed three or four times per day. Ruohonen et al. (1998) determined that in order to achieve maximum growth rainbow trout (*Oncorhynchus mykiss*) should be fed at least three times per day and that feeding higher nutrient dense diets reduces the feeding frequency required to achieve maximum growth. Jobling (1983) reported that dominance hierarchy effects increased as access to food became more limiting in Arctic charr (*Salvelinus alpinus*). The authors observed that feeding by the majority of the fish was inhibited by the presence of larger individuals. Thia-Eng and Seng-Keh (1978) determined the optimal feeding frequency for food intake, weight gain and feed conversion efficiency of estuary grouper (*Epinephelus tauvina*) to be every 48 h or every other day.

Clearly, there are species specific differences related to appropriate feeding frequencies in fish. However, there are also some generalities that seem to be common to all species. Generally, younger fish perform better when fed more often than do older, larger fish. Smaller fish have higher energy demands than larger fish and usually their stomachs are too small to hold all the feed they require during one feeding a day. Herbivorous species and grazers (tilapia) require more frequent feedings than predatory species (grouper) due to inherent differences in gut length associated with the breakdown of lower nutrient dense feedstuffs.

As a robust predator largemouth bass have relatively large mouths and stomachs designed for swallowing large prey items and consequently do not need to be fed as often as some other species. Additionally, largemouth bass are often fed highly nutrient dense diets, such as Skretting's Classic Bass formulation with 48% protein and 18% fat (Skretting, Utah, USA), further reducing the necessity of multiple daily feedings. Under commercial culture conditions, fry and small largemouth bass fingerlings (< 7.5 cm) are fed up to eight times a day or as few as two times a day provided they are thoroughly satiated. During the feed training stage largemouth bass are often fed several times per day; although the feed is poorly utilized until the fish are habituated. Larger fingerlings (5.0–25 cm) seem to benefit from two feedings per day (morning and evening) during the first summer growing season. Largemouth bass >25 cm are typically fed only one time per day for further growout to food-fish size.

To avoid the effect of dominance hierarchy on feeding, some largemouth bass producers use feed blowers mounted to a truck (Figure 9.1) or utility vehicle to quickly spread feed over the entire length of the pond levee (personal communication, Robert Mayer, Bardstown, Kentucky, USA). The most aggressive fish in the pond tend to swim alongside the vehicle as the feed is being spread allowing for subordinate fish to feed freely. This is difficult to achieve when feeding by hand. Additionally, largemouth bass feed best early in the morning (30 min after sunrise) and late in the evening (30 min before sunset). During the hottest months of the summer it may be preferable to feed in the morning when the water temperatures are cooler.

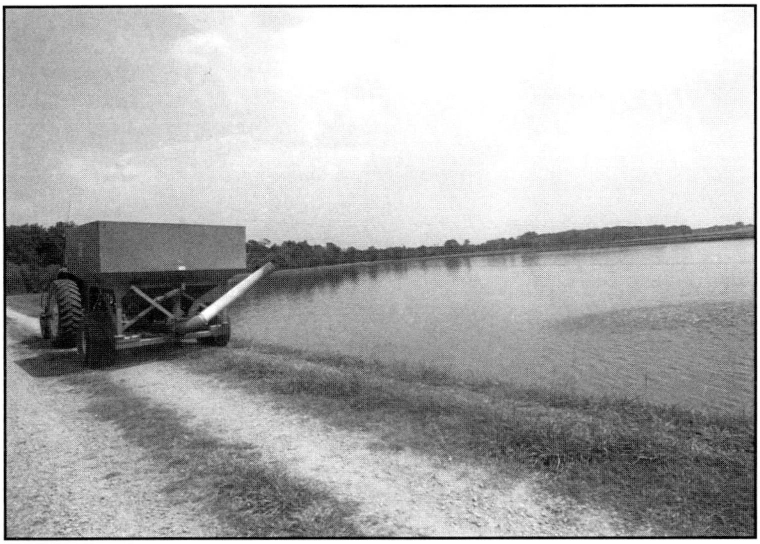

Figure 9.1 A truck mounted feed blower. It allows feed pellets to be uniformly spread over the pond surface.

9.4 Types of pellets

A single type of feed is not fed all the way through a fish's growout. As a fish grows, usually the pellet size increases and the protein content decreases. Also, as a fish grows, the feeding rate as a percentage of bodyweight decreases while the actual amount of feed fed increases. Other factors involved in efficient feeding include the correct choice of pellets with the proper physical characteristics. There are a number of pellet forms and manufacturing options to produce them.

9.5 Fry and fingerling feeds

Meal type feeds are fine particles used to feed first feeding fry in species that go directly from endogenous feeding (relying on nutrition in the yolk sac) to accepting artificial diets immediately upon switching to exogenous feeding (utilizing external sources of food). Largemouth bass fry do not readily accept artificial feeds at these early stages, so meal type feeds are not currently utilized in their production. During the feed-training process for largemouth bass, the artificial diets that the fish are transitioned to are usually pellets of 1.0–2.5 mm. These may be sinking pellets (steam pelleted) or sometimes floating pellets (extruded pellets). As the fish train to the feed and grow, pellet sizes are increased gradually to 5.5 mm during the first year of growth.

9.6 Development of practical growout/production diets

In early work on feed-trained largemouth bass at the Marion Fish Hatchery, Snow (1968) utilized a ration composed of 80% ground frozen fish, 10% dry commercial trout feed, and 10%

ground beef liver. Snow (1968) fed this mixture at rates up to 100 kg/ha/d and estimated this to be 5.3 to 11.2% of total BW (biomass) per day. The author also reported that artificially fed bass readily adjusted back to consuming forage fish if needed and that artificially fed largemouth bass achieved spawning success similar to broodfish raised on natural foods.

As noted previously, Snow and colleagues at the Marion, Alabama, National Fish Hatchery in 1968 began trials evaluating the OMP for use in largemouth bass production. The OMP was based on 10 years of research and was successfully tested in several salmonids including chinook, coho, and sockeye salmon and steelhead trout. The OMP proved to be more economical (34% savings compared to ground fish diets) and relatively efficient (food conversion ratio [FCR] 2.3). They also reported less disease problems with largemouth bass raised on OMP. Snow and Maxwell (1970) reported that largemouth bass in ponds fed the OMP "were more consistent" with respect to yield, feed conversion, survival, and rate of gain than ponds receiving other diets. Consistency of production is very important to both hatchery managers and commercial producers.

However, the OMP had some disadvantages, a primary one being it had to be stored under refrigeration (Hublou, 1963). This is due to moisture contents of 30–35%. To achieve longer shelf life dry pelleted feeds usually contain less than 10% moisture. Reducing moisture also reduces weight, resulting in substantial savings in shipping and handling costs. Piper et al. (1982) recommended a moist feed, such as OMP for largemouth bass, but also said a quality dry feed such as W-7 coolwater fish feed could be used. They also presented a feeding rate chart for largemouth bass on dry feeds (Table 9.1).

Much of the work referenced up to this point was still focused on producing fish for stocking programs and sizes (≤ 100 g). However, demand for larger fish increased during the 1980s (Brandt, 1991), based largely on increasing utilization of larger largemouth bass in fee-fishing (JSA, 1983), managed trophy fisheries (Dupree and Huner, 1984), and as live food products in ethnic markets. In the USA in 1983, the Joint Subcommittee on Aquaculture (JSA) listed research priorities for developing largemouth bass aquaculture. These priorities included

Table 9.1 Bass feed chart: percent body weight fed per day in raceway culture for formulated dry feeds (Piper et al., 1982).

	Size (inches)				
	1–2	2–3	3–4	4–5	5+
	Weight (pounds)				
Water temperature (°F)	0.002	0.002–0.015	0.015–0.03	0.03–0.06	0.06
65	4.4%	4.0%	3.2%	2.4%	1.6%
70	5.5%	4.7%	2.5%	2.2%	2.0%
75	6.0%	5.0%	4.0%	3.0%	2.0%
80	6.5%	5.4%	4.3%	3.3%	2.2%
85	7.1%	5.9%	4.7%	3.5%	2.4%
90	7.5%	6.3%	5.1%	3.9%	2.7%
Feedings per hour	4	4	2	1	1

Note: Winter feeding rate: 1% body weight per day.

determination of efficient growout procedures, evaluation of effects of water quality (metabolic wastes) under intensive culture conditions, and development of species-specific, cost-efficient, diets utilizing practical feed ingredients (JSA, 1983). The Joint Sub-Committee proposed that if this information can be generated, there appears to be a favorable financial potential for commercial production of this species.

Beginning in 1995, researchers at Kentucky State University (KSU) began a series of studies focused on (1) developing species specific-feeds for largemouth bass and (2) culture methods to produce large harvest sizes (≥ 500 g) intensively in ponds. Tidwell et al. (1996) stocked advanced juvenile (122 g) largemouth bass at 12,350/ha and fed three dietary protein levels (42, 44, and 47%) once daily for a full 12 months. This allowed feed consumption, water quality, and fish growth to all be monitored monthly over four seasons of growth.

In terms of water quality, overall means (over the full 12 months) for total ammonia-nitrogen (TAN), were significantly different among ponds in which fish were fed the 42, 44, and 47% protein diets, averaging 0.62, 0.83, and 1.3 mg/1, respectively (Figure 9.2). Differences in concentrations of TAN at individual sampling dates occurred primarily during periods of low water temperatures, especially December, January, and February. Concentrations of TAN during those periods reflected the same relationships to dietary protein levels as did overall TAN means (47% > 44% > 42% diets).

Overall nitrite concentrations for the 12 month culture period also reflected dietary protein levels (47% > 44% > 42%), though these differences were not statistically significant. There were significant treatment differences in nitrite concentrations at some individual sampling dates (Figure 9.3), primarily during periods of rapidly decreasing (November–December), and increasing (February–March) water temperatures, with ponds in which fish were fed the 47% protein feed having higher levels.

In terms of growth and production, at final harvest largemouth bass fed the 47% protein diet had significantly higher average weights (436 g), gains (351 g), survival (99%), and total biomass (4,252 kg/ha), and significantly lower feed conversion ratios (FCR; 2.0), than bass fed the 42% protein diet (Table 9.2). Bass fed the 44% protein diet were not significantly different from those fed 42–47% protein diets in any of these variables. Significant differences in average weights developed by 2 months post-stocking. Bass fed 47% protein gained approximately 202% during

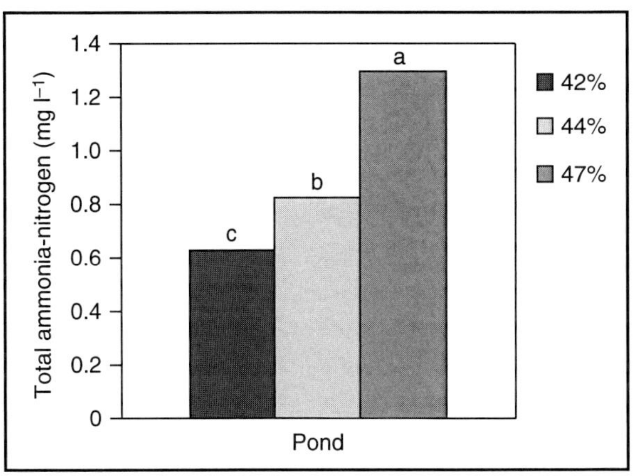

Figure 9.2 Overall means of total ammonia-nitrogen (mg l^{-1}) in ponds in which juvenile largemouth bass were fed diets containing 42, 44, or 47% protein. Each bar represents a mean of 52 weekly samples per pond in three replicate ponds per diet. Different letters above bars indicate significant differences among treatment means ($P < 0.05$).

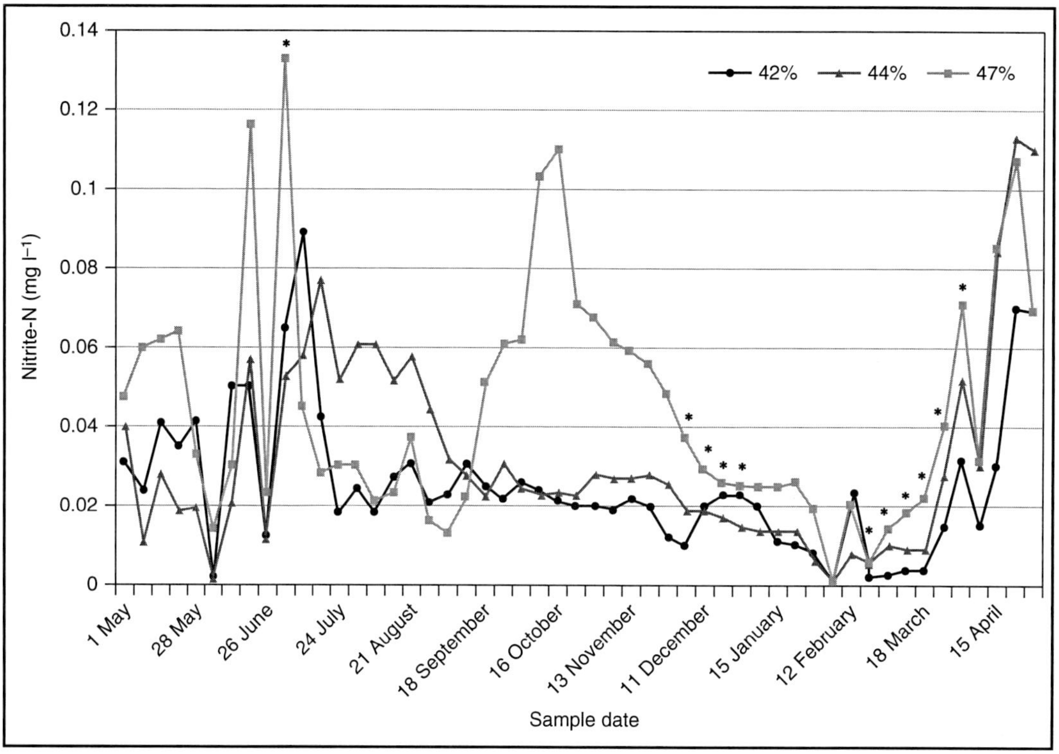

Figure 9.3 Weekly means of nitrite-nitrogen (mg l^{-1}) in ponds in which juvenile largemouth bass were fed diets containing 42, 44, or 47% protein. Each point represents four weekly samples per pond in three replicate ponds. An asterisk indicates a difference among treatments ($P < 0.05$).

Table 9.2 Individual weight, weight gain, percentage survival, feed conversion ratio (FCR), and unit production of largemouth bass fed diets containing three protein percentages.

Production variable	Dietary protein		
	42%	44%	47%
Harvest weight (g)	374 ± 19b	406 ± 23ab	436 ± 38a
Total individual gain (g)	313 ± 22b	331 ± 18ab	351 ± 25a
Survival (%)	86 ± 6b	92 ± 7ab	99 ± 1a
Total FCR	2.6 ± 0.3a	2.3 ± 0.2ab	2.0 ± 0.2b
Gross yield (kg ha^{-1})	3972 ± 325b	4613 ± 469ab	5330 ± 505a
Summer individual gain (%)	162.5 ± 14.8b	157 ± 7.0b	201.7 ± 6.2a
Summer specific growth rate (%)	0.54 ± 0.04b	0.53 ± 0.02a	0.62 ± 0.01a
Summer FCR	2.2 ± 0.1ab	2.4 ± 0.2a	1.9 ± 0.0b
Winter individual gain (%)	19.6 ± 11.0	28.5 ± 5.4	17.3 ± 5.1
Winter specific growth rate (%)	0.09 ± 0.6	0.12 ± 0.03	0.09 ± 0.03
Winter FCR	4.2 ± 1.9	2.4 ± 0.4	3.9 ± 1.0

Notes: Values are means of ± s.e. of three replicate ponds. Means in the same row with different letters are significantly different ($P < 0.05$).

the summer period and 17% during the winter (Table 9.2). There were no significant differences between fish in the three treatments in winter individual gains, winter specific growth rate (SGR), or winter FCR.

Dressout percentages, and head, fillet, and gut weights (as a percentage of BW) did not differ significantly among bass fed the three diets. Moisture, lipid, protein, and ash averaged 71.2, 6.0, 18.9, and 3.8% in the whole body and 76.9, 1.3, 20.6, and 1.1% in the fillet.

In terms of feeding patterns, the bass were active feeders, especially in early summer (June) and slowed later in the summer (Figure 9.4). Feeding continued until temperatures dropped below approximately 8°C. In the spring, bass began to feed actively again as temperatures rose above 8°C. This response is similar to those reported for the hybrid bluegill (*Lepomis cyanellus* × *L. macrochirus)* (Tidwell et al., 1994).

Largemouth bass feeding and growth slowed during the winter months, but winter gains (October–March) averaged approximately 22% over all three diets. When compared with another centrarchids, winter gains were similar to results for small (40 g) hybrid bluegill (28%) (Tidwell et al., 1992), and higher than winter gains of larger (100 g) hybrid bluegill (17%) (Tidwell et al., 1994). Total weight gains over the 12 month period (257%) were higher than those reported for hybrid bluegill (167%) stocked at the same density for a similar culture period (Tidwell et al., 1994). Feed conversion ratios were superior to those for hybrid bluegill, averaging 2.0 for largemouth bass, while hybrid bluegill averaged 5.7 (Tidwell et al., 1994).

Currently several fish feed manufacturers produce formulations designed specifically for largemouth bass. Commercially available largemouth bass diets typically contain relatively high levels of protein (45–48%) and lipids (16–22%) and low levels of carbohydrate (<21%) compared to diets for other commercially important fish species. These highly nutrient dense diets are considered to be necessary for health maintenance of largemouth bass and are typically formulated using high levels of animal source proteins, primarily fish meal.

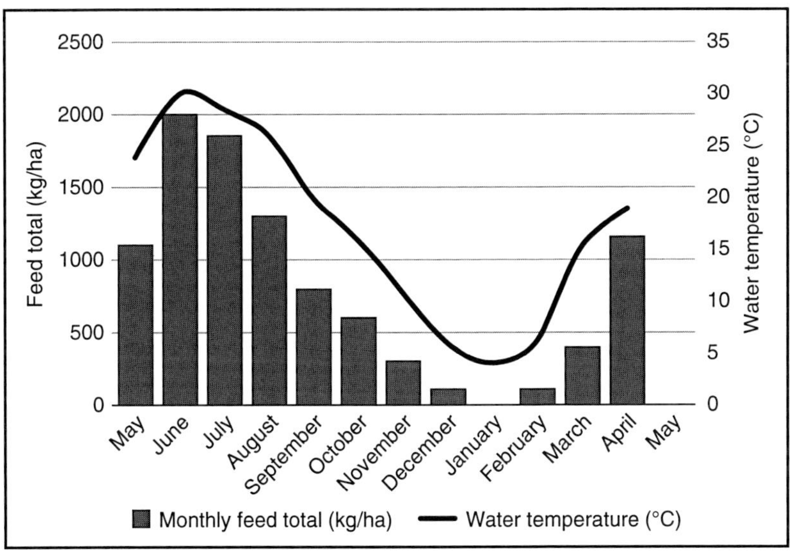

Figure 9.4 Overall monthly feed totals per pond for all diets at different water temperatures over a 1 year culture period.

9.7 Effects of stocking density on feed response and feed conversion

In an associated study, Tidwell et al. (1998a) also evaluated the impact of stocking density on growth and feed conversion of advanced largemouth bass fingerlings. Feed-trained fingerlings (122 g) were stocked in May at either 6,175 or 12,350/ha and fed a 44% protein diet once daily to satiation for a full 12 months. At harvest, there was no significant difference in weight gain or average weight of largemouth bass stocked at 6,175 or 12,350 fish/ha (Table 9.3). These data differ from those reported by Tidwell et al. (1994) for hybrid bluegill (also a centrarchid) for whom increasing stocking density from 6,175 to 12,350/ha significantly decreased weight gain and average weight at harvest. Tucker and Robinson (1990) stated that for channel catfish increasing fish density normally decreases average fish size. Total yield was greater for largemouth bass stocked at 12,350/ha than at 6,175/ha (4,598 and 2,354 kg/ha, respectively). At the higher stocking density, feed was more efficiently utilized, as indicated by a significantly lower FCR (2.3) compared to the low stocking density (3.3). Results differ from those for catfish, where higher stocking densities usually result in higher feed conversion ratios due to reduced feed intake and decreased efficiency of feed conversion (Tucker and Robinson, 1990).

Tidwell et al. (1996) reported that the most active feeding period for largemouth bass was June–July (> 25°C). However, in this study largemouth bass stocked at the lower density consumed more feed and gained weight more rapidly during the fall period of declining water temperatures (September–November), while those stocked at high density consumed more feed and gained weight more rapidly during the rising water temperatures of spring (March–May) (Figure 9.5). At final harvest, average weights of fish in the two treatments were similar. Stocking largemouth bass juveniles at the higher density (12,350/ha) resulted in higher net and gross yields and more efficient feed conversion than stocking at low density, without decreasing average individual weights or reducing survival.

There is demand for large (> 500 g) largemouth bass for corrective stocking in sport-fish ponds, fee-fishing, and managed trophy fisheries. A study was conducted at KSU to evaluate

Table 9.3 Initial individual weight (mean ± SE), final individual weight, final lengths, percentage, survival, average individual gain, total yield, and feed conversion ratio (FCR) for largemouth bass fed prepared diets for one year in ponds. Means within a row followed by the different letters are significantly different ($P < 0.05$).

	Stocking rate (fish/ha)	
	6,175/ha	12,350/ha
Stocking weight (g)	124 ± 4	122 ± 2
Final weight (g)	406 ± 32	406 ± 22
Weight gain (%)	282 ± 29	283 ± 23
Final length (cm)	29.3 ± 0.8	29.1 ± 0.5
Survival (%)	93.9 ± 8.5	91.7 ± 6.7
Total yield (kg/ha)	2354 ± 242b	4598 ± 418a
FCR	3.3 ± 0.3a	2.3 ± 0.2b

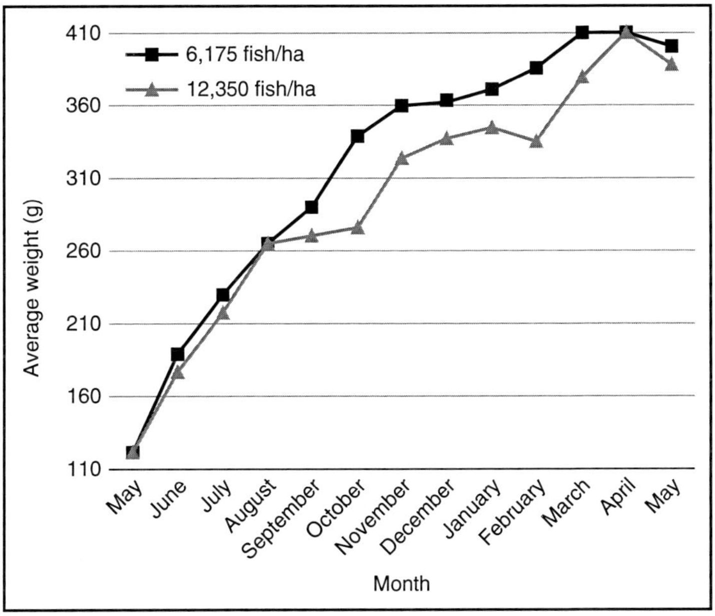

Figure 9.5 Mean sample weights of largemouth bass stocked at 6,175 or 12,350 fish/ha. There were no significant differences ($P \geq 0.05$) in average weight at any sampling date.

the effects of stocking density on third-year growth of feed-trained largemouth bass raised in ponds (Tidwell et al., 1998b). Lovell (1989) observed that feed consumption, growth rate, and feed conversion efficiencies generally decrease as fish size increases. Busch (1985) demonstrated in channel catfish that growth slowed and feed conversion ratios increased during third-year growth. Tidwell et al. (1998b) reported that during second-year growth largemouth stocked at higher density had significantly lower FCRs than those stocked at low density. The objective of this study was to evaluate the effects of stocking density on growth and feed conversion of largemouth bass during third-year growth.

Juvenile largemouth bass (383 g) were stocked in May at either 3,750/ha or 7,500/ha and fed a 44% protein diet once daily to satiation for 334 days. In terms of weight gain the pattern of weight gain in this third-year study (Figure 9.6) differs from that reported in Tidwell et al. (1998a) for second-year largemouth bass. The primary difference was during the period of August to November in second year fish those stocked at low density gained more weight, while in third-year fish those stocked at high density gained more weight. Production data are presented in Table 9.4. There was no significant difference in individual weight gain, with an overall average harvest weight of 536 g and average individual gain of 40%. This compares to 113% individual weight gain for channel catfish during third-year growth (Busch, 1986). Since increased density did not reduce average fish size, treatment densities resulted in large differences in pond production data, with the high-density treatment producing significantly greater total yields and pond unit production rates than the low-density treatment (Table 9.4).

When we look at feeding activity and efficiency of feed utilization, the differences in feed conversion ratios were large (9.6 and 3.8 in low- and high-density third-year ponds, respectively) but not statistically significant due to high within-treatment variation. Feed conversion ratios for third-year bass at high densities (3.8) were much higher than those reported for second-year bass at high densities (2.3; Tidwell et al., 1998a, 1998b). These data agree with

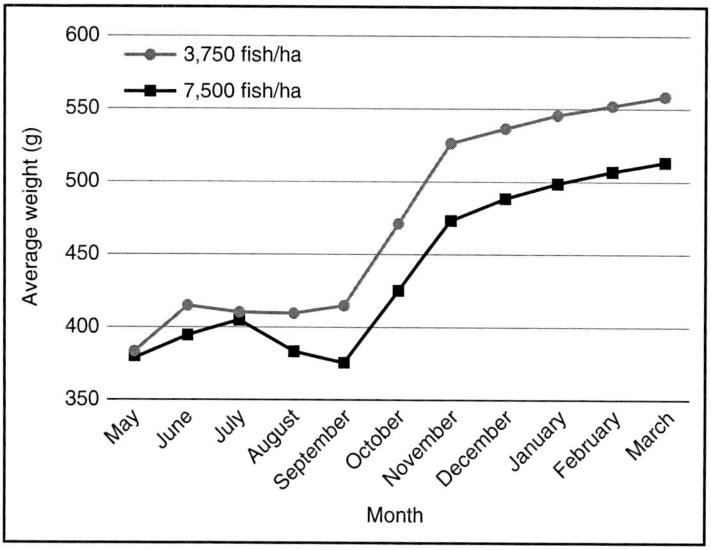

Figure 9.6 Mean sample weights of largemouth bass stocked at 3,750 and 7,500 fish/ha. There were no significant differences ($P \geq 0.05$) in average weight at any sampling date.

Table 9.4 Initial individual weight (mean ± SE), final individual weight, final lengths, percentage, percent survival, average individual gain, total yield, and feed conversion ratio (FCR) for largemouth bass fed prepared diets for one year in ponds. Means within a row followed by the different letters are significantly different ($P < 0.05$).

	Stocking rate (fish/ha)	
	3,750/ha	7,500/ha
Stocking weight (g)	380 ± 24a	366 ± 5a
Final weight (g)	514 ± 38a	559 ± 7a
Weight gain (%)	35 ± 5a	47 ± 5a
Final length (cm)	92.3 ± 4.0a	82.7 ± 16.1a
Survival (%)	341 ± 123b	1,040 ± 66a
Total yield (kg/ha)	1,758 ± 230b	3,909 ± 19a
FCR	9.6 ± 4.0a	3.8 ± 0.4a

Lovell (1984) who stated that growth rate and feed conversion efficiencies generally decrease as fish size increases. Busch (1986) reported an FCR of 2.2 for third-year channel catfish. Average individual gains and FCRs averaged over both treatments (58% and 7.3, respectively), were similar to those reported for third-year walleye production in ponds (45% and 9.1, respectively) (Coyle and Tidwell, 1997). High FCRs are usually indicative of overfeeding, inefficient utilization of consumed feed, or both. In this study feeding rates were based on fish response. This required that some feed be presented to fish in each pond to allow the opportunity to feed. On days when fish did not respond, this feed was wasted. This was especially true during the winter. During summer months, fish normally consumed feed but apparently did not convert efficiently.

9.8 Effect of reduced fish meal levels on feed consumption and growth

Other factors are known to affect feed acceptance and feeding rate in fish. As a carnivore, largemouth bass do not always readily accept diets with low levels of fish meal. Cochran et al. (2009) fed diets containing varying levels of fish meal (8, 24, and 45%) to largemouth bass under practical production conditions in ponds. They reported that the average daily feed consumption, average harvest weight, survival, and total production did not differ among fish fed the experimental diets. The feed conversion ratio was very good for fish fed all three diets and was significantly lower (1.34) in fish fed the 24% FM diet than in fish fed the 45% FM (1.43) diets.

The authors in Cochran et al. (2009) noted that the custom manufactured pellets were "slow sink" and were more readily consumed than the commercial floating pellets (used as a commercial control reference diet) especially on bright sunny days. This indicates that physical pellet characteristics might still be a factor to be evaluated in largemouth bass.

The trend toward reducing fish meal in diets for carnivore fishes, such as largemouth bass continues. As discussed, Cochran et al. (2009) demonstrated that practical diets containing 8% fish meal were still consumed well and performed well in ponds. Tidwell et al. (2005) evaluated largemouth bass diets containing 0% fish meal in tanks. Poultry by-product meal (PBM) successfully replaced all fish meal with no significant impacts on growth, survival, or feed conversion ratio. However, PBM is an animal source protein. All plant protein diets were not successfully evaluated.

9.8.1 *Feed attractants*

One approach to improve the consumption of plant protein-based diets in other species has been the use of chemoattractants or feed enhancers. For the hybrid striped bass, (*Morone saxatilis*) certain amino acids (alanine, serine, glycine, and proline) have been reported to be efficient feed attractants as were fish solubles (Papatryphon and Soars, 2000). Fish solubles (FS) were reported to increase feed intake in red drum (*Sciaenops ocellatus*) fed a soybean based diet (McGoogan and Gatlin, 1997) but were not beneficial for red drum fed diets containing fish meal (Davis et al., 1995).

Kubitza and Lovshin (1997) conducted a series of trials to identify feed enhancers for largemouth bass. In their Trial 1, fish meal (FM) was decreased (60, 40, 20, and 0%) and replaced by 20, 40, and 60% soybean meal (SBM). As the fish meal was decreased and SBM increased, feed intake declined. In Trial 2, the 0% FM diet was then used as a Control diet to test candidate feed enhancers (including eight amino acids, two nucleotides, and betaine). The betaine and amino acids did not affect feed consumption but nucleotides increased feed intake by 45% compared to the Control diet. A third trial identified the nucleotide inosine-5-monophosphaate (IMP05') as the most effective chemical feed enhancer tested. However, including even 10% fish meal in the formulation was more effective than adding the nucleotide.

A study evaluating attractants in largemouth bass fed 100% plant protein diets compared soluble fish protein (SFP), Fisharon (a commercial product; FA), and fish silage (FS) (Oliveira and Cyrino, 2004). Only the Fisharon produced positive results. Identifying products with feed attractant properties is not always an intentional process. Y.-J. Chen et al. (2012) conducted a study to evaluate possible detrimental effects of oxidized (rancid) dietary lipid on the growth and health of largemouth bass. Unexpectedly, they found that the oxidized oils actually enhanced feed intake, fish growth, and the efficiency of feed conversion. This is unusual as use of rancid oils in fish diets is usually associated with poor palatability of the diet and reduced feed intake (Kestemont and Baras, 2001; Fontagne et al., 2006).

9.9 Pellet characteristics

Early commercial fish diets were manufactured by steam pelleting into densely compressed particles that sink. Later, extrusion processed feeds that float on the water surface became more common. Floating feed is a valuable management tool because it allows the farmer to see how much, and how actively, the fish eat (Mgbenka and Lovell, 1984). Extrusion can also increase the water stability of the pellet (Lovell, 1984). However, the energy costs to produce extruded feeds are higher. In the manufacture of extruded feeds, the ingredient mix is heated to a higher temperature. Also, extruded feeds require heat in drying, while pelleted feeds do not (Mgbenka and Lovell, 1984). However, in some species the lower nutrient density and greater pellet stability of extruded diets prolonged gastric emptying time compared with steam pellets and consequently reduced feed intake (Hilton et al., 1981; Venou et al., 2009) and even growth (Booth et al., 2000, 2002; Honorato et al., 2010).

The size and shape of the feed pellet may also affect the amount of feed consumed (Jobling, 2001). The pellet size of fish feeds should be as large as possible to minimize nutrient leaching (Lovell, 1989). Optimally, pellet size should be 25–50% of the species, mouth width (Jobling, 2001). Kubitza and Lovshin (1997) fed age 1 largemouth bass (initial weight, 62 g) a 7 mm trout pellet and reported that pellet size may have been too small. They indicated that largemouth bass strike at individual pellets and many strikes would be required to satiate a fish. Kubitza and Lovshin (1997) proposed that by feeding a large pellet to largemouth bass, less feeding energy would be expended per meal and faster growth might be attained.

To evaluate the relative performance of largemouth bass fed feeds with different pellet characteristics (sinking or floating and pellet size) under practical pond conditions, Tidwell et al. (2015) produced three experimental diets, all containing 43% protein and 17% lipid. Floating pellets were produced with diameters of 5.5 mm (control) and 13.0 mm (large). Sinking pellets were produced at 5.5 mm. Nine 0.0-ha ponds (three replicates per treatment) were stocked with largemouth bass averaging 185 g at 10,000 bass/ha. Fish were fed once daily (0800) to apparent satiation for 151 days.

9.9.1 Effect of pellet size

Both pellet sizes of the floating diet were well utilized by the fish throughout the experiment. Harvest data indicated that standard size (control, 5.5 mm) versus large (13.0) floating pellets produced no significant impact on production characteristics during second year growth of largemouth bass in ponds. Although Kubitza and Lovshin (1997) proposed that largemouth bass might benefit from increased pellet sizes, they did not conduct a controlled comparison. While Tidwell et al. (2015) showed no benefit in feeding larger pellets, Nortvedt and Tuene (1995) reported that feeding larger pellets had improved feed conversion efficiencies in Atlantic halibut *Hippoglossus hippoglossus*. Linner and Brannas (1994) reported that in Arctic Char *Salvelinus alpinus* responded more rapidly to larger pellets, but pellet consumption was better at intermediate sizes.

9.9.2 Effect of floating versus sinking pellets

The largemouth bass fed the 5.5 mm sinking pellets were significantly larger at harvest (629 g) than those fed a similar size floating pellet (566 g). Specific growth rate was also significantly higher ($P \leq 0.05$) in fish fed the sinking pellet (206 g/d) than in those fed the floating pellet (2.2 g/d). There was no significant difference ($P > 0.05$) in survival (>90%), total yield, condition factor, FCR, or average daily feed consumption among fish fed the similar size floating or sinking diets. Total yields in our study were higher than for the largemouth bass reported by Cochran et al. (2009), who compared diets containing different fish meal levels but stocked at a lower density (8,650/ha versus 10,000/ha). Fish fed the 5.5 mm sinking pellets, compared with those fed the large (13 mm) floating pellets, had production metric differences similar to the differences between the 5.5 mm sinking versus floating pellets.

The larger average size at harvest and higher SGR of largemouth bass fed sinking pellets are in agreement with findings of Booth et al. (2000, 2002) for silver perch *Bidyanus bidyanus* and with Honorato et al. (2010) for pacu *Piaractus mesopotamicus*. According to Sorensen (2012), the lower bulk density (less weight per unit volume) of floating pellets compared with sinking pellets would result in fish fed floating pellets becoming physically satiated at a lower energy intake. This is supported by Mgbenka and Lovell (1984), who reported that sinking feeds had less bulk per unit of weight (that is, were denser) and less digestible energy. Dense pellets with low energy concentrations would allow fish to consume more of the nutrients essential to growth before becoming satiated by energy intake or stomach fullness.

There are also behavioral aspects associated with feeding sinking pellets versus floating. Kubitza and Lovshin (1997) proposed that use of sinking pellets might result in more wasted feed (that is, higher FCR) because largemouth bass were not likely to pick up pellets off the bottom. However, we found FCR was not different among fish fed floating or sinking pellets, indicating the efficient use of sinking pellets. Both studies utilized satiation feeding. Other behavioral traits might also affect the suitability of different pellet characteristics. Kubitza and Lovshin (1997) also observed that, when using floating pellets, largemouth bass were reluctantly forced into surface waters with high light levels and temperatures (≥ 30°C). Cochran et al. (2009) also observed that largemouth bass were hesitant to feed on floating pellets at the surface on bright sunny days, but would readily consume pellets that would "slow-sink" through the water column.

Another potential positive aspect of the use of sinking feeds for largemouth bass is that the manufacture of sinking pellets allows lower dietary carbohydrate levels. To product floating pellets a formulation must contain ≥ 20% carbohydrate for proper expansion (Lovell, 1989). However, as a strict carnivore, largemouth bass have been found to be negatively impacted by carbohydrate levels of 20% (Goodwin et al., 2002; Amoah et al., 2008). Use of sinking pellets would allow more flexibility in feed formulation and reduction of carbohydrate content. Also, it would increase the potential of more localized feed production because steam pelleting facilities are more common and less complex than extruders.

A potential approach to capitalize on the positive results of sinking pellets, without sacrificing the positive feed management characteristics of floating pellets, could be to feed primarily sinking feed but mix in some floating pellets as "indicator pellets" to assist in monitoring feeding activity and consumption, as evaluated by Mgbenka and Lovell (1984) in channel catfish *Ictalurus punctatus*. They proposed the feeding of a 15 : 85 ratio of extruded to pelleted diets to reduce costs while providing the same management benefits of feeding observation.

9.9.3 Effect of water temperature on feed consumption

Largemouth bass, as are other fish, are very much influenced by their environment. As poikilothermic animals, water temperature is one of the most powerful environmental variables, largely controlling their metabolic rate and as such, their feed consumption rate. Johnson and Charlton (1960) evaluated the effects of water temperature on the metabolism and activity of fingerling largemouth bass (6–10 g). They reported that food consumption, swimming speed, and scope-for-activity rose steadily from 5°C to level off over the range of 22–29°C. They reported that the maximum scope-for-activity to be approximately 25°C, the physiological limit of the fish to be approximately 28–30°C and the upper lethal limit to be around 35°C. According to Johnson and Charlton (1960) largemouth bass are unusual in that their activity rate continues to increase right up to the upper end of their temperature tolerance. In many species, the activity rate drops off well below the upper lethal level.

As part of a series of studies evaluating largemouth bass as a culture species Tidwell et al. (2003) evaluated feeding activity, growth, survival, and body composition of largemouth bass raised at three temperatures (20, 26, and 32°C). Feed-trained juvenile largemouth bass (9 g) were stocked into nine 3,610 l tanks at 140 fish/m^3 (500 fish/tank). The bass were fed a salmonid diet (45% protein, 16% lipid) to apparent satiation twice daily for 12 weeks.

The growth pattern of bass raised at different culture temperatures is shown in Figure 9.7. Consistent differences were established by the first sample date. After 97 d, the average weight of bass cultured at 20°C was significantly lower than fish in the 26 and 32°C treatments, which were not significantly different from each other (Table 9.5). Bass grown at 26 and 32°C had significantly higher weight gain (%), SGR (%), condition factors (K), and production (kg/m^3) than those in the 20°C treatment. There was no significant difference in survival among treatments, which averaged 96.5% overall. However, fish in the 32°C treatment suffered an outbreak of *Aeromonas* sp. This epizootic in the high temperature treatment may indicate that 32°C is high enough to represent stressful conditions for largemouth.

Bass in the 26°C treatment had significantly lower FCR indicating a more efficient feed utilization. Fish raised at 26°C also had a higher percentage protein deposited (PPD) than bass raised at 20 and 32°C, which were not significantly different (Table 9.5). These data indicate that largemouth bass gain weight and convert feed and dietary protein more efficiently at 26°C than at 20 or 32°C. Largemouth bass will feed at 20°C and convert feed efficiently, though appetite is reduced compared to higher temperatures. As culture temperature is increased to 26 and 32°C, appetite and growth both increase. At higher end of that range, feed and protein efficiencies decrease. At 32°C food intake did not increase further, while energy demands for maintenance and activity increase (Weatherly and Gill, 1987) as evidenced by reduced oxygen concentrations

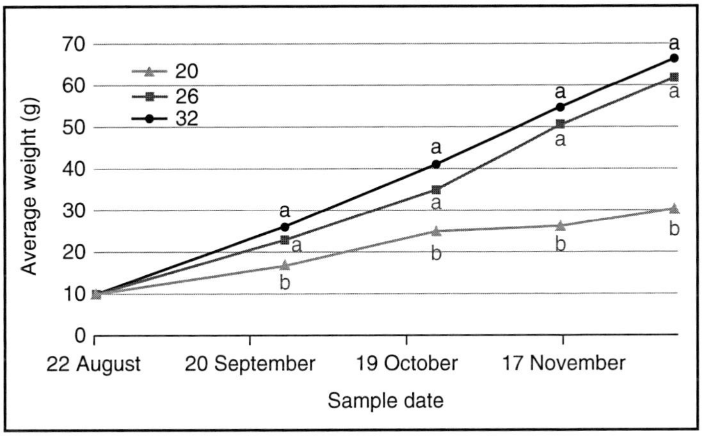

Figure 9.7 Relationship between largemouth bass body weight and sample date when raised at three culture temperatures (22, 26, and 32°C). Each symbol represents the mean of three replicate tanks. Sample means with different letters are significantly different (*P* < 0.05).

Table 9.5 Final average weights, production, feed conversion, survival, weight gains, specific growth rates, and protein efficiency ratio, condition factory (K), and hepatosomatic index (HSI) for largemouth bass raised at three temperatures for 97 d. Values are mean ± SE of three replicates. Means within a row followed by different letters are significantly different (*P* < 0.05) by ANOVA.

	Culture temperature (°C)		
	20	26	32
Average weight (g)	30.5 ± 0.8b	61.9 ± 0.6a	66.1 ± 3.6a
Production (kg/m3)	2.8 ± 0.2b	7.12 ± 0.04a	6.63 ± 0.61a
FCR	1.2 ± 0.0a	1.0 ± 0.0b	1.1 ± 0.1a
Survival (%)	96.8 ± 1.9a	97.7 ± 1.3b	86.5 ± 9.8a
Weight gain (%)	325.1 ± 1.8b	666.2 ± 2.9b	627.4 ± 48.9a
Specific growth rate (%/d)	1.3 ± 0.0b	2.0 ± 0.0a	1.9 ± 0.1a
Percent protein deposited	33.4 ± 1.0	39.9 ± 1.6a	32.5 ± 3.5b
K factor	1.3 ± 0.1b	1.4 ± 0.0a	1.4 ± 0.1a
HSI	2.6 ± 0.4a	2.3 ± 0.2a	2.0 ± 0.34a

in 32°C tanks. Dissolved oxygen concentrations were reduced below levels accounted for by direct effects on the water's ability to dissolve oxygen. These factors could explain the decreased feed conversion efficiency at the high temperature treatment. Other possible explanations may be shifts of enzyme activities to different isozymes, and stress reactions due to increased occurrence of disease (that is, *Aeromonas* sp.) (Keembiyehetty and Wilson, 1998).

While it is well known that changes in culture temperature can influence the body composition of fish, reactions among species vary, increasing the need to evaluate impacts on individual species (Cui and Wootton, 1988). In Tidwell et al. (2003) there was no significant difference in the protein, lipid, or ash content of whole body or white muscle of largemouth bass raised at the three treatment temperatures. This differs from channel catfish *Ictalurus punctatus* in which lipid deposition has been shown to increase as culture temperature increases (Andrews and Stickney, 1972). Moisture content of bass tissues was affected by temperature. However, the actual magnitude of changes in moisture levels were quite small and are not likely biologically significant.

Hepatosomatic index (HSI) consistently decreased as culture temperatures increased, though differences were not statistically significant. This agrees with Heidinger and Crawford (1977) who reported increased temperature lowered HSI in largemouth bass. Keembiyehetty and Wilson (1998) reported that in sunshine bass liver metabolism was altered between the two study temperatures (26.7 and 32.2°C) with increased temperatures shifting lipid from the liver to visceral storage. They reported that this may have indicated stress at the higher temperature. In Tidwell et al. (2003) there appeared to be the opposite trend in largemouth bass. Lipid concentrations in the liver were significantly increased at 32°C (Table 9.5) while whole body lipid concentrations showed a decreasing trend with temperature. Since lipid concentrations in white muscle were low (<0.05%), and did not change with temperature, this indirectly indicates decreased visceral storage. In largemouth bass visceral fat stores are tightly bound to pyloric cecae and accurate direct measurements are extremely difficult.

In Tidwell et al. (2003) at a water temperature near 26°C, feeding, growth, survival, feed conversion, and protein retention appear near optimal. At 20°C, feed conversion and survival remain good but feeding activity and growth rate is reduced approximately 35%. At 32°C, feeding is active and growth is similar to that at 26°C, but feed conversion efficiency and protein retention is decreased. Also, fish may be under chronic stress conditions and more susceptible to disease outbreaks.

Brandt and Flickinger (1987) recommended feeding largemouth bass a semi-moist sinking feed at 1% of BW/day when pond water temperatures are below 10°C every 5–7 d. However, this is seldom practiced in commercial production of largemouth bass.

9.10 Effect of photoperiod on feeding

Photoperiod is also known to influence feed intake and growth of fish. Petit et al. (2003) stated that the largemouth bass is a diurnal species whose activity pattern is based on day-night alterations, and if presented with continuous light, will remain active. They conducted a study to evaluate food intake and growth of largemouth bass held under a 12L : 12D alternating cycle or continuous light. At the end of 12 weeks largemouth bass under continuous light conditions had significantly higher feed consumption, higher average weight, and higher feed conversion efficiency than fish held under day–night alteration.

9.11 Effects of artificial feeding on morphology and fitness

It is accepted that largemouth bass of advanced sizes can be raised much more intensively and cost effectively on formulated feeds than using live forage. However, there have been reports of pellet-raised largemouth bass having morphological differences from those raised on live forage (Wintzer and Motta, 2005). These changes could negatively affect fitness if used in a sport-fish stocking. However, the morphology of the skulls of pellet-reared fish were observed to converge toward wild largemouth bass after being provided with live forage for a period. In a recent study, Keretz et al. (2018) compared survival of pellet-raised largemouth bass with pellet raised which had been "naturalized" by feeding live forage for different periods (1–12 weeks), with all forage fed wild largemouth bass. Fish from these backgrounds were subjected to a series of sublethal stressors. Under the conditions of this study, pellet-reared bass survived as well as naturalized and wild largemouth bass.

9.12 Conclusion

Although the body of research concerning largemouth bass aquaculture continues to grow slowly, there still remains a considerable amount of work to be done. A complete understanding of appropriate feeds and feeding technologies for largemouth bass is still lacking. Fish producers and feed manufacturers still struggle with the notion of the dietary connection to long-term health in largemouth bass. As researchers begin to better understand the relationship between nutrition and health in largemouth bass thus allowing feed manufacturers more flexibility in diet formulations the cost of raising largemouth bass for the food-fish market should decrease over time.

References

Amoah, A., Coyle, S.D., Webster, C.D., Durborow, R.M., Bright, L.A. and Tidwell, J.H. (2008) Effects of graded levels of carbohydrate on growth and survival of largemouth bass, *Micropterus salmoides*. *Journal of the World Aquaculture Society* 39 (3), 395–405.

Andrews, J.W. and Stickney, R.R. (1972) Interactions of feeding rates and environmental temperature on growth, food conversion, and body composition of channel catfish. *Transactions of the American Fisheries Society* 101, 94–99.

Booth, M.A., Allan, G.L. and Warner-Smith, R. (2000) Effects of grinding, steam conditioning and extrusion of practical diet on digestibility and weight gain of silver perch *Bidyanus bidyanus*. *Aquaculture* 182, 287–299.

Booth, M.A., Allan, G.L., Evans, A.J. and Gleeson, V.P. (2002) Effects of steam pelleting or extrusion on digestibility and performance of silver perch *Bidyanus bidyanus*. *Aquaculture Research* 33, 1163–1173.

Boyd, C.E. (1990) *Water Quality in Ponds for Aquaculture*. Birmingham Publishing Co., Birmingham, AL.

Brandt, T. (1991) Temperate basses, (*Morone* spp.), and black basses, (*Micropterus* spp.). In: Wilson, R.P. (ed.) *Handbook of Nutrient Requirements of finfish*. CRC Press, Baca Raton, FL.

Brandt, T.M. and Flickinger, S.A. (1987) Feeding largemouth bass during cool and cold weather. *The Progressive Fish Culturist* 49 (4), 286–290.

Busch, R.L. (1985) Channel catfish culture in ponds. In: Tucker, C.S. (ed.) *Channel Catfish Culture: Developments in Aquaculture and Fisheries Science*, Vol. 15. Elsevier Science Publishers B.V., Amsterdam, pp. 13–84.

Busch, R.L. (1986) Third year growth on channel catfish. *Progressive Fish-Culturist* 48, 188–189.

Chen, Y.-J., Lui, Y.-J., Yang, H.-J., Yuan, Y., Liu, F.-J., Tian, L.-X., Liang, G.-Y. and Yuan, R.-M. (2012) Effect of dietary oxidized fish oil on growth performance, body composition, antioxidant defense mechanism and liver histology of juvenile largemouth bass *Micropterus salmoides*. *Aquaculture Nutrition* 18 (3), 321–331.

Cochran, N.J., Coyle, S.D. and Tidwell, J.H. (2009) Evaluation of reduced fish meal diets for second year growth of the largemouth bass, *Micropterus salmoides*. *Journal of the World Aquaculture Society* 40, 735–743.

Coyle, S.D. and Tidwell, J.H. (1997) A summary of walleye research at KSU. *Kentucky Fish Farming* 10 (3/4), 6–7.

Cui, Y. and Wootton, R.J. (1988) Effects of ration, temperature and body size on the body composition, energy content and condition of the minnow, *Phoxinus phoxinus* (L.). *Journal of Fish Biology* 32 (5), 749–764.

Davis, D.A., Jirsa, D. and Arnold, C.R. (1995) Evaluation of soybean proteins as replacements for menhaden fish meal in practical diets for red drum (*Sciaenops ocellatus*). *Journal of the World Aquaculture Society* 26, 48–58.

Davis, J.T. and Lock, J.T. (1997) *Culture of largemouth bass fingerlings.* Southern Regional Aquaculture Center Publication No. 201, Southern Regional Aquaculture Center, Mississippi State, MS.

Dupree, H.K. and Huner, J.V. (1984) Propagation of black bass, sunfishes, tilapias, eels, and hobby fishes. In: Dupree, H.K. and Huner, J.V. (eds) *Third Report to the Fish Farmers.* U.S. Department of the Interior, Fish and Wildlife Service, Washington, DC, pp. 119–135.

Engle, C.R., Stone, N. and Xie, L. (2013) Feasibility of pond production of largemouth bass, *Micropterus salmoides*, for a filet market. *Journal of the World Aquaculture Society* 44 (6), 805–813.

Fontagne, S., Bazin, D., Breque, J., Vachot, C., Bernarde, C., Rouault, T. and Bergot, P. (2006) Effects of dietary oxidized lipid and vitamin A on the early development and antioxidant status of Siberian sturgeon (*Acipenser baeri*) larvae. *Aquaculture* 257 (1–4), 400–411.

Goodwin, A.E., Lochmann, R.T., Tieman, D.M. and Mitchell, A.J. (2002) Massive hepatic necrosis and nodular regeneration in largemouth bass fed diets high in available carbohydrate. *Journal of the World Aquaculture Society* 33 (4), 466–477.

Heidinger, R.C. (2000) A white paper on the status and needs of largemouth bass culture in the north central region. *NCRAC White Papers* 4. Available at: http://lib.dr.iastate.edu/ncrac_whitepapers/4.

Heidinger, R.C. and Crawford, S.D. (1977) Effect of temperature and feeding rate on the liver-somatic index of the largemouth bass, *Micropterus salmoides. Journal of the Fisheries Board of Canada* 34 (5), 633–638.

Hilton, J.W., Cho, C.Y. and Slinger S.J. (1981) Effect of extrusion processing and steam pelleting diets on pellet durability, pellet water absorption, and the physiological response of rainbow trout (*Salmo gairdneri* R.). *Aquaculture* 254 (2–3), 185–194.

Honorato, C.A., Almeida, L.C., DaSilva Nunes, C., Carneiro, D.J. and Moraes, G. (2010) Effects of processing on physical characteristics of diets with distinct levels of carbohydrates and lipids: the outcomes on the growth of pacu (*Piaractus mesopotamicus*). *Aquaculture Nutrition* 16 (1), 91–99.

Hublou, W.F. (1963) Oregon pellets. *The Progressive Fish-Culturist* 25 (4), 175–180.

Jobling, M. (1983) Effect of feeding frequency on food intake and growth of Arctic charr, *Salvelinus alpinus L. Journal of Fish Biology* 23 (2), 177–185.

Jobling, M. (2001) Nutrient partitioning and the influence of feed composition on body composition. In: Houlihan, D., Boujard, T. and Jobling, M. (eds) *Food Intake in Fish*, Blackwell, Oxford, pp. 354–375.

Johnson, M.G. and Charlton, W.H. (1960) Some effects of temperature on the metabolism and activity of the large-mouth bass, *Micropterus salmoides* Lacépède. *The Progressive Fish-Culturist* 22 (4), 155–163.

JSA (Joint Subcommittee on Aquaculture) (1983) Largemouth bass species plan. In: *National Aquaculture Development Plan*, Vol. II. Department of the Interior, Washington, DC.

Keembiyehetty, C.N. and Wilson, R.P. (1998) Effect of water temperature on growth and nutrient utilization of sunshine bass (*Morone chrysops* x *Morone saxatilis*) fed diets containing different energy/protein ratios. *Aquaculture* 166, 151–162.

Keretz, K.R., Dinken, C.P., Allen, P.J. and Schramm, Jr., H.L. (2018) Survival of pellet-reared, naturalized, and wild advanced-size largemouth bass exposed to angling and handling stressors. *North American Journal of Aquaculture* 80, 52–58.

Kestemont, P. and Baras, E. (2001) Environmental factors and feed intake: mechanisms and interactions. In: Houlihan, D., Boujard, T. and Jobling, M. (eds.) *Food Intake in Fish*, Blackwell, Oxford, pp. 131–156.

Kubitza, F. and Lovshin L.L. (1997) Pond production of pellet-fed advanced juvenile and food-size largemouth bass. *Aquaculture* 149 (3–4), 253–262.

Langlois, T.H. (1932) Problems of pondfish culture. *Transactions of the American Fisheries Society* 62 (1), 156–166.

Langlois, T.H. (1933) More problems of pond-fish culture. *Transactions of the American Fisheries Society* 63 (1), 391–403.

Linner, J. and Brannas, E. (1994) Behavioral response to commercial food of different sizes and self-initiated food size selection by Arctic char. *Transactions of the American Fisheries Society* 123 (3), 416–422.

Lovell, T. (1984) Effect of size on feeding responses of catfish in ponds. *Aquaculture Magazine* 10, 35–36.

Lovell, T. (1989) *Nutrition and Feeding of Fish*. Van Nostrand Reinhold, New York.

McCraren, J.P. (1974) Hatchery production of advance largemouth bass fingerlings. *Proceedings of the Annual Conference of Western Association of State Game and Fish Commissioners LV* 36, 260–270.

McGoogan, B.B. and Gatlin III, D.M. (1997) Effects of replacing fish meal with soybean meal in diets for red drum (*Sciaenops ocellatus*) and potential for palatability enhancement. *Journal of the World Aquaculture Society* 28 (4), 374–385.

Mgbenka, B.O. and Lovell, R.T. (1984) Feeding combinations of extruded and pelleted diets to channel catfish in ponds. *The Progressive Fish-Culturist* 46 (4), 245–248.

Nortvedt, R. and Tuene, S. (1995) Multivariate evaluation of feed for Atlantic halibut. *Chemometrics and Intelligent Laboratory Systems* 29 (2), 271–282.

Oliveira, A.M.B.D.M. and Cyrino, J.E.P. (2004) Attractants in plant protein-based diets for the carnivorous largemouth bass *Micropterus salmoides*. *Scientia Agricola* 61 (3), 326–331.

Papatryphon, E. and Soars, Jr., J.H. (2000) Identification of feeding stimulants for striped bass, *Morone saxatilis*. *Aquaculture* 185 (3–4), 339–352.

Petit, G., Beauchaud, M., Attia, J. and Buisson, B. (2003) Food intake and growth of largemouth bass (*Micropterus salmoides*) held under alternated light/dark cycle (12L : 12D) or exposed to continuous light. *Aquaculture* 228, 397–401.

Piper, R.G., McElwain, I.B., Orme, L.E., McCraren J.P., Gowler, L.G. and Leonard, J.R. (1982) *Fish Hatchery Management*. U.S. Department of the Interior, Fish and Wildlife Service, Washington, DC.

Riche, M., Haley, D.I., Oetker, M., Garbrecht, S. and Garling, D.L. (2004) Effect of feeding frequency on gastric evacuation and the return of appetite in tilapia *Oreochromis niloticus* (L.). *Aquaculture* 234 (1–4), 657–673.

Ruohonen, K., Vielma, J. and Grove, D.J. (1998) Effects of feeding frequency on growth and food utilization of rainbow trout (*Oncorhynchus mykiss*) fed low-fat herring or dry pellets. *Aquaculture* 165 (1–2), 111–121.

Simco, B.A., Williamson, J.H., Carmichael, G.J. and Tomasso, J.R. (1986) Centrarchids. In: Stickney, R.R. (ed.) *Culture of Nonsalmoid Freshwater Fishes*. CRC Press, Boca Raton, FL, pp. 73–89.

Snow, J.R. (1963) Results of further experiments on rearing largemouth bass fingerlings under controlled conditions. *Proceedings of the Annual Conference Southeastern Association Game Fish Commission* 17, 191–203.

Snow, J.R. (1968) Production of six- to eight-inch largemouth bass for special purposes. *The Progressive Fish-Culturist* 30 (3), 144–152.

Snow, J.R. and Maxwell, J.I. (1970) Oregon moist pellet as a production ration for largemouth bass. *The Progressive Fish-Culturist* 32 (2), 101–102.

Sorensen, M. (2012) A review of the effects of ingredient composition and processing conditions on the physical qualities of extruded high-energy fish feed as measured by prevailing methods. *Aquaculture Nutrition* 18 (3), 233–248.

Thia-Eng, C. and Seng-Keh, T. (1978) Effects of feeding frequency on the growth of young estuary grouper, *Epinephelus tauvina* (Forskal), cultured in floating net-cages. *Aquaculture* 14 (1), 31–47.

Tidwell, J.H, Webster, C.D. and Clark, J.A. (1992) Growth, feed conversion, and protein utilization of female green sunfish x male bluegill hybrids fed isocaloric diets with different protein levels. *Progressive Fish-Culturist* 54, 234–239.

Tidwell, J.H., Webster, C.D., Clark, J.A. and Brunson, M. (1994) Pond culture of female sunfish (*Lepomis cyanellus)* x male bluegill (*L. macrochirus*) hybrids stocked at two sizes and densities. *Aquaculture* 126, 305–313.

Tidwell, J.H, Webster, C.D. and Coyle, S.D (1996) Effects of dietary protein level on second year growth and water quality for largemouth bass (*Micropterus salmoides*) raised in ponds. Aquaculture 145 (1–4), 213–223.

Tidwell, J.H., Coyle, S.D. and Webster, C.D. (1998a) Effects of stocking density on third-year growth of largemouth bass, (*Micropterus salmoides*), fed prepared diets in ponds. *Journal of Applied Aquaculture* 8 (4), 39–45.

Tidwell, J.H., Webster, C.D., Coyle, S.D. and Schulmeister, G. (1998b) Effect of stocking density on growth and water quality for largemouth bass (*Micropterus salmoides*) growout in ponds. *Journal of the World Aquaculture Society* 29, 88–92.

Tidwell, J.H., Coyle, S.D. and Woods, T.A. (2000) Species profile – largemouth bass. *Publication Number 732*, Southern Regional Aquaculture Center, Stoneville, MS.

Tidwell, J.H., Coyle, S.D., Bright, L.A., VanArnum, A. and Yasharian, D. (2003) Effect of water temperature on growth, survival and biochemical composition of largemouth bass *Micropterus salmoides. Journal of the World Aquaculture Society* 34 (2), 175–183.

Tidwell, J.H., Coyle, S.D., Bright, L.A. and Yasharian, D. (2005) Evaluation of plant and animal source proteins for replacement of fish meal in practical diets for the largemouth bass *Micropterus salmoides.* Journal of the World Aquaculture Society 36 (4), 454–463.

Tidwell, J., Coyle, S. and Bright, L.A. (2015) Effect of feed pellet characteristics on growth and feed conversion efficiency of largemouth bass raised in ponds. *North American Journal of Aquaculture* 77, 55–58.

Tucker, C.S. and Robinson, E.H. (1990) *Channel Catfish Farming Handbook.* Van Nostrand Reinhold, New York.

Venou, B., Alexis, M.N., Fountoulaki, E. and Haralabous, J. (2009) Performance factors, body composition and digestion characteristics of gilthead sea bream (*Sparus aurata*) fed pelleted or extruded diets. *Aquaculture Nutrition* 15 (4), 390–401.

Weatherly, A.H. and Gill, H.S. (1987) *The Biology of Fish Growth.* Academic Press, New York.

Wintzer, A.P. and Motta, P.J. (2005) Diet-induced phenotypic plasticity in the skull morphology of hatchery-reared Florida largemouth bass, *Micropterus salmoides floridanus. Ecology of Freshwater Fish* 14 (4), 311–318.

CHAPTER 10

Common diseases of largemouth bass

Kathryn M. Mitchell and Robert M. Durborow

Kentucky State University, Aquaculture Research Center, Frankfort, Kentucky, USA

10.1 Introduction

The largemouth bass (*Micropterus salmoides*) is native to North America and is the largest member of the Centrarchidae family. Historically, the primary culture focus has been stock enhancement for the sport-fish industry, but it has also become a popular food-fish sold live in ethnic Asian markets (Brandt, 1991; Cochran et al., 2009). Fish in aquaculture are in much higher densities than in wild populations and suboptimal environments generate a physiological stress response that weakens the immune system. A compromised immune system increases the chance of a disease outbreak; therefore, stress must be minimized throughout production to reduce disease occurrences, but not to the point where the production level becomes unprofitable. Therapeutants applied to the water are used to treat external parasite and bacterial infections. Potassium permanganate ($KMnO_4$) and copper sulfate ($CuSO_4$) are commonly used for this purpose because they are on "deferred status" by FDA and are, therefore, legal for use on food-fish. In the case of a bacterial disease outbreak, necessitating the use of antibiotics (which are formulated in or sprayed on commercial feed), it is important for bass to be feed trained in order to receive medication.

This chapter provides an overview of the maladies and diseases found in largemouth bass, as well as treatment and prevention methods. As of January 2017, in the USA, a Veterinary Feed Directive (VFD) is required to treat fish with antibiotics and a section of this chapter is dedicated to information pertaining to VFDs. This chapter will close with a 28 year record of largemouth bass disease diagnoses from the archives of the Kentucky State University Fish Disease Diagnostic Laboratory (KSU-FDDL).

10.2 Bacterial diseases

10.2.1 Motile Aeromonas septicemia

One of the most common and problematic bacterial diseases found in farm-raised fish is motile *Aeromonas* septicemia (MAS), also referred to as red sore disease or hemorrhagic septicemia (Huizinga et al., 1979; Hazen et al., 1981). This disease is most often caused by *Aeromonas hydrophila,* however *A. caviae, A. veronii,* and *A. sobria* (all part of the *Aeromonas* Complex bacteria) are also responsible for mortalities. Poor water quality increases the chance of disease, and this is especially true during times of low dissolved oxygen, high ammonia, high water temperatures, or pH instability. Stress caused by overcrowding, spawning, high organic loads, seining, parasite infestation, and transportation also increases disease occurrence (Camus et al., 1998). MAS outbreaks normally occur when water temperatures are between 18°C and 29°C (65°F and 85°F) but occurrences have been reported in a wider temperature range. Clinical signs of *Aeromonas* infections are nonspecific, making it challenging to identify and distinguish from other diseases. However, common signs are exophthalmia and hemorrhagic lesions on the skin and at the base of fins (Figure 10.1a). Lesions can develop into hemorrhagic septicemia (Noga, 2010). Fish may also exhibit a distended abdomen due to ascites (Figure 10.1b). Internal organs are usually swollen and appear mottled or hemorrhagic. In systemic infections, fish may swim erratically due to infection within the nervous system and brain. Fish can be asymptomatic carriers of *Aeromonas* bacteria.

Aeromonads are gram-negative rods that are facultative aerobes with motility from a single, polar flagellum (Terhune and Beck, 2015). Growth occurs between 5°C and 37°C on complex culture media (tryptic soy agar enhanced with 5% sheep blood is commonly used). Individual colonies are visible within 24 h and this rapid growth may explain the fast onset of disease. When infections are limited to the skin, a treatment with 2 to 4 parts per million (milligrams/liter) of potassium permanganate ($KMnO_4$) is effective, if the organic load in the water is not excessive. A demand test should first be used to determine the rate of potassium permanganate

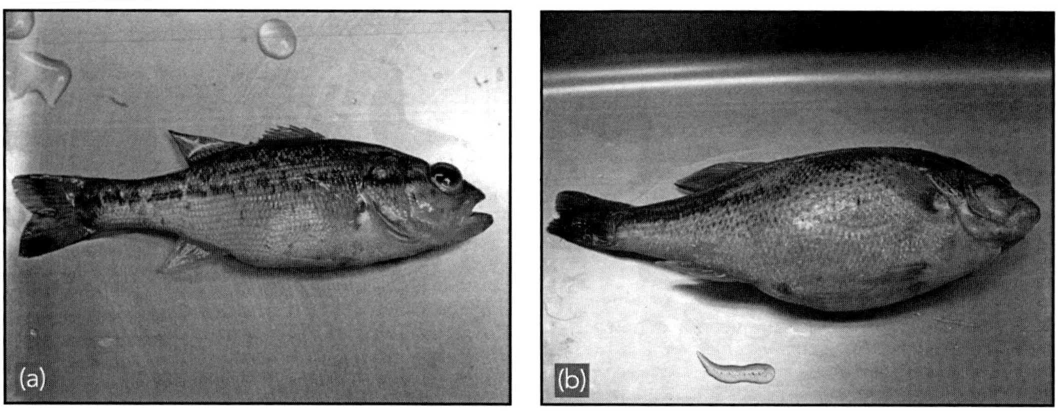

Figure 10.1 (a) Largemouth bass with exophthalmia due to aeromonas infection. (b) Largemouth bass with distended abdomen due to ascites caused by aeromonas.

that needs to be applied to prevent the organic content of the water from neutralizing the treatment. Camus et al. (1998) reported that *Aeromonas* is frequently resistant to Romet® 30 and oxytetracycline (Terramycin®) but usually sensitive to florfenicol (Aquaflor®); this, however, can be quite variable. An antibiotic susceptibility analysis should be conducted to select the most effective treatment.

Other disease-causing bacteria that have been isolated from largemouth bass with etiologies similar to *Aeromonas* Complex bacteria include *Pseudomonas* spp., *Plesiomonas shigelloides*, *Vibrio* spp., *A. salmonicida*, *Citrobacter freundii*, *Salmonella* spp., *Acinetobacter calcoaceticus*, and *Proteus* spp.

10.2.2 Columnaris

Columnaris is a bacterial disease caused by *Flavobacterium columnare* and most commonly affects the gills, fins, and mucous layer (Figure 10.2a). Primarily an epithelial disease, columnaris causes skin erosion with mold-like growth and gill lesions that can become necrotic (Figure 10.2b). Clinical signs are whitish plaques with a red perimeter that are mainly present on the head, fins, and back. It is frequently referred to as saddleback disease because of the saddle-like appearance when it occurs on the back (Noga, 2010). Columnaris outbreaks have been reported in most freshwater fish and are typically pathogenic in the spring, summer, and fall when temperatures range from 25 to 32°C and become more severe with increasing temperatures (Durborow et al., 1998b; Noga, 2010). Poor water quality and stress increase the chance of an outbreak and this is especially true when largemouth bass are being feed trained. Bass that are not successfully feed trained become more susceptible to columnaris due to starvation (Figure 10.3) (Bebak et al., 2009).

Flavobacterium columnare is characterized by gram-negative rods ranging from 3 to 10 nm long, visible at 200× magnification and higher. It is aerobic, nonflagellated and uses a flexing or gliding movement for motility. The key diagnostic feature is bacterial cells forming columns or "haystacks" that can be observed microscopically. Bacteria can be grown on low-nutrient media (such as Hsu-Shotts, modified Shieh, cytophaga, or tryptone yeast extract salts [TYES] medias)

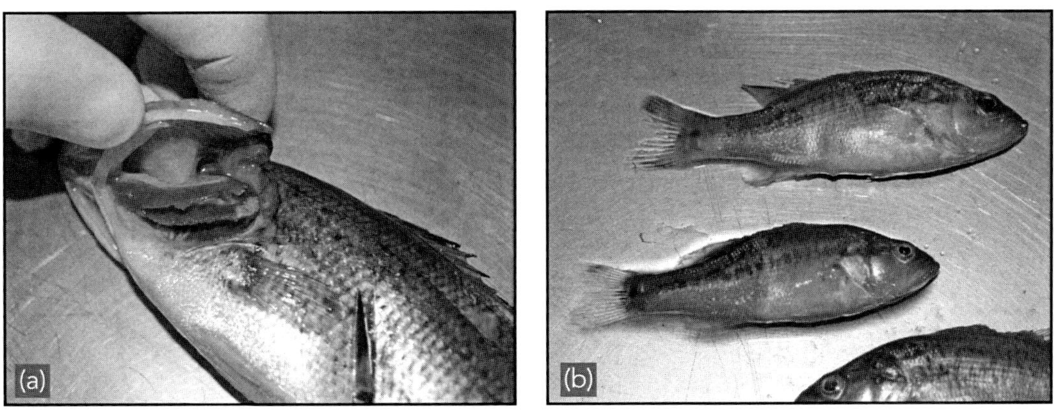

Figure 10.2 (a) Largemouth bass with columnaris infection on the gills. (b) Cotton-like growth on skin of largemouth bass due to columnaris infection.

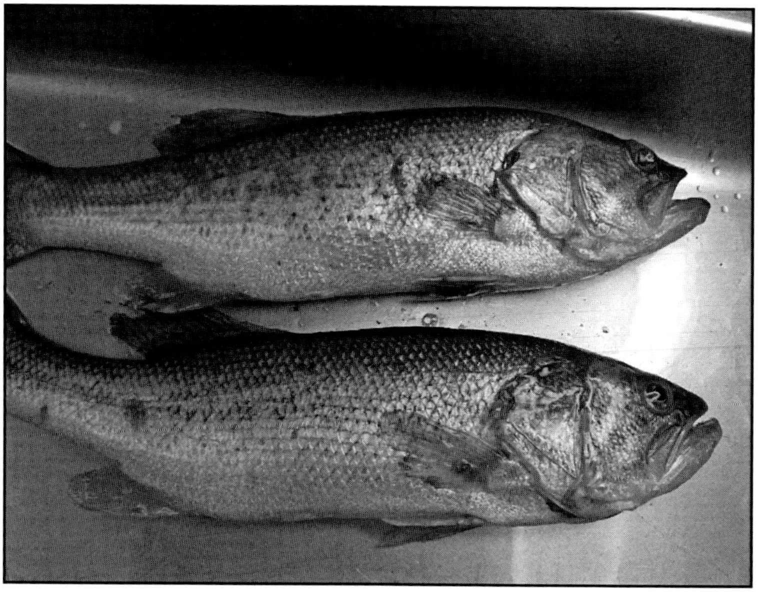

Figure 10.3 Emaciation in largemouth bass caused by internal columnaris infection.

(LaFrentz et al., 2014) at an optimal temperature of 25°C, but growth occurs between 4 and 30°C. Colonies are dry, yellowish, and rhizoid (Terhune and Beck, 2015).

Columnaris is opportunistic and can be a primary or secondary pathogen. In one case example, largemouth bass from Kentucky State University case F08–8 were infected with both *Flavobacterium columnare* and *Aeromonas hydrophila*, and florfenicol (Aquaflor®) was successfully used to treat. Other treatment options include oxytetracycline bath, Halamid® Aqua (Chloramine-T), copper sulfate ($CuCO_4$), and $KMnO_4$. Another approach is preventive; Bebak et al. (2009) demonstrated the efficacy of a commercial vaccine for largemouth bass against *Flavobacterium columnare* when challenged naturally (compared to sham-vaccinated bass). Vaccinated largemouth bass had a 43% lower risk of dying from the natural exposure to columnaris bacteria. Lange (2003) also showed effectiveness of a commercially made autogenous vaccine (developed from *Flavobacterium columnare* isolated from the facility where the study was performed) when the largemouth bass were immerse-vaccinated at 6 grams in size but not when the bass were vaccinated at 1 g. An oxytetracycline (OTC) bath at 20 mg/l every third day for the duration of the feed-training period, however, conferred better protection from columnaris infection than the vaccinated or OTC-fed bass for both sizes (1 and 6 g fish; Lange, 2003).

10.2.3 Edwardsiellosis

Edwardsiellosis, caused by *Edwardsiella tarda*, elicits muscle tissue necrosis and is often referred to as fish gangrene due to gas filled pockets that produce a foul odor. *Edwardsiella tarda* is a gram-negative anaerobe that produces hydrogen sulfide and is normally treated with either Terramycin or Romet. The bacterium is an opportunistic and facultative pathogen that has been reported in both saltwater and freshwater warmwater fishes. Disease epizootics involving *E. tarda* normally occur during hot temperatures (above 30°C) and are associated with polluted and stressful environments (Noga, 2010). Infected fish appear listless or lethargic. External hemorrhaging occurs around the abdomen and at the base of the fins, and the anal vent may become swollen and red.

10.2.4 Epitheliocystis

Epitheliocystis has been observed in largemouth bass cases submitted to the KSU-FDDL; it is a tumor-like proliferation of cells occurring on various skin and gill surfaces of fish and is caused by a chlamydia-like bacterium (Draghi et al., 2004). It has been found in otherwise healthy fish but it can cause mortality when hyperinfection occurs. In healthy fish, epitheliocystis is in a benign form but in severe cases, infected cells can cover the gills and produce an inflammatory response. Goodwin et al. (2005) reported successfully treating this disease with a 25 mg/l oxytetracycline tank treatment.

10.3 Viral diseases

10.3.1 Largemouth bass virus

Largemouth bass virus (LMBV) is an iridovirus that was first discovered in Florida and has since been found in other areas of the southeastern USA, Michigan, and Indiana. LMBV is the only known virus that has caused widespread mortalities in wild largemouth bass populations (Grizzle and Brunner, 2003). A study by Maceina and Grizzle (2005) found that LMBV was most prevalent in young to intermediate-age bass ranging from 1.5 to 6 years old (25 to 40 cm in length) and rare in fish smaller than 10 cm and larger than 50 cm. This study indicated that the absence of LMBV in fish greater than 50 cm may be due to larger and older fish dying prior to collection in the Alabama reservoirs that were surveyed. Hanson et al. (2000), however, did not find a correlation between age/size and LMBV occurrence in a Mississippi reservoir, but they were able to detect LMBV in a third of the bass they sampled even 13 months after the outbreak. They also reported a yellow waxy substance (a fibrin clot consisting of erythrocytes and eosinophils) in the swim bladder of infected bass. Southard et al. (2009) also noticed a swim bladder anomaly associated with infected largemouth bass in a Texas lake. Mortalities in adult largemouth bass due to LMBV occur during the summer months when temperatures are greater than 20°C (68°F) but subclinical infections can occur year-round, and higher temperatures (30°C [86°F]) cause greater mortalities compared to when temperatures are at 24°C (75°F) (Grant et al., 2003). The only clinical signs are gross lesions on the swim bladder and/or an overinflated swim bladder. Infected fish appear lethargic, experience a loss of equilibrium, and swim near the surface.

The largemouth bass virus can be identified by using polymerase chain reaction (PCR) (Plumb et al., 1999) and a more recent qPCR (quantitative PCR, or real-time PCR) has been developed by Getchell et al. (2007). The American Fisheries Society (2016) Fish Health Section Blue Book approves BF-2 (bluegill *Lepomis macrochirus* fry) cell line as one of the acceptable cell lines for detecting LMBV (Getchell et al., 2014). In 2014, Getchell et al. reported success in identifying LMBV with a new cell line derived from the largemouth bass ovary. Other cell lines susceptible to the LMBV include fathead minnow (FHM), epithelioma papulosum cyprinid, and channel catfish ovary (CCO) cells (McClenahan et al., 2005). McClenahan et al. (2005) also worked out many of the details for optimizing the detection of LMBV such as how long to allow virus samples to absorb on cell lines and the use of orbital shakers and blind passages to increase the level of detection of the virus. Leis et al. (2018) found that using mucus collected nonlethally from largemouth bass by swabbing and testing it for LMBV in traditional cell culture was just as effective in detecting the virus as when bass tissue samples were inoculated onto the cell cultures (after lethally extracting the tissues from the bass). The mucus samples proved to be more reliable than the conventional tissue samples when conventional and quantitative PCR testing was used to detect the LMBV (Leis et al., 2018).

Beck et al. (2006) showed that LMBV enters largemouth bass quickly (within an hour) and can be found in various organs even when the fish are not moribund or showing clinical signs, but antibody titers were shown to be highest in the swim bladder (Woodland et al., 2002). The virus is capable of infecting bass by an oral route (Woodland et al., 2002). The infection can become undetectable within a month after exposure (Beck et al., 2006). LMBV outbreaks can be caused by holding largemouth bass in fishing boat live wells after they are captured during tournaments. Incidence of LMBV resulting from tournament stress was almost 50% in a study by Schramm et al. (2011), explained in more detail below in the Stress section.

Nath et al. (2010) addressed the potential for LMBV to associate with bacterial biofilms, thus gaining protection from topical disinfectants. Researchers demonstrated that when LMBV is entrapped in *Pseudomonas fluorescens* biofilm it is resistant to sodium hypochlorite (bleach) and povidone iodine (Betadine™) disinfectants but not to ethanol (Nath et al., 2010). They were not able to demonstrate that LMBV is able to exist in natural aquatic environments in association with biofilms.

Boonthai et al. (2018) demonstrated (using experimental infections) that LMBV causes mortality as well as clinical signs in young-of-the-year smallmouth bass (clinical signs consistent to those observed in smallmouth bass die-offs in natural bodies of water, including skin hemorrhaging; a broken, hemorrhaged, and ulcerated mandible; exophthalmia and corneal opacity; ruptured eye with vitreal loss; abdominal distension; enlarged, edematous, mottled, and friable livers; a dark, edematous spleen; and hemorrhaged kidneys and gonads). Higher mortalities were noted at 28 than at 23 or 11°C, and mortalities were compounded when *Flavobacterium columnare* co-infections occurring concurrently with LMBV were "devastating" to the young smallmouth bass even though *A. salmonicida* is a pathogen that prefers cool temperatures (Boonthai et al., 2018).

10.3.2 Viral hemorrhagic septicemia

Viral hemorrhagic septicemia virus (VHSV) has caused mortality and morbidity in multiple species of farmed and wild fish. Kim and Faisal (2010, 2011) demonstrated that muskellunge and largemouth bass were more affected in disease severity and cumulative mortality by VHSV (genotype IVb) compared to other fish species (even at low infection doses). There are VHSV genotypes I through IV with several subtypes. In North America, aside from genotype IVb, all other VHSV genotypes affecting freshwater fish (genotypes Ia, Ic, Id, Ie, and III) affect only trout species. The genotype IVb virus is the genotype that has caused the greatest alarm nationwide in recent years due to large-scale die-offs of many different fish species (28 species) in the Great Lakes region. It has not yet caused a disease outbreak in aquaculture fish and has not been reported south of the states bordering the Great Lakes (Illinois, Indiana, Michigan, Minnesota, New York, Ohio, Pennsylvania, and Wisconsin) and is not usually found in southern parts of these states.

Some states require VHSV-free certification for transportation and sale of live fish. Typically, 60 fish per lot or body of water are required for testing and results must be negative for VHSV in order to legally transport live fish.

10.3.3 Other viruses

In 2008, a ranavirus causing skin and muscle ulcerations and mortality in largemouth bass in China was isolated and sequenced; it was genetically identical to doctor fish virus and closely related to largemouth bass virus (Deng et al., 2011). Gao and Chen (2018) describe a relatively new virus *Micropterus salmoides* rhabdovirus (MSRV) that causes bass to exhibit a crooked body with an irregular, corkscrew swimming pattern. They found that it causes apoptosis in fish skin cells, and they uncovered the transcriptomic profiles using RNA sequencing.

10.4 Parasite infections

10.4.1 Protists

The most common parasites found in cultured fish are single-celled organisms or protist ectoparasites, which have a direct life cycle and can occur on the host for the entire or partial life cycle. Common signs of protist ectoparasites are damage to the skin and gills caused by parasitic feeding activity, this irritation can also cause behavioral changes. A photograph from case F08–30 (Figure 10.4) is a largemouth bass with an *Ichthyobodo* spp. infection; irritation and sloughing

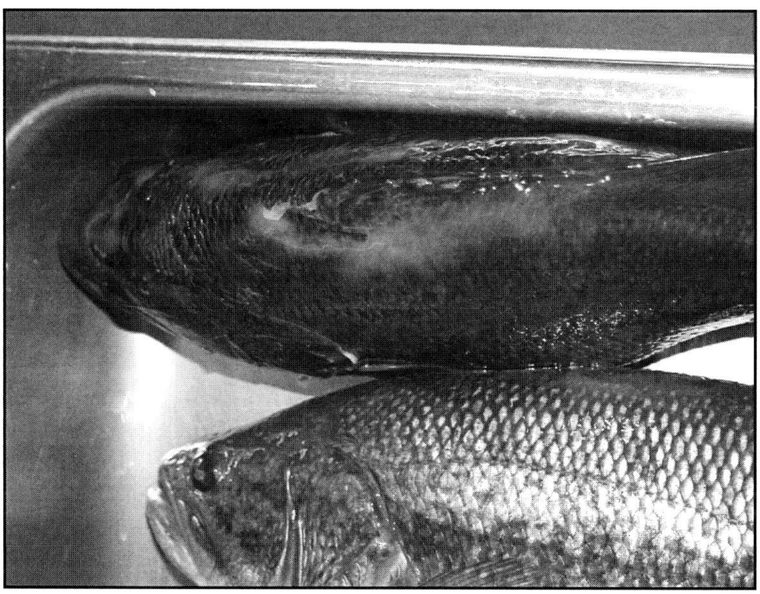

Figure 10.4 Largemouth bass infected with *Ichthyobodo* spp., which can be seen around the dorsal fin and on the head.

of mucus can be seen around the dorsal fin. This disease is often called "blue slime" disease. Obligate parasites such as *Ichthyobodo* spp. and *Ichthyopthirius* spp. actively feed on the host epithelium and others such as *Trichodina* spp. and *Ambiphyra* spp. have a commensal relationship with the host but are still capable of causing morbidity and mortality in host fish, especially if their concentrations are heavy enough (MacMillan, 1991). This can lead to irritation of the fish's skin and/or gills and partial obstruction of oxygen flow to the fish. Although *Trichodina* typically causes problems in an aquaculture setting where fish are much more crowded than in the wild, it can also be a problem in wild fish. A *Trichodina* epizootic in wild largemouth bass from a North Carolina river was reported by Huh et al. (2005). Initial reports from anglers were of a "jelly like slime coat" on the skin. Follow-up electrofishing by these researchers found that 10% of captured bass had trichodinosis clinical signs (a bluish-white mucoid layer characterized by a very thick hyperplastic epidermis with relatively few mucous cells). No other disease organisms besides *Trichodina* were reported (Huh et al., 2005).

10.4.2 Ichthyophthirius multifiliis

Ichthyophthirius multifiliis causes "Ich," which is the most infamous fish parasite. It is highly nonspecific and affects all species of freshwater fish. Ich is recognized by white spots or pustules sprinkled on the skin that are visible to the naked eye. This is the source of the common names of white spot or salt-and-pepper disease. It is found on the skin, gills, and fins and can cause excess mucus production and sloughing of the skin, however, sometimes the only indicator of an Ich outbreak is the presence of dead or dying fish. Fish infected with Ich are often seen rubbing on the pond bottom or hard objects. This is called "flashing" because of the sporadic exposure of the light-colored belly of the fish. In the later stages of the disease, fish may gather around inflowing water, appear lethargic, and stop eating. Microscopically, Ich is sphere shaped and moves around in a rolling motion using cilia and mature Ich have a C-shaped nucleus.

Ich is usually transmitted by a carrier fish, other animals, humans, or from a contaminated water source. Ich has a life cycle that requires 52 or more hours to complete, which slows in cooler weather and cannot reproduce properly above 29°C. Ich leaves the infected fish as a tomont and attaches to the pond bottom or other surface and develops a thin-walled cyst. The tomont divides many times within the cyst, forming as many as 2,000 tomites. Tomites are released from the cyst and elongate into theronts or swarmers. Theronts have a day or two to find a fish host and infiltrate the fish's epithelium using a penetrating gland and ciliary action. When Ich enters the epithelium, it is referred to as a trophont. Trophonts then feed and mature on the fish's epithelium until leaving the fish as a tomont and the cycle continues.

Fish mortality is due to Ich eroding the epithelial tissue, irritation from theront penetration, abrasions from flashing, not eating, anemia, and/or excess mucus production on gills that obstruct oxygen transfer. Ich can be prevented by eliminating entry of wild fish, quarantining new fish, putting filters on water inlets in ponds, and drying or dipping equipment in disinfectant before using between ponds.

Not all stages of the Ich life cycle are susceptible to chemical treatments. Trophonts are protected by the fish's epithelium, therefore chemical treatments are only effective on theronts and tomonts. In order to treat these vulnerable stages, multiple treatments must be administered and depending on temperature, three to seven treatments may be needed to be effective. Chemical drugs approved to treat Ich in food-fish are formalin (Formalin-F™), copper sulfate, and potassium permanganate. In ponds, formalin should be administered at a rate of 15 to 25 ppm, which is equivalent to 4.5 to 7.5 gallons of formalin per acre-foot (or 13.5–22.5 l of formalin per 1,000m^3 of water). Copper Sulfate ($CuSO_4$) is used as an indefinite treatment and treatment rate is dependent on the total alkalinity of the water. Therefore, the treatment rate of copper sulfate in ppm is equal to the total alkalinity of the water being treated divided by 100 (Durborow et al., 1998a).

Copper sulfate is not typically used when total alkalinity is less than 40 ppm or greater than 300 ppm; copper sulfate is more toxic to fish in low alkalinity waters. In high alkalinity waters, copper may precipitate out of the solution making treatment ineffective. Algae blooms may be killed during copper sulfate treatments so dissolved oxygen concentrations must be monitored. Before stocking a pond, copper sulfate can be applied to kill any theronts or tomonts in the water as a preventive. Potassium permanganate is usually used as an indefinite treatment; it oxidizes organic materials in the water and a demand test should be performed to determine the effective dose for a body of water. The minimum dose recommended is 2 ppm, therefore 2 ppm of potassium permanganate should be added at a time until a wine-red color is attained and to be considered effective, this color should persist for at least 8 h.

10.4.3 Epistylis spp.

Epistylis spp. are facultative colonial ciliates with non-contractile stalks. Reproduction occurs by simple binary fission or by formation of teletrochs. Bell-shaped cells form a ring of cilia that flatten to form the teletroch which attaches to hard parts of the fish such as scales, fins, and spines. At the point of attachment, red ulcerative sores develop and the tissue develops a furry white fungus-like growth. The attachment points usually become infected with bacteria that can dissolve spines and scales. Extensive infestations typically indicate polluted waters with poor water quality (Terhune and Beck, 2015). The most common treatment in food-fish is 0.1 to 1.0% salt and/or 15–25 mg/l formalin as an indefinite treatment.

10.4.4 Cestodes (tapeworms)

Cestodes or tapeworms affect all vertebrates, are widely distributed, and normally demonstrate a high degree of host specificity. The bass tapeworm has a complex life cycle that involves two intermediate hosts and a final host. The adult tapeworm lives in the intestinal tract and releases eggs that reach the outside environment through the feces. The eggs then infect cyclopoid copepods and develop into proceroids, the first larval form. When the copepod is consumed by another fish (including bass), the larval tapeworms migrate out of the intestinal tract into the abdominal cavity of the intermediate host and forms the plerocercoid larvae. When the intermediate fish host is eaten by the final host (largemouth bass), the adult tapeworms develop and attach to the host intestinal wall with its head or scolex. Here, it absorbs nutrients and undergoes reproduction (Terhune and Beck, 2015). Adult tapeworms cause minimal damage in light infestations, however, severe infections can lead to nutritional deficiencies or intestinal blockage. Host fish severely affected are more susceptible to other diseases and stressors.

The bass tapeworm, *Proteocephalus ambloplitus*, is of most concern due to the damage and sterilization of reproductive organs in largemouth bass hosts. Bass tapeworm infections can lead to sterilization of largemouth bass broodstock, a result of bass tapeworm plerocercoids (larval stage) migrating through the bass ovaries and causing destructive connective tissue formation. However, bass tapeworms are not a significant problem in largemouth bass fed a pelleted diet. Boonyaratpalin and Rogers (1984) found that mebendazole (methyl-5-benzoyl benziraidazole-2-carhamate) at 200 mg/kg/d (injected or by capsular implant) reduced the tapeworm infection by 95% after six weeks, while 100 mg/kg/d administered orally for 14 consecutive days reduced infection by 90%. These doses did not interfere with reproductive success of the bass brooders but increasing the mebendazole injection dose to 300 mg/kg led to the absence of fry production.

In some molecular-based work, Durborow et al. (1988) demonstrated competitive exclusion interaction between bass tapeworms in largemouth bass and the acanthocephalan *Neoechinorhynchus* sp. High numbers of either parasite significantly reduced the infection rate of the other parasite due to cross-protective immunity/cross-resistance (antibodies against either parasite reacted with antigens of the other). Cross-resistance in largemouth bass's reaction to various species of mussel glochidia has also been observed (Dodd et al., 2005). Durborow (1986) also characterized the molecular weights of largemouth bass antibodies (immunoglobulins) including the heavy and light chains that comprise the bass immunoglobulin.

10.4.5 Crustaceans

Lernaea sp. (Lernaeidae) are parasitic copepods in the order Cyclopoida. These parasites undergo multiple free-swimming life stages before attaching to the host fish and reproducing. Attachment to the host fish normally occurs on the fish abdomen or around the base of the fins and only the females penetrate the skin and mature into adults. Light infestations are normally not of concern unless the fish is small but heavy infestations or infestations around vital organs are problematic. Also, the attachment point can become infected with fungal pathogens or opportunistic bacteria (Noga, 2010). Anchor parasites (*Lernaea cruciata*) were described as a problem in 55% of large (> 100 mm) largemouth bass collected from the Chowan River in North Carolina from May to October (Noga, 1986). The infestation was compounded by secondary bacterial and fungal infections. This parasite was also reported by Timmons and Hemstreet (1980) on bass from a reservoir on the Alabama–Georgia border.

10.4.6 Monogenea

Monogenea or monogenes (phylum Platyhelminthes) are small flatworms that are commonly referred to as skin or gill flukes (although, technically, they are not flukes). Dactylogyroidea and Gyrodactyloidea are the most economically important monogenes in cultured fish; they attach to the epidermal surfaces using a haptor that include 2–4 hamuli (anchors) and 12–16 marginal hooks (Hoffman, 1999). Reproduction varies depending on the family but only one host is required for all monogenes. Gyrodactylids are viviparous and attach to the skin and gills, however, dactylogyrids are oviparous and primarily attach to the gills. Monogenes are problematic when infestations become heavy, which can cause mucus production, respiratory impediment, and inappetence in fish, leading to anorexia. Heavy infestations are more common in waters with poor water quality and high organic content (Noga, 2010).

10.4.7 Digenea

Digenea or digenes (phylum Platyhelminthes) are referred to as grubs and have a complex life cycle that utilizes both asexual and sexual reproduction. Beginning in the definitive host, the adult digene releases a fertilized egg into the water column where it hatches and becomes a free-swimming miracidium. The miracidium is ingested by the second host, a mollusk (snail), and forms a sporocyst. From sporocysts, cercariae develop and leave the snail and have a limited amount of time to find a second intermediate host (fish). The cercariae become metacercariae in the fish. Infected fish are then consumed by a mammal, bird, or another fish, where the digene develops into an adult and the cycle continues. Digenes can be controlled by eliminating snails and/or birds. Snail population can be reduced by removing aquatic vegetation and by targeting snails along the pond margins with copper sulfate or hydrated lime applications. The presence of birds can be discouraged by various scare tactics or by selective killing (with the proper federal permit).

Common digenes found in largemouth bass are yellow grub (*Clinostomum marginatum* or *C. complanatum*), white grub (*Posthodiplostomum minimum*), eye fluke (*Diplostomum spathaceum*), and black spot (*Uvulifer ambloplitis*). Eye fluke cercariae can enter anywhere on the body of the fish and travel to the lens of the eye, causing blindness if infestations are heavy enough (Hoffman, 1999). In most cases, when the cercariae penetrate the fish there is minor damage and minimal stress response. However, heavy infestations may kill the host fish, which is especially true for small fish. In chronic cases, opportunistic bacteria may be able to infect the host through the opening created by the cercariae.

10.4.8 Leeches

Although of limited importance in aquaculture, reports of leech infestations are found in pond-raised and wild bass populations. Leeches feed on a range of aquatic and terrestrial animals and reports of leech infestations of largemouth bass have been documented in the United States. Largemouth bass living in an estuarine environment in coastal North Carolina were observed by Noga et al. (1990) to have bacterially infected mouth ulcerative lesions caused by an infestation of the leech *Myzobdella lugubris* (formerly *Illinobdella moorei*). They attributed the leech infection to the stressful, high-salinity environment, and regarded the concurrent bacterial infection as secondary (Noga et al., 1990).

10.4.9 Fungi

Winter saprolegniasis (winter "fungus" or winter mortality) is the most common fungal pathogen found in largemouth bass. It usually occurs between October and March when water temperatures drop below 15°C (59°F), however, the disease has been reported as early as September and as late as April and is associated with a sudden drop in temperature that causes immune suppression. *Saprolegnia* spp. are facultative pathogens that obtain nutrients from dead organic matter. Diseased fish have brownish patches of cottony or wooly fungus, skin lesions, endophthalmia, and hemorrhaging around the infection. Lesions start out in small circular, depigmented areas but can become ulcerative and break the skin exposing the muscle tissue. Bacteria can enter

Table 10.1 Diseases of importance found in largemouth bass.

Disease	Temperature range (°C)	Reference
Aeromonas	18–20	Camus et al., 1998
Columnaris	25–32	Durborow et al., 1998
Edwardsiellosis	> 30	Noga, 2010
LMBV	> 20	Grizzle and Brunner, 2003
VHS	~3–18	Kim and Faisal, 2011
Winter Fungus	< 15	Durborow et al., 2003
Ich	20–25	Durborow et al., 1998
Protozoan Parasites		Durborow et al., 2003

through lesions resulting in septicemia or blood poisoning, though death is thought to be associated with the loss of osmoregulation (Durborow et al., 2003). Prevention is the best treatment method, and reducing stress, minimizing handling, and maintaining good water quality, especially during late summer and early fall, can minimize the effect of winter fungus.

Table 10.1 provides a list of the most frequently diagnosed diseases, their respective temperature ranges, and references to find additional information.

10.5 Stressors in largemouth bass

Stress in fish leads to impaired reproductive success and decreased survival (Ostrand et al., 2002). Stressors include improper handling, crowding, and poor water quality. Largemouth bass water quality requirements and tolerances are covered in Chapter 4. In general, largemouth bass can tolerate dissolved oxygen (DO) as low as 1.4 mg/l, but DO less than 3–4 mg/l should be avoided. The largemouth bass has a high tolerance to nitrite; the 96 h LC_{50} for nitrite is 460 mg/l in largemouth bass compared to 25 mg/l in channel catfish (Tidwell et al., 2000). However, largemouth bass are similar to channel catfish in ammonia tolerance, with a 24 h un-ionized ammonia LC_{50} of 1.69 mg/l. Additional stressors to largemouth bass include inadequate diet, rough handling, and high levels of waste solids.

The ideal temperate range for largemouth bass is 20–30°C. Seining and handling should be avoided when temperatures are above 27°C to prevent stress-related secondary infections. Soft mesh netting should be used to prevent scale loss and infection when fish are seined or netted. A treated net/seine should never be used on largemouth bass because the stiff nature of treated netting causes abrasion. Fish should be purged from feed two days before transport to reduce stress. When transporting largemouth bass, tank water temperature should be between 5 and 15°C, salt concentration should be 3–5 ppt, and stocking density should be 120–240 g of fish per liter of water. Fish can be anesthetized prior to loading; a legal anesthesia for food-fish is a mixture of 1 l of acetic acid (concentrated vinegar) and 1.8–3.6 kg of sodium bicarbonate (baking soda) in 3,785 ml of water. Bass should be adequately sedated for safe handling after 6 min and can safely remain in the solution up to 1 h.

A somewhat related stressor is the holding of largemouth bass in fishing boat live wells after being captured during tournaments. Plumb et al. (1988) demonstrated that survival of largemouth bass caught under tournament conditions and held in live wells was higher (98.9%) when the bass were caught and released (within 30 min) compared to those held for 3 to 9 h (90.8% survival). Schramm et al. (2011) investigated 12 summer tournaments and found that reducing water temperature and increasing salt content in live well holding tank water significantly increased survival of largemouth bass (from 93% to 97%) that were caught and held in these live wells. However, after these captured fish were held for 5 d in net pens after the tournaments, survival averaged 24% regardless of improved live tank holding conditions. Incidence of largemouth bass virus during the five-day post-tournament holding period ranged from 64% to 70%, while LMBV occurrence post-electrofishing during the same holding period was 47%. Survivals were 24% and 41% for the post-tournament and post-electrofishing groups, respectively, showing a correlation between stress and disease/mortality, especially in a lake infected with largemouth bass virus (Schramm and Davis, 2006; Schramm et al., 2011). High mortalities were not observed during bass tournaments in lakes not infected with LMBV.

10.6 Treatments and Veterinary Feed Directive (VFD)

As of 1 January 2017, a VFD must be issued by a licensed veterinarian and a valid veterinarian–client–patient relationship (VCPR) must be established in order to legally treat fish with antibiotics in the USA. A VFD has an expiration date and antibiotics cannot be administered after that date. If there is not an expiration date specified on the product label then it will expire 6 months after the date of issuance, however, the veterinarian can assign a shorter expiration date. Currently no refills are allowed for VFD drugs and if another outbreak occurs, it is up to the treating veterinarian to decide if a new VFD is needed. Medicated drugs approved for use in aquaculture are Aquaflor® (florfenicol), Terramycin® (oxytetracycline), and Romet® TC/Romet-30 (sulfadimethoxine/ormetoprim). Immersion drugs approved for use in aquaculture are Halamid® Aqua (chloramine-T), Formalin-F™/Formacide-B/Parasite-S® (formalin), 35% Perox-Aid® (hydrogen peroxide), and Tricaine-S (tricaine methanesulfonate). Potassium permanganate ($KMnO_4$) and copper sulfate ($CuSO_4$), mentioned earlier in the chapter are often used to treat external bacteria and parasites.

Information on usage and treatment rate for approved aquaculture drugs can be found on the FDA website (https://www.fda.gov/AnimalVeterinary/DevelopmentApprovalProcess/Aquaculture/ucm132954.htm).

The Kirby–Bauer antibiotic testing or agar diffusion test determines the antibiotic susceptibility of bacteria. Bacteria are streaked on a Mueller–Hinton agar plate and antibiotic susceptibility discs are dispensed onto the plate. Bacterial growth up to or close to the disc indicates that the bacteria are resistant to that antibiotic but a zone of growth inhibition around the antibiotic disc indicates that the bacteria are susceptible to that antibiotic.

10.7 Diagnostic case history at Kentucky State University

The KSU-FDDL has diagnosed 355 largemouth bass disease cases over the past 28 years (1990–2017; see Figure 10.5). The most frequent disease diagnosed (75 out of 355 cases) was

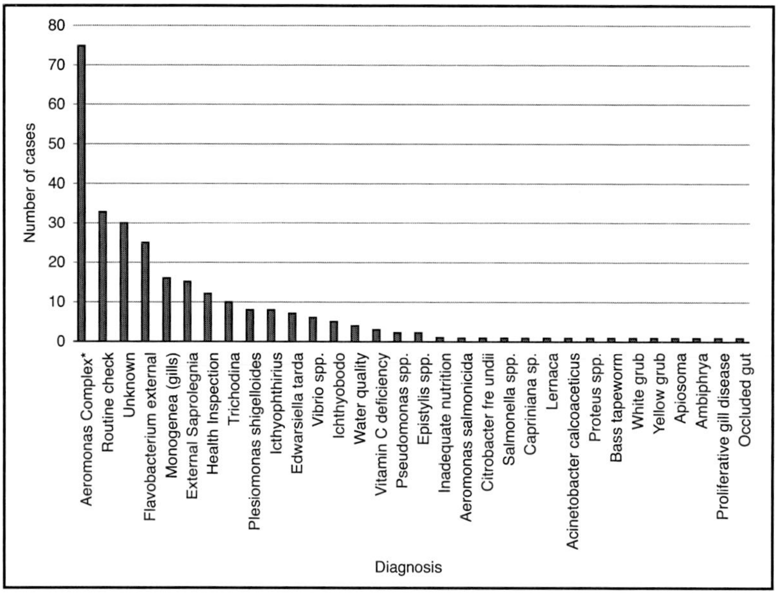

Figure 10.5 Diagnosis of largemouth bass (*Micropterus salmoides*) cases submitted to the Kentucky State University Fish Disease Diagnostic Lab from 1990–2017.

Note: *Aeromonas complex includes *Aeromonas hydrophila, A. caviae, A. veronii,* and *A. sobria.*

Table 10.2 Bacterial diseases diagnosed in largemouth bass cases submitted to the KSU-FDDL.

Bacteria	Frequency of Occurrence
Aeromonas hydrophila	60
Flavobacterium columnare	21
Aeromonas sobria	8
Plesiomonas shigelloides	8
Edwarsiella tarda	7
Vibrio spp.	6
Aeromonas veronii	4
Aeromonas spp.	3
Pseudomonas spp.	2
Aeromonas salmonicida	1
Citrobacter freundii	1
Salmonella spp.	1
Unidentified bacteria	30

Aeromonas complex, which includes *Aeromonas hydrophila, A. caviae, A. sobria,* and *A. veronii. Columnaris* was the second most common bacterial disease diagnosed at KSU with 25 cases (Table 10.2). Gill monogenes were the most frequently occurring parasite with 16 cases diagnosed, followed by 9 cases of *Trichodina* and 8 cases of Ich (Table 10.3). Of the 355 cases diagnosed, 33 cases were routine checks and 30 cases were diagnosed as unidentified bacteria as cause of death.

Table 10.3 Parasites that have been found on largemouth bass submitted to the KSU-FDDL.

Parasites	Frequency of Occurrence
Monogenea (gills)	16
External *Saprolegnia*	15
Trichodina	9
Icthyophthirius	8
Ichthyobodo	5
Epistylis sp.	2
Capriniana sp.	1
Lernaea sp.	1
Bass tapeworm	1
White grub	1
Yellow grub	1
Apiosoma	1
Ambiphrya	1

10.8 Interesting cases

10.8.1 Copper sulfate overdose

In late winter 2006, largemouth bass mortalities (about 30 fish per day) were reported from a 0.4 ha aquaculture pond, averaging 1.2 m deep. Copper sulfate at a rate of about 1.1 mg/l was initially used to prevent aquatic weeds from becoming established in the pond. This treatment rate was double the conventional rate (the pond's total alkalinity was 51 mg/l, and the usual treatment would be 0.51 mg/l for $CuSO_4$ if total alkalinity were divided by 100 to get the recommended rate). Because of this overdose, the bass were exhibiting stressed behavior; this behavior, however, was interpreted by the farmer to be a sign of a disease in the bass that required more $CuSO_4$ treatment. So, another 1.1 mg/l of $CuSO_4$ were added to the pond, adding to the stress on the fish. The cold water also exacerbated the problem; Marple et al. (2001) demonstrated that free copper in the water persisted much longer at cold water temperatures than at warmer temperatures. The compounded overtreatment (4 times the normal rate) led to mortalities and a very peculiar reaction of the bass to loud banging on a plastic five-gallon bucket at the pond's edge. Bass startled by the noise went into convulsions, became stiff with mouth agape and died instantly. The Kentucky Division of Water found dissolved copper concentrations of 57 μg/l in the pond water indicating that high copper levels played a role in the bass mortalities. Gill histopathology revealed an edematous gill epithelium consistent with pathology caused by a water-borne irritant.

10.8.2 Acid sulfate soil in watershed of largemouth bass ponds

In an Ohio fish kill case submitted to the KSU-FDDL in 2006, 12,000 out of 15,000 largemouth bass died in a series of five ponds receiving water sequentially (water originating from a watershed composed of acid-sulfate soil). The water in these ponds was poorly buffered (total alkalinity values between 0 and 4 mg/l), so the rain runoff from the iron-sulfide-containing soil in the watershed quickly brought water pH values down to 4.1, a level lethal to fish. Soil in the watershed not only contained high levels of iron sulfide, but the soil itself was disturbed during deforestation in this watershed, leaving the iron-sulfide soil exposed to the air, forming sulfuric acid. Rain run-off water acquired an elevated sulfuric acid content as it percolated over this exposed soil, and then ran directly into the top pond. The top pond flowed into the second pond and so on, gradually diluting as it eventually flowed into the last (bottom) pond. The first three ponds in the series had 100% mortality of the largemouth bass; the fourth and fifth ponds had 80% and 60% mortality, respectively; while the last two ponds (sixth and seventh ponds) had no mortalities. The affected water had a reddish orange precipitate characteristic of ferric hydroxide, ferric oxide, and ferric oxyhydroxide that all originate from ferrous iron in the soil. Treating all the ponds with 4,500 to 9,000 kg/ha of pelletized lime and applying 2,250 kg/ha of pulverized lime to the watershed hillside elevated total alkalinity to 20 mg/l and the pH to 7, ending the fish mortalities.

References

American Fisheries Society (2016) Fish Health Section Bluebook (https://units.fisheries.org/fhs/fish-health-section-blue-book-2016/).

Bebak, J., Matthews, M. and Shoemaker, C. (2009) Survival of vaccinated, feed-trained largemouth bass fry (*Micropterus salmoides*) during natural exposure to *Flavobacterium columnare*. *Vaccine* 27, 4297–4301.

Beck, B.H., Bakal, R.S., Brunner, C.J. and Grizzle, J.M. (2006) Virus distribution and signs of disease after immersion exposure to largemouth bass virus. *Journal of Aquatic Animal Health* 18 (3), 176–183.

Boonthai, T., Loch, T.P., Yamashita, C.J., Smith, G.D., Winters, A.D., Kiupel, M., Brenden, T.O. and Faisal, M. (2018) Laboratory investigation into the role of largemouth bass virus (ranavirus, iridoviridae) in smallmouth bass mortality events in Pennsylvania Rivers. *BMC Veterinary Research* 14, 62.

Boonyaratpalin, S. and Rogers, W.A. (1984) Control of bass tapeworm, *Proteocephalus ambliplitis* (Leidy), with mebendazole. *Journal of Fish Diseases* 7 (6), 449–456.

Brandt, T. (1991) Temperate basses, *Morone* spp., and black basses, *Micropterus* spp. In: Wilson, R.P. (ed.) *Handbook of Nutrient Requirements of Finfish*, CRC Press, Boca Raton, FL, pp. 161–168.

Camus, A.C., Durborow, R.M., Hemstreet, W.G., Thune, R.L. and Hawke, J.P. (1998) *Aeromonas Bacterial Infections – Motile Aeromonad Septicemia*. Southern Regional Aquaculture Center, Publication 478.

Cochran, N.J., Coyle, S.D. and Tidwell, J.H. (2009) Evaluation of reduced fish meal diets for second year growth of largemouth bass, *Micropterus salmoides*. *Journal of the World Aquaculture Society* 40, 735–743.

Deng, G., Li, S., Xie, J., Bai, J., Chen, K., Ma, D., Jiang, X., Lao, H. and Yu, L. (2011) Characterization of a ranavirus isolated from cultured largemouth bass (*Micropterus salmoides*) in China. *Aquaculture* 312, 198–204.

Dodd, B.J., Barnhart, M.C., Rogers-Lowery, C.L., Fobian, T.B. and Dimock Jr., R.V. (2005) Cross-resistance of largemouth bass to glochidia of Unionid mussels. *Journal of Parasitology* 91 (5), 1064–1072.

Draghi II, A., Popov, V.L., Kahl, M.M., Stanton, J.B., Brown, C.C., Tsongalis, G.J., West, A.B. and Frasca Jr., S. (2004) Characterization of "*Candidatus Piscichlamydia salmonis*" (Order Chlamydiales), a chlamydia-like bacterium associated with epitheliocystis in farmed Atlantic Salmon (*Salmo salar*). *Journal of Clinical Microbiology* 42 (11), 5286–5297.

Durborow, R.M. (1986) Partial characterization of largemouth bass immunoglobulin and immune response of largemouth bass against bass tapeworms. PhD dissertation, Auburn University.

Durborow, R.M., Rogers, W.A. and Klesius, P.H. (1988) Interaction of bass tapeworm *Proteocephalus ambloplitis*, and *Neoechinorhynchus* sp. (Acanthocephala) in largemouth bass, *Micropterus salmoides*. *Journal of Parasitology* 74 (6), 1056–1059.

Durborow, R.M., Mitchell, A.J. and Crosby, M.D. (1998a) *Ich (White Spot Disease)*. Southern Regional Aquaculture Center, Publication 476.

Durborow, R.M., Thune, R.L., Hawke, J.P. and Camus, A.C. (1998b) *Columnaris disease: a bacterial infection caused by* Flavobacterium columnare. Southern Regional Aquaculture Center, Publication 479.

Durborow, R.M., Wise, D.J. and Terhune, J.S. (2003) *Saprolegniasis (winter fungus) and Branchiomycosis of commercially cultured channel catfish*. Southern Regional Aquaculture Center, Publication 4700.

Gao, E.B. and Chen, G. (2018) *Micropterus salmoides* rhabdovirus (MSRV) infection induced apoptosis and activated interferon signaling pathway in largemouth bass skin cells. *Fish Shellfish Immunology* 76, 161–166.

Getchell, R.G., Groocock, G.H., Schumacher, V.L., Grimmett, S.G., Wooster, G.A. and Bowser, P.R. (2007) Quantitative polymerase chain reaction assay for largemouth bass virus. *Journal of Aquatic Animal Health* 19 (4), 226–233.

Getchell, R.G., Groocock, G.H., Cornwell, E.R., Schumacher, V.L., Glasner, L.I., Baker, B.J., Frattini, S.A., Wooster, G.A. and Bowser, P.R. (2014) Development and characterization of a largemouth bass cell line. *Journal of Aquatic Animal Health* 26 (3), 194–201.

Goodwin, A.E., Park, E. and Nowak, B.F. (2005) Successful treatment of largemouth bass, *Micropterus salmoides* (L.), with epitheliocystis hyperinfection. *Journal of Fish Diseases* 28, 623–625.

Grizzle, J.M. and Brunner, C.J. (2003) Review of largemouth bass virus. *Fisheries* 28 (11), 10–14.

Grant, E.C., Philipp, D.P., Inendino, K.R. and Goldberg, T.L. (2003) Effects of temperature on the susceptibility of largemouth bass to largemouth bass virus. *Journal of Aquatic Animal Health* 15 (3), 215–220.

Hanson, L.A., Hanson, L.P., Meals, K.O., Chinchar, V.G. and Rudis, M. (2000) Persistence of largemouth bass virus infection in a northern Mississippi reservoir after a die-off. *Journal of Aquatic Animal Health* 13 (1), 27–34.

Hazen, T.C., Esch, G.W. and Raker, M.L. (1981) Agglutinating antibody to *Aeromonas hydrophila* in wild largemouth bass. *Transactions of the American Fisheries Society* 110 (4), 514–518.

Hoffman, G.L. (1999) Parasites of North American freshwater fishes. Cornell University Press, Ithaca, New York.

Huh, M.D., Thomas, C.D., Udomkusonsri, P. and Noga, E.J. (2005) Epidemic *trichodinosis* associated with severe epidermal hyperplasia in largemouth bass, *Micropterus salmoides*, from North Carolina, USA. *Journal of Wildlife Diseases* 41 (3), 647–653.

Huizinga, H.W., Esch, G.W. and Hazen, T.C. (1979) Histopathology of red-sore disease (*Aeromonas hydrophila*) in naturally and experimentally infected largemouth bass *Micropterus salmoides* (Lacépède). *Journal of Fish Diseases* 2 (4), 263–277.

Kim, R. and Faisal, M. (2010) Experimental studies confirm the wide host range of the Great Lakes viral hemorrhagic septicemia virus genotype IVb. *Journal of Fish Diseases* 33, 83–88.

Kim, R. and Faisal, M. (2011) Emergence and resurgence of the viral hemorrhagic septicemia virus (novirhabdovirus, rhabdoviridae, mononegavirlaes). *Journal of Advanced Research* 2, 9–23.

LaFrentz, B.R., Goodwin, A.E. and Shoemaker, C.A. (2014) Columnaris disease. In: American Fisheries Society Fish (ed.) *Health Section Bluebook.* https://units.fisheries.org/fhs/fish-health-section-blue-book-2016/.

Lange, M.D. (2003) Methodologies to reduce mortalities due to *Flavobacterium columnare* during the feed-training and cage-culture of largemouth bass (*Micropterus salmoides*). MS thesis, Kentucky State University.

Leis, E., McCann, R., Standish, I., Bestul, A., Odom, T., Finnerty, C. and Bennie, B. (2018) Comparison of lethal and nonlethal sampling methods for the detection of largemouth bass virus (LMBV) from largemouth bass in the upper Mississippi River. *Journal of Aquatic Animal Health* 30 (3), https://doi.org/10.1002/aah.10029.

Maceina, M.J. and Grizzle, J.M. (2005) The relation of largemouth bass virus to largemouth bass population metrics in five Alabama reservoirs. *Transactions of the American Fisheries Society* 135 (2), 545–555.

MacMillan, J.R. (1991) Biological factors impinging upon control of external protozoan fish parasites. *Annual Review of Fish Diseases* 1, 119–131.

Marple, S.L., Davis, E.R. and Larimore, M.S. (2001) Monitoring free copper to determine application rates of copper sulfate: A case study. In: *Proceedings of the Annual Conference of the Southeastern Association of Fish and Wildlife Agencies* 55: 235–242.

McClenahan, S.D., Beck, B.H. and Grizzle, J.M. (2005) Evaluation of cell culture methods for detection of largemouth bass virus. *Journal of Aquatic Animal Health* 17 (4), 365–372.

Nath, S., Aron, G.M., Southard, G.M. and McLean, R.J.C. (2010) Potential for largemouth bass virus to associate with and gain protection from bacterial biofilms. *Journal of Aquatic Animal Health* 22, 95–101.

Noga, E.J. (1986) The importance of *Lernaea cruciate* (Le Sueur) in the initiation of skin lesions in largemouth bass, *Micropterus salmoides* (Lacépède), in the Chowan River, North Caroline, USA. *Journal of Fish Diseases* 9 (4), 295–302.

Noga, E.J., Bullis, R.A. and Miller, G.C. (1990) Epidemic oral ulceration in largemouth bass (*Micropterus salmoides*) associated with the leech *Myzobdella lugubris*. *Journal of Wildlife Diseases* 26 (1), 132–134.

Noga, E.J. (2010) *Fish Disease: Diagnosis and Treatment*, 2nd edn. Iowa State Press, Ames, IA, pp. 185–186.

Ostrand, K.G., Cooke, S.J. and Wahl, D.H. (2002) Effects of stress on largemouth bass reproduction. *North American Journal of Fisheries Management* 24 (3), 1038–1045.

Plumb, J.A., Grizzle, J.M. and Rogers, W.A. (1988) Survival of caught and released largemouth bass after containment in live wells. *North American Journal of Fisheries Management* 8 (3), 325–328.

Plumb, J.A., Noyes, A.D., Graziano, S., Wang, J., Mao, J. and Chinchar, V.G. (1999) Isolation and identification of viruses from adult largemouth bass during a 1997–1998 survey in the southeastern United States. *Journal of Aquatic Animal Health* 11, 391–399.

Schramm Jr., H.L. and Davis, J.G. (2006) Survival of largemouth bass from populations infected with largemouth bass virus subjected to stimulated tournament. *North American Journal of Fisheries Management* 26, 826–832.

Schramm Jr., H.L., Walters, A.R., Grizzle, J.M., Beck, B.H., Hanson, L.A. and Rees, S.B. (2011) Effects of live-well conditions on mortality and largemouth bass virus prevalence in largemouth bass caught during summer tournaments. *North American Journal of Fisheries Management* 26 (4), 812–825.

Southard, G.M., Fries, L.T. and Terre, D.R. (2009) Largemouth bass virus in Texas: distribution and management issues. *Journal of Aquatic Animal Health* 21, 36–42.

Terhune, J.S. and Beck, B.H. (2015) Common diseases of black bass: implications for conservation and management. *American Fisheries Society Symposium* 82, 333–350.

Tidwell, J.H., Coyle, S.D. and Woods, T.A. (2000) *Species profile: largemouth bass.* Southern Regional Aquaculture Center, Publication 722, Stoneville, Mississippi.

Timmons, T.J. and Hemstreet, W.G. (1980) Prevalence rate of *Lernaea cyprinacea* (Copepoda: Lernaeidae) on young-of-the-year largemouth bass, *Micropterus salmoides* (Lacépède), in West Point Reservoir, Alabama-Georgia, U.S.A. *Journal of Fish Diseases* 3 (6), 529–530.

Woodland, J.E., Brunner, C.J., Noyles, A.D. and Grizzle, J.M. (2002) Experimental oral transmission of largemouth bass virus. *Journal of Fish Diseases* 25 (11), 669–672.

CHAPTER 11

Harvest and transport of largemouth bass

Shawn D. Coyle

Kentucky State University, Aquaculture Research Program, Frankfort, Kentucky, USA

Todd S. Harmon

Walt Disney World, Animal Programs, Lake Buena Vista, Florida, USA

11.1 Introduction

Largemouth bass (*Micropterus salmoides*) are produced to supply recreational sport-fish for stocking throughout much of North America and regionally in Europe and Asia, notably Japan. Market demand for largemouth bass as a sportfish encompasses all sizes from fry to trophy size fish (Figure 11.1). Largemouth bass are also produced extensively as food-fish, which are primarily marketed live in major cities with large ethnic Asian populations. Fresh-on-ice largemouth bass can also be found in parts of Mexico. Market demand for the food-fish market is typically for 0.45–0.90 kg fish with a desired minimum market size of 0.6 kg in the USA. The production of food-fish largemouth bass in temperate regions typically involves three production phases: nursery/feed training, first summer growth and second year grow out. Each phase of production involves: harvest, handling, grading and some degree of live transportation. This chapter

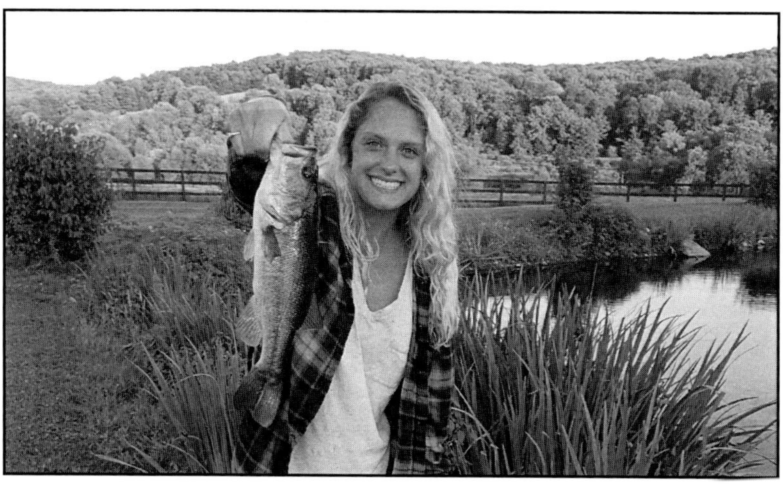

Figure 11.1 A largemouth bass caught from a privately owned pond.

will primarily focus on the practice of harvesting and live transport of food-size largemouth bass in the USA; although many of the considerations and recommendations are also applicable to smaller sizes of fish and other regions.

11.2 Fish response to the capture and transport process

Handling of fish cannot be avoided in aquaculture and plays a major role in the success of transport. Fish are subject to aerial exposure, crowding, net handling, and environment changes during harvest, sorting, and loading for transport. These handling processes have the potential to cause stress and possible mortality of the fish (Yeager et al., 1990). Fish react to stress with a series of physiological changes. During the primary response, catecholamine and cortisol levels increase. The release of these hormones induces a number of secondary stress responses including: elevated blood glucose (Mazeaud et al., 1977), elevated blood lactic acid (Wedemeyer, 1970), increased glycogen metabolism (Schwalme and MacKay, 1991), and osmoregulatory disturbances (Weirich et al., 1992).

If these biological disturbances are too great or too numerous and the fish is unable to recover, mortality may result. Fish have physiological mechanisms that allow them to cope with stress at a metabolic cost associated with diverting energy from normal metabolic functions. However, these response actions can be forced beyond their normal limits, thus becoming detrimental to the fish and ultimately resulting in mortality (Barton and Iwama, 1991). The severity of the stress response and the length of time before homeostasis is regained are directly related to the duration of the stressor and the characteristics of the recovery water (Reubush and Heath, 1997).

Stressors that affect fish can be categorized into acute (short term) and chronic (long term) stressors (Davis, 2006). Acute stressors include handling, confinement, abrupt changes in water quality and improper acclimation; while chronic stressors include extended periods of poor water quality, improper stocking densities, and improper diets (Harmon, 2009). Severe acute stress might result in immediate mortality, presumably through ion loss (McDonald and Milligan, 1997), whereas chronic stress often results in severely compromised immune system and/or decreased energy stores (Portz et al., 2006). Immunosuppressed fish allow pathogens to initiate a disease that would otherwise normally be resisted by the fish (Wedemeyer, 1997).

"Delayed mortality" can occur days or even weeks after transport depending on the underlying cause and severity (Harmon, 2009). This can make it difficult to verify the exact mechanisms responsible, but generally are considered as mortality due to the transport process. This process starts as the fish are removed from the pond and includes the transport itself and then the acclimation into their new environment. Utilizing good husbandry practices throughout this process is important in the success of harvest and transport.

Relatively little work has been conducted specifically on largemouth bass in documenting the effects of physiological stress. Carmichael et al. (1984a) characterized normal values for blood parameters and evaluated the effects of net confinement and water quality induced stress (oxygen depletion and elevated ammonia levels) in largemouth bass. They reported that plasma glucose and corticosteroid values were good indicators of stress during application of acute stressors, whereas chloride and osmolality were more useful indicators of long-term stress or as stress-recovery indicators.

During the transport and harvesting process reducing the number of stressors is important in getting a good product to the buyer or consumer. Because there is not one large event to focus on, many small practices can prove invaluable in providing healthy fish as an end product.

11.3 Harvest

The food-fish market for largemouth bass is somewhat unique in that the fish are typically marketed live to the consumer. This requires that the physiological condition of the fish following harvest and transport to market is strong enough to endure several days or weeks in retail display tanks. Conversely, channel catfish (*Ictalurus punctatus*) and rainbow trout (*Oncorhynchus mykiss*) harvest and transport procedures are primarily based on live delivery to a nearby processing plant. At the time of writing there is no known commercial processing of largemouth bass in the USA. Since largemouth bass are marketed live, they should be thought of as a perishable product with a shelf life similar to that of produce. As with produce, the clock starts at the time of harvest and even when maintained under optimal conditions the product quality can slowly deteriorate over time. This situation requires that stress be minimized at every step from harvest to retail sale.

Stress from various handling practices associated with harvesting weakens fish that can make them susceptible to disease outbreaks and adverse physiological imbalances (Wedemeyer, 1970). The sensitivity of fish to handling varies among species; where some species are more tolerant while others are delicate and sensitive to what would be generally considered a minor stress (Jensen and Brunson, 1992). The largemouth bass is considered a relatively stress sensitive species with a limited ability to tolerate net confinement, temperature change, or periods of low oxygen or high ammonia concentrations (Williamson and Carmichael, 1986; Suski et al., 2007; Vanlandeghem et al., 2010).

As poikilothermic animals, water temperature and temperature change have a great effect on the physiological stress response in fishes. Largemouth bass do not tolerate rapid changes in water temperature as well as some other commercial aquaculture species such as channel catfish or rainbow trout (Currie et al., 1998). However, the stress response is attenuated at lower water temperatures. Carmichael et al. (1984a) reported a significant reduction in plasma glucose and corticosteroid levels following abrupt temperature change in largemouth bass previously acclimated to lower water temperatures of 10–16°C than for those acclimated to 23°C.

During the summer months, largemouth bass are typically not harvested for food-fish sales due to increased stress and mortality associated with warmer waters in conjunction with harvest, holding and transport. This limits the market window for sale of live largemouth bass. Producers primarily market their fish only when pond water temperatures have stabilized for a couple of weeks below 18°C. Poor survival following harvest at higher water temperatures is thought to be primarily due to an elevated stress response followed by disease outbreaks within days after handling, resulting in financial losses for the buyers. This is of great economic importance to the customer (retail grocer) as the market value of iced fish is less than 20% of the live value in ethnic Asian markets. Some producers cool ponds using ground water or spring water to access live markets during the summer months but at this time accounts for a small percentage of total sales.

Over the past 20 years, the average price paid by live haulers for live largemouth bass picked up at the farm has remained relatively stable at US$8.80–13.20/kg (personal communication, Robert Mayer, Kentucky, 2017). This suggests that, at this time, supply has not surpassed demand. However, the temperature constrained opportunity for sale and distribution creates a seasonal oversupply as producers attempt to reduce pond holdings before the onset of the coldest months of winter. This generally results in a period of lower prices. This can happen again as the water warms in the spring if producers still have significant holdings of fish for sale. Some producers hold inventory and wait for the price to increase and stabilize, typically around mid-December. They may harvest ponds during ice cover. This is accomplished by breaking the ice around the perimeter of the pond and seining under the ice to an area of the pond where the ice has been melted sufficiently to extract the seine and harvest the fish. Melting of ice in a pond can be accomplished when the air temperatures are > 3°C by use of a surface aerator or tractor powered power take-off (PTO) aerator.

Largemouth bass are usually harvested from ponds by seining the pond with a seine net that is ≥150% of the length and depth of the pond. Different fish species vary greatly in their susceptibility to capture by seine. In purpose built ponds with few obstructions, largemouth bass are relatively easy to capture by seining. Generally, > 90% of the population can be captured in one haul provided the seine is appropriately sized for the pond (personal communication, Robert Mayer, Kentucky, 2017). In contrast, Nile tilapia (*Oreochromis niloticus*) are particularly difficult to seine with reported catch rates of 15–23% in a single haul and with great differences reported between strains (Sifa et al., 1999). Steeby and Lovshin (1993) reported cumulative average harvest efficiencies of 57, 75 and 83% for three seine hauls with channel catfish.

A sufficiently sized collection bag in the seine is necessary as largemouth bass will readily jump over the seine. Seines for largemouth bass should be constructed of the softest knotless mesh available to reduce abrasion to the mucosal layer of the epidermis and underlying scales. Seines designed for channel catfish should not be used as they are coated to prevent their spines from penetrating and can be abrasive. The fish's mucus and skin is the first line of defense against pathogens and disease and any disruption provides an entryway. Largemouth bass do not tolerate skin abrasion associated with rough handling well.

When seining, it is important that the producer captures only the number of fish that they can load into a pond-side transport or holding tank, supplied with pure oxygen, within 30 min. It may be necessary to intentionally only capture a portion of the fish in the pond at one time. Hauling tanks mounted to a tractor or front-end loader that can be lowered into the pond during harvest greatly improves harvest efficiency and reduces aerial exposure time of harvested fish. Largemouth bass should not be overloaded into nets and/or baskets during harvest to prevent fish from bruising and abrading one another. Rubber nets are becoming more popular because they reduce skin injuries to the fish and tend not to rub off the mucous on the skin and limit eye injuries. If handling trophy bass, moving them in water can provide an added layer of protection. Water bags (such as ones used in tournaments) or vinyl fish stretchers can benefit by limiting abrasions and loss of mucous in larger fish, but this process can be time consuming since you are only handling a few fish at a time.

11.4 Holding tanks

Pond harvested largemouth bass food-fish are often moved into holding tanks where they are maintained prior to pick up. Transport from the pond to the holding tank is a crucial first step. Holding densities in pond-side transport tanks should not exceed 240 g/l, and should contain 2–3 g/l salinity and the duration in the tank should be limited to 30 min before they are transferred into larger long-term holding tanks. When water temperatures are > 18°C and when handling smaller fish, it is beneficial to anesthetize largemouth bass using tricaine methanesulfonate (MS-222) in the pond once the seine net is pulled up to reduce the stress associated with handling.

Most producers of food-fish largemouth bass sell to specialty live haulers that distribute live fish to Asian markets. Live haulers generally prefer the fish to be harvested a couple of days ahead of time and "hardened" in tanks prior to over the road transport. This holding period allows the fish time to purge their stomachs and recover from the stressors of pond harvest. It also allows the producer to inspect the fish for disease and be sure the full number of fish will be available when the live-hauler arrives. When fish are held in tanks prior to transport it is also much easier to grade out undersize fish when loading the truck.

Holding tanks vary in size and shape but are generally supplied with flow through water from either wells, springs or surface water. The quality of the water source and supply dictates many variables associated with successfully holding fish. Temperature change is one of the most important variables to consider, even when water temperatures are within the acceptable range for transport of 3–18°C. It is important to not abruptly change the water temperature more than 4°C/h and no more than 12°C over a 24 h period. This can be difficult to achieve in situations where the ground water temperature is much higher than the surface water temperature. In the coldest periods of winter, it may be beneficial to use surface water to supply water to holding tanks to more closely align with pond water temperatures from which the fish are harvested.

Water temperature also dictates the allowable biomass densities that can be held with minimal stress. For example, for a farmer using surface water to supply water to holding tanks, as water temperatures decrease from 18 to 3°C over the course of the winter; the allowable stocking densities in holding tanks may increase from 10 kg/m^3 (10 g/l) to 40 kg/m^3 (40 g/l). Note that the densities in holding tanks are much lower than those often used during live hauling as the duration is often much longer. The holding tank period should be considered a recovery period from the stress of harvest prior to the upcoming stress of live hauling.

The acceptable duration for holding largemouth bass should also be related to water temperature. When water temperatures are at or near the maximum of 18°C bass should only be held for ≤ 2–3 d before live hauling to market. However, when water temperatures are 3–5°C bass can be held for up to 2 weeks.

Prophylactic chemical treatments to alleviate stress and prevent disease prior to transport is a common practice. Carmichael et al. (1984b) recommended daily copper sulfate treatments for 10 consecutive days prior to transport of juvenile largemouth bass. Producers routinely use salt (2–10 g/l), copper sulfate (1–3 mg/l), diquat (2–4 mg/l) or formalin (20 mg/l) as daily treatments during holding. Check with your local aquaculture extension agent to ensure compliance with state and federal regulations before administering chemical treatments on fish even if they are not considered food-fish.

11.5 Fish "quality"

The "quality" of fish to be transported is a crucial criterion. The fish must be healthy and in good condition. Weakened individuals and fish with signs of disease or parasites should be eliminated from the consignment, particularly when the temperature during shipment is high or transport times are long. When fish are of poor quality, even reducing biomass densities may not prevent mortality. It is ultimately the responsibility of the live hauler to accept or reject a load of fish before they are loaded for shipment. However, the poor reputation associated with the delivery of undersize or sick fish will ultimately reside with the farm from which they originated. When moving fish from the holding tanks to the truck it is important to recognize unhealthy individuals and not include them in the transport.

The size of the fish is also an important factor considered in the quality of the fish. The live market for food-fish in the USA currently requires largemouth bass to be a minimum size of 560 g. Owing to inherent size variability within largemouth bass cohorts generally the average individual weight of the population has to be > 600 g in order for the smaller fish in the group to achieve the minimum acceptable weight requirement. If a significant number of fish are undersize (> 5%), the producer should remove the submarket size fish from the lot. Graded-off fish can either be restocked for another year of growth or marketed as sportfish for pond stocking. It is important to communicate with the buyer regarding the acceptable percentage of submarket fish. Sometimes the seller or buyer may negotiate a reduced price for the ungraded lot to negate the additional stress associated with grading the fish prior to transport.

Ethnic Chinese customers place a high priority on healthy fish at the point of sale (Jia et al., 2016). Fish quality is generally visually determined by the consumer with main criteria being clear eyes and bright shiny scales. Brandt et al. (1986) evaluated the incidence of corneal cloudiness in transported largemouth bass. After 6 to 28 h of simulated transport, 46 to 83% of fish had cloudy eyes. Generally, opacity increased as the length of the simulated transport increased. Overall mortality in the study was < 1%. The condition was deemed reversible as > 75% of affected fish had recovered within 48 h after the stress was removed and 100% recovered within 7 d. The authors reported that they had not added salt to the water during the simulation which likely increased the occurrence of the abnormality.

11.6 Live transport

11.6.1 Live hauling

Transportation of live fish is a common practice in fish culture operations and the ultimate goal is keeping the fish alive and healthy during and after distribution. The greatest challenge with live fish transport is to minimize stress on the fish. Stress in fish associated with transport is related to disturbances in the normal physiological state as a result of various factors (Francis-Floyd, 2002). Transported fish are often, within a short time period, exposed to multiple stressors such as: high density confinement, physical handling, unfavorable water quality and conditioning to a new environment. Transport associated mortality might be the result of one severe stressor, several mild stressors or infectious disease (Harmon, 2009). Even if the fish are carefully handled and transported, a combination of mild stressors might act together and cause mortality (Carmichael et al., 2001).

Freshwater finfish farmed in China are primarily marketed live to the domestic market where annual mortality of transported fish averages about 7% of the total production (Bureau of Fisheries of Ministry of China, 2013, in Jia et al., 2016). A recent study quantified customer claims of mortality of transported live fish in Beijing, China (Jia et al., 2016). Although physiological and transport conditions were not described, the authors reported an average of 16.1% mortality of largemouth bass. The store managers stated that substandard conditions of transportation were the primary cause. Some mortality during and following fish transport is common and generally accepted as "the nature of the business" as long as mortalities are less than 0.5–1% of the total load. Producers frequently add 1–2% extra fish by weight to compensate for losses due to mortality and "shrinkage" associated with bodily waste elimination.

The primary objectives of the commercial live hauler are to keep the fish alive and healthy but also to deliver them economically. Commercial live haulers desire to haul as many fish as possible as load hauled is directly proportionate to the revenue generated. This creates a situation where fish are often hauled at maximum carrying capacity based on water conditions, distance and experience. The number or weight of fish that can be successfully transported depends on the water quality, the duration of the transport, water temperature, fish size and the species (Harmon, 2009). Piper et al. (1982) suggested that loading rates can be increased 25% for each 5°C decrease in water temperature, but if the duration exceeds 12 h, the loading rate should be decreased by 25%. If environmental conditions are constant, the carrying capacity during transport depends primarily on the species and the size of the fish. Piper et al. (1982) suggested that with trout the maximum permissible weight is directly proportional to their length. Thus, if a tank can hold 10 kg of 5 cm trout, then it can hold 20 kg of 10 cm trout. Similarly, Carmichael (1984) recommended maximum shipping densities of 90 g/l for 12.7 cm largemouth bass and 180 g/l for 20.3 cm fish for long-haul shipping (up to 30 h).

Much of the research conducted on live transport of fish is related to work at government run hatcheries where the transport times are generally < 10 h and the fish are small fingerlings for stocking. Largemouth bass fingerlings are often transported during mid to late summer when water temperatures are relatively warm which decreases acceptable loading densities. Piper et al. (1982) provided recommended carrying capacities for commonly cultured fish and reported that 100 g channel catfish and rainbow trout could be similarly hauled at 400–500 g/l for up to 10 h. The authors reported that transport densities for largemouth bass of similar size and duration should be limited to 240 g/l. Similarly, McCraren and Millard (1978) suggested that advanced fingerling (15–25 cm) largemouth bass could be transported at densities up to 240 g/l for up to 10 h with the use of agitators, bottled oxygen, and circulators (Table 11.1). Wilson (1950) reported that biomass densities during transport of 10 cm largemouth bass should be limited to 120 g/l for up to 16 h at water temperatures ranging from 18 to 24°C (Table 11.1). However, the duration of the transport can exceed 24 h to reach the West Coast of the USA from the South Central region where the majority of largemouth bass production occurs.

Carmichael (1984) and Carmichael et al. (1984a, 1984b) conducted a series of experiments to improve the success of long distance transport of largemouth bass for stock enhancement.

Table 11.1 Maximum loading densities based on average length for largemouth bass fingerlings transported for 10–16 hours at water temperatures ranging from 18 to 24°C (Wilson, 1950).

Fish length cm (inches)	Number of fish per kg (lb)	Number of fish per l (gal)	Density of fish g/l (pounds/gal)
2.5 (1)	2,200 (1,000)	1265 (333)	40 (0.33)
5.0 (2)	880 (400)	760 (200)	60 (0.50)
7.5 (3)	220 (100)	255 (67)	80 (0.66)
10.0 (4)	55 (25)	95 (25)	120 (1.0)
20.0 (8)[a]	8 (3.6)	16 (7.2)	240 (2.0)

Note: [a]McCraren and Millard (1978).

Carmichael (1984) showed that lower biomass densities of 80–90 g/l were necessary for long distance transport (> 30 h) of largemouth bass fingerlings (12 cm). Carmichael et al. (1984a, 1984b) evaluated various chemical treatments and methods for alleviation of stress associated with hauling largemouth bass. Stress was reduced significantly and mortality was eliminated when fish were treated for diseases, held 72 h without food prior to transport, anesthetized before they were loaded, hauled at a cool temperature in physiological concentrations of salts with an antibiotic and a mild anesthetic, and allowed to recover in the same medium without the anesthetic.

Carmichael and Tomasso (1988) conducted a survey of public and private hatcheries to assess transportation techniques used, which were highly variable for all species. Largemouth bass were the third most commonly transported species, behind rainbow trout and channel catfish, respectively. Largemouth bass were most commonly transported for durations of < 5 h at water temperatures of 21–26°C and biomass densities of < 60 g/l. All respondents reported using salt at 1–5 g/l, 49% of respondents reported using some type of antibacterial compound, and 8.2% used an anesthetic. The highest reported transport density with largemouth bass was 286 g/l. Generally, densities hauled (g/l) were lower for smaller fish, warmer water, and longer transport times.

Commercial live haulers of largemouth bass food-fish often haul at lower water temperatures and higher loading densities than those found in the literature. Assuming that all other parameters are suitable in regards to the quality of the fish, water and equipment; a maximum transport density of 360 g/l can be successfully achieved with food-fish size largemouth bass provided that the water temperature is 3–8°C and the duration of the trip is ≤14 h (personal communication, Robert Mayer, Kentucky, 2017) (Table 11.2). Water temperature and trip duration

Table 11. 2 Maximum loading densities based on water temperature and trip duration for food-size (0.45–0.9 kg average individual weight) largemouth bass (Piper et al., 1982).

Water temperature		Trip duration	
°C	g/l @ ≤ 14 h	g/l @ 15–20 h	g/l @ 21–25 h
3–8	360[a]	270	180
9–13	270	180	135
14–18	180	135	90

Note: [a]Personal communication, Robert Mayer, Kentucky, 2017.

should be used to decide allowable transport densities of market-size food-fish within the range of 80–360 g/l for 3–18°C (Table 11.2). For every 5°C increase in water temperature the density should be reduced by 25% (Piper et al., 1982). Similarly, for every 6 h increase in transport duration the biomass density should be reduced by 25%. These are estimates based on experience and communications with live haulers and fish farmers; however, there are many unforeseen circumstances that can arise, such as a truck or equipment failure, so it is always advisable to error on the conservative side if possible.

11.6.2 Fry transport

Largemouth bass fry are sensitive to environmental changes. Oxygen levels should be monitored carefully during transport. Colt (2006) recommends avoiding oxygen concentrations above 25 ppm in culture systems. Matthews et al. (2017) showed significant mortality in Guadalupe bass *Micropterus treculii* at 200% saturation and recommend staying below 15 ppm dissolved oxygen when transporting fry of all black bass species. Maintaining dissolved oxygen levels between 10 and 12 ppm is recommended for newly hatch fry. Do not add salt to the water when transporting largemouth bass fry. Transporting fry over distances in hauling boxes is not typically hindered by hauling densities as 1,000,000 largemouth bass fry weigh only 3.64 kg (0.0036 g average weight; 275 fry/g). For on-site moving of fry from the hatchery building out to ponds a density of 1,000 fry/l (4–5 g/l) is acceptable. Oxygen should be checked frequently and turned off once concentrations reach 15 ppm. These densities are intentionally low to enable a slow controlled acclimation. Agitators should not be run due to the physical damage potential to the fry. Largemouth bass fry can be successfully shipped at 10 g/l for 36 h and up to 18 g/l for 24 h in standard plastic fish transport bags containing 10 l of water within Styrofoam shipping boxes. Time in shipping boxes should not exceed 36 h with best results at shipping times of < 24 h. Although fry can tolerate a wide range of water temperatures extra care and time should be taken during acclimation.

11.6.3 Transport water preparation

Several mitigation techniques are commonly used to lessen the severity of the stress response induced by handling, including: a 3 d pre-stress fasting period, anesthetic treatment prior to handling, increasing water hardness, and the addition of salt mixtures (Tomasso et al., 1980). The addition of salts is perhaps the most common technique used with freshwater fish to alleviate the severity of the stress response. Salts passively diffuse from areas of high concentration in the blood to areas of low concentration in fresh water. Therefore, salts are slowly but continuously lost to the environment.

The gills and skin are coated with a thin layer of mucus which helps reduce the loss of salts to the surrounding fresh water. However, netting and handling removes some of the protective mucus coating from fish. Additionally, during excitement and in stressful conditions, epinephrine (adrenaline) is released into the bloodstream increasing the permeability of water across the gill epithelia in fish (Moyle and Cech, 1988). This increases the water gain and blood ion loss in freshwater fish resulting in disturbance of osmoregulatory homeostasis (Portz et al., 2006). Lost salts must be replaced by re-absorbing them from the water or during food digestion; these are active processes requiring significant energy. Ion regulation in fish is physiologically costly accounting for up to 20% of resting metabolism (Febry and Lutz, 1987).

The addition of salt to the transport water limits the loss of salt during transport by reducing or eliminating the concentration gradient between fish blood and the water environment. This reduces energy demands and diffusion leakage while providing a supply of environmental salts for re-absorption and replacement of lost blood salts. Weirich and Tomasso (1991) demonstrated that red drum (*Sciaenops ocellatus*) tolerate confinement and transport stress best in water that is nearly isosmotic with their blood plasma. The authors suggested that fish in the nearly isosmotic solutions were faced with smaller ionic and osmotic gradients and presumably required less energy to maintain proper water and ion balances during confinement.

Sodium chloride is not the only salt important to fish physiology; for example, potassium salts are critical for the normal function of heart, nerve and muscle tissue (Lovell, 1989). The blood of most freshwater fish has a salinity of approximately 9 g/l and the relative percentages of ionic concentrations of plasma fluid are: sodium 47.4, chloride 45.6, potassium 1.1, magnesium 0.44, and calcium 0.76 (Karnaky, 1997). Vanlandeghem et al. (2010) reported that rapid temperature change and exposure to low dissolved oxygen affect potassium balance in largemouth bass suggesting that the addition of potassium chloride to hauling tank water may be advantageous.

Carmichael (1984) described largemouth bass in poor condition following long-distance transport and suggested the cause to be osmoregulatory dysfunction. Carmichael (1984) described the fish as appearing discolored with opaque eyes. The fish were unable to move normally and stiff. Necropsy showed cloudy eyes and turgidity of the body was likely due to osmotic shock. The scales around the caudal peduncle appeared distended and rough to the touch with some hemorrhaging present along the caudal and anal fins. The plasma chloride levels of the fish remained low for 95 h after loading for transport. The turgid condition of affected fish indicates a probable influx of water and loss of the ability to retain homeostasis. Due to their weakened condition a secondary stressor would likely overcome their compensatory ability resulting in death.

Traditionally, 0.5 to 2 g/l sodium chloride solutions have been used to reduce stress during transport of freshwater fish (Tomasso et al., 1980). However, higher salinities may be beneficial when transporting largemouth bass. Carmichael et al. (1984b) reported a reduced stress response and increased survival in largemouth bass exposed to simulated transport conditions when using transport water with a isosmotic salt content (8 g/l) containing salts similar to those in plasma by addition of sodium chloride, potassium chloride, potassium phosphate and magnesium sulfate. Carmichael (1984) used a 5 g/l mixture of salts that closely resembled plasma values for long distance transport of largemouth bass fingerlings and reported better survival rates than in previous trials where the salinity was only 3.8 g/l.

In an unpublished study (Coyle and Tidwell, Kentucky State University), addition of a commercial marine salt premix was found to be effective in reducing mortality and improving osmoregulation of largemouth bass following 24 h of simulated transport. The trial evaluated 0, 8, and 16 g/l salinity and resulted in higher whole blood concentrations of sodium, potassium, chlorine, and lower blood glucose levels in fish at 16 g/l. Results also showed lower oxygen and higher ammonia concentrations in the blood of fish transported at 16 g/l than for fish subjected to 8 g/l, possibly indicating that 16 g/l salinity is too high for largemouth bass. Susanto and

Peterson (1996) determined from physiological measurements that largemouth bass adapt well to salinities up to 8 g/l, but reported that higher levels caused measurable osmoregulatory dysfunction. The use of marine premixes should more closely match fish blood chemistries than pure salt and may improve osmoregulatory function, but are also much more expensive.

Live haulers typically add evaporated salt or water softener salt to hauling containers at 2–3 g/l (ppt) to aid in osmoregulation and reduce hauling stress during the transport of largemouth bass. The use of higher rates of salinity of 5–8 g/l are generally used only for short periods of up to one hour following harvest and handling procedures such as weighing for sampling and as a prophylactic treatment when bass are held in tanks supplied with flow through water. Increasing salinity also increases foam production in hauling tank water, which may be considered undesirable. However, based on the reported literature higher concentrations of salt (5–8 g/l) could be beneficial during transport of largemouth bass.

11.6.4 Dissolved oxygen

Ideally dissolved oxygen (DO) should be maintained at or near 100% saturation throughout transport. Saturation is the amount of dissolved gas when the water and atmospheric phases are in equilibrium (Piper et al., 1982). The solubility of oxygen is dependent on water temperature, gas composition, salinity and total pressure. The solubility of oxygen decreases as the water temperature, salinity and altitude increase. Gas supersaturation can occur when the dissolved gases are greater than the equilibrium concentration. The gases of importance are nitrogen and oxygen which, in the atmosphere, are at partial pressures of approximately 78% nitrogen and 21% oxygen. However, oxygen is twice as soluble as nitrogen, so in water oxygen (35%) is approximately half as plentiful as nitrogen (65%) (Harvey, 1975).

DO is often the single most limiting factor in any fish-holding and transport system. The initial 30–60 min in the transport container is the most critical for monitoring DO levels because of the increased activity of the fish (Piper et al., 1982). Therefore, it is important to saturate or supersaturate the water with oxygen prior to placing a heavy load of fish into a transport tank. Various methods have been used to achieve and maintain proper DO levels throughout fish transport including compressed oxygen gas, agitators, aerators, circulation pumps equipped with spray bars and liquid oxygen. Commercial fish haulers use pure oxygen injection systems employing either compressed oxygen gas bottles or liquid oxygen Dewar's. Most commercial live haulers use liquid oxygen due to increased volume and reduced refill frequency. However, liquid oxygen Dewar's lose approximately 2% by volume daily so may be economically impractical in situations of long periods of inactivity (Timmons et al., 2002).

Fine pore ceramic diffusers greatly improve the efficiency of using pure oxygen due to the greater air to water surface area of the small bubbles produced. Carmichael et al. (1992) compared efficiencies of oxygen diffusers in fish-hauling tanks and reported oxygen transfer efficiencies of less than 15% for all air diffusers tested at the time. More recently, the development of micro bubble diffusers has greatly increased oxygen transfer efficiency or absorption rates to approximately 50% at 1 m depth and increasing linearly with increased water depth. Most micro bubble diffusers require 25–40 psi (172– 275 kilopascal) to operate but are susceptible to cracking at pressures > 50 psi (345 kilopascal). This limits oxygen flow rate potential (l/min) to the surface area of the diffuser so it is important to size the diffuser to the desired flow rate or carrying capacity. Also, since the oxygen flows only from one side of the diffuser it is very important to ensure the diffuser does not flip over during transport thus causing the bubbles to coalesce; this is easily accomplished by attaching a piece of rebar horizontally across the diffuser with a cable tie.

Some live hauling systems use agitation devices, circulation pumps or aeration in combination with pure oxygen injection to strip excess gas and maintain oxygen levels at or near solubility. The primary disadvantage of using agitators and circulation pumps is the heat generated from their operation increases the water temperature of the hauling tanks (0.5°C/h for aerators and 1°C/ha for pumps; Piper et al., 1982). Fries et al. (1993) evaluated aeration systems during high density (521 g/l) transport of channel catfish and reported that after 4 hours water temperatures rose from 21.5 to 23.5°C. Agitators can also cause increased foaming in water containing salt (Carmichael et al., 2001). Carmichael et al. (1992) recommended a combination of agitators and pure oxygen for high density transport of largemouth bass. The advantages of including aeration equipment include carbon dioxide stripping as well as backup in the event of a failure of the primary oxygenation system. However, the associated water temperature increase accompanying the operation of aeration devises is considered a problem for long distance transport of largemouth bass.

While using pure oxygen during transport it is very easy to supersaturate the water. Fish species vary in their ability to tolerate supersaturation of DO which can affect the mechanics and equipment needs during transport. When fish are exposed to supersaturated water the excess gas can form bubbles in various fish tissues which is referred to as gas bubble disease and can result in high mortality. Gas bubble disease can be identified by the appearance of gas bubbles or blisters on the fins and other external surfaces of fish. Bubbles frequently occur behind the cornea and in the connective tissue of the eyes, producing severe exophthalmia or "pop-eye" (Noga, 2000). Piper et al. (1982) suggested maintaining DO levels at just under saturation when transporting salmonids to prevent this condition. Much of the work on gas supersaturation and the resulting gas bubble disease has been conducted on salmonids (Weitkamp and Katz, 1980). Total gas pressure (TGP) and nitrogen (N_2) supersaturation should be maintained below 110% to avoid mortality in salmonids. Largemouth bass are more tolerant to TGP and N_2 supersaturation than salmonids and reportedly tolerate levels up to 120% of saturation (Blahm et al., 1976).

Since oxygen is assimilated metabolically it is less likely than other gases (such as nitrogen) to form persistent bubbles (Noga, 2000). Wiebe and McGavock (1932) reported no mortality in rainbow trout exposed to supersaturation of DO at 300% for 14 d or at 580% for 24 h. Wedemeyer (1996) noted that mortality from gas bubble disease normally does not occur if oxygen (using pure oxygen) supersaturation is $\leq$200%. Vanlandeghem et al. (2010) evaluated the physiological response of largemouth bass exposed to oxygen stress. The authors reported that largemouth bass acclimated to 20°C water displayed signs of physiological stress at oxygen levels of 4 mg/l (44% of saturation), however, hyperoxic conditions of 18 mg/l (200% of saturation) did not result in any changes relative to control values. It is likely that largemouth bass are well adapted to conditions of hyperoxia which occurs naturally in eutrophic waters having high amounts of photosynthetic algae often resulting in oxygen supersaturation. As a good practice, live haulers using pure oxygen should maintain 100–150% of oxygen saturation, although 200% of saturation is not likely to cause damage.

11.6.5 Carbon dioxide

Elevated carbon dioxide levels are detrimental to fish and can be a limiting factor in fish transportation. Carbon dioxide is produced as a by-product of respiration. In transport containers carbon dioxide levels slowly increase relative to the density and respiration of the fish. For each 1ml of oxygen a fish consumes approximately 0.9 ml of carbon dioxide is produced (Piper et al., 1982). Increasing levels of carbon dioxide acidifies the tank water thus lowering the pH, which reduces ammonia toxicity (Piper et al., 1982). However, elevated carbon dioxide levels also lowers the oxygen carrying capacity of the blood, further necessitating the importance to maintain DO levels at or above saturation.

Severely elevated levels of carbon dioxide can result in hypercapnia and acidosis leading to narcosis and death (Wedemeyer, 1997). Aeration or agitation are sometimes used to reduce carbon dioxide buildup, however, the friction caused by the operation of electric motors causes an increase in water temperature. Also, if the tank lids are tight fitting without ventilation carbon dioxide gas that has been stripped from the water can build up in the air space between the water and the tank cover reducing the efficiency of using aeration to remove carbon dioxide (Harmon, 2009). Some live haulers, especially long-distance haulers, will have “air stacks” that allow for gases to escape the hauling box, thus not allowing for a build-up of carbon dioxide in the airspace above the water and top of the tank.

As with all water quality parameters, different fish species have different thresholds of tolerance for carbon dioxide. Trout appear to tolerate carbon dioxide at levels less than 15.0 mg/l under the conditions of adequate DO and appropriate temperature but become distressed when carbon dioxide levels reach 25 mg/l (Piper et al., 1982). Wedemeyer (1996) recommended, as a general rule, maintaining carbon dioxide levels below 30–40 mg/l during fish transport but warned that if DO is not saturated this level might be reduced. Carmichael et al. (1984a) evaluated water quality induced stress in largemouth bass by exposing them to elevated carbon dioxide levels for 24 h and measuring their secondary stress response. The authors reported that largemouth bass tolerate moderate levels of carbon dioxide (35 mg/l) with no apparent ill effects and that very high levels of carbon dioxide (135 mg/l) altered plasma corticosteroids and glucose, but had little effect on plasma chloride and osmolality.

11.6.6 Ammonia

When fish are transported, their excretory products accumulate in the tank water. Ammonia is a highly toxic waste product produced by plants and animals and is also generated by the decomposition processes of microorganisms. Ammonia is the primary by-product of metabolic processes in fish and is mainly excreted through the gills. During conditions of live transport largemouth bass may be exposed to higher than normal concentrations of ammonia for prolonged periods. Water temperature and time of last feeding are important factors regulating ammonia excretion. Water temperature during shipping should be as low as can be tolerated by the fish being handled (Piper et al., 1982). The accumulation of ammonia can be minimized by fasting fish prior to transport. Fasting fish for at least 24 h is recommended to reduce the accumulation of feces and ammonia in the tank. Carmichael et al. (1984b) recommended to withhold food from largemouth bass for 72 h before hauling. Wedemeyer (1996) reported that when transporting salmonids a typical protocol is to fast the fish for 48–72 h prior to transport. Piper et al. (1982) noted that trout fasted for 63 h produced one-half the amount of ammonia as recently fed fish.

Suski et al. (2007) evaluated sublethal ammonia toxicity in largemouth bass acclimated to 25°C and reported that total ammonia-nitrogen (TAN) levels as low as 1.7 mg/l cause physiological disturbances that can impair the recovery from exercise. Exposure to 17 mg/l caused significant reductions in ventilation rates and increases in erratic swimming. As a rule of thumb, un-ionized ammonia concentrations should be maintained below 0.2 mg/l during transport to reduce stress.

In water, toxic ammonia (NH^3) exists in equilibrium with non-toxic dissolved ammonium ions (NH^{4+}). TAN is the total amount of nitrogen in the forms of toxic ammonia and non-toxic dissolved ammonium ions. The proportion of toxic ammonia in TAN increases as the pH and temperature of water increases. Lowering of the water temperature not only slows the metabolic activity in the fish but also directly reduces the toxicity of ammonia by decreasing the percentage of un-ionized (toxic) ammonia. Lowering the pH of the water will also reduce the percentage of un-ionized ammonia, however, this is seldom practiced. Maintaining high oxygen levels and low water temperature are the best ways to reduce ammonia toxicity during transport. Chemical agents which stabilize pH and remove ammonia are commercially available and are widely used in the transport of fish (Harmon, 2009). However, before using any chemical agent on food-fish, including small sportfish which may at some point be consumed, it is necessary to check the U.S. FDA regulatory guidelines for food-fish. Your local aquaculture extension agent is usually a good source of information for these regulations.

11.6.7 Water temperature

Maintaining water temperature during transport within a desired range is probably the second most import factor after oxygen. Controlling water temperature fluctuations is generally achieved through the use of insulated hauling tanks and the addition of ice to the transport water; however, temperature controlled box trucks and chillers are also used. Tank materials can have a large impact on maintaining temperature, particularly if the water temperature and the air temperature are very different. Most hauling tanks are made of either aluminum, fiberglass or polyurethane with an insulated layer between the inner and outer surfaces of the tank. Polyurethane has the best insulation properties of the commonly used materials (Harmon, 2009). Because temperature is such an important factor it should be continuously monitored and controlled (Piper et al., 1982).

Since fish are cold blooded, lowering water temperatures reduces metabolic activity, oxygen consumption and waste excretion and also increases the oxygen carrying capacity of water. However, when fish are exposed to lowering of water temperature, the safety margin is quite small and mortality can occur if the temperature is lowered too far or too quickly. Carmichael et al. (1984a) found that abrupt temperature change, above all other factors evaluated, caused the greatest physiological stress response in largemouth bass. Rapid water temperature changes of 12°C resulted in 20% mortality immediately and 100% mortality during subsequent handling. It is well documented that fish may initially survive temporary changes in water quality, temperature or handling but later die of disease (Wedemeyer, 1970; Lewis, 1971). Fish mortalities due to temperature shock have also been attributed to osmoregulatory dysfunction (Maetz and Evans, 1972).

Vanlandeghem et al. (2010) evaluated the physiological effects of immediate temperature shock in largemouth bass acclimated to 20°C. They reported that a large cold shock (12°C) resulted in a six-fold increase in cortisol and a doubling of glucose levels but that a small cold shock (5°C) had no effect on these parameters. Heat shock from 20 to 32°C was not as severe in terms of the cortisol increase, but did produce an increase in plasma glucose similar to that reported for largemouth bass following exhaustive exercise (Suski et al., 2006). Changes in cortisol are considered to be of particular importance because they have lethal and sublethal consequences for fish. Iversen and Eliassen (2009) reported that a 2–3-fold increase in cortisol levels in Atlantic salmon (*Salmo salar*) one hour after transport resulted in a 10-fold increase in 6 d cumulative mortality compared to fish showing no changes in cortisol.

Largemouth bass sold as food-fish are typically only transported live to market when water temperatures are between 4–18°C to reduce stress, disease outbreaks and subsequent mortality (Table 11.2). Largemouth bass marketed as sport-fish are often transported for stocking purposes as soon as the appropriate size is available from production ponds; which is typically during periods of warmer water temperatures (18–28°C) greatly reducing applicable loading densities (Table 11.1). Natural ice is often added to transport tanks to cool the water. Dry ice produced from carbon dioxide or carbonic acid should be avoided. Twenty-five kilograms of ice will cool 1,000 l of water by 2°C. If the ice used is made from chlorinated water add 7.4 mg/l sodium thiosulfate ($Na_2S_2O_3$) for every 1 mg/l chlorine for neutralization (Wedemeyer, 1996). If the water contains fish during the cooling process the temperature drop should not be faster than 4°C/h and not exceed 12°C over a 24 h period for food-size largemouth bass. As a general protocol the water temperature should not be reduced more than 1°C every 15 min.

11.6.8 Use of anesthetics

Anesthetics are chemical agents that calm animals and cause them to progressively lose their mobility, equilibrium, consciousness and finally their reflex action. Anesthetizing fish prior to transport can reduce metabolic rate and associated oxygen demand, reduce general activity, increase the ease of handling and mitigate the stress response (Coyle et al., 2004). Light anesthesia that permits fish to maintain equilibrium and swimming activity can be effective for mitigating stress associated with fish handling and fish transport (Piper et al., 1982). When using anesthetics during transportation it is important that the level of anesthesia is limited to mild sedation so that fish are not physically damaged resulting from collision with the tank walls (Cooke et al., 2004). Chemical anesthetics have been demonstrated to improve transport survival by reducing oxygen consumption and stress in largemouth bass (Carmichael et al., 1984a, 1984b; Cooke et al., 2004).

Tricaine methanesulfonate (MS-222) is the only approved anesthetic registered for use with food-fish in the USA with the condition of a 21 d withdrawal period before the fish can be sold as food. This makes MS-222 impractical for use as an anesthetic for fish en route to market. However, based on increased survival and a reduction in the measured stress response, Carmichael et al. (1984b) suggested that the most effective method for hauling subadult largemouth bass involved anesthetizing fish before capture (50 mg/l MS-222) and the use of a mild anesthetic (15 mg/l MS-222) during transport. Due to use restrictions, MS-222 can only be used for the rested harvest and transportation of broodfish or small fish that are not immediately destined for the food-fish market.

Other popular anesthetics for sedating fish are clove oil and Quinaldine which have been used as substitutes for MS-222 in the baitfish and tropical fish industries as well as for fisheries management and research procedures. Clove oil and Quinaldine both have a greater margin of safety over MS-222 and are considerably less expensive (Coyle et al., 2004). Quinaldine does not produce deep anesthesia necessary for surgical procedures where clove oil does but has a longer recovery time than either Quinaldine or MS-222. Cooke et al. (2004) reported that 60 mg/l clove oil was sufficient to produce deep anesthesia for surgical procedures in largemouth bass where 5 to 9 mg/l was effective for producing light sedation for handling and transport purposes.

Sodium bicarbonate (baking soda) when mixed with a weak acid will produce carbon dioxide gas; which has been used to produce anesthesia in fish. Durborow and Mayer (unpublished data) found that largemouth bass reached stage 2–3 anesthesia after 6 min when exposed to 0.67 g/l $NaHCO_3$ solution (30 l water, 20 g $NaHCO_3$, and 7.5 ml acetic acid) and recovered 10–15 min after being anesthetized for 1 h. The main advantage of carbon dioxide is that it is not a controlled substance in the USA and is "generally recognized as safe" (GRAS) by the FDA. This permits its use on food-fish with no withdrawal time; which at this time is the only chemical method available for use when harvesting or transporting food-fish to market.

Many factors can affect the efficacy of anesthetic treatments; therefore, experimental doses should be tested on a small group of non-critical animals before any large-scale anesthetizing is done. For environmental and human safety, the production, sale and use of chemicals is regulated by government agencies. In the USA, FDA regulates the use of chemicals on food-fish. Currently, the only chemical anesthetic approved by the FDA for use on food-fish is MS-222; it requires a 21 d withdrawal period. These regulations are subject to change and users are encouraged to check with local extension specialists regularly for new information.

11.6.9 Other chemical treatments

Chemicals designated as bactericides, bacteriostats, therapeutants, herbicides, and water conditioners are commonly used in aquaculture for routine management practices. It is well known that handling fish predisposes them to attack by various forms of bacteria and protozoans that are seemingly ubiquitous in nature (Maule et al., 1988; Davis, 2006). As a result, disease treatments are at times necessary to treat identified pathogens and sometimes prophylactically used to eliminate disease causing agents on the surface of fish prior to or following a known stressor such as harvest and transport. Prophylactic treatment is a common practice to reduce stress and the subsequent occurrence of disease to mitigate mortality and economic loss.

The use of unapproved drugs or misuse of approved drugs in aquacultured fish poses a potential human health hazard. Chemicals for use in food-fish generally must be approved or conditionally approved by the FDA. Under certain conditions a new drug may be index listed as a legally marketed unapproved new animal drug which may be used in early nonfood life stages of food-producing-species. FDA also restricts the manner in which drugs are used and provides dosage restrictions of their use. These regulations are subject to change at any time, so it is very important to continually review updates prior to using any drug in aquaculture on the FDA website (http://www.fda.gov/AnimalVeterinary/DevelopmentApprovalProcess/Aquaculture/defaul.htm).

The following review of chemicals previously used successfully as treatments for largemouth bass does not imply that they are legal for use on fish produced for either the sport or food markets.

Carmichael et al. (1984b) evaluated protocols to alleviate stress associated with live transport of juvenile largemouth bass for governmental stocking programs. The most effective method involved prophylactic treatment for disease with copper sulfate (10 mg/l) for 1 h/d for 10 consecutive days prior to hauling; anesthetizing before handling with MS-222 (50 mg/l); hauling in water containing: isosmotic salt content (8–10 g/l), a mild anesthetic (15–25 mg/l MS-222) and an antibacterial compound (3 mg/l acriflaven or 10 mg/l oxytetracycline). The post-hauling recovery tanks also contained salts similar to those in plasma by addition of sodium chloride, potassium chloride, potassium phosphate and magnesium sulfate. Post-hauling the prophylactic disease treatment of adding copper sulfate to the recovery tanks at 10 mg/l per day for 10 consecutive days was repeated. The copper sulfate treatments used in this study are greater than normally recommended, however, the alkalinity was also relatively high at 320 mg/l. These treatments reduced hauling-induced mortality to an average of 5% compared to an average mortality of 88% in fish hauled in untreated well water.

Piper et al. (1982) recommended several chemical treatments for external bacteria and parasites of warmwater fish. Diquat (37% active ingredient) has been used effectively at 8.4 to 16.8 mg/l (2–4 mg/l active cation) for columnaris and fungus control. Oxytetracycline is effective as a prolonged bath at 15–20 mg/l active ingredient for columnaris disease. Copper sulfate can be used at whatever concentration is safe in the existing water chemistry. Generally, copper sulfate is safe at 1 mg/l for every 100 mg/l of total alkalinity (that is, if the total alkalinity is 50 mg/l than only 0.5 mg/l of copper sulfate should be used). Potassium permanganate is effective at 2 mg/l in clear water with little organic load; if the color changes in less than one hour it may be necessary to repeat the treatment. Formalin is effective at 125–250 mg/l for 1 h or 15–25 mg/l indefinitely for control of protozoan diseases. More recently Florfenicol, Chloramine-T and hydrogen peroxide have been evaluated to control mortality caused by columnaris (Bowker et al., 2013; Mathews et al., 2013).

Water conditioners are sometimes used during fish transport to aid in osmoregulation, stabilize pH, remove ammonia, as anti-foaming agents or as probiotics to inhibit the growth of pathogenic micorganisms. For example, the hardness and alkalinity of the water is an important consideration during live fish transport. Alkalinity should be ≥100 mg/l to stabilize pH and can be increased by addition of baking soda. Ideally the calcium concentration should be ≥100 mg/l for holding and transporting fish to enable the fish to maintain osmotic balance (Grizzle et al., 1985). The use of calcium chloride in low calcium water is an inexpensive means of improving success in fish handling and transportation. Potassium chloride can also be used as an aid in osmoregulation to relieve stress and prevent shock (Carmichael et al., 1984a).

11.6.10 Vitamin C

Vitamin C (ascorbic acid; AA) is essential in the immune responses in fish and is necessary for wound repair (Navarre and Halver, 1989). One of the physiological alterations that occur due to stress is the rapid depletion of interrenal ascorbic acid (Wedemeyer and Yasutake, 1977). Vitamin C deficiency signs are often related to hyperplasia of support cartilage in the gills, spines and fins (Klontz, 1995); which is often observed in largemouth bass after transport when held in retail display tanks for 7–10 d. Since vitamin C is depleted during the initial stress associated with harvest and transport, it is therefore in short supply for normal physiological functions during the live holding period prior to sale.

Halver (Halver et al., 1969, Halver, 2002) suggested that when fish are exposed to stress or are inflicted with muscular wounds, the ascorbic acid requirement would double or triple to aid in physiological stress mechanisms and wound repair. Inadequate dietary vitamin C levels have also been attributed to reduced resistance to bacterial disease (Lovell, 1989). In many cases, physical handling of largemouth bass particularly in warmwater is followed within 2–3 d by a severe episode of a systemic bacterial or viral disease. Given the importance of vitamin C in the stress response of fish, providing a mega dose to largemouth bass just prior to harvest may help alleviate the effects of stress associate with harvest and transport. The protective effect of vitamin C on the innate stress response is an area of research that should be investigated.

11.7 Acclimation

By the time largemouth bass food-fish reach the retail market, they have gone through more than three adjustments in physical and chemical environmental conditions related to pond harvest, holding tanks, transport, and retail display tanks. Fish can become stressed if not acclimated properly to the conditions of the receiving tank. This can be a crucial step in successful delivery as the fish have already been exposed to a series of stressors and stress is known to be cumulative; poor acclimation will likely result in immunosuppressed fish, possibly leading to delayed mortality (Harmon, 2009). Abrupt changes in water quality variables such as temperature, pH, hardness, and salinity should be avoided. If the gradient differential between these parameters is too great the fish should be slowly acclimated to receiving waters to reduce stress. It may be necessary to adjust the receiving water to match as closely as possible the conditions during transport if there is known to be great variation. For example, when holding live bass in retail display tanks for sale it may be preferable to ice the holding tanks down to match the conditions of the hauling tank and let the fish slowly acclimate up to ambient temperature.

Timmons et al. (2002), in a general statement, recommended that temperature change should not exceed 5.5°C in 20 min and if the pH differs by more than one unit to exchange 10% of the tank water every 10–20 min with the receiving water until it is similar. Fish species are known to vary greatly in their tolerance to abrupt changes in water chemistry. Most fish seem to tolerate a rapid decrease in temperature better than an increase in temperature of similar magnitude (Noga, 2000). Salmonids are reported to tolerate a 10°C change in water temperature with only mild stress provided that the fish are healthy and all other parameters are optimal (Wedemeyer, 1996). Carmichael et al. (1984b) reported that following an abrupt 12°C increase in temperature, from 10 to 22°C, 20% of largemouth bass died immediately followed by subsequent 100% mortality of the group following sampling. However, the authors reported that a rapid 6°C change resulted in no mortality and no significant changes in plasma values of corticosteroids, glucose, chloride and osmolality. Because of each unique situation (number of stressors, duration, fish health and so on) even the same species can have various outcomes to acclimation. One has to be practical, but cautious at the same time.

As a general protocol, water temperature change should be limited to 4°C/h and not more than 12°C over 24 h. Even within this recommendation it is preferable to change the water temperature slowly (1°C/15 min) to allow the body of the fish time to acclimate. One thing to consider is that as cold-blooded animals the body temperature of the fish must equilibrate to that of the water environment. Owing to a greater body mass, larger fish may take longer to physically acclimate to changes in water temperature than smaller fish.

Carmichael (1984) described five separate long distance (> 30 h) shipments of largemouth bass fingerlings and made several important observations. The conditions during transport were similar with water temperatures 15–18°C and the addition of 3.8–5 g/l salt. The first two shipments were successful with little mortality; however, fish began dying soon after arrival and mortality peaked 3 to 4 d after shipment with few survivors after 2 weeks of holding in tanks (13 and 2.5% survival). The third lot of fish were significantly larger than the previous shipments (20.3 cm compared to 12.7 cm). This resulted in better survival (55%). Owing to the sequence of unsuccessful stockings, the fourth shipment was tracked by taking blood samples from fish before, during and following transport. Results indicated that plasma corticosteroids and plasma glucose remained high for 24 h and that plasma chloride levels did not return to normal levels until 64 h after transport. Long periods of time (more than 64 h) appear necessary for largemouth bass to fully recover from hauling stress. When the fish are not permitted to recover completely a second, normally nonfatal, stressful occurrence, might now be fatal. Carmichael (1984) recommended following transport that the receiving waters should also contain 3–5 g/l salt to help alleviate transport induced osmoregulatory imbalance. This is not always practical and achievable, however, if it is possible it should be practiced.

11.8 Legal considerations of transport

Restrictive regulations are necessary to protect the interests and safety of humans and the environment. Aquaculture is regulated at various levels of government in the USA. Regulations vary greatly from state-to-state and there is no central source where all such regulations are available. Within the states, local laws may be different in certain municipalities or geographical areas. Additionally, the agencies responsible for aquaculture regulation vary widely between states creating a perplexing combination of regulations with little or no consistency (Rumley, 2012). Different federal agencies are responsible for particular areas of aquaculture regulation: the FDA regulates food safety, the Environmental Protection Agency (EPA) regulates pollution and water discharge and the Fish and Wildlife Service (FWS) regulates injurious wildlife and the Lacey Act. Of particular interest to fish transportation is the Lacey Act.

The Lacey Act is a federal statute regulating the importation and interstate transport of wildlife in the USA with special emphasis on wildlife determined to be injurious and/or endangered species. The original intent of the Lacey Act was to prevent poaching and the illegal commercial trade in wildlife by making interstate commerce of illegally taken wildlife a federal violation, thus removing jurisdictional boundaries for prosecution and levying harsher penalties than imposed by the individual states. Currently, commercially produced aquatic animals legally owned by private fish farmers are considered "wildlife" by FDA and interstate transportation is regulated under the Lacey Act. Since state laws differ greatly regarding species which are considered injurious, this creates a situation where a farmer transporting a legal species in one state into another where they are illegal, can be in violation of federal regulations under the Lacey Act.

Concern over the establishment of nonindigenous species into areas outside of their native range has increased over time leading to increased enforcement and scrutiny over their movement from state to state as well as within specific geographical regions within states. This is further complicated due to the potential for accidental contamination of a load of fish by a species considered indigenous or established in one region and then transported into another region where that species is regulated as nonindigenous and may be listed as injurious.

Regulatory complexity and a lack of clarity in state regulations for interstate transport of fish greatly increases the legal risks associated with transporting largemouth bass to distant markets.

Since largemouth bass are popular as both food-fish and sport-fish, they are commercially shipped live to virtually all states across the continental USA. As a result, farms producing largemouth bass are heavily impacted by regulations related to transporting live fish into the states where their buyers are located as well as through states en route to end markets. Most small and medium sized largemouth bass food-fish producers rely on independent live haulers to transport their product to distant markets. Thus, shifting the responsibility of regulation compliance to the live haulers which act as middleman usually supplying several independent grocery stores in one or more cities. Sport-fish producers are more likely to deliver small quantities of live fish regionally to other farms and to stock private ponds and lakes.

Extreme care when loading fish for transport is necessary to prevent accidental contamination of a load of fish which may result in a Lacey Act violation. The risks associated with the Lacey Act can be minimized by shipping only in-state; however, this may not be feasible for some businesses. Producers involved in interstate transport should know the risks and take steps to mitigate them by having proper documentation for each load and by exercising due care in ensuring compliance with the laws of all states that the shipment passes through.

References

Barton, B.A. and Iwama, G.K. (1991) Physiological changes in fish from stress in aquaculture with emphasis on the response and effects of corticosteroids. *Annual Review of Fish Diseases* 1, 3–26.

Blahm, T.H., McConnell, B. and Snyder, G.R. (1976) Gas supersaturation research. In: Fickeisen, D.H., and Schneider, M.J. (eds) *Gas Bubble Disease*. Technical Information Center, Energy Research and Development Administration, Oak Ridge, TN, pp. 11–19.

Bowker, J.D., Carty, D., Trushenski, J.T., Bowman, M.P., Wandalear, N. and Matthews, M. (2013) Controlling mortality caused by external columnaris in largemouth bass and bluegill with chloramine-T or hydrogen peroxide. *North American Journal of Aquaculture* 75, 342–351.

Brandt, T.M., Jones Jr., R.M. and Koke, J.R. (1986) Corneal cloudiness in transported largemouth bass. *The Progressive Fish Culturist* 48, 199–201.

Carmichael, G.J. (1984) Long distance truck transport of intensively reared largemouth bass. *Progressive Fish-Culturist* 46, 111–115.

Carmichael, G.J. and Tomasso, J.R. (1988) Communications: Survey of fish transportation equipment and techniques. *The Progressive Fish Culturist* 50, 155–159.

Carmichael, G.J., Tomasso, J.R., Simco, B.A. and Davis, K.B. (1984a) Confinement and water quality-induced stress in largemouth bass. *Transactions of the American Fisheries Society* 113, 767–777.

Carmichael, G.J., Tomasso, J.R., Simco, B.A. and Davis, K.B. (1984b) Characterization and alleviation of stress associated with hauling largemouth bass. *Transactions of the American Fisheries Society* 113, 778–785.

Carmichael, G.J., Jones, R.M. and Morrow, J.C. (1992) Comparative efficacy of oxygen diffusers in a fish-hauling tank. *The Progressive Fish Culturist* 54, 35–40.

Carmichael, G.J., Tomasso, J.R. and Schwelder, T.E. (2001) Fish transportation. In: Wedemeyer G.A. (ed.) *Fish Hatchery Management.* American Fisheries Society, Bethesda, MD, pp. 641–660.

Colt, J. (2006) Water quality requirements for reuse systems. *Aquacultural Engineering* 34:143–156.

Cooke, S.J., Suski, C.D., Ostrand, K.G., Tufts, B.L. and Wahl, D.H. (2004) Behavioral and physiological assessment of low concentrations of clove oil anaesthetic for handling and transporting largemouth bass (*Micropterus salmoides*). *Aquaculture* 239, 509–529.

Coyle, S.D., Durborow, R.M. and Tidwell, J.H. (2004) Anesthetics in Aquaculture. Southern Regional Aquaculture Center. Publication Number 3900, Stoneville, MS.

Currie, R.J., Bennet, W.A. and Beitinger, T.L. (1998) Critical thermal minima and maxima of three freshwater game-fish species acclimated to constant temperatures. *Environmental Biology of Fishes* 51, 187–200.

Davis, K.B. (2006) Management of physiological stress in finfish aquaculture. *North American Journal of Aquaculture* 68, 116–121.

Febry, R. and Lutz, P. (1987) Energy partitioning in fish: the activity related cost of osmoregulation in a euryhaline cichlid. *Journal of Experimental Biology* 128, 63–85.

Francis-Floyd, R. (2002) Stress – Its Role in Fish Disease. University of Florida IFAS Extension circular 919, University of Florida, Gainsville, FL.

Fries, J.N., Berkhouse, C.S., Morrow, J.C. and Carmichael, G.J. (1993) Evaluation of an aeration system in a loaded fish-hauling tank. *The Progressive Fish Culturist* 55, 187–190.

Grizzle, J.M., Mauldin II, A.C., Young, D. and Henderson, E. (1985) Survival of juvenile striped bass (*Morone saxatilis*) and *Morone* hybrid bass (*Morone chrysops* and *M. saxatilis*) increased by addition of calcium to soft water. *Aquaculture* 46, 167–171.

Halver, J.E. (2002) The vitamins. In: Halver, J.E. and Hardy, R.W. (eds) *Fish Nutrition*, third edition, Academic Press, San Diego, California, pp. 61–141.

Halver, J.E., Ashley, L.M. and Smith, R.R. (1969) Ascorbic acid requirement of coho salmon and rainbow trout. *Transactions of the American Fisheries Society* 98, 762–771.

Harmon, T.S. (2009) Methods for reducing stressors and maintaining water quality associated with live fish transport in tanks: a review of the basics. *Reviews in Aquaculture* 1, 58–66.

Harvey, H.H. (1975) Gas disease in fishes-a review. In: Adams, W.A. (ed.) *Chemistry and Physics of Aqueous Gas Solutions.* The Electrochemical Society, Princeton, NJ, pp. 450–485.

Iversen, M. and Eliassen, R.A. (2009) The effects of AQUI-S sedation on primary, secondary, and tertiary stress responses during salmon smolt, *Salmo salar* L., transport and transfer to sea. *Journal of the World Aquaculture Society* 40, 216–225.

Jensen, G.L. and Brunson, M.W. (1992) Harvesting warmwater fish. Southern Regional Aquaculture Center. Publication Number 394, Stoneville, MS.

Jia, B., St-Hilaire, S., Styhn, H., Yu, J., Groman, D.B. and Gardner, I.A. (2016) Analysis of transaction records of live freshwater finfish in China: a case study of customers' claims of fish mortality using cross-classified modeling. *Aquaculture Reports* 4, 150–155.

Karnaky, K.J. (1997) Osmotic and ionic regulation. In: Evans, D.H. (ed.) *The Physiology of Fishes*, second edition. CRC Press, Boca Raton, FL, pp. 157–176.

Klontz, G.W. (1995) Care of fish in biological research. *Journal of Animal Science* 73, 3485–3492.

Lewis, S.D. (1971) The effect of salt solutions on osmotic changes associated with surface damage to the golden shiner, *Notemigonus crysoleucas. Dissertation Abstracts, B, Sciences and Engineering* 31, 6346.

Lovell, T. (1989) *Nutrition and Feeding of Fish*. Van Nostrand Reinhold, New York.

Maetz, J. and Evans, D.H. (1972) Effects of temperature on branchial sodium-exchange and extrusion mechanisms in the seawater-adapted flounder, *Platichthys flesus* L. *Journal of Experimental Biology* 56, 565–582.

Matthews, M.D., Bowker, J.D., Carty, D.G., Wandfelear, N., Bowman, M.P. and Sakmar, J.C. (2013) Efficacy of Aquaflor (50% Florfenicol)-medicated feed to control mortality associated with *Flavobacterium columnare* infection in Florida largemouth bass and bluegill. *North American Journal of Aquaculture* 75, 329–454

Matthews, M.D., Prangnell, D. and Glenewinkel, H. (2017) Sensitivity of Guadalupe Bass swim-up fry to hyperoxia. *North American Journal of Aquaculture* 79:289–298.

Maule, A.G., Schreck, C.B., Bradford, C.S. and Barton, B.A. (1988) Physiological effects of collecting and transporting emigrating juvenile Chinook salmon past dams on the Colombia River. *Transactions of the American Fisheries Society* 117, 245–261.

Mazeaud, M.M., Mazeaud, F. and Donaldson, E.M. (1977) Primary and secondary effects of stress in fish: some new data with a general review. *Transactions of the American Fisheries Society* 106, 201–212.

McCraren, J.P. and Millard, J.L. (1978) Transportation of warmwater fishes. In: *Manual of Fish Culture.* U.S. Fish and Wildlife Service, Washington, DC, pp. 43–88.

McDonald, G. and Milligan, L. (1997) Ionic, osmotic and acid-base regulation in stress. In: Iwama G.W., Pickering A.D., Sumpter J.P., and Schreck C.B. (eds) *Fish Stress and Health in Aquaculture*, Cambridge University Press, New York, pp. 119–144.

Moyle, P.B. and Cech Jr., J.J. (1988) *Fishes: An Introduction to Ichthyology*. Prentice Hall, Englewood Cliffs, NJ.

Navarre, O. and Halver, J.E. (1989) Disease resistance and humoral antibody production in rainbow trout fed high levels of vitamin C. *Aquaculture* 79, 207–221.

Noga, E.J. (2000) *Fish Disease: Diagnosis and Treatment.* Iowa State University Press, Ames, IA.

Piper, R.G., McElwain, I.B., Orme, L.E., McCraren, J.P., Fowler, L.G. and Leonard, J.R. (1982) Fish Hatchery Management. American Fisheries Society, Bethesda, MD.

Portz, D.E., Woodley, C.M. and Cech, J.J. (2006) Stress-associated impacts of short-term holding on fishes. *Reviews in Fish Biology and Fisheries* 16, 125–170.

Reubush, K.J. and Heath, A.G. (1997) Effects of recovery water salinity on secondary stress responses of hybrid striped bass fingerlings. *The Progressive Fish Culturist* 59, 188–197.

Rumley, E.R. (2012) Aquaculture and the Lacey Act. Southern Regional Aquaculture Center. Publication Number 5005, Stoneville, MS.

Schwalme, K. and MacKay, W.C. (1991) Mechanisms that elevate the glucose concentration of muscle and liver in yellow perch (*Perca flavescens* Mitchill) after exercise-handling stress. *Canadian Journal of Zoology* 69, 456–461.

Sifa, L., Chenhong, L., Dey, M. and Dunham, R. (1999) Seinability of four strains of Nile tilapia, *Oreochromis niloticus*, in Chinese ponds. *Aquaculture* 174(3–4), 223–227.

Steeby, J.A. and Lovshin, L.L. (1993) Comparison of seines equipped with rubber roller or gathered-netting mud lines for harvesting channel catfish in earthen ponds. *The Progressive Fish-Culturist* 55 (2), 133–136.

Suski, C.D., Killen, S.S., Kieffer, J.D. and Tufts, B.L. (2006) The influence of environmental temperature and oxygen concentration on the recovery of largemouth bass from exercise: implications for live-release angling tournaments. *Journal of Fish Biology* 68, 120–136.

Suski, C.D., Kieffer, J.D., Killen, S.S. and Tufts, B.L. (2007) Sub-lethal ammonia toxicity in largemouth bass, *Comparative Biochemistry and Physiology* Part A 146, 381–389.

Susanto, G.N. and Peterson, M.S. (1996) Survival, osmoregulation and oxygen consumption of YOY costal largemouth bass, *Micropterus salmoides* (Lacépède) exposed to saline media. *Hydrobiologia* 323 (2), 119–127.

Timmons, M.B., Ebling, J.M., Wheaton, F.W., Summerfelt, S.T. and Vinci, B.J. (2002) *Recirculating Aquaculture Systems*. Cayuga Aqua Adventures, Ithaca, NY.

Tomasso, J.R., Davis, K.B. and Parker, N.C. (1980) Plasma corticosteroid and electrolyte dynamics of hybrid striped bass (white bass × striped bass) during netting and hauling. *Proceedings of the World Mariculture Society* 11, 303–310.

Vanlandeghem, M.M., Wahl, D.H. and Suski, C.D. (2010) Physiological responses of largemouth bass to acute temperature and oxygen stressors. *Fisheries Management and Ecology* 17, 414–425.

Wedemeyer, G.A. (1970) The role of stress in the disease resistance of fishes. *American Fisheries Society Special Publication* 5, 30–35.

Wedemeyer, G.A. and Yasutake, W.T. (1977) Clinical methods for the assessment of the effects of environmental stress on fish health. Technical paper no. 89, U.S. Fish and Wildlife Service, U.S. Department of the Interior, Washington, DC.

Wedemeyer, G.A. (1996) *Physiology of Intensive Culture Systems*. Chapman and Hall, New York.

Wedemeyer, G.A. (1997) Effects of rearing conditions on the health and physiological quality of fish in intensive culture. In: Iwama, G.W., Pickering, A.D., Sumpter, J.P. and Schreck, C.B. (eds) *Fish Stress and Health in Aquaculture*. Cambridge University Press, New York, pp. 119–144.

Weirich, C.R. and Tomasso, J.R. (1991) Confinement- and transport-induced stress on red drum juveniles: effect of salinity. *The Progressive Fish-Culturist* 53, 146–149.

Weirich, C.R., Tomasso, J.R. and Smith, T.I. (1992) Confinement and transport-induced stress in white bass *Morone chrysops* × striped bass *M. saxatilis* hybrids: effects of calcium and salinity. *Journal of the World Aquaculture Society* 23, 49–57.

Weitkamp, D.E. and Katz, M. (1980) A review of dissolved gas supersaturation literature. *Transactions of the American Fisheries Society* 109, 659–702.

Wiebe, A.H. and McGavock, A.M. (1932) The ability of several species of fish to survive on prolonged exposure to abnormally high concentrations of dissolved oxygen. *Transactions of the American Fisheries Society* 62, 267–274.

Williamson, J.H. and Carmichael, G.J. (1986) Differential response to handling stress by Florida, northern, and hybrid largemouth bass. *Transactions of the American Fisheries Society* 115 (5), 756–761.

Wilson, A.J. (1950) Distribution units for warm-water fish. *The Progressive Fish-Culturist* 12 (4), 211–213.

Yeager, D.M., Van Tassel, J.E. and Wooley, C.M. (1990) Collection, transportation, and handling of striped bass brood stock. In: Harrell R.M., Kerby, J.H. and Minton, R.V. (eds) *Culture and Propagation of Striped Bass and its Hybrids*. American Fisheries Society, Bethesda, MD, pp. 39–42.

CHAPTER 12

Major markets for largemouth bass

Angela Caporelli

Kentucky Department of Agriculture, Frankfort, Kentucky, USA

12.1 Introduction

The largemouth bass (*Micropterus salmoides*) is a difficult species to secure hard data on in terms of both production statistics, and market scope and characteristics. A number of US states have not allowed the raising or the selling of largemouth bass into the live food markets. It has been considered by many a sport-fish only species, coveted and protected by trophy anglers and sport angler's clubs. It is one of the most popular freshwater fish in North America due to both its wide distribution and reputation as a tough and entertaining fighter (Figure 12.1). As a farmed species, the largemouth bass is one of the highest value freshwater aquaculture species. Competing markets for both sport-fish stocking and as a food-fish help maintain a high selling price.

Largemouth bass are produced by private hatcheries to supply recreational sport-fish stocking throughout much of North America as well as parts of Europe and Asia. In fact, the world record largemouth bass was caught in Japan in 2009 weighing in at 10.12 kg. Market demand for largemouth bass as a sport-fish encompasses all sizes from small fingerlings to trophy-size fish. Millions of largemouth bass fingerlings are also produced by federal and state public hatcheries

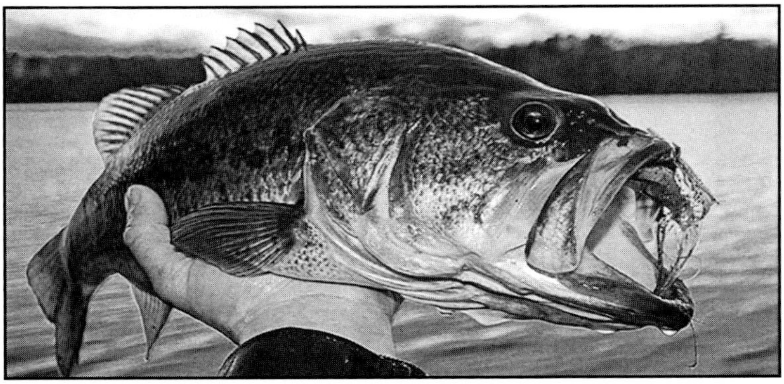

Figure 12.1 The largemouth bass as a sport-fish.

throughout the USA to meet the demand for recreational use. In the USA, largemouth bass are also produced as food-fish, which are primarily marketed live in major cities with large ethnic Asian populations. In Mexico, largemouth bass are raised and sold fresh-on-ice in certain regions. In China, the species is highly regarded and their production and marketing there are covered in Chapter 3. In the USA, the food-fish market is typically for 0.45–0.90 kg fish with a desired minimum market size of 0.6 kg.

Since the 1970s, there has been market research conducted on both wild caught and farmed fish. These studies have involved both academia and private research entities. The information generated on composition, pricing, and delivery has helped several sectors of the aquaculture industry expand. However, little market related research has been conducted on largemouth bass marketing opportunities to help guide the development of the industry.

Largemouth bass has an optimal growing temperature of 24–28°C. This environmental factor largely defines the geographic regions suitable for production. However, optimal production areas are not always within economical driving distances to the available live food-fish markets or recreational waters for stocking. This marketing consideration is one of several factors affecting the decision to produce them and can have a large impact on farm profitability.

12.2 Sport-fish market

The largemouth bass was scientifically described in 1802 by Lacépède and were harvested commercially and recreationally as a food-fish without oversight until 1871, when the U.S. Fish Commission was created. The Commission sanctioned fish stocking programs by the US government and by 1900, largemouth bass had been stocked far outside of their native range including 26 states and several other countries.

Largemouth bass fingerlings have been produced by state and federal hatcheries since the 1890s (Lydell, 1903; Turner and Kraatz, 1920). Today, state fish hatcheries stock tens of millions of largemouth bass fingerlings into public waters to support the recreational demand. The Texas Parks and Wildlife Department (TPWD) alone reportedly stocks 6 to 8 million largemouth bass in lakes across Texas in a typical year.

Before the 1960s, hatcheries primarily relied solely on live feeds. Unlike channel catfish (*Ictalurus punctatus*) and rainbow trout (*Oncorhynchus mykiss*), newly hatched largemouth bass fry (swim-up stage) cannot be easily trained to accept prepared diets (Brandt et al., 1987; Williamson et al., 1993). Therefore, bass fry is usually raised in fertilized nursery ponds until they reach 25–50 mm TL (1–2 g). These small fingerlings are either sold directly following the nursery phase (untrained) or are habituated to feed on commercially available dry fish-feed (Tidwell et al., 2000). Feed-training increases their value by approximately 30% (Engle and Southworth, 2008). Almost all larger sizes are produced using "feed-trained" fingerlings as it is much more cost effective than using forage fish to support growth (Engle and Southworth, 2008).

The popularity of largemouth bass as a sport-fish in the USA led to the establishment of the Bass Anglers Sportsman Society (BASS) in 1968. They and other clubs persuaded state fish and wildlife agencies to not allow the farming or sale of largemouth bass as a food-fish in several states. These clubs feared that if allowed, there would be fishing, whether legal or not, in public waters and that "trophy" fish would be sold in the market. This was supported by the estimated value of privately produced fish in 1983 at US$393 million compared to the US$17.3 billion sport-fishing industry which increased to US$28.2 billion by 1985 (personal communication, BASS).

Angler clubs have tripled in number since 1980 and fishing clubs in high schools have increased five times since then. Adding to the public awareness of largemouth bass, professional bass and club tournaments are now widely televised. While this has tended to inhibit the growth of food-fish production, it has likely increased the demand for largemouth bass to stock private and public lakes and ponds. In conversations with several live haulers, it is estimated that the demand for largemouth bass for stocking in sport-fish applications increased by 200% between 2000 and 2017 and suggests that the market continues to grow. They also estimate that demand for large (0.5 to 1.0 kg) largemouth bass for sport-fish stocking will double by 2025 (personal communication, Adam Hatter, Ohio, 2018).

Largemouth bass fingerlings are typically sold into the sport-fish market according to their approximate length. For example, common sizes are 2.5–5 cm (1–2"), 5–10 cm (2–4"), 10–15 cm (4–6"), 15–20 cm (6–8") and 20–25 cm (8–10"). Sizes larger than 25 cm are typically sold by weight. Many sport-fish suppliers purchase adult largemouth bass from food-fish producers. The retail price of largemouth bass sold as sport-fish is typically much higher (~100%) than the wholesale price received for food-fish.

Private hatcheries primarily sell largemouth bass to landowners wishing to enhance recreational opportunities on their lands and increasingly into managed trophy fisheries and pay lake operations. Some state agencies also contract live fish purchases through private producers in addition to or instead of public hatcheries. The actual scale of commercial sales into the sport-fish market is difficult to quantify due to the inherent problems of knowing the ultimate use of a fish, which may be sold multiple times before reaching the end user. However, the number of small largemouth bass fingerlings produced by private hatcheries for recreational purposes is very small compared to the millions produced by state and federal hatcheries for stocking into public and private waters in the USA.

The United States Department of Agriculture (USDA) periodically conducts a Census of Aquaculture in the USA. They have published data sets for 2005 and 2013 (USDA, 2014). Between 2005 and 2013 the total sales of sport-fish increased 32%. In 2013, total sales of sport-fish in the US was US$23,849,000. Of that, US$14,452,000 was generated by largemouth bass, representing 61% of total sport-fish sales. Small fingerlings or fry were raised on 66 farms and 1,964,000 small fingerlings or fry were produced. Average sizes and prices were not reported. Stocker size fingerlings were produced on 52 farms. Sales were 1,122,000 fish with an average weight of 272 g. They generated US$1,868,000 and averaged a selling price of US$10/kg.

12.3 Food-fish market

Largemouth bass has long been prized for not only their recreational but also their culinary qualities. Long et al. (2015) gave a historical perspective of black bass management in the USA. In this article, the authors provide historical reference to the overexploitation of the fishery in the 1800s and the rebuilding efforts that followed. Perhaps the first reference to the food-fish market is from an excerpt from the magazine *Forest and Stream*, which indicated that largemouth bass from Virginia were selling for 18 cents at fish markets in 1875 (Anonymous, 1875). Shortly after, it was reported in the *New York Times* that lakes in Pennsylvania were being "depopulated of its fish" by those wishing to "fill his boat" through the use of dynamite (Anonymous, 1884). The food-fish market for largemouth bass has changed dramatically over the years both in the manner of which they are obtained and the ethnicity of the consumer groups.

State laws differ widely in the USA in their approaches and statutes to protect and regulate fish and wildlife resources. This can have dramatic effects on the market factors for aquacultured species which can also be considered sport-fish. For example, in Mississippi it is illegal to sell sport-fish, including largemouth bass, as a food-fish. Producers are only permitted to sell small fingerlings. However, Mississippi has the largest pond-based aquaculture infrastructure in the USA. The ponds were constructed for channel catfish production, but that industry has contracted approximately 40% in recent years leaving substantial pond acreage unused. Should future state legislation allow Mississippi farmers to produce largemouth bass for sale as food, the scale and pricing structure of largemouth bass production in the USA could change dramatically.

State fish and wildlife agencies' concerns regarding the sale of largemouth bass for food are based on an assumption that anglers would attempt to harvest fish illegally for black market sales. However, as recently as 2013, New York State legislation took effect permitting the sale of largemouth bass as food-fish. The legislation requires that individual farms obtain a permit from the New York State Department of Environmental Conservation and that the seller must provide a bill of sale to the purchaser and retain a copy of the same. The seller must also provide the purchaser a fish health inspection report certifying the fish to be disease free. The shipping container must also be marked "black bass". Sellers must retain copies of their purchase and sales records for 2 years and sellers (the fish market) are required to kill the fish before transferring possession to the final customer. With this change in regulations, New York City had been the largest market for largemouth bass food-fish in North America. This demonstrates the dramatic effect that state legislation can have on the market potential and growth of the aquaculture industry.

From roughly 2005 to 2016, Toronto, Canada was the largest outlet for US farm-raised largemouth bass sold as food-fish. In recent years, fewer largemouth bass have been sold into Canada (personal communication, Charlie Conklin, Idaho, 2018). Part of this was due to changes in currency exchange rates. Largemouth bass are the most expensive commercially available cultured freshwater fish. When the exchange rate is above 1.2 (US$1 equals CAN$1.2) Canadian buyers often chose to purchase cheaper alternatives, such as tilapia and carp species. Between 2014 and 2018 the exchange rate increased from 1.0 to 1.33. It is quite fortunate that the New York market was opening up, and distribution channels were developing, just as the Canadian market constricted. This created a situation where regulation change in New York essentially provided a safety net for US largemouth bass producers. The fickle and complex nature of the market for live fish, and for largemouth bass in particular, necessitates that producers develop good relationships and maintain open lines of communication with their buyers and regulators so they can quickly adapt to the changing environment.

The food-fish market for largemouth bass is somewhat unique in that the fish are typically marketed live to the consumer. This requires that the physiological condition of the fish be sufficient to tolerate the steps from harvest to marketing, including holding in retail display tanks over a period of several days to weeks. For other fishes, such as channel catfish (*Ictalurus punctatus*) and rainbow trout (*Oncorhynchus mykiss*), harvest and transport procedures are based only on live delivery to a processing plant, which is usually in relatively close proximity. At the time of the writing of this chapter, there were no known commercial processing of largemouth bass in the USA. Since largemouth bass are marketed live, they should be thought of as a perishable product with a shelf life similar to that of produce. As with produce, the clock starts at the time of harvest and even when maintained under optimal conditions the product quality can slowly deteriorate over time. This situation requires that stress be minimized at every step from harvest to retail sale.

The largemouth bass is a somewhat stress sensitive species with a limited ability to tolerate net confinement, temperature change, periods of low oxygen, or of high ammonia concentrations (Williamson and Carmichael, 1986). Harvesting requires special considerations to limit unhealthy fish being sent to market and subsequent stress associated mortality. As poikilothermic animals, water temperature and temperature change have great effects on the physiological stress response in fishes. Largemouth bass may not tolerate rapid changes in water temperature as well as other aquaculture species such as channel catfish or rainbow trout (Currie et al., 1998). However, the overall stress response of handling is reduced at lower water temperatures.

During the summer months, largemouth bass are typically not harvested for food-fish sales due to increased stress and subsequent mortality. Harvest at high water temperatures likely produces an elevated stress response, followed by disease outbreaks. High mortality is usually seen a few days after delivery to market, resulting in financial losses for the buyers. This is of great economic importance to the customer (retail grocer) as the market value of a dead fish on ice is less than 20% of the live value of the same fish in ethnic Asian markets. Some producers cool ponds using ground water or spring water to access live markets during the summer months but at this time accounts for a small percentage of total sales. Producers primarily market their fish only when pond water temperatures have stabilized for a couple of weeks below 18°C.

The USDA 2013 Aquaculture Census does not list the largemouth bass being produced under its food-fish category. It only lists them under sport-fish production. However, it does have a largemouth bass size category under sport-fish of food-size or market sized. It is safe to assume that most of those fish are not going to be stocked but are actually going to market as a food-fish. The census lists 60 farms raising 1,664,000 food-size largemouth bass, producing a total weight of 975,455 kg. The average individual weight was 590 g. With an average selling price of US$11.70/kg, they generated US$11,424,000. That is six times the income generated for stocker largemouth bass.

Over the past 20 years, the average price paid by live haulers for live largemouth bass picked up at the farm has remained relatively stable at US$8.80–13.20/kg (personal communication, Robert Mayer, Kentucky, 2017). This suggests that, at this time, supply has not surpassed demand. However, the temperature constrained period for sale and distribution creates a temporary oversupply at the beginning of fall harvest season as producers attempt to reduce pond holdings before the onset of the coldest months of winter. This generally results in a lower price during late fall and early winter. Some producers hold inventory and wait for the price to increase and stabilize, typically around mid-December. This may require that they harvest ponds during ice cover. The vast majority of food-size largemouth bass are sold into the ethnic Asian markets during the months of January and February as they are very popular for use in the traditional Chinese style steamed fish, especially during Chinese New Year celebrations which last for 15 days. Largemouth bass, called "mang cho" in Cantonese, are considered a sign of wealth and prosperity, which promotes continued good fortune into the coming year. If producers still have a significant inventory of fish, a temporary price drop can occur again in spring as water temperatures increase.

Most producers of food-fish largemouth bass sell to specialty live haulers that distribute live fish to Asian markets. Live haulers generally prefer the fish to be harvested a couple of days ahead of time and "to harden" in tanks prior to over the road transport. This holding period allows the fish time to purge and recover from the stressors of pond harvest. It also gives the producer an opportunity to inspect the fish for disease signs and be sure that the number of fish contracted for purchase will be available when the live hauler arrives. When fish are held in tanks prior to transport it is also much easier to grade out undersized fish.

Ethnic Chinese customers place a high priority on healthy fish at the point of sale (Jia et al., 2016). Fish quality is generally visually determined by the consumer with main criteria being clear eyes, bright shiny scales, and vibrant red gills. Weakened individual fish with signs of disease or parasites should be eliminated from the lot. When fish are of poor quality, even reducing biomass densities may not prevent mortality during transport. It is the responsibility of the live hauler to accept or reject a batch of fish before they are loaded for shipment. However, a poor reputation gained from selling undersize or sick fish will ultimately reside with the farm from which they originated.

The size of the fish is an important factor. The live market for food-fish in the USA currently requires largemouth bass to be a minimum size of 0.6 kg. However, because of inherent size variability the average individual weight of the population has to be > 0.6 kg to ensure that the smaller fish in the group also achieve the minimum acceptable weight. If a significant number of fish are undersize (> 5%), the producer should grade and remove the submarket size fish from the lot in order to maintain a high level of quality. Undersized fish can either be restocked for another year of growth or marketed for sport-fish pond stocking. It is important to communicate with the buyer regarding the acceptable percentage of submarket fish. Sometimes the seller or buyer may negotiate a reduced price for the ungraded lot to negate the additional stress associated with grading the fish prior to sale.

There have been some reports of producers selling submarket size largemouth bass to high end restaurants where they are purchased seasonally in small volumes and typically processed by hand in the restaurants (personal communication, Rocky Allen, Kentucky, 2018). Producers often look for another outlet for submarket fish. This situation creates a seasonal opportunity for the sale of pan-sized (400–500 g) largemouth bass at a reduced price, possibly allowing for entry into a fresh-on-ice sales to restaurants at a more competitive price.

12.4 Fillet market

As a carnivorous species, largemouth bass currently have a higher cost of production than some other aquaculture species, such as catfish and tilapia. Largemouth bass require relatively high levels of dietary protein. Engle et al. (2013) estimated the cost of production for largemouth bass to be US$7.27–9.36/kg compared to US$1.21–1.32/kg for channel catfish. Engle et al. (2013) estimated the profit margin typical of catfish food-fish producers to be approximately US$0.11–0.55/kg. Currently the sale prices of largemouth bass food-fish are US$11.02–13.22/kg (personal communication, Robert Mayer, Bardstown, Kentucky, 2018) representing a profit margin of US$1.66–5.95/kg for largemouth bass food-fish producers using production cost data provided by Engle et al. (2013).

Engle et al. (2013) evaluated whole-dress (head and viscera removed) and fillet (shank fillet without belly meat) yield of largemouth bass. Whole-dressed yield from 61–62% of the weight of the whole fish and fillets yield averaged and 34–35% of the original fish weight. Tidwell et al. (1996) reported whole dress and fillet yields (fillet with belly meat) for largemouth bass of 61.2 and 37.5% of the whole weight, respectively. These reported dress-out yields for largemouth bass are basically similar to channel catfish, better than tilapia (with 30% fillet yield) but less than salmon which typically yield fillet weights of > 60%.

Dasgupta and Caporelli (unpublished data) surveyed restaurants in Kentucky to examine chefs' perceptions of farm raised largemouth bass. Two fish, sourced from a commercial farm in Kentucky and a questionnaire were provided to 33 restaurants with 12 restaurants providing responses. The preferred form of largemouth bass was fillets (53%), followed by gutted fish (23%), with 18% preferring whole fish, and 6% desiring live fish. The majority (83%) of respondents indicated that they were unsure whether they would buy the fish. The most preferred product form and price was fillets at US$13.76/kg, the lowest price offered for fillets. Price seemed to be the most important factor. Only 3% of respondents indicated that they would pay US$39.65/kg for largemouth bass fillets, the highest price offered, but also the only price that would be similar to that currently obtained by the live market, considering the cost of processing, a fillet yield of 34–38% and a current sale price of US$11.02–13.22/kg for live largemouth bass sold as food-fish.

12.5 Market research

In the 1970s, increasing demand within the food-fish industry particularly for live fish resulted in increased popularity of commercial production of largemouth bass. Several states, which formerly prohibited the culture of largemouth bass due to their sport-fish status, now allow the sale of largemouth bass raised responsibly under licensed aquaculture methods. By the 1990s, aquaculture research expenditure in the USA was US$1.04 billion with catfish accounting for 57% of the total. This has led to great returns on investment, as the industry is valued at over US$29 billion. Recently, research expenditures have diversified into several other promising species including largemouth bass (Figure 12.2). Furthermore, the realization that US produced aquaculture products cannot efficiently compete with commodity fish products in the global marketplace has led research and production strategies in the US to focus on supplying live products directly to the consumer and particularly to ethnic Asian markets.

Increases in food-fish demand since the 1980s are partially due to the US population becoming more health conscious as well as more food savvy through more national and international travel and domestic restaurants using more exotic proteins. Ethnic diversity also has become a big factor. There is an increased demand for species that were unheard of in fish markets prior to 1980. Fish farming has expanded the availability of diverse species, but not without struggles. Fish farming has been the target of several environmental groups stating that the feed fed to fish is toxic and those fish raised should not be eaten, and only wild caught fish are healthy. This has been challenged through research (Mozaffarian and Rimm, 2006). They reviewed data

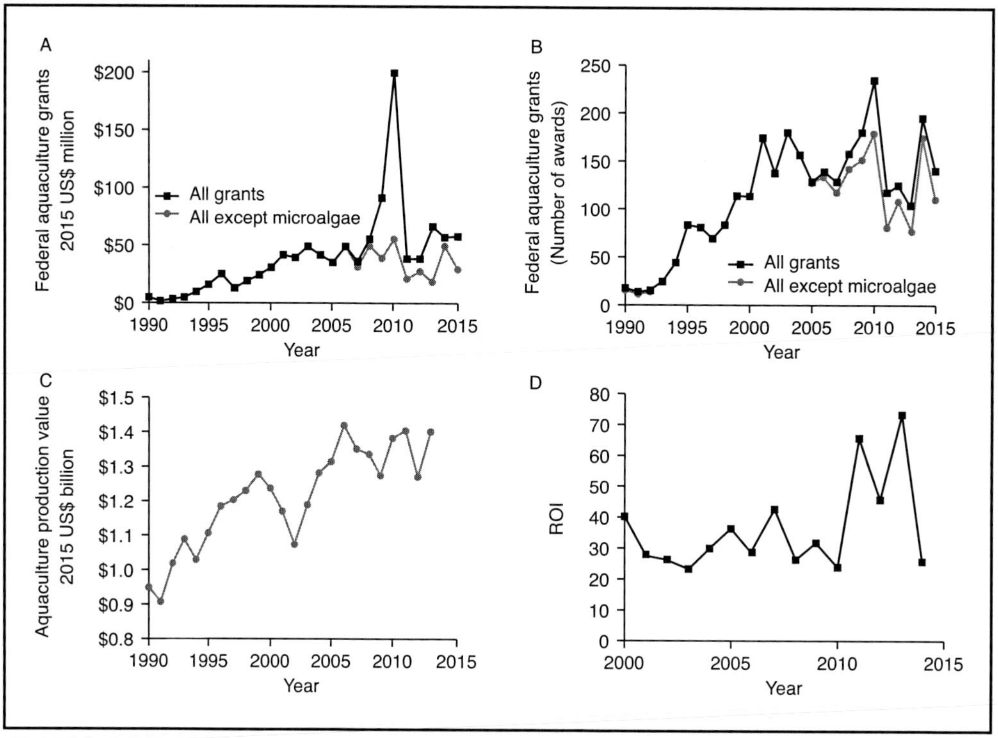

Figure 12.2 Aquaculture research expenditures in the USA. (a) Total grant spending per year, 1990–2015 (cumulative total US$1.04 billion); (b) total number of grant awards, 1990–2015; (c) aquaculture value per year, 1990–2013 (cumulative total US$29.13 billion); (d) return on investment, 2000–2014 (total gain minus total investment divided by the total cost of investment), federal grant funding for aquaculture has had a 37-fold return on investment since 2000.

Source: An Analysis of Nearly One Billion Dollars of Aquaculture Grants Made by the US Federal Government from 1990 to 2015, David C. Love, Irena Gorski, Jillian P. Fry, *Journal of the World Aquaculture Society*, Volume 48, Issue 5, October 2017, pages 689–710.

from the Environmental Protection Agency (EPA) and calculated that if 100,000 people ate farmed salmon twice a week for 70 years, the extra polychlorinated biphenyl (PCB) intake could potentially cause 24 extra deaths from cancer – but would prevent at least 7,000 deaths from heart disease. They also found that levels of PCBs and dioxins in fish are very low, similar to levels in meats, dairy products, and eggs, and moreover 90% of the PCBs and dioxins in the US food supply come from such non-seafood sources, including meats, dairy, eggs, and vegetables. Therefore, the thought of PCBs and dioxins in fish should not influence any decision about which fish or any other food source to consume. It is all about balance.

Cargill (2017) surveyed 1000 US residents in August 2017, led by Grant Murray of Duke University, in their *Feed4Thought Sustainable Seafood Survey* report. The survey found that 72% believed seafood is an important part of a healthy diet and a source of good nutrition. Over 61% agreed that sustainability of source was important when purchasing seafood. They found that 93% of millennials born between 1980–2000 would pay more if certified as sustainably raised and sourced. However, 80% of those surveyed held sensory qualities as most important.

As stated previously, people are becoming much more food savvy and experienced. This in large part due to increased national and international travel. Reynolds (2017) found that in 1974, 2.4 million adults traveled overseas, in 1980 over 3 million and in 2015 over 24 million or 3.5% of the adult population traveled internationally. Most of these travelers are looking for authentic experiences and tasting the real culture. They are bringing these culinary experiences back home and demanding more seafood choices and cultural food experiences.

Fish offerings on menus have changed drastically since the 1970s and 1980s. Gone are the days of breaded fried catfish as the only fish option. Chefs have included squid or calamari to almost every menu. Tilapia, which were not available in the USA until the early 1990s, as of 2018 is the third most popular seafood product in the USA and is available wherever there are more than two fish choices. Inclusion of more exotic species such as squid, whiting, monkfish, and ocean pout (formerly yellow eel) was a direct result of the chef/fisherman collaborative campaign in the 1990s to "Serve By-Catch" in the UK and the "Bite-Back" campaign in the USA. These species were then promoted heavily and served at top restaurants. For the first time ever, commercial fishermen, aquaculturists, regulators, NGOs, and famous chefs came together to help with the overfishing solution that would benefit all by filling the gaps for now regulated wild fish and promoting aquaculture. The marketing campaigns that followed were well thought out and very successful in steering chefs and consumers to think more about their fish and seafood choices. These campaigns also lead to more support for aquaculture and the development of alternative species, such as the largemouth bass.

In order to introduce lesser known species, or seasonally available species, to the public and chefs, a good marketing plan needs to be in place and consistent supply of product needs to be available. As a young industry, aquaculture in the USA is facing the same problems that poultry faced 75 years ago; distribution, processing, quality, consistency and demand. The efforts that have been in place are catching hold through states and grass roots organizations to educate consumers on the benefits of locally raised agriculture products, of which largemouth bass is a valuable one.

The Slow Foods International movement or Buy Local programs in many states have proven to have a positive impact on small farm sales. Both these marketing strategies lend themselves to influencing the consumer that "If it is local, it is fresher and healthier" and has less of an environmental impact than imported products. This is a great advantage for largemouth bass farmers to use these marketing programs to assist them in promoting their products and developing a consistent customer base.

Consumers also want to know the story of where their food comes from and the story of the farmers and the farm history. Several states are employing incentive programs to assist in the marketing and distribution for local producers of all agriculture products including aquaculture. This is especially important for live aquaculture products, as fish sourced from local waters experience less stress, ultimately leading to a better product with a longer shelf life (personal communication, Leo Ray, Idaho, 2018).

Live haulers and grocers offering live food-fish indicate that issues with inconsistent supply and delivery are the main limiting factors to expansion of the market for largemouth bass food-fish (personal communication, Mark Eikenberry, Indiana, 2018). A limited number of farmers can handle and deliver the fish well enough to yield good survival and appearance (personal communication, Adam Hatter, Ohio, 2018). Most live haulers have established relationships with suppliers and are very reluctant to try new suppliers, even when demand requires more product. The primary objectives of the commercial live hauler are keeping the fish alive and healthy and delivering them economically (Figure 12.3). Commercial live haulers of largemouth bass need to haul as many fish as possible as the weight transported is directly proportional to revenue generated. However, this can also potentially contribute to unnecessary stress and mortality. Research is being done on the academic level but farmers and live haulers are often not aware of the best management practices. Any farmer wanting to enter live fish marketing needs to ensure high quality fish, responsible transport and a long shelf life, especially in ethnic markets.

Ethnic diversity is a large reason for the increase in live food-fish demand, especially for largemouth bass. In 2007, the demand for live fish in Ethnic Asian markets was primarily for tilapia and hybrid striped bass (Carlberg et al., 2007). However, was this truly based on demand or primarily availability of these two species as live products? The sale of largemouth bass was not legally permitted in New York State until 2013. Clearly, demand for largemouth bass has increased significantly since 2007.

Myers et al. (2009) conducted a survey of ethnic live seafood market operators in the Northeastern US catering specifically to East Asian customers (Figure 12.4). The study evaluated

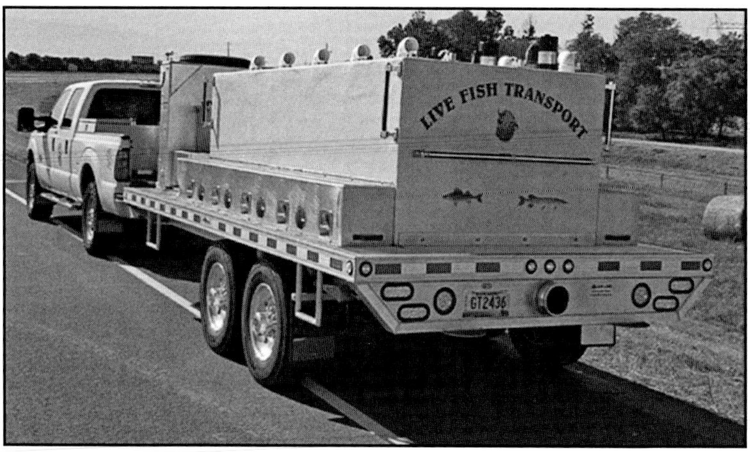

Figure 12.3 A live haul trailer.

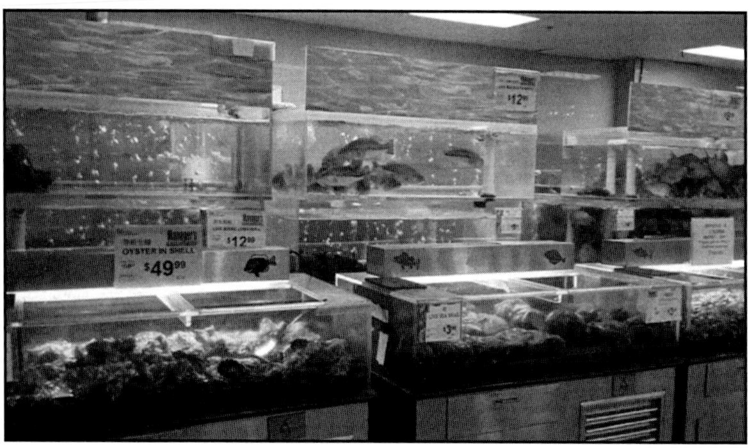

Figure 12.4 Live largemouth bass for sale in a market catering to East Asian customers.

live fish markets in New York, New Jersey, and Pennsylvania. There had previously been little market research on the retail markets selling live seafood. They examined factors that influence live fish sales, expansion opportunities, and characteristics of these businesses and markets. The goal was to develop scenarios that would help local US producers with production and distribution strategies to address these live food-fish markets. A second goal was to identify issues affecting future growth including geographic distribution issues, associated costs and net returns, and risk comparisons. There were 160 markets visited with a 27% response rate of the written survey (35). Thirty-eight percent of the markets used one to three vendors for live-fish supply; half of those were local distributors and 44% were out of state suppliers. Over 90% become associated with their supplier by word of mouth or one-on-one visits from the farmers or live haulers. Tilapia and hybrid striped bass were the top two live finfish species sold (58%). Results indicate that due to demographic changes and trends in seafood demand, growth in the live seafood market is expected. Twenty-four percent of these respondents stated that they plan to expand live-fish sales and tanks in the near future. The unique findings of the study were that: (1) freshness and quality were valued over price; and (2) fish that show good appearance and are energetic will have better quality flesh and longer life in the tanks. Within these ethnic markets, locality or origin was not valued as high or as important as freshness or quality. Sixty-five percent of respondents stated that availability was very important with only 15% stating that regular availability was not important. One-on-one negotiations were the mode of buying from producers or haulers and quality, freshness, and availability were triggers to start price negotiations.

Of the markets responding to Myers et al. (2009), 64% stated that ethnic Asians composed 50–80% of their customers and another 32% of markets stated Asians composed 20–50% customers. Other ethnic groups also purchasing live fish were Hispanic and African Americans. Seasonality was a factor affecting live food-fish sales with June through September having the least sales, and colder months of November through February having the most. Fidler (2000) reported that because of seasonality trends of live seafood, recreational stocking demand and food-fish demand could complement each other. Producers could choose what sector to sell into during different times and profits could increase by restricting supply to one sector over another.

According to the 2010 US Census (U.S. Census Bureau, 2010), the Asian population grew 45.6% between 2000–2010, much more than the 9.7% of the overall US population. Of the total US population, 14.7 million or 4.8%, were Asian and 2.6 million reported Asian combined with another race. This means that 17.3 million or 5.6 % of the US population is Asian or a combination of Asian and another race. Asian populations grew 30% in each state and equate to 50% of the population in Hawaii. Among the 20 metropolitan statistical areas with the largest Asian, alone-or-in-combination, ethnic Chinese was the largest detailed Asian group in 6 of the 20 metro areas (New York City, Los Angeles, San Francisco, San Jose, Boston, and Seattle). The Asian Indian population was also the largest detailed Asian group in six of the 20 metro areas (Chicago, Washington, Dallas-Fort Worth, Philadelphia, Atlanta, and Detroit). The New York /New Jersey area alone had 1.1 million Asian immigrants migrate into the area in the decade 2000–2010.

Research by Puduri and associates (2010) was conducted to characterize the Asian population's preferences in purchasing live seafood products, as well as the availability and the ability of producers to supply these growing markets. Information from producers has been difficult to accrue due to concerns over competition; however, Puduri et al. (2010) found that most producers see the benefit of cooperation to grow the live fish market and increase demand.

Five markets within New York, New Jersey, and Pennsylvania participated in this study and all had over 227 kg (500 lb) of live seafood product sales. A total of 252 consumers were interviewed collecting data on: awareness and perception of live fish sales, importance on availability or seasonality, freshness, quality, health concerns, source of product and characteristics such as size and whether wild or farm raised. In terms of most important attributes, 78% indicated quality and freshness. Another 23% indicated quality and health concerns were important. Hybrid striped bass was preferred by 47% of respondents, 36% wanted wild caught, 26% wanted smaller fish, 53% scaled fish and 45% wanted shellfish. Other findings were on average consumers traveled eight miles, six times per month and spent an average of US$15.19/visit on live food-fish. Ninety-nine percent of the respondents were 20–50 years old with 42% between 21–35 years old and 45% 36–50 years old, 53% had up to college level education, 35% of those had post grad education and 58% of respondents were female. In summation, consumers in the live fish markets prefer year-round availability, if the consumers are more quality and health driven, have college educations, are between age 20–50 and have household incomes of between US$25–75,000 supporting 3.7 people/per household.

The Asian tradition of fresh fish, as the highlight of protein within their daily meals equates to consumption of 21–32 kg/person/year (Degner et al., 1994; Sechena et al., 1999) as compared to non-Asian populations of 7.4 kg/person/year (NMFS, 2008). This along with the fact that in several large cities, Asian communities are growing and their traditional meals and demand for fresh fish will be on the rise. This is a great opportunity for live fish producers to gain market access.

Quagrainie et al. (2011a, 2011b) surveyed shoppers for live seafood products in the Midwestern US, including Chicago, Indianapolis, West Lafayette, Fort Wayne, Evansville, Columbus, Fairfield, Cincinnati, and Cleveland. The study assessed the decisions of shoppers of live seafood and the influence of various factors using binary choice and latent class profit model. The study included 28 ethnic Asian stores. A US$3 coupon was given to participants of which 365 of the 461 approached completed the survey (79%) in person. Results indicated that consumer preferences for live fish species vary by ethnic group in the Midwest and there were two distinct groups of consumers: traditional shoppers and occasional shoppers. Product appearance and weekly frequency of purchase were not important variables to traditional shoppers who were motivated by ethnic traditions and price. Occasional shoppers purchased live seafood less frequently and were more influenced by appearance and distance travelled, as opposed to price.

Thapa et al. (2015) used a binary logit model to study the factors influencing preferences for live and fresh fish products in Asian ethnic markets. This study, conducted in select markets in New York, New Jersey, and Pennsylvania during the summer of 2009, found that market demand varied by ethnic group, but was dominated by the East Asian communities consisting of Chinese, Korean and Japanese. These shoppers visited live fish markets two or three times per week and spent US$16–20 per visit on medium-sized live fish (less than 1 kg live weight). Freshness and appearance of eyes, gills and skin were the most important attributes influencing consumer purchases. Of the ethnic groups within the East Asian communities, Japanese had the highest consumption of fresh fish at 65 kg/person/year, Malaysians at 45 kg/person/year, Thai at 33 kg/person/year, Filipinos 27 kg/person/year, Chinese 25 kg/person/year with an overall average of 27 kg/person/year (Dey et al., 2008). Overall, these are about four times higher than Caucasian consumption of 8 kg/person/year (NMFS, 2008).

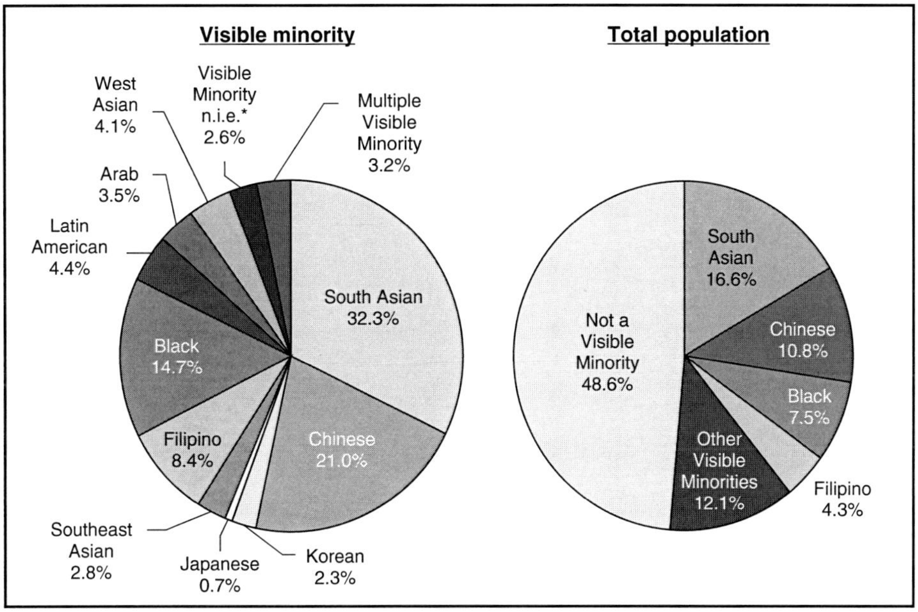

Figure 12.5 Ethnicity of populations in Toronto, Canada as reported by Statistics Canada.
Note: *n.i.e, not identified elsewhere.

Other interesting findings by Thapa et al. (2015) were that the East Asian purchasers of live fish were 83% female, primarily between the ages of 25–55, 34% completed college and 73% were employed full time with 50% making between $40,000–100,000/year. Ninety-one percent preferred to buy live fish at an Asian grocery. However, this last data point may be biased as all participants were surveyed in an Asian grocery. The importance of this research is that in recent decades, a large number of people have come to Canada and large urban areas of the USA from India and other South Asian countries. As of 2011, South Asians alone make up over 15% of the Greater Toronto Area's population and are projected to make up 24 percent of the region's population by 2031 (Gee, 2011).

According to Gee (2011), Toronto, Canada is an ever-changing South-East Asian community. This dramatic growth in Toronto's Indian community and other groups from South Asia are already the biggest visible-minority group in the Greater Toronto Area. There were 684,000 as of the 2006 census, a couple of hundred thousand more than the second biggest group: Chinese. These populations are expected to nearly triple by 2031, reaching around 2.1 million. By that time, a Statistics Canada report said that in 2016 close to one in four people in the Toronto area will be of South Asian heritage (Figure 12.5) and that the Chinese population will expand to 1.1 million, double the current figure.

12.6 Conclusion

Through ethnic migration, future migration and the high amount of live fish demand by this group, we can assume the market will also grow for largemouth bass and other high-quality fish.

These markets can be met by existing farmers that want to expand and/or new farmers that may want to diversify or start raising largemouth bass. However, farmers entering into the market need to be well versed in how to raise and handle these fish to ensure only high-quality, healthy fish enter the live market.

References

Anonymous (1875) Sea and river fishing: fish in season in January. *Forest and Stream* 3 (24), 378.

Anonymous (1884) Killing fish with dynamite. *New York Times* (August 31), 3.

Brandt, T.M., Jones, R.M. Jr. and Anderson, R.J. (1987) Evaluation of prepared feeds and attractants for largemouth bass. *The Progressive Fish-Culturist* 49, 198–203.

Cargill (2017) https://www.cargill.com/2017/survey-says-americans-will-splurge-on-sustainable-seafood.

Carlberg, J.M., Massingill, M.J. and Van Olst, J.C. (2007) Twenty-one years of hybrid striped bass culture in the U.S. (1987–2007). Striped Bass Growers Association, Hybrid Striped Bass 2007 Statistics Report. http://www.stripedbassgrowers.org/Publications/HSB2007FINAL.ppt (accessed 1 April 2008).

Currie, R.J., Bennet, W.A. and Beitinger, T.L. (1998) Critical thermal minima and maxima of three freshwater game-fish species acclimated to constant temperatures. *Environmental Biology of Fishes* 51, 187–200.

Degner, R.L., Adams, C.M., Moss, S.D. and Mack, S.K. (1994) Per capita fish and shellfish consumption in Florida. http://www.agmarketing.ifas.ufl.edu/downloads/SEAFOOD.pdf.

Dey, M.M, Garcia, Y.T., Kumar, P., Piumsombun, S., Haque, M.S., Li, L., Radam, A., Senaratne, A., Khiem, N.T. and Koeshendrajana, S. (2008) Demand for fish in Asia: a cross-country analysis. *The Australian Journal of Agricultural and Resource Economics* 51, 321–338.

Engle, C. and Southworth, B. (2008) *Cost of Raising Largemouth Bass Fingerlings.* Publication ETB260, University of Arkansas at Pine Bluff, Cooperative Extension Service, Pine Bluff, AK.

Engle, C.R., Stone, N. and Xie, L. (2013) Feasibility of pond production of largemouth bass, *Micropterus salmoides*, for a filet market. *Journal of the World Aquaculture Society* 44(6), 805–813.

Fidler, F.H. (2000) Economic feasibility of trout production in West Virginia: a mixed integer and quadratic-programming analysis. Master's thesis, West Virginia University, Morgantown, WV.

Gee, M. (2011) South Asian immigrants are transforming Toronto. *The Globe and Mail, http://www.dfo-mpo.gc.ca/aquaculture/farmed-elevage/listing-eng.htm.*

Jia, B., St-Hilaire, S., Styhn, H., Yu, J., Groman, D.B. and Gardner, I.A. (2016) Analysis of transaction records of live freshwater finfish in China: a case study of customers' claims of fish mortality using cross-classified modeling. *Aquaculture Reports* 4, 150–155.

Long, J. M., Allen, M.S., Porak, W.F. and Suski, C.D. (2015) A historical perspective of black bass management in the United States. *American Fisheries Society Symposium* 82, 99–122.

Lydell, D. (1903) *The Habits and Culture of the Black Bass.* U.S. Fish Commission Bulletin for 1902, Government Printing Office, Washington, DC.

Mozaffarian, D. and Rimm, E.B. (2006) Fish intake, contaminants, and human health: evaluating the risks and the benefits. *Journal of the American Medical Association* 296, 1885–99.

Myers, J.J., Govindasamy, R., Ewart, J.W., Liu, B., You, Y., Puduri, V.S. and O'Dierno, L.J. (2009) Survey of ethnic live seafood market operators in the Northeastern USA. *Aquaculture Economics and Management* 13, 222–234.

National Marine Fisheries Service (NMFS) (2008) *Fisheries of the United States 2007.* Fisheries Statistic Division, Silver Spring, MD.

Puduri, V.S., Govindasamy, R., Myers, J.J. and O'Dierno, L. (2010) Demand for live aquatic products in the Mid-Atlantic States: an ordered probit analysis towards consumers' preferences. *Aquaculture Economics and Management* 14, 30–42.

Quagrainie, K.K., Xing, A. and Hughes, K.G. (2011a) Factors influencing the purchase of live seafood in the North-Central region of the United States. *Marine Resource Economics* 26, 59–74.

Quagrainie, K.K., Hughes, K.G. and Xing, A. (2011b) Delineating shoppers of live seafood in the Midwestern United States. *Aquaculture Economics Management* 15 (3), 155–165.

Reynolds, J. (2017) Travel Trends by Age Demographics, *Groups Today* magazine. https://groupstoday.com/business/404-travel-trends-by-age-demographic.

Sechena, R., Nakano, C., Liao, S., Polissar, N., Lorenzana, R., Truong, S. and Fenske, R. (1999) Asian and Pacific Islander: seafood consumption study. http://www.epa.gov/r10earth/offices/oea/risk/a&pi.pdf.

Thapa, G., Dey, M.M. and Engle, C. (2015) Consumer preferences for live seafood in the northeastern region of USA: results from Asian ethnic fish market survey. *Aquaculture Economics and Management* 19 (2), 210–225.

Tidwell, J.H., Coyle, S.D. and Woods, T.A. (2000) *Species Profile Largemouth Bass*. Southern Regional Aquaculture Center (SRAC). SRAC Publication No. 722, Stoneville, MS.

Tidwell, J.H, Webster, C.D. and Coyle, S.D (1996) Effects of dietary protein level on second year growth and water quality for largemouth bass (*Micropterus salmoides*) raised in ponds. *Aquaculture* 145 (1–4), 213–223.

Turner, C.L. and Kraatz, W.C. (1920) Food of young largemouth bass in some Ohio waters. *Transactions of the American Fisheries Society* 50, 372–380.

U.S. Census Bureau (2010) U.S. Bureau of the census, county population estimates by demographic characteristics – age, sex, race, and Hispanic origin; updated annually for states and counties. http://www.census.gov/popest/counties/asrh/.

United States Department of Agriculture (USDA) Census of Aquaculture (2013). Volume 3. Special Studies. Part 2. AC-12-SS-4. National Agriculture Statistics Service, Washington, DC.

Williamson, J.H. and Carmichael G.J. (1986) Differential response to handling stress by Florida, northern, and hybrid largemouth bass. *Transactions of the American Fisheries Society* 115 (5), 756–761.

Williamson, J.H., Carmichael, G.J., Graves, K.G., Simco, B.A. and Tomasso, J.R. (1993) Centrarchids. In: Stickney, R.R. (ed.) *Culture of Non-Salmonid Freshwater Fishes*, 2nd edn. CRC Press, Boca Raton, FL, pp. 145–197.

CHAPTER 13

Composition and product forms

James H. Tidwell

Kentucky State University, Aquaculture Research Center, Frankfort, Kentucky, USA

13.1 Introduction

While today we primarily think of the largemouth bass as a sport-fish, it may actually have a longer history in the USA as a food-fish. Long et al. (2015) cited an 1874 document that reported "large numbers of black bass" were harvested "chiefly with nets" from the Delaware River for food. They also cited a publication stating that in 1875, largemouth bass were selling in fish markets for 18 cents. Later, the Black Bass Act 1926 was promulgated to control market fishing and bootlegging of largemouth bass across state lines. The valuable largemouth bass were known to be smuggled in barrels by sandwiching them between layers of less valuable rough fish.

Even after the Black Bass Act shut down the commercial harvest of largemouth bass, early sport-fishing activities primarily focused on catching the bass for food and their palatability was highly regarded. The concept of "catch and release" had not yet developed. People went fishing for fun, but to also put food on the table. In many areas, the thought of catching fish just to turn it loose would still be regarded as a ridiculous act. In the Great Depression–Dust Bowl years of the later 1930s and early 1940s, when the newly formed US Soil Conservation Service began to promote and support the construction of farm ponds, one of the main purposes of the pond was as a self-supporting source of food. The largemouth bass was one of the species emphasized in the stocking programs.

As we moved into the 1960s and 1970s, sport-fishing of largemouth bass for food was replaced by a greater emphasis on "catch and release" fishing purely for sport. As the most popular sport-fish in North America, there has long been an interest in producing the fish in hatcheries for stock enhancement of sport-fisheries. Robbins and MacCrimmon (1974) reported that > 35 million largemouth bass were stocked annually from 1966 to 1970. Most of these were small fish (5–7.5 cm). Later work showed that larger stocker fish (18–23 cm) survived and performed better. Growing fingerlings to these larger sizes may be well justified as it may take five times as many 5 cm fish to make the same lasting contribution to an age group as it does 10 cm fish

(Lochmann, 2013). This demand for large numbers of large largemouth bass stockers led to specialized hatchery and feed-training procedures (see Chapters 6 and 7).

While many of these stocker fish are produced by public hatcheries (state and federal), large numbers are also produced by private aquaculture enterprises. In fact, during the Reagan administration there was a push to shift fingerling production for use in stocking public waters from public to private hatcheries. The 2013 Census of Aquaculture shows, in terms of sport-fish sales, the largemouth bass was produced on more farms (176) and yielded more sales (US$14,452,000) than any of the other sport-fish. Lochmann (2013) indicated that 5 cm fish sold for US$0.46–0.75 each while 10–15 cm fish sold for US$0.81–1.60 each. Heidinger (2000) stated that the wholesale values of small lots of largemouth bass fingerlings were priced individually at US$0.35 for 2.5–5 cm fish, US$0.68 for 5–10 cm fish, US$0.94 for 10–15 cm fish, US$2.07 for 15–20 cm fish, and US$3.74 each for 20–25 cm fish.

Heidinger (1976) referred to largemouth bass being raised as food-fish. However, he said the fish were largely the result of polyculture schemes where they were used to control the populations of large forage organisms. Based on the high prices received for large sizes of largemouth bass, it was a natural progression for some producers to follow fish beyond the 20–25 cm advanced stockers size and carry fish onto larger sizes. In the 1980s and 1990s a demand for these larger fish was identified among urban ethnic markets in the USA and Canada (Figure 13.1). The largemouth bass was highly regarded in those markets and it was proposed that it resembles the Chinese bass or Mandarin fish (*Siniperca chuatsi*) that the immigrants were familiar with back home (Figure 13.2). Tidwell et al. (2002) estimated that > 500,000 kg of market size largemouth bass (400–700 g) were being sold annually as food-fish. Heidinger (2000) reported that these fish were bringing US$6.60–11/kg live weight for those markets. Most growers do not sell directly to the end user but actually sell to a live-hauler. Some small live-haulers service both markets (food-fish or stocking). However, large-scale haulers tend to focus on food-fish.

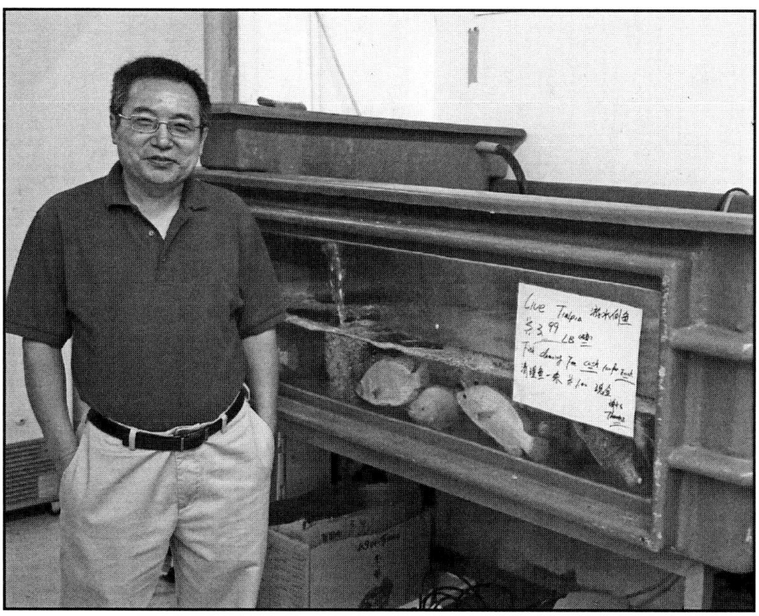

Figure 13.1 An ethnic Asian market for live largemouth bass.

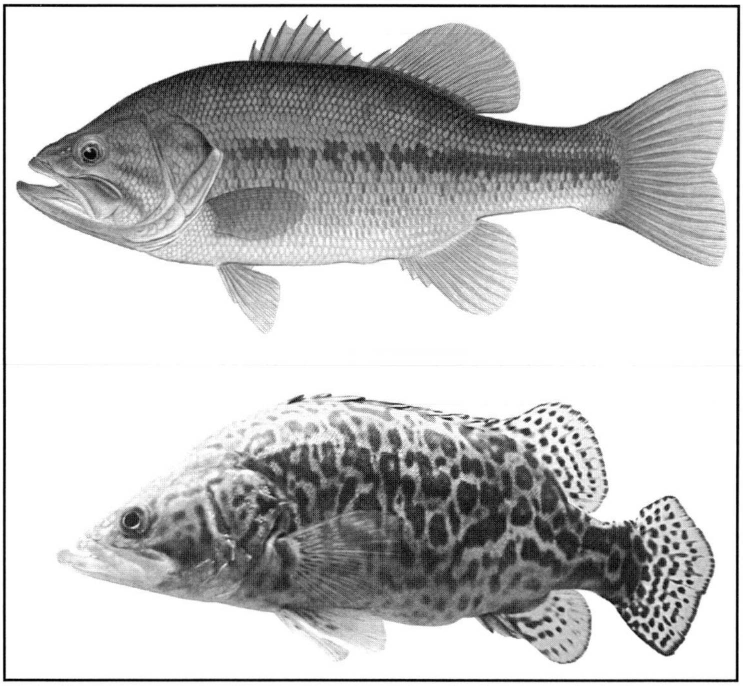

Figure 13.2 The largemouth bass, *Micropterus salmoides* (top) and the Mandarin fish, *Siniperca chuatsi* (bottom).

In the USA, most largemouth bass food-fish are marketed live. As with many things this is both good and bad. The "good" is that it protects domestic production. While well over 90% of the seafood in the USA is imported, primarily from Asia, live is a product form not readily transported such long distances. The "bad" aspect is that it limits the growth of largemouth bass production in the USA. In North America, consumers willing to purchase live fish are largely limited to persons of Asian descent. Outside of this group, North American producers prefer processed product forms, such as fillets. In fact, a shift away from the live whole product forms occurs generationally even among those of Asian descent.

13.2 Proximate composition

In an earlier work, Chatfield and Adams (1940) reported the chemical composition of wild largemouth bass to be 76.7% moisture, 26.6% protein, 1.8% lipid, and 1.2% ash. Proximate analysis of largemouth bass raised to food-fish sizes on feed were reported in Tidwell et al. (1996). For the whole body, values were 71.2% moisture, 6.0% lipid, 18.9% protein, and 3.8% ash. For the fillet portion only they averaged 76.9% moisture, 1.3% lipid, 20.6% protein, and 1.1% ash. Ash was higher in the whole-body analysis as it includes the frame (skeleton), which is primarily composed of minerals that are retained as ash. The lipid concentration is higher in the whole body than in the fillet as this fish tends to store lipid in the abdomen, in the mesentery and around the pyloric caeca, rather than in the fillet.

Trushenski and DeKoster (2017) compared the dry matter proximate composition of fillets from wild versus pond-raised largemouth bass. Protein, lipid, fiber, and ash average 89.1, 5.1, and 5.8%, respectively, in the wild largemouth bass and 81.8, 10.3, and 5.0% in the farmed largemouth bass. Brecka et al. (1996) evaluated six commercial diets and found that only body lipid and moisture were affected by diet while protein and ash were not. Body lipid decreased and moisture content increased as protein content in the diets increased. Tidwell et al. (1996) reported that the proximate composition of the fish was not significantly affected by dietary protein levels of 42, 44, and 47%.

13.3 Composition by sex

In a study evaluating non-invasive methods to estimate body composition in largemouth bass, Barziza and Gatlin (2000) analyzed 85 fish over a broad range of water bodies, culture systems, body sizes, and various seasons. On a percent wet basis, whole body moisture, lipid, protein, and ash for all fish collected averaged 70.0, 6.8, 17.9, and 4.4%, respectively. When analyzed by sex, males average 69.9, 6.7, 17.9, and 4.6%, respectively, while females averaged 70.1, 6.9, 17.8, and 4.3%, respectively. The authors stated that there were no significant differences between male and female bass in any of the proximate body composition variables when expressed as a percentage of total body weight. It should also be noted that largemouth bass are known to be sexually dimorphic, with females being larger. In the non-selective sampling used by Barziza and Gatlin (2000) to collect the body composition data, males averaged 662 g while females averaged 1,300 g, an almost two-fold increase.

13.4 Lipid characteristics

Lipid characteristics affect many aspects of the final sellable product. For largemouth bass being sold as a sport-fish, "stocker" body lipids can represent stored energy to give the fish time to adapt to the new environment and begin to capture prey. For broodstock, stored lipids again represent stored energy important to enduring the rigors of reproduction. For broodfish, the particular lipids available are also important as they are used to develop the yolk sac which is the sole source of food for the developing larvae during a critical period of growth.

Stored lipids are also important in terms of nutritional attributes of the final product, as well as storage stability. Tidwell et al. (1996) reported that largemouth bass had very high levels of docosahexaenoic acid (DHA) (22:6 n-3) in eggs and muscle tissue. Along with eicosapentaenoic acid (EPA) (20A:5n-3), these are the two primary fatty acids associated with human health benefits (Swanson et al., 2012). The concentration of these important fatty acids as a percentage of total fatty acids is actually higher in largemouth bass than it is in species such as salmon, which are recommended as good dietary sources. However, since salmon have higher total fat levels in the edible portion, salmon can deliver more EPA and DHA per standard portion (85 g). According to USDA analyses (2018), an 85 g portion of Atlantic salmon delivers 1.564 g of EPA and DHA, while largemouth bass delivers 0.206 g for farmed largemouth bass versus 0.197 g for wild largemouth bass (Trushenski and DeKoster, 2017). In terms of storability indicators, there were few if any meaningful differences in farmed versus wild largemouth bass in terms of shelf-life or physical characteristics (Trushenski and DeKoster, 2017).

13.5 Product forms

13.5.1 Frozen whole

Heidinger (2000) stated that to expand largemouth bass production, there was a need to develop frozen and iced food-fish markets. Mraz et al. (1978) reported that largemouth bass, as a frozen product, can be kept for long periods because of its low fat content. However, as stated previously, most food-fish are sold live in ethnic Asian markets in urban areas. In most of these retail outlets, whole frozen largemouth bass (Figure 13.3) are also available but at prices significantly lower than live fish of similar size. These frozen fish likely represent fish stressed by transport or holding conditions and are a "salvage" product. Whole frozen largemouth bass are available for sale on seafood oriented websites (www.cportnet). The country of origin for this product is listed as Taiwan.

13.5.2 Fillet

To expand into more of a mass market in North America, product forms such as fillets (Figure 13.3) or even value-added and/or ready to cook type products would need to be developed. Tidwell et al. (1996) reported that dressout and fillet percentages for largemouth bass (61% and 38%, respectively) were similar to those reported for channel catfish (59% and 40%) (Ammerman, 1985). Engle et al. (2013) investigated the feasibility of producing largemouth bass for a fillet market. They reported that individual fillets of 85–142 g or 142–198 g were the

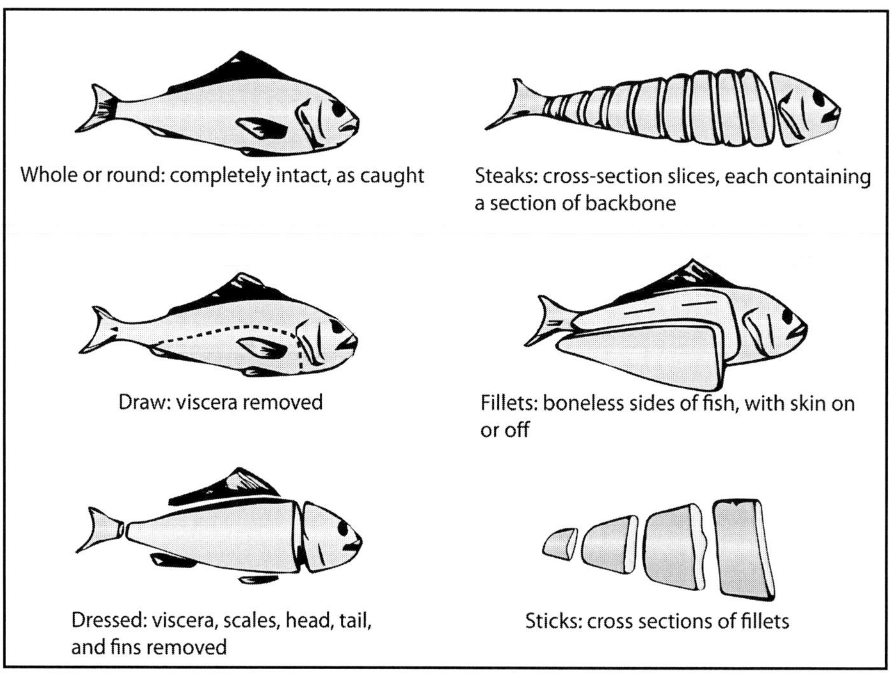

Figure 13.3 Different product forms derived from whole fish.

primary sizes utilized in the USA. At 38% fillet yield reported by Tidwell et al. (1996) that would require whole fish weights of 447–474 g for the smaller fillet category and 747–1,042 g for the larger fillets. While total fish harvest weights required for the smaller fillet category are achievable, efficient growth to sizes required for the larger fillets has proven difficult (Tidwell et al., 1998). Steps in filleting a largemouth bass can be found online (such as http://www.wildharvesttable.com/2016/07/14/processing-a-large-mouth-bass/).

Economic analysis by Engle et al. (2013) determined that production costs for largemouth bass fillets would be US$7.26–9.34/kg and that those prices would likely be too high for a feasible fillet market. They indicated that the primary drivers of the high production costs were fingerlings (their budget used US$1.60/fish at a size of 57 g) and feed (US$1,323/MT). It is likely that both of these costs can be significantly reduced with additional research and development efforts.

13.6 Organoleptic traits

With prescience to the future potential of largemouth bass as a food-fish, Snow and Lovell (1974) compared the organoleptic quality of largemouth bass raised on live forage with those raised on an artificial diet. Hatchery reared largemouth bass were raised from an initial size of 5 mm TL to age classes 2, 3, and 4 on either Oregon Moist Pellets (OMP) or live forage (primarily goldfish and tilapia). Fish were whole dressed and frozen. After thawing, fish were filleted and unseasoned fillets were wrapped in foil and baked at 200°C for 20 min. Two evaluations were made. First was a triangle difference test (Larmond, 1977). If a difference was indicated, a, 10-point hedonic rating test was used to evaluate the intensity of differences in flavor, texture, or appearance. The eight evaluators were trained in detecting off-flavors in fish.

The dressing percentage (whole dressed) reported by Snow and Lovell (1974) was 47.6%. This is lower than the 61% reported by Tidwell et al. (1996). One possible difference is that Snow and Lovell (1974) weights were with the skin removed, while Tidwell et al. (1996) included skin. The fish evaluated by Snow and Lovell (1974) also included a very large range of sizes (481–1,492 g). Large fish are known to have lower dress out percentages due to greater weight losses in mature gonads and larger heads.

Organoleptic evaluations readily distinguished between largemouth bass fed the OMP and those raised on live forage (Snow and Lovell, 1974). The largemouth bass raised on forage received higher scores on the 10-point hedonic scale (higher indicating greater preference) than fish fed the OMP. Judges comments indicated that the OMP fed largemouth bass had a "fish-oil" flavor. Other flavor comments included "strong" and "pond-like." Comments on the forage fed largemouth bass were usually "mild", "sweet", and "typical good bass flavor."

The authors proposed that the undesirable flavors in the fish fed the artificial diet were due to the very high levels of marine fish oils present in the OMP formula. Texture and appearance were not negatively affected. The researchers proposed that new formulations of artificial diets for largemouth bass be investigated with an emphasis on the organoleptic quality of the largemouth bass being produced.

While aspects of the diet, especially dietary lipids, can affect the taste of the fish being produced, off-flavors can also be absorbed from the culture environment (Tucker and Hargreaves, 2004).

Most off-flavors in pond raised fish are caused by naturally occurring organic compounds produced by aquatic algae or bacteria and absorbed into the fish through the skin, gills, or intestines. The most common off-flavor compounds are produced by cyanobacteria (aka blue-green algae) and include geosmin and 2-methylisoborneol (MIB) (Tucker and Hargreaves, 2004). These compounds are known to cause off-flavors in many fish, and even in the water itself.

Although off-flavors are often thought to primarily be associated with pond production environments, fish raised in recirculation systems can also develop off-flavors. These off-flavors are thought to originate in the biofilter (Losordo et al., 2004). Schrader et al. (2005) reported "earthy" and "musty" off-flavors in fillets from largemouth bass cultured in recirculating systems. Instrumental analysis using solid-phase microextraction-gas chromatography-mass spectrometry indicated that these off-flavors were due to geosmin and MIB.

13.7 Conclusion

The primary marketing form for largemouth bass at the present time is live fish in ethnic Asian markets in large metropolitan centers. These markets also offer some whole frozen largemouth bass. The American market is heavily biased toward boneless fillet product forms. Current production costs may make these product forms very expensive. However, developments in fingerling production costs and species-specific feeds could help to address those variable costs in the future.

References

Ammerman, G.R. (1985) Processing. In: C.S. Tucker (ed.) *Channel Catfish Culture.* Elsevier Science Publishing, Amsterdam, pp. 569–620.

Barziza, D.E. and Gatlin, D.M. (2000) An evaluation of total body electrical conductivity to estimate body composition of largemouth bass, *Micropterus salmoides. Aquatic Living Resources* 13 (6), 439–447.

Brecka, B.J., Wahl, D.H. and Hooe, M.L. (1996) Growth, survival, and body composition of largemouth bass fed various commercial diets and protein concentrations. *The Progressive Fish-Culturist* 58 (2), 104–110.

Chatfield, C. and Adams, G. (1940) Proximate composition of American food materials. *United States Department of Agriculture*, (549).

Engle, C.R., Stone, N. and Xie, L. (2013) Feasibility of pond production of largemouth bass, *Micropterus salmoides*, for a filet market. *Journal of the World Aquaculture Society* 44 (6), 805–813.

Heidinger, R.C. (1976) Synopsis of biological data on the largemouth bass *Micropterus salmoides. FAO Fisheries Synopsis* 115.

Heidinger, R.C. (2000) A white paper on the status and needs of largemouth bass culture in the North Central Region. *North Central Regional Aquaculture Center Whitepapers*, (4).

Larmond, E. (1977) *Laboratory Methods for Sensory Evaluation of Food.* Research Branch, Canada Dept. of Agriculture 1284.

Lochmann, S. (2013) Stock enhancement as a fishery management tool for largemouth bass. University of Arkansas at Pine Bluff – Cooperative Extension Publication FSA 9612.

Long, J.M., Allen, M.S., Porak, W.F. and Suski, C.D. (2015) A historical perspective of black bass management in the United States. *American Fisheries Society Symposium* 88, 99–122.

Losordo, T.M., Ray, L.E. and DeLong, D.P. (2004) Flow through and recirculating systems. In: C.S. Tucker and J.H. Hargreaves (eds) *Biology and Culture of Channel Catfish*. Elsevier Publishing Co., San Diego, CA, pp. 545–560.

Mraz, D., Kmiotek, S. and Frankenberger, L. (1978) The largemouth bass: its life history, ecology and management. Department of Natural Resources, publications of the Wisconsin Conservation Department 232.

Robbins, W.H. and MacCrimmon, H.R. (1974) *The Black Bass in America and Overseas*. Publications Division, Biomanagement and Research Enterprises. Sault Ste, Marie, Ontario.

Schrader, K.K., Rubio, S.A., Piedrahita, R.H. and Rimando, A.M. (2005) Geosmin and 2-methylisoborneol cause off-flavors in cultured largemouth bass and white sturgeon reared in recirculating-water systems. *North American Journal of Aquaculture* 67 (3), 177–180.

Snow, J.R. and Lovell, R.T. (1974) Comparison of organoleptic quality of largemouth bass fed natural and artificial diets. *Progressive Fish Culturist* 36 (4), 216–218.

Swanson, D., Block, R. and Mousa, S.A. (2012) Omega-3 fatty acids EPA and DHA: health benefits throughout life. *Advances in Nutrition* 3 (1), 1–7.

Tidwell, J.H., Webster, C.D. and Coyle, S.D. (1996) Effects of dietary protein level on second year growth and water quality for largemouth bass (*Micropterus salmoides*) raised in ponds. *Aquaculture* 145 (1–4), 213–223.

Tidwell, J.H., Coyle, S.D. and Webster, C.D. (1998) Effect of stocking density on third-year growth of largemouth bass *Micropterus salmoides*, fed prepared diets in ponds. *Journal of Applied Aquaculture* 8 (4), 39–45.

Tidwell, J.H., Coyle, S.D., and Webster, C.D. (2002) Centrarchids: Largemouth Bass, *Micropterus salmoides*. In: Webster, C.D. and Lim, C. (eds) *Nutrient Requirements and Feeding of Finfish for Aquaculture*, CABInternational, New York, pp. 374–380.

Trushenski, J. and DeKoster, T. (2017) Comparing nutritional values of wild and farmed whitefish. *The Global Aquaculture Advocate*, January 23.

Tucker, C.S. and Hargreaves, J.H. (2004) *Biology and Culture of Channel Catfish*. Elsevier Publishing Co., San Diego, CA.

USDA (2018) National nutrient database for standard reference legacy release. http://ndb.nal.usda.gov/ndb/foods/show/15209. Accessed 22/8/2018.

CHAPTER 14

Economics

Carole R. Engle

Engle-Stone Aquatic$, LLC, Adjunct Faculty, Virginia Seafood AREC, Virginia Polytechnic Institute and State University, Blacksburg, Virginia, USA

14.1 Introduction

The economics of fish production varies a great deal depending on the level of capital investment in different production systems and scales of production, the types of feeds used, and the production performance (for example, yield, growth, survival, feed conversion ratio [FCR]) of different species in different production systems. Largemouth bass are carnivorous fish that require a relatively high protein and high fat diet as compared to many other cultured species. Such a diet is also a higher-cost diet, due to the more expensive ingredients. In addition, largemouth bass fingerlings are more expensive than fingerlings of many other commonly raised warmwater species. The combination of greater feed and fingerling costs results in different cost structures for production of largemouth bass when compared to species such as catfish, baitfish/sport-fish, hybrid striped bass, and trout. The greater feed and fingerling costs also result in relatively greater production costs than for many other commercial warmwater species.

Greater overall costs of production will require careful attention to effective marketing strategies for commercial production of largemouth bass to be profitable. The marketing plan for the business will need to focus on strategies to receive greater market prices that more than cover the relatively greater production costs. Careful thought needs to be given to developing a very comprehensive marketing plan to ensure that adequate numbers of customers are willing and able to purchase a sufficient volume of largemouth bass at prices high enough to result in a profit for farmers raising largemouth bass.

This chapter will focus on the economics of producing largemouth bass. Chapter 12 focuses on a description of major markets for largemouth bass. Those considering investing in and starting a for-profit largemouth bass farm should include both the marketing information from Chapter 12 and the cost information presented in this chapter in developing their overall business plan. Given the general lack of information on the economics of producing largemouth bass, the estimated production costs used in this chapter are those from a number of production studies conducted in ponds in the USA and reflect US prices and costs. Those raising largemouth bass in other countries are encouraged to use what is presented here as guidance only and change prices and line-item costs to reflect economic realities of their production location.

14.2 Food-fish production costs

The majority of food-fish raised in the USA are produced in earthen ponds. According to the 2013 Census of Aquaculture, 48% of all US aquaculture farms (including shellfish and other marine species) use ponds for production (USDA-NASS, 2014). Thus, a great deal is known about farm-level costs associated with raising a variety of food-fish species in the USA (see Engle, 2010, for examples). However, much less is known about the costs of producing largemouth bass, particularly for sale as a food-fish product. Moreover, there are few commercial farms producing largemouth bass as food-fish in the USA, and hence there are no farm-level data from which to draw industry-wide costs.

Several research studies conducted in the USA have measured production parameters for various stocking densities and feeds in research-scale earthen ponds. These studies provide some data on relative production performance characteristics such as yield (kilogram per hectare of fish produced), FCRs, and survival rates. This section will draw upon the data from those studies that have focused on management strategies to produce largemouth bass as food-fish in the USA. Clearly, the information presented here will need to be updated with prices and line-item costs appropriate for their country and location.

It is important to understand that care must be taken in extrapolating research data, such as that used in this chapter, to project expected costs and returns on commercial farms. Reported yields (kilogram per hectare produced) often are greater in research studies, FCRs lower, and survival rates greater than on commercial farms. These differences stem primarily from the necessity for researchers to control and standardize as many variables as possible (other than the treatments being tested) to isolate and identify effects of the specific variable under study. Under commercial farming conditions, many variables that affect fish production cannot be controlled by the farmer and lead to lower yields, higher FCRs, and lower survival rates. Thus, those planning to raise largemouth bass for food-fish should select yields, FCRs, and survival rates that are more conservative than those used in the following analysis. This analysis is intended primarily to show the relative differences among alternative management strategies, although the results perhaps provide some indication of the most optimistic economic outcomes that may be possible.

The five US research studies found in the literature that include pond production performance data were: Tidwell et al. (1996), Tidwell et al. (1998), Cochran et al. (2009), Engle et al. (2013), and Tidwell et al. (2015). Tidwell et al.'s (1996, 1998, 2015) and Cochran et al.'s (2009) studies were conducted in Kentucky while Engle et al.'s (2013) study was conducted in Arkansas, a more southerly state with a longer growing season for warmwater fish. The Tidwell et al. (1998) study compared effects of two stocking densities (6,175 and 12,350 largemouth bass per hectare) of fingerlings stocked at a mean individual weight of 122 to 124 g (Table 14.1). Engle et al. (2013) followed up on the Tidwell et al. (1998) study and added a higher stocking density of 18,525/ha, but stocked a smaller 57 g fish. Tidwell et al. (1998) compared three protein levels (42%, 44%, and 48% protein) in feed fed to 122 g fish stocked at 12,350 fish/ha. The days to harvest were similar across these three studies with trials lasting approximately one year. However, the

Table 14.1 Key production performance data from production studies to produce largemouth bass food-fish.

Production parameter	Engle et al. (2013)[a]			Tidwell et al. (1998)[a]		Tidwell et al. (1996)[b]	Cochran et al. (2009)[c]	Tidwell et al. (2015)[d]
Stocking density (head/ha)	6,175	12,350	18,525	6,175	12,350	12,350	8,650	10,000
Mean individual weight fish stocked (g)	57	57	57	124	122	122	210	185
Feed conversion ratio	3.6	2.5	2.5	9.6	3.8	2.3	1.36	1.7
Days to harvest (days)	372	372	372	365	365	365	179	151
Mean final weight harvested (g)	896	827	744	406	406	406	527	566
Survival (%)	71	74	65	92	83	92	95	94
Gross yield (kg/ha)	3,989	7,434	9,096	2,354	4,598	4,613	4,670	5,321

Notes: [a]Stocking density trial. [b]Trial of three protein levels in feed. Used 44% protein feed that had best economic outcome. [c]Trial of three diets. Control did not result in market-sized fish, but diet treatments did. Used mean of dietary treatments. [d]Compared forms of feed. No significant differences due to form. Used values for standard floating pellet.

Cochran et al. (2009) and Tidwell et al. (2015) studies were stocked in the spring and harvested in the fall of the same year. Cochran et al. (2009) evaluated replacing fishmeal content in the diet by stocking 8,650 largemouth bass per ha at an average size of 210 g, whereas Tidwell et al. (2015) compared various forms of feed pellets to 185 g bass stocked at 10,000/ha.

It is important to note that the minimum market size of largemouth bass sold as food-fish was achieved only in three of these studies: the Arkansas study, in the three treatment diets of the Cochran et al. (2009) study in Kentucky, and in the Tidwell et al. (2015) study of pellet form. The Arkansas production study produced the largest fish (individual mean weights ranged from 744 to 896 g/fish across the three stocking density treatments) of the five studies. Average weights of individual fish in the four Kentucky studies ranged from 406 g to 566 g (Table 14.1). The two most recent Kentucky studies (Cochran et al., 2009; Tidwell et al., 2015) were the only Kentucky studies to achieve average weights of individual fish harvested greater than 500 g, the size considered the minimum market size for largemouth bass food-fish (Watts et al., 2016). The greater growth in the Arkansas study likely reflects a longer growing season with more favorable water temperatures for growth of largemouth bass. All but the Cochran et al. (2009) and Tidwell et al. (2015) studies lasted for approximately 1 year. While the largemouth bass in the Arkansas study were stocked at a smaller size, they still grew to market size in that one-year growing period. While fish in the Cochran et al. (2009) and Tidwell et al. (2015) studies did reach minimum market size in a 6 month period, the starting sizes were larger stockers, 210 g and 185 g, respectively. The greatest gross yield (kg/ha) values were obtained at the two greater densities in the Arkansas study, 7,434 kg/ha and 9,096 kg/ha as compared to gross yields of 2,354 to 4,598 kg/ha in the Kentucky density studies. Survival rates were greater in the Kentucky studies, ranging from 83 to 95% as compared to 65 to 74% in the Arkansas study. While the reasons for such differences are not clear, lower survival rates in Arkansas may have been due to the greater summer temperatures in Arkansas during which there was some degree of chronic mortality observed across all ponds. FCRs were generally better in Arkansas as well, ranging from 2.5 to 3.6 as compared to 3.8 to 9.6 in the Kentucky density studies. However, the best FCRs (1.36 and 1.7) were obtained in the Cochran et al. (2009) and Tidwell et al. (2015) Kentucky studies. Such low FCRs in these two most recent studies may be due to the lack of a winter period in those studies as compared to the three other studies.

To compare cost of production across these four studies, whole-farm enterprise budgets were developed for eight management scenarios for a 32 ha (surface water ha) farm composed of eighty 0.4 ha ponds. Given that the fixed costs associated with land, pond construction, and equipment are similar for pond production of largemouth bass as for production of catfish, the fixed costs were established based on recent fixed cost values from surveys of catfish farms in the south (Kumar, 2017). Fixed costs were held constant across the management strategies to allow for comparison of the effects of the varying yields, survival rates, and FCRs. Representative US costs were used for all line items in the budgets.

Table 14.2 compares annual costs of production associated with results from the four largemouth bass production studies under standardized assumptions related to the overall farm business. The greatest costs to produce largemouth bass were those of feed and fingerlings. For most of the management strategies evaluated, fingerling cost was greater than that of feed cost. Fingerling costs were proportionately greater in the studies in which larger sizes of largemouth bass were stocked (such as the 210 g fish stocked in Cochran et al. (2009) and the 122 g fish stocked in Tidwell et al., 1996, 1998) as compared to the 57 g fingerlings stocked in Engle et al. (2013).

Total annual ownership costs were held constant across all studies and included farm insurance, legal and accounting costs, and annual depreciation on all depreciable assets such as ponds, vats, buildings, and equipment, and interest on the investment of capital in land as well as the other capital assets (Table 14.2). Total costs are presented with and without the value of the time spent by family labor and management to produce largemouth bass food-fish. While labor and management are necessary inputs to the production of largemouth bass, many operators of small-scale farms, such as a 32 ha farm, do not pay themselves a wage or a salary. However, the value of the time spent by the owner/operator and his/her family is important to consider (Engle, 2017). If those who do the work and make management decisions are not adequately compensated, economics shows that they will not continue in the business. Thus, a cost for family labor and management is included. Total costs were greatest for the strategies with the greatest stocking densities, as would be expected.

Breakeven prices represent the cost per kilogram of largemouth bass produced. Breakeven prices above total costs include all costs necessary to produce largemouth bass food-fish and are calculated on a per kilogram basis. Breakeven prices represent the price per kilogram that must be received for the farm to just break even (above variable costs and fixed costs). It is important to understand that the price received must be greater than the breakeven price for there to be any profit. Another key consideration in interpreting these values is that the quantity of fish used in the calculation must be the weight sold, not the weight produced. Most commercial farms produce more than they are able to sell.

Breakeven prices for the eight research-based scenarios analyzed show that the cost of production ranged from a low of US$7.64/kg to a high of US$14.48/kg (Table 14.2). Given that the often-quoted market price of largemouth bass food-fish is US$10/kg, and that the breakeven prices estimated did not include costs associated with grading, transportation, and other

Table 14.2 Key production costs and breakeven prices for largemouth bass food-fish production, based on experimental production results, but without any costs associated with marketing. Costs are total farm costs for a 32 ha farm with eighty 0.4 ha ponds.

Item	Engle et al. (2013)[a]			Tidwell et al. (1998)[a]		Tidwell et al. (1996)[b]	Cochran et al. (2009)[c]	Tidwell et al. (2015)[d]
Variable costs								
Feed	653,744	840,000	985,600	262,027	355,442	357,025	194,040	294,896
Fingerlings	400,000	800,000	1,200,000	540,000	1,080,000	1,080,000	980,000	1,004,152
Seining and hauling	22,338	41,630	50,938	11,766	22,988	23,061	23,341	26,600
All other variable costs[e]	68,400	69,280	69,920	68,400	69,280	69,280	68,400	69,280
Int. on oper. capital	114,488	175,091	230,646	88,219	152,771	152,937	126,578	139,493
Total variable costs	1,258,931	1,926,001	2,537,103	970,412	1,680,481	1,682,302	1,392,359	1,534,421
Total fixed costs[f]	103,421	103,421	103,421	103,421	103,421	103,421	103,421	103,421
Total costs w/out labor and mgmt.	1,362,351	2,029,422	2,640,524	1,073,833	1,783,902	1,785,723	1,452,406	1,637,842
Unpaid labor, mgmt.	30,000	30,000	30,000	30,000	30,000	30,000	30,000	30,000
Total annual costs	1,392,351	2,059,422	2,670,524	1,103,833	1,813,902	1,815,723	1,482,406	1,667,842
Breakeven price above total costs	9.62	7.64	8.09	14.48	12.18	12.15	9.80	9.68

Notes: All figures US$. [a]Stocking density trial. [b]Trial of three protein levels in feed. Used 44% protein feed that had best economic outcome. [c]Trial of three diets. Control did not result in market-sized fish, but diet treatments did. Used mean of dietary treatments. [d]Compared forms of feed. No significant differences due to form. Used values for standard floating pellet. [e]Includes electricity, fuel, pond amendments like salt, repairs and maintenance, predator control, telephone, office supplies. [f]Includes farm insurance, legal and accounting expenses, interest on investment of all capital assets, including land and annual depreciation of all depreciable assets such as ponds, office and storage building, wells, and equipment.

marketing functions, it appears that profit margins for largemouth bass food-fish are fairly thin. The lowest breakeven prices were those estimated from the Engle et al. (2013) study done in Arkansas. This study achieved greater yields than the Kentucky studies, even at similar stocking densities. The greater yields from the Arkansas study likely resulted from the generally warmer weather in Arkansas as compared to Kentucky. However, greater yields do not always result in greater profits. In Engle et al. (2013), the lowest (most profitable) breakeven prices were found in the 12,350/ha density in spite of the greater yields measured in the 18,525/ha treatment. The increased fingerling cost in the highest density was proportionately greater than the increased revenue in that treatment which resulted in a greater breakeven price in the high-density treatment. Breakeven prices were consistently lower at the 12,350/ha density when compared with the 6,175/ha density in both the Arkansas and Kentucky density studies (Tidwell et al., 1998; Engle et al., 2013). Across the Kentucky studies, the lowest breakeven costs were those of the Cochran et al. (2009) and Tidwell et al. (2015) studies. Both these studies resulted in mean weights of fish greater than the minimum market size of 500g (Watts et al., 2016), but importantly, also achieved the lowest FCRs among all eight experimental scenarios.

Table 14.3 presents results related to the relative importance of the various line item inputs used (in terms of costs) in production of largemouth bass from the eight scenarios analyzed. Feed costs ranged from 13% to as much as 47% of total costs. By way of comparison with catfish production costs, feed costs constituted from 43 to 47% across ten different catfish management strategies on a 32 ha catfish farm (Kumar, 2017).

The most striking cost percentage in Table 14.3 is that of fingerlings. The cost of largemouth bass fingerlings constituted from 29 to 66% of total costs. Compared with catfish food-fish production, catfish fingerling costs constituted from 7 to 10% of total costs across five different

Table 14.3 Percentage of production costs of key inputs for production of largemouth bass food-fish production, based on experimental production results, but without any costs associated with marketing. Costs are for a 32 ha farm with eighty 0.4 ha ponds.

Item	Engle et al. (2013)[a]			Tidwell et al. (1998)[a]		Tidwell et al. (1996)[b]	Cochran et al. (2009)[c]	Tidwell et al. (2015)[d]
Feed	47%	41%	37%	24%	20%	20%	13%	18%
Fingerlings	29%	39%	45%	49%	60%	59%	66%	60%
Seining and hauling	2%	2%	2%	1%	1%	1%	2%	2%
All other variable costs[e]	5%	3%	3%	6%	4%	4%	5%	4%
Interest on operating capital	8%	9%	9%	8%	8%	8%	9%	8%
Total variable costs	90%	94%	95%	88%	93%	93%	94%	92%
Total fixed costs[f]	7%	5%	4%	9%	6%	6%	4%	6%
Unpaid family labor, management	2%	1%	1%	3%	2%	2%	2%	2%

Notes: [a]Stocking density trial. [b]Trial of three protein levels in feed. Used 44% protein feed that had best economic outcome. [c]Trial of three diets. Control did not result in market-sized fish, but diet treatments did. Used mean of dietary treatments. [d]Compared forms of feed. No significant differences due to form. Used values for standard floating pellet. [e]Includes electricity, fuel, pond amendments like salt, repairs and maintenance, predator control, telephone, office supplies. [f]Includes farm insurance, legal and accounting expenses, interest on investment of all capital assets, including land and annual depreciation of all depreciable assets such as ponds, office and storage building, wells, and equipment.

management strategies for channel catfish and from 12 to 15% for five different hybrid catfish management strategies (Kumar, 2017), including split-pond production (Kumar et al., 2016). Such high costs of largemouth bass fingerlings result, in large part, from the great variability in survival and yields of largemouth bass fingerlings from pond to pond. This results in the necessity for a bass hatchery to charge a sufficiently high price to cover what can be nearly total losses in some ponds on the farm.

Such high feed and fingerling costs for largemouth bass food-fish production resulted in percentages of variable costs that ranged from 88 to 95%. In comparison with catfish production costs, variable costs constituted from 80 to 87% of total costs of production (Kumar, 2017).

Indoor production of largemouth bass in recirculating aquaculture systems (RAS) has been conducted on an experimental basis but studies conducted to date have not resulted in market-sized (> 500 g) largemouth bass (Watts et al., 2016). Thus, no economics work has been done to develop reliable estimates of production costs of largemouth bass produced in RAS. The lack of commercial-scale RAS production of largemouth bass makes it difficult to develop relevant cost estimates. Production costs per kilogram tend to be greater in RAS than in outdoor earthen ponds, given the much greater proportion of capital costs in tanks and equipment that leads to greater annual fixed costs than in ponds. For example, with hybrid striped bass, the cost to produce fingerling hybrid striped bass in indoor tanks was more than three times greater than the production cost in ponds (Eklund et al., 2012). Thus, while it may become possible to produce market-sized largemouth bass food-fish indoors in RAS systems, it is likely that the production cost per kg will be greater than that of largemouth bass produced in ponds.

Clearly, the two drivers of the high production costs of largemouth bass food-fish in the USA are the costs of the fingerlings and the feed. The Cochran et al. (2009) and Tidwell et al. (2015) studies were encouraging in their low FCRs that contributed to lower production costs. Ongoing research efforts to develop lower cost diets for largemouth bass that still result in good growth and production performance are important lines of research that may help to reduce production costs of largemouth bass in the future.

However, there is an even greater need for research efforts to target ways to reduce the cost of producing largemouth bass fingerlings. The next section of this chapter will explore the underlying cost structures for production of largemouth bass fingerlings to shed light on the factors that contribute to this high fingerling cost.

14.3 Fingerling production costs

Largemouth bass fingerlings are produced by a number of public and private hatcheries in the United States, mostly for state-managed stocking programs and for stocking private fishing ponds. However, increased demand for largemouth bass fingerlings for growout to food-fish may increase the proportion of fingerlings sold to food-fish producers over time.

Engle and Southworth (2013) surveyed public and private hatchery producers of largemouth bass fingerlings in 15 southern states in the USA: Alabama, Arkansas, Florida, Georgia, Kentucky, Louisiana, Maryland, Mississippi, Missouri, Oklahoma, North Carolina, South Carolina, Tennessee, Texas, and Virginia. The production data obtained from the survey of these hatcheries was used to develop the cost estimates that will be presented in this chapter. Given the substantial differences found between management strategies used in public and private hatcheries, many of which affect the costs of production, only private hatchery results will be used in this analysis. The northern strain of largemouth bass was the principal strain raised by private hatcheries, and the data used reflect those of northern-strain largemouth bass. Given that most private hatcheries fed pelleted feeds, the following costs will focus on production of feed-trained bass fingerlings for stocking on food-fish growout production. Since these costs were based on US prices, the values presented for fingerling production will need to be adapted to reflect realistic prices in other countries.

Fingerling production begins, of course, with broodstock. Hatcheries need to maintain broodstock in good condition throughout the year to obtain quality eggs and fry. Various sizes of ponds were found in the Engle and Southworth (2013) study to be used to hold broodstock throughout the year. However, this analysis is based on the use of a 0.4 ha pond for holding and maintaining broodstock throughout the year. The cost to hold and maintain broodstock represents an annual cost that needs to then be included in the cost of fry production. The annual holding costs for broodstock on a largemouth bass farm were found to constitute a relatively substantial cost for the hatchery. Table 14.4 shows that the annual costs to hold, feed, and maintain broodstock in good spawning condition was US$11,226/0.40 ha pond, or US$16.86/broodfish. This cost is related primarily to the relatively high cost of feed (45% of total annual costs) required to hold broodfish and the costs of maintaining the entire pond for a relatively low weight of fish.

Largemouth bass can be spawned in ponds, as the more traditional method, or in raceways. Pond spawning costs include the cost of the broodstock stocked into that pond for spawning, fertilizer to promote a phytoplankton bloom, and feed (including the shipping cost) for the broodfish. For the 2 month spawning period, total annual costs were estimated to be US$2,558 per 0.4 ha pond, or US$0.051 per fry (Table 14.5). The cost to hold and maintain broodstock throughout the year constituted 66% of the total costs of fry produced from pond spawning. Some largemouth bass hatcheries spawn largemouth bass in raceways. Raceway spawning costs also include the costs of the broodfish and feed, but include additional costs of the spawning mats, spawning hormones, labor, and other variable costs of electricity, fuel, pumping, and repairs and maintenance. Annual fixed costs of raceway spawning include the annual depreciation and interest on the investment of the raceways that would need to be constructed. Table 14.6 shows that the cost per fry spawned in raceways was much less than in ponds, at US$0.00082 per fry. In raceways, the cost to hold and maintain broodstock throughout the year were only 26% of the total cost to spawn fry due to the greater number of fry produced per broodfish in raceway spawning as compared to pond spawning. Total fixed costs were 28% of the total costs of fry production, as compared to only 6% in pond spawning due largely to the capital investment in concrete raceways. Labor costs were low for pond spawning, constituting only 1% of total costs in pond spawning to obtain fry, but were greater with raceway spawning, constituting 10% of total costs of fry production.

Fry harvested from spawning ponds are typically stocked into fertilized ponds until they reach a size of approximately 5 cm when they can be feed trained. This stage of production was characterized by widely varying survival and yield in the Engle and Southworth (2013) survey, with survival rates that ranged from 0% to 123%, and yields that ranged from 0 to 296,400 fingerlings

Table 14.4 Holding costs for largemouth bass broodstock, for one 0.4 ha pond stocked at 1,645 broodstock per ha with an average weight of 1.13 kg for 10 months.

Item	Unit	Cost/unit (US$)	Quantity	Total cost 0.4 ha pond (US$)
Variable costs				
Feed	lb/pond/year	0.7	4,996	3,497
Shipping feed	Total	0.3	4,996	1,499
Treatment for filamentous algae	US$/pond	17	1	17
Labor	US$/pond/month	13.75	10	138
Electricity	US$/pond/month	8.00	10	80
Fuel	US$/pond/month	10.83	10	108
Pumping	US$/pond/month	17.58	10	176
Repairs and maintenance	US$/pond/month	8.08	10	81
Bird depredation	US$/pond/month	8.33	10	83
Office supplies	US$/pond/month	0.92	10	9
Interest on operating capital		0.0833[a]	5,687	474
Total variable costs				6,162
Fixed costs				
Telephone	US$/pond/month	1.42	10	14
Farm insurance	US$/pond/month	3.63	10	36
Legal/accounting	US$/pond/month	1.57	10	16
Land				
Interest on average investment	US$/pond/month	18.75	10	188
Ponds				
Annual depreciation	US$/pond/month	13.43	10	134
Interest on average investment	US$/pond/month	13.43	10	134
Equipment – Ponds				
Annual depreciation	US$/pond/month	15.88	10	159
Interest on average investment	US$/pond/month	5.41	10	54
Broodstock				
Annual depreciation	US$/pond/year	3,330	1	3,330
Interest on average investment	US$/pond/year	9,990	0.1	999
Total fixed costs				5,064
Total annual costs				11,226
Annual cost/kg of broodstock to hold for 10 months (breakeven price/kg) ($/kg)				14.86
Annual cost per broodfish to hold for 10 months (breakeven price per broodfish)($/fish)				16.86

Note: [a]Monthly rate, based on 10% annual percentage rate.

per hectare and 20 to 481 kg/ha. Respondents attributed these wide ranges to the variability and quality of the phytoplankton bloom produced in ponds following fertilization.

The cost to produce 5-cm fingerlings in fertilized ponds was estimated to be US$4,356 per 0.4 ha pond with a per-fingerling cost of US$0.118 (Table 14.7). For largemouth bass to accept pelleted feeds requires that the fish be trained to accept a pelleted feed. Feed training is best done in concrete vats where it is possible to crowd the fish and ensure that feed is available to all fish frequently throughout the day. Total costs per vat for feed training were US$1,161 for each 5,700 l vat, and feed training added US$0.0206 per fingerling to the cost (Table 14.8). The greatest costs of feed training were that of krill and krill meal. It should be

Table 14.5 Pond spawning annual costs for one 0.4-ha pond; pond used for this purpose for two months.

Item	Unit	Cost/unit (US$)	Quantity	Total cost (US$)
Variable costs				
Broodstock costs	US$/broodfish for holding	16.85	100	1,685
Fertilizer				
Cottonseed meal	US$/pond/application	0.212	200[a]	42.4
Inorganic fertilizer	US$/pond/application	0.54	100[a]	54
Feed	kg	1.54	6.12	9.45
Shipping feed	kg	0.66	6.12	4.05
All other operating costs				577
Interest on operating capital		0.0083[b]	2,372	39
Total variable costs				2,411
Total fixed costs				147
Total annual costs				2,558
Annual cost/kg of Fry (breakeven price/kg) ($/kg)				39.36
Annual cost/Fry (breakeven price/fry) ($/fry)				0.051

Notes: [a]Four applications per year. [b]Monthly rate, based on 10% annual percentage rate.

noted that the costs estimated were based on 100% of the 5 cm fingerlings being trained successfully to feed on artificial diets. Some percentage of these fish will not learn to eat feed; the cost per feed-trained 5 cm fingerling will increase as the percentage of fingerlings that do not learn to eat feed increases.

Rearing feed-trained fingerlings to 10 cm on feed cost US$4,226 per 0.4 ha pond and fingerlings cost US$0.241 each, with reported yields of 224 kg/ha (data not shown). For production of larger 15 cm fingerlings, respondents reported yields of 2,240 kg/ha (data not shown). Production of 15 cm feed-trained fingerlings cost US$10,826 per 0.4 ha pond, and fingerlings cost US$0.541 per fingerling (Table 14.9). The greatest annual cost of producing 15 cm fingerlings was that of the feed (including its shipping), that constituted 56% of the total costs of production. The second-greatest cost of a 15 cm fingerling was that of the 5 cm fingerlings stocked, that constituted 32% of the cost of producing 15 cm fingerlings.

The fingerling production cost values used in this analysis were based on average yields, survival rates, and FCRs from Engle and Southworth (2013). Largemouth bass hatcheries that sell fingerlings will need to charge a sufficiently high price to recoup losses occurred in various ponds across their farm. The Engle and Southworth (2013) survey documented very high fluctuations in yields and survivals on largemouth bass hatcheries that result in financial risk for hatcheries that must be recovered in prices charged for the fingerlings sold.

14.4 Proportion of farm used for broodstock and fingerling production

For the 32 ha farm modeled for largemouth bass food-fish production, 1.2 ha would be required for broodstock, 8.1 ha for spawning, 5.7 ha for production of 5 cm bass for feed training, and

Table 14.6 Vat/raceway annual costs of spawning; vats used for two months.

Item	Unit	Cost/unit (US$)	Quantity	Total cost (US$)
Variable costs				
Broodfish costs	Broodfish	16.86	240	4,046
Feed – forage fish	Kg	8.82	272.1	2,400
Spawning mats	Each	5	120	600
Spawning hormone	Thousand IU	0.10896	1309	143
Labor	$/hr	9.0	168	1,512
Electricity	US$/vat/month	20	2	400
Fuel	US$/vat/month	27	2	540
Pumping	US$/vat/month	44	2	880
Repairs and maintenance	US$/vat/month	20	2	400
Office supplies	US$/vat/month	0.19	2	3.80
Interest on operating capital	US$	0.0083[a]	10,925	181
Total variable costs				11,106
Fixed costs				
Telephone	US$/month	28	2	56
Farm insurance	US$/month	73	2	146
Legal/accounting	US$/month	31	2	62
Raceways				
Annual depreciation	US$/month	534	2	1,068
Interest on average investment	US$/month	534	2	1,068
Equipment				
Annual depreciation	US$/month	673	2	1,346
Interest on average investment	US$/month	282	2	564
Total fixed costs				4,310
Total annual costs				15,416
Annual cost/kg of Fry (breakeven price/kg) (US$/kg)				0.62
Annual cost/Fry (breakeven price/fry) (US$/fry)				0.00082

Note: [a]Monthly rate, based on 10% annual percentage rate.

Table 14.7 Fry rearing to 5 cm, annual costs in one 0.4 ha pond; pond used for two months.

Item	Unit	Cost/unit (US$)	Quantity	Total cost (US$)
Fry	each	0.051	74,000	3,774
Fertilizer				
Cottonseed meal		0.212	550[a]	117
Inorganic fertilizer		0.54	275[a]	149
Interest on operating capital		0.0083[b]	4,177	69
Total variable costs				4,246
Total fixed costs				110
Total annual costs				4,356
Annual cost/kg, 5-cm fingerlings (breakeven price, 5-cm fingerlings (US$/kg)				67.65
Annual cost/5-cm fingerling (breakeven price, 5-cm fingerling) (US$/fish)				0.118

Notes: [a]Twice a week for 3 weeks, then once per week. [b]Monthly rate, based on 10% annual percentage rate.

Table 14.8 Feed training annual costs. Costs are for a unit of eight vats used for 0.5 months.

Item	Unit	Cost/unit (US$)	Quantity	Total cost (US$)
Variable costs				
Feed				
Krill	kg	43.00	82.35	3,541.20
Krill meal	kg	20.95	151.86	3,181.55
Crumbles	kg	1.76	146.36	257.60
2.0 mm, 3/32 in	kg	1.76	25.45	44.80
2.5 mm pellet, 1/8 in	kg	1.65	25.45	42
Shipping feed	kg	0.66	432.05	285.15
Labor	US$/h	9.0	96	864
Electricity	US$/month	160	0.5	80
Fuel	US$/month	217	0.5	108
Pumping	US$/month	351.7	0.5	175.8
Repairs and maintenance	US$/month	162	0.5	81
Oxygen	US$/month	25	0.5	12.5
Bags to move fry	US$/month	60	0.5	30
Office supplies	US$/month	18	0.5	9
Interest on operating capital	US$	0.0083[a]	8,713	36.16
Total variable costs				8,749
Fixed costs				
Telephone	US$/month	28	0.5	14
Farm insurance	US$/month	73	0.5	36.5
Legal/accounting	US$/month	31	0.5	15.5
Vats				
Annual depreciation				13
Interest on average investment				13
Holding shed				
Annual depreciation				62.50
Interest on average investment				62.50
Equipment				
Annual depreciation				223
Interest on average investment				96
Total fixed costs				536
Total annual costs				9,285
Annual cost per kg (breakeven price per pound) (US$/kg)				15.90
Annual cost per feed-trained fish (breakeven price per feed-trained fish) (US$/fish)				$0.0206

Note: [a]Monthly rate, based on 10% annual percentage rate.

8.1 ha for production of 15 cm bass for stocking, leaving only 9.3 ha for final growout. Thus, 71% of the water surface area on the farm is needed to produce enough fingerlings to stock into final growout. The only ponds that generate revenue for the farm would be those used for final growout. With on-farm production of largemouth bass fingerlings, then, only 29% of the water area on the farm would generate direct revenue. It appears that it is not feasible for small-scale producers to raise their own fingerlings. The opportunity cost of on-farm fingerling production is the revenue that would have been received from sale of the food-fish grown in the same ponds

Table 14.9 Rearing feed-trained fingerlings to 15 cm, annual costs, in one 0.4 ha pond; pond used for 6 months.

Item	Unit	Cost/unit (US$)	Quantity	Total cost (US$)
Variable costs				
Fingerlings, 5 cm		0.118	25,000	2,950
Feed training		0.0206	25,000	515
Feed (2.4mm)	kg	1.65	909.09	1,500
Feed (3.2mm)	kg	1.54	1,818.2	2,800
Shipping feed		0.66	2,727.27	1,800
Fertilizer				
Cottonseed meal	US$/pond	0.212	50	11
Inorganic fertilizer	US$/pond	0.54	25	13
All other operating costs				409
Interest on operating capital		0.0083[a]	9,998	498
Total variable costs				10,496
Total fixed costs				330
Total annual costs				10,826
Annual cost/kg (breakeven price/kg) (US$/kg)				11.93
Annual cost per 15-cm fish (breakeven price/15-cm fish) (US$/fish)				0.541

Note: [a]Monthly rate, based on 10% annual percentage rate.

used for fingerlings. It is clear that most largemouth bass food-fish producers, unless operating on a very large scale, will need to purchase fingerlings from hatcheries that specialize in production of fingerlings.

14.5 Financial risk of producing largemouth bass

There are a variety of types of risk inherent in any business, especially in a farming business. Production losses due to predators (such as birds and otters), disease, or extreme temperatures clearly result in reduced revenue and income for fish farmers. Similarly, market risks such as fluctuations in price, or changes in demand (that make it difficult to sell volumes sold in the past) will result in reduced revenue for the business. Such risks affect all fish farming businesses.

However, the financial risk in largemouth bass farming appears to be greater than in other pond-based fish farming businesses. The greater risk stems largely from the high cost of fingerlings and feed for bass, market risks associated with live food-fish markets, and uncertainties related to commercial production of a new type of fish crop.

Total production costs estimated in this chapter from research experiments show that per-ha costs ranged from 33,557 to US$82,516/ha. Such per hectare costs are several times greater than those for pond-raised catfish. While the market price for bass is greater than that for catfish, the total amount of capital required per ha represents a greater financial risk. If a pond of largemouth bass is lost due to disease or predators, the amount of that financial loss is greater than that for catfish because more money was spent on the fingerlings and feed. The potential for greater losses is a financial risk that prospective producers must consider carefully.

Cost of feed is a major cost of largemouth bass production. Thus, achieving feed efficiencies is important to the cost of producing largemouth bass food-fish. For example, the FCRs reported in various research studies ranged from a low of 1.36 to a high of 9.6. The higher FCRs reported were from studies in which the fish were carried over the winter. In some of these cases, the hatcheries that supplied fingerlings for the study only sold the appropriate sizes of fingerlings in the fall; thus, fingerlings purchased in the fall would need to be carried over the winter and possibly subjected to the same conditions that likely resulted in higher FCRs. If possible, it clearly would be preferable to avoid stocking fingerlings prior to the winter and wait to stock growout ponds until spring as a strategy to reduce risks associated with higher overwintering FCRs. The studies that did avoid a winter period (Cochran et al., 2009; Tidwell et al., 2015) reported feed conversions of 1.36 and 1.7, respectively. However, given the limited number of hatcheries that produce largemouth bass fingerlings, it may not always be possible to wait until spring to stock ponds. If so, the farmer will need to plan for greater feed costs from poorer FCRs over the winter.

Additional improvements in FCRs during the main production season will also result in reduced production costs and financial risk. For example, the breakeven price in the scenario with a 1.7 FCR was US$9.68/kg. A 25% reduction in the FCR would reduce the breakeven price to US$9.22/kg. Such a reduction in the production cost would increase the profit margin but as importantly would reduce the economic risk by providing a greater buffer against a sudden and unexpected decrease in market price.

The other major cost of producing largemouth bass food-fish is that of fingerlings. While the fingerling production cost also reflects the high cost of feed, the production risk in fingerling production is another contributor to this high cost. Fingerling producers, to be profitable and stay in business, need to cover their risk also. The Engle and Southworth (2013) survey showed widely varying survival rates and yields (kilogram per hectare), particularly in the phase that involves rearing fry to a size of 5 cm. Survivals in this stage of production were reported to range from 0% to 123%. As an example of how this variability can affect production costs, if the yield of 5 cm fingerlings decreases to 24,700/ha from the reported average of 123,500 fingerlings/ha, the cost of 15 cm fingerlings will more than double per fish. The unexplained production losses in the 5 cm production stage were reported by a number of respondents to occur on a frequent basis and are a contributing factor to the high cost of largemouth bass fingerlings. The risk associated with poor production in the 5 cm production phase increases the overall fingerling cost because hatchery operators must earn enough to cover those types of losses. Widely varying yields and survivals that create financial risk were also documented for other stages of largemouth bass fingerling production.

Market risks are also greater when selling into live food-fish markets. In more well-established food-fish industries, there has been increased use of contracts between farmers and processing plants that provide some degree of stability in terms of price and the volume of fish that will be sold. However, live fish markets typically operate as cash markets with few options for contracts, especially those that specify price and volume. Moreover, to maintain market share, a business must maintain adequate supplies to meet the needs of their customers throughout the year. It often is difficult to accurately estimate what demand will be in live fish markets. Thus, many farms end up producing more fish than they can sell. When the farm cannot sell the more expensive largemouth bass, the financial losses are greater than they would be for less-expensive catfish.

14.6 Research needed to reduce the cost of producing largemouth bass

While much research has been done to develop technologies to successfully rear largemouth bass to a marketable size, there are some key gaps in the research that is currently available. Addressing these research gaps has potential to reduce the costs and risk of producing largemouth bass for food-fish. The primary areas of greatest need include production studies that would lead to reduced farm-level costs of largemouth bass fingerlings and feed, managing strategies to overwinter largemouth bass, and marketing studies that lead to strategies that would reduce market risk.

There is a strong need to identify the causes of variability in yields in the production stage in which fry are stocked into fertilized ponds and raised to a size of 5 cm. This is the size that is appropriate for feed training. On the one hand, there is evidence that it is possible to obtain high yields in this stage of production. Yields of 296,400 fish/ha were reported in some ponds by respondents in the Engle and Southworth (2013) survey. However, total losses in other ponds that were managed in a similar fashion substantially increase production risk associated with this stage of production. Hatchery managers attribute this extreme variability to the variable nature of the types of phytoplankton blooms that develop in different ponds. Work is clearly needed to develop efficient production systems to produce 5-cm fingerlings with much more reliable survival rates and yields.

There also is insufficient research data on production of 15–18 cm largemouth bass fingerlings. If yields in these ponds could be doubled, to 3,570 kg/ha, the cost per fingerling would be cut in half. Hatchery managers reported generally good survival rates and growth in this phase of production (Engle and Southworth, 2013). Given the food-fish production yields above 4,500 kg/ha, it would seem that yields of 3,570 kg/ha in the 15–18 cm production stage should be achievable. However, there is insufficient research data from which to judge what yields are realistic for this stage of production. Additional production trials for this stage of production would also generate additional data related to FCRs. Improvements in feed conversion rates will also reduce costs of 15–18 cm bass fingerlings.

There will be times in temperate regions when largemouth bass need to be in ponds over the winter. There have been no studies to identify optimal management strategies for the winter period. Yet research studies that have included a winter period have shown much poorer FCRs than those conducted within a single growing period.

Largemouth bass currently are sold into live food-fish markets. While there is some evidence of growth in these markets (Thapa et al., 2015), the overall volume of fish sold in live markets is small in the U.S. The growth rates that have been measured in these markets are such that growth will not absorb major increases in production volumes without substantially decreasing prices received by producers. Additional research is needed to understand key factors driving demand for live fish in the USA, including the extent to which this demand is tied to strong preferences for specific species or to a more generic preference for live seafood. If the latter, preferences may be more for a wide variety of live fish, and customers may be more likely to readily substitute among various species. Research is also needed to explore opportunities to develop much larger markets for largemouth bass that may have potential to absorb larger volumes of production without depressing price. In the U.S. and in many countries around the world, the major product form preferred by consumers is that of fillet products. Additional work is needed to explore the potential to market largemouth bass as a fillet product. Such a step would likely require additional decreases in the cost of production, or, alternatively, the creation of market products with strong appeal to specific market segments where a higher price can be achieved. While current price points likely make this difficult, there has been insufficient market research in the USA to understand various market segments well enough to know if there are segments where a fillet product might be introduced successfully. Market prices in other countries will reflect the demand of the relevant consumer groups and will need to be used in economic analyses of largemouth bass production.

14.7 Hidden costs of small-scale production

Small-scale production of an aquaculture crop often entails costs that are not accounted for in the initial plan for the business. As a result, when the need to make these expenditures does arise, the effect on the business may be severe. The hidden costs that are most often omitted from financial planning for aquaculture businesses frequently are those associated with capital assets, such as land, existing farm equipment and buildings. Not accounting for land results in lack of consideration for its opportunity costs. However, it is well understood in economics that if someone can make more from their land from some activity other than raising largemouth bass, they will not continue to raise largemouth bass. Rather, they will switch at some point to the more profitable use of land. If farm equipment such as a truck, tractor, or building already exists on the farm, that investment is considered a "sunk" cost. However, if the farmer does not account for the value of such assets, in proportion to their use in largemouth bass production, then it is not possible to see if the business is generating sufficient revenue to be able to replace those items when they wear out (Engle and Stone, 2014). If they cannot be replaced, then the business will likely fail.

The labor and management skills of the largemouth bass producer and family must also be accounted for in financial planning whether or not the owner pays him/herself or family members a salary or wage. Aquaculture producers must earn enough from their largemouth bass production to be able to save for retirement, to pay for their children's college education, and for an occasional vacation (Engle, 2017). Otherwise, they are unlikely to continue to spend such long hours raising and selling bass.

A common error in budgeting is to assume that all fish produced are, in fact, sold when that often is not the case. In many cases, fish produced are not always in the size range desired by customers. Market demand varies from year to year and producers often overestimate what the demand may be for the coming year. At the same time, it is important for a business to be certain to have an adequate supply on hand so that customers do not begin to search for other suppliers. Thus, there often are fish produced that are not sold. Revenue projections must be based on very conservative projections of volumes of fish that realistically will be sold, with plans for disposing of inventory not sold in that year.

Other common errors when planning a startup aquaculture business are based on use of data from research studies. This most commonly takes the form of applying the yields from research studies as the quantity of fish expected to be sold in financial planning instruments. While the cost estimates presented in this chapter have relied heavily on experimental results from research studies, these should be interpreted by prospective bass farmers with great caution. There is no database of production data from commercial bass farms from which to draw more realistic values. The analysis presented in this chapter did rely on commercial-scale pond-based fish farm data for fixed capital costs and variable costs such as utilities, repairs and maintenance. However, the all-important values for the yield to be sold, FCRs, and survival rates, for food-fish production were based on research data. Yields from research studies and FCRs typically are much better than what commercial farmers can obtain. This has to do with the way that research studies are conducted. Such methods are appropriate for research, but these studies control for many factors that are outside the control of an aquaculture producer. Thus, it is best to use values that are more conservative than what is published in the research literature, especially for yield, FCRs, and survival rates.

14.8 Marketing costs

The estimated costs per kilogram of production of largemouth bass food-fish presented in this chapter do not include costs of selling and marketing live food-fish. The primary markets for live largemouth bass are in urban areas in the northern tier of the USA and in Canada. Thus, for customers to have the opportunity to purchase farm-raised largemouth bass, the fish must be held, size graded, and transported, often to wholesale facilities in cities that have tanks to maintain fish in good condition. From the wholesale facilities, the fish are distributed on smaller transport tanks to the various supermarkets where sold.

Clearly, there are a variety of costs associated with these intermediate market functions of wholesaling, transportation, and distribution. These functions require holding or grading sheds that can be large, open buildings that cover series of concrete vats used to hold, sort, and size grade the fish. These sheds and vats require a supply of oxygen (often oxygen saturators that are installed on each vat), electrical service, and adequate space for farm trucks to offload fish brought in from ponds and to load the larger trucks used to transport live fish to the cities that constitute key markets. Equipment necessary to sell fish thus includes the trucks, oxygen systems on the trucks, nets, and baskets to load and unload fish.

While no studies have been done that estimate these costs for selling live largemouth bass, there are estimates of marketing costs for catfish. Engle and Stone (2014) estimated that annual marketing costs of catfish for direct sales were approximately 0.066 to US$0.2/kg for the equipment and supplies needed to support direct sales. The cost of transporting live fish to markets would be an additional cost. Additional research is needed to estimate the costs of marketing to live food-fish markets in the USA and Canada.

14.9 Conclusion

The research that has been done on production of largemouth bass for sale as a live food-fish has demonstrated that it is possible to raise these fish to an acceptable market size in the USA. There is evidence that it may be possible to do so profitably, although additional work is needed to more fully understand marketing costs, consumer demand, and trends in live fish markets. However, at current production costs, the profit margins appear to be fairly thin. It is also clear that there is considerable financial risk involved in raising largemouth bass, due to the greater costs per ha of feed and fingerlings. Additional research is needed that leads to reduced financial risk in the form of reducing overall farm costs of feed and fingerlings for largemouth bass food-fish producers.

References

Cochran, N.J., Coyle, S.D. and Tidwell, J.H. (2009) Evaluation of reduced fish meal diets for second year growout of the largemouth bass, *Micropterus salmoides. Journal of the World Aquaculture Society* 40 (6), 735–743.

Eklund, P., Engle, C. and Ludwig, G. (2012) Comparative cost analysis of hybrid striped bass fingerling production in ponds and tanks. *North American Journal of Aquaculture* 74 (1), 39–53.

Engle, C.R. (2010) *Aquaculture Economics and Financing: Management and Analysis.* Blackwell Scientific, Ames, IA.

Engle, C.R. (2017) The cost of time in aquaculture and aquaponics businesses. *Aquaculture Magazine* 43 (6), 56–58.

Engle, C.R. and Southworth, B. (2013) *Costs of raising largemouth bass fingerlings.* ETB 260, Cooperative Extension Service, University of Arkansas at Pine Bluff, Pine Bluff, Arkansas.

Engle, C.R. and Stone, N.M. (2014) *Costs of small-scale catfish production for direct sales.* Southern Regional Aquaculture Center Publication No. 1800, Mississippi State University, MS.

Engle, C.R., Stone, N. and Xie, L. (2013) Feasibility of pond production of largemouth bass, *Micropterus salmoides*, for a fillet market. *Journal of the World Aquaculture Society* 44 (6), 805–813.

Kumar, G. (2017) Economics of various catfish production strategies. National Warmwater Aquaculture Center, Annual Producer Seminar Series, November 16, 2017, Stoneville, MS.

Kumar, G., Engle, C.R. and Tucker, C.S. (2016) Costs and risk of catfish split-pond systems. *Journal of the World Aquaculture Society* 47 (3), 327–340.

Thapa, G., Dey, M. and Engle, C.R. (2015) Consumer preferences for live seafood in the Northeastern region of USA: results from Asian ethnic fish market survey. *Aquaculture Economics & Management* 19 (2), 210–225.

Tidwell, J., Coyle, S. and Bright, L.A. (2015) Effect of feed pellet characteristics on growth and feed conversion efficiency of largemouth bass raised in ponds. *North American Journal of Aquaculture* 77 (1), 55–58.

Tidwell, J.H., Webster, C.D. and Coyle, S.D. (1996) Effects of dietary protein level on second year growth and water quality for largemouth bass (*Micropterus salmoides*) raised in ponds. *Journal of the World Aquaculture Society* 145, 213–223.

Tidwell, J.H., Webster, C.D., Coyle, S.D. and Schulmeister, G. (1998) Effect of stocking density on growth and water quality for largemouth bass *Micropterus salmoides* growout in ponds. *Journal of the World Aquaculture Society* 21 (1), 79–83.

USDA-NASS (2014) *2013 Census of Aquaculture.* National Agricultural Statistics Service, United States Department of Agriculture, Washington, DC.

Watts, C., Bright, L.A., Coyle, S. and Tidwell, J. (2016) Evaluation of stocking density during second-year growth of largemouth bass, *Micropterus salmoides*, raised indoors in a recirculating aquaculture system. *Journal of the World Aquaculture Society* 47 (4), 538–543.

CHAPTER 15

Future prospects

James H. Tidwell

Kentucky State University, Aquaculture Research Center, Frankfort, Kentucky, USA

Previous chapters have shown how the largemouth bass was highly regarded as a food-fish in the 1800s and the culture of largemouth bass developed as early as the mid-1800s. Production of large numbers of largemouth bass fingerling expanded during the 1930s to stock new waters being developed during the "New Deal" programs of the Franklin Roosevelt administration in the USA. Most culture activity was based on supporting largemouth bass sport fisheries. Much of the sport-fish management of the 1960s, 1970s, and 1980s relied on supplemental stocking programs using small fingerlings. However, the effectiveness of sport-fish stocking began to be questioned and evaluated. It was shown that the use of larger fingerlings was more effective in terms of long-term impact on the fishery. In the 1970s, Snow and associates developed the Marion Method to produce large numbers of large fingerlings by training the fish to accept artificial diets. During that same decade, largemouth bass began to be sold into ethnic Asian markets as a live food-fish. The production of largemouth bass as a food-fish is now probably 1,000,000 kg in the USA and likely exceeds 150,000,000 kg in China. So where does largemouth bass production go from here?

The current major constraint to the expansion of the largemouth bass as a culture species is summed up as high production costs. This affects almost all considerations as we discuss future directions. In fact, high production costs have a large impact on the current situation. In Chapter 2, a large largemouth bass food-fish producer in the USA described how a shift in currency exchange rates basically caused most Canadian largemouth bass buyers to shift to cheaper alternatives, demonstrating the fragility of the market and constraints of high production costs.

Maybe largemouth bass producers should expand beyond the live-fish markets and into processed markets, such as fillets. Engle et al. (2013) conducted a production and economics study. Their conclusion was that with "production costs of \$7.26-\$9.34/kg (total costs), that largemouth bass production for a fillet market is unlikely to be feasible" (Engle et al., 2013: 805).

So how might production costs of largemouth bass be lowered? Engle et al. (2013) reported that at the test density (12,500/ha) similar to commercial densities, the largest single cost item was the cost of feed (41–45% of total costs). Their economic analyses were based on a feed cost of US$1,323/MT. Their sensitivity analysis showed that for every US$100/MT decrease in the price of feed, the breakeven price would decrease by US$0.66/kg. A study by Cochran et al. (2009) demonstrated a reduced fish meal diet (24% FM) that lowered feed costs per unit of gain almost 30%. Lowering the feed cost used in Engle et al. (2013) by even 22% would represent a reduction of US$300/MT and decrease the breakeven price by US$1.98/kg.

Studies have shown that the largemouth bass is able to utilize alternative protein sources, especially animal source proteins (Tidwell et al., 2005). The largemouth bass also does not appear to have significant dietary requirements for the long-chain highly unsaturated fatty acids found in fish oil (AA, EPA, DHA) and perform well on alternative lipids (Tidwell et al., 2007). These traits also make it more likely that feed costs can in fact be substantially reduced.

In the analyses of Engle et al. (2013) fingerling costs were the second largest cost (27–37% of total costs). Their analyses were based on a cost of US$1.60 each for 15 cm fingerlings. Sensitivity analysis showed that for every US$0.10/fingerling decrease in fingerling price, breakeven price would decrease US$0.16–0.22/kg, depending on stocking density.

Part of the relatively high cost of largemouth bass fingerlings is due to the feed training step which is not required for many other culture species such as channel catfish, rainbow trout, and tilapia. However, there is a definite trend in largemouth bass toward this being less of an issue.

Heidinger (2000) reported that after 7–10 d of intensive training (freeze dried krill) ≥ 60% of the fingerlings would have learned to accept a prepared diet. However, if fingerlings are produced from hatchery-reared, feed-trained broodstock, feed-training success increases to > 90%. This is almost certainly the result of domestication. According to information presented in Chapter 6, in the past few years, fingerlings during feed-training are more readily adapting to prepared diets without the stimulant feeds of ground fish, carp eggs, or freeze-dried krill. Fingerlings are also adapting to artificial feeds at smaller sizes. Most largemouth bass feed-training procedures recommend initiating training at 3.8–5.0 cm. However, according to information in Chapter 3, in China fingerlings are being feed trained at < 2 cm. Research also indicates that the nursery pond phase can be skipped entirely (Skudlarek et al., 2007). This leads to the potential of scale-up of intensive fingerling production as discussed in Chapter 6.

Another potential improvement would be reducing the growout period from two years to one. Engle et al. (2013) stated that largemouth bass can reach sizes of 426–515 g in the first year of production. Their sensitivity analysis indicates that this would decrease the breakeven price by US$0.26/kg compared to 2 year production costs.

Not all of these potential improvements would be directly additive. However, it might be useful to consider hypotheticals. As stated earlier, changes in feed costs indicated by Cochran et al. (2009) could lower breakeven costs by US$1.98/kg of live-weight fish. A lowering of fingerling costs from US$1.60 per 15 cm fingerling to US$1.20/fingerling could decrease the breakeven cost by US$0.78/kg. Growout in one year rather than 2 years could lower the breakeven cost by US$0.26/kg. If additive, these changes could lower the breakeven cost by US$3.00/kg, approaching a breakeven cost of US$4.25/kg.

It seems that the changes in feed costs could be accomplished in the relative short-term. However, long-term reductions in feed costs, fingerling costs, improved feed conversion ratios, and shortened growout period could all be positively impacted by improved genetics. Documented improvements in feed-training success of fingerlings is largely the result of undirected inadvertent genetic changes through the "Unnatural Selection" of domestication. Just by keeping several generations of a fish in a farm environment, the fish genetically unsuited for that environment do not pass on their genes, while those that are better suited contribute to the subsequent generations.

Through active intervention and selection, strains of largemouth bass could likely be developed which more readily accept artificial diets at first feeding, efficiently utilize lower protein levels and/or higher inclusions of plant source proteins. Strains could also be developed which are disease resistant, grow uniformly, and grow fast enough to achieve market sizes in 1 year. A percentage of fish in the USA already achieve sizes > 500 g in one year, indicating that the genetic potential exists.

The impact of improved genetics is already documented. In China (Chapter 3) the development of an improved largemouth bass strain "Youlu No. 1" was developed by the Pearl River Fisheries Institute. This genetic variety has a good body confirmation, low rate of deformities, good growth with minimal individual size variation, and high production rates. It has already been widely adopted across China and allowed largemouth bass production to expand into new regions as well as into new types of production systems.

Overall, the largemouth bass has already developed from a large public and small private enterprise for producing large numbers of small fish for sport-fish stocking into generating over 150,000 MT of food-fish worldwide. Almost all of this without the research support devoted to other aquaculture food-fish species. With proper support, the fish could be a major contributor to aquaculture growth and diversification in the future.

References

Cochran, N.J., Coyle, S.D. and Tidwell, J.H. (2009) Evaluation of reduced fish meal diets for second year growth of the largemouth bass, *Micropterus salmoides. Journal of the World Aquaculture Society* 40, 735–743.

Engle, C.R., Stone, N. and Xie, L. (2013) Feasibility of pond production of largemouth bass, *Micropterus salmoides*, for a filet market. *Journal of the World Aquaculture Society* 44 (6), 805–813.

Heidinger, R.C. (2000) A white paper on the status and needs of largemouth bass culture in the north central region. *NCRAC White Papers* 4. The North Central Regional Aquaculture Center, East Lansing, MI.

Skudlarek, N.A., Cochran, N.J., Larimore, M., Marple, S., Coyle, S. and Tidwell, J.H. (2007) Alternatives to freeze–dried krill in the feed training phase of largemouth bass. *North American Journal of Aquaculture* 69, 395–399.

Tidwell, J.H., Coyle, S.D., Bright, L.A. and Yasharian, D. (2005) Evaluation of plant and animal source proteins for replacement of fish meal in practical diets for the largemouth bass *Micropterus salmoides. Journal of the World Aquaculture Society* 36 (4), 454–463.

Tidwell, J.H., Coyle, S.D. and Bright, L.A. (2007) Effect of different types of dietary lipids on growth and fatty acid composition of largemouth bass. *North American Journal of Aquaculture* 69 (3), 257–264.

Index